Textbook of

Kidney Transplantation

Textbook of Kidney Transplantation

Editors

Vinant Bhargava
DNB (Medicine) DNB (Nephrology) MNAMS
FASN FRCP (Edinburgh) FACP MBA (HCM)
Senior Consultant
Department of Nephrology
Sir Ganga Ram Hospital
New Delhi, India

Manisha Sahay
MD (Pediatrics) DNB (Pediatrics) DM (Nephrology)
DNB (Nephrology) FRCP
Professor and Head
Department of Nephrology
Osmania Medical College and General Hospital
Hyderabad, Telangana, India

Priti Meena
MD (Medicine) DrNB (Nephrology) FASN
Assistant Professor
Department of Nephrology
All India Institute of Medical Sciences
Bhubaneswar, Odisha, India

Vinay Sakhuja
MD (Medicine) DM (Nephrology) MNAMS (Nephrology)
Director
Department of Nephrology and Transplant Medicine
Max Hospitals, Mohali, Punjab, India
Former Head
Department of Nephrology
Postgraduate Institute of Medical Education and Research
Chandigarh, India

Amit Gupta
MD (Medicine) DNB (Nephrology) FRCP (London)
Director and Head
Department of Nephrology and Renal Transplantation
Apollomedics Hospital, Lucknow
Former Head
Department of Nephrology
Sanjay Gandhi Postgraduate Institute of Medical Sciences
Lucknow, Uttar Pradesh, India

Forewords

DS Rana
AK Bhalla
V Jha

JAYPEE

JAYPEE BROTHERS MEDICAL PUBLISHERS
The Health Sciences Publisher
New Delhi | London

JAYPEE **Jaypee Brothers Medical Publishers (P) Ltd**

Headquarters
EMCA House
23/23-B, Ansari Road, Daryaganj
New Delhi 110 002, India
Landline: +91-11-23272143, +91-11-23272703
+91-11-23282021, +91-11-23245672
E-mail: jaypee@jaypeebrothers.com

Corporate Office
4838/24, Ansari Road, Daryaganj
New Delhi 110 002, India
Phone: +91-11-43574357
Fax: +91-11-43574314
E-mail: jaypee@jaypeebrothers.com

Overseas Office
J.P. Medical Ltd.
83, Victoria Street, London
SW1H 0HW (UK)
Phone: +44 20 3170 8910
E-mail: info@jpmedpub.com

EU GPSR Authorised Representative
Logos Europe, 9 rue Nicolas Poussin
17000, La Rochelle, France
Phone: +33 (0) 6 67 93 73 78
E-mail: contact@logoseurope.eu

Website: www.jaypeebrothers.com
Website: www.jaypeedigital.com

Textbook of Kidney Transplantation

First Edition: 2023

Reprint: **2025**

ISBN: 978-93-5465-946-1

Printed in India

Contributors

Abhijit Taraphder
MD (Medicine) DM (Nephrology)
WHO Fellow
Senior Consultant
Department of Nephrology
Apollo Multispecialty Hospitals
Kolkata, West Bengal, India

Ajay Kumar Baranwal
MD (Pathology) PhD
Professor and Head
Department of Immunohematology and Blood Transfusion
Armed Forces Medical College
Pune, Maharashtra, India

Ajaypal Singh MBBS
Fellow
Department of Psychiatry
Postgraduate Institute of Medical Education and Research
Chandigarh, India

Ajit S Narula
MD (Medicine) DM (Nephrology)
Director of Nephrology and Kidney Transplant
Department of Nephrology
Fortis Escorts Kidney and Urology Institute
New Delhi, India

Akhilesh Sharma MD (Psychiatry)
Associate Professor
Department of Psychiatry
Postgraduate Institute of Medical Education and Research
Chandigarh, India

Akshay Kriplani
MS MCh (Urology) Fellowship Renal Transplantation (SGPGI, Lucknow)
Assistant Professor
Department of Urology
Jawaharlal Nehru Medical College
Wardha, Maharashtra, India

Alan Almeida
MD (Medicine) MNAMS (Nephrology)
Consultant Nephrologist
Section Coordinator
Director of Clinical Research
Department of Nephrology
PD Hinduja Hospital
Mumbai, Maharashtra, India

Aman Jha MD (Medicine)
Nephrology Postgraduate Fellow
Department of Nephrology
Apollo Hospital
Hyderabad, Telangana, India

Amit Gupta
MD (Medicine) DNB (Nephrology) FRCP (London)
Director and Head
Department of Nephrology and Renal Transplantation
Apollomedics Hospital, Lucknow
Former Head
Department of Nephrology
Sanjay Gandhi Postgraduate Institute of Medical Sciences
Lucknow, Uttar Pradesh, India

Aneesh Srivastava
MS (Surgery) MCh (Urology)
Head
Department of Urology and Renal Transplantation
Sanjay Gandhi Postgraduate Institute of Medical Sciences
Lucknow, Uttar Pradesh, India

Aniket Hase
DNB (Medicine) DNB (Nephrology)
Consultant Nephrologist
Department of Nephrology
Jupiter Hospital
Thane, Maharashtra, India

AK Bhalla
MD (Medicine) DM (Nephrology) MNAMS FISN FASN (USA) FRCP (Edinburgh) FISOT
Professor and Chairman
Department of Nephrology
Sir Ganga Ram Hospital
New Delhi, India

Anna Gupta
MD (Medicine) DM (Nephrology)
Consultant Nephrologist
Fortis Hospital
Mohali, Punjab, India

Anshul Bhalla MD (Medicine) FASN
Transplant Nephrologist
Assistant Professor
Department of Surgery
University of Tennessee Health Science Center
James D Eason Transplant Institute at Methodist University Hospital
Memphis, TN, USA

Anurag Gupta
MD (Medicine) DM (Nephrology)
Senior Consultant
Department of Nephrology
Sir Ganga Ram Hospital
New Delhi, India

Anwitha Varmudy
MD (Medicine) DM (Nephrology)
Assistant Professor
Department of Nephrology
Nizam's Institute of Medical Sciences
Hyderabad, Telangana, India

Arpana Iyengar
MD (Medicine) DNB FPN FRCP
Professor
Department of Pediatric Nephrology
St John's National Academy of Health Sciences
Bengaluru, Karnataka, India

Arpita Ray Chaudhury
MD (Medicine) DM (Nephrology) DNB
Professor
Department of Nephrology
Institute of Post Graduate Medical Education and Research
Kolkata, West Bengal, India

Aruna V Vanikar
MD FICPath PhD D Litt
President
Undergraduate Medical Education Board
National Medical Commission
Former I/C Vice Chancellor
Gujarat University of Transplantation Sciences, Ahmedabad
Professor and Head
Department of Pathology, Lab Medicine, Transfusion Services and Immunohematology
Department of Stem Cell Therapy and Regenerative Medicine
GR Doshi and KM Mehta Institute of Kidney Diseases and Research Centre
Dr HL Trivedi Institute of Transplantation Sciences
Ahmedabad, Gujarat, India

Arunkumar S
MD (Medicine) DM (Nephrology) MRCP (UK) SCE (Nephrology)
Assistant Professor
Department of Nephrology
All India Institute of Medical Sciences
New Delhi, India

Arvind Bagga MD (Pediatrics)
Professor and Head
Division of Nephrology
Department of Pediatrics
All India Institute of Medical Sciences
New Delhi, India

Arvind Canchi
MD (Medicine) DM (Nephrology)
Consultant Nephrologist and
Transplant Physician
The Bangalore, Sagar and Trustwell
Hospitals, Bengaluru
Co-Founder
Bloom Value Corporation
Bengaluru, Karnataka, India

Ashish Kumar
MD (Medicine) DM (Gastroenterology)
FACP FISG FINASL
Professor and Senior Consultant
Department of Gastroenterology
Sir Ganga Ram Hospital
New Delhi, India

Ashwani Gupta
MD (Medicine) DM (Nephrology) FISN FASN
Professor and Co-Director
Department of Nephology
Sir Ganga Ram Hospital
New Delhi, India

Atim Pajai
MD (Medicine) DNB (Nephrology)
Associate Professor
Department of Nephrology
Topiwala National Medical College and
BYL Nair Charitable Hospital
Mumbai, Maharashtra, India

Ayan Dey
DNB (Medicine) DNB (Nephrology)
FCCCM (Critical Care) Fellowship in Adult
Nephrology Transplantation (Toronto)
Consultant Nephrologist
Department Nephrology
PD Hinduja Hospital
Mumbai, Maharashtra, India

B Karthikeyan
MD (Medicine) DM (Nephrology)
Consultant Nephrologist
Department of Nephrology
Dr Rela Institute and Medical Centre
Chennai, Tamil Nadu, India

B Ramesh Kumar
MD (Medicine) DM (Gastroenterology)
Professor and Head of the Department
Osmania General Hospital
Hyderabad, Telangana, India

Chacko Korula Jacob
MD (Medicine) DM (Nephrology)
MNAMS (Nephrology)
Consultant Nephrologist
Department of Nephrology
Annasawmy Mudaliar General Hospital
Bengaluru, Karnataka, India
Former Head
Department of Nephrology
Christian Medical College
Vellore, Tamil Nadu, India

Chandani Bhagat
MD (Medicine) DM (Nephrology)
Consultant
Department of Nephrology and
Kidney Transplant
Institute of Liver and Biliary Sciences
New Delhi, India

D Bhaumik
MD (Medicine) DM (Nephrology)
Professor
Department of Nephrology
All India Institute of Medical Sciences
New Delhi, India

Dharmendra Bhadauria
MD (Medicine) DM (Nephrology) FASN
Additional Professor
Department of Nephrology and
Renal Transplantation
Sanjay Gandhi Postgraduate Institute of
Medical Sciences
Lucknow, Uttar Pradesh, India

Dinesh Khullar
MD (Medicine) DM (Nephrology)
FACP FRCP (Edinburgh) FISOT
Chairman and Head
Department of Nephrology and Renal
Transplant Medicine
Max Super Speciality Hospital
New Delhi, India

Divya Bajpai
MD (Medicine) DM (Nephrology)
Associate Professor
Department of Nephrology
Seth Gordhandas Sunderdas
Medical College and
King Edward Memorial Hospital
Mumbai, Maharashtra, India

Divyanshu Malhotra
MD (Medicine) FASN
Transplant Nephrologist
Assistant Professor
Department of Medicine
Johns Hopkins University
Johns Hopkins Hospital
Baltimore, MD, USA

Edwin Fernando
MD (Medicine) DM (Nephrology)
Professor and Head
Department of Nephrology
Government Stanley Medical College
Chennai, Tamil Nadu, India

Georgi Abraham MD (Medicine) FRCP
Professor
Department of Nephrology
MGM Health Care
Chennai, Tamil Nadu, India

Gokulnath
BSc MD (Medicine) DM (Nephrology)
DNB (Nephrology) FISN FRCP (London)
Director Nephrology Services and
Senior Consultant
Department of Nephrology
Apollo Hospitals
Bengaluru, Karnataka, India

Govardhan Gupta
DNB (Medicine) DNB (Nephrology)
Consultant Nephrologist
Department of Nephrology
Narayana Multispecialty Hospital
Kolkata, West Bengal, India

Harbir S Kohli
MD (Medicine) DM (Nephrology)
FRCP (London) FAMS FISN
Professor and Head
Department of Nephrology
Postgraduate Institute of Medical
Education and Research
Chandigarh, India

Hari Shankar Meshram
MD (Medicine) DM (Nephrology)
Assistant Professor
Department of Nephrology
Institute of Kidney Diseases and
Research Center and
Dr HL HL Trivedi Institute of
Transplantation Sciences
Ahmedabad, Gujarat, India

Indira Menon
DNB (Medicine) MRCP (UK) FRCP (London)
Senior Consultant and Head
Department of Critical Care Medicine
Bangalore Baptist Hospital
Bengaluru, Karnataka, India

Jasmine Sethi
MD (Medicine) DM (Nephrology)
Assistant Professor
Department of Nephrology
Postgraduate Institute of Medical
Education and Research
Chandigarh, India

Jayasurya R
MD (Pediatrics) DM (Nephrology)
Consultant Nephrologist
Department of Nephrology
Apollo Multispeciality Hospital
Kolkata, West Bengal, India

Jeethu Joseph Eapen
MD (Medicine) DM (Nephrology)
Associate Professor
Department of Nephrology
Christian Medical College
Vellore, Tamil Nadu, India

Jony Agarwal
MD (Medicine) DM (Nephrology)
Associate Consultant
Department of Nephrology
Apollomedics Superspeciality Hospital
Lucknow, Uttar Pradesh, India

Joyita Bharati
MD (Medicine) DM (Nephrology)
Assistant Professor
Department of Nephrology
Postgraduate Institute of Medical Education and Research
Chandigarh, India

K Sampathkumar
MD (Medicine) DM (Nephrology) FRCP FISN FASN
Senior Consultant Nephrologist
Department of Nephrology
Meenakshi Mission Hospital
Madurai, Tamil, Nadu, India

Kalpana Shailesh Mehta
MD (Medicine) DNB (Nephrology)
Professor and Head
Department of Nephrology
Topiwala National Medical College and BYL Nair Charitable Hospital
Mumbai, Maharashtra, India

Kapil N Sejpal
MD (Medicine) DM (Nephrology)
Assistant Professor
Department of Nephrology
Jawaharlal Nehru Medical College
Wardha, Maharashtra, India

Krishan Lal Gupta
MD (Medicine) DM (Nephrology)
Dip NB FAMS FRCP FASN
Professor and Former Head
Department of Nephrology
Postgraduate Institute of Medical Education and Research
Chandigarh, India

Krishna Kumar Agrawaal
MD (Medicine) DM (Nephrology) FACP FASN
Associate Professor and Head
Department of Nephrology
Universal College of Medical Sciences
Bhairahawa, Lumbini, Nepal

Kristin George
MD (Medicine) DM (Nephrology)
Assistant Professor
Department of Nephrology
Sapthagiri Institute of Medical Sciences and Research Institute
Bengaluru, Karnataka, India

Manish Malik
MD (Medicine) DNB (Nephrology)
Senior Consultant
Chairman (Dialysis Services)
Department of Nephrology
Sir Ganga Ram Hospital
New Delhi, India

Manisha Sahay
MD (Pediatrics) DNB (Pediatrics)
DM (Nephrology) DNB (Nephrology) FRCP
Professor and Head
Department of Nephrology
Osmania Medical College and General Hospital
Hyderabad, Telangana, India

Mastakim A Mazumder
MD (Medicine) DM (Nephrology)
Associate Consultant
Department of Nephrology and Kidney Transplant
Kidney and Urology Institute
Fortis Escorts
New Delhi, India

Mayuri Trivedi
MD (Medicine) DM (Nephrology)
Senior Consultant and Head
Department of Nephrology
Lokmanya Tilak Municipal General Hospital
Mumbai, Maharashtra, India

Mehakinder Singh
MD (Medicine) DM (Nephrology) ESENeph
Consultant Nephrologist and Renal Transplant Physician
SGHS Sohana Hospital
Mohali, Punjab, India

N Gopalakrishnan
MD (Medicine) DM (Nephrology) MRCP (UK) FRCP
Professor and Head
Department of Nephrology
Madras Medical College
Chennai, Tamil Nadu, India

Narayan Prasad
MD DNB (Medicine) DM DNB (Nephrology)
MNAMS FISN FISOT FASN (Nephrology)
FRCP (London)
Professor and Head
Department of Nephrology
Sanjay Gandhi Postgraduate Institute of Medical Sciences
Lucknow, Uttar Pradesh, India

Nikhil Saxena
MD (Medicine) DM (Nephrology)
DrNB (Nephrology)
Assistant Professor
Department of Nephrology
Lokmanya Tilak Municipal Medical College and General Hospital
Mumbai, Maharashtra, India

Niwrutti Hase
MD (Medicine) DNB (Nephrology) FICP
Director
Department of Nephrology
Jupiter Hospital, Thane
Former Professor and Head
Department of Nephrology
Seth Gordhandas Sunderdas Medical College and King Edward Memorial Hospital
Mumbai, Maharashtra, India

Noble Gracious
MD (Medicine) DM (Nephrology)
Associate Professor
Department of Medicine
Government Medical College
Thiruvananthapuram, Kerala, India

Padmini Sirkanungo
DNB (Medicine) DNB (Nephrology) ISN ANIO CNC
Consultant
Department of Nephrology
Medica Superspeciality Hospital
Kolkata, West Bengal, India

Pallav Gupta
MD (Medicine) PDCC (Renal and Transplant Pathology) MAMS ISN-ANIO Scholar (Renal Pathology)
Associate Professor
Department of Pathology
Sir Ganga Ram Hospital
New Delhi, India

Pallavi Prasad
MD (Medicine) DNB (Nephrology)
Assistant Professor
Department of Nephrology and Renal Transplant Medicine
Vardhman Mahavir Medical College and Safdarjung Hospital
New Delhi, India

Pankaj R Shah
MD (Medicine) DNB (Nephrology) FISOT (Transplantation) FRCPEDIN (London)
Ex-Head
Department of Nephrology and Transplantation Medicine
Institute of Kidney Diseases and Research Centre
Institute of Transplantation Sciences
Ahmedabad
Ex-Dean
Gujarat University of Transplantation Sciences
Ahmedabad, Gujarat, India

PP Varma
AVSM SM VSM (Retd) MD (Medicine) DM (Nephrology) MNAMS FICP FACP FRCP (Edinburgh) FISOT FISN FASN FAMS
Chairman
Department of Nephrology
Primus Hospital
New Delhi, India

Prabhjyot Singh Chowhan
DM (Interventional Radiology)
Department of Radiology
Postgraduate Institute of Medical Education and Research
Chandigarh, India

Pranaw K Jha
MD (Medicine) DNB (Nephrology) FASN
Senior Consultant and Head
Department of Nephrology
Arihant Multispeciality Hospital
Nagpur, Maharashtra, India

Prashant C Dheerendra
MD (Medicine) DM (Nephrology)
ISN Fellow (Interventional Nephrology)
Consultant Nephrologist
Department of Nephrology
Apollo Hospitals
Bengaluru, Karnataka, India

Prateek Kumar
MD (Medicine) DrNB (Nephrology)
Consultant Nephrologist
Department of Nephrology
Capitol Hospital
Jalandhar, Punjab, India

Praveen Kumar Etta
MD (Medicine) DM (Nephrology)
Senior Consultant Nephrologist
Department of Nephrology
Olive Hospital
Hyderabad, Telangana, India

Priti Meena
MD (Medicine) DrNB (Nephrology) FASN
Assistant Professor
Department of Nephrology
All India Institute of Medical Sciences
Bhubaneswar, Odisha, India

PS Priyamvada
MD (Medicine) DM (Nephrology)
Professor
Department of Nephrology
Jawaharlal Institute of Postgraduate Medical Education and Research
Puducherry, India

Rahul Grover
MD (Medicine) DM (Nephrology)
Associate Director
Department of Nephrology
Max Super Speciality Hospital
New Delhi, India

Raj Kumar Sharma
MD (Medicine) DNB (Nephrology)
Professor
Director and Head
Department of Nephrology and Kidney Transplant Medicine
Kidney and Urology Institute
Medanta Hospital, Lucknow
Former Head of the Department
Sanjay Gandhi Postgraduate Institute of Medical Sciences
Lucknow, Uttar Pradesh, India

Raja Ramachandran
MD (Medicine) DM (Nephrology)
Associate Professor
Department of Nephrology
Postgraduate Institute of Medical Education and Research
Chandigarh, India

Rajendra Prasad Mathur
MD (Medicine) DM (Nephrology) FRCP (London) FICP FISN ISN Scholar
Senior Consultant and Head
Department of Nephrology and Renal Transplant Medicine
Institute of Liver and Biliary Sciences
New Delhi, India

Rakesh Kumar Ambati
DNB (Medicine) DNB (Nephrology)
Fellow
Department of Nephrology
Virinchi Hospital
Hyderabad, Telangana, India

Ratan Jha
MD (Medicine) DM (Nephrology)
DNB (Nephrology) DTCD (Gold Medalist)
FISN (India)
Senior Consultant
Nephrologist and Transplant Physician
Department of Nephrology
CARE Hospitals
Hyderabad, Telangana, India

Ruju Gala MD (Medicine) DM (Nephrology)
Assistant Professor
Department of Nephrology
Topiwala National Medical College and BYL Nair Hospital
Mumbai, Maharashtra, India

Sabina Yusuf
MD (Medicine) DNB (Nephrology)
Associate Professor
Christian Medical College
Vellore, Tamil Nadu, India

Sandeep Guleria
MS DNB FRCS (England) FRCSEd FRCS (Glasgow) FRCP (Edinburgh)
Senior Consultant Surgeon
Department of General Surgery
Gastrointestinal Surgery and Transplantation
Indraprastha Apollo Hospitals
New Delhi, India

Sandeep Mahajan
MD (Medicine) DM (Nephrology)
FASN FRCP FISN
Professor
Department of Nephrology
All India Institute of Medical Sciences
New Delhi, India

Sanjay K Agarwal
MD (Medicine) DNB FRCP (Edinburgh)
Professor and Head
Department of Nephrology
All India Institute of Medical Sciences
New Delhi, India

Sanshriti Chauhan
MD (Medicine) DM (Nephrology)
Assistant Professor
Department of Nephrology
Institute of Kidney Diseases and Research Center and
Dr HL Trivedi Institute of Transplantation Sciences
Ahmedabad, Gujarat, India

Santosh Varughese
MD (Medicine) DM (Nephrology)
FRCP (London) MBA (BITS)
Professor and Head
Nephrology Unit
Department of Nephrology
Christian Medical College
Vellore, Tamil Nadu, India

Saugat Dasgupta
MD (Medicine) DM (Nephrology)
Fellow
Department of Nephrology
Institute of Post Graduate Medical Education and Research
Kolkata, West Bengal, India

Shahzad Alam
MD (Medicine) DM (Nephrology)
Consultant Nephrologist
Department of Nephrology
Apollomedics Hospital
Lucknow, Uttar Pradesh, India

Shiv Chadha
MD (Medicine) DM (Nephrology)
Associate Consultant
Department of Nephrology
Sir Ganga Ram Hospital
New Delhi, India

Shruti Tapiawala
MD (Medicine) DNB (Nephrology)
Consultant Nephrologist and Transplant Physician
Director ATDI Lab Pvt Ltd., Mumbai
Global Hospitals, Mumbai
Sir HN Reliance Foundation Hospital and Research Center
Mumbai, Maharashtra, India

Shyam Bansal
MD (Medicine) DM (Nephrology) FISN FASN FRCP (London)
Director
Department of Nephrology and Kidney Transplantation
Medanta—The Medicity
Gurugram, Haryana, India

Sonia Mehrotra PhD (Biochemistry)
Senior Scientist (Molecular Biology and Immunology)
Department of Nephrology and Kidney Transplant Medicine
Kidney and Urology Institute
Medanta Hospital
Lucknow, Uttar Pradesh, India

Soumita Bagchi
MD (Medicine) DM (Nephrology)
Additional Professor
Department of Nephrology
All India Institute of Medical Sciences
New Delhi, India

Sree Bhushan Raju
MD (Medicine) DM (Nephrology) DNB MNAMS (Nephrology) MBA FASN FISN FACP FICP FISOT FIACM
Professor and Unit Head
Department of Nephrology
Nizam's Institute of Medical Sciences
Hyderabad, Telangana, India

Sreejith Parameswaran
MD (Medicine) DM (Nephrology) DNB (Medicine)
Professor
Department of Nephrology
Jawaharlal Institute of Postgraduate Medical Education and Research
Puducherry, India

Suceena Alexander
MD (Medicine) DM (Nephrology) FRCP (London) FASN PhD
Professor
Christian Medical College
Vellore, Tamil Nadu, India

Suchita Jogale MSc
Quality Manager and Technical Head
ATDI Lab Pvt Ltd
Mumbai, Maharashtra, India

Sukanya Bhrugumalla
MD (Medicine) DM (Gastroenterology)
Associate Professor
Department of Medical Gastroenterology
Nizam's Institute of Medical Sciences
Hyderabad, Telangana, India

Sukanya Govindan
MD (Pediatrics) DM (Nephrology) FISN (UK)
Consultant Nephrologist
Department of Nephrology
Mehta's Multispeciality Hospital
Chennai, Tamil Nadu, India

Sunil Shroff
MS (Surgery) FRCS (Glasgow) D Urol (UK)
Senior Consultant
Department of Urology and Renal Transplantation
Madras Medical Mission Hospital
Chennai, Tamil Nadu, India
Trustee, MOHAN Foundation

Surendra K Mattoo MD (Psychiatry)
Former Professor and Head
Department of Psychiatry
Postgraduate Institute of Medical Education and Research
Chandigarh, India

Susan Uthup
MD (Pediatrics) DM (Nephrology) DNB (Pediatrics) DNB (Nephrology)
Professor and Head
Department of Pediatric Nephrology
SAT Hospital, Government Medical College
Thiruvananthapuram, Kerala, India

Swarnalata Gowrishankar
MD (Pathology)
Senior Consultant Pathologist
Apollo Hospitals, Jubilee Hills
Hyderabad, Telangana, India

Swarnalatha Guditi
MD (Medicine) DM (Nephrology) FRCP FISN FISOT
Professor and Unit Head
Department of Nephrology
Nizam's Institute of Medical Sciences
Hyderabad, Telangana, India

Tanuj M Lamech
MD (Medicine) DM (Nephrology)
Assistant Professor
Department of Nephrology
Institute of Nephrology
Madras Medical College
Chennai, Tamil Nadu, India

Tukaram Jamale
MD (Medicine) DM (Nephrology)
Professor and Head
Department of Nephrology
Seth Gordhandas Sunderdas Medical College and King Edward Memorial Hospital
Mumbai, Maharashtra, India

Ujjwal Gorsi MD (Radiodiagnosis)
Associate Professor
Department of Radiodiagnosis
Postgraduate Institute of Medical Education and Research
Chandigarh, India

Uma Kanga MSc (Hons) PhD (AIIMS)
Associate Professor
Department of Transplant Immunology and Immunogenetics
All India Institute of Medical Sciences
New Delhi, India

Umapati Hegde
MD (Medicine) DNB (Nephrology) FISN
Vice Chairman
Department of Nephrology
Muljibhai Patel Urological Hospital
Nadiad, Gujarat, India

Urmila Anandh
MD (Medicine) DM (Nephrology) DNB (Medicine) DNB (Nephrology)
Senior Consultant and Head
Department of Nephrology
Amrita Hospital
Faridabad, Haryana, India

Vaibhav Tiwari
MD (Medicine) DM (Nephrology) MRCP SCE
Associate Consultant
Department of Nephrology
Sir Ganga Ram Hospital
New Delhi, India

Venkatesh Arumugam
MD (Pediatrics) DM (Nephrology)
Post-Doctoral Fellow (Pediatric Nephrology)
Assistant Professor
Madras Medical College
Rajiv Gandhi Government General Hospital
Chennai, Tamil Nadu, India

Venu Madhav Thumma
MS (Surgery) DNB (Surgical Gastroenterology) MRCS (Edinburgh)
Additional Professor
Department of Surgical Gastroenterology
Nizam's Institute of Medical Sciences
Hyderabad, Telangana, India

Vijay Kher
MD (Medicine) DM (Nephrology) FAMS FRCPE FIMAS
Chairman
Department of Nephrology and Transplant Medicine
Epitome Kidney and Urology Institute
New Delhi, India

Vinant Bhargava
DNB (Medicine) DNB (Nephrology) MNAMS FASN FRCP (Edinburgh) FACP MBA (HCM)
Senior Consultant
Department of Nephrology
Sir Ganga Ram Hospital
New Delhi, India

Vinay Sakhuja
MD (Medicine) DM (Nephrology) MNAMS (Nephrology)
Director
Department of Nephrology and Transplant Medicine
Max Hospitals
Mohali, Punjab, India
Former Head
Department of Nephrology
Postgraduate Institute of Medical Education and Research
Chandigarh, India

Vivek Kumar
MD (Medicine) DM (Nephrology)
Associate Professor
Department of Nephrology
Postgraduate Institute of Medical Education and Research
Chandigarh, India

Vivek Kute
MD (Medicine) DM (Nephrology)
Professor and Unit Head
Department of Nephrology
Institute of Kidney Diseases and Research Center and
Dr HL Trivedi Institute of Transplantation Sciences
Ahmedabad, Gujarat, India

Foreword

At the outset, we wish to declare that the field of organ transplantation excites us sheerly because of its impact in improving survival in patients with end-stage kidney disease. With emerging medical technologies and improved understanding of immunobiology, this field has seen progress from the era of splenectomy to the era of the use of biological agents and immunoadsorption to reduce allosensitization pre- as well as post-transplantation. However, we are now dealing with agents that have their own set of long-term problems such as infections (pertinent to our subcontinent), slow graft loss, malignancies and systemic side effects. On the overall we have to develop newer methods to achieve immune tolerance and to find to hone our understanding of xenotransplantation as well as lab cultivated organs. Till we reach unto this stage, we must ensure that we are able to allocate each kidney disease patient an appropriate organ (live/deceased) to remove the stigma associated with this disease. We hope, that you find this *Textbook of Kidney Transplantation* as a handy weapon to guide your endeavor in the future. I wish the contributors of this masterpiece, which has been specially crafted for the Indian readers (students/physicians/transplant surgeons), success in their endeavor to spread knowledge and bust myths regarding this subject.

Padma Shree DS Rana
MD MNAMS
Professor
Department of Nephrology
Chairman, Institute of Renal Sciences
Chairman, Sir Ganga Ram Trust Society
New Delhi, India
Dr BC Roy awardee

Padma Shree AK Bhalla
MD DM MNAMS FISN FASN (USA) FRCP (Edinburgh) FISOT
Professor and Chairman
Department of Nephrology
Sir Ganga Ram Hospital
New Delhi, India
Dr BC Roy awardee

Foreword

The first successful kidney transplantation between identical twins in December 1954 at the Peter Bent Brigham Hospital, Boston, USA, opened a new door to the world of increased survival and vastly improved quality of life for patients with end-stage kidney failure.

Much water has flown down many rivers around the world over the last 68 years, with improvement in patient and graft survival, thanks to refinements in surgical techniques, the development of never more specific and less toxic immunosuppressive agent, and improved monitoring ability to detect and pre-empt complications and institute early treatment.

The global transplantation community continues to look for ways to further improve the survival and life experience of people who have received a kidney transplantation. Contraindications to transplantation have progressively diminished, as has access to organs. Given the transformative nature of transplants, increasing access to potentially life-saving donor organs to all subjects eligible to receive an allograft is an important goal. Efforts towards the latter require engaging with societies, policymakers and patient groups to expand the scope of deceased organ donation in all parts of the world.

A number of challenges still remain—in particular, our quest to improve the long-term outcomes of transplantation and better understand as well as manage the vexed issue of allosensitization that can limit the life of an allograft. Immune tolerance that might permit successful transplants without the need for additional immunosuppression remains an aspirational goal. Progress in the field of xenotransplantation and/or the development of kidney organoids might ultimately be the answer, but at this stage seems not ready for prime time. Also critical is to minimize infection risk and have access to tools that allow early identification and appropriate management of this critical complication.

In this context, I am pleased to write this foreword for a very relevant and comprehensive work—one that looks at all elements of kidney transplantation that one could encounter in clinical practice. What is notable that all this has been written by Indian experts, so provides the right context for all practicing transplanters. It is important to use such a work to bust myths and develop a framework that allows us to provide not only the best evidence-based care under resource limited situations, but also pushing the envelope to improve the standard of practice in the country that makes them uniform and eliminates the wide disparities that exist in our society and ability of patients with kidney failure to access the best care possible.

A number of challenges remain—an important one is for kidney transplantation to be included in the ambit of universal health coverage that takes away the financial barrier that limits access to this wonderful miracle of medical care to all who can benefit from it. Work is also needed to improve the organ donation environment in the country—which will also require community engagement, enabling legislative reforms and removal of differential access.

I congratulate the authors and the editors on their tremendous work and hope that improved knowledge will translate into efficient action leading to meaningful change.

Vivekanand Jha MD DM
Chair
Global Kidney Health Imperial College, London
Conjoint Professor of Medicine
University of New South Wales
Sydney, Australia
Ex-Professor
Department of Nephrology
Postgraduate Institute of Medical Education and Research
Chandigarh, India

Preface

Kidney transplantation as we now understand is the most superior form of renal replacement therapy in end-stage kidney disease patients. A successful kidney transplant provides a better quality of life as well as prolongs survival in such patients. However, only a handful of this population is fortunate enough to receive a kidney transplant. Hence, in several parts of the world, this modality still remains a privilege and a large proportion of this population is dependent on dialysis. Furthermore dialysis facilities are still largely inadequate to make up for the deficits.

Transplantation has been an attractive and a novel concept for many years now. In 1945, three young surgeons at the Peter Brigham Hospital in Boston, Charles Hufnagel, Ernest Lansteiner and David Hume, anastomosed the brachial vessels of a comatose young woman with acute renal failure to the vessels of a cadaver kidney. The graft and patient outcome was good, however the patient recovered from her acute renal failure and had functioning native kidneys. The allograft was later on removed from this patient. This provided the desired impetus towards transplantation in patients with chronic kidney disease and especially so those who were prescribed dialysis.

Initial attempts were experimental animal models by the Dr Emerich Ulman (1902) in Vienna, and then by Dr Alecia Carrel (1903) in the United States of America. The vascular anastomosis technique by Carrel continues to be used in the present date. The concept of rejection was not very well discussed during this time. However, Dr Carl Williamson of the Mayo Clinic was very clear on autograft and homograft (1923) when he described the concept of rejection in the allograft.

Despite all these shortcomings, Dr David Hume in Boston, performed a cadaveric kidney transplant where he placed the organ on the thigh of the patient. However, in spite of performing many surgeries, only one kidney survived for nearly 6 months, raising the expectation for a longer successfully functional allograft. This was performed without immunosuppressive medication. Dr Morton Simonsen in Copenhagen and Dr William Dempster in London demonstrated problems with rejection in animal models. Thereafter, in 1953, Drs Rupert Billingham, Lesley Brent and Peter Medawar demonstrated that tolerance to an allogeneic skin graft in an adult animal could be produced by injecting the fetus with donor strain tissue, thus confirming experimentally the clonal selection hypothesis of Burnet and Fenner in the recognition of self and non-self. This provided a major thrust to the field of research in transplantation medicine. Achieving immune tolerance has always remained the ultimate goal of transplant immunologists ever since.

In 1954, following the successful transplantation of identical twins at Peter Bent Brigham Hospital, Boston, USA by Joseph Murray and his team, led to many more such transplants. Richard and Ronald Herrick were the identical twins, but Richard was dying of kidney disease. Ronald donated one of his kidneys, and it was successfully transplanted into Richard. Because they were identical twins, the organ did not appear foreign to Richard's body, which did not reject it. This confirmed Peter Medawars work on skin allograft.

Despite all this, the dilemma of rejection of any kidney other than an identical-twin kidney still persists. Dr Merril's group in Boston attempted to suppress the immune response to a kidney allograft with total body irradiation of the recipient under the direction of Drs Kuss, Hamburger from Paris and by Professor Shackman's group in London. Rejection of a graft could be suppressed by irradiation, but the complications of the irradiation were not conducive to accepting this as a valid approach. However, an occasional relatively long-term acceptance of a graft provided encouragement for the future.

Then came the discovery of 6-mercaptopurine in 1959 by Drs Schwartz and Dameshek. This was shown to suppress the immune response of rabbits to human serum albumin. Shortly afterwards, they showed that the survival of skin allografts in rabbits was significantly prolonged. Roy Cale in London and Charles Zukoski working with David Hume showed that this same drug markedly prolonged the survival of kidney allografts in dogs. 6-mercaptopurine was first used in a patient in Boston in 1960. Elion and Hitchings of the Burroughs Wellcome Research Laboratories in New York State then developed azathioprine, which quickly replaced the 6-mercaptopurinein clinical practice as it was less toxic. With the advent of steroids, a combination of these two drugs laid the path for the present day immunosuppression protocol. Calcineurin inhibitors, induction agents (Thymoglobulin, basiliximab, daclizumab, alemtuzumab) the scenario of immunosuppression began to change worldwide. These new agents enabled high immunological risk transplantation. Thereafter, co-stimulatory blockers such as CTLA-4 fusion molecules such as belatacept enabled CNI-free regimens in low-risk transplantation. Further advances in immunoadsorption therapies have eased transplantation in blood group mismatch conditions.

Not just immunosuppressants, the next era aimed at developing new techniques for detecting antibodies so as to decrease the level of immunosuppression in patients. Human leukocyte antigen (HLA)-based matching techniques between donor and recipient were developed. With the advent of solid antigen-based assays detecting selective antibodies that might induce immune injury by rejection has enabled the incidence of rejections to be at the lowest possible as compared to the past few decades. However, the persistent endeavor of achieving immune tolerance and minimal immunosuppression will be the next level of achievement for mankind.

In this book, we have tried to cover pertinent topics related to renal transplantation bearing in mind renal fellows, practicing physicians, immunologists, and transplant surgeon. We have a special emphasis on case-based discussions and summaries at the end of chapters. We have in addition to renal transplantation covered combined organ transplantation also. We have a special emphasis on cadaver transplant and how to setup cadaver transplant program in the country. The Cadaver transplantation program has immense potential in this country and has a long way to go to help the end-stage renal disease patient. We hope this book is of value to all those who read it. We will be open to suggestions if any, to improvise our next edition.

Vinant Bhargava
Manisha Sahay
Priti Meena
Vinay Sakhuja
Amit Gupta

Acknowledgments

To our mentors in nephrology.

To our colleagues, well-wishers and contributors whose work has paved the path forward for the future generations.

To our parents, wives and families who have endured with us with their patience and unfailing support during the preparation of this edition.

To our God, our patients, without whom we would not have the privilege to cure and care.

Contents

CHAPTER 1

Immunobiology and Evaluation Techniques

1.1 Transplant Immunobiology

Shruti Tapiawala, Suchita Jogale

INTRODUCTION

Transplantation is the preferred option of treatment for patients suffering from end-stage organ diseases. The immune system is directed to distinguish self from nonself and destroy the nonself. Rejection of a transplanted organ, tissue, or cell is a process in which the immune system identifies the transplanted organ, tissue, or cells as nonself/foreign and initiates a response to destroy it. The challenge to maintain the function of the transplanted organ and prevent rejection is the Achilles heel of transplantation medicine. Understanding the immune responses to the new organ is the basis of evolution of drugs and strategies to prevent rejection of the transplanted organ.

This chapter will explain the terminologies used in immunobiology of transplantation, concepts of transplant immunobiology, key cells and chemicals which are important in the immune response to a transplanted organ, and the mechanisms of rejection and tolerance.

TERMINOLOGIES USED IN TRANSPLANT IMMUNOBIOLOGY

The transplanted organ/tissue is called a graft and based on the origin of the graft, different terms are used **(Fig. 1)**. When an organ or tissue is transplanted from one site to another in the same individual, the graft is termed autograft. If the graft is transplanted into an identical individual, it is termed an isograft. If the graft is transplanted into a nonidentical individual from the same species, the graft is termed an allograft. If a transplanted organ is taken from different species, it is termed xenograft.[1]

The immune response to an allograft is termed allo-immune response which is initiated by T-cell recognition termed allorecognition of transplantation antigens or

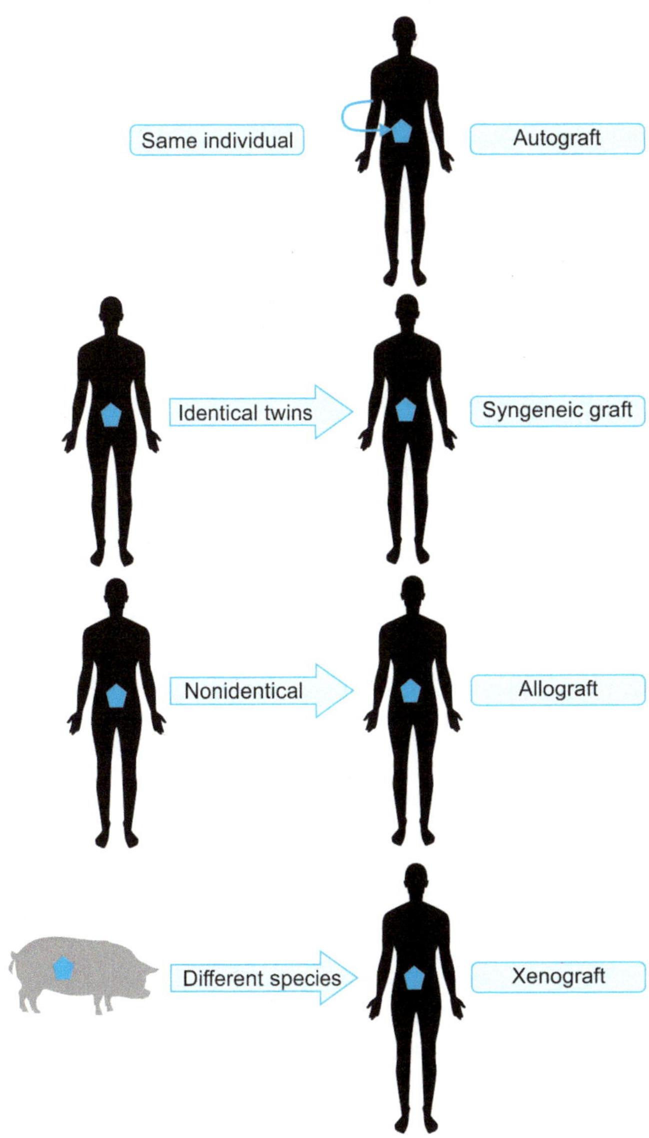

Fig. 1: Types of grafts.

alloantigens which are unidentical in recipient and donor and may be responsible for graft rejection.

MAJOR HISTOCOMPATIBILITY COMPLEX (FIG. 2)

The major histocompatibility complex (MHC) is a gene family that produces membrane proteins and is found on the short arm of chromosome 6 (6p21.3). It is the most variable gene cluster in the human genome. In 1958, Jean Dausset (1916–2009) discovered the first human leukocyte antigen (HLA), which he named "MAC" after the three letters of three of his volunteers' first names. HLA-A2 was the name given to it later. HLA class I and II antigens were discovered via lymphocytotoxicity tests (LCT) and mixed lymphocyte culture (MLC). MHC antigens relevant to clinical transplantation were broadly divided into two classes—classes I and II. Each class is encoded by several loci.[2,3]

The MHC class I molecules are expressed on almost all nucleated cells and platelets. The MHC class I proteins are subdivided into classical loci HLA-A, HLA-B, and HLA-C. HLA-E, HLA-F, HLA-G, MHC class I polypeptide-related sequence A (MICA) and B (MICB), etc., are classified as nonclassical MHC class I genes. MHC class II molecules are expressed on antigen-presenting cells (APCs) such as B cells, dendritic cells, and macrophages. The clinically relevant HLA class II loci are HLA-DR, -DP, and -DQ.[1,4]

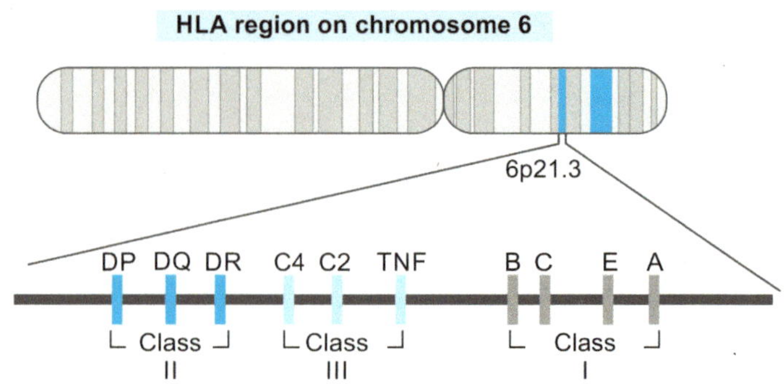

Fig. 2: Major histocompatibility complex. (HLA: human leukocyte antigen)

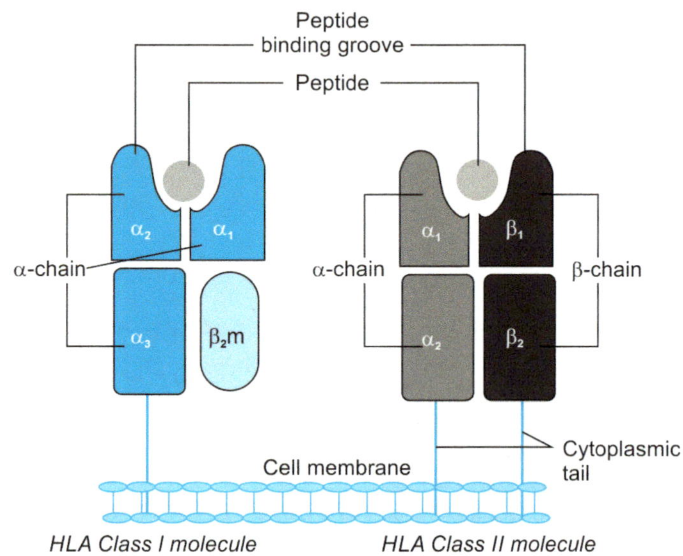

Fig. 3: Human leukocyte antigen (HLA) molecular structure. (β_2m: β_2-microglobulin)

HUMAN LEUKOCYTE ANTIGEN STRUCTURE (FIG. 3)

Human Leukocyte Antigen Class I

Class I molecules consist of glycosylated heavy chains encoded by the HLA class I genes and noncovalently bound to extracellular β_2-microglobulin (β_2m). Heavy chain (45,000 kD) consists of three α domains, namely α_1, α_2, and α_3. The HLA specificity is conferred due to the polymorphic regions in α_1 and α_2 domains. The light chain, β_2m molecule (12,000 kD), is associated with a heavy chain, not covalently bound to it and not attached to the cell membrane.[5]

Human Leukocyte Antigen Class II

Human leukocyte antigen class II (cell surface glycopeptides) has a molecular weight of approximately 63,000 kD and consists of two structurally similar α and β transmembrane glycoprotein chains.

These chains have two amino acid domains, the outermost domain containing the variable region of class II alleles. The peptide-binding groove in class I and class II molecules is critical for functional aspects of HLA molecules.[6]

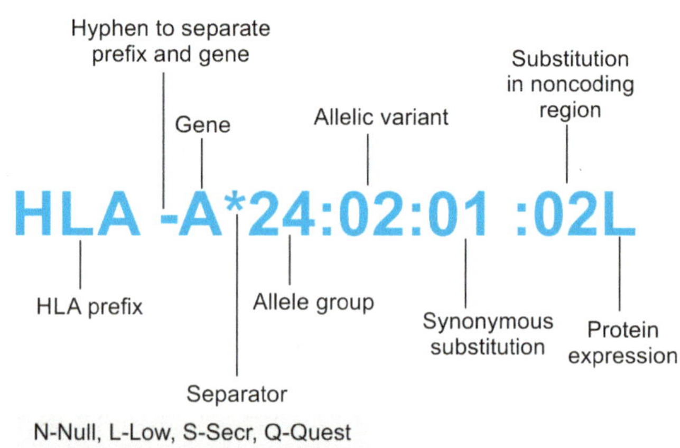

Fig. 4: Human leukocyte antigen (HLA) nomenclature.

NOMENCLATURE (FIG. 4)

All alleles begin with the letters "HLA," indicating that they are part of the human *MHC* genes. The following part (HLA-A) tells which gene the allele is a variant of. The first two numbers (HLA-A*24) indicate the antigen type of that specific allele, which usually indicates the serological antigen present. The next two numbers (HLA-A*24:**02**) indicate the allele code of protein, and these are numbered in the order in which they were discovered. The third digit (HLA-A*24:02:**01**) indicates an allele variant that has a different deoxyribonucleic acid (DNA) sequence than the normal gene but generates the same protein. The fourth digit (HLA-A*24:02:01:**01**) indicates single or multiple nucleotide polymorphisms in a noncoding region. Finally, the suffix (HLA-A*24:02:01:**01N**) denotes changes in expression.[7,8]

FUNCTION

Although HLA molecules are best known as transplantation antigens, their primary biological function is to regulate immune response.

Human Leukocyte Antigen Class I

The function of class I MHC is to present endogenous antigens to T cells. Peptide antigens derived from proteins that may be self-protein, altered self-proteins such as those found in cancer cells, and viral proteins found in viral infected cells fit into peptide-binding groove of HLA molecules. These antigens are degraded by large multifunctional proteases (LMPs) and transported to the endoplasmic reticulum (ER) by a transporter associated with antigen processing (TAP) inside the cell. Then, they are transported to cell surface. They interact with CD8+ T cells. There is an inflammatory response if the T-cell receptor (TCR) of a T lymphocyte can bind antigenic peptide.[4]

Human Leukocyte Antigen Class II

In contrast to class I, class II molecules are synthesized in the ER, but peptide antigens are not placed in the peptide-binding groove. Instead, an invariant chain (Ii) is placed as a stopper combined class II–invariant chain is carried to the endosome. In endosome, another molecule called DM first removes the invariant chain, followed by insertion of class II antigenic peptide. Exogenous proteins, which can be normal self-proteins or microorganisms, are used to make these peptides. Class II molecules are delivered to the cell surface, where they interact with $CD4^+$ T cells, causing antibodies to be produced.[4]

Table 1 shows the difference between HLA class I and class II.

RELEVANCE IN RENAL TRANSPLANTATION

Foreign peptides are presented by the mismatched HLA present on the allograft to the immune system of the recipient. Once presented to the immune system, donor-specific antibodies (DSAs) are produced. A higher number of HLA mismatches between recipient and donor have consistently been noted to increase rates of early rejections and inferior allograft survival in multiple studies.[9]

Donor-specific antibodies have been proven to be causative of immune events in the allograft and can cause allograft loss. Preformed DSAs and de novo DSAs formed post-transplant are risk factors for graft loss in organ transplants. With advancing technology, HLA antibodies can be identified by means of sensitive HLA crossmatches and virtual crossmatch, which take into account the donor HLA and HLA antibody specificities identified by solid-phase assays in the patient's serum.[10,11]

HLA-A, -B, and DR have the most polymorphism, and their mismatching has been seen to be associated with a higher risk of HLA sensitization. Recently, studies have shown that HLA-DQ antibodies commonly develop de novo DSA among post-transplants, and a strong positive correlation exists between the development of donor-specific HLA-DQ antibodies and a higher risk of allograft rejection.[4] (*See* Chapter 1.4 "Donor-specific Antibodies in Kidney Transplantation.)

MINOR HISTOCOMPATIBILITY ANTIGENS

The minor histocompatibility antigens (MiHA) are proteins which are expressed in some individuals in the population. This creates potential antigenic differences between donors and recipients. In theory, a polymorphism of any protein

TABLE 1: Differentiating features between HLA class I and class II.

	HLA class I	*HLA class II*
Structure	Contains three α domains, namely α_1, α_2, and α_3 One β_2-microglobulin	Consists of two structurally similar α and β transmembrane glycoprotein chains
Peptide (number of AA)	9–11	12–28
Present on	All nucleated cells	Antigen-presenting cells such as B cells, dendritic cells, and macrophages
Peptide-binding region	α_1 and α_2	α_1 and β_1
Antigen source	Present endogenous antigens to T cells	Present exogenous antigens to T cells
Peptide generation	By cytosolic proteasome	By endosomal and lysosomal proteases
Interact with	CD8+ T cells	CD4+ T cells

(HLA: human leukocyte antigen)

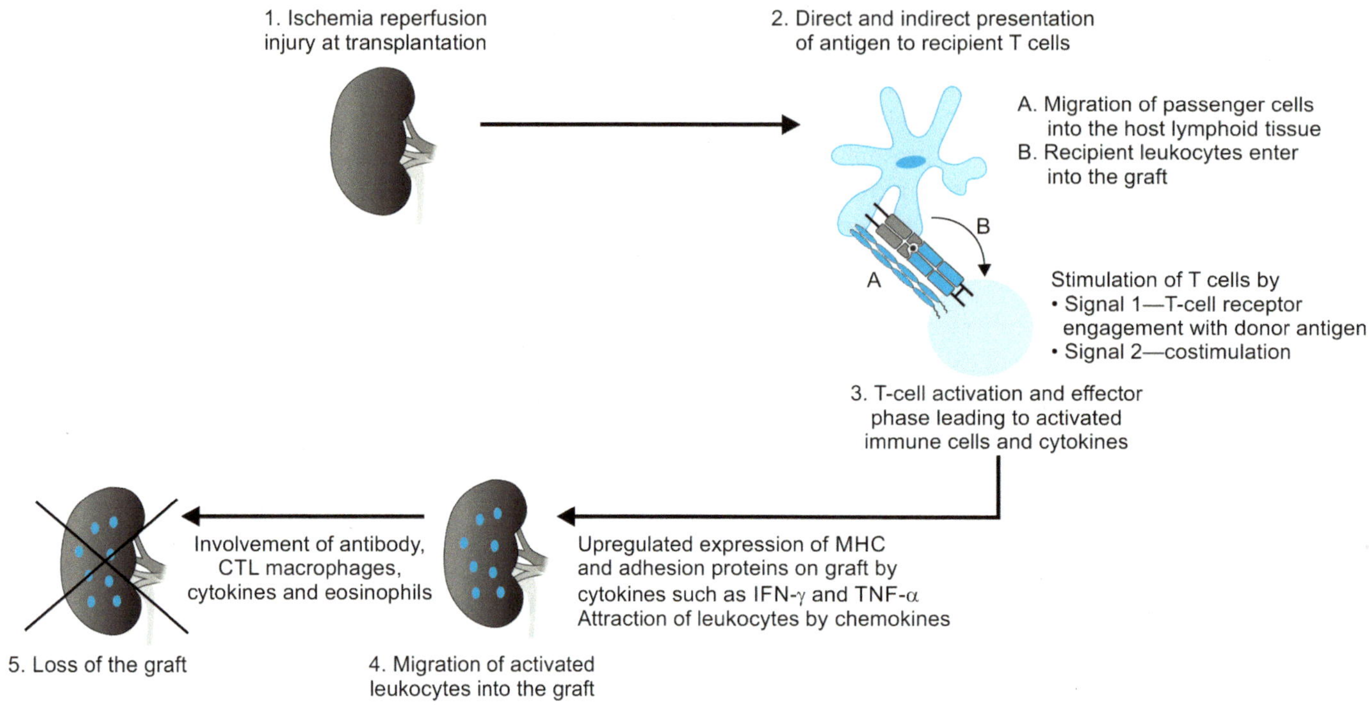

Fig. 5: Evolution of immune response after kidney transplant recipients (KTR). (CTL: cytotoxic T lymphocyte; IFN: interferon; MHC: major histocompatibility complex; TNF: tumor necrosis factor)

between donor and recipient, e.g., certain cell surface receptors and enzymes that can be processed and presented, can elicit a rejection response. These antigens are recognized by the CD8+ cytotoxic T cells, leading to rejection.[1,10]

Transplant immunology is an evolving field, and antigenic stimuli have been identified in various proteins over the last five decades. In case of bone marrow transplants, where a well-matched graft has been transplanted, the MiHA play an important role in causing graft versus host disease. Another MiHA noted is the Y-MiHA, produced when a male allograft is transplanted into a female. Here, protein coded by Y-chromosome elicits an immune response. Other non-HLA antibodies that can cause rejection are antiangiotensin-2 receptor, antiglutathione S-transferase T1, antiendothelial antibodies, and antibodies to MHC class I-related chains A and B (MICA and MICB). Some antigens may come from mitochondrial proteins and enzymes.[1,4] (*See* Chapter 1.4 "Donor-specific Antibodies in Kidney Transplantation.)

IMMUNE RESPONSE TO A TRANSPLANTED GRAFT

The rejection process has two parts: (1) An afferent/initiation or sensitization limb where recognition of foreign antigens takes place and (2) an effector limb which destroys the allograft **(Fig. 5)**.[12,13]

Recognition of Foreign Antigens

Allorecognition (recognition of allograft MHC antigen) is the trigger for allograft rejection. T cells recognize alloantigens via direct and indirect pathways **(Figs. 6A and B)**, which are mutually exclusive.

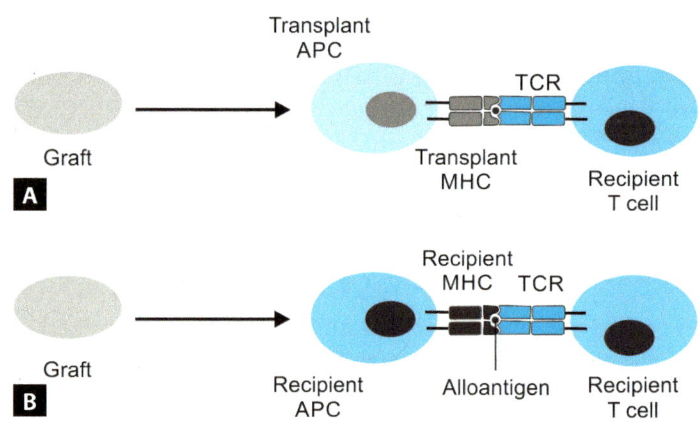

Figs. 6A and B: (A) Direct allorecognition; and (B) Indirect allorecognition. (APC: antigen-presenting cell; MHC: major histocompatibility complex; TCR: T-cell receptor)

Direct recognition occurs when recipient T cells recognize intact donor HLAs expressed by donor cells.

In contrast, indirect recognition occurs when the recipient APC processes the donor-HLA antigens prior to presentation to the recipient's T cells.

The direct pathway plays an important role in the immediate post-transplant period and can put forth a strong alloresponse, which occurs primarily due to recipient T cells recognizing the mismatched/nonself-graft antigens. This can cause acute cellular rejection. The indirect pathway may also participate in early acute rejections, but this mechanism predominantly causes late-onset acute and chronic rejections. Due to the constant presence of an allograft which is in itself a self-antigen, the APC itself picks up alloantigens which are shed from the allograft and this initiates an alloimmune response.

Semidirect pathway: Dendritic cells (DCs) acquire intact MHC–peptide complexes from other DCs and endothelial cells (ECs) and present them to alloreactive T cells. This pathway involves the uptake and surface expression of intact foreign MHC+ peptide complexes by the recipient APC.

Activation of T Cells

T-cell activation is central to the immune response to an allograft. Tissue destruction occurs due to direct T cell-mediated lysis of graft cells, activation of accessory cells, and alloantibody production with or without complement activation. Three distinct signals are involved from T-cell activation to production of effector T cells and alloantibodies, which ultimately result in damage of the allograft. These include (1) antigen recognition, (2) costimulation, and (3) cytokine-mediated differentiation and expansion of pool of alloreactive effector cells that participate in graft injury and destruction **(Figs. 7A and B)**.[1,10,13]

Signal 1

The interaction between the antigen-specific T cells and APCs acts as the first signal for T-cell activation. The interaction leads to phosphorylation of the immunoreceptor tyrosine-based activation motifs (ITAMs) of the TCR/CD3 complex.[1,10]

Signal 2—Costimulatory Signal (Fig. 8)

In addition to the formation of MHC–peptide complex, a costimulatory signal is necessary. In the absence of the costimulatory signal, the T cells become anergic or unresponsive.[14,15] Although there are many costimulatory molecules on T cells, the focus of clinical transplantation has been on CD28 and CD154 pathways.

The CD28/B7 costimulatory pathway is involved in allo T-cell activation. CD28 is expressed on the resting T cells, and its ligands are expressed on the activated APCs, the ligands being B7.1 (CD80) and B7.2 (CD86). CD28 signaling reduces the threshold of TCR signaling, which further promotes T-cell proliferation, cytokine production, and differentiation.

CD4 and CD8 T cells play a major role in rejections of grafts mismatched for MiHA. CD4 T cells facilitate CD8 T cells differentiation by direct cell-to-cell contact or by producing cytokines such as interleukin-2 (IL-2) and interferon-gamma (IFN-γ). These, in turn, will help CD8 T-cell proliferation and killing of graft tissue.[16,17]

The CD154/CD40 costimulatory pathway has also been researched in animal transplantation models. CD154 is expressed on activated T cells, while CD40 is expressed on APCs and B cells.

Blockade of these signals leads to inactivation/anergy of the antigen-specific T cells. T cells also possess cytotoxic T-lymphocyte-associated antigen 4 (CTLA4), a protein that is a negative regulator of the immune response that can compete for binding with CD80 and CD86. Belatacept (LEA29Y), a second-generation humanized fusion protein that binds CTLA4, has been used with a promise to suppress rejection and improve long-term graft survival. Blocking CD28/B7 and CD154/CD40 therapeutically works synergistically to prevent acute and chronic rejections.[18]

Signal 3 and Effector Phase of Graft Rejection

The costimulatory response after T-cell interaction (signal 1) activates three signal transduction pathways: calcineurin pathway, activated protein kinase pathway, and IκB kinase (IKK)—nuclear factor κB (NK-κB). This initiates the effector phase of rejection. The effector phase of the graft rejection involves the entry of activated T cells into the allograft and the production of cytokines.[1,10]

CD8+ T cells require cytokine signals produced by macrophages and/or DCs for the generation of effector and memory cells population and to survive to take the cascade further. The CD8+ T cells that do not receive the cytokine signals after signals 1 and 2 are devoid of cytolytic function and become unresponsive.

Once signals 1 and 2 are received, generation of cytokines including CD25, CD154, IL-2, and IL-15 is induced. These interleukins then release growth signals (signal 3) through the mammalian target of rapamycin pathway and phosphoinositide-3-kinase pathway. These subsequently trigger the T-cell growth cycle and proliferation. The completely activated T cells undergo clonal expansion and release cytokines and effector T cells. These eventually produce CD8+ cytotoxic T cells, which help macrophage-induced delayed-type hypersensitivity response with the help of CD4-T helper cells 1. They further help B cells to produce antibodies with $CD4^+$ T helper cells 2.

Complement system also plays a major role in the effector mechanism of rejection. Signals 1 and 2 augment the intracellular cleavage of complement C3. The fragments are transported to the cell membrane, which bind to their corresponding receptors and further amplify the activation signal of T cells. Complement-dependent cytotoxicity remains a crucial step in the lysis of donor cells.[19]

The effector elements, as mentioned above, are responsible for the clinical manifestations of allograft rejection. A subset of the activated T cells further goes on to become alloantigen-specific memory T cells.[1,10,20-23]

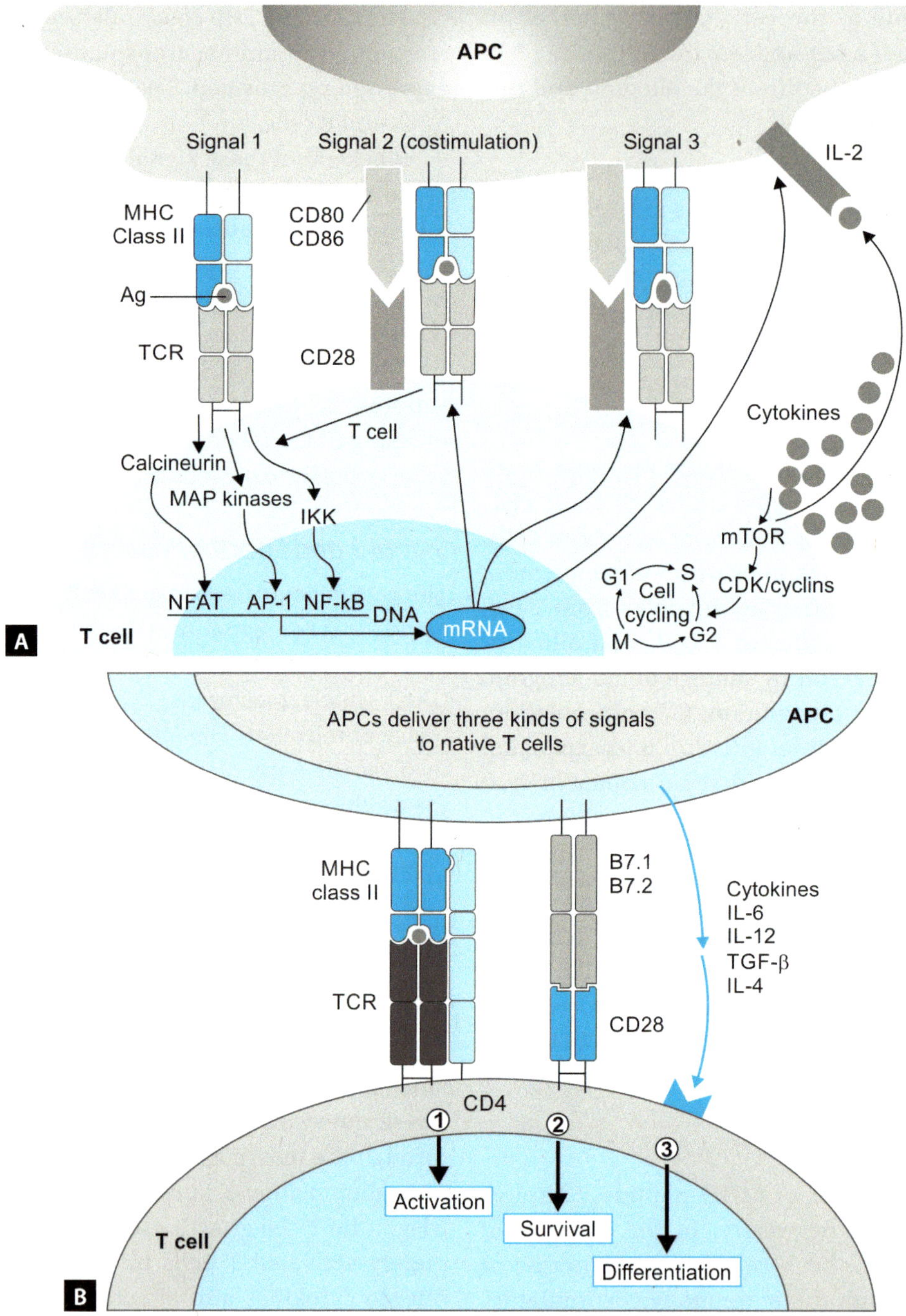

Figs. 7A and B: (A) The three-signal model; (B) The three-signal model with effectors. (APC: antigen-presenting cell; CDK: cyclin-dependent kinase; DNA: deoxyribonucleic acid; IKK: IκB kinase; IL: interleukin; MAP: mitogen-activated protein; MHC: major histocompatibility complex; mRNA: messenger ribonucleic acid; mTOR: mammalian target of rapamycin; NF-κB: nuclear factor kappa B; NFAT: nuclear factor of activated T cells; TCR: T-cell receptor)

Termination of Immune Response

Transplant rejection is a vicious cycle where release of donor antigens, production of alloreactive T cells, and infiltration of the allograft with effector T cells leads to further shedding of graft antigens and further alloimmune activation till the graft is destroyed.

Effector lymphocytes are generated during an immune response, but most undergo activation-induced cell death (AICD) by apoptosis as the response progresses. Few effector lymphocytes that survive give rise to memory T lymphocytes (Tm). Exhaustion occurs when the effector or memory T lymphocytes repeatedly encounter a persistent antigen as would occur in the case of an allograft. Repeated antigenic stimulation induces the expression of inhibitory molecules that make T cells hypo- or unresponsive.

CD4$^+$ Foxp3+ regulatory T cells (Tregs) are a subset of helper T cells, which help control the response by secreting cytokines (e.g., IL-10 and TGFβ) and inhibitory

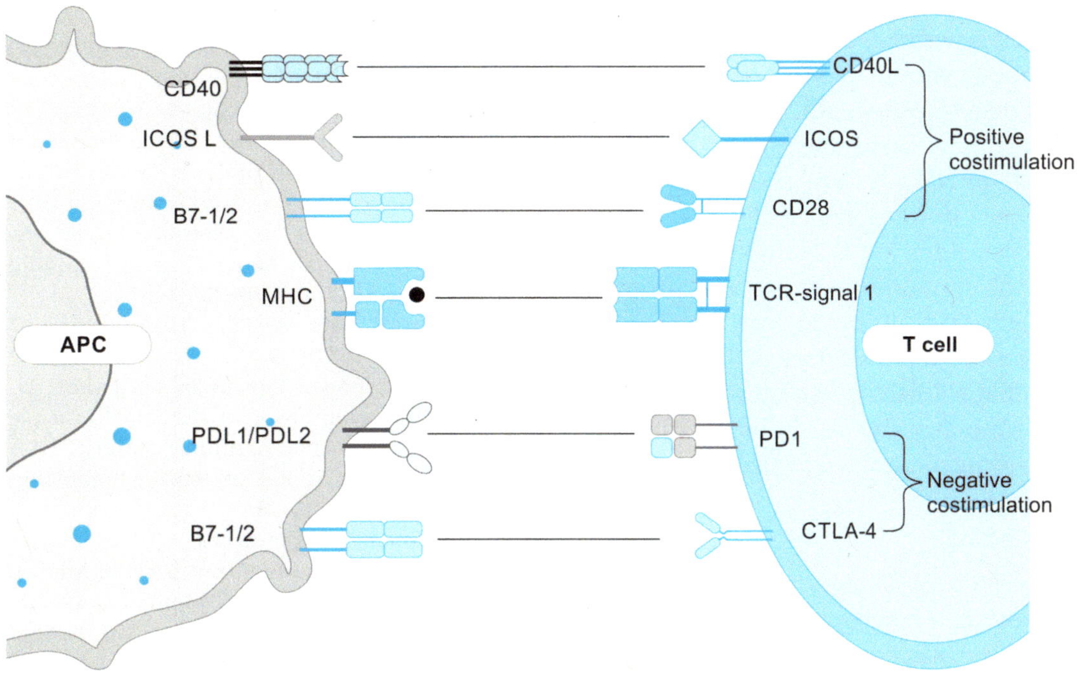

Fig. 8: Costimulatory molecules. (APC: antigen-presenting cell; MHC: major histocompatibility complex; TCR: T-cell receptor; ICOS: inducible co-stimulator; PDL: programmed death ligand; PD: programmed death; CTLA: cytotoxic T lymphocyte antigen)

membrane molecules (e.g., CTLA-4), which inhibit immune responses and prevent the immune response from continuing indefinitely and control inflammation. These cells also suppress effector cells and modulate dendritic cell maturation.[1,23,24]

B CELLS

The role of B cells and their progeny, plasma cells, lies in the production of anti-HLA antibodies, which have been implicated in both acute and chronic rejection. B cells express antigen-specific receptors on their surfaces. When these immunoglobulin receptors bind to the respective antigens from the donor with assistance from T helper cells (CD4$^+$TH2), activation occurs. Some activated B cells generate plasma cells, which secrete antibodies and some become memory B cells.[25-27] B-cell activation is facilitated by membrane contact involving receptors and ligands such as CD40 and CD154 or with the help of secreted cytokines such as IL-4. Plasma cells and CD20+ B cells have been seen infiltrating the allografts. These have been identified to be markers of irreversible acute rejection episodes.[28,29]

The donor-specific HLA antibodies bind to antigens and cause allograft injury by complement-dependent cytotoxicity or through Fc receptors on natural killer (NK) cells. B cells also participate in the indirect allorecognition pathway where they present allograft-derived antigens to T cells, activate T cells, and further amplify T cell-mediated damage.[1,10]

NATURAL KILLER CELLS

Natural killer cells represent a specific population of lymphocytes (5–10% of circulating lymphocytes), which are involved in the innate immune response in an individual, which is involved in antitumor and antiviral defense of an individual. NK cells are naturally cytotoxic and do not require antigen exposure to mediate their effects.[30,31]

The NK cells exert their lytic effect through direct lysis and antibody-dependent cellular cytotoxicity (ADCC). Recognition of self-HLA molecules by inhibitory receptors, namely the killer cell immunoglobulin-like receptors (KIRs), inhibits the lytic effect of NK cells. Direct lysis happens when the NK cells fail to detect self-HLA molecules on the target cells. ADCC happens when the Fc receptor (FcγRIII) of the NK cell interacts with the Fc fragment of the HLA antibody, recognizing foreign antigen on the target cell and inducing lysis. NK cells, once activated, kill their targets by secreting enzymes such as granzyme, perforin, and IFN-γ. NK cells can prime the adaptive immune system and facilitate the migration of dendritic cells, which can cause an alloimmune response and loss of allograft.[30-32]

The presence of NK cells and donor-specific HLA antibodies (DSAs) has been shown to facilitate rejection. The mere presence of DSAs in the absence of NK cells does not induce rejection, although it can lead to late graft failure. The pathogenic function of NK cells causing antibody-mediated rejection (ABMR) is mediated through the expression of CD16. The pathogenicity can be triggered by the presence of DSAs and can cause graft injury.

NK cells have been identified in the peritubular capillaries of tissues with ABMR. It is postulated that DSAs bind to the EC where they can interact with the FcγRIII receptors present on NK cells and cause lysis by ADCC. NK cells have also been associated with chronic rejection.[1,32-34]

Specific subsets of NK cells are associated with the induction of tolerance in transplant recipients. Activated NK cells can kill donor-derived DCs through direct lysis, thus dampening the immune response and promoting tolerance of the allograft.[1] It is unclear which factors move the NK cells toward donor-derived dendritic cells. It can be thought that NK cells might be able to integrate stimulatory and inhibitory signals, influenced by T-cell behavior, causing the outcome of rejection or tolerance.[33]

DENDRITIC CELLS

Dendritic cells are APCs found in tissues such as skin and mucosal membranes. Their functions are to process antigens and present them to the immune system and are the bridge between innate and adaptive immunity. Their importance lies in the induction of a protective immune response against pathogens. The key role of DCs in transplantation is in the activation and maintenance of immune responses to allografts. Once the DCs are activated, they move to the lymphatic tissues to further interact with T and B cells to make an adaptive response. Due to their ability to regulate both innate and adaptive immunity, DCs are considered to potentially direct immune responses toward rejection or tolerance. Allograft rejection is initiated at the allograft EC layer and forms an immunogenic barrier for migrating DCs. The DC/EC interactions play an important role in the rejection. Direct and indirect pathways are used by donor DCs and host DCs, respectively, to activate alloreactive T cells and mediate rejection.[35]

It is thought that clonal deletion, induction of T regulatory cells, and inhibition of memory cell responses help achieve tolerance. These properties have encouraged research to use tolerogenic DC as a therapeutic strategy to promote tolerance in a transplant patient. Infusions of donor/recipient-derived tolerogenic DCs have helped achieve tolerance in murine models.[36]

CONCLUSION

An understanding of transplant immunobiology and its orchestra consisting of cells and their effector elements helps us form the basis of transplantation and immunosuppression used to prevent rejection and maintain an allograft. It further helps us work toward therapies and immunomodulation to establish tolerance and accommodations in transplantation.

REFERENCES

1. Danovitch GM. Handbook of Kidney Transplantation, 6th edition. New Delhi: Lippincott Williams and Wilkins a Wolters Kluwer Business; 2017.pp. 21-45.
2. Degos L. Jean Dausset a scientific pioneer: Intuition and creativity for the patients (1916–2009). Haematologica. 2009;94:1331-32.
3. Bach FH, Amos DB, Whitmore FC, Emery KO, Cooke HBS, Swift DJP. Hu-1: Major Histocompatibility Locus in Man. Science. 1967;156:1506-8.
4. Klein J, Sato A. The HLA system. N Engl J Med. 2000;343(10):702-9.
5. Orr HT, López de Castro JA, Lancet D, Strominger JL. Complete amino acid sequence of a papain-solubilized human histocompatibility antigen. HLA-B7.2 Sequence determination and search for homologies. Biochemistry. 1979;18(25):5711-25.
6. Kaufman JF, Strominger JL. The extracellular region of light chains from human and murine MHC Class II antigens consists of two domains. J Immunol. 1983;130(2):808-17.
7. Bodmer JG, Marsh SG, Albert ED, Bodmer WF, Dupont B, Erlich HA, et al. Nomenclature for factors of the HLA system. Vox Sang. 1992;63:142-57.
8. Marsh SGE, Albert ED, Bodme WFr, Bontrop RE, Dupont B, Erlich HA, et al. Nomenclature for factors of the HLA system 2010. Tissue Antigens. 2010;75(4):291-455.
9. Cecka JM, Qiuheng JZ, Raja R, Reed E. Chapter 3: Histocompatibility Testing, Crossmatching, Immune Monitoring. Handbook of Kidney Transplantation, 6th edition. New Delhi: Lippincott Williams and Wilkins a Wolters Kluwer Business; 2017.pp. 46-75.
10. Kumbala D, Zhang R. Essential concepts of transplant immunology for clinical practice. World J Transplant. 2013;3(4):113-8.
11. Kramer CSM, Roelen DL, Heidt S, Claas FHJ. Defining the immunogenicity and antigenicity of HLA epitopes is crucial for optimal epitope matching in clinical renal transplantation. HLA. 2017; 90:5-16.
12. Colvin RB. Cellular and molecular mechanisms of allograft rejection. Annu Rev Med. 1990;41:361-75.
13. Rao KV. Mechanism, pathophysiology, diagnosis and management of renal transplant rejection. Med Clin North Am. 1990;74(4):1039-57 .
14. Jenkins MK, Pardoll DM, Mizuguchi J, Chused TM, Schwartz RH. Molecular events in the induction of a nonresponsive state in interleukin 2-producing helper T-lymphocyte clones. Proc Natl Acad Sci USA. 1987;84(15):5409-13.
15. Jenkins MK, Shwartz RH. Antigen presentation by chemically modified splenocytes induces antigen-specific T cell unresponsiveness in vitro and vivo. J Exp Med. 1987;165:302.
16. Filatenkov AA, Jacovetty EL, Fischer UB, Curtsinger JM, Mescher MF, Ingulli E. CD4 T cell-dependent conditioning of dendritic cells to produce IL-12 results in CD8-mediated graft rejection and avoidance of tolerance. J Immunol. 2005;174:6909-17.
17. Shrikant P, Khoruts A, Mescher MF. CTLA-4 blockade reverses CD8+ T cell tolerance to tumor by a CD4+ T cell- and IL-2-dependent mechanism. Immunity. 1999;11:483-93.

18. Larsen CP, Elwood ET, Alexander DZ, Ritchie SC, Hendrix R, Tucker-Burden C, et al. Long-term acceptance of skin and cardiac allografts after blocking CD40 and CD28 pathways. Nature. 1996;381:434-8.
19. Cravedi P, Leventhal J, Lakhani P, Ward SC, Donovan MJ, Heeger PS. Immune Cell-Derived C3a and C5a Costimulate Human T Cell Alloimmunity. Am J Transplant. 2013;13(10):2530-9.
20. Curtsinger JM, Mescher MF. Inflammatory cytokines as a third signal for T cell activation. Curr Opin Immunol. 2010;22:333-40.
21. Mescher MF, Curtsinger JM, Agarwal P, Casey KA, Gerner M, Hammerbeck CD, et al. Signals required for programming effector and memory development by CD8+ T cells. Immunol Rev. 2006; 211:81-92.
22. Fiorentino L, Austen D, Pravtcheva D, Ruddle FH, Brownell E. Assignment of the interleukin-2 locus to mouse chromosome. Genomics. 1989;5:651-3.
23. Tsaur I, Gasser M, Aviles B, Lutz J, Lutz L, Grimm M, et al. Donor antigen-specific regulatory T-cell function affects outcome in kidney transplant recipients. Kidney Int. 2011;79:1005-12.
24. Ingulli E. Mechanism of cellular rejection in transplantation. Pediatr Nephrol. 2010;25(1):61-74.
25. Mills DM, Cambier JC. B lymphocyte activation during cognate interactions with CD4+ T lymphocytes: molecular dynamics and immunologic consequences. Semin Immunol. 2003;15:325-9.
26. Richards S, Watanabe C, Santos L, Craxton A, Clark EA. Regulation of B-cell entry into the cell cycle. Immunol Rev. 2008;224:183-200.
27. Gatto D, Martin SW, Bessa J, Pellicioli E, Saudan P, Hinton HJ, et al. Regulation of memory antibody levels: the role of persisting antigen versus plasma cell life span. J Immunol. 2007;178: 67-76.
28. Hippen BE, DeMattos A, Cook WJ, Kew CE, 2nd, Gaston RS. Association of CD20+ infiltrates with poorer clinical outcomes in acute cellular rejection of renal allografts. Am J Transplant. 2005; 5:2248-52.
29. Lehnhardt A, Mengel M, Pape L, Ehrich JH, Offner G, Strehlau J. Nodular B-cell aggregates associated with treatment refractory renal transplant rejection resolved by rituximab. Am J Transplant. 2006;6:847-51.
30. Morvan MG, Lanier LL. NK cells and cancer: you can teach innate cells new tricks. Nat Rev Cancer. 2016;16:7-19.
31. Beilke JN, Grill RG. Frontiers in nephrology: the varied faces of natural killer cells in transplantation—contributions to both allograft immunity and tolerance. J Am Soc Nephrol. 2007;18:2262-7.
32. Yagisawa T, Tanaka T, Miyairi S, Tanabe K, Dvorina N, Yokoyama WM, et al. In the absence of natural killer cell activation donor-specific antibody mediates chronic, but not acute, kidney allograft rejection. Kidney Int. 2019;95: 350-62.
33. Hadad U, Martinez O, Krams SM. NK cells after transplantation: friend or foe. Immunol Res. 2014;58:259-67.
34. Yazdani S, Callemeyn J, Gazut S, Lerut E, de Loor H, Wevers M, et al. Natural killer cell infiltration is discriminative for antibody-mediated rejection and predicts outcome after kidney transplantation. Kidney Int. 2019;95:188-98.
35. Schlichting CL, Schareck WD, Kolfer S, Weis M. Involvement of dendritic cells in allograft rejection, new implications of dendritic cell-endothelial cell interactions. Mini Rev Med Chem. 2007;7(4):423-8.
36. Raimondi G, Thomson AW. Dendritic cells, tolerance and therapy of organ allograft rejection. Contrib Nephrol. 2005;146:105-20.

1.2 Immunologic Evaluation of Kidney Transplant Candidates

Ajay Kumar Baranwal, Uma Kanga

CASE VIGNETTE 1

A 32-year-old multiparous woman with end-stage renal disease, secondary to lupus nephritis, was being worked up for live donor renal transplantation. She had been on hemodialysis for the last 3 years. There was no history of blood transfusions or transplantation. Apart from renal failure, she had no major comorbidities. Potential donor has a 3/6 mismatch. Flow crossmatch was positive. Single antigen beads (SAB) assay was negative for donor-specific antibody (DSA). What would be your approach in such a case?

Discussion: The patient is a case of lupus nephritis, an autoimmune disease. She has the propensity to produce autoantibodies. Keeping in mind her history, clinical picture, and SAB assay negative for DSA in a background of flow crossmatch positivity, the most likely possibility for discordant flow crossmatch and SAB result is the presence of autoantibodies. Auto-crossmatch was done in this case and turned out to be positive. She underwent transplantation and doing well 1 year after transplantation.

CASE VIGNETTE 2

A 48-year-old male patient with end-stage renal disease secondary to hypertension and diabetes mellitus was being worked up for the second transplant. First transplant was done 9 years ago. The recipient had a history of multiple transfusions. Potential donor has a 4/6 mismatch. Panel reactive antibody (PRA) is 78% and a prospective flow crossmatch is performed using a freshly drawn specimen. The crossmatch is T-cell negative and B-cell positive at 80 mean channel shift (MCS) (cutoff > 50 MCS). This result is most likely explained by what type of antibody?

- *A: Class I and II human leukocyte antigen (HLA) antibodies*
- *B: Class I only HLA antibodies*
- *C: Class II only HLA antibodies*
- *D: Autoimmune antibodies*

Discussion: The patient was sensitized, having PRA 78% with risk factor of previous transplantation and multiple transfusions. T-cell flow crossmatch is negative while B-cell flow crossmatch is positive. In such a scenario with sensitization history, the patient is most likely to have anti-HLA class II antibodies. The patient may also have low titer anti-HLA class I antibodies. SAB assay was done in this patient. The patient had class II DSA with mean fluorescence intensity (MFI) of 9,300 and class I MFI of 1,400. The patient later on underwent kidney paired donation and is doing well after 6 months.

INTRODUCTION

The human leukocyte antigen (HLA) complex located on the short arm of chromosome 6 is the 4 Mb long, complex genomic region comprising hundreds of genes that are functionally relevant. These genes are highly polymorphic, display linkage disequilibrium, and are inherited en bloc. The antigens encoded by the *HLA* genes are divided into class I (HLA-A, -B, and -C) and class II (HLA-DR, -DQ, and -DP). According to the latest Immuno Polymorphism Database-ImMunoGeneTics (IPD-IMGT)/HLA database version 3.50 (http://www.ebi.ac.uk/ipd/imgt/hla), approximately 36,016 allelic variants have been reported and this number is growing exponentially. HLA compatibility between recipient and donor is of major clinical relevance in both hematopoietic stem cell and solid organ transplantation.

Human leukocyte antigen laboratory in a setting of organ transplantation is entrusted with two main responsibilities: (1) HLA typing to determine the degree of mismatch between the recipient and donor and (2) detection of HLA antibodies, particularly those directed against donor HLA. Several technologies have been established for accurate HLA typing and detection of anti-HLA antibodies, and these are discussed in detail in subsequent sections.

HUMAN LEUKOCYTE ANTIGEN TYPING TECHNOLOGIES

In 1964, Terasaki and McClelland first introduced the serological HLA typing, which has been the mainstay of HLA typing technology.[1] In the 1980s, the deoxyribonucleic acid (DNA)-based methodology was initiated and restriction fragment length polymorphism (RFLP) established for HLA typing. Since the advent of polymerase chain reaction (PCR) in 1986, DNA-based tissue typing techniques have become routine in the histocompatibility laboratories. The PCR-based assays include sequence-specific primers (SSP), sequence-specific oligonucleotide probe (SSOP), reverse SSO, sequence-based typing (SBT), real-time PCR, and next-generation sequencing (NGS).[2,3] A brief description of various methods for HLA typing and their advantages and disadvantages are given below.

SEROLOGICAL TECHNIQUE: COMPLEMENT-DEPENDENT MICROLYMPHOCYTOTOXICITY TEST

The serology-based HLA typing or the microlymphocytotoxicity assay is a technique that applies the principle of complement-dependent cytotoxicity (CDC). For this assay, the lymphocytes of an individual are separated and incubated with a set of HLA-specific alloantisera and/or monoclonal antibodies, and later the reaction starts with the addition of rabbit serum, which is used as a source of complement. The method enables identification of HLA alleles expressed on lymphocyte surface. Based on this principle, when the antibody binds to HLA antigen on the cell surface, it activates the complement and forms a membrane attack complex that damages the cell membrane and makes it permeable to vital dyes. Results are visualized on addition of the fluorochrome-based dyes (ethidium bromide/acridine orange) or supravital dye (eosin Y). The staining distinguishes live and dead cells, as the live cells look unstained, refractile, and small round shiny structures while the dead cells look large, dark structures. The results can be evaluated by counting the percentage of dead cells on an inverted fluorescence microscope.[1,4] The HLA allele is assigned for the particular cell/sample depending on the antibody to which the binding was observed. Several HLA antigens share antigenic determinants (polymorphic epitopes); therefore, one antibody can react with a number of HLA antigens. Extensive quality checks, i.e., good screening of alloantisera or use of monoclonal antibodies, are important for this CDC-based technique.

Advantages and disadvantages of serology: This assay is simple and easy to perform, does not require expensive equipment, and can be performed in a short duration of 3–4 hours. Presently, this technique is not routinely used for HLA typing but is used as an adjunct to molecular methods, i.e., to identify the "N" null alleles or the nonexpressed HLA alleles. However, this conventional method has certain limitations, such as cell viability, need for fresh sample in large volume, dependence on surface expression of HLA alleles, complexity in interpretation due to cross-reactivity of antisera, and cannot be used for high-resolution typing or detection of rare alleles. Therefore, alternative technologies were developed for HLA typing.

DEOXYRIBONUCLEIC ACID-BASED HUMAN LEUKOCYTE ANTIGEN TYPING TECHNOLOGIES

Molecular techniques have an advantage over the serological methods as fresh blood/live lymphocytes are not required, and DNA can be extracted from any nucleated cell and stored for long durations. This helps in high throughput testing and also repeat testing if required. All of the DNA-based methods utilize the PCR to identify the genomic region of interest. For most DNA-based methodologies, the PCR process is used only as an amplification step to acquire the required target DNA. The HLA typing process then requires a postamplification step to discriminate between the different alleles. These molecular techniques are employed for low-, intermediate-, and high-resolution typing and are commonly used in laboratories performing clinical testing for diagnostics and/or donor selection for transplantation.

Although HLA typing can be performed by using a single molecular technique, ambiguities can arise depending on the primers and probes used for the region being analyzed. The three possible reasons for the generation of ambiguities are: (1) If the polymorphic sites distinguishing the alleles in question are located outside the amplified region, (2) when multiple allele pairs display identical heterozygous sequences, and (3) when part of the sequence is incomplete within the genomic region being analyzed. The ambiguities can usually be resolved by utilizing multiple molecular techniques. The molecular techniques for HLA typing are described below.

Polymerase Chain Reaction

Sequence-specific Primer

In this technology, SSP pairs selectively amplify target sequences that are specific for a single allele or allele groups present on the target DNA within the locus of interest.[5] Several allele-specific primers for the locus of interest are utilized, and multiple individual PCR amplifications are performed.[6,7] The synthesis of a new strand is dependent on binding between the genomic DNA and the 3′ end of the primer, as the 3′ end confers specificity to the primers to anneal and thus amplify the target sequence. Furthermore, each reaction is multiplexed with a nonpolymorphic "housekeeping" gene serving as an internal control. Presence of an amplicon, i.e., a positive reaction with one or more allele-specific primer sets, is detected by agarose gel electrophoresis, and the HLA allele is assigned based on the amplification pattern. This technique is unlikely to detect a new unidentified allele unless the primer picks the variation at a specific site and results in an unexpected or unique reaction pattern.

Advantages and disadvantages: Most commercial PCR-SSP assays utilize common thermal cycling conditions for amplification of both HLA class I and II alleles. This is the preferred technology for laboratories requiring results in short duration of 4–5 hours and have lower throughput. This is an effective alternative to serology-based testing. However, this method usually requires a large quantity of DNA, is cumbersome to perform, and generates low-resolution information. Furthermore, intermediate/high-resolution information can be generated by using primers for all alleles within a particular allelic family, but the assay is expensive. This methodology is useful for cadaveric donor typing or for diagnostic and pharmacogenomic screening tests of single alleles such as HLA-B*27 (ankylosing spondylitis), HLA-B*51 (Behcet's disease), B*57:01 (abacavir hypersensitivity), B*15:02 (carbamazepine hypersensitivity), and HLA-DQA/DQB (celiac disease).

Sequence-specific Oligonucleotide Probes

Polymerase Chain Reaction Sequence-specific Oligonucleotide Probes

This method employs locus-specific PCR amplification followed by immobilization of the PCR amplicon on the nylon membrane and hybridization with allele-specific oligonucleotide probes. The HLA typing is obtained depending on the binding of each oligo probe with the complementary sequence in the PCR amplicon. Use of radioactive probes was a limitation of PCR-SSOP that was overcome by the development of the option to use biotinylated oligoprobes. Although longer hybridization protocols and the need to employ a large number of probes increased the test duration, SSOP was often used for HLA typing of a large number of samples. Depending on the primers and probes used, PCR-SSOP was employed for both low- and high-resolution HLA typing.[8,9] This technology is no longer in regular use as several advanced technologies are now available.

Reverse Line Strip Assay Sequence-specific Oligonucleotide

The above mentioned SSOP technology was further modified with the use of biotinylated PCR primers (specific for exons 2 and 3 for class I and exon 2 for class II) and immobilization of locus- and allele-specific oligos on nylon strips. Therefore, the technique is named reverse line strip (RLS) assay. It is based on three major processes: PCR target amplification of an HLA locus, hybridization of the amplified products to an array of immobilized SSOPs, and detection of the probe-bound amplified product by color formation. Amplicon binding is detected via streptavidin horseradish peroxidase (HRP) and a chromogenic substrate, which generates a blue line at the position of positive probe **(Fig. 1)**. The technology utilizes a combination of probes for polymorphisms that are shared between large numbers of alleles. This leads to significant limitation, i.e., either precise identification of alleles, or generates allelic strings, thus resulting in low- to intermediate-resolution HLA typing and is unlikely to detect a new undefined HLA allele.

Luminex Sequence-specific Oligonucleotide

The SSO assays were further improvised with development of Luminex® xMAP technology.[10] The basic principle involves measurement of multiple analytes simultaneously. A series of probes are immobilized on microbeads that are color coded

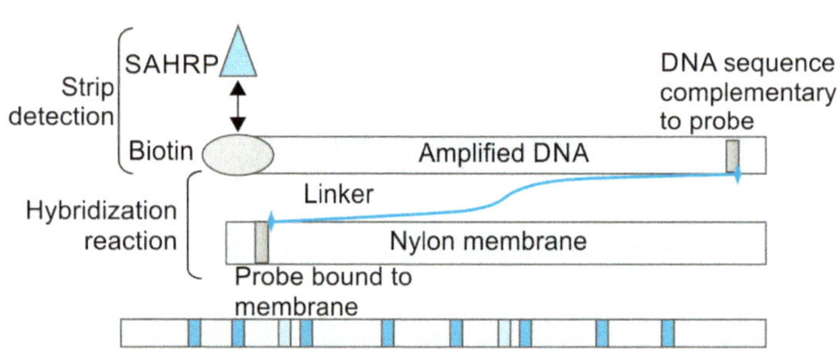

Fig. 1: Reverse line strip blot sequence-specific oligonucleotide (SSO) assay representation. (DNA: deoxyribonucleic acid; SAHRP: streptavidin-horseradish peroxidase)
Source: Smith L, Fidler S. HLA typing technologies. In: Mehra NK (Ed). The HLA Complex in Biology and Medicine: A Resource Book. Jaypee Brothers Medical Publishers (P) Ltd; 2010.

using a blend of fluorescent intensities of two dyes. Target genomic regions of HLA loci (exons 2 and 3 for HLA class I and exon 2 for HLA class II) are amplified and biotinylated PCR amplicons are hybridized with beads carrying locus-specific probes. The binding was detected using streptavidin-conjugated phycoerythrin (SAPE) **(Fig. 2)**. The fluorescent signals are detected using Luminex flow analyzer platform and interpretation software detects the bead reaction pattern assigned to the HLA allele. More than 100 individual beads, i.e., >100 different probes, are available for each assay, which improves the resolution of HLA typing.

Although this technique requires longer execution time, it has selected advantages, namely rapid kinetics reduce incubation times, requires less quantity of DNA, can be applied for high-throughput testing, and provides intermediate- to high-resolution results. Additionally, this technique has been improved for last several years by the addition of a large number of probes; therefore, high-resolution-level HLA typing information can also be obtained using high-definition beads with a larger number of probes. The development of 500 bead system associated with LabScan 3D has helped in reducing allele ambiguities by using powerful software for assessment of reaction patterns and thus improving the reliability of results.[11] Therefore, currently, this is the most preferable technique for generic and high-resolution HLA typing of all loci.

Real-time Polymerase Chain Reaction

This DNA-based HLA typing technology was developed for rapid detection of specific HLA alleles with increased sensitivity and utilized the TaqMan assay.[12] This approach was applied for typing of single HLA alleles.[13] Further advancements in combining the PCR-SSP and SYBR green principles led to the development of the real-time PCR (RT-PCR) assay that can detect PCR products without postamplification manipulation. The PCR is performed with SYBR green in the buffer, and both thermal cycling and melting curve analysis are performed on the quantitative PCR (qPCR) equipment.[14] After thermal cycling, PCR amplicons are heated across a temperature range and they melt (become single stranded) at a certain temperature depending on the size, guanine-cytosine content, and sequence motif captured within the DNA fragment. When each amplicon melts, the SYBR green fluorescence decreases rapidly, which is captured by the instrument. This technology helps identify HLA alleles at a low–intermediate resolution in few hours. This approach has considerable advantages for rapid HLA typing required for deceased donor testing in solid organ transplantation.[15]

Sequencing-based Typing

This technology is based on locus- or group-specific PCR amplification, followed by cycle sequencing using dye terminator technology.[16] Usually, the HLA sequencing

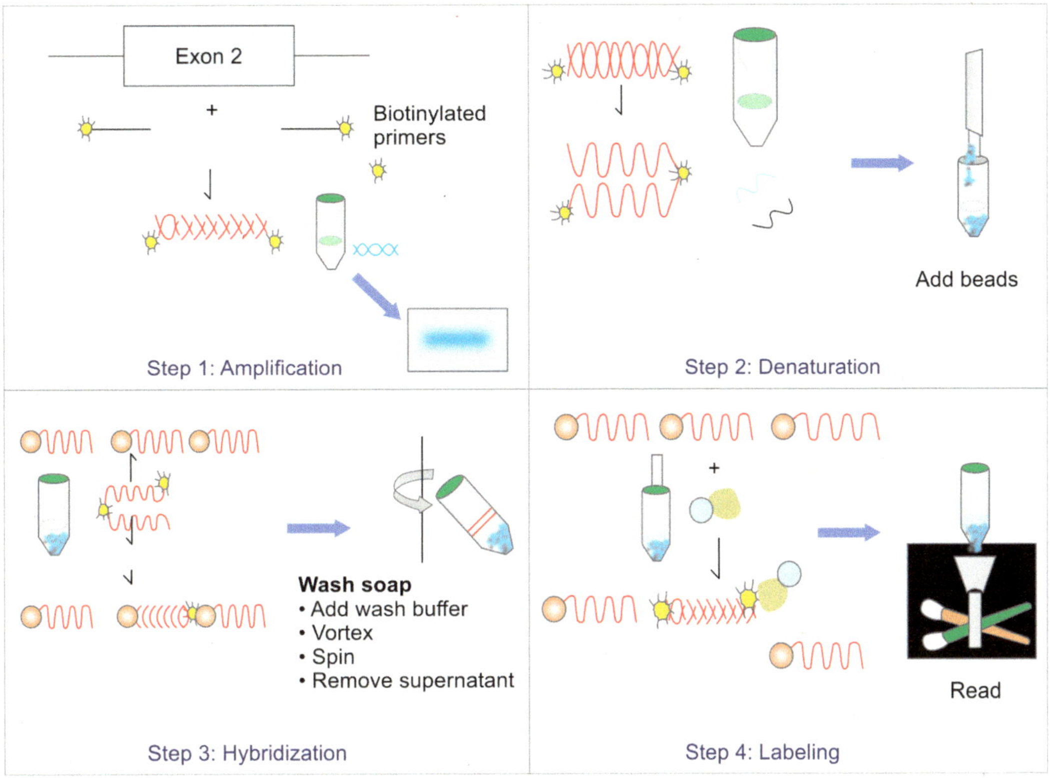

Fig. 2: Principle of Luminex-based reverse sequence-specific oligonucleotide (SSO) method.
Source: Smith L, Fidler S. HLA typing technologies. In: Mehra NK (Ed). The HLA Complex in Biology and Medicine: A Resource Book. Jaypee Brothers Medical Publishers (P) Ltd; 2010.

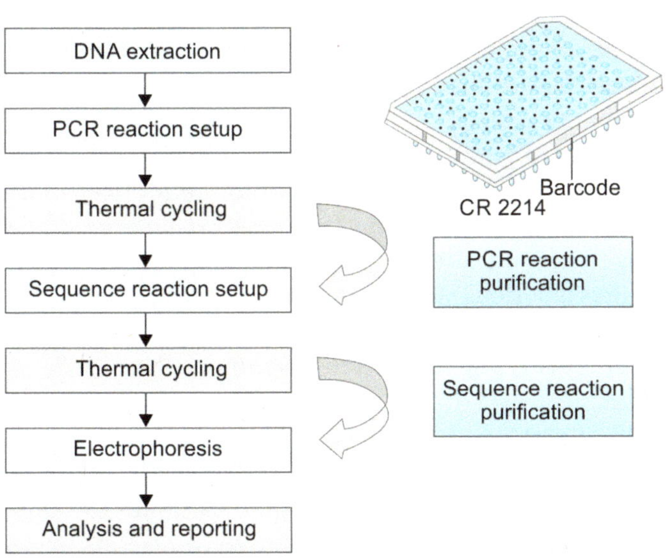

Fig. 3: Sequenced-based human leukocyte antigen (HLA) typing general workflow. (DNA: deoxyribonucleic acid; PCR: polymerase chain reaction)
Source: Smith L, Fidler S. HLA typing technologies. In: Mehra NK (Ed). The HLA Complex in Biology and Medicine: A resource book. Jaypee Brothers Medical Publishers (P) Ltd; 2010.

is restricted to exons 2 and 3 for HLA class I alleles and exon 2 for HLA class II alleles. Initial amplicons generated are purified to remove unincorporated nucleotides, and product is sequenced using multiple sequencing primers in separate reactions **(Fig. 3)**. The four different

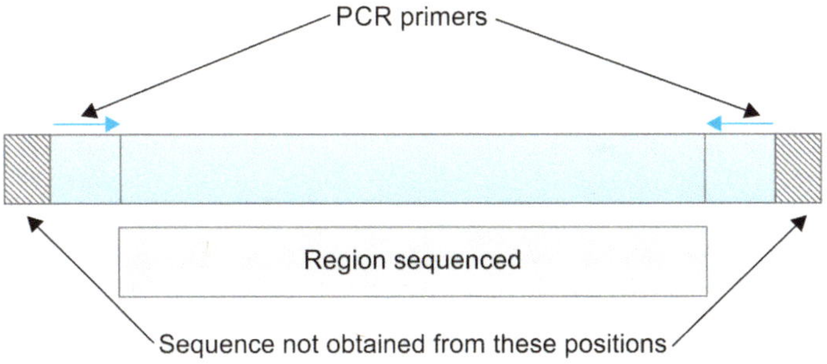

Fig. 4: Genomic region sequenced based on primer location. (PCR: polymerase chain reaction)
Source: Smith L, Fidler S. HLA typing technologies. In: Mehra NK (Ed). The HLA Complex in Biology and Medicine: A Resource Book. Jaypee Brothers Medical Publishers (P) Ltd; 2010.

2′,3′-dideoxyribonucleotides, once incorporated in the growing sequence, cause a stop of elongation and emit light at different wavelengths. After PCR, the DNA fragments are sequenced on an automated capillary sequencer and the nucleotides at the end of fragments are identified by the fluorescence emitted.

The sequence generated depends on the primer design for initial PCR and can vary, i.e., (1) primer located within the exon of interest, (2) in flanking introns, and (3) on adjacent exons. Use of primers within introns results in complete exon sequence **(Figs. 4 and 5)**, but can lead to allele dropout due to lack of intron sequences. An alternate approach is the use of multiplexing allele/group-specific primers **(Fig. 6)**.

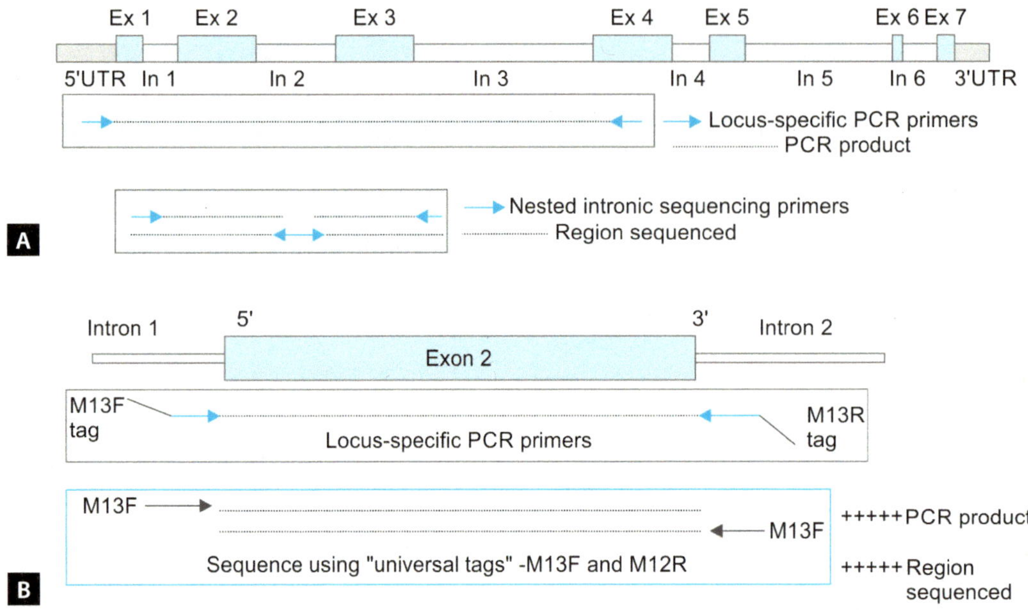

Figs. 5A and B: Polymerase chain reaction (PCR) strategy for sequencing of (A) Human leukocyte antigen (HLA) class I genes (nested sequencing primer); and (B) HLA class II (with universal tags). (UTR: untranslated region)
Source: Smith L, Fidler S. HLA typing technologies. In: Mehra NK (Ed). The HLA Complex in Biology and Medicine: A resource book. Jaypee Brothers Medical Publishers (P) Ltd; 2010.

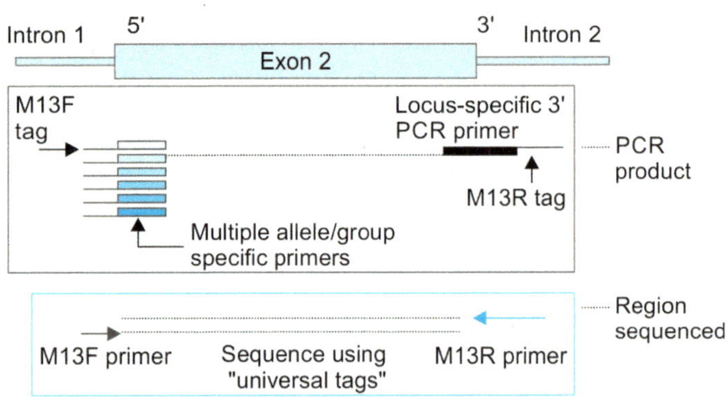

Fig. 6: Multiplex group/allele-specific polymerase chain reaction (PCR) strategy for human leukocyte antigen (HLA) class II sequencing.
Source: Smith L, Fidler S. HLA typing technologies. In: Mehra NK (Ed). The HLA Complex in Biology and Medicine: A Resource Book. Jaypee Brothers Medical Publishers (P) Ltd; 2010.

To resolve ambiguities located outside the amplified regions stated above, additional regions such as exon 4 for class I and exon 3 for class II alleles are also sequenced. HLA typing by SBT was initially employed as a tool to resolve ambiguities arising in other molecular methods; however, despite sequencing, several factors lead to ambiguities. The sequenced region can be shared by several HLA alleles; thus, a pair of common HLA alleles or several less common allelic pairs can be assigned. The ambiguous result due to identical heterozygote sequences can be resolved by group-specific primary amplification and each allele amplified and sequenced.[17,18]

The advantage of determining the complete nucleotide sequence promoted SBT as the gold standard for high-resolution HLA typing. This technology is not dependent on known polymorphisms and picks up new alleles that are not recognized by existing primers and probes. Additionally, SBT enables evaluation of the synonymous and nonsynonymous mutations. These approaches have enabled identification of thousands of HLA alleles, and these observations have helped in updating the commonly well-defined (CWD) catalog. This technology is expensive and time consuming, but use of capillary-based automated sequencers increased the efficiency and decreased the cost to some extent. However, expertise in interpreting sequenced-based typing results is crucial for final interpretation and allele assignment. Resolving ambiguous allele combinations requires laborious efforts and does not remain cost effective as it has to be combined with other molecular methods and requires many high-resolution workflows.[19,20]

Next-generation Sequencing

The true innovations, i.e., technological advancements such as NGS, have revolutionized the characterization of polymorphic *HLA* genes as this technology generates a massive amount of data for a large number of different target DNA sequences in parallel in a single reaction. This technology is based on the monitoring of sequential addition of nucleotides to immobilized DNA templates arranged spatially. NGS provides careful characterization of *HLA* genes by high-resolution genotyping with relatively simple and cost-effective protocols. The NGS process generally involves few steps: Sample preparation and locus-specific amplification, DNA library preparation, normalization, sequencing, data acquisition, and bioinformatics. Different NGS platforms, such as Ion Torrent, Illumina, Pacific

Biosciences, and Oxford Nanopore, all differ in terms of sequencing approach and have variable processing time ranging from few hours to days. The manufacturers have now developed varying processes to acquire sequence data from amplified single DNA fragments in their platforms.

As the sequences are generated from single molecules, complications associated with cis/trans ambiguities get rectified at a cost comparable to SBT.[21] The benefits and feasibility of NGS approaches as an alternate HLA sequencing methodology have been evaluated using large reference panels previously tested by PCR-SSP/SSO/SBT.[22,23] NGS could contribute to expand the knowledge about the biological relevance of both coding and noncoding HLA sequences in solid organ and stem cell transplantation.[24-26] The clinical efficacy of NGS has been successfully validated, and most histocompatibility testing laboratories define the standards for clinical typing by the different sequencing platforms.[27] NGS allows sequencing of multiple HLA loci, i.e., 6–11 loci, and the laboratories can perform high-throughput HLA typing as multiple samples can be barcoded and pooled into one library and sequenced together.

The laboratory's choice of technology to be employed differs and is based on clinical need, throughput, urgency, infrastructure, and staff skills. There are several advantages and disadvantages for each technology **(Table 1)**. Most laboratories employ combinations of methods for perfect assignment of HLA alleles and for resolving ambiguities arising by any single methodology.

IMMUNOLOGICAL ASSESSMENT FOR TRANSPLANTATION

The main aim of testing for HLA antibody in allograft recipients is to determine the donor–recipient compatibility and to evaluate the ongoing immune status of the recipient before and after transplantation in order to assess the potential risk for graft loss. This information enables clinicians to make logical decisions regarding donor selection, immunosuppression regimens, and post-transplant patient care. Thus, an accurate, sensitive, and HLA-specific detection of these antibodies becomes very important. In pursuit to achieve this, several methodologies have been developed since the introduction of the original cell-based cytotoxicity assay. Currently, anti-HLA antibodies can be detected by target donor cell-based assays, such as CDC or flow cytometry and HLA protein-based (solid phase) assays, such as an enzyme-linked immunosorbent assay (ELISA) or HLA-antigen-coated fluorescence bead assay system. Importantly, evaluation of assay results depends on understanding the characteristics of each assay, the theoretical principles involved, and the technological or biophysical limitations of the reagents, instrumentation, and analytical methods employed. The methods for detecting HLA antibodies are used in two distinct clinical applications: (1) As a crossmatch method to determine if a patient has antibodies directed against donor and (2) as a screening assay to determine the level of sensitization. The specific

TABLE 1: Advantages and disadvantages of human leukocyte antigen (HLA) typing technologies.

Technique	*Advantages*	*Disadvantages*
Serology	• Rapid and inexpensive • Assesses HLA cell surface expression • Time taken 3–4 hours	• Cross-reactivity • Limited polymorphism detection • Low resolution • Requires viable lymphocytes • HLA cell surface expression critical
PCR-SSP	• Resolution is better than serology • Specific allele can be identified • DNA can be stored • Low and high resolution possible • Time taken 4–5 hours	• Low throughput • Labor intensive • High DNA quantity required • Several PCR reactions for each locus • 24 reactions HLA-A; 48 reactions HLA-B; 24 reactions HLA-DRB1
PCR-SSO	• Locus-specific amplification • Generic and high resolution possible • Low DNA quantity • High throughput 96 tests at once • Time taken 6–7 hours	• Sequence of allele must be known • Hybridization is critical • At times ambiguities issue
SBT	• More reliable and specific • Allele sequence detected • Low DNA quantity required • Novel alleles can be detected	• Huge infrastructure required • Expensive than other techniques • Time taken 24–36 hours
NGS	• Most reliable and specific • Allele sequence detected • Low DNA quantity required • Novel alleles can be detected	• Infrastructure is expensive • Cost effective if high throughput • Bioinformatics expertise required • Time taken 3–4 days

(DNA: deoxyribonucleic acid; NGS: next-generation sequencing; PCR: polymerase chain reaction; PCR-SSO: PCR-sequence-specific oligonucleotide; PCR-SSP: PCR-sequence-specific primers; SBT: sequence-based typing)

features and limitations of the available techniques for detection of anti-HLA antibodies are discussed in detail in the subsequent paragraphs, and their evolution is depicted in **Figure 7**.

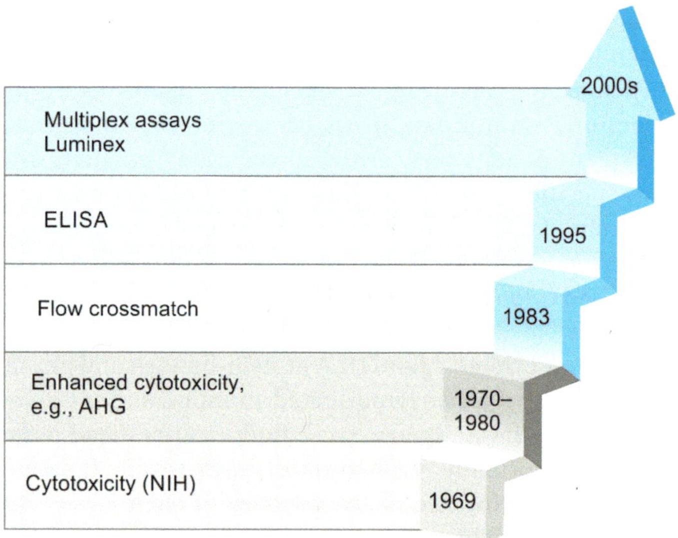

Fig. 7: Evolution of antihuman leukocyte antigen (HLA) antibody testing. (AHG: antihuman globulin; ELISA: enzyme-linked immunosorbent assay; NIH: National Institutes of Health)

HUMAN LEUKOCYTE ANTIGEN ANTIBODY DETECTION ASSAYS

Cell-based Assays

Complement-dependent Cytotoxicity

The complement-dependent microcytotoxicity (CDC) is a lymphocyte-based biological assay that requires antibody binding, complement activation, and cellular damage to register a positive reaction **(Figs. 8A and B)**. The results are scored using a standardized ranking system introduced by Terasaki and later adopted by the National Institutes of Health (NIH).[4] The technology for performing the test and association of positive crossmatch transplant with hyperacute rejection in renal allografts was described by Terasaki et al.[1,28] Soon, it became a working paradigm to perform CDC crossmatch (CDCXM) test before proceeding for renal transplantation and positive CDCXM was considered a contraindication to transplantation.

Modified Lymphocytotoxicity Assays

Several modifications to the original method have been introduced in order to increase the sensitivity and specificity. These modifications as given in **Table 2** include the addition

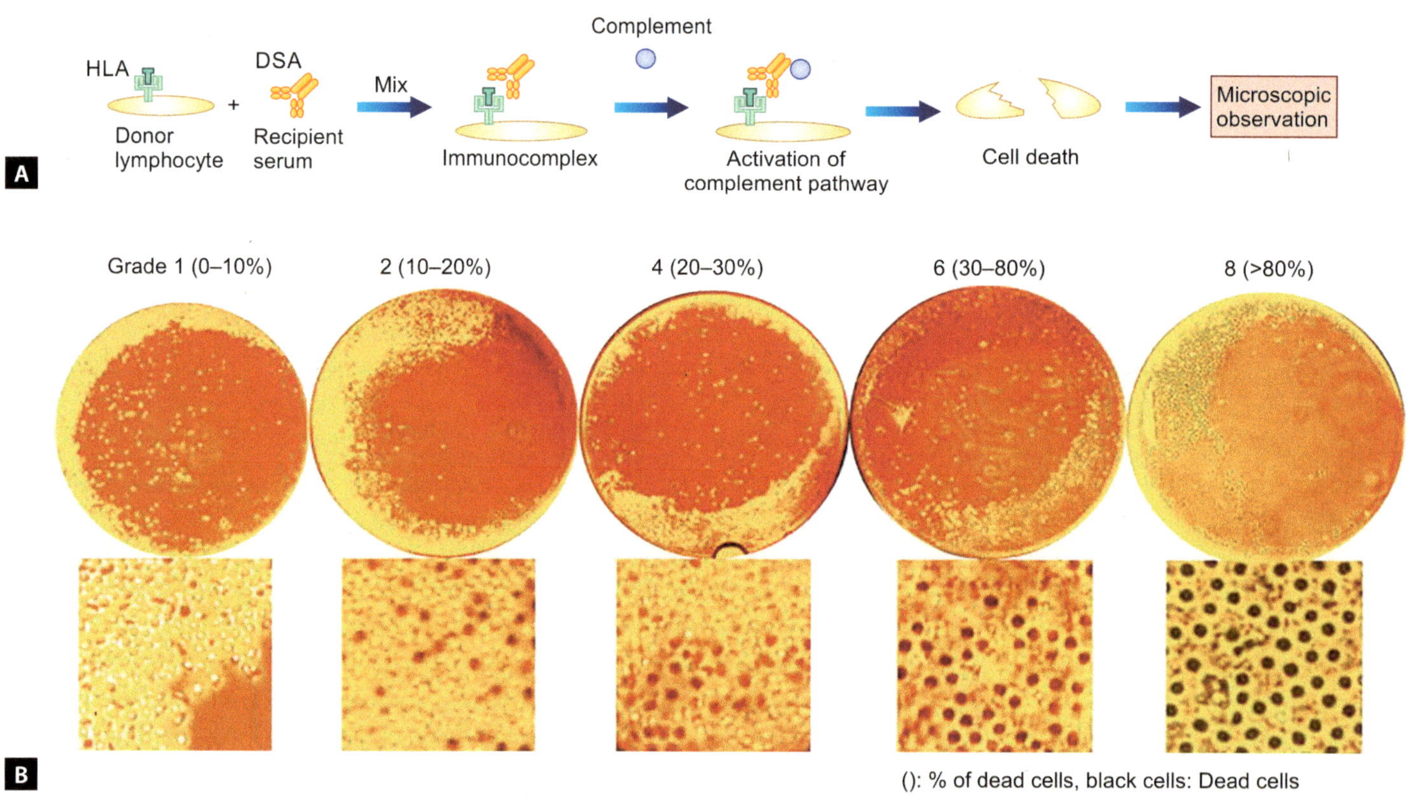

Figs. 8A and B: Standard complement-dependent cytotoxicity (CDC) test. (A) Schematic presentation of CDC; and (B) Representative results of CDC. Dead cells are shown as black by eosin dye. Negative reaction (grades 1–2) and positive reaction (grades 4–8). (DSA: donor-specific antibody; HLA: human leukocyte antigen)

Source: Nakamura T, Ushigome H, Shirouzu T, Yoshimura N. Donor-specific anti-HLA antibodies in organ transplantation: transition from serum DSA to intra-graft DSA. In: Mahdi BM (Ed). Human Leukocyte Antigen (HLA). London: IntechOpen; 2018. [online] Available from https://www.intechopen.com/chapters/62771. [Last accessed September, 2022].

TABLE 2: Modifications of lymphocytotoxicity assay over standard complement-dependent cytotoxicity (CDC).

Modification over standard CDC (NIH)	*Modification detail*	*Remarks*
Amos	One wash prior to complement	To remove anticomplementary factors
Amos (modified)	Three to four washes prior to complement	To remove anticomplementary factors
Antihuman globulin (AHG) enhanced	Addition of AHG prior to complement over Amos (modified) technique	To increase the ability to detect low titer antibodies
Extended incubation	60 minutes serum/cell; 120 minutes complement; no washes	To increase the binding of low avidity antibodies
DTT treatment	Treatment of serum with DTT	To reduce IgM pentamers to monomers, rendering them incapable of fixing complement

(DTT: dithiothreitol; IgM: immunoglobulin M; NIH: National Institutes of Health)

of wash steps to eliminate anticomplementary factors,[29] the use of an antihuman globulin (AHG) to increase the ability to detect low-titer and/or noncomplement fixing antibodies,[30] extended incubation to increase the binding of low avidity antibodies,[31] and the use of separate T and B lymphocyte target cells.[32] Of all the modifications mentioned above, the most widely utilized is the use of AHG-CDC to enhance the sensitivity of complement fixing alloantibody detection.[33]

Complement-dependent cytotoxicity assays detect both immunoglobulin M (IgM) and IgG classes of antibodies. Clinically, greater emphasis is put on IgG antibodies rather than IgM antibodies. Moreover, most of the autoantibodies are IgM antibodies and can interfere with the detection of IgG antibodies. To negate the effects of IgM antibodies, it is an accepted laboratory practice to pretreat the test serum with heat or reducing agents such as dithiothreitol (DTT).

The CDC assay was further modified as an antibody screening assay by using cell panels composed of randomly selected HLA-typed donor lymphocytes in an effort to mimic the natural distribution of HLA antigens within a population. The results are expressed as %PRA (percent of cells in the panel giving a positive reaction). PRA is a measure of sensitization. However, the %PRA for a given serum sample could vary significantly depending on the antigen composition of the test panel. This means a high %PRA could either be because of serum containing several different specificities or just a single specificity corresponding to an overrepresented antigen on the test panel. Later, commercial cell panels became available, providing a limited degree of consistency in PRA testing. CDC-based PRA testing has several important drawbacks, such as it neither reflects the complex array of antibodies that could be present nor reflects the specificity of the antibody. In addition, non-HLA antibodies could give CDC-positive results, thus further skewing the %PRA result.

Flow Cytometry Crossmatch

The flow crossmatch technique was first introduced in 1983 by Garovoy et al. primarily to address some of the problems inherent to the CDC assay.[34] The assay involves incubation of purified donor mononuclear cells with the patient's serum and then adding fluorescein conjugated, secondary antihuman immunoglobulin antibody to detect antibody in the patient's serum bound to the cellular targets **(Figs. 9A to D)**. Subsequently, it was modified to employ two-color analysis of T and B cells in separate tubes and a three-color analysis of T and B cells in a single tube to permit the simultaneous evaluation of T- and B-cell reactivities.[35,36] This involved an additional incubation step with anti-CD3 PerCP/CD19-PE to identify the T- and B-cell populations, respectively.[37] Moreover, by varying the type of secondary antibody used, one can test for IgG, IgM, or IgA immunoglobulin isotypes. The amount of cell-bound antibody is quantified by fluorescence intensity and the degree of positivity is expressed as channel shift. A 40-channel shift for T cells and an 80-channel shift for B cells are generally considered a positive test.[38] However, it is apt for the laboratories to set their own criteria. The possible combination of CDC and flow crossmatch reactivity and their interpretation is shown in **Table 3**.

Even though flow cytometry crossmatch (FCXM) is much more sensitive to CDCXM, it is not free of limitations. Most notably, nonspecific binding of immunoglobulins to Fc receptors can be mistaken as positive result. Non-HLA antibodies as well as monoclonal antilymphocyte antibodies such as thymoglobulin, rituximab, and alemtuzumab used for immunosuppression can also interfere with the assay giving a false-positive result.[39,40] Unlike CDCXM, it is a binding assay and not a functional test because it only provides information on the binding of the DSA to its potential donor target and not on the killing of the target cells. Furthermore, it does not discriminate between complement and noncomplement fixing antibodies. The use of pronase has been utilized to reduce the rate of false-positive B-cell crossmatch due to nonspecific binding of immunoglobulins to Fc receptors as well as reactivity with therapeutic antibodies specific for CD20.

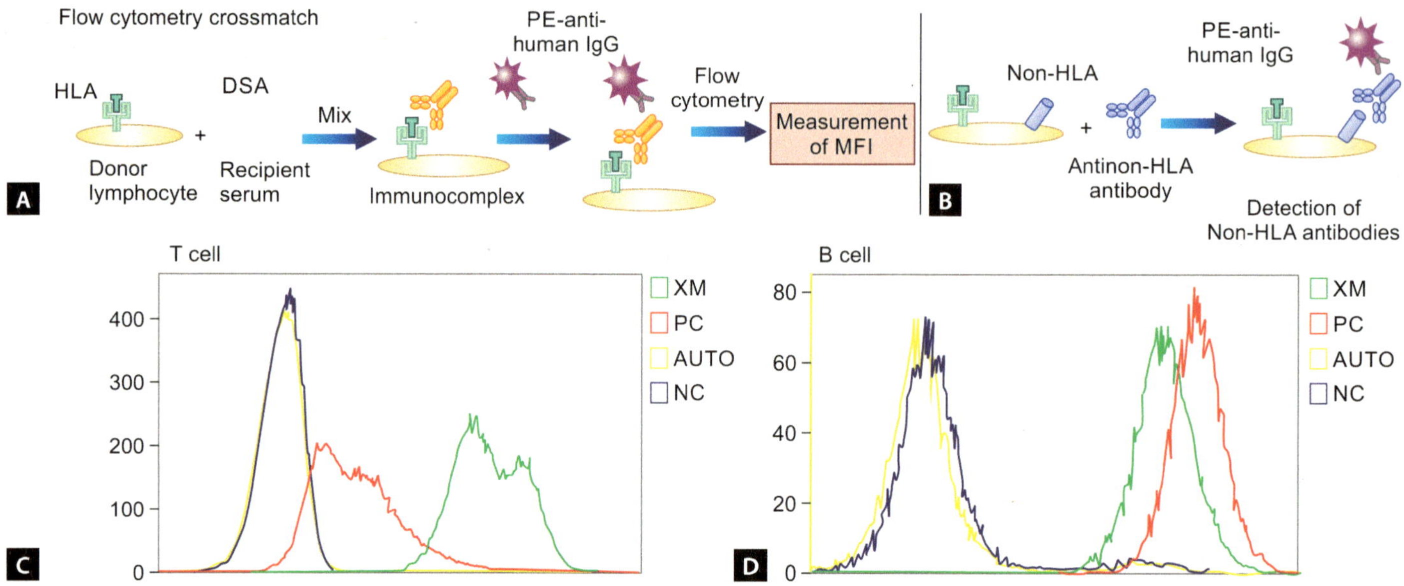

Figs. 9A to D: Flow cytometry crossmatch (FCXM). (A) Schematic presentation of FCXM; (B) An example of positive reaction by non-human leukocyte antigen (HLA) antibodies; Representative results of FCXM using (C) T cell or (D) B cell. (AUTO: auto cross match sample; DSA: donor-specific antibody; IgG: immunoglobulin G; MFI: mean fluorescence intensity; NC: negative control; PC: positive control; PE: phycoerythrin; XM: cross match sample)

Source: Nakamura T, Ushigome H, Shirouzu T, Yoshimura N. Donor-specific anti-HLA antibodies in organ transplantation: transition from serum DSA to intra-graft DSA. In: Mahdi BM (Ed). Human Leukocyte Antigen (HLA). London: IntechOpen; 2018. [online] Available from https://www.intechopen.com/chapters/62771. [Last accessed September, 2022].

TABLE 3: Different combinations of complement-dependent cytotoxicity (CDC) and flow crossmatch reactivity and its interpretation.

	CDC crossmatch		***Flow crossmatch***		
Scenarios	***T cell***	***B cell***	***T cell***	***B cell***	***Interpretation***
Scenario 1	Neg	Neg	Pos	Pos	Anti-HLA class I (low titer)
Scenario 2	Neg	Pos	Pos	Pos	Anti-HLA class I (low titer) ± anti-HLA class II
Scenario 3	Neg	Pos	Neg	Pos	Anti-HLA class II ± anti-HLA class I (low titer) or therapeutic antibodies
Scenario 4	Pos	Pos	Pos	Pos	Anti-HLA class I (high titer) ± anti-HLA class II
Scenario 5	Pos	Pos	Neg	Neg	Autoantibodies (IgM antibody)
Scenario 6	Pos	Neg	Pos	Neg	Likely T-cell-specific non-HLA antibody

(HLA: human leukocyte antigen; IgM: immunoglobulin M; Neg: negative; Pos: positive)

Solid-phase Assays

Enzyme-linked Immunosorbent Assay

Kao et al. developed an ELISA-based HLA antibody detection method using affinity-purified HLA class I from platelets as the target antigens for the detection of HLA antibodies in patient sera.[41] Subsequently, several ELISA-based assays to detect HLA antibodies were introduced in the 1990s, and all were more sensitive than CDC assay but less sensitive than the FCXM. The viability of this assay as a clear indicator of the amount of antibody detected is questionable, since the test uses quantities of HLA antigens much greater than the normal biologic expression on the immune cell. Undoubtedly, ELISA was a significant step forward, but it was cumbersome to perform and has been superseded by the bead-based assays.

Flow Cytometry-based Panel Reactive Antibody

This technique was first developed by Pei et al. in 1998 to address the issues associated with ELISA such as sensitivity and separate test required to discriminate HLA class I and II antibodies.[42] This approach utilized isolation and purification of HLA class I and II proteins from Epstein–Barr virus (EBV) transformed cell lines and their subsequent coupling to microparticles that could easily pass through a flow cytometer. This assay combined 30 individual beads for class I and 30 individual beads for class II with each bead coated with either HLA class I or class II phenotype. Two distinct properties, namely bead size and inherent bead fluorescence, help to discriminate beads expressing HLA class I antigens from class II antigens. The class I beads are smaller and nonfluorescent while the class II beads are

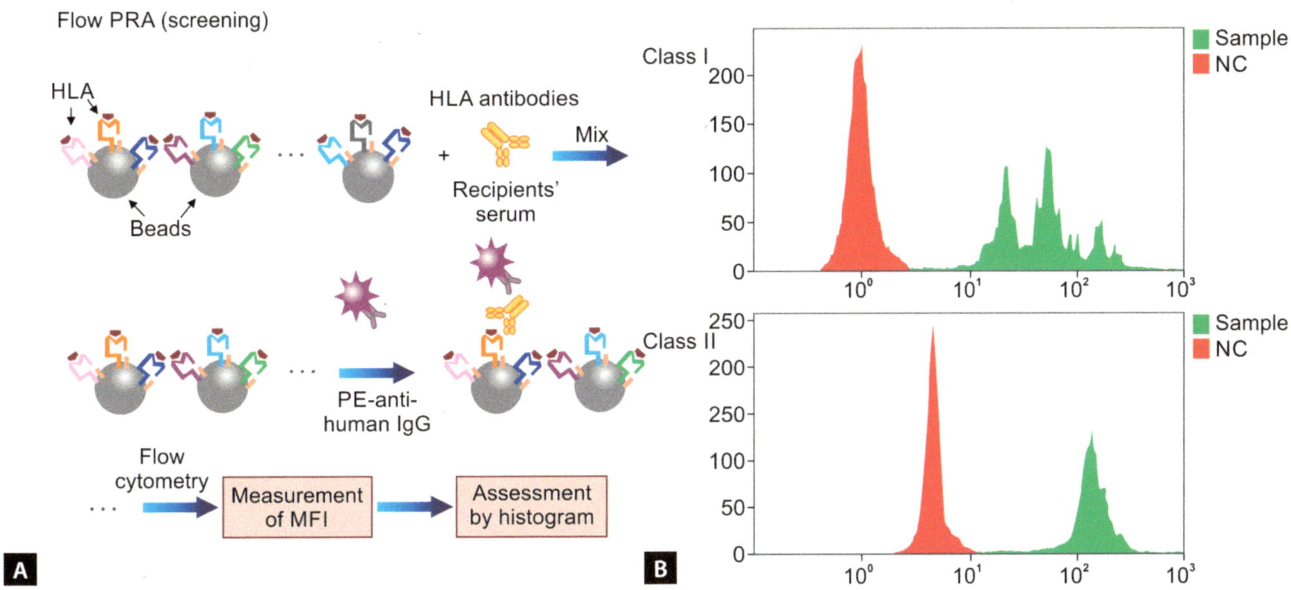

Figs. 10A and B: FlowPRA screening. (A) Schematic presentation of FlowPRA screening; (B) Examples of positive FlowPRA screening results about class I (upper) and class II (lower). (HLA: human leukocyte antigen; IgG: immunoglobulin G; MFI: mean fluorescence intensity; NC: negative control; PE: phycoerythrin)

Source: Nakamura T, Ushigome H, Shirouzu T, Yoshimura N. Donor-specific anti-HLA antibodies in organ transplantation: transition from serum DSA to intra-graft DSA. In: Mahdi BM (Ed). Human Leukocyte Antigen (HLA). London: IntechOpen; 2018. (online) Available from https://www.intechopen.com/chapters/62771. [Last accessed September, 2022].

slightly larger and are impregnated with a fluorescent dye that has excitation/emission properties similar to phycoerythrin (PE). A positive reaction is determined by the number and fluorescence intensity of beads. Beads that exhibit increased fluorescence [fluorescein isothiocyanate (FITC) antihuman, IgG] compared to background controls are considered positive. These differences permit simultaneous testing for both class I and II HLA antibodies. The %PRA is calculated as the percentage of beads that demonstrate a significant positive fluorescence shift above background **(Figs. 10A and B)**. It has been shown that the FlowPRA can detect HLA antibodies 10–20% more frequently than ELISA or cytotoxicity.[43]

In addition to increased sensitivity and simultaneous detection of antibodies against HLA class I and class II, the assay has additional advantages of being specific for HLA antigens without significant interference from non-HLA antibodies. It is not affected by subjective microscopic readings or cell viability and gives a semiquantitative assessment of antibody binding but failed to determine individual HLA specificities. Subsequently, it was modified to coat microparticles with individual HLA molecules.[44] This assay used panels of 8 or 11 individual beads, each identified by their unique level of red fluorescence signature. Green fluorescence indicates the quantity of HLA antibody that is bound. Hence, a broadly sensitized patient could have all his/her HLA antibodies identified, thereby making it possible to predict compatibility with specific donors. Although extremely useful, the assay was cumbersome requiring up to 15 tubes per patient, with each tube containing 8 or 11 individual, single HLA-antigen-coated beads. This proved to be a major drawback and a significant technical handicap. Thus, the high degree of HLA diversity and the challenges of highly sensitized patients made its use limited.

Luminex Platform-based Assays

This technology has completely transformed the histocompatibility laboratory's approach and ability to detect HLA antibodies. Its usefulness lies in the characterization of HLA antibody specificities in highly reactive sera.[45,46] The technique has been successfully applied to monitor patient antibody profiles in relation to particular specificities, such as following desensitization treatment at pretransplant stage and therapeutic monitoring of antibody removal therapies.

The Luminex assay is a semiquantitative bead-based array system that utilizes polystyrene microbeads coated with purified HLA class I or class II antigens. These beads are impregnated with a unique blend of different intensities of two fluorescent dyes that are simultaneously excited by red laser at 635 nm. The emitted light can be detected at wavelengths of 660 nm (red) and 730 nm (infrared) using a dedicated footprint flow cytometer. By measuring the composition of emission intensities for both channels, up to 100 distinct microbead sets can be identified concomitantly (classifier parameters). These microbeads act as molecular carriers that capture samples. The detection of HLA antibody is achieved by using a secondary antibody conjugated with the reporter fluorophore R-PE, which is excited by green laser (532 nm) and detected at 576 nm. The fluidics of the Luminex cytometer aligns the microbeads in a single file as occurs with a flow cytometer. The optics then focuses on each

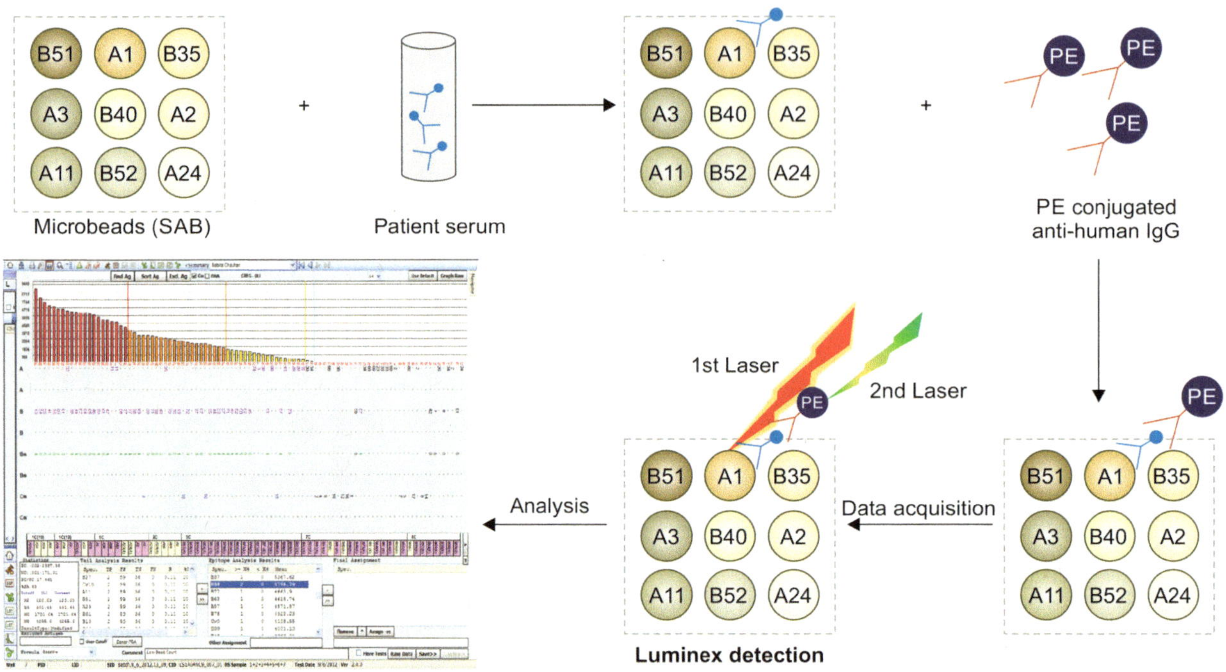

Fig. 11: Schematic presentation of human leukocyte antigen (HLA) antibody testing using single antigen bead (SAB) assay. Recombinant HLA bound to "single antigen" microbeads bind with anti-HLA antibody present in patient serum and are stained by a secondary antihuman immunoglobulin G (IgG) antibody conjugated with phycoerythrin (PE). Data acquisition is done on Luminex platform wherein red laser identifies the bead being examined and green laser measure the assay result on its surface.

bead to generate and collect the fluorescent signals, while the electronics convert and digitize the signals for computer analysis. **Figure 11** schematically shows the principle of HLA antibody screening using Luminex technology.

Based on the composition of target antigens, there are three versions of the test, namely pooled antigen, phenotype panels, and SAB in the order of increasing resolution. The "pooled antigen panels" are typically used as a preliminary screening test to detect the presence or absence of class I and II antibodies in a single test. The bead set is composed of 10–17 beads, and each of them is coated with affinity-purified HLA antigens obtained from multiple individual cell lines. Although this is relatively less expensive with a very high negative predictive value, it is unable to specify possible antigen and is purely qualitative. The "phenotype panels" detect antibodies and their specificity against HLA class I and II antigens separately. The class I panel contains approximately 55 beads, while class II contains 35 beads. Each bead is coated with class I or class II HLA antigen derived from a single individual cell line. Since there is more than one HLA specificity present on each bead, greater expertise is required for the interpretation of results as compared to the pooled or single antigen panel.[47,48]

One of the major advantages of this technique is that through single antigen test panels, it enables detection of epitope-specific antibodies to individual and specific HLA alleles and thus provides information on the virtual crossmatch (VXM).[49] Moreover, it permits identification of antibodies to HLA loci that were not amenable to detection by traditional cell-based assays. These include HLA-C antigens that are poorly expressed on the lymphocyte surface, DQ and DP antigens, as well as DRB3, 4, and 5, which were difficult to distinguish from DRB1 antigens coexpressed on the surface of B cells. This technology also enables detection and characterization of antibodies against major histocompatibility complex (MHC) class I-related chain A (MICA). The MFI of the beads is a measure of the degree of saturation of the total antigens present on the beads by antibodies and is used as a surrogate marker for the level of antibody titers. There is no recommended cutoff value for MFI positivity and most laboratories set their own cutoff levels. In our center, MFI > 1,000 is taken as relevant.

This widely accepted assay is not free of limitations, and there are important critical factors that should be considered while analyzing the data. Being highly sensitive, the technology provides false-positive results, leading to unnecessary delays on the waiting list. The current panel of single HLA beads does not cover the whole diversity of HLA alleles. Hence, populations such as Asian Indians that are characterized by many novel alleles and unique HLA haplotypes will be at a disadvantage because antibodies raised against such HLA alleles are likely to be missed. Luminex beads accommodate both intact and denatured HLA molecules. The immobilization procedure of the HLA molecules on beads may alter the tertiary structure of the molecule exposing neoepitopes which may lead to false-negative and/or -positive reactions. Morales-Buenrostro et al. described the presence of naturally occurring antibodies to HLA class I and II molecules, which may be produced as a result of cross-reactivity with epitopes on vaccines or with epitopes on environmental proteins such as microbes or ingested foods.[50] Epitope analyses have revealed that these natural HLA antibodies react with polymorphic amino acid residues that are usually not exposed to the molecular surface.[51]

The relative density of a particular antigen, especially HLA-Cw, -DQ, and -DP on SAB, is higher as compared to phenotype beads and human cells. As a consequence, antibodies directed against these antigens run the risk of being overestimated yet may represent only a low immunologic risk for renal transplant rejection.[52] Conversely, antibodies against public epitopes such as Bw4 or Bw6 may appear underrepresented because a single antibody may be dispersed across many beads underestimating its actual level (peanut butter effect).[53] Disparities in relative antigen quantity exist across the different bead formats and different HLA molecules on the SAB.

The technique remains susceptible to the interference caused by substances inherent to serum or by exogenous substances. This may lead to the potential underestimation of HLA antibodies due to false-negative reactions or may give false-positive results. Similar to the prozone or Hook phenomenon, the serum appears weak or negative when tested neat and becomes more strongly reactive upon dilution, especially in highly sensitized patients. The main reason for this prozone-like effect using Luminex beads is attributed to the presence of IgM antibodies and complement component C1. Dilution or hypotonic dialysis of serum as well as treatment of sera with DTT, ethylenediaminetetraacetic acid (EDTA), or heat activation helps to overcome this phenomenon.[54] Therapeutics such as intravenous immunoglobulin (IVIg), antithymocyte globulin (ATG), bortezomib, and eculizumab also cause interferences for detection of HLA antibodies. High-dose IVIg (2 g/kg) interferes with the assays using an antiglobulin reagent. It leads to more than fivefold increase in reactivity with negative control beads. Treatment with ATG results in misleading HLA-specific reactivity. Treatment with bortezomib and eculizumab leads to significant reduction in the strength of antibody. However, hypotonic dialysis of sera prevents any such reduction in antibody strength.[55]

Parameters that indicate interferences in Luminex-based assays include:[48]

- High reactivity with the negative control bead
- Low reactivity with the positive control bead
- Sudden change in the pattern of reactivity in sequential sera from a patient in the absence of any specific treatment or event
- Reactivity that does not reconcile with the results of CDC or FCXM tests
- Reactivity with the patient's own HLA antigens.

The specific features along with the limitations of the available techniques based on cell and solid phase assays for the detection of anti-HLA antibodies are summarized in **Figure 12.**

Luminex Crossmatch

Luminex crossmatch (LUXM) detects donor-specific anti-HLA IgG antibodies against class I and/or class II antigens in single well. Donor lymphocytes isolated from peripheral blood are solubilized with a nonionic detergent to obtain a lysate and are used as the source material for HLA. Two of the beads in a single blend of Luminex beads are coated with mouse antibodies with specificity for nonpolymorphic sequence on HLA class I and II molecules. Beads capture HLA molecules of the donor from donor lysate cells. Capture beads are then reacted with recipient sera, and the bound antibody, if present, is detected with fluorescently labeled secondary antibody, and results are read as per the conventional bead assay **(Fig. 13)**. The blend of Luminex beads also includes background and conjugate control beads. The main advantage of the technique is that the donor lysate can be stored frozen for future testing and avoids the cell viability issues. This makes it ideal to use both for pre- and post-transplant testing. Bacterial contamination of the samples as well as the presence of immune complexes or other immunoglobulin aggregates in the sample may cause an increased nonspecific binding and produce erroneous results in this assay. Several studies have demonstrated the failure to detect class II antibodies especially against DQ and DP antigens. LUXM is not recommended to be used as a stand-alone method for transplant decisions.[56]

Virtual Crossmatch

Luminex SAB assay and DNA-based HLA typing at high resolution have permitted the concept of VXM gain acceptance worldwide. The VXM is defined as "An assessment of immunological compatibility based on the patient's alloantibody profile compared to the donor's histocompatibility antigen."[57] The VXM takes into account the HLA antibody profile of the patient to predict crossmatch negative donors. In other words, it gives an insight into acceptable mismatches. In majority of cases, VXM correlated with FCXM. Disagreement between FCXM and VXM should be considered with much deliberation rather than disregarding the results as false.[58-61] **Table 4** highlights the discordant scenarios of FCXM and VXM, factors responsible for such discordance and further evaluation to confirm or negate such factors.

CALCULATED PANEL REACTIVE ANTIBODY

The degree of sensitization as measured by PRA is imprecise and highly variable as it is dependent on panel cell construction and not true representation of donor pool. In 2007, the United Network of Organ Sharing (UNOS) approved a proposal by the Histocompatibility Committee to use calculated PRA (cPRA). It is based on antibody specificity, not from positive reactions on a panel, and is computed from HLA frequencies in different ethnic populations. It takes into consideration the frequency of unacceptable HLA

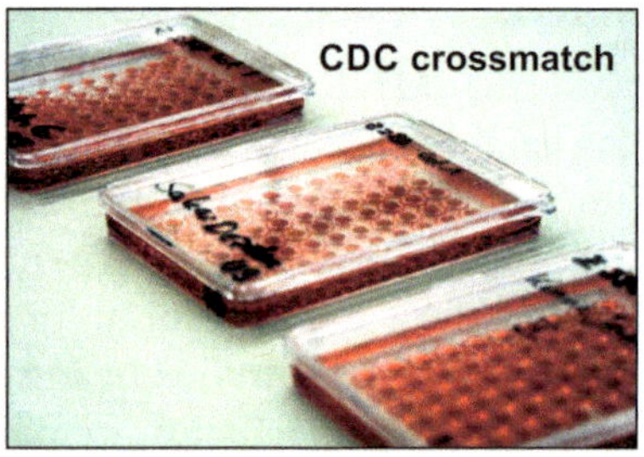

- Low sensitivity and specificity
- No distinction between IgG and IgM antibodies
- False positivity due to the detection of non-HLA antibodies/autoantibodies or high background reading due to spontaneous cell death
- Cumbersome procedure; time-consuming
- Detection of complement-fixing antibodies only
- Dependent on cell surface expression of HLA antigen

Flow cytometry

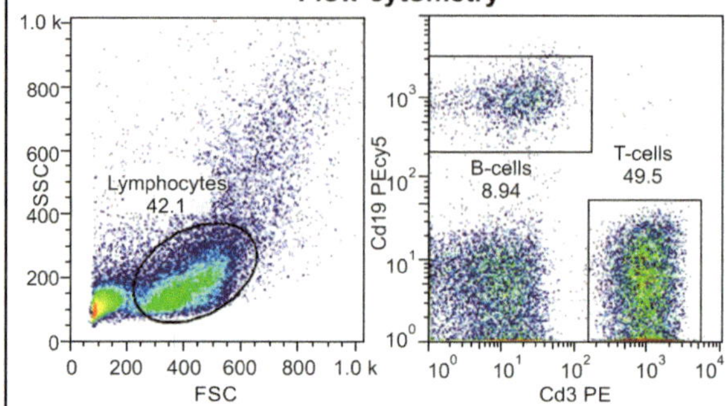

- More sensitive than CDC
- False positivity due to nonspecific binding of immunoglobulins to Fc receptors or detection of non-HLA antibodies
- Optimal channel shift an issue
- Difficult to standardize due to variability among cytometers, fluorochromes, antiglobulin reagents and variation in cell to serum ratio

Luminex-based technology

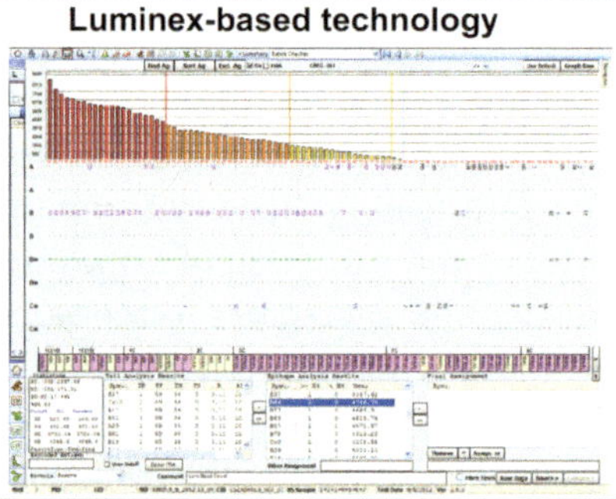

- Highly sensitive; semi-quantitative and enables precise definition of anti-HLA antibodies
- Detection and characterization of anti-MICA antibodies
- Lack of consensus on optimum MFI cutoffs
- Questionable utility as a stand-alone test for antibody detection
- Problems of false positivity due to exposure to cryptic epitopes and reaction to denatured HLA molecules
- Problems of false negativity
- Remains susceptible to the interferences caused by substances inherent to serum or by exogenous substances
- Disparities in relative antigen quantity across the different bead formats and among different HLA molecules
- Do not cover the whole diversity of HLA alleles

Fig. 12: A summarized view of the cell-based [complement-dependent cytotoxicity (CDC) crossmatch and flow cytometry] and solid phase-based assays (Luminex-based technology) for the detection of antihuman leukocyte antigen (HLA) antibodies, highlighting main advantages and disadvantages. (IgG: immunoglobulin G; IgM: immunoglobulin M; MFI: mean fluorescence intensity; MICA: major histocompatibility complex class I-related chain A)

Source: Mehra NK, Baranwal AK. Clinical and immunological relevance of antibodies in solid organ transplantation. Int J Immunogenet. 2016;43(6):351-68. Reproduced with permission from John Wiley & Sons.

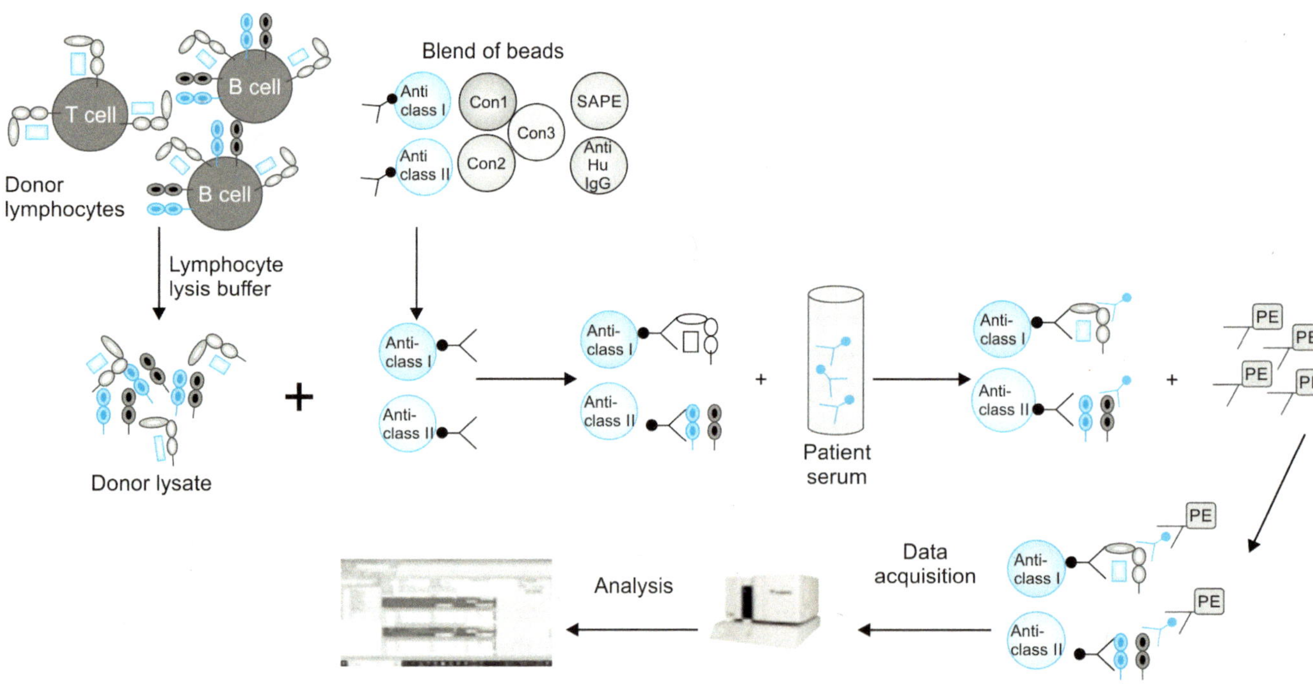

Fig. 13: Schematic presentation of Luminex crossmatch. Donor lysate is prepared from donor lymphocytes using lysis buffer. Lysate is mixed with DSA beads to capture donor class I and II human leukocyte antigen (HLA) on to beads. Donor-specific antibodies present in patient serum binds with HLA on capture beads and is then stained by a secondary antihuman immunoglobulin (IgG) antibody conjugated with phycoerythrin (PE). Data acquisition is done on Luminex platform and the results are analyzed. (Con: control)

TABLE 4: Discordant scenarios based on flow cytometry crossmatch (FCXM) and virtual crossmatch (VXM) results, factors responsible, and further evaluation.

Scenarios	*Flow crossmatch (FCXM)*	*SAB for DSA (VXM)*	*Factors responsible*	*Further evaluation*
Scenario 1	Positive	Negative	Autoantibodies	Auto-flow crossmatch
			Nonspecific binding	Pronase treatment
			Alloantibody to shared epitopes ("peanut butter effect")	–
			Non-HLA antibody	Test for non-HLA antibody
			Donor allele/antigen not covered by SAB	Check for allele representation on bead
			Prozone/Hook effect	Pretreat sera with EDTA/heat or dilution of sera with repeat assay
			Incomplete/incorrect HLA typing	Ensure complete and correct typing
Scenario 2	Negative	Positive	Antibody toward denatured HLA	Acid treat SAB
			DSA with low affinity/avidity	–
			Low HLA expression	–

(DSA: donor-specific antibody; EDTA: ethylenediaminetetraacetic acid; HLA: human leukocyte antigen; SAB: single antigen bead)

Flowchart 1: Algorithm for candidates with potential living donor.

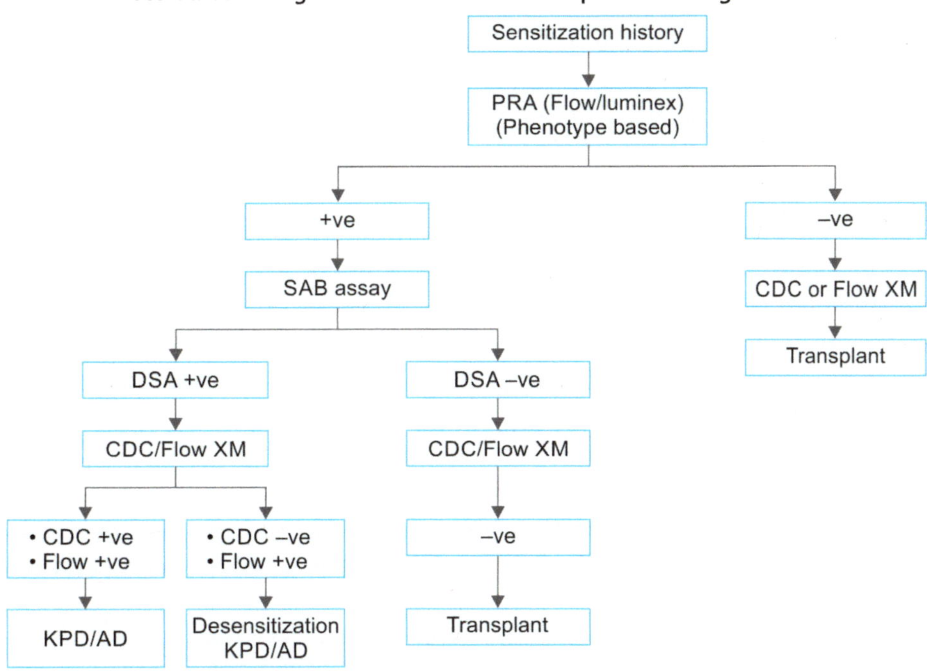

(AD: alternate donor; CDC: complement-dependent cytotoxicity; DSA: donor-specific antibody; KPD: kidney paired donation; PRA: panel reactive antibody; SAB: single antigen bead; XM: crossmatch)

in the donor pool. The computer software system uses an established formula and HLA frequencies derived from the HLA types of that population to calculate the cPRA value. Different countries have different calculators suited to their ethnic population. It provides a more representative estimate of sensitization not only because of the use of more accurate HLA frequencies, but also includes both class I and II antigens in the calculation, unlike that of traditional PRA, where class I and II specificities are measured separately.[62]

ALGORITHM FOR PATIENTS WITH POTENTIAL LIVING DONOR

Proper history-taking of a sensitizing event is critical for the correct interpretation of the crossmatch and antibody detection assays. **Flowchart 1** highlights the algorithm for the candidates with potential living donors. It may differ among different setups based on the preferences and availability of the assays.

CONCLUSION

The Luminex-based SAB assay coupled with HLA sequencing data provides a platform to identify epitopes against which HLA antibodies are directed. This in turn leads to a better opportunity for clinical decision-making with accuracy and maximizes the success of transplant. In view of intricacies associated with rapid development of techniques, it is imperative for the transplant physicians to communicate with transplant immunologists on an individual patient basis.

REFERENCES

1. Terasaki P, McClelland JD. Microdroplet assay of human serum cytotoxins. Nature. 1964;204:998-1000.
2. Eng HS, Leffell MS. Histocompatibility testing after fifty years of transplantation. J Immunol Methods. 2011;369:1-21.
3. Dunn PP. Novel approaches and technologies in molecular HLA typing. Methods Mol Biol. 2015;1310:213-30.
4. Terasaki PI, McClelland JD, Park MS, McCurdy B. Microdroplet lymphocyte cytotoxicity test. In: Ray JG, Hare DB, Pedersen PD, Kayhoe DE (Eds). Manual of Tissue Typing Techniques. Bethesda: National Institutes of Health; 1974. pp. 67-74 (DHEW Publication NIH 75-545).
5. Olerup O, Zetterquist H. HLA-DR typing by PCR amplification with sequence-specific primers (PCR-SSP) in 2 hours: an alternative to serological DR typing in clinical practice including donor-recipient matching in cadaveric transplantation. Tissue Antigens. 1992;39:225-35.
6. Bunce M, O'Neill CM, Barnardo MC, Krausa P, Browning MJ, Morris PJ, et al. Phototyping: comprehensive DNA typing for HLA-A, B, C, DRB1, DRB3, DRB4, DRB5 and DQB1 by PCR with 144 primer mixes utilising sequence-specific primers (PCR-SSP). Tissue Antigens. 1995;46:355-67.
7. Olerup O, Zetterquist H. HLA-DR typing of polymerase chain reaction amplification with sequence-specific primers (PCR-SSP). In: Hui KM, Bidwell JL (Eds). Handbook of HLA Typing Techniques. Boca Raton, FL: CRC Press, Inc.; 1993. pp. 149-74.
8. Wordsworth P. Techniques used to define human MHC antigens: polymerase chain reaction and oligonucleotide probes. Immunol Lett. 1991;29:37-9.
9. Cao K, Chopek M, Fernandez-Vina MA. High and intermediate resolution DNA typing systems for class I HLA-A, B, C genes by hybridisation with sequence-specific oligonucleotide probes (SSOP). Rev Immunogenet. 1999;1:177-208.
10. Dunbar SA. Applications of Luminex xMAP technology for rapid, high-throughput multiplexed nucleic acid detection. Clin Chim Acta. 2006;363(1-2):71-82.
11. Testi M, Andreani M. Luminex-based methods in high-resolution HLA typing. Methods Mol Biol. 2015;1310:231-4.
12. Danzer M, Polin H, Pröll J, Hofer K, Fae I, Fischer GF, et al. High-throughput sequence-based typing strategy for HLA-DRB1 based on real-time polymerase chain reaction. Hum Immunol. 2007;68:915-7.
13. Fan W, Huang L, Zhou Z, Zeng X, Li G, Deo P, et al. Rapid and reliable genotyping of HLA-B*27 in the Chinese Han population using a duplex real-time TaqMan PCR assay. Clin Biochem. 2012;45:106-11.
14. Hammond E, Mamotte C, Nolan D, Mallal S. HLA-B*5701 typing: evaluation of an allele-specific polymerase chain reaction melting assay. Tissue Antigens. 2007;70:58-61.
15. Erali M, Voelkerding KV, Wittwer CT. High resolution melting applications for clinical laboratory medicine. Exp Mol Pathol. 2008;85:50-8.
16. Sanger F, Nicklen S, Coulson AR. DNA sequencing with chain-terminating inhibitors. Proc Natl Acad Sci U S A. 1977;74(12):5463-7.
17. Dunn PP. Human leucocyte antigen typing: techniques and technology, a critical appraisal. Int J Immunogenet. 2011;38:463-73.
18. Erlich H. HLA DNA typing: past, present, and future. Tissue Antigens. 2012;80:1-11.
19. Adams SD, Barracchini KC, Chen D, Robbins F, Wang L, Larsen P, et al. Ambiguous allele combinations in HLA class I and class II sequence-based typing: when precise nucleotide sequencing leads to imprecise allele identification. J Transl Med. 2004;2:30.
20. Paunić V, Gragert L, Madbouly A, Freeman J, Maiers M. Measuring ambiguity in HLA typing methods. PLoS One. 2012;7:e43585.
21. Lind C, Ferriola D, Mackiewicz K, Heron S, Rogers M, Slavich L, et al. Next-generation sequencing: the solution for high-resolution, unambiguous human leukocyte antigen typing. Hum Immunol. 2010;71:1033-42.
22. Kong D, Lee N, Dela Cruz ID, Dames C, Maruthamuthu S, Golden T, et al. Concurrent typing of over 4000 samples by long-range PCR amplicon-based NGS and rSSO revealed the need to verify NGS typing for HLA allelic dropouts. Hum Immunol. 2021;82(8):581-7.
23. Shiina T, Suzuki S, Ozaki Y, Taira H, Kikkawa E, Shigenari A, et al. Super high resolution for single molecule-sequence-based typing of classical HLA loci at the 8-digit level using next generation sequencers. Tissue Antigens. 2012;80:305-16.
24. De Santis D, Dinauer D, Duke J, Erlich HA, Holcomb CL, Lind C, et al. 16th IHIW: review of HLA typing by NGS. Int J Immunogenet. 2013;40:72-6.
25. Monos D, Maiers MJ. Progressing towards the complete and thorough characterization of the HLA genes by NGS (or single-molecule DNA sequencing): consequences, opportunities and challenges. Hum Immunol. 2015;76:883-6.
26. Mayor NP, Wang T, Lee SJ, Kuxhausen M, Vierra-Green C, Barker DJ, et al. Impact of previously unrecognized HLA mismatches using ultrahigh resolution typing in unrelated donor hematopoietic cell transplantation. J Clin Oncol. 2021;39(21):2397-409.
27. Duke JL, Lind C, Mackiewicz K, Ferriola D, Papazoglou A, Gasiewski A, et al. Determining performance characteristics of an NGS-based HLA typing method for clinical applications. HLA. 2016;87:141-52.
28. Patel R, Terasaki PI. Significance of a positive crossmatch test in kidney transplantation. N Engl J Med. 1969;280:735-9.
29. Amos DB, Bashir H, Boyle W, MacQueen M, Tiilikainen A. A simple micro cytotoxicity test. Transplantation. 1969;7:220-3.
30. Johnson AH, Rossen RD, Butler WT. Detection of alloantibodies using a sensitive antiglobulin microcytotoxicity test: identification of low levels of pre-formed antibodies in accelerated allograft rejection. Tissue Antigens. 1972;2(3):215-26.

31. Cross DE, Whittier FC, Weaver P, Foxworth J. A comparison of the antiglobulin versus extended incubation time crossmatch: results in 223 renal transplants. Transplant Proc. 1977;9(4):1803-6.
32. Povlsen JV, Madsen M, Rasmussen A, Strate M, Graugaard BH, Birkeland SA, et al. Clinical applicability of the immunomagnetic beads technique for serological crossmatching in renal transplantation. Tissue Antigens. 1991;38:111-6.
33. Zachary AA, Klingman L, Thorne N, Smerglia AR, Teresi GA. Variations of the lymphocytotoxicity test. An evaluation of sensitivity and specificity. Transplantation. 1995;60(5):498-503.
34. Garovoy MR, Rheinschmidt MA, Bigos M, Perkins H, Colombe B, Feduska N, et al. Flow cytometry analysis: a high technology crossmatch technique facilitating transplantation. Transplant Proc. 1983;15:1939-44.
35. Bray RA, Lebeck LK, Gebel HM. The flow cytometric crossmatch. Dual-color analysis of T cell and B cell reactivities. Transplantation. 1989;49:834-40.
36. Bray RA, Nickerson PW, Kerman RH, Gebel HM. Evolution of antibody detection: technology emulating biology. Immunol Res. 2004;29(1-3):41-53.
37. Bray RA, Gebel HM. Clinical utility of flow cytometry in allogeneic transplantation. In: Keren D (Ed). Clinical Flow Cytometry. Chicago, IL: ASCP Press; 2007. pp. 275-92 [Chapter 14].
38. Graff RJ, Duffy B, Xiao H, Radell J, Lentine KL. The role of the crossmatch in kidney transplantation: past, present and future. J Nephrol Ther. 2012;(Suppl. 4):002.
39. Ettenger RB, Jordan SC, Fine RN. Cadaver renal transplant outcome in recipients with auto-lymphocytotoxic antibodies. Transplantation. 1983;35:429-31.
40. Wagenknecht D, Sizemore J, House K, Birhiray RE, McIntyre JA. Humanized monoclonal Campath-H1 can mimic alloantibodies in CDC and flow cytometry crossmatches. Hum Immunol. 2004;65:S73.
41. Kao KJ, Scornik JC, Small SJ. Enzyme-linked immunoassay for anti-HLA antibodies—an alternative to panel studies by lymphocytotoxicity. Transplantation. 1993;55:192-6.
42. Pei R, Wang G, Tarsitani C, Rojo S, Chen T, Takemura S, et al. Simultaneous HLA class I and class II antibodies screening with flow cytometry. Human Immunol. 1998;5:313-22.
43. Gebel HM, Bray RA. Sensitization and sensitivity: defining the unsensitized patient. Transplantation. 2000;69:1370-4.
44. Pei R, Lee JH, Shih NJ, Chen M, Terasaki PI. Single human leukocyte antigen flow cytometry beads for accurate identification of human leukocyte antigen antibody specificities. Transplantation. 2003;75;43-9.
45. Gibney EM, Cagle LR, Freed B, Warnell SE, Chan L, Wiseman AC. Detection of donor-specific antibodies using HLA-coated microspheres: another tool for kidney transplant risk stratification. Nephrol Dial Transplant. 2006;21:2625-9.
46. Vaidya S, Partlow D, Susskind B, Noor M, Barnes T, Gugliuzza K. Prediction of crossmatch outcome of highly sensitized patients by single and/or multiple antigen bead Luminex assay. Transplantation. 2006;82(11):1524-8.
47. Tait BD, Hudson F, Brewin G, Cantwell L, Holdsworth R. Solid phase HLA antibody detection technology—challenges in interpretation. Tissue Antigens. 2010;76(2):87-95.
48. Tait BD, Süsal C, Gebel HM, Nickerson PW, Zachary AA, Claas FHJ, et al. Consensus guidelines on the testing and clinical management issues associated with HLA and non-HLA antibodies in transplantation. Transplantation. 2013;95:19-47.
49. El-Awar N, Lee JH, Tarsitani C, Terasaki PI. HLA class I epitopes: recognition of binding sites by mAbs or eluted alloantibody confirmed with single recombinant antigens. Hum Immunol. 2007;68(3):170-80.
50. Morales-Buenrostro LE, Terasaki PI, Marino-Vazquez LA, Lee JH, El-Awar N, Alberu J. "Natural" human leukocyte antigen antibodies found in nonalloimmunized healthy males. Transplantation. 2008;86:1111-5.
51. El-Awar N, Terasaki PI, Nguyen A, Sasaki N, Morales-Buenrostro LE, Saji H, et al. Epitopes of human leukocyte antigen class I antibodies found in sera of normal healthy males and cord blood. Hum Immunol. 2009;70:844-53.
52. Taylor CJ, Kosmoliaptsis V, Summers DM, Bradley JA. Back to the future: application of contemporary technology to long-standing questions about the clinical relevance of HLA-specific alloantibodies in renal transplantation. Hum Immunol. 2009;70:563-8.
53. Garcia-Sanchez C, Usenko CY, Herrera ND, Tambur AR. The shared epitope phenomenon—a potential impediment to virtual crossmatch accuracy. Clin Transplant. 2020;34(8):e13906.
54. Greenshields AL, Liwski RS. The ABCs (DRDQDPs) of the prozone effect in single antigen bead HLA antibody testing: lessons from our highly sensitized patients. Hum Immunol. 2019;80(7):478-86.
55. Jaramillo A, Ramon DS, Stoll ST. Technical aspects of crossmatching in transplantation. Clin Lab Med. 2018;38(4):579-93.
56. Tait BD. Detection of HLA antibodies in organ transplant recipients—triumphs and challenges of the solid phase bead assay. Front Immunol. 2016;7:570.
57. Bray RA. The acceptability and application of virtual crossmatching in lieu of serologic crossmatching for transplantation. Virtual Crossmatch Workgroup Report, CDC2014.
58. Schinstock CA, Gandhi MJ, Stegall MD. Interpreting anti-HLA antibody testing data: a practical guide for physicians. Transplantation. 2016;100(8):1619-28.
59. Desoutter J, Apithy MJ, Guillaume N. Unexpected positive prospective crossmatches in organ transplant. Exp Clin Transplant. 2017;15(3):253-9.
60. Morris AB, Sullivan HC, Krummey SM, Gebel HM, Bray RA. Out with the old, in with the new: virtual versus physical crossmatching in the modern era. HLA. 2019;94(6):471-81.
61. Bhaskaran MC, Heidt S, Muthukumar T. Principles of virtual crossmatch testing for kidney transplantation. Kidney Int Rep. 2022;7(6):1179-88.
62. Cecka JM. Calculated PRA (CPRA): the new measure of sensitization for transplant candidates. Am J Transplant. 2010;10(1):26-9.

1.3 Donor-specific Antibodies in Kidney Transplantation

Rahul Grover, Narayan Prasad

CASE VIGNETTE

Ms EM, 45/F, k/c/o ADPKD, on dialysis w.e.f. 7/8/21, came for renal transplant with husband as prospective donor. She had one child delivered via lower segment cesarean section (LSCS) in 2001. There was no h/o any blood transfusion or other sensitizing event. There was ABO incompatibility [blood group B→A, anti-B titer 1:16]. Her CDC crossmatch was found to be week positive, however her flow crossmatch was detected to be –ve. HLA 12 antigen by NGS and Luminex SAB Class I and Class II were ordered to further assess immunological risk. Non-DSA anti-HLA antibody were detected against Class I antigens and moderate titer Class II DSA were detected [SAB Class I non-DSA: A 80:01-5552, rest Class I [<1000 MFI], Class II: DSA DQB1:05:01 2656, 1288 MFI]. She underwent desensitization with following protocol: rituximab 200 mg [day-16], MFS [day-16], tacrolimus [day-4], MP 125 mg [day-2], MP 250 mg [day-1], PLEX [1.5 volume exchange day-2, day-1], IVIG 1 g/kg [POD-1], IL2RA induction, MP 500 mg POD 0, MP 250 mg POD1,2; MP 125 mg POD 3,4, f/b prednisolone 25 mg OD. She underwent Robotic RAR + Right ovarian cystectomy + Subserosal fibroid excision—23/11/2021. She had immediate graft function and was discharged on POD 7 with creatinine of 0.8 mg/dL and continues to be around 1.2–1.3 mg/dL at last f/u in September 22. Post-transplant DSA monitoring was discussed but not done in view of economical concerns.

INTRODUCTION

The report by Patel and Terasaki in 1969 regarding the significance of positive crossmatch in kidney transplant, "24 of 30 with positive crossmatch versus just 8 of 195 with negative crossmatch failed to function," made screening for preformed cytotoxic antibodies against donor an integral part of transplant evaluation.[1] Since then, the methods for assessing circulating donor-specific antibodies (DSA) have undergone many refinements. DSA either maybe present pretransplant or may develop anytime post-transplant. The presence of DSA predisposes to the development of antibody-mediated rejection (AMR), which is considered the leading cause of graft loss. Pretransplant evaluation for DSA to assess the degree of sensitization as well as post-transplant monitoring of DSA to predict, prevent, and manage rejections and prevent graft loss continues to evolve.[2]

HUMAN LEUKOCYTE ANTIGENS AND PATHWAYS TO ALLOIMMUNE RECOGNITION

Human Leukocyte Antigens

Human leukocyte antigens (HLA) are dimeric glycoprotein molecules that are present on nucleated cells and perform the role of antigen presentation through their highly polymorphic peptide-binding groove.[3] Class I HLA molecules (HLA A, B, and C) are dimers of alpha-chain and beta 2-microglobulin. They present intracellular peptides to CD8$^+$ T cells. Class II HLA molecules (DR, DP, and DQ) are dimers made of a constant alpha chain (DR) or polymorphic alpha chain (DQ, DP) with polymorphic beta chains (DP, DQ, and DR). They are constitutively expressed on B cells and antigen-presenting cells (APC). Their expression can be induced on endothelial cells (ECs) and activated T cells. They present endocytosed extracellular peptides which get loaded via phagolysosomes to CD4$^+$ T cells.

The genes encoding HLA molecules reside on the short arm of chromosome 6 in the major histocompatibility complex (MHC) region. They show a high degree of polymorphism (>16,000 alleles reported). This polymorphism while being a protective mechanism against infectious organisms acts as a barrier for organ transplantation. Exposure to nonself HLA leads to allorecognition via direct, semidirect, or indirect immunological pathways.[4] *See* **Table 1** for terms and definitions.

Direct Pathway of Allorecognition

Direct pathway involves donor APC [passenger cells] presenting nonself [donor] HLA peptide complex to recipient CD4$^+$ T cell. CD4$^+$ cells then provide T cell help for the effector function of CD8$^+$ cells. This occurs in early post-transplantations and lasts till the donor APCs become depleted. This pathway is considered to be responsible for early acute cellular rejections.

Indirect Pathway of Allorecognition

Indirect pathway involves recipient APC phagocytosing and processing donor allopeptide and presenting them on self-MHC class II molecules to CD4 +ve T cells. These CD4 +ve T cells provide help to de novo allospecific CD8 +ve T cells. This leads to allorecognition and initiation of chronic allograft rejection.

Semidirect Pathway of Allorecognition

It is recognized that intact MHC class I and class II molecules are transferred between recipient and donor APC. This is accomplished by either direct cell to cell contact [trogocytosis] or through extracellular vesicles [exosomes] that are engulfed by APCs. In this way, recipient APCs acquire and present intact [unprocessed] donor peptide MHC complex on their surface [referred to as crossdressing].

Recipient APC thus has ability to express simultaneously on their surface 'self-HLA molecule with processed donor

TABLE 1: Terms and definitions.

DSA	Donor-specific antibodies, usually against HLA	
Non-HLA DSA	DSA to non-HLA	
HLA	Human leukocyte antigens	
AMR	Antibody-mediated rejection	
MHC	Major histocompatibility complex	A highly polymorphic region on short-arm chromosome 6 contributes to the immunological repertoire, autoimmunity, sensitization
Class I HLA molecules	HLA A, B, and C	Present on all nucleated cells
Class II HLA molecules	HLA DR, DP, DQ	Present on antigen-presenting cells, B cells
APC	Antigen-presenting cells	
$CD4^+$ T cells	T helper cells	
$CD4^+$ Tfh	T follicular helper cells	
$CD8^+$ T cells	Effector T cells	
CDR	Complementarity-determining region	Part of the variable region of B-cell receptor, antibodies, T-cell receptor that binds to the antigen
Epitope	Part of antigen that is recognized by the immune system	
Paratope	Part of the antibody that recognizes epitope	
Eplet	Clusters of two to three amino acid sequences (out of the 15–22 that make the epitope) that are recognized by HLA antibodies	Can be considered as functional epitopes
CREG	Cross-reactive epitope groups	Defined by the presence of cross-reactive HLA antibodies due to the presence of shared epitopes
Immunologically naive	No previous exposure to alloantigen	Absence of DSA does not mean immunologically naive status
Immunological sensitization	Previous exposure to alloantigen	DSA maybe present
PRA	Panel-reactive antibody	• A method to assess the degree of sensitization • Patients' serum tested against around 100 representative blood donors

peptides [class II] to CD4 +ve Th cells' as well as intact [unprocessed] donor peptide expressing donor HLA molecule [class I] to CD8 +ve T cells. This constitutes the three cell model or linked model of allorecoginition. This model is considered pertinent in development of alloantibodies. **(Figs. 1A and B)**.

ANTIBODY GENERATION

Naïve B cells carry a huge preimmune antibody repertoire with complementarity-determining regions (CDR) that help them recognize varied non-self HLA epitopes. On encountering the non-self HLA, the cognate naive B cell undergoes activation, proliferation, and maturation to DSA-specific memory B cells and long-lived plasma cells. The antigen-stimulated rapidly proliferating B cells in the germinal center of lymphoid tissues undergo somatic hypermutations in variable regions of their B-cell receptors (BCR). A subset of allospecific $CD4^+$ T cells that gets activated via the indirect or semidirect pathway moves to the

CHAPTER HIGHLIGHTS

- DSA are generated as a result of affinity-based maturation of B cells in germinal centers with $CD4^+$ T follicular helper (TFh) cells providing appropriate co-stimulation.
- A de novo response to HLA and non-HLA is generated post-transplantation due to epitope mismatches between donor and recipient. These responses ultimately lead to allograft dysfunction and graft loss.
- The DSA cause tissue injury by complement activation and antibody-dependent cellular cytotoxicity (ADCC). Additionally, sublethal injury by DSA causes endothelial cell activation and phenotype change contributing to vasculopathy, glomerulopathy, and fibrosis.
- Preformed DSA predict the possibility of an early acute rejection. The prevalence of de novo DSA increases over time and is a predictor of acute and chronic AMRs and graft loss.
- Prevention of generation of DSA with good HLA matching remains a desirable goal to improve long-term graft outcomes.
- Molecular mismatch algorithms analyzing mismatches at eplet or amino acid level may help overcome limitations of current HLA serological matching.

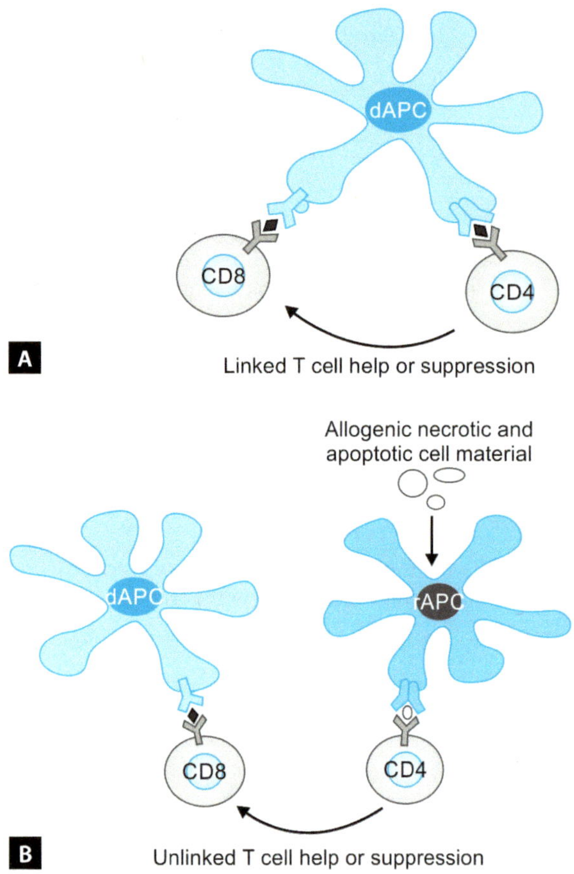

Figs. 1A and B: (A) Traditional three-cell model T cells cross talk, also called linked model, in which donor APCs activate both CD4 and CD8 T cells; (B) In four-cell models, recipient $CD8^+$ T cells stimulated through the direct pathway by donor APC can receive T-cell help or suppression from $CD4^+$ T cells activated via the indirect pathway by recipient dendritic cells. (APC: antigen-presenting cell)

T-cell zones in the lymphoid follicle. These $CD4^+$ Tfh cells help complementary B cells in cross switching from short-lived immunoglobulin M (IgM)-producing B cells to long-lived immunoglobulin G (IgG)-producing B cells as a part of affinity-based maturation—a method of negative selection so that only cells with highest antigen affinity proliferate. DSA are thus generated as a consequence of alloimmune recognition and close interaction of APC, B cells, and T cells.[5,6] These are regulated by a host of co-stimulatory or subordinate signaling pathways including cytotoxic T-lymphocyte-associated protein 4 (CTLA4), CD28, CD40L to B7, and CD40 on T and B cells, respectively. Interaction of CD28–B7 promotes interleukin-2 (IL-2) release causing proliferation and differentiation of B cells and CD40L–CD40 interaction promotes class switch.

While these DSA show high specificity to respective HLA molecules, they also show cross-reactivity with groups of non-self HLA molecules (cross-reactive epitope groups or CREGs). This is explained by the presence of shared epitopes (antigenic/immunogenic domains of HLA) or shared eplets [configuration of polymorphic amino acid determinant (usually three to five amino acid long) of epitope]. It is realized that it is the eplets to which the DSA actually bind and epitopes of different HLA molecules may also have shared eplets.[7,8]

While DSA against the non-self HLA are the chief cause of AMRs, non-HLA DSA are also generated and can be responsible for some of the rejections. These non-HLA antibodies include those against MHC class I chain-related molecule A (MICA), anti-protein kinase C (PKC) zeta, angiotensin II type I receptor (ATR1), antiendothelial cell antibodies (AECA), anti-peroxisomal trans-2-enoyl-CoA reductase (PERC), antiendoglin, MIG, ITAC, etc.

H-Y minor histocompatibility antigen encoded by Y chromosome can be a target for alloimmune response against male kidneys transplanted in female recipients.

IMMUNOLOGICAL MEMORY: NAÏVE VERSUS SENSITIZED RECIPIENT

Exposure to non-self HLA by sensitizing events such as blood product transfusions, pregnancy, previous transplant, and implants [ventricular assist device (VAD), homografts, etc.] leads to host mounting an immunological response. This response is both cellular, i.e., "generation of donor-reactive memory T and B cells" and humoral, i.e., generation of anti-HLA antibodies. Alloreactive immune T-cell response may also arise due to cross-reactivity of infectious pathogens with donor antigens. Individuals with these exposures are considered to be sensitized and are likely to pose an anamnestic immunological response post solid organ transplant leading to allograft rejection. A person not exposed to the above can be considered to be immunologically naive and is unlikely to host an anamnestic immune response against allograft.

No single laboratory test can determine the sensitization status of a patient. Cellular memory responses are difficult to assess; tests such as interferon-γ enzyme-linked immunosorbent spot (ELISpot) assay do provide some insight.

Donor-specific antibodies are the most readily used laboratory tests to determine sensitization.

Circulating HLA antibodies both donor specific and non-donor specific give an idea about the presence of sensitization. Sensitization is usually measured by detecting the presence of antibodies against a panel of representative HLAs from the general population. These antibodies are called the panel-reactive antibodies. The more the number of antibodies present, the more the sensitization.

There are, however, limitations in defining the specificity of measured DSA. On one hand, complement-dependent cytotoxicity (CDC) is very specific. On the other hand, single antigen bead (SAB) on Luminex platforms is highly sensitive. SAB assays pick up a lot of noise due to the detection of DSA to cryptic epitopes of HLA (that are not clinically significant) that get exposed due to the limitations in the technical process of synthesizing and loading HLA on

TABLE 2: Immunological workup for renal transplant.

Assessment of immune memory	**Table 4**
HLA typing and DSA: Laboratory assessment	**Table 6**
Clinical attributes of DSA	**Tables 3 and 5**
Molecular mismatch analysis	**Table 7**

(DSA: donor-specific antibodies; HLA: human leukocyte antigen)

the beads. As such, the tests have to be interpreted in terms of clinical history.

Evaluation of sensitization involves documenting the history of HLA-sensitizing events, inflammatory events that may boost alloimmune memory (such as major surgery, infections, and vaccinations), and non-DSA and DSA documented at any time pretransplant. DSA appearing within 2 weeks and up to 3 months post-transplant may still suggest the presence of immunological memory rather than de novo antibody responses. Autoantibody assessment as well as determination of non-HLA antibodies is also mandated.

Key points for Immunological workup for renal transplant are provided in **Table 2**.

DE NOVO DONOR-SPECIFIC ANTIBODIES

Alloimmune recognition of the engrafted organ leads to the generation of de novo DSA. Risk factors for the development of de novo DSA include a high number of HLA mismatches, inadequacy of immunosuppression, and factors that increase graft immunogenicity such as viral infections, ischemia-reperfusion injury, etc. They often develop against class II antigens, especially against DQ due to its highly polymorphic beta chain. New-onset DSA develop commonly in the first year post-transplant but can develop at any time post-transplantation.

Donor-specific Antibodies

Class I Donor-specific Antibodies

These are formed against the alpha chain of HLA A, B, and C. They are usually of IgG1 and IgG3 subclass and are complement-binding antibodies. Preformed class I DSA may result in positive T-cell crossmatch contraindicating transplant. De novo class I antibodies develop relatively early post-transplant and can cause acute AMR and graft dysfunction. C4d positivity is seen and rejections are often responsive to treatment.

Class II Donor-specific Antibodies

These are formed against the alpha and beta chains of DR, DQ, and DP antigens. They are usually of IgG2 and IgG4 subclass, and complement activation is weak. They result in a positive B-cell crossmatch and are responsible for chronic and subclinical rejections. They are difficult to desensitize and less amenable to treatment.

Nonhuman Leukocyte Antigen Donor-specific Antibodies

These are usually formed by humoral response toward non-HLA on ECs. They came into recognition as causative antibodies for unexpected hyperacute AMR in identical twin donations. A wide variety of antibodies are now recognized and they play a role in acute and chronic allograft rejections. Their routine detection, attributable risk, and pathogenic role on graft outcomes continue to be evaluated.[9]

PATHOGENESIS OF TISSUE INJURY

The ECs constitutively express class I antigens (with HLA A, B finding greater expression than class C). Class II antigens expression gets induced in the presence of events promoting inflammation (such as ischemia-reperfusion injury, delayed graft function, etc.). DSA bind to expressed HLA depending on the avidity of eplet–antibody interaction that determines their pathogenicity.

The DSAs cause graft injury by one of the following mechanisms—by promoting complement activation, by ADCC, or by inducing modifications in endothelium.[10]

Occasionally the DSAs bind to endothelial antigen without any inflammation or endothelial injury, a process referred to as accommodation.

Immunoglobulin M, IgG1, and IgG3 classes of antibodies are complement fixing. Their binding activated the classical complement pathway leading to the activation of MAC and lysis of antibody-coated cells. The by-products of the complement pathway additionally participate in the recruitment of inflammatory cells. Tissue deposits of C4d are histological markers for the activation of complement pathway.

Antibody-dependent cell-mediated cytotoxicity is induced by the interaction of Fc-gamma receptors of natural killer (NK) cells (as well as neutrophils and macrophages) with Fc-gamma region of DSA. This results in the formation of synapses and release of granzymes and perforins leading to apoptosis of the target cell. The release of chemokines further enhances HLA expression and inflammation. All classes of DSA including noncomplement activating DSA (IgG2, IgG4) participate in ADCC. Histologically, it is characterized by microvascular inflammation in the absence of C4d deposits.

Additionally, DSA binding to class I HLA on ECs induces intracellular signaling cascades. These lead to EC activation and phenotype modifications enhancing cell proliferation and survival. This contributes to the development of intimal proliferation, fibrosis, transplant glomerulopathy, and vasculopathy **(Fig. 2)**.

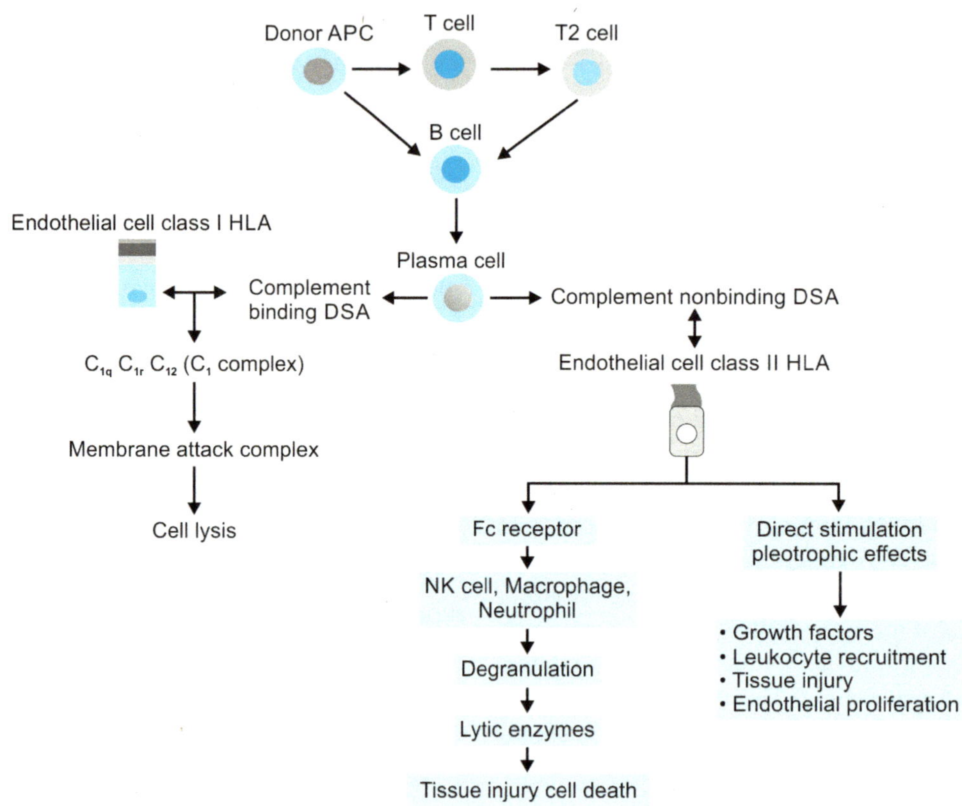

Fig. 2: Pathogenesis of complement-binding donor-specific antibodies (DSA) and complement nondependent binding of DSA.

ASSESSMENT OF DONOR-SPECIFIC ANTIBODIES

Presence of DSA is tested by one of the following methods: Classical cytotoxicity crossmatch, flow crossmatch, and solid phase assays (beads conjugated with single antigen or multiple HLA). The SAB assays are very sensitive, while cytotoxic crossmatch is very specific.

The DSA are assessed for their strength, complement-fixing ability, and subclass.[11]

The strength is measured in terms of mean fluoresce intensity (MFI) on Luminex assays. Higher MFI increases the likelihood of complement activation and tissue injury. However, the correlations between MFI and tissue injury are not definitive. There is often a high coefficient of variance (CV%) in MFI value, different DSAs may have similar MFI but may not cause similar tissue injury. The affinity for the beads may not correspond to the in vivo antigen binding on the ECs. DSAs targeting shared epitopes may get diluted on the multiple beads. Inhibitors, prozone effects, and denatured beads may affect interpretation.

C1q-binding DSAs help to improve specificity. C1q-binding DSAs show higher odds in predicting tissue injury compared to DSA that do not bind C1q. C3d- and C4d-binding DSA serve to assess more downstream complement activation. C3d and C4d assays used alone or along with C1q-binding assays serve to be a better predictor of AMR. However, there are limitations in these approaches. Complement fixation strongly correlates with MFI titers and as such often is only a surrogate of high MFIs. Also, it is recognized that c4d staining is seen histologically in AMRs in which DSA were not fixing complement in vitro.

Donor-specific antibody IgG subclasses give an insight into the maturity of immune response. Sequential IgG subclass switching occurs during immune response from IgG3 → IgG1 → IgG2 → IgG4. IgG3 and IgG1 tend to activate complement, while IgG2 does so minimally and IgG4 does not activate the complement cascade. The presence of IgG2 and IgG4 thus represents a more advanced stage of immune response. These DSA recruit effector cells via Fc-gamma receptor. IgG3-dominant AMR occurs earlier and is associated with C1q positivity, microcirculation injury, and C4d positivity. IgG4-dominant AMR maybe more subclinical and is associated with transplant glomerulopathy, interstitial fibrosis, and tubular atrophy.

MONITORING OF DONOR-SPECIFIC ANTIBODIES

Donor-specific antibodies are monitored as a part of pretransplant risk stratification, monitoring efficacy of desensitization, and post-transplant to predict AMR.

Risk Stratification

Risk is stratified on the basis of two types of immune responses: (1) The immune memory that leads to anamnestic response and (2) HLA mismatch that leads to the development of de novo alloimmune recognition. Features and outcomes of AMR related to memory versus de novo responses may vary.

All HLA immunizing events are not equal. The alloimmune response varies depending on the type of immunizing event. There maybe differences in response between a term pregnancy, miscarriage, blood product transfusion, previous transplant, etc. The antibody titers or MFI can be measured serially to assess strength and trends. DSA measurements have limitations, MFI does not always correlate with titers, the absence of DSA/calculated panel-reactive antibody (cPRA) does not necessarily mean immunologically naive status, acceptable antigens used in the listing may also have alloimmune sensitization but below thresholds used for listing, pretransplant titers do not necessarily correlate with post-transplant antibody responses, and c1q negative DSA can still mount c4d +ve AMR [at least six c1q DSA molecules in close proximity are required to activate complement, lower titers of complement fixing antibody can thus go undetected]. Thus, there remains significant unpredictability in the assessment of memory for risk stratification. Also, measuring memory cell responses remains difficult adding to unpredictability.

Similarly, assessing for de novo alloimmune response is also challenging. An HLA epitope has six CDRs out of that the third region of the variable heavy-chain antibody-binding site (CDR H3) is the eplet. This three to five amino acid region binds most strongly and represents the "functional epitope" for antibody specificity, while all the six CDRs together represent "structural epitope" and determine antibody avidity. HLA serological matches do predict the development of DSA and long-term graft outcomes. Those with the higher number of HLA mismatches have higher chances of development of DSAs and deterioration of graft function over time. However, serological assessment of HLA mismatches has inherent immunogenicity of organ transplanted (kidney vs. liver), adequacy of immunosuppression, and type of induction also need to be considered for risk stratification.[2,12]

The recommendations from Sensitization in Transplantation: Assessment of Risk (STAR) working group meeting reports (2017 and 2019) regarding DSA assessment and monitoring are summarized in **Tables 3 to 7**.

Desensitization

Currently, HLA antibody titers are used to assess desensitization protocol. Beyond that assessment of the effect on immunological memory in desensitization protocols like

TABLE 3: Comparison of class I and II donor-specific antibodies (DSA).

	Class I DSA	*Class II DSA*
HLA	A, B, and C	DR, DQ, and DP
Epitopes' location	α-Chain	α- and β-chains
Expression	All nucleated cells	Antigen-presenting cells
Preformed DSA:		
Positive crossmatch	T cells	B cells
De novo DSA:		
• Detection	• Sooner	• Later
• IgG subclasses	• IgG1, IgG3	• IgG2, IgG4
• Complement binding	• Strong	• Weak/no
• Frequency	• Fewer	• Common, especially DQ
Antibody-mediated rejection:		
• Phenotypes	• Acute	• Chronic/subclinical
• Presentation	• Early	• Later
• Graft dysfunction	• Rapidly	• Slowly
• C4d deposit	• Positive	• Negative
• Treatment	• More responsive	• Less responsive
• Graft loss	• Early	• Later

(HLA: human leukocyte antigens; IgG: immunoglobulin G)

TABLE 4: Assessment for immune memory.[2,12]

History		*Immune memory*	
HLA-sensitizing events	• Pregnancy transfusions • Previous transplant implants (VAD, homografts, etc.)	Latent potential for alloimmune memory response	• History of sensitizing event • Non-DSA HLA antibody detected at one or more time prior to transplant • Non-DSA detected pretransplant
Inflammatory events that boost preexisting alloimmune memory	• Major surgery • Major infection • Recent vaccination	Active potential for alloimmune response	DSA present at the time of transplantation or in the historical sample
		Alloimmune memory response	DSA response post-transplant or pretransplant DSA or new DSA within 2 weeks post-transplant

Notes: Patients without HLA-sensitizing events to be considered low risk for immunological memory.
Immunological memory status should be used for risk stratification, determining the frequency of DSA testing post-transplant.
(DSA: donor-specific antibodies; HLA: human leukocyte antigens; VAD: ventricular assist device)

TABLE 5: Attributes of donor-specific antibodies (DSA).[2,12]

	Attributes	***Consequence***
DSA	• High MFI • High antibody titers • Complement-fixing antibodies	Increased risk of AMR
	IgG subclass	• IgG1, IgG3—acute AMR • IgG2, IgG4—chronic active AMR
	DSA-associated cell signaling	Endothelial cell modifications
Memory cell alloimmunity	T- and B-cell assays (donor HLA-specific IFN gamma-secreting T cells, panel reactive T cells, T follicular helper cells, frequency of HLA-binding memory B cells, etc.)	At research level

(AMR: antibody-mediated rejection; IFN: interferon; HLA: human leukocyte antigens; IgG: immunoglobulin G; MFI: mean fluoresce intensity)

TABLE 6: Human leukocyte antigen (HLA) laboratory assessment.[2,12]

HLA typing	Should be comprehensive	HLA A, B, C, DRB1, DRB3/4/5, DQA1/DQB1, DPA1/DPB1
HLA antibody assessment	Solid-phase assays	Report up to allele level
	Inhibitors should be removed	DTT, EDTA, titration studies, heat inactivation
	Epitope sharing to be analyzed	Stacking antibodies against CREGs
	MFI cut-off 1,000–1,500	Possible false negative if it belongs to CREG False positive if against denatured/cryptic epitopes, autoantigen/allele, nonspecific patters (hot beads)
	Differences in MFI <25% not significant	High coefficient of variance in MFI

(CREG: cross-reactive epitope group; DTT: dithiothreitol; EDTA: ethylenediaminetetraacetic acid; HTA: human leukocyte antigens; MFI: mean fluoresce intensity)

TABLE 7: Molecular mismatch analysis.[2,12]

HLA matchmaker	Donor–recipient amino acid sequences to determine continuous and discontinuous eplets that maybe recognized by antibody CDRs	• Focus on polymorphic regions • All mismatched eplets are given same value • Generates an eplet mismatch score	• Verified and unverified eplet terms used to define detected eplets not serologically confirmed • Immune response does not work on total loads
Electrostatic mismatch score	Electrostatic surface value of amino acids on HLA molecules	Tries to add physiochemical properties over and above the number of mismatches	
• Predicted indirectly recognizable HLA • Epitopes presented by recipient HLA-class II • Antigens = PIRCHE-II	Focus on HLA DR presentable antigens	T-cell help for B-cell maturation is needed	
Amino acid sequence comparison	Looks at number of amino acid mismatches (rather than eplet mismatch)	No prior assumptions regarding the relevance of mismatched amino acids make it less biased	

(CDR: complementarity-determining region; HLA: human leukocyte antigens)

limitations and does not predict de novo alloimmune responses accurately. For a given HLA serotype, there are differences at epitope and eplet levels. Also, there may exist immunodominant HLA epitopes. A good matching at HLA, especially at epitope or eplet levels, remains a desirable goal. Computerized algorithms for molecular mismatch load analysis, eplet matching are being evaluated for risk stratification for de novo alloimmune response and clinical outcomes.

Risk stratification also depends on factors other than preexisting immune memory and epitope/eplet mismatches. Factors such as age of the recipient (young vs. old), effects on memory B or T cells remains difficult to assess. The impact of attributes of DSA such as complement-binding ability, antibody class, and isotype switch remains undefined.

Post-transplant Monitoring

The frequency of screening for DSA post-transplant should be based on immunological risk (immunological memory, HLA serology/epitope/eplet mismatches, and factors such as age and type of organ transplanted). However, the cost–benefit for these approaches needs to be evaluated.

REFERENCES

1. Patel R, Terasaki PI. Significance of the positive crossmatch test in kidney transplantation. N Engl J Med. 1969;280(14): 735-9.
2. Tambur AR, Campbell P, Chong AS, Feng S, Ford ML, Gebel H, et al. Sensitization in transplantation: assessment of risk (STAR) 2019 Working Group Meeting Report. Am J Transplant. 2020;20(10):2652-68.
3. Williams TM. Human leukocyte antigen gene polymorphism and the histocompatibility laboratory. J Mol Diagn. 2001; 3(3):98-104.
4. Afzali B, Lombardi G, Lechler RI. Pathways of major histocompatibility complex allorecognition. Curr Opin Organ Transplant. 2008;13(4):438-44.
5. Clatworthy MR, Espeli M, Torpey N, Smith KGC. The generation and maintenance of serum alloantibody. Curr Opin Immunol. 2010;22:669-81.
6. Alberts B, Johnson A, Lewis J, Raff M, Roberts K, Walter P. The generation of antibody diversity. Molecular Biology of the Cell, 4th edition. New York: Garland Science; 2002.
7. El-Awar N, Jucaud V, Nguyen A. HLA epitopes: the targets of monoclonal and alloantibodies defined. J Immunol Res. 2017;2017:3406230.
8. Bezstarosti S, Bakker KH, Kramer CSM, de Fijter JW, Reinders MEJ, Mulder A, et al. A comprehensive evaluation of the antibody-verified status of eplets listed in the HLA Epitope Registry. Front Immunol. 2022;12:800946.
9. Matsuda Y, Sarwal MM. Unraveling the role of allo-antibodies and transplant injury. Front Immunol. 2016;7:432.
10. McCaughan J, Xu Q, Tinckam K. Detecting donor-specific antibodies: the importance of sorting the wheat from the chaff. Hepatobiliary Surg Nutr. 2019;8(1):37-52.
11. Zhang R. Donor-specific antibodies in kidney transplant recipients. Clin J Am Soc Nephrol. 2018;13:182-92.
12. Tambur AR, Campbell P, Claas FH, Feng S, Gebel HM, Jackson AM, et al. Sensitization in transplantation: assessment of risk (STAR) 2017 Working Group Meeting Report. Am J Transplant. 2018;18(7):1604-14.

1.4 Role of non-HLA Antigen in Kidney Transplantation

Jasmine Sethi, Vivek Kumar

CASE VIGNETTE

*A 25-year-old male underwent retransplantation (Basic disease being IgA nephropathy) with a human leukocyte antigen (HLA) negative cross matched deceased donor kidney. He had lost his first kidney transplant to chronic rejection three years prior and had underwent allograft nephrectomy. The pretransplant cytotoxic and flow crossmatches (T and B lymphocyte) were negative. Furthermore, pretransplant HLA antibody testing by solid phase luminex testing showed no antidonor HLA antibodies. He was induced with antithymocyte globulin and maintained on prednisone, tacrolimus and mycophenolate mofetil. He had a stable postoperative course and was discharged on postoperative day seven with serum creatinine of 0.7 mg/dL. One month post-transplant, the patient presented with oliguria and serum creatinine of 3.5 mg/dL. He was treated with solumedrol pulses and allograft biopsy was performed. Biopsy revealed Banff type IIB ACR and ABMR with C4d negativity. Donor specific antibodies (DSA) were repeated and found to be negative. Further investigations for non-HLA antibodies revealed that the recipient had donor specific MICA antibody directed against MICA*012. Evaluation of the bio-banked pretransplant serum revealed preformed MICA*012 antibodies with levels that were elevated even before transplant (MFI = 15,782). The levels at the time of rejection were also elevated (MFI = 15,743). The patient was treated with antithymocyte globulin along with 7 sessions of plasmapharesis followed by IVIG (2g/kg). The patient partially responded to therapy with a serum creatinine of 1.6 mg/dL at 2 months.*

BACKGROUND

Kidney transplantation is a modern scientific achievement that has transformed the lives of patients with end-stage kidney disease (ESKD). Over the last few decades, remarkable progress has been made to prevent acute rejection of the kidney allograft. However, preventing immunologic allograft loss in the long term is still considered the "Achilles' heel" in management of kidney transplant recipients. Despite best efforts, most kidney transplant recipients would develop varying degrees of chronic allograft rejection in the long term.

Traditionally, the concept of "self versus other" has centered around the human leukocyte antigens (HLAs). These are encoded by the major histocompatibility complex (MHC) on the short arm of chromosome 6. These are considered the most important alloantigens as presence of anti-HLA antibodies directed against donor (also called donor-specific antibodies or DSAs) is strongly associated with acute or chronic rejection and decreased allograft survival. The presence of DSAs is an important characteristic of antibody-mediated rejection (ABMR). However, there has been increasing recognition of the fact that rejection of the kidney allograft can also occur in recipients who do not have demonstrable or clinically significant DSAs. With the advent of molecular typing techniques that allow epitope- and eplet-level resolution of HLA mismatches, the role of non-HLA antibodies has gained more significance. Although adsorption of DSA within the allograft has been proposed to explain the occurrence of ABMR in DSA-negative recipients, mounting evidence point to possible role of non-HLA antibodies in allograft rejection.[1] The first indirect evidence for the involvement of non-HLA antibodies in allograft outcome came from reports of allograft rejection in HLA-identical sibling transplants that had a negative crossmatch for anti-HLA antibodies. In the 2017 update on the Banff classification scheme for allograft histology, testing for non-HLA antibodies was strongly advised in cases where ABMR occurred in the absence of detectable or clinically significant DSAs.[2]

MINOR HISTOCOMPATIBILITY (NONHUMAN LEUKOCYTE ANTIGEN) ANTIGENS IN KIDNEY TRANSPLANTATION

Definition

As is suggested by the name, any non-MHC-encoded polymorphic protein that is sufficiently antigenic to induce an immune response against the allograft will qualify as a non-HLA. Such antigens may initiate cascade of immunologic damage to the kidney allograft in the absence of anti-HLA antibodies or DSAs. These are also known as minor histocompatibility antigens (mHA). These are likely to be transmembrane or extracellular or cell surface proteins which are polymorphic and hence could be different between different individuals of the same species. Nonself alloantigens are identified by either direct or indirect allorecognition. It is the indirect allorecognition by the recipient's immune system that is primarily responsible for recognition of non-HLA and development of antibodies against mHA.[3]

The allograft endothelium is the first interface of contact between recipient immune system and donor tissue antigens. HLAs are constitutively expressed on endothelial cell surface. Therefore, it is not surprising that non-HLA or proteins expressed on allograft endothelium are considered as primary culprits behind DSA-negative allograft rejection.

However, we must remember that not all proteins that may be different between recipient and donor are likely to be expressed on the endothelial surface. Some of the potential antigens may be cryptic, i.e., their usual location and conformation prevent access by the immune system. Tissue damage due to various reasons may create permissive conditions that may lead to exposure and presentation of such cryptic antigens to the recipient's immune system. This in turn may lead to development of alloantibodies (if the protein is polymorphic) or autoantibodies (if the protein is monomorphic). Binding to these antibodies to antigenic targets may start a cascade of vascular inflammation and allograft injury.[1] The specificity of these could be broad and mechanisms are currently not very clear.

Why is Routine Evaluation Negative?

Detection of specific antibodies is dependent on characterization of specific antigens. In the case of DSAs, this is facilitated by decades of extensive research into high-resolution characterization of different types and subtypes of HLA in various populations. The current methods of routine identification and quantitation of DSAs are targeted exclusively against HLA. Therefore, allograft rejections in the setting of negative DSAs represent the clinical phenotype of non-HLA-mediated immunologic injury provided falsely negative interpretations of DSAs are taken care of. Antibodies against non-HLA are not usually detected by methods routinely used for crossmatching since these antigens may not be expressed on the lymphocytes.[4]

Classifying Nonhuman Leukocyte Antigen Antibodies

There is no formal classification of antibodies against non-HLA in kidney transplantation. However, these can be broadly classified into three different types:[5]

1. *Alloantibodies direct against polymorphic antigens:* These antigens differ between the recipient and donor, e.g., antimajor histocompatibility complex class I-related chain A (MICA) antibody.
2. *Autoantibodies that recognize self-antigens which are usually cryptic:* These constitute the majority of currently characterized non-HLA antibodies. A significant proportion of these react with autoantigens expressed by vascular endothelial cells (VECs). These antiendothelial cell antibodies (AECAs) include a spectrum of different antibodies depending on antigenic specificity such as anti-angiotensin-II type 1 receptor (AT1R) antibody, anti-endothelin-1 type A receptor (ETAR) antibody, anti-perlecan/three laminin-like globular domains (LG3) antibody, and antiagrin antibody.
3. *Natural antibodies that exist in the absence of exogenous antigen exposure:* These are polyreactive, e.g., anti-apoptotic cell antibody.

CHAPTER HIGHLIGHTS

- Non-HLA antibodies can lead to antibody mediated rejection without C4d deposition.
- Various forms of non-HLA Abs play an important role in acute or chronic allograft rejection and portend a negative long-term graft outcome.
- The incorporation of non-HLA antibodies into the immunological risk assessment needs evaluation. Research is needed to identify patients who would benefit from this kind of evaluation.

Detection of Antibodies against Nonhuman Leukocyte Antigens

More than 10% of cases with C4d-positive ABMR fail to show circulating anti-HLA antibodies or DSAs. Causes of DSA-negative ABMR could be falsely negative DSAs due to technical issues (variations in assay sensitivity or reporting threshold), rare donor HLA not represented in the assay kits, DSAs' sequestration within the allograft, or presence of antibodies against non-HLA donor antigens. As of now, there are no commercially available methods for the reliable detection of antibodies against non-HLA donor antigens. Different testing approaches have been used to detect these.[6] As VECs are considered the primary interface, extracts or preparations of endothelial cells have been used as substrates for broad or specific antibody screening assays. Detection of antibodies targeted against specified antigens can be done through commercially available assays for antibodies against MICA, AT1R, and ETAR. Proteomic and genomic approaches have also been advocated and tested to ascertain variations between recipients and donors. Genome-wide incompatibility and development of allo-genomics mismatch score have been shown to add value to HLA incompatibility with respect to allograft outcomes in small studies. However, lack of extensive data and limited availability of such approaches forbid routine applications at present.

Pathogenic Mechanisms

Mechanisms for production of non-HLA antibodies and associated allograft injury have been described, though these are still not fully understood.[5,7,8] The process of pathogenic antibody production starts with allograft injury. Allograft injury by insults such as ischemia reperfusion injury (IRI), chronic inflammation, surgical trauma, infection, nephrotoxicity, or rejection exposes the cryptic non-HLA.[9] It induces the production of non-HLA antibodies and their binding to now exposed or expressed cryptic antigens. Some non-HLA antibodies (e.g., antiperlecan) are present in the body even prior to transplant and bind to their targets following tissue injury in the post-transplantation period.[10] Vascular access creation and manipulation may also play a role in the production of non-HLA antibodies prior to transplant.

Allograft injury leads to release of extracellular vesicles (EVs) in circulation that express autoantigens on the surface. These EVs can be exosomes, microparticles, or apoptotic bodies and may contain numerous autoantigens. These are then presented, most likely, by the recipient's antigen presenting cells (APC) to the recipient's autoreactive T cells. This indirect alloreactive pathway is considered to be more important in context of non-HLA histocompatibility antigens. CD4 T cells indirectly stimulate autoreactive B cells and thus lead to autoantibody production. Activation of autoreactive T cells results in production of proinflammatory cytokines and local allograft injury. Tertiary lymphoid tissue (TLT) along with Th17 support the formation and proliferation of autoreactive B cells and autoantibodies. Interleukin (IL)-17 produced by Th17 leads to leukocyte recruitment and allograft damage. Finally, autoreactive B cells escape apoptosis in TLT due to sustained local production of IL-21 which promotes B-cell survival. These autoantibodies act through both complement-dependent and complement-independent cytotoxicity. These can also induce lysis of target cells through activation of natural killer (NK) cells, by a process known as antibody-dependent cell-mediated cytotoxicity (ADCC). These can also induce vascular endothelial call activation/injury and subsequent immune dysfunction.

There may be a complex relationship between tissue injury, anti-HLA, and non-HLA immunity in enhancing allograft damage. Inflammatory response induced by non-HLA antibodies could upregulate HLA expression and increase the risk of developing anti-HLA DSAs.[11]

Specific Nonhuman Leukocyte Antigens

The important non-HLA against which antibodies have been described are as follows **(Table 1)**:

- *Major histocompatibility complex class I-related chain A (MICA):* MICA antigens are expressed on the surface of dendritic cells, fibroblasts, VECs, and monocytes but not on lymphocytes. Since MICA is not expressed on resting lymphocytes, it cannot be detected with classical lymphocyte-based crossmatching techniques. Normally, MICA antigens are not expressed on the surface of quiescent VECs. However, stressful conditions such as infection, inflammation, and hypoxia induce MICA expression on the surface of these cells. MICA gene locus is highly pleomorphic and is located on chromosome 6 in close linkage equilibrium to HLA-B locus. Antibodies against MICA antigens may form due to the cross-reactivity with other antigens such as in infections. MICA sensitization can also occur through mechanisms similar to HLA, such as previous transplants, pregnancy, or transfusion. Anti-MICA antibodies have been associated with both ABMR and acute cellular rejection (ACR).[12-14]
- *Angiotensin-II type 1 receptor (AT1R):* AT1R is a transmembrane G-protein coupled receptor (GPCR), which has seven transmembrane domains and is expressed on VECs, podocytes, and other kidney tissues. Aldosterone acts through AT1R and regulates salt and water retention, inflammation, and vascular remodeling. IRI may modulate AT1R and facilitate interaction with AT1R antibodies. AT1R antibodies are agonistic and lead to increased production of proinflammatory cytokines and further stimulate T cells. AT1R antibodies have been associated with severe acute vascular rejection and malignant hypertension.[15] Compared to DSA-mediated rejection, AT1R Ab-associated rejection is associated with higher prevalence of hypertension, more vascular rejection, and lack of complement deposition. Angiotensin II receptor blockers represent an interesting therapeutic option in patients with AT1R-mediated rejection in combination with plasmapheresis. However, their clinical utility remains unproven.

TABLE 1: Common nonhuman leukocyte antigens.[8]

Perlecan/LG3	Heparin sulfate proteoglycan and a major component of vessel wall
Vimentin	Intermediate filament protein present in the cells of mesenchymal origin, including endothelial cells
Endothelin 1 type A receptor (ETAR)	Receptor for endothelin 1
Major histocompatibility complex class I-related chain A (MICA)	Expressed on endothelial cells, keratinocytes, monocytes, dendritic cells, fibroblasts, and epithelial cells
Angiotensin-II type 1 receptor (AT1R)	G protein-coupled receptor that mediates the action of angiotensin II
Vimentin	Type III intermediate filament protein, expressed by lymphocytes and macrophages
Collagen I, Collagen V, and α-tubulin	Collagens are extracellular matrix proteins, and tubulin is the major constituent of microtubules
RSP4Y protein	This is located on Y chromosome, may induce alloreactivity in gender mismatched transplants

(LG3: three laminin-like globular domains)

- *Endothelin-1 type A receptor (ETAR):* It is also a transmembrane GPCR that acts as a receptor for endothelin 1 (ET1). Similar to AT1R antibodies, ETAR antibodies are also agonistic antibodies. Binding of ET1 to ETAR induces vasoconstriction and its mitogenic and proinflammatory effects lead to obliterative vasculopathy and progressive tissue fibrosis. Anti-ETAR antibodies are associated with vasculopathy and arteritis.[16]
- *Perlecan/LG3:* It is a heparin sulfate proteoglycan and a component of the vascular basement membrane (VBM). Its C terminal domain contains LG3. The LG3 domain can be released by caspase-dependent cleavage during apoptosis and might act as neoantigen and promote antibody production. High levels of anti-LG3 antibodies in both pre- and post-transplant periods are associated with increased risk of vascular rejection.[17] Bortezomib can block the production of anti-LG3 autoantibodies triggered by exosome-like vesicles and may prove useful for preventing autoantibody production before transplantation.[18]
- *Collagen-IV, vimentin, and fibronectin:* Autoantibodies to collagen-IV and fibronectin have been associated with transplant glomerulopathy (TG).[19] Autoantibodies to vimentin have been found to be elevated in patients with interstitial fibrosis and tubular atrophy and those with previously failed renal allografts.[20]

CONCLUSION

Immune mechanisms that lead to non-HLA antibody formation are complex and poorly understood. Mounting evidence has shown that various forms of antibodies against non-HLA play an important role in acute or chronic allograft rejection and portend a poor long-term allograft outcome. Identification of these antibodies by advanced molecular techniques, integration of proteomics or genomics data to further refine alloincompatibility beyond HLA mismatch, and standardization of testing platforms for widespread applicability are required to make progress in this field.

REFERENCES

1. Cardinal H, Dieude M, Hebert MJ. The emerging importance of non-HLA autoantibodies in kidney transplant complications. J Am Soc Nephrol. 2017;28(2):400-6.
2. Haas M, Loupy A, Lefaucheur C, Roufosse C, Glotz D, Seron D, et al. The Banff 2017 kidney meeting report: revised diagnostic criteria for chronic active T cell-mediated rejection, antibody-mediated rejection, and prospects for integrative endpoints for next-generation clinical trials. Am J Transplant. 2018;18(2):293-307.
3. Reindl-Schwaighofer R, Heinzel A, Gualdoni GA, Mesnard L, Claas FHJ, Oberbauer R. Novel insights into non-HLA alloimmunity in kidney transplantation. Transpl Int. 2020; 33(1):5-17.
4. Matsuda Y, Sarwal MM. Unraveling the role of allo-antibodies and transplant injury. Front Immunol. 2016;7:432.
5. Zhang Q, Reed EF. The importance of non-HLA antibodies in transplantation. Nat Rev Nephrol. 2016;12(8): 484-95.
6. Regele H. Non-HLA antibodies in kidney allograft rejection: convincing concept in need of further evidence. Kidney Int. 2011;79(6):583-6.
7. Tinckam KJ, Chandraker A. Mechanisms and role of HLA and non-HLA alloantibodies. Clin J Am Soc Nephrol. 2006; 1(3):404-14.
8. Zhang X, Reinsmoen NL. Impact of non-human leukocyte antigen-specific antibodies in kidney and heart transplantation. Front Immunol. 2017;8:434.
9. Dragun D, Catar R, Philippe A. Non-HLA antibodies in solid organ transplantation: recent concepts and clinical relevance. Curr Opin Organ Transplant. 2013;18(4):430-5.
10. Etta PK, Madhavi T, Parikh N. The multifaceted role of non-human leukocyte antigens' immune response in renal allograft rejection. Saudi J Kidney Dis Transpl. 2021; 32(3):622-36.
11. Dragun D, Catar R, Philippe A. Non-HLA antibodies against endothelial targets bridging allo- and autoimmunity. Kidney Int. 2016;90(2):280-8.
12. Zou Y, Stastny P, Susal C, Dohler B, Opelz G. Antibodies against MICA antigens and kidney-transplant rejection. N Engl J Med. 2007;357(13):1293-300.
13. Chowdhry M, Makroo RN, Singh M, Kumar M, Thakur Y, Sharma V. Role of anti-MICA antibodies in graft survival of renal transplant recipients of India. J Immunol Res. 2018; 2018:3434050.
14. Baranwal AK, Mehra NK. Major histocompatibility complex class I chain-related A (MICA) molecules: relevance in solid organ transplantation. Front Immunol. 2017;8:182.
15. In JW, Park H, Rho EY, Shin S, Park KU, Park MH, et al. Anti-angiotensin type 1 receptor antibodies associated with antibody-mediated rejection in patients without preformed HLA-donor-specific antibody. Transplant Proc. 2014;46(10):3371-4.
16. Banasik M, Boratynska M, Koscielska-Kasprzak K, Krajewska M, Mazanowska O, Kaminska D, et al. The impact of non-HLA antibodies directed against endothelin-1 type A receptors (ETAR) on early renal transplant outcomes. Transpl Immunol. 2014;30(1):24-9.
17. Cardinal H, Dieude M, Brassard N, Qi S, Patey N, Soulez M, et al. Antiperlecan antibodies are novel accelerators of immune-mediated vascular injury. Am J Transplant. 2013; 13(4):861-74.
18. Dieude M, Bell C, Turgeon J, Beillevaire D, Pomerleau L, Yang B, et al. The 20S proteasome core, active within apoptotic exosome-like vesicles, induces autoantibody production and accelerates rejection. Sci Transl Med. 2015;7(318): 318ra200.
19. Angaswamy N, Klein C, Tiriveedhi V, Gaut J, Anwar S, Rossi A, et al. Immune responses to collagen-IV and fibronectin in renal transplant recipients with transplant glomerulopathy. Am J Transplant. 2014;14(3):685-93.
20. Lopez-Soler RI, Borgia JA, Kanangat S, Fhied CL, Conti DJ, Constantino D, et al. Anti-vimentin antibodies present at the time of transplantation may predict early development of interstitial fibrosis/tubular atrophy. Transplant Proc. 2016; 48(6):2023-33.

1.5 Tolerance and Accommodation in Renal Transplantation

Aruna V Vanikar, Pankaj R Shah

INTRODUCTION WITH HISTORICAL PERSPECTIVE

Lord Ganesha with an elephant's head transplanted over a human body is the first example of successful xeno-transplantation accepted by the human race. Subsequently, examples in other civilizations involving transplantation of limbs, heart, and the spirit have been recorded. This chapter briefly discusses the immunology of rejection, tolerance, and different modes of inducing and measuring it. It also touches upon accommodation.

NEED FOR TOLERANCE IN KIDNEY TRANSPLANTATION

Successful kidney transplantation was achieved simultaneously by Merrill and Murray in identical twins in Boston, and by Hamburger who transplanted kidney from sister to brother in Paris. Surgical skills were established by the 17th century AD.[1] However, immunological success is still not achieved in the 21st century. A transplanted kidney being a foreign body gets rejected by the immune system of the host. The advent of immunosuppressants/immune modulators beginning from 6-mercaptopurine, calcineurin inhibitors (CNI), or mammalian target of rapamycin (m-TOR) inhibitors supported by mycophenolate, azathioprine, and steroids have helped in controlling acute rejections.[2-5] However, none could usher in immunosuppression-free normal life. Immunosuppressants have toxic side effects of suppressing the general immune response of the recipient making him susceptible to bacterial, viral, and fungal infections, malignancies/diabetes mellitus, and a myriad of other problems in the long run. In spite of optimum immunosuppression, eventually, the graft is lost to chronic attrition after an enormous financial burden to the system/family.[4,6,7] Striking a balance between prevention of rejection and drug toxicity is still elusive.

REJECTION AND TOLERANCE

The introduction of an antigen is recognized as a foreign invasion by the host immune system evoking a cellular or humoral immune response involving T-cell/B-cell activation. Immunity protects the human body from infections/malignancy; paradoxically, the same immune system is responsible for the rejection of a graft. Hence, for the survival of transplanted graft, the host immune system needs to be suppressed/downregulated.

Tolerance

Immune tolerance or immunological tolerance is a state of absence of a destructive immune response by the recipient immune system toward a well-functioning donor organ/graft in the absence of maintenance immunosuppression and with a fully intact immune system.[8]

Clinical/Operational Tolerance

Tolerance has been achieved anecdotally in renal transplant recipients by the successful withdrawal of immunosuppressive medications.[9] Although such withdrawal was not planned in most cases, a number of trials were conducted for immunosuppression withdrawal.[9-17] These trials were not without risk; in renal transplant patients, acute rejection episodes correlated strongly with the development of chronic allograft nephropathy and reduced graft function was recognized as a risk factor for cardiovascular death.[12,18] Selection of ideal patients before transplantation by immunological and molecular phenotypic analyses, coupled with aggressive immune monitoring post-transplantation, is of paramount importance for successful tolerance induction. Thus, the term "operational tolerance" evolved, which is defined as stable graft function without clinical features of chronic rejection and in the absence of any immunosuppressive drugs, usually for >1 year.[19,20] It has been observed in liver transplant patients more than in other allograft recipients. Biopsy was not a requisite for operational tolerance.

Propè Tolerance

After substantial efforts by many groups, immune or even operational tolerance was emerging as a Utopian dream. This led to the addition of one more term to the tools defining transplantation tolerance called "Propè tolerance." Propè (or almost) tolerance was described as a state in which graft acceptance is maintained by a low, nontoxic dosage of maintenance immunosuppression, which may not be required indefinitely.[21]

Mechanisms of Tolerance

In 1938, Gorer identified immune rejection of transplanted tissue.[22,23] He believed that the humoral arm of immunity was responsible for rejection and if this was arrested, tolerance would be achieved. Billingham et al. established the concept of chimeric tolerance (cellular arm of immunity) through Owen's model of natural tolerance induction in bovine twins, which they extrapolated in the neonatal mice model.[24,25] This was revived with bone marrow (BM) and liver transplantation in the clinic.[26]

Tolerance is believed to be induced by two basic pathways: Central or thymic tolerance and peripheral tolerance. In central tolerance, the double positive T cells ($CD4^+$ $CD8^+$) are selected to become either $CD4^+$ if the T-cell receptors (TCR) react with major histocompatibility complex (MHC) class II antigens or $CD8^+$ if the TCR react with MHC class I antigens on antigen-presenting cells (APCs) (dendritic cells, macrophages, thymic medullary epithelium). They may undergo apoptotic deletion if this engagement fails. A negative selection follows in which most self-reactive $CD4^+$ or $CD8^+$ cells undergo TCR-induced death if they interact with MHC molecules on APCs carrying self-peptides. Alloreactive cells can also undergo negative selection in the thymus during the interaction of antigen-specific T cells with "tolerogenic" dendritic cells expressing varying levels of co-stimulatory molecules.

In peripheral tolerance, autoreactive/alloreactive cells that escape thymic deletion may be deleted or controlled in circulation by activation-induced cell death, by programmed cell death, or by the suppressive action of Tregs and cytokines. Alloreactive cells repeatedly stimulated with alloantigen can undergo activation-induced cell death by "death receptors" (Fas) cross-linking Fas ligand, leading to caspase cascade activation and cell apoptosis. This pathway is critical to the inhibition of cell proliferation as well as to the development of tolerance[27-29] **(Fig. 1)**.

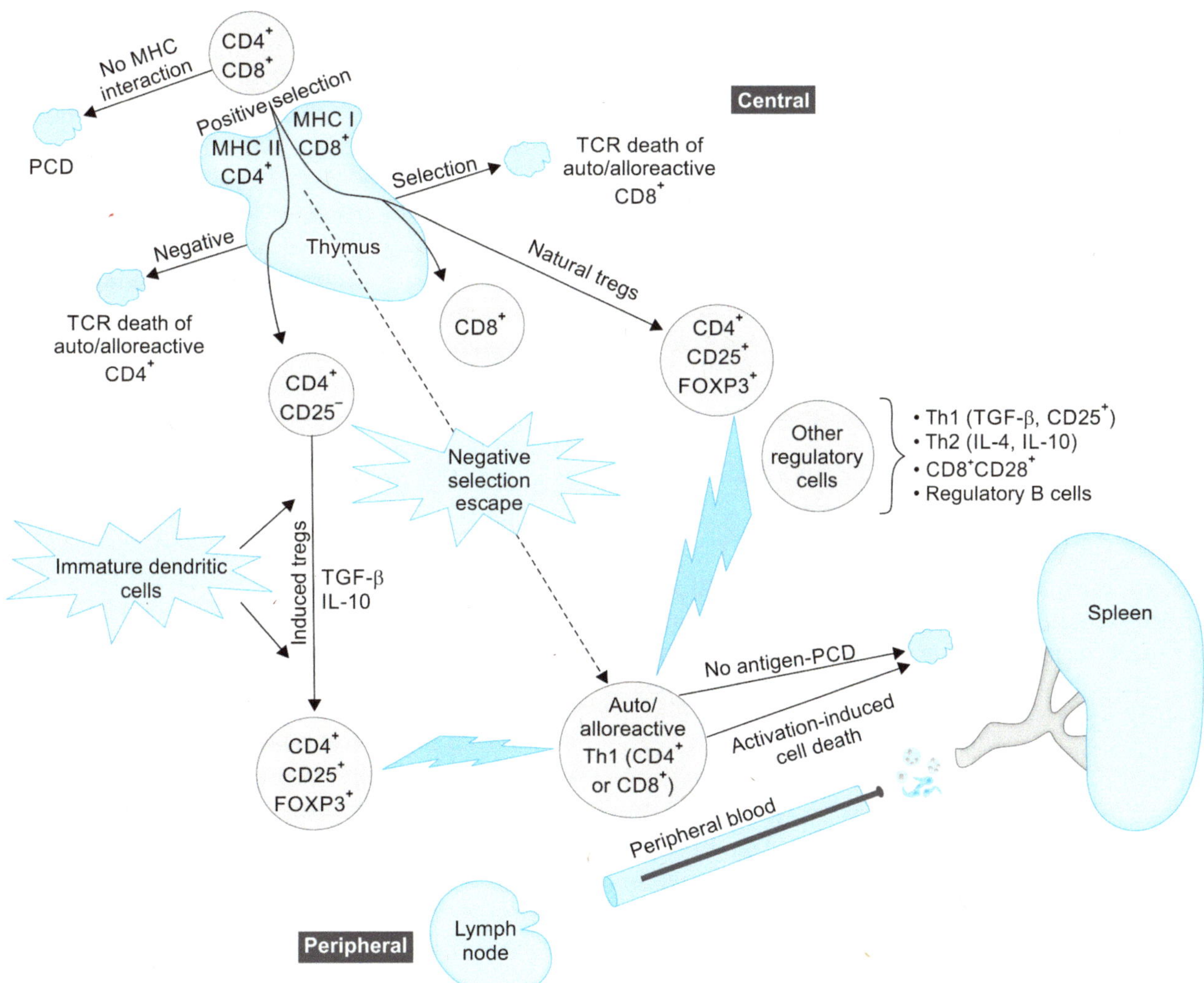

Fig. 1: Proposed mechanism of tolerance. The figure displays the central and peripheral mechanisms for regulation of autoimmune/alloimmune responses. CD3þ cells that are initially double positive for CD4 and CD8 first undergo positive selection to become either $CD4^+$ [major histocompatibility complex (MHC) class II interaction] or $CD8^+$ (MHC class I interaction) followed by deletion or negative selection if autoreactive/alloreactive. However, some $CD4^+$ and $CD8^+$ cells can escape negative selection and become autoreactive/alloreactive Th1 cells in the periphery (lymph nodes, blood, spleen). Mechanisms to regulate these peripherally reactive T cells that can cause autoimmune diseases and transplant rejection are displayed: (1) Immunoregulation from natural (thymic-derived) or induced (in the context of proregulatory cytokines/dendritic cells) regulatory T cells (Tregs) or other regulatory cells; (2) Activation-induced cell death; and (3) No activation resulting in programmed cell death. (IL-10: interleukin-10; PCD: programmed cell death; TCR: T-cell receptors; TGF-β: tumor growth factor-beta)

The mechanisms proposed for peripheral tolerance induction include:[9,18,30-35]

- Chimeric tolerance (simultaneous peaceful existence of two different kinds of cells in one host)
- Clonal deletion (removal of rejecting cell groups)
- Clonal anergy
- Regulation/suppression (of these rejecting clones)

Long-lasting tolerance is believed to involve multiple mechanisms with the goal of profound reduction in clonal T-cell expansion along with active immune regulation.[9,10] Multiple receptors, ligands, and signaling intermediates have been identified to serve therapeutic targets for tolerance induction strategies including co-stimulatory blockade, TCR targeting, and profound T-cell depletion.[36] Animal and human data suggest that administration of donor antigens concurrent with these immunomodulatory agents may be an important adjuvant therapy for successful tolerance strategies.

CHAPTER HIGHLIGHTS

- Tolerance in transplantation is referred to as a state in which there is the absence of a destructive immune response in the recipient toward a functioning *allograft*, while the immune system is fully intact with no use of exogenous immunosuppression.
- Principle mechanisms involved in T-cell tolerance are deletion, anergy, clonal ignorance, and suppression.
- The adaptive immune response to any stimulus involves recruitment and activation of effector T and B cells in addition to regulatory T cells (Tregs). Tregs have an indispensable role in achieving tolerance.

ROLE OF DONOR-SPECIFIC TRANSFUSION VERSUS STEM CELL THERAPY IN TOLERANCE INDUCTION

Importance of the blood transfusion effect gets diminished with the introduction of cyclosporine.[37-39] Suppression of alloimmune responses after blood transfusion could be partly attributed to induction of regulatory CD4$^+$ T cells, which appears to be dependent on recognition of an allopeptide shared between blood/organ donor and recipient in the context of self-human leukocyte antigen (HLA) class II.[40] Presentation in this manner induces hypo-responsiveness to other alloantigens presented on the same APC bearing the shared class II molecule, a phenomenon called linked suppression.[41] These and similar studies provide a better understanding of the mechanisms of beneficial effect, which should also help to prevent one of the most feared complications of this form of therapy, i.e., recipient sensitization.

ROLE OF MESENCHYMAL STEM CELLS AND REGULATORY T CELLS IN TRANSPLANT TOLERANCE

Mesenchymal stem cells (MSCs) have immunomodulatory, immunosuppressive, and tolerogenic effects, and also enhance the action of hematopoietic stem cells (HSCs). MSCs are a potential "homeostatic niche" for Tregs and play role in Treg recruitment, regulation, and maintenance in vitro.[42-44] Immunoregulatory functions of MSC are not fixed, but are rather consequences of the microenvironment they encounter in vivo.[45]

Tregs are a large group of Regulatory T cells (with various markers), known to use a variety of mechanisms to mediate cell-mediated suppression effects. In addition, Tregs can produce copious amounts of immune-suppressive cytokines, including tumor growth factor-beta (TGF-β), interleukin (IL)-10, and IL-35 known for inhibiting a wide spectrum of cellular activities **(Fig. 2)**. CD4$^+$CD25$^+$ Tregs at the time of transplantation were shown to be capable of suppressing rejection initiated by a 100-fold excess of donor-alloantigen-specific CD8$^+$ TCR-transgenic T cells demonstrating the potency of CD4$^+$CD25$^+$ T cells.[46,47] Treg pool contains a population of committed Tregs and a small fraction of uncommitted Tregs. Such uncommitted Tregs can lose their expression and become T-effector cells. Ex vivo expanded Tregs exhibit a signature similar to T-effector cells rather than Tregs.[48] This may be one of the key reasons for the instability of Tregs and, therefore, there is paucity of Tregs in vivo in transplant recipients, even under tolerizing conditions. Subclinical rejection of renal allografts refers to histological patterns of acute rejection despite stable renal function. For finding out whether the presence of Tregs could help determine the functional importance of tubulointerstitial infiltrates observed in protocol biopsies, cases of subclinical rejection were also evaluated. The presence of Treg discriminated harmless from injurious infiltrates, evidenced by independently predicting better graft function 2 and 3 years after transplantation.[49] Furthermore, the Treg/CD3$^+$ T-cell ratio positively correlated with graft function at 2 years post-transplantation, suggesting that an increasing proportion of Treg within the global T-cell infiltrate may facilitate renal engraftment; therefore, immunostaining for Treg in patients with subclinical rejection on protocol biopsies may ultimately be useful to identify patients who may require alterations in their immunosuppressive regimens. In vitro studies have shown that Tregs are capable of suppressing the proliferation of syngeneic alloactivated T cells.[50] Treatment of positively selected CD4$^+$CD25$^+$ cells enabled them to prevent acute graft-versus-host disease (GVHD).[51]

STRATEGIES AND PROTOCOLS OF TOLERANCE INDUCTION IN RENAL TRANSPLANTATION

Stanford University and the association between the Universities of Louisville and Northwestern Harvard University in the United States and Trivedi et al. in India have attempted tolerance induction in renal transplant recipients using stem cell (SC) transplantation **(Fig. 3)**.[52,53]

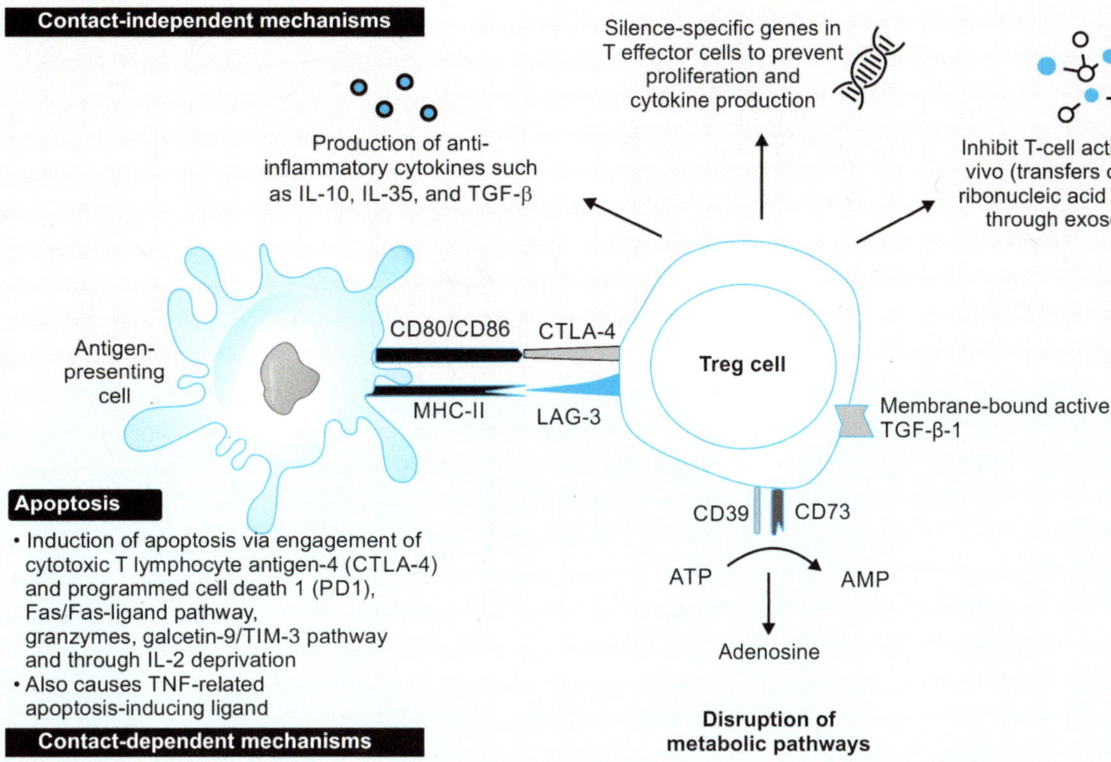

Fig. 2: Mechanisms of regulatory T cell (Treg) suppression. (AMP: adenosine monophosphate; ATP: adenosine triphosphate; IL: interleukin; MHC: major histocompatibility complex; TGF-β: tumor growth factor-beta; TNF: tumor necrosis factor)

- Stanford group attempted tolerance in 12 HLA-matched recipients who received donor $CD34^+$ selected cells [5–16 × 10^6/kg bodyweight (BW)] and $CD3^+$ T cells (1–10 ×10^6/kg BW), intravenously (IV) on day 11.[54] Conditioning regimen was total lymphoid irradiation (TLI) (10 doses, 80–120 cGy) to spleen, lymph nodes, thymus plus anti-T-cell antibodies [five doses of rabbit antithymocyte globulin (r-ATG)] during the first 10 days after kidney transplantation. Immunosuppression of mycophenolate mofetil (MMF) (2 g/day) × 1 month; cyclosporine discontinued 6–17 months after transplantation. Chimerism persisted for at least 6 months according to short-tandem-repeat analysis of deoxyribonucleic acid (DNA) from blood granulocytes and lymphocytes and there was no evidence of GVHD or rejection (clinical/biopsy).[55] They succeeded in 8 out of 12 patients and had a mean follow-up of 25 months. Recurrence of focal segmental glomerulosclerosis (FSGS) was observed in one patient. Subsequently, more patients were added. The last report states that 24/29 recipients have been taken off immunosuppression.[52]
- The association of the Northwestern group attempted it in eight patients.[56] Salient features in their protocol were HLA-mismatched kidneys and infusion of tolerogenic graft facilitating cells (FCs) with HSC. Conditioning was with fludarabine, total body irradiation (TBI; 200 cGy), and cyclophosphamide. Immunosuppression was with tacrolimus and MMF. The absolute neutrophil counts reached a nadir 1 week after transplant, with recovery by 2 weeks. Multilineage chimerism was observed at 1 month (6–100%). Conditioning was well tolerated. Transient chimerism was noted in two out of eight patients who were maintained on low-dose tacrolimus monotherapy. One patient had viral sepsis 2 months post-transplant. Five patients displayed durable chimerism, immunocompetence, and donor-specific tolerance by in vitro proliferative assays and were weaned off all immunosuppression 1 year after transplant. None of the recipients produced donor-specific antibodies (DSA)/GVHD. They concluded that their protocol was a safe, practical, and reproducible means of inducing durable chimerism and donor-specific tolerance in solid-organ transplant recipients.
- Trivedi et al. attempted tolerance induction in 69 recipients across HLA barriers.[57] Renal transplantation was performed from living donors after a TLI-based clonal deletion protocol with no post-transplant maintenance immunosuppression planned. If needed, immunosuppression was started on a patient-specific basis, adding one drug at a time, a strategy named "DAWN" (drugs added when needed). Following this strategy, at the last follow-up, 40 of the 69 patients (58%) had to be rescued by conventional immunosuppression, 23 (33%) had to be started on daily prednisone, and

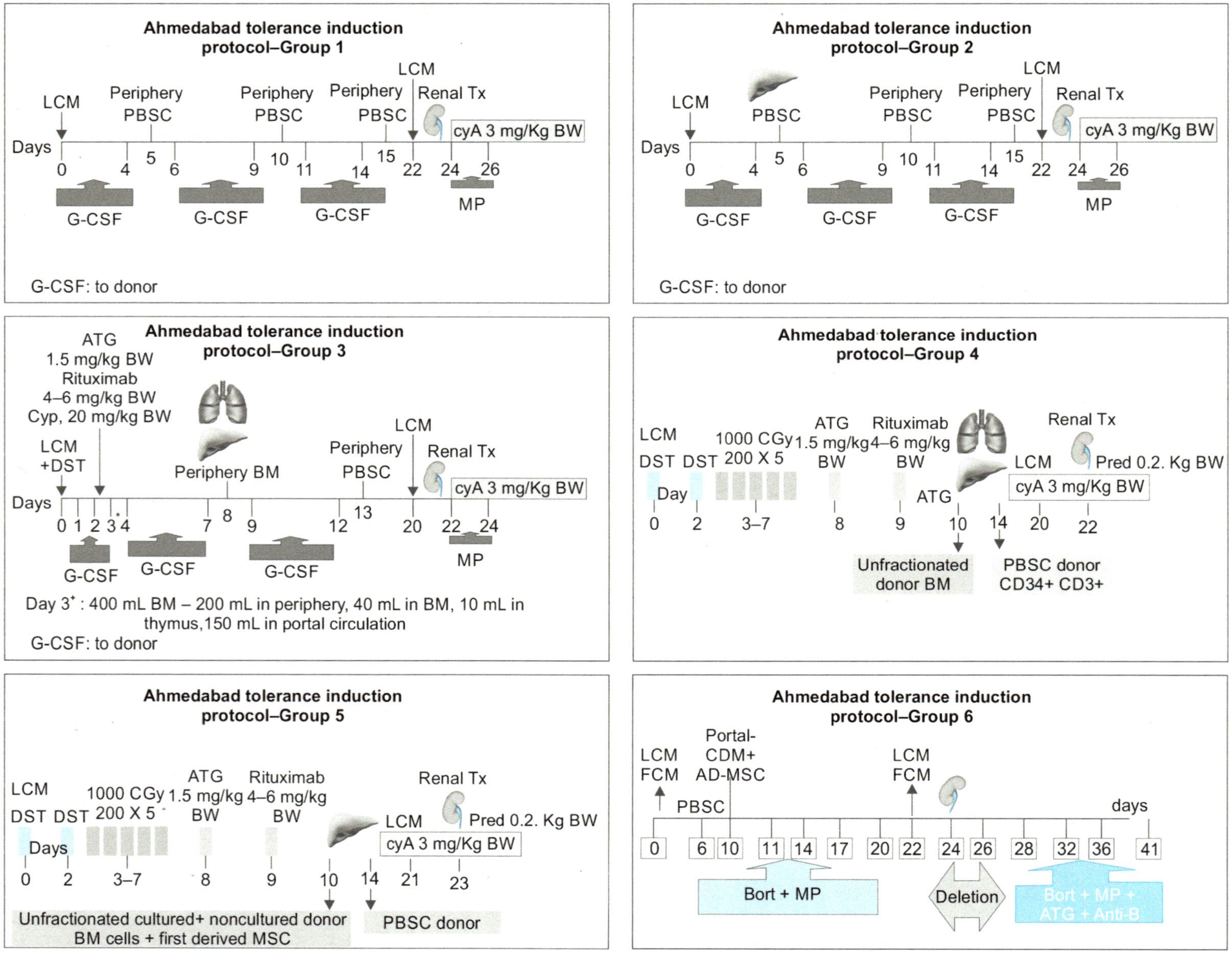

Fig. 3: The Ahmedabad tolerance induction protocol. (ADMSC: adipose tissue-derived mesenchymal stem cells (donor); ATG: antithymocyte globulin; Bort: bortezomib; CBM: cultured donor bone marrow; FCM: flow crossmatch; LCM: lymphocytotoxicity crossmatch; PBSC: donor-derived peripheral blood stem cell infusion cyclophosphamide + ATG)

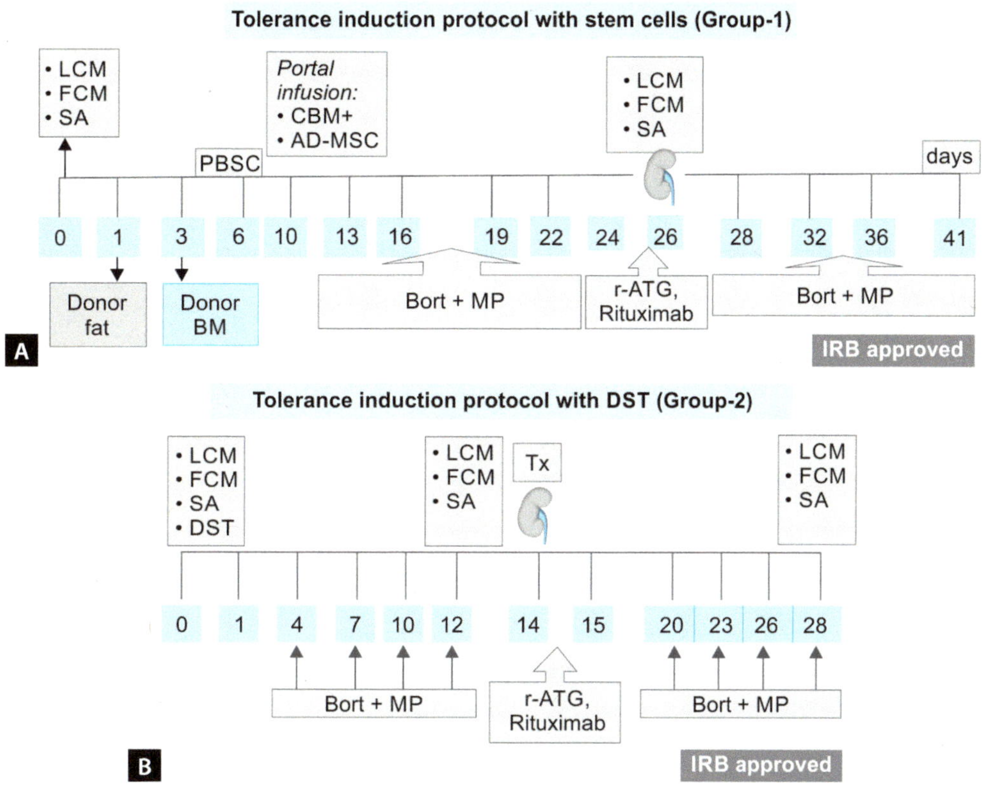

Figs. 4A and B: Follow-up of tolerance induction protocol using stem cell therapy (SCT)-representative cartoon. (ADMSC: adipose tissue-derived mesenchymal stem cells (donor); Bort: bortezomib; CBM: cultured donor bone marrow; DST: donor-specific transfusion; FCM: flow crossmatch; IRB: institutional review boards; LCM: lymphocytotoxicity crossmatch; MP: methylprednisone; PBSC: donor-derived peripheral blood stem cell infusion; r-ATG: rabbit antithymocyte globulin; SA: single antigen)

6 (9%) remained with no maintenance immunosuppression. The overall rate of de novo DSA produced was 36% (in 25/69 patients), at a mean time of about 4 months. Acute rejection episodes with humoral components were noted in 19 cases (27%), of which 14 were pure antibody-mediated rejection, 5 combined antibody- and T-cell-mediated rejection, and 6 episodes (9%) of pure T-cell-mediated rejection. Although complete clonal deletion was not achieved, 42% (29/69) were on prednisone alone/with no immunosuppression for a total mean follow-up of 13.3 months. The mean serum creatinine of 16 patients was 1.33 ± 0.2 mg/dL, over a mean follow-up of 19.3 months. It was concluded that clonal deletion can be used to transplant patients without maintenance immunosuppression, adding drugs only as needed.

- The only successful tolerance induction protocol (TIP) starting from zero conventional immunosuppression was performed by the Ahmedabad group at Institute of Kidney Diseases and Research Centre–Institute of Transplantation Sciences (IKDRC–ITS) **(Figs. 4A and B)**.[36] They undertook open-labeled two armed clinical trials comparing the role of donor-specific transfusion (DST) with SC infusion pretransplant to induce tolerance in living-related renal transplantation. Both the arms, the SC arm and DST arm, had 10 patients each, across HLA barriers. SC arm included infusion of adipose-derived MSC (ADMSC), BM-HSC, and peripheral blood stem cells (PBSC) in liver. DST arm included DST in the peripheral circulation of recipients. Conditioning was with bortezomib methylprednisone (125 mg IV), one cycle, pre- and post-transplant, and r-ATG at the end of transplantation surgery followed by rituximab on day 1 of transplantation. No conventional immunosuppression was given. Immune monitoring included DSA, T- and B-cell flow crossmatch and antihuman globulin (AHG) crossmatch pretransplantation. Post-transplant monitoring was with DSA weekly for the first 3 months and 3 monthly along with monitoring of Tregs (CD $127^{low/-}/CD4^{+}/25^{high}$) (representative **Figs. 5A and B**). There was 100% patient and graft survival 1-year posttransplant in the SC arm. One graft was lost to chronic graft dysfunction with the biopsy revealing unexplained interstitial fibrosis and tubular atrophy (IF/TA) and absence of DSA. Two patients were lost, one to pneumonia at 33 months post-transplant and one to sudden cardiac arrest at 38 months post-transplant. At 6 years post-transplant, out of seven patients, five were on no conventional immunosuppression and two on mycophenolate sodium

PT.5–GA, 29/F (father; 54/M) Tx: 2 August 2010 | 9 Aug 13 | POD: 1070

	A		B		Cw		DRB 1		DRB 345		DQ		Bw	
PT	11	24	27	37	6	15	10	15	–	51	5	6	4	6
DN	2	24	27	40	–	15	–	15	–	51	–	6	4	6

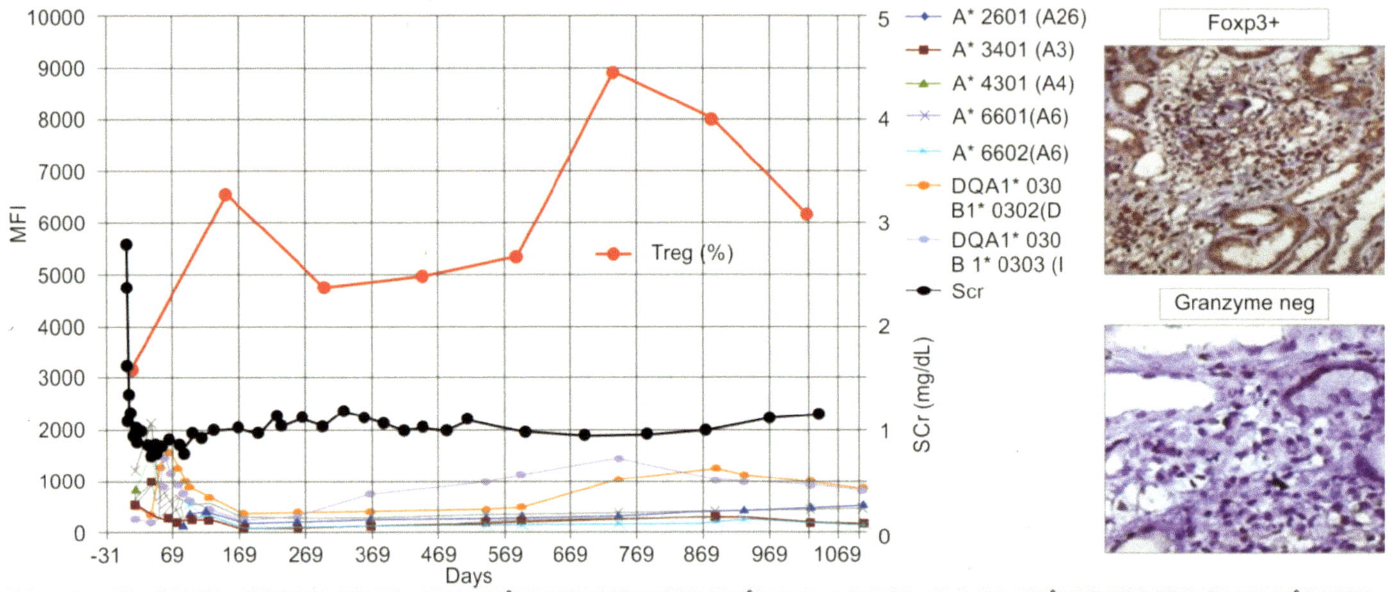

No. of cells infused: PBSC- 176 mL, 19.9 x 10^8/kg BW, CD34: 6.96 x 10^6/kgBW, CBM: 95 mL, 0.33 x 10^8/kg BW, CD34: 0.06 x 10^6/kg BW, ADMSC: 3 mL, 4.0 x 10^4, CD45-/90+: 2.3 x 10^4 CD73+: 0.93 x 10^4/kg BW

A Current SCr -1.4 mg/dL, IS- Prednisone 5 mg OD

Ms: 29/M (Father donor) Tx: 25 June,'10 | 20-June-13 | POD-1089

	A		B		Cw		DRBI		DRB345		DQ		BW	
PT	2	33	27	44	7	12	7	15	51	53	2	6	4	–
DN	11	33	40	44	7	12	7	15	51	53	2	6	4	6

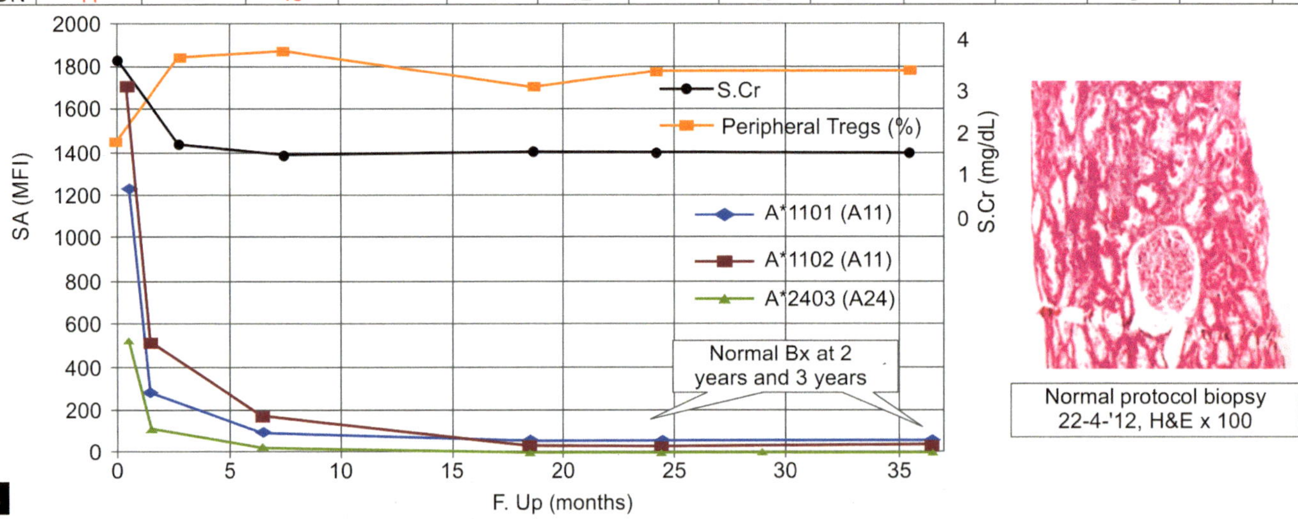

B

Figs. 5A and B: Tolerance induction protocols with (A) Stem cell therapy (SCT); and (B) Donor-specific transfusion (DST). (ADMSC: adipose-derived mesenchymal stem cells; BW: bodyweight; CBM: cultured donor bone marrow; Treg: regulatory T cell; PBSC: peripheral blood stem cells)

(360 mg BD) and prednisone (5 mg/day).[56] In the DST arm, one patient was lost to de novo FSGS and associated complications at 10 months post-transplant, two grafts were lost, one at 17 months to chronic graft dysfunction and the second at 40 months post-transplant to IF/TA. Both had developed DSA. Out of seven patients on follow-up at 6 years, four were on no conventional immunosuppression, two on mycophenolate sodium, and one on triple immunosuppression of tacrolimus, mycophenolate, and prednisone.

- The other reports are mentioned in **Table 1**.[58-66]

TABLE 1: Tolerance trials across the globe.

Center	Number of recipients	HLA-matched status (n/6)	Protocol	References
MGH, USA	10-b	Match	Full/mixed chimerism	58
	12-b	Mismatch	Transient mixed chimerism	59
Stanford, USA	29-c	Match	Mixed chimerism	60
	19-b	Mismatch	Mixed chimerism	60
CIRM, USA	22-d	Mismatch	DHSC and recipient Tregs (mixed chimerism)	Yet to start
Northwestern, USA	20-b	Match	Alemtuzumab and donor HSC infusion	61
	37-b	Mismatch	Durable chimerism, FCRx	62
	09-b + 120-d	Mismatch	Treg (TRACT therapeutics)	63
Johns Hopkins, USA	1	Mismatch	Full chimerism (FCRx)	
UCSF, USA	3-c	Mismatch	Tregs	64
The One Study (combined)	6	Mismatch	Donor-alloantigen-reactive Tregs (UCSF)	https://clinicaltrials.gov/ct2/show/NCT02244801?term=NCT02244801&rank=1
	11	Mismatch	Autologous tolerogenic dendritic cells	https://clinicaltrials.gov/ct2/show/NCT02252055?term=NCT02252055&rank=1
	08	Mismatch	Donor-derived regulatory macrophage	https://clinicaltrials.gov/ct2/show/NCT02085629?term=NCT02085629&rank=1
	15-c	Mismatch	Tregs (UK)	https://clinicaltrials.gov/ct2/show/NCT02129881?term=NCT02129881&rank=1
	09-c	Mismatch	Tregs (Germany)	https://clinicaltrials.gov/ct2/show/NCT02371434?term=NCT02371434&rank=1
	08-c	Mismatch	Tregs + belatacept (Boston)	https://clinicaltrials.gov/ct2/show/NCT02091232?term=NCT02091232&rank=1
IRCCS, Italy	04+	Mismatch	MSC	65
Talaris	120-d	Mismatch	Full chimerism (FCRx)—multicenter	Yet to be started
Sam Sang University, South Korea	09-c	Mismatch	Mixed chimerism	66
Trivedi–Terasaki	69-b	Across HLA barriers	TLI-based DAWN protocol with SCT	56
IKDRC–ITS, Ahmedabad, India	10-b	Mismatch	Combined MSC + HSC administration in thymus, liver + conditioning with bortezomib, r-ATG + rituximab	57
	10-b	Mismatch	DST + conditioning with bortezomib, r-ATG + rituximab	36

(b: completed; c: ongoing; CIRM: California Institute of Regenerative Medicine; d: to be initiated soon; DAWN: drugs added when needed; DHSC: donor hematopoietic stem cells; DST: donor-specific transfusion; FCRx: DHSC plus facilitating cells; HLA: human leukocyte antigen; HSC: hematopoietic stem cells; IKDRC–ITS: Institute of Kidney Diseases and Research Centre–Institute of Transplantation Sciences, Ahmedabad, India; IRCCS: Istituto di Ricovero eCura a Carattere Scientifico; MGH: Massachusetts General Hospital; MSC: mesenchymal stem cells; r-ATG: rabbit antithymocyte globulin; SCT: stem cell therapy; TLI: total lymphoid irradiation; Treg: regulatory T cell; TRACT: Treg adoptive cellular transfer; UCSF: University of California at San Francisco)

BIOMARKERS FOR MEASURING TOLERANCE

The absence of DSA in patients with established tolerance has been noted and their reappearance with rising in serum creatinine or subclinical rejections has been observed by Trivedi et al.[57] Thus, measurement of antibodies by the luminex platform can be one of the best-established biomarkers currently that has fulfilled the litmus test of proving the absence of antibodies in subjects with tolerance.

TABLE 2: Biomarkers in operational tolerance in kidney transplantation.

Parameter	*Technique of measurement*
NK cells	
Peripheral NK cells	Flow cytometry
T cells	
Peripheral T cells	Flow cytometry
T-cell alloreactivity	• IFN-γ ELISpot • Trans-vivo DTH assay
Whole blood gene expression	RT-PCR
B cells	
Peripheral B-cell phenotype	Flow cytometry
B-cell cytokine production	IC cytokine staining
PBMC/B-cell gene expression	RT-PCR
Whole blood gene expression	Microarray/RT-PCR
Urinary gene expression	RT-PCR
Serum HLA antibodies	Luminex

(DTH: delayed-type hypersensitivity; IC: intracellular; HLA: human leukocyte antigen; IFN: interferon; NK: natural killer; PBMC: peripheral blood mononuclear cell; RT-PCR: reverse transcription polymerase chain reaction)

Normal graft biopsy, although invasive can still be considered as the gold standard of tolerance, provided the graft function is normal with maintained immune status in absence of immunosuppression.

Mixed chimerism although being used as markers for tolerance, the studies have established that transient chimerism has been observed in patients with sustained tolerance. Hence, chimerism may not be considered as biomarker for testing tolerance.

Tregs ($CD4^+/25^{high}/127^{low}$) in peripheral blood can be established as both immunomodulators, helping in establishing tolerance as well as biomarkers for tolerance.[67-69]

Some examples of biomarkers in operational tolerance in kidney transplantation are provided in **Table 2.**[70]

ROLE OF B CELLS IN TOLERANCE[71]

Previously B cells were only considered to have pathogenic role in kidney transplantation, but now there are growing evidence showing that B cells also have important role in the induction and maintenance of transplant tolerance. Regulatory B cells (Bregs) are characterized by secretion of IL-10 and other cytokines such as TGF-β and IL-35. The two important subsets of Bregs are $CD5^+CD19^+CD1d^{hi}$ B10 and $CD19^+CD21^{hi}CD23^{hi}$ $CD24^{hi}$ transitional-2 (T2) Bregs. The main functions of Bregs are given below:

- Suppression of $CD8^+$ effector T-cell function
- T-cell apoptosis induction via binding the FAS and programmed cell death 1 (PD-1) receptors
- Induction of Tregs
- Suppression of antigen-presenting and cytokine secretion by dendritic cells and M1 macrophages
- Natural killer (NK) cells and neutrophils suppression

ACCOMMODATION

Accommodation is a state of acquired resistance of a grafted organ to immune-mediated damage.[72] It was first observed in ABO-incompatible kidney transplants, which survived and functioned normally in recipients with high titers of anti-blood group antibodies that were directed against the graft antigens.[73] The mechanism of development of tolerance is being understood a little better than that of accommodation. Accommodation differs from tolerance in that the immune system retains the capability to reject fresh tissue from the same donor, but accommodated donor tissue remains protected even if retransplanted into a new recipient.[74] Moreover, biopsies of normal functioning grafts revealed ABO antigens on their endothelial surfaces.[75] Hallmark of these biopsies is CD4 deposition on peritubular capillaries without rejection, unlike intolerance.

CONCLUSION

Tolerance induction is feasible, and TIP described above is safe. The important arms of sustained tolerance induction are clonal deletion and stem cell therapy (SCT), which may induce chimeric tolerance initially and link suppression with infectious tolerance subsequently. Moreover, financially tolerance induction is proving cost-effective. SCT under safe and effective nonmyeloablative conditioning does not lead to GVHD. If transplantation with zero immunosuppression is not feasible, the initial protocols of immunosuppression minimization can be practiced safely.

REFERENCES

1. Murray JE, Merrill JP, Harrison JH, Wilson RE, Dammin GJ. Prolonged survival of human kidney homografts by immunosuppressive drug therapy. New Engl J Med. 1963;268: 1315-23.
2. Chung-Wen CP, Hricik DE. What are immunosuppressive medications? How do they work? What are their side effects? In: McKay DB, Steinberg SM (Eds). Kidney Transplantation: A Guide to the Care of Kidney Transplant Recipients, 1st edition. Vol. XIV. Springer Publisher; 2011. p. 119.
3. Wiseman AC, Cooper JE. Optimizing immunosuppression. In: McKay DB, Steinberg SM (Eds). Kidney Transplantation: A Guide to the Care of Kidney Transplant Recipients, 1st edition. Vol. XIV. Springer Publisher; 2011. p. 137.
4. Starzl TE. Experience in Renal Transplantation. Philadelphia, London: W.B. Saunders; 1964.
5. Calne RY. Inhibition of the rejection of renal homografts in dogs by purine analogues. Transplant Bull. 1961;28:445-61.
6. Morozumi K, Takeda A, Uchida A, Mihatsch MJ. Cyclosporine nephrotoxicity: how does it affect renal allograft function and transplant morphology? Transplant Proc. 2004;36: 251S-6S.

7. Christians U, Reisdorph N, Klawitter J, Schmitz V. Biomarkers of immunosuppressive drug toxicity. Curr Opin Organ Transplant. 2005;10:284-94.
8. Salama AD, Womer KL, Sayegh MH. Clinical transplantation tolerance. Many rivers to cross. J Immunol. 2007;178:5419-23.
9. Trivedi HL, Vanikar AV, Gumber MR, Patel HV, Shah PR, Kute VB. Abrogation of antibodies improves outcome of renal transplantation. Transplant Proc. 2012;44:241-7.
10. Anderson D, Bilingham RE, Lampkin GH, Medawar PB. The use of skin grafting to distinguish between monozygotic and dizygotic twins in cattle. Heredity. 1951;5:379-97.
11. Calne RY. The rejection of renal homografts: inhibition in dogs by using 6-meracaptopurine. Lancet. 1960;1:417-8.
12. Zukoski CF, Lee HM, Hume DM. The prolongation of functional survival of canine renal homografts by 6-mercaptopurine. Surg Forum. 1960;11:470-2.
13. Roussey-Kesler G, Giral M, Moreau A, Subra JF, Legendre C, Noel C, et al. Clinical operational tolerance after kidney transplantation. Am J Transplant. 2006;6:736-46.
14. Owens ML, Maxwell JG, Goodnight J, Wolcott MW. Discontinuance of immunosuppression in renal transplant patients. Arch Surg. 1975;110:1450-1.
15. Zoller KM, Cho SI, Cohen JJ, Harrington JT. Cessation of immunosuppressive therapy after successful transplantation: a national survey. Kidney Int. 1980;18:110-4.
16. Starzl TE, Murase N, Demetris AJ, Trucco M, Abu-Elmagd K, Gray EA, et al. Lessons of organ-induced tolerance learned from historical clinical experience. Transplantation. 2004;77: 926-9.
17. Christensen LL, Grunnet N, Rudiger N, Moller B, Birkeland SA. Indications of immunological tolerance in kidney transplantation. Tissue Antigens. 1998;51:637-44.
18. Calne RY, Friend PJ, Moffatt S, Bradley A, Hale G, Firth J, et al. Propè tolerance, perioperative campath 1H, and low dose cyclosporine monotherapy in renal allograft recipients. Lancet. 1998;351:1701-2.
19. Devlin J, Doherty D, Thomson L, Wong T, Donaldson P, Portmann B, et al. Defining the outcome of immunosuppression withdrawal after liver transplantation. Hepatology. 1998;27:926-33.
20. Takatsuki M, Uemoto S, Inomata Y, Egawa H, Kiuchi T, Fujita S, et al. Weaning of immunosuppression in living donor liver transplant recipients. Transplantation. 2001;72:449-54.
21. Calne RY. Propè tolerance: the future of organ transplantation—from the laboratory to the clinic. Transplantation. 2004;77(6):930-2.
22. Gorer PA. The antigenic basis of tumor transplantation. J Pathol Bacteriol. 1938;47:231.
23. Gorer PA, Lyman S, Snell GD. Studies on the genetic and antigenic basis of tumor transplantation: linkage between a histocompatibility gene and "fused" in mice. Proc R Soc Lond. 1948;136:499-505.
24. Owen RD. Immunogenic consequences of vascular anastomosis between bovine twins. Science. 1945;102:400-1.
25. Billingham RE, Brent L, Medawar PB. Actively acquired tolerance to foreign cells. Nature. 1953;172:603-6.
26. Auchincloss H. In search of the elusive Holy Grail: the mechanisms and prospects for achieving clinical transplantation tolerance. Am J Transplant. 2001;1:6-12.
27. Pan TL, Goto S, Lin YC, Lord R, Chiang KC, Lai C, et al. The fas and fas ligand pathways in liver allograft tolerance. Clin Exp Immunol. 1999;118:180-7.
28. Desbarats J, Duke RC, Newell MK. Newly discovered role for Fas ligand in the cell-cycle arrest of CD4+ T cells. Nat Med. 1998;4:1377-82.
29. Desbarats J, Freed JH, Campbell PA, Newell MK. Fas (CD95) expression and death-mediating function are induced by CD4 cross-linking on CD4+ T cells. Proc Natl Acad Sci USA. 1996;93:11014-8.
30. Schwartz R, Damashek W. Drug induced immunologic tolerance. Nature. 1959;183:1682.
31. Kawai T, Cosimi B, Spitzer TR, Tolkoff-Rubin N, Suthanthiran M, Saidman SL, et al. HLA-mismatched renal transplantation without maintenance immunosuppression. N Engl J Med. 2008;358:353-61.
32. Kawai T, Sachs DH, Sprangers B, Spitzer TR, Saidman SL, Zorn E, et al. Long-term results in recipients of combined HLA-mismatched kidney and bone marrow transplantation without maintenance immunosuppression. Am J Transplant. 2014;14(7):1599-611.
33. Kirk AD, Mannon RB, Kleiner DE, Swanson JS, Kampen RL, Cendales LK, et al. Results from a human renal allograft tolerance trial evaluating T-cell depletion with alemtuzumab combined with deoxyspergualin. Transplantation. 2005; 80:1051-9.
34. Scandling JD, Busque S, Dejbakhsh-Jones S, Benike C, Sarwal M, Millan MT, et al. Tolerance and withdrawal of immunosuppressive drugs in patients given kidney and hematopoietic cell transplants. Am J Transplant. 2012;12: 1133-45.
35. Spitzer TR, Delmonico F, Tolkoff-Rubin N, McAfee S, Sackstein R, Saidman S, et al. Combined histocompatibility leukocyte antigen matched donor bone marrow and renal transplantation for multiple myeloma with end stage renal disease: the induction of allograft tolerance through mixed lymphohematopoietic chimerism. Transplantation. 1999;68:480-4.
36. Vanikar AV, Trivedi HL, Gopal SC, Kumar A. Tolerance in allogeneic living-related renal transplantation: Comparison of pre-transplantation donor specific leucocyte infusion versus stem cell transplantation. KGPH; 2015; Éditions universitaires européennes. (May 2, 2017).
37. Salvatierra Jr O, Vincenti F, Amend W, Potter D, Iwaki Y, Opelz G, et al. Deliberate donor-specific blood transfusions prior to living related renal transplantation. A new approach. Ann Surg. 1980;192(4):543-52.
38. Borel JF, Feurer C, Gubler HU, Stähelin H. Biological effects of cyclosporine A: a new antilymphocytic agent. Agents Actions. 1976;6:468-75.
39. Calne RY, White DJG. Cyclosporin A—a powerful immunosuppressant in dogs with renal allografts. IRCS Med Sci. 1977;5:595.
40. Trivedi HL, Vanikar AV, Modi PR, Shah VR, Vakil JM, Trivedi VB, et al. Allogeneic hematopoietic stem-cell transplantation, mixed chimerism, and tolerance in living related donor renal allograft recipients. Transplant Proc. 2005;37: 737-42.
41. Frasca L, Carmichael P, Lechler R, Lombardi G. Anergic T cells effect linked suppression. Eur J Immunol. 1997:27: 3191-7.

42. Aggarwal S, Pittenger MF. Human mesenchymal stem cells modulate allogeneic immune cell responses. Blood. 2005; 105:1815-22.
43. Bartholomew A, Sturgeon C, Siatskas M, Ferrer K, McIntosh K, Patil S, et al. Mesenchymal stem cells suppress lymphocyte proliferation in vitro and prolong skin graft survival in vivo. Exp Hematol. 2002;30:42-8.
44. Koc ON, Gerson SL, Cooper BW, Dyhouse SM, Haynesworth SE, Caplan AI, et al. Rapid hematopoietic recovery after coinfusion of autologous-blood stem cells and culture-expanded marrow mesenchymal stem cells in advanced breast cancer patients receiving high-dose chemotherapy. J Clin Oncol. 2000;18:307-16.
45. Casiraghi F, Perico N, Remuzzi G. Mesenchymal stromal cells to promote solid organ transplantation tolerance. Curr Opin Organ Transplant. 2013;18:51-8.
46. Maurik VA, Wood KJ, Jones N. Cutting edge: CD4+CD25+ alloantigen-specific immunoregulatory cells that can prevent CD8+ T-cell-mediated graft rejection implications for anti-CD154 immunotherapy. J Immunol. 2002;169: 5401-4.
47. Lin CY, Graca L, Cobbold SP, Waldmann H. Dominant transplantation tolerance impairs CD8+ T-cell function but not expansion. Nat Immunol. 2002;3:1208-13.
48. Lal G, Bromberg JS. Epigenetic mechanisms of regulation of Foxp3 expression. Blood. 2009;114:3727-35.
49. Oriol B, Josep MC, Inés R, Torras J, Goma M, Seron D, et al. Presence of FoxP3+ regulatory T cells predicts outcome of subclinical rejection of renal allografts. J Am Soc Nephrol. 2008;19:2020-6.
50. Zheng SG, Wang JH, Koss MN, Quismorio Jr F, Gray JD, Horwitz DA. CD4+ and CD8+ regulatory T cells generated ex vivo with IL-2 and TGF-beta suppress a stimulatory graft-versus-host disease with a lupus like syndrome. J Immunol. 2004;172:1531-9.
51. Taylor PA, Lees CJ, Blaza BR. The infusion of ex vivo activated and expanded CD4+CD25+ immune regulatory cells inhibit graft-versus-host disease lethality. Blood. 2002;99:3493-9.
52. Leventhal JR, Mathew JM. Outstanding questions in transplantation: tolerance. Am J Transplant. 2019;20:348-54.
53. Schnitzler MA, Skeans MA, Axelrod DA, Lentine KL, Randall HB, Snyder JJ, et al. OPTN/SRTR 2016 annual data report: economics. Am J Transplant. 2018;18(Suppl 1): 464-503.
54. Scandling JD, Busque S, Shizuru JA, Engleman EG, Strober S. Induced immune tolerance for kidney transplantation. N Engl J Med. 2011;365(14):1359-60.
55. Leventhal J, Abecassis M, Miller J, Gallon L, Ravindra K, Tollerud DJ, et al. Chimerism and tolerance without GVHD or engraftment syndrome in HLA-mismatched combined kidney and hematopoietic stem cell transplantation. Sci Transl Med. 2012;4(124):124-8.
56. Vanikar AV, Trivedi HL, Thakkar UG. Six years' experience of tolerance induction in renal transplantation using stem cell therapy. Clin Immunol. 2018;187:10-4.
57. Trivedi HL, Kaneku H, Terasaki PI, Feroz A, Vanikar AV, Trivedi VB, et al. Clonal deletion using total lymphoid irradiation with no maintenance immunosuppression in renal allograft recipients. Clin Transpl; 2009. pp. 265-80.
58. Spitzer TR, Sykes M, Tolkoff-Rubin N, Kawai T, McAfee SL, Dey BR, et al. Long-term follow-up of recipients of combined human leukocyte antigen-matched bone marrow and kidney transplantation for multiple myeloma with end-stage renal disease. Transplantation. 2011;91(6):672-6.
59. Sasaki H, Oura T, Spitzer TR, Chen YB, Madsen JC, Allan J, et al. Preclinical and clinical studies for transplant tolerance via the mixed chimerism approach. Hum Immunol. 2018; 79(5):258-65.
60. Scandling JD, Busque S, Lowsky R, Shizuru J, Shori A, Engleman E, et al. Macrochimerism and clinical transplant tolerance. Hum Immunol. 2018;79(5):266-71.
61. Leventhal JR, Mathew JM, Salomon DR, Kurian SM, Friedewald JJ, Gallon L, et al. Nonchimeric HLA identical renal transplant tolerance: regulatory immunophenotypic/genomic biomarkers. Am J Transplant. 2016;16(1):221-34.
62. Leventhal JR, Ildstad ST. Tolerance induction in HLA disparate living donor kidney transplantation by facilitating cell-enriched donor stem cell Infusion: the importance of durable chimerism. Hum Immunol. 2018; 79(5):272-6.
63. Mathew JM, Voss JH, LeFever A, Konieczna I, Stratton C, He J, et al. A phase I clinical trial with ex vivo expanded recipient regulatory T cells in living donor kidney transplants. Sci Rep. 2018;8(1):7428.
64. Chandran S, Tang Q, Sarwal M, Laszik ZG, Putnam AL, Lee K, et al. Polyclonal regulatory T cell therapy for control of inflammation in kidney transplants. Am J Transplant. 2017; 17(11):2945-54.
65. Casiraghi F, Perico N, Remuzzi G. Mesenchymal stromal cells for tolerance induction in organ transplantation. Hum Immunol. 2018;79(5):304-13.
66. Lee K, Park J, Chung Y, Kim S. Tolerance induction with hematopoietic stem cells in kidney transplantations. Am J Transplant. 2019;19(Suppl 3):349-50.
67. Mathew JM, Leventhal JR. Clinical transplant tolerance: coming of age. Hum Immunol. 2018;79(5):255-7.
68. Vanikar AV, Trivedi HL. T-regulatory cells: the recently recognized players of immunomodulation. J Stem Cell Res Ther. 2014;4(10):1-6.
69. Trivedi HL, Vanikar AV, Patel HV, et al. Regulatory T-cells support stem cell therapy in safe minimization of immunosuppression in living donor renal transplantation. J Stem Cell Res Ther. 2014;4(10):1-8.
70. Heidt S, Wood KJ. Biomarkers of operational tolerance in solid organ transplantation. Expert Opin Med Diagn. 2012;6(4):281-93.
71. Schmitz R, Fitch ZW, Schroder PM, Choi AY, Jackson AM, Knechtle SJ, et al. B cells in transplant tolerance and rejection: friends or foes? Transpl Int. 2020;33(1):30-40.
72. Lynch RJ, Platt JL. Accommodation in renal transplantation: unanswered questions. Curr Opin Organ Transplant. 2010; 15:481-5.
73. Chopek MW, Simmons RL, Platt JL. ABO-incompatible renal transplantation: initial immunopathologic evaluation. Transplant Proc. 1987;19:4553-7.
74. Rother RP, Arp J, Jiang J, Ge W, Faas SJ, Liu W, et al. C5 blockade with conventional immunosuppression induces long-term graft survival in presensitized recipients. Am J Transplant. 2008;8:1129-42.
75. Bannett AD, McAlack RF, Morris M, Chopek M, Platt JL. ABO incompatible renal transplantation: a qualitative analysis of native endothelial tissue ABO antigens after transplant. Transplant Proc. 1989;21:783-5.

CHAPTER 2

Evaluation of Living Kidney Donors

Ajit S Narula, Mastakim A Mazumder

CASE VIGNETTE 1

A 45-year-old male kidney donor on urinalysis was found to have three to five red blood cells per high-power field (RBC/HPF) on more than two occasions. There was no albuminuria and the estimated glomerular filtration rate (eGFR) was normal. Urological assessment and a kidney biopsy were done. Would he make a suitable kidney donor?

Microscopic hematuria is typically defined as presence of more than two to five RBC/HPF of urinary sediment on two to three separate occasions unrelated to exercise, trauma, sexual activity, or menstruation. To assess the suitability of such kidney donors, it is recommended to do a urine culture to assess for infection. Cystoscopy and imaging should be done to look for nephrolithiasis or urinary tract malignancy. A 24-hour urine stone panel to assess for high-risk stone formers, and a kidney biopsy to look for glomerular diseases. Donors with microscopic hematuria which resolves after treatment of urinary infection or those with thin basement membrane disease on a kidney biopsy may be accepted as kidney donors.

CASE VIGNETTE 2

A 27-year-old woman wishes to donate a kidney to her brother. In an earlier pregnancy, she has history of preeclampsia. Her blood pressure now is 120/70 mm Hg, eGFR 100 mL/1.73 m^2 body surface area (BSA), and albuminuria is undetected. In the future, she plans to have a second child. Can she be accepted as a kidney donor?

In women donors in the reproductive age groups, prior hypertensive disorders of pregnancy or the desire for future pregnancies should be enquired. Women with a prior hypertensive disorder of pregnancy may be acceptable for donation if their otherwise long-term postdonation risks are acceptable. Early small studies did not identify any increased risk of pregnancy complications in women after donation. However, in subsequent larger series, an increased risk of gestational hypertension and preeclampsia has been reported after kidney donation. To reduce the risk of complications in postdonation pregnancies, several dietary and lifestyle interventions including interventions to reduce or prevent obesity have the potential to reduce the risk of preeclampsia.

INTRODUCTION

Recent publications have described the long-term medical risks of kidney donors. In order to properly select donors who are at minimal risk of developing future kidney disease or other medical complications, numeric thresholds of various risk parameters have been suggested. The risks due to a specific abnormal parameter should be assessed in the context of other potential risk factors and not in isolation. In this chapter, we review the evaluation of the living kidney donors and various risk factors[1] for a living kidney donation **(Table 1)**. The contraindications to living kidney donation[2,3] are given in **Box 1**, and the usual kidney-specific, history, examination, and laboratory investigations are given in **Table 2**.

TABLE 1: Risk factors for living kidney donation.

Diabetes mellitus	HbA1c ≥6.5%, fasting plasma glucose ≥126 mg/dL, random plasma glucose of ≥200 mg/dL, plasma glucose concentration ≥200 mg/dL 2 hours after a 75-g anhydrous glucose load in an oral glucose tolerance test
Prediabetes	Fasting plasma glucose of 110–125 mg/dL and 1-hour post 75-g anhydrous glucose load, a plasma glucose of 140–199 mg/dL
Hypertension	BP ≥140/90 mm Hg on at least two occasions or mean ABPM or home measurements of SBP of 135 mm Hg or greater or DBP of 85 mm Hg or greater or history of hypertensive medications
Persistent hematuria	>2–5 red blood cells per high-power field of urinary sediment on 2–3 separate occasions
Pyuria	Presence of 10 or more white cells/mm^3 in an unspun urine specimen or three or more white cells per high-power field of unspun urine
BMI	A measure of weight scaled for height, as: • Underweight (<18.5 kg/m^2) • Normal weight (18.5–24.9 kg/m^2) • Overweight (25–29 kg/m^2) • Obese (30–34.9 kg/m^2); morbidly obese (>35 kg/m^2)

(ABPM: ambulatory blood pressure monitoring; BMI: body mass index; BP: blood pressure; DBP: diastolic blood pressure; HbA1c: hemoglobin A1c; SBP: systolic blood pressure)

BOX 1: Contraindications for living kidney donation.

- Age <18 years
- Uncontrolled hypertension or hypertension with end-organ damage
- BMI ≥35 kg/m^2 (Relative)
- Active malignancy,* active infection
- High-risk kidney stone formers
- Untreated psychiatric conditions
- Albuminuria >100 mg/g creatinine, glomerular pathology†
- GFR less than accepted threshold
- Bilateral renal artery atherosclerosis or fibromuscular dysplasia involving the orifices of both renal arteries
- Donor coercion, unable to give consent

*Cancers with low risk of transmission may be considered.
†Thin basement membrane nephropathy is acceptable.
(BMI: body mass index; GFR: glomerular filtration rate)

TABLE 2: Evaluation of living kidney donors.

History	• Hypertension, diabetes, kidney stones • Proteinuria, hematuria • Recurrent urinary tract infections • Cancers • Family history of kidney diseases
Examination	• Blood pressure-two readings and if high normal or if >140/90 mm Hg, then AMBP monitoring • BMI • Psychosocial evaluation by a psychiatrist
Laboratory investigations	• eGFR, confirmed by mGFR or 24-hour creatinine clearance • Spot albumin/creatinine ratio, confirmed with AER • Urinalysis and culture • Fasting glucose, HbA1c and/or oral GTT if high risk • Serological/molecular tests for hepatitis B and C, HIV, CMV • EB virus, COVID-19 • 24-hour urine calcium, oxalate, uric acid, citrate, creatinine, sodium in those with present/history of kidney stones • Pregnancy test (if indicated) • Complete blood count and coagulation profile, electrolytes, and liver function tests • Cancer screening as for general population • Echocardiography, stress test if indicated
Radiology investigations	• Confirm Kidney size, asymmetry, masses/cysts/ stones, hydronephrosis • Isotope kidney scans • Anatomy of renal arteries and veins • Patency of iliofemoral vessels
Compatibility tests	• ABO blood grouping • HLA testing and crossmatch for anti-HLA antibodies

(AER: albumin excretion rate; BMI: body mass index; CMV: cytomegalovirus; EB: Epstein–Barr; eGFR: estimated glomerular filtration rate; GTT: glucose tolerance test; HbA1c: hemoglobin A1c; HIV: human immunodeficiency virus; HLA: human leukocyte antigen; mGFR: measured glomerular filtration rate)

INFORMED CONSENT

A psychiatric evaluation is recommended to confirm that the donor has the mental capacity to provide informed consent for evaluation and organ donation. The components of informed consent include information on the process of evaluation, the short- and long-term risks of organ donation, and the freedom to withdraw consent at any stage of the evaluation.[4]

AGE

The lower age limit of 18 years for living kidney donation is the age accepted for giving a legally valid consent. No upper age limit has been defined. Many centers are accepting donors over the age of 60 years and even 70 years on a case-by-case basis. Rather than the chronological age, donor glomerular filtration rate (GFR) and other coexisting medical conditions are important determinants for accepting kidney donors. Young potential donors with borderline risk factors are at relatively higher risk for developing medical complications or end-stage kidney disease (ESKD) in the long term, when compared to older donors with the same abnormality. For example, unlike in young donors, older donors with impaired glucose tolerance may not have enough years in their life to progress to diabetes or ESKD. Studies looking at perioperative outcomes such as operative time, blood loss, and hospital length of stay have reported similar outcomes in selected elderly donors when compared to younger donors.[5-8]

GLOMERULAR FILTRATION RATE

Glomerular filtration rate can be calculated by using estimating equations (eGFR), creatinine clearances (CrCl), or measured by exogenous filtration markers such as iohexol/chromium 51-labeled ethylenediaminetetraacetic isotopes (^{51}CrEDTA).[9] Measured GFR (mGFR) most closely reflects the true GFR. 24-hour urine creatinine clearance as a measure of GFR tends to overestimate it by 10–20%.[2] eGFR using creatinine, cystatin, or both is not an accurate measure of GFR but is often used as the first step in estimating GFR because of the ease of use, followed by confirmatory test using CrCl or mGFR. To reduce interpatient variability and facilitate donor selection, GFRs are expressed standardized to BSA of 1.73 m^2.[9] The differential kidney function is determined by technetium-99m dimercaptosuccinic acid (^{99m}TcDMSA) scanning.[10] The evaluation of GFR in living kidney donors is given in **Table 3**.[9] In cases where there is an asymmetry in GFR, parenchymal abnormalities, vascular abnormalities, or urological abnormalities, which do not preclude donation, the more severely affected kidney should be used for transplantation.[10]

TABLE 3: Guideline recommendations for glomerular filtration rate (GFR) assessment in living kidney donor candidates.

Guideline	*GFR*	*GFR-based criteria*
British Transplantation Society (2018)[10]	mGFR in everyone after initial screening using eGFR	Provides age- and sex-specific GFR criteria
KDIGO (2017)[1]	eGFR, followed by confirmation with mGFR, CrCl	Donor candidates with GFR ≥90 mL/min/1.73 m^2 should be considered acceptable, and those with GFR ≤60 mL/min/1.73 m^2 should be excluded. Decision to approve donor candidates with GFR 60–89 mL/min/1.73 m^2 should be individualized on the basis of demographic and health profile in relation to the transplant program's acceptable risk threshold
OPTN (2021)[48]	mGFR or 24-hour CrCl	No specific recommendations provided
Canadian KPD Protocol (2015)[49]	GFR on two separate occasions, followed by 24-hour CrCl on two separate occasions or mGFR	Provides age-specific criteria
ERBP (2013)[11]	eGFR; mGFR when more exact knowledge of GFR is needed or where there is doubt regarding the accuracy of eGFR	Recommends age-dependent GFR cut-offs such that the GFR of the remaining kidney will be 37.5 mL/min/1.73 m^2 at the time the donor reaches the age of 80 years
CARI (2010)[50]	eGFR, at least on two separate occasions or CrCl; mGFR if there is doubt regarding the accuracy or eGFR or CrCl	Recommends against accepting kidneys from donors with GFR <80 mL/min/1.73 m^2
Amsterdam forum (2005)[51]	eGFR or CrCl; mGFR may be used in patients with borderline GFR determination	• GFR <80 mL/min/1.73 m^2 or body surface area-adjusted GFR, 2 SD below normal on the basis of age and sex generally preclude donation • Additionally noted successful transplantation from some, usually elderly living donors with GFR as low as 65–70 mL/min/1.73 m^2 indicating a need for individualization in donors with GFR <80 mL/min/1.73 m^2

(CrCl: creatinine clearance; eGFR: estimated glomerular filtration rate; mGFR: measured glomerular filtration rate; SD: standard deviation)
Source: With permission from Garg N, Poggio ED, Mandelbrot D. Evaluation of kidney function in living kidney donor candidates. Kidney360. 2021;2:1523-30.

URINARY ABNORMALITIES: ALBUMINURIA/ MICROSCOPIC HEMATURIA/PYURIA

Albuminuria is a sign of an underlying kidney disease. The initial screening is performed using a spot urine albumin-to-creatinine ratio and confirmed by either using albumin excretion rate (AER) expressed as mg/day or albumin creatinine ratio (ACR) expressed as mg/g in a timed urine specimen. The acceptable threshold of AER for kidney donation is <30 mg/day or ACR of 30 mg/g of creatinine. AER >100 mg/day or ACR >100 mg/g is a contraindication to donation. Orthostatic albuminuria and transient exercise-induced albuminuria are benign conditions and do not preclude a donation.[1,3] For albuminuria in the range of 30–100 mg/day, the decision to accept a donor is based on age, GFR, and other risk factors.[1,11]

Persistent hematuria indicates a kidney or a urological disease. A urine culture, urine cytology, and renal imaging are done routinely. Cystoscopy is indicated in patients aged 35 years or older to exclude urinary tract malignancy.[12] Donors with uroepithelial malignancy are unfit for donation. In the absence of an identified cause, for the urinary abnormality, a kidney biopsy is advised. Donors with thin basement membrane nephropathy may be accepted as kidney donors.[13]

Donors with pyuria due to urinary tract infection, which has been treated, are acceptable while those with sterile pyuria need further investigations.[14]

DIABETES MELLITUS/PREDIABETES

Donors with diabetes mellitus are commonly excluded from living donation. In prediabetes, there is a risk of progression to diabetes and there are conflicting recommendations for accepting prediabetics as kidney donors. This is due to low-quality evidence examining new-onset proteinuria, hypertension, rate of decline of GFR, and end-stage renal disease (ESRD) between donors with and without prediabetes.[1] The risk of developing diabetes and subsequent renal impairment in a young potential kidney donor with prediabetes may not be acceptable, but elderly prediabetic donors who may not develop diabetes during their lifetime may be accepted as kidney donors.[10]

OBESITY

Obesity is considered a relative contraindication to living kidney donation because of the increased risk of surgical complications and the adverse impact of obesity on renal function in the longer term. Multiple guidelines recommend body mass index (BMI) >35 kg/m^2 as an absolute or relative contraindication to donation. In donors with BMI >30 kg/m^2, a careful evaluation of other comorbidities is recommended.[1,15,16]

HYPERTENSION

Hypertension contributes to causation of chronic kidney disease (CKD). GFR reduction from kidney donation may accelerate the risk or progression of hypertension over time to a greater extent than expected from normal aging. Ambulatory blood pressure monitoring or home monitoring is recommended to exclude white coat or masked hypertension. If blood pressure is not controlled to <140/90 mm Hg on one or two antihypertensive drugs or there is evidence of end-organ damage (retinopathy, left ventricular hypertrophy, proteinuria, and previous cardiovascular disease) or there is an unacceptable risk of lifetime incidence of ESRD, then donors are excluded from donation.[10,17-20]

KIDNEY STONES

Kidney stones are a common cause of CKD. However, a current small single stone <1.5 cm may be acceptable in a donor. A kidney donation is not accepted in the presence of an uncorrectable metabolic cause for kidney stones (cystinosis or hyperoxaluria), in presence of struvite stones, bilateral kidney stones, multiple stones, nephrocalcinosis, and from those who have a high risk of recurrence of kidney stones (age <40 years, recurrent kidney stones in past and a family history of kidney stones).[21] In accepted donors, it is preferable to remove the kidney containing the stone. If the stone is very small, it may be left in situ or may be removed, ex vivo, by uretero-nephroscopy before implanting the donor's kidney.[22]

HEREDITARY RENAL DISEASES

The possibility of inherited kidney disease or a genetic predisposition should be suspected in every kidney donor with a positive family history of kidney disease. However, a negative family history does not exclude a hereditary renal disease.[13] With the exception of autosomal dominant polycystic kidney disease (ADPKD), most familial renal diseases are rare in a transplant program.

Donors with ADPKD should not donate, but donors with a family history of ADPKD in a first-degree relative may be acceptable for donation if they meet age-specific imaging or genetic testing criteria that reliably exclude ADPKD. Age-dependent ultrasound criteria for diagnosis and disease exclusion have been established for at-risk adults with unknown ADPKD gene type. In the absence of any cyst or with one cyst, ultrasound has a negative predictive value (NPV) of 100% in patients aged older than 40 years, but only 96% for younger kidney donors.[23,24] Using a total of >10 cysts as a test criterion in subjects younger than 30 years of age, an MRI provides a sensitivity and specificity of 100% in excluding ADPKD.[25] Gene testing can also sometimes help to diagnose or exclude ADPKD.[26]

ALPORT SYNDROME

Alport syndrome in majority is inherited as an X-linked trait. Most heterozygote Alport women will have microscopic hematuria and are at low risk to progress to kidney failure, though ESKD has been reported. In males, urinary abnormalities appear in childhood with progression to kidney failure in adulthood. The outcome after kidney donation is uncertain in Alport women, and it is recommended to use alternative kidney donors. In a small series of women Alport donors, new-onset hypertension, proteinuria, and reduced renal function during a follow-up period of 2–14 years were reported. An X-linked heterozygous Alport mother over 45 years of age who has no clinical manifestation of the disease may be considered a kidney donor as a rare event.[27,28]

APOLIPOPROTEIN L1 RISK ALLELES

Individuals of African ancestry carrying both the risk alleles of the apolipoprotein L1 (*APOL1*) gene are associated with focal segmental glomerulosclerosis, HIV-associated nephropathy, CKD, and adverse donor and recipient outcomes after living kidney donation. However, the precise risk for kidney failure in an affected individual after kidney donation is unknown. Given the potential impact of *APOL1* variants on the safety of living kidney donation, the American Society Transplant Expert Group opined that all African-American living donors should be informed about the associations of *APOL1* risk alleles.[29-31]

MALIGNANCY

In donors with history of treated cancers, there is a risk of recurrence of cancers and transmission of latent cancers. The Ad Hoc Disease Transmission Advisory Committee (DTAC) of the Organ Procurement and Transplantation Network/ United Network for Organ Sharing (OPTN/UNOS) has categorized six levels of risk for donor cancer transmission to the recipient.[32] Donors with active or treated cancers with less than minimal (0–0.1%) lifetime risks of recurrence or transmission (basal cell carcinoma skin, squamous cell carcinoma skin, resected renal cell carcinoma <1 cm, in situ cervical carcinoma, vocal cord carcinoma, solitary papillary thyroid carcinoma ≤0.5 cm, minimally invasive follicular carcinoma thyroid ≤1.0 cm) may be accepted for donation.[1]

RENAL CYSTS

A common finding in donors of increasing age is kidney cysts. A small simple single (Bosniak I) cyst is acceptable for kidney donation. Donation of a kidney with a Bosniak II renal cyst should proceed only after assessment to exclude a cystic renal cell carcinoma. A kidney with high-grade Bosniak renal cysts (III or higher) or small (T1a) renal cell carcinoma which can be resected prior to implantation may be acceptable on a case-by-case basis.[33]

INFECTIONS

Screening for latent infections in the donor minimizes the risk of transmitting infections to the recipient. Kidney donors are usually screened for tuberculosis, hepatitis B virus (HBV), hepatitis C virus (HCV), human immunodeficiency virus (HIV), cytomegalovirus (CMV), Epstein–Barr virus (EBV), and lately for COVID-19 infections.

In endemic areas, there are no reliable methods to diagnose latent tuberculous infection. The tuberculin skin test and interferon gamma release assay are of limited use.[34] Screening for latent tuberculosis is limited to a medical history and X-ray/computed tomography (CT) scan of chest.

According to the regional epidemiology and individual-based history, donor candidates should undergo testing for strongyloidiasis, *Trypanosoma cruzi*, West Nile virus, histoplasmosis, and/or coccidioidomycosis. To screen donor candidates for emerging infections, transplant program centers should develop their own protocols.

Screening of HIV, HBV, and HCV should ideally be performed within 28 days of donation.

In all donor candidates, testing for immunoglobulin G (IgG) hepatitis B core antibody (anti-HBcAb) and hepatitis B surface antigen (HBsAg) should be done. HBV deoxyribonucleic acid (DNA) nucleic acid testing (NAT) can be performed in donor candidates from HBV endemic areas with anti-HBcAb+, suspected to have possible mutant HBV infections, with abnormal liver function tests or have a past history of liver disease of unknown etiology. Transplantation of kidneys from HBsAg+ donors with active viral replication is contraindicated[35] and so also transplanting kidneys from HBsAg+ donors into nonvaccinated HBV-naive recipients.[1,10,36] The proposed management for several types of donor and recipient pairs according to the results of HBV serology tests is shown in **Flowchart 1**. The presence of HBV-DNA positivity increases the risk of transmission in immunized recipients.[35] (Read Chapter 12.2.4 for details.)

Hepatitis C virus testing involves testing for anti-HCV antibody and HCV-RNA.[37] With the advent of new direct-acting antiviral drugs, donation from anti-HCV+ donors is no longer considered a contraindication irrespective of the recipient HCV status. (Read Chapter 12.2.3 for details.)

All donor candidates (living or deceased) should be screened for HIV by testing antibodies to HIV [i.e., anti-HIV 1/2 Ab or HIV antigen/antibody (Ag/Ab) combination assay]. (Read Chapter 12.2.5 for details.)

The other common latent/past infections screened in the donor–recipient pair are CMV and EBV infections.[38] (Read Chapters 12.2.1 and 12.2.6 for details.)

PREGNANCY RISKS

Women should not be excluded from donation solely because they desire to conceive children after donation. They need to be counseled about the risk of gestational hypertension or preeclampsia and on how to reduce the risk of complications in future pregnancies by maintaining a healthy prepregnancy weight.[39]

LIVING MARGINAL DONORS

To meet the shortage of organs the selection criteria for living donors have been widened to include the use of marginal donors (MDs) who would have otherwise been unsuitable to donate. While a clear definition of living marginal donors

Flowchart 1: Proposed management of HBV donor and recipient pairs.

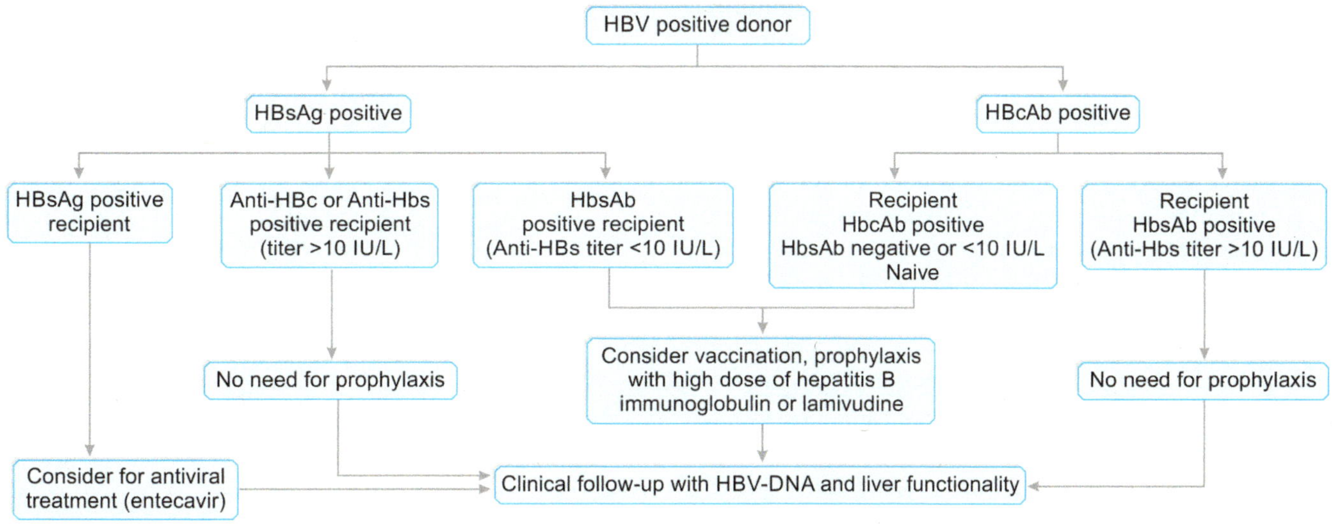

(DNA: deoxyribonucleic acid; HBcAb: hepatitis B core antibody; HBsAb: hepatitis B antibody; HBsAg: hepatitis B surface antigen; HBV: hepatitis B virus)

Source: With permission from Massimiliano V, Vincenzo A, Daniela C, Giaquinta A, Ekser B, Sinagra N, et al. Kidney transplantation from donors with hepatitis B. Med Sci Monit. 2016;22:1427-4.

also known as Expanded Criteria Living Donors (ECLDs)[40] is lacking, donors are generally of older age, have diabetes, hypertension, microalbuminuria, nephrolithiasis, border line eGFRs, and kidney cysts. The functioning grafts from marginal donors appears comparable to that of grafts from standard deceased donors, but inferior to that of standard living donors. The concerns regarding the use of these organs are related more to the potential harm to the donor rather than the quality of the graft.[41,42]

There is limited data on living kidney donors older than 70 years, but it is shown that donor nephrectomy is safe and postdonation survival and recovery is similar to that of younger donors. In accepting marginal donors rather than actual age itself, the presence of other comorbidities determines whether an older living kidney donor should be accepted. Impaired kidney function may be considered more acceptable for older donors than for younger ones because of shorter life expectancy. Rather than a single comorbidity like hypertension or high normal albuminuria, the combination of both increases the postdonation risk of impaired kidney function.[40]

Decisions on how to approach potential marginal donors are complicated by the lack of postdonation long-term follow-up studies hence the choice to accept a marginal donor often becomes subjective.

OUTCOMES IN THE LIVING KIDNEY DONOR

In living kidney donation, there are risks related to the surgery and long-term health risk related to the development of hypertension, proteinuria, and preeclampsia in women donors.

An annual check of blood pressure, albuminuria, serum creatinine with eGFR estimates, and BMI measurements is recommended.[1]

The reduction in renal mass increases the risk of kidney failure in donors when compared to the nondonor population with similar demographic and risk factors. This risk is nonlinear with younger donors at a higher lifetime risk of developing kidney failure. In an analysis, the 15-year kidney failure risk was 30.8 per 10,000 donors whereas it was 3.9 per 10,000 in their matched healthy nondonors.[43] The risk is higher in subgroups with hypertension, diabetes, obesity, moderate albuminuria, lower eGFRs, and history of smoking.[44] Risk prediction tools that combine the effects of demographic and health factors are available at www.transplantmodels.com. To improve the kidney risk stratification, genetic markers are being incorporated.

Surgical complications are reported in 6–29% donors, with <3% experiencing a major complication.[45,46] The risk of death within 90 days of donation is reported at 0.03%.[47] The most common causes of death after living donation are pulmonary emboli, hepatitis, and cardiac events.[10] In an Indian study using the Kocak-modified Clavien–Dindo system to grade and report the severity of complications in 1,430 patients who had undergone live donor nephrectomy, the overall complication rate was 8.6% with 0.06% mortality rate.[43]

To summarize, living kidney donation may increase the risk to donors for some adverse outcomes. Understanding the acceptable thresholds of these risks and taking care of the living donors are important for donor safety and the success of a transplant program.

REFERENCES

1. Lentine KL, Kasiske BL, Levey AS, Adams PL, Alberú J, Bakr MA, et al. KDIGO Clinical Practice Guideline on the evaluation and care of living kidney donors. Transplantation. 2017;101:S1-109.
2. Bailey P, Edwards A, Courtney AL. Living kidney donation. BMJ. 2016;354:i4746.
3. Kher A, Mandelbrot DA. Living kidney donor evaluation: focus on renal issues. Clin J Am Soc Nephrol. 2012;7:366-71.
4. Organ Procurement and Transplantation Network. Guidance for the informed consent of living donor. [online] Available from: https://optn.transplant.hrsa.gov/resources/guidance/guidance-for-the-informed-consent-of-living-donors. [Last accessed October, 2021].
5. Dols LFC, Kok NFM, Roodnat JI, Tran TCK, Terkivatan T, Zuidema WC, et al. Living kidney donors: impact of age on long-term safety. Am J Transplant. 2011;11:737-42.
6. Neipp M, Jackobs S, Jaeger M, Schwarz A, Lueck R, Gwinner W, et al. Living kidney donors >60 years of age: is it acceptable for the donor and the recipient? Transpl Int. 2006;19:213-7.
7. Kumar A, Kumar RV, Srinadh ES, Bhandari M, Sharma RK, Gupta A, et al. Should elderly donors be accepted in live related renal transplant programs? Clin Transplant. 1994;8:523-6.
8. Grams ME, Sang Y, Levey AS, Matsushita K, Ballew S, Chang AR, et al. Kidney-failure risk projection for the living kidney-donor candidate. N Engl J Med. 2016;374:411-21.
9. Garg N, Poggio ED, Mandelbrot D. Evaluation of kidney function in living kidney donor candidates. Kidney360. 2021;2:1523-30.
10. British Transplant Society (BTS). (2018). United Kingdom Living Kidney Donor Guidelines. Assessment of Renal Function. [online] Available from: https://bts.org.uk/wp-content/uploads/2018/01/.pdf. [Last accessed October, 2020].
11. European Renal Best Practice Transplantation Guideline Development Group. ERBP guideline on the management and evaluation of the kidney donor and recipient. Nephrol Dial Transplant. 2013;28(Suppl. 2):ii1-71.
12. Davis R, Jones JS, Barocas DA, Castle EP, Lang EK, Leveillee RJ, et al. Diagnosis, evaluation and follow-up of asymptomatic microhematuria (AMH) in adults: AUA guideline. J Urol. 2012;188:2473-81.
13. Lee YM, Baek SY, Kim JH, Kim DS, Lee JS, Kim PK. Analysis of renal biopsies performed in children with abnormal findings in urinary mass screening. Acta Paediatr. 2006;95:849-53.
14. Wise GJ, Schlegel PN. Sterile pyuria. N Engl J Med. 2015;372:1048-54.
15. Andrews PA, Burnapp L, Manas D, Bradley JA, Dudley C, British Transplantation Society/Renal Association. Summary of the British Transplantation Society/Renal Association

UK guidelines for living donor kidney transplantation. Transplantation. 2012;93:666-73.
16. DeMaria EJ, Carmody BJ. Perioperative management of special populations: obesity. Surg Clin North Am. 2005;85: 1283-9.
17. Textor SC, Taler SJ, Larson TS, Prieto M, Griffin M, Gloor J, et al. Blood pressure evaluation among older living kidney donors. J Am Soc Nephrol. 2003;14:2159-67.
18. O'Brien E, Parati G, Stergiou G, Asmar R, Beilin L, Bilo G, et al. European Society of Hypertension position paper on ambulatory blood pressure monitoring. J Hypertens. 2013;31:1731-68.
19. Chobanian AV, Bakris GL, Black HR, Cushman WC, Green LA, Izzo Jr JL, et al. Seventh report of the Joint National Committee on prevention, detection, evaluation, and treatment of high blood pressure. Hypertension. 2003;42:1206-52.
20. Stergiou GS, Asayama K, Thijs L, Kollias A, Niiranen TJ, Hozawa A, et al. Prognosis of white-coat and masked hypertension: International Database of Home blood pressure in relation to cardiovascular outcome. Hypertension. 2014; 63:675-82.
21. Thomas SM, Lam NN, Welk BK, Nguan C, Huang A, Nash DM, et al. Risk of kidney stones with surgical intervention in living kidney donors. Am J Transplant. 2013;13:2935-44.
22. Olsburgh J, Thomas K, Wong K, Bultitude M, Glass J, Rottenberg G, et al. Incidental renal stones in potential live kidney donors: prevalence, assessment and donation, including role of ex vivo ureteroscopy. BJU Int. 2013;111: 784-92.
23. Pei Y, Hwang YH, Conklin J, Sundsbak JL, Heyer CM, Chan W, et al. Imaging-based diagnosis of autosomal dominant polycystic kidney disease. J Am Soc Nephrol. 2015;26:746-53.
24. Pei Y, Obaji J, Dupuis A, Paterson AD, Magistroni R, Dicks E, et al. Unified criteria for ultrasonographic diagnosis of ADPKD. J Am Soc Nephrol. 2009;20:205-12.
25. Zand MS, Strang J, Dumlao M, Rubens D, Erturk E, Bronsther O. Screening a living kidney donor for polycystic kidney disease using heavily T2-weighted MRI. Am J Kidney Dis. 2001;37:612-9.
26. Simms RJ, Travis DL, Durkie M, Wilson G, Dalton A, Ong ACM. Genetic testing in the assessment of living related kidney donors at risk of autosomal dominant polycystic kidney disease. Transplantation. 2015;99:1023-29.
27. Gross O, Weber M, Fries JW, Müller GA. Living donor kidney transplantation from relatives with mild urinary abnormalities in Alport syndrome: long-term risk, benefit and outcome. Nephrol Dial Transplant. 2009;24:1626-30.
28. Kashtan CE. Women with Alport syndrome: risks and rewards of kidney donation. Nephrol Dial Transplant. 2009; 24:1369-70.
29. Limou S, Nelson GW, Kopp JB, Winkler CA. APOL1 kidney risk alleles: population genetics and disease associations. Adv Chronic Kidney Dis. 2014;21:426-33.
30. Kopp JB, Nelson GW, Sampath K, Johnson RC, Genovese G, An P, et al. APOL1 genetic variants in focal segmental glomerulosclerosis and HIV-associated nephropathy. J Am Soc Nephrol. 2011;22:2129-37.
31. Newell KA, Formica RN, Gill JS, Schold JD, Allan JS, Covington SH, et al. Integrating *APOL-1* gene variants into renal transplantation: considerations arising from the American Society of Transplantation expert conference. Am J Transplant. 2017;17:901-11.
32. Nalesnik MA, Woodle ES, Dimaio JM, Vasudev B, Teperman LW, Covington S, et al. Donor-transmitted malignancies in organ transplantation: assessment of clinical risk. Am J Transplant. 2011;11:1140-7.
33. Israel GM, Bosniak MA. An update of the Bosniak renal cyst classification system. Urology. 2005;66:484-8.
34. Saha S, Kumar A, Saurabh K, Shankar SH, Kashyap A, Nischal N, et al. Current status of treatment of latent tuberculosis infection in India. Indian J Med Sci. 2019;71:54-9.
35. Srisuwarn P, Sumethkul V. Kidney transplant from donors with hepatitis B: a challenging treatment option. World J Hepatol. 2021;13:853-67.
36. Massimiliano V, Vincenzo A, Daniela C, Giaquinta A, Ekser B, Sinagra N, et al. Kidney transplantation from donors with hepatitis B. Med Sci Monit. 2016;22:1427-4.
37. Pagan J, Ladino M, Roth D. Should my patient accept a kidney from a hepatitis C virus–infected donor? Kidney360. 2020;1:127-29.
38. Len O, Garzoni C, Lumbreras C, Molina I, Meije Y, Pahissa A, et al. Recommendations for screening of donor and recipient prior to solid organ transplantation and to minimise transmission of donor-derived infections. Clin Microbiol Infect. 2014;20:10-8.
39. Ibrahim HN, Akkina SK, Leister E, Gillingham K, Cordner G, Guo H, et al. Pregnancy outcomes after kidney donation. Am J Transplant. 2009;9:825-34.
40. Plage H, Pielka P, Liefeldt L, Budde K, Ebbing J, Sugünes N, et al. Extended criteria donors in living kidney transplantation including donor age, smoking, hypertension and BMI. Ther Clin Risk Manag. 2020;16:787-93.
41. Cantarelli C, Cravedi P. Criteria for living donation from marginal donors: one, no one, and one hundred thousand. Nephron. 2019;142(3):227-32.
42. Maggiore U, Cravedi P. The marginal kidney donor. Curr Opin Organ Transplant. 2014;19(4):372-80.
43. Muzaale AD, Massie AB, Wang MC, Montgomery RA, McBride MA, Wainright JL, et al. Risk of end-stage renal disease following live kidney donation. JAMA. 2014;311:579-86.
44. Lentine KL, Lam NN, Segev DL. Risk of living kidney donation. Current state of knowledge on outcomes important to donors. Clin J Am Soc Nephrol. 2019;14:597-608.
45. Srivastava A, Bansal A, Sureka SK, Yadav P, Srivastava D, Jena R, et al. A retrospective analysis of complications of laparoscopic left donor nephrectomy using the Kocak's modification of Clavien-Dindo system. Indian J Urol. 2018;34:133-9.
46. Clavien PA, Barkun J, de Oliveira ML, Vauthey JN, Dindo D, Schulick RD, et al. The Clavien-Dindo classification of surgical complications: five-year experience. Ann Surg. 2009;250:187-96.
47. Segev DL, Muzaale AD, Caffo BS, Mehta SH, Singer AL, Taranto SE, et al. Perioperative mortality and long-term survival following live kidney donation. JAMA. 2010;303: 959-66.
48. Organ Procurement and Transplantation Network/UNOS (United Network for Organ Sharing). (2021). OPTN Policies, Policy 14: Living Donation. [online] Available from http://optn.transplant.hrsa.gov/ContentDocuments/OPTN_Policies.pdf. [Last accessed May, 2022].
49. Richardson R, Connelly M, Dipchand C, Garg AX, Ghanekar A, Houde I, et al. Kidney paired donation protocol for participating donors 2014. Transplantation. 2015;99:S1-88.
50. Cohney S, Kanellis J, Howell M, CARI. The CARI guidelines. Donor renal function. Nephrology (Carlton). 2010;15:S137-45.
51. Delmonico F, Council of the Transplantation Society. A report of the Amsterdam forum on the care of the live kidney donor: data and medical guidelines. Transplantation. 2005;79:S53-66.

CHAPTER 3

Evaluation of Kidney Transplant Recipients

Edwin Fernando, Sukanya Govindan

CASE VIGNETTE

Evaluation of a patient with chronic Hepatitis C infection on dialysis

A 45-year-old male patient is on maintenance hemodialysis for 1.5 years. At the time of initiation on dialysis he tested positive for Hepatitis C infection. He had no episodes of jaundice, ascites, hematemesis or melaena. He is now being worked up for a live related renal transplant with his mother as prospective blood group matched donor. He undergoes the following evaluation for Hepatitis C infection: Anti-HCV antibodies by ELISA—positive, HCV RNA quantitative PCR—1,84,000 copies, Ultrasound abdomen—shows altered coarse liver echotexture, normal portal vein wedge pressure and no splenic enlargement. A fibro scan was ordered by the hepatologist for this patient which showed stage F1. The patient was advised therapy with sofosbuvir-velpatasvir regimen for 12 weeks. After completion of therapy the patient had attained sustained virologic response (SVR). The patient was cleared for renal transplant as there was no decompensation of liver disease, no portal hypertension and patient had SVR following directly acting antiviral (DAA) therapy.

INTRODUCTION

There is a constant increase in the number of patients with end-stage kidney disease (ESKD) receiving renal replacement therapy with over 3.5 million people currently on dialysis globally. The cost of delivering life-long dialysis therapy is enormous. In addition, dialysis patients have high requirements for elective or emergency admission to hospital, further increasing costs. Kidney transplantation both is cost effective and confers better survival and quality of life compared to dialysis treatment. There is, therefore, a strong motivation to counsel patients with irreversible kidney failure for renal transplantation.

Suitability of candidates for transplantation is determined by the relative risk of transplantation in comparison to staying on dialysis treatment. Hence, a thorough workup is often needed for estimation of risk in a prospective transplant recipient. After a decision to proceed to transplantation is made, strategies to minimize risks and maximize the chances of a successful outcome are undertaken as part of the candidate-evaluation process. The evaluation should be as efficient and cost effective as possible.[1]

TIMING OF TRANSPLANTATION REFERRAL

The optimal timing of transplantation is not known with certainty. All patients with ESKD who are medically stable should be referred for kidney transplant. Possible preemptive transplantation can be planned at least 6–12 months ahead of anticipated dialysis initiation for identification and workup of living donors.[2]

INITIAL EVALUATION

All prospective renal transplant recipients were subjected to screening tests to assess their suitability for transplantation.

Initial workup includes:

- *Review of native kidney biopsy:* (1) To determine the cause of ESKD in candidates whenever possible; and (2) To inform risks of recurrence of native disease and management post-kidney transplantation and the resultant risk of graft loss.
- *Testing for genetic kidney disease:* In appropriate patients
- Full blood count (hemoglobin, leukocytes, platelets) and renal function tests (Cr, urea, electrolytes, Ca, P)
- Urine culture
- Liver function test [LFT (liver enzymes, serum proteins)], hemoglobin A1c (HBA1c), parathyroid hormone (PTH)
- International normalized ratio (INR)/prothrombin time (PT)/activated partial thromboplastin time (APTT)
- Serology for hepatitis B, hepatitis C, human immunodeficiency virus (HIV) and cytomegalovirus (CMV), COVID reverse transcription-polymerase chain reaction (RT-PCR)

- Coronary artery disease (CAD) screening
- Chest X-ray
- Ultrasound of kidneys and Doppler of iliac vessels
- Electrocardiogram (ECG) and echocardiography
- *Cancer screening:* Pap smear and mammogram for prospective female recipients, serum prostate-specific antigen (PSA) and digital rectal examination (DRE) in those >50 years in males.
- Regular visit to dentist and ENT (ear, nose, and throat) team to look into focal sepsis
- Voiding cystogram and urodynamics study in selected patients
- Psychiatric and psychological evaluation
- Pregnancy test to be done and pregnancy ruled out
- *Potential sensitization risks:* History of blood product (packed red cells, platelets) transfusion, pregnancies, and prior transplants
- *In retransplantation candidates:* Prior transplantation courses and cause of graft loss, medication adherence, and previous transplant complications.[1]

CHAPTER HIGHLIGHTS

- Pretransplant evaluation should assess the perceived risks of transplantation relative to the risks of not receiving a transplant.
- Pretransplant evaluation should be done in all eligible patients on dialysis and ideally should start 6–12 months before the anticipated start of dialysis.
- A detailed workup of all systems with special focus on native kidney disease, infections, cardiac status, and urogenital system should be done.
- Patients with pre-existing comorbid conditions should undergo a thorough evaluation of specific organ systems to assess reversibility, damage, and the possibility of affecting graft function and life after transplant.
- Surgical assessment of all recipients should be done, including iliac vessel dimensions, bladder assessment and need for pretransplant nephrectomy.

CONTRAINDICATIONS TO RENAL TRANSPLANTATION ALONE

- Multiple myeloma, light chain deposition disease, or heavy chain deposition disease unless they have received a potentially curative treatment regimen and are in stable remission
- Amyloid light-chain (AL) amyloidosis with significant extrarenal involvement
- Decompensated cirrhosis (consider for combined liver-kidney transplant)
- Severe irreversible obstructive or restrictive lung disease
- Severe uncorrectable and symptomatic cardiac disease that is deemed by a cardiologist to preclude transplantation, namely ejection fraction <30%
- Progressive central neurodegenerative disease[1]
- Acute hepatitis.

WORKUP FOR RENAL TRANSPLANTATION CAN BE DELAYED

- Patients with uncontrolled psychiatric illness which could affect decision-making or puts the recipient at an unacceptable level of post-transplant risk.
- Ongoing substance—use disorder that affects decision-making or puts the candidate at an unacceptable level of post-transplant risk.
- Nonadherent behavior despite education and counseling
- Active infection (excluding hepatitis C virus infection) that is not properly treated.
- Active malignancy except for those with indolent and low-grade cancers such as prostate cancer (Gleason score ≤6) and incidentally detected renal tumors (≤1 cm in maximum diameter).
- Currently, active or symptomatic cardiac disease (angina, arrhythmia, heart failure, valvular heart disease), which has not been evaluated by cardiologist.
- Active peripheral arterial disease.
- Recent cerebrovascular events.
- *Active symptomatic:* Peptic ulcer disease; diverticulitis, acute pancreatitis, gallstone/gallbladder disease inflammatory bowel disease.[1]

EVALUATION OF A RENAL TRANSPLANT CANDIDATE

Evaluation of a renal transplant candidate should include:

- Referral to a nephrologist and a surgeon/urologist with expertise in kidney transplantation.
- Candidates should be assessed for medical conditions that inhibit wound healing and/or preclude hernias including obesity, undernutrition, tobacco use, and prior abdominal surgeries. Detailed evaluation is needed for prospective recipients with previous known urological malignancy, dysfunctional voiding, recurrent urinary infections, urinary diversions or augmented bladder, significant structural anomalies of urinary tract, and/or renal stone disease.
- Detailed history to assess infectious, cardiac, urological, and psychological risks.
- A thorough physical examination of all the systems including cardiovascular and peripheral vascular, abdominal, and urogenital systems[1].

ADDITIONAL EVALUATION OF COMORBID CONDITIONS

Cardiovascular Disease

All patients with chronic kidney disease (CKD) are at high risk of cardiovascular disease compared with individuals who do not have CKD. *All* patients with angina symptoms, cardiomyopathy with reduced ejection fraction, or diabetes mellitus with diabetic nephropathy as the cause of their CKD *or* patients with a positive noninvasive stress test are considered to be at high risk for CAD. The decision to proceed with angiography and possible angioplasty or surgery is made in conjunction with the patient's cardiologist. Noninvasive tests such as dobutamine stress echocardiogram (ECHO) or myocardial perfusion study have limitations in their ability to detect CAD in patients with CKD, particularly those with diabetes.

In patients without history of angina or any other abnormalities on ECG and echocardiography, the following should be considered as risk factors for invasive cardiac testing: age >60 years, hypertension, dyslipidemia, peripheral vascular disease, previous history of CAD, left ventricular hypertrophy, family history of heart disease, dialysis vintage greater than 1 year, prolonged duration of CKD, and history of smoking. The optimal choice of cardiac testing is generally based upon the expertise of the particular center and patient characteristics.[3]

Pulmonary Hypertension

Pulmonary hypertension in ESKD patients is associated with time on dialysis, systolic/diastolic heart dysfunction, obstructive sleep apnea, pulmonary embolism, and tobacco use. Patients with pulmonary hypertension should be treated, if possible, prior to transplantation. Select patients that are otherwise acceptable transplant candidates may become eligible if pulmonary hypertension is successfully controlled with pulmonary vasodilator therapy. Patients with irreversible moderate-to-severe pulmonary hypertension should be excluded from transplantation.

Neurological Disease

Kidney transplant reduces the risk of cerebrovascular events and ameliorates peripheral neuropathy due to uremia. Hence, transplant should be offered to all patients with nonprogressive neurological illness and peripheral neuropathy. Patients with a recent history of stroke should wait for at least 6 months after transient ischemic attack (TIA) provided there is no progressive or dense neurological deficit.[4]

Patients with previous history of cerebrovascular accidents, diabetes, hypertension, smoking, and hyperlipidemia are at risk of future cerebrovascular disease. However, currently no routine neurological evaluation is recommended in asymptomatic patients prior to renal transplant. However, a thorough and focused clinical examination should be done in all prospective transplant recipients.

Evaluation in Neurological Disease

Patients with a history of *stroke or TIA* should undergo cardiac evaluation including ECG and echocardiogram to rule out treatable causes of stroke such as atrial fibrillation (AF) and cardiac emboli due to valvular heart disease prior to transplant. Carotid artery imaging is also suggested to rule out carotid artery stenosis in these patients.

Patients with *autosomal dominant polycystic kidney disease (ADPKD)* should be screened for intracranial aneurysms (ICA) if they have positive family history of ICA or prior aneurysmal bleeding.[5]

Patients with *seizure disorder* on anticonvulsant therapy should be evaluated to assess the need for continuation of therapy. Drug interactions of anticonvulsant drugs with calcineurin inhibitors should be kept in mind before prescribing or continuing these medicines.[4]

Gastrointestinal and Liver Disease

A focused history and clinical examination of the GI system should be done in all prospective kidney transplant recipients. Commonly encountered GI diseases in CKD patients include peptic ulcer disease, diverticulitis, pancreatitis, and cholelithiasis. Many of these illnesses if present and not treated can be exacerbated in the post-transplant period.[1]

Symptomatic patients with *diverticulitis* will need evaluation with barium enema or colonoscopy, and renal transplant should be postponed till symptoms resolve. Asymptomatic patients, however, need not be routinely screened for diverticulitis. Prophylactic colectomy is not advocated nowadays for patients with history of diverticulitis.

The incidence of *peptic ulcer disease* has decreased considerably in recent years. Active peptic ulcer disease can cause perforation and bleeding in the post-transplant period. Hence, an active disease should be looked for and treated medically before transplant.

History of chronic *pancreatitis* is not a contraindication for renal transplant. However, transplant should be postponed for a minimum of 3 months after an episode of acute pancreatitis. Reversible or treatable causes of pancreatitis such as hyperparathyroidism, hyperlipidemia, cholelithiasis, and alcohol intake should be addressed before transplant. Medications such as steroids and azathioprine increase the risk of pancreatitis post-transplant. Patients with history of pancreatitis are at risk of developing post-transplant diabetes and should be monitored.[4]

Symptomatic *cholelithiasis or cholecystitis* warrants treatment prior to transplant and cholecystectomy should be offered to all these patients. Transplant should also be postponed till acute cholecystitis is resolved.

Liver Disease

All prospective kidney transplant recipients should be screened for liver disease with total bilirubin, alanine aminotransferase, INR, and albumin. Patients with suspected cirrhosis should be referred for specialist evaluation and isolated kidney transplant should be offered to only patients with compensated liver disease. Patients with decompensated cirrhosis should be offered combined or sequential liver–kidney transplant.

All prospective transplant recipients should be screened for *chronic hepatitis B* with hepatitis B surface antigen (HBsAg), hepatitis B surface antibody (anti-HBs), and hepatitis B core antibody (anti-HBc) and for *chronic hepatitis C* infection with immunoassay. All candidates with hepatitis B virus (HBV) and hepatitis C virus (HCV) infection should be evaluated for severity of liver disease and presence of portal hypertension prior to acceptance for kidney transplantation.[1,4]

Hematologic Disease

Patients with history of thrombotic events should undergo evaluation for thrombophilia and all patients with known antiphospholipid antibody (APLA) syndrome and/or systemic lupus erythematosus (SLE) should have APLA checked before transplant. Patients receiving regular single antiplatelet therapy have little risk of bleeding and these agents can be continued. Patients on dual antiplatelet therapy and directly acting oral anticoagulants (DOACs) should have preoperative assessment and plan for anticoagulant therapy use perioperatively with monitoring. Treatment should be aimed at balancing and reducing the risk of thromboembolism and preventing excessive bleeding. For patients on vitamin K antagonist, the anticoagulant effect will be reduced for several days after stopping and similar levels have to be established perioperatively. Hence shorter acting agents, such as heparin, should be considered during this time. The DOACs have shorter half-lives, making them easier to discontinue and resume rapidly.

Monoclonal gammopathy of undetermined significance (MGUS) and smouldering myeloma are not contraindications for renal transplant. However, these patients have a higher risk of lymphoproliferative disorders and the same should be discussed with patients prior to transplant. Patients with acute leukemia and high-grade lymphomas should be cancer free before transplant. The decision to do transplant after recovery from acute leukemia and in a patient with chronic leukemia or lymphoma should be made in discussion with a hematologist.[1]

Psychiatric Disease

Psychosocial assessment should be done in all prospective transplant recipients by a psychiatrist or psychologist or social worker familiar with renal transplant issues. Transplant should not be offered to patients with an unstable psychiatric illness or an ongoing substance-abuse disorder which interferes with decision making. Patients with history of pretransplant nonadherence or graft loss due to nonadherence should receive counseling before transplant.[1,4]

INFECTIONS

Tuberculosis (TB): Candidates from intermediate and high TB prevalence areas should be screened for latent TB as per local guidelines and need increased vigilance in the post-transplant period for active TB.

Hepatitis C virus (HCV): Patients with HCV infection and compensated cirrhosis (without portal hypertension) can undergo isolated kidney transplantation. Direct-acting antiviral (DAA) therapy can be given either before or after transplantation. Combined liver–kidney transplantation should be offered to patients with HCV and decompensated cirrhosis deferring HCV treatment until after transplantation.[1]

Hepatitis B (HBV): HBsAg positive and/or HBV deoxyribonucleic acid (DNA) positive candidates can undergo isolated kidney transplantation if they do not have decompensated cirrhosis and are stable on antiviral therapy after specialist evaluation.

COVID-19 evaluation RT-PCR test of potential recipients and donors should be undertaken prior to transplant surgery in accordance with local guidelines.

VACCINATIONS

Vaccinations against hepatitis B, pneumococcal vaccines, annual influenza, varicella, *Haemophilus*, and COVID-19 should be done. All live vaccines should be completed at least 6 weeks prior to transplantation.

Transplant recipients scheduled for transplantation should be given any COVID-19 vaccine that is authorized or approved by their health regulators/agencies vaccine 2 weeks prior to surgery or 1–6 months post-transplant.

MALIGNANCY

Routine cancer screening as per local guidelines for general population should be done for all prospective recipients. No waiting time is required for candidates with curatively treated skin malignancies such as nonmetastatic basal cell and squamous cell carcinoma, melanoma in situ, small renal cell carcinoma (<3 cm), prostate cancer (Gleason score ≤6), carcinoma in situ (ductal carcinoma in situ, cervical, others), thyroid cancer (follicular/papillary <2 cm of low-grade histology), and superficial bladder cancer.

Decisions about transplantation for candidates in remission from cancer should be made collaboratively with oncologists, transplant nephrologists, patients, and their caregivers.[1]

SURGICAL EVALUATION

Pretransplant surgical evaluation should be done in all patients to identify obesity/frailty, vascular anatomy, native kidney size in polycystic kidney disease, previous abdominal surgeries, presence of hernia, and bladder assessment.

Obesity is a relative contraindication to transplant, and weight loss interventions should be offered. The risk of increased postoperative complications such as delayed wound healing and increased mortality should be explained to patients.

The renal allograft is placed extraperitoneally in the iliac fossa and anastomosed to the external iliac vessels. *Iliac vessel dimension* is assessed by ultrasound Doppler and additional imaging such as contrast computed tomography (CT) or venography to assess vessel patency and health might be needed in patients with peripheral vascular disease and lower extremity catheters or grafts as dialysis access.[4]

Pretransplant nephrectomy is a consideration in patients with polycystic kidney disease and a noncontrast CT is done to evaluate native kidney size. Pretransplant nephrectomy is also performed when necessary in pediatric patients with heavy proteinuria, recurrent native kidney infections, in patients with high risk of native kidney malignancy such as nephroblastoma.[1,4]

Bladder assessment: Although an abnormal lower urinary tract is not a contraindication to kidney transplant, a compliant bladder with safe bladder pressures is necessary for preventing graft dysfunction post-transplant. Bladder function assessment with preliminary clinical history, focussed clinical examination, and ultrasound of the bladder with postvoid residue measurement in patients with residual urine output should be done in all prospective transplant recipients. History of lower urinary tract symptoms, urinary and fecal incontinence, recurrent urinary infections, and basic kidney disease must be taken in all patients. Focussed clinical examination should be done for overdistended bladder, symmetry of gluteal folds, anal sphincter tone, lower limb tone, and reflexes. Additional functional assessment with micturating cystourethrogram with or without invasive urodynamics would be necessary in patients with reflux nephropathy, neurogenic bladder, and posterior urethral valves. The need for bladder augmentation prior to transplant must be discussed with the urologist if the native bladder is unlikely to be safe for transplant.

Parathyroidectomy: Parathyroidectomy for patients with severe refractory hyperparathyroidism (PTH levels >800 pg/mL) and moderate-to-severe symptoms may be considered. Some centers do not perform parathyroidectomy for this indication, prior to transplant as it is believed that the symptoms will resolve after transplant.

BASIC KIDNEY DISEASE

Renal diagnosis: The clinician should be aware that many diseases can recur in the allograft and, in some cases, are more likely to lead to graft failure.[1]

Focal segmental glomerulosclerosis (FSGS): In view of increased risk of recurrent disease in the allograft, genetic testing should be performed in children and young adults with a clinical course consistent with genetic FSGS.

Membranous nephropathy (MN): Autoantibodies to phospholipase A2 receptor (PLA2R) should be measured pretransplant to predict recurrence post-transplant.

C3G, including dense deposit disease (DDD) and C3 glomerulonephritis (C3GN): The risk of high recurrence should be considered and discussed with the patient. Patients with C3G to be screened for genetic or acquired causes for the dysregulation of the complement alternative pathway to guide treatment and transplant decisions.

Antiglomerular basement membrane (anti-GBM) disease: Anti-GBM antibody titers to be measured in candidates and that transplantation is only performed when antibodies are undetectable.

Hemolytic-uremic syndrome (HUS): It is mandatory to assess patients with suspected atypical HUS (aHUS) for a genetic or acquired defect in complement regulation or other genetic causes of aHUS to inform risk of recurrence. Any abnormality in complement regulation places them at high risk of recurrence, and renal transplantation should not proceed unless a complement inhibitor can be administered or combined liver-kidney transplant can be performed.

REFERENCES

1. Chadban SJ, Ahn C, Axelrod DA, Foster BJ, Kasiske BL, Kher V, et al. KDIGO clinical practice guideline on the evaluation and management of candidates for kidney transplantation. Transplantation. 2020;104(4S1 Suppl 1):S11-103.
2. Bunnapradist S, Danovitch GM. Evaluation of adult kidney transplant candidates. Am J Kidney Dis. 2007;50(5):890-8.
3. Lentine KL, Costa SP, Weir MR, Robb JF, Fleisher LA, Kasiske BL, et al. Cardiac disease evaluation and management among kidney and liver transplantation candidates: a scientific statement from the American Heart Association and the American College of Cardiology Foundation. J Am Coll Cardiol. 2012;60(5):434-80.
4. Danovitch GM. Handbook of Kidney Transplantation. Philadelphia: Wolters Kluwer; 2017.
5. International Study of Unruptured Intracranial Aneurysms Investigators. Unruptured intracranial aneurysms—risk of rupture and risks of surgical intervention [published correction appears in N Engl J Med. 1999;340(9):744]. N Engl J Med. 1998;339(24):1725-33.

CHAPTER 4

Surgical Techniques of Kidney Transplantation

Sandeep Guleria

INTRODUCTION

More than 60 years ago, the first successful kidney transplant (KT) was performed, and now, thanks to considerable breakthroughs in immunosuppressive medication, KT is the preferred modality of treatment in end-stage renal disease (ESRD) patients.[1] The kidney was the first organ to be transplanted, and it is still the most common. For most persons with ESRD, transplantation increases survival, improves the quality of life, and saves costs when compared to chronic dialysis. Most people with ESRD should be considered candidates because there are few absolute contraindications.[2] The surgical procedure of KT involves both vascular and urological procedures. **Figure 1** shows the evolution of surgical technique in kidney transplantation. The safety and success of the procedure are based on an effective approach for vascular and ureteric anastomoses, which serves as the foundation for many types of KT (open, laparoscopic, and robotic).[3]

PREPARATION OF RECIPIENT[2]

The preoperative evaluation is divided into:

- Medical
- Surgical
- Immunologic
- Psychosocial.

The *surgical examination* looks for vascular or urologic abnormalities that could interfere with the transplant process. To further investigate signs of vascular disease if disclosed in the history (e.g., history of claudication or rest discomfort) or physical examination (e.g., decreased or missing pulse, bruit), Doppler investigations or angiography should be performed. In circumstances where a severe aortoiliac disease makes transplantation technically impossible, revascularization with an aortobifemoral graft before the transplant may be an option.

In areas of severe stenosis near the targeted implantation site, preoperative balloon angioplasty or stenting

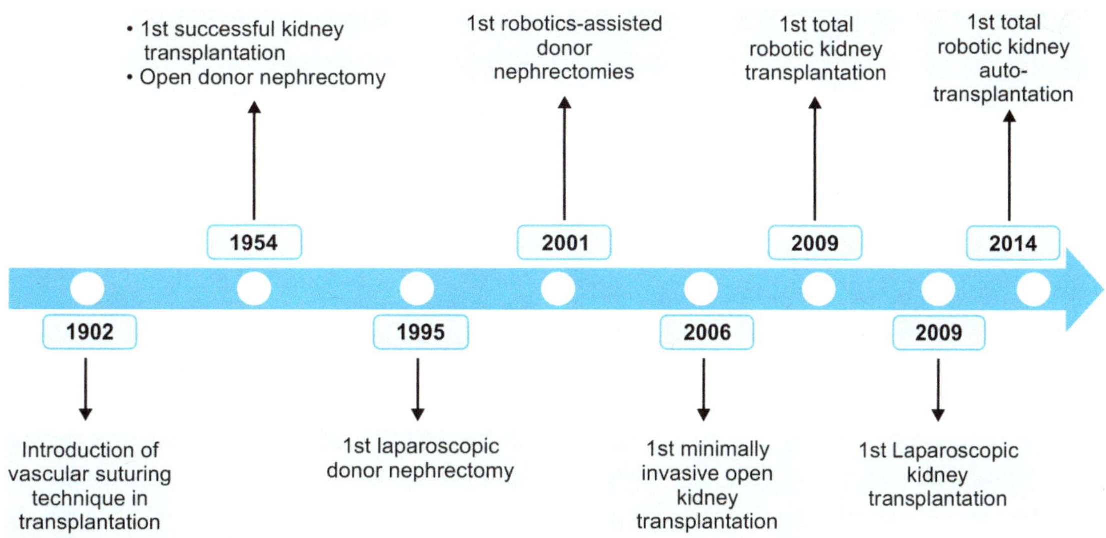

Fig. 1: Evolution of surgical technique in kidney transplantation.[3]

Source: The Evolution of Kidney Transplantation Surgery Into the Robotic Era and Its Prospects for Obese Recipients Transplantation 2018;102:1650-65.

may be required. Prior to the KT, nephrectomy of the native kidney may be required for causes such as large polycystic kidneys, persistent renal infection significant reflux, or suspected malignancy. To rule out reflux and bladder outlet obstruction, a full genitourinary tract examination is especially crucial for youngsters.

DONOR NEPHRECTOMY

Traditional open access, mini-incision, pure or hand-aided laparoscopy (transperitoneal or retroperitoneal), supported by robots, single site [laparoendoscopic single-site surgery (LESS)], and natural orifices [natural orifice transluminal endoscopic surgery (NOTES)] are all options for living donor nephrectomy.[3] Whichever approach is used, the kidney chosen must meet stringent anatomical requirements. The healthier kidney should be kept in the donor. In circumstances when both kidneys are of equal health, the left kidney is removed first because of its more favorable anatomy. It is more accessible and has longer vessels, making subsequent transplantation less difficult from a technical standpoint.

Laparoscopic right donor nephrectomy[4] is a rare procedure, with success rates ranging from 1 to 4%. When compared to left kidneys, the initial technical hurdles with laparoscopic right nephrectomy resulted in more vascular complications. These outcomes can be improved by modifying donor procedures to preserve donor vein length and recipient techniques to mobilize the iliac venous system. Multiple renal arteries and abnormal renal venous architecture, on the other hand, are not contraindications to left donor nephrectomy. The presence of stones, cysts, or abnormalities in the right kidney strongly suggests right-sided nephrectomy rather than left-sided nephrectomy. The requirement for liver retraction alters the surgical strategy. Limited right lobe mobilization is combined with the use of a liver retractor to lift the liver above the superior pole of the right kidney.

The operation is compounded further by the need to divide the right gonadal vein, which runs straight into the vena cava. Because the right adrenal vein is independent of the right renal vein, it usually does not need to be separated. The shorter right renal vein necessitates special care when stapling with vascular stapling instruments, whether cutting or noncutting. To allow installation of the stapling device for maximum vein length, the kidney is retracted to its greatest length and the vena cava is exposed.

Steps of a traditional open nephrectomyare as follows:

- The patient is positioned in a lateral decubitus.
- An oblique lumbar incision is made.
- The peritoneum is split bluntly and reflected medially to obtain access to the retroperitoneal region and kidney.

OPEN NEPHRECTOMY THROUGH MINI-INCISION

The same previous position of the patient is used. Mini-incision can be subcostal, horizontal, or vertical. In the muscle section, separation without making an incision is advisable. Rib resection should be avoided. Muscle splitting is less painful than muscle cutting. When we opt for a transperitoneal laparoscopic nephrectomy, after the complete separation of the kidney, ureter, and renal vessels, a mini-Pfannenstiel incision is made, through which the organ will be removed. Renal vessels should be, preferably, connected using, at least, two clamps on each of them.

RETROPERITONEAL LAPAROSCOPIC NEPHRECTOMY

The lateral decubitus position is used, and the creation of the workspace is done through digital or balloon dilation. The trocars are placed, and renal and vascular dissection is performed.

Hand-assisted laparoscopic nephrectomy can be performed via a trans- or retroperitoneal approach. The surgery begins with an incision to place the device and introduce the hand. The kidney and the vessels are laparoscopically dissected with manual aid. Renal extraction is made through the hand-insertion device.

In robot-assisted laparoscopic nephrectomy, the donor is laterally positioned, and four portals are used—two for the surgeon, one for the camera, and another for the assistant. The surgeon operates outside the surgical field, with a magnified three-dimensional (3D) view, and the robotic arms offer an amplitude of movements similar to those of the human fist. Surgery lengths are the same and the kidney can be removed through a midline incision. Single-site (LESS) or natural orifices (NOTES) laparoscopic nephrectomy, with fewer or no scars, has also been used in living donor nephrectomy.

Several randomized studies comparing living donor nephrectomy using mini-incision against conventional and laparoscopic open surgery has been published. The mini-incision can be made in any of three places: Anterior, flank, or posterior. When compared to traditional lumbotomy, the mini-incision has more operation time ($p = 0.02$), less blood ($p = 0.01$), less painkiller use, and a shorter hospital stay ($p < 0.0001$). After up to 30 days, no difference was found in postoperative problems or serum creatinine value in the recipient. In two trials, there was a rise in the use of analgesics, the length of operation and recovery, as well as warm ischemia time ($p < 0.05$) for all comparisons when compared to laparoscopic surgery. In a recent retrospective cohort research, compared to laparoscopic surgery, the mini-incision reduced the length of operation

[53.9 minutes (40–75) vs. 93.7 minutes (75–140); $p < 0.001$], warm ischemia time (2.14 vs. 2.66 minutes; $p < 0.001$), and length of hospital stay (2.44 vs. 3.28 days; $p < 0.001$). There were no significant differences in pain, graft function, or quality of life assessments between the two groups.

GRAFT PREPARATION[5]

The viability of the graft must be preserved during the interval between explanation and implantation. KT teams consist of a minimum of two different groups. One group prepares the donor, while the other group performs surgery on the recipient simultaneously or with a slight delay, depending on the time required to carry the graft from the donor to the recipient.

Warm ischemic time: It is the time from cessation of circulation to removal of organ and perfusion with cold preservation solution (<60 minutes).

Cold ischemic time: It is the time from initiation of cold preservation solution to the restoration of warm circulation after transplantation (<24 hours ideal).

Static cold storage lowers the temperature of the graft from 0 to 4°C with the aim of preventing ischemic reperfusion injury.

The ischemia duration of the graft should be kept as brief as possible. Long-term ischemia depletes adenosine triphosphate levels, resulting in a build-up of reactive oxygen species, inflammation, and coagulation following reperfusion, causing renal tubular cell injury and increasing the chance of graft injury.

Simple hypothermia is not sufficient to keep the graft viable, so removal of the blood from the graft and its replacement with a preservation solution are must during graft preparation.

In the deceased donors, graft cold irrigation is done during the harvesting operation by irrigation of the clamped aorta.

Examples of pre-prepared solutions used for irrigation are:

- Belzer University of Wisconsin's (UW)
- Histidine-Tryptophan-Ketoglutarate (HTK, Bretschneider or Custodiol)
- Euro-Collins, Celsior
- Other newer solutions such as Biolasol®.

Irrigation of the graft in living donors is mostly done by more simple solutions such as lactated Ringer's solution. Published literature showed that if the total ischemic time is <60 minutes (as observed in most living donor programs), there is no difference in long-term graft survival using simple solutions as compared to complex solutions. After administration of anesthesia, a central catheter is placed into the internal jugular vein or the subclavian vein. Sometimes, the insertion of a central line is also required to maintain a central venous pressure of 7–10 cmH_2O.

STEPS OF THE SURGERY

A balloon catheter is inserted into the bladder using a full aseptic technique. Then, the skin is properly prepared, commencing with the removal of all hair with clips and the application of an antibacterial agent such as povidone-iodine or chlorhexidine gluconate to the skin of the abdomen wall. Because the original incision may need to be enlarged or abandoned, and the opposite iliac fossa opened, it is best to prepare the entire abdomen from the nipples to the midthighs, especially in a vascular patient.

Site

Some important factors that impact the surgeon's decision on which site the kidney graft should be implanted are described in **Table 1**.

When all the factors are equivocal, the graft kidney is usually placed in the right iliac fossa.[4-8] Currently, the common practice is to place the left kidney in the right iliac fossa and the right kidney in the left iliac fossa. In this approach, the pelvis and ureter are positioned anteriorly, which aids in urological tract rebuilding to some extent, especially if a subsequent urological condition needs surgery.

Special scenarios:

- In patients with autosomal dominant polycystic kidney disease (ADPKD), the kidney is transplanted on the smaller polycystic kidney side, if there is room below it. If indicated, it is easy to remove a large polycystic kidney by a transperitoneal approach. Although it is advisable to do this as a distinct surgical procedure prior to the transplant surgery, however, it can also be performed concurrently with the transplant operation, utilizing the same retroperitoneal approach (mostly extended) or a midline incision with implanting the graft kidney in the extraperitoneal region.

TABLE 1: Important factors determining the preference for the site of kidney graft implantation.

Factors to consider	*Preferred site for graft implantation*
Large graft size as compared to the recipient	Abdominal fossa
Previous surgeries	Opposite iliac fossa
Short ureter	Retrovesical area
Donor kidney laterality	It is always better to use the right iliac fossa; however, some surgeons also use the opposite site
Simultaneous pancreas–kidney transplantation	The pancreas is transplanted in the right iliac fossa; thus, the kidney is transplanted to the contralateral iliac fossa

- *Children:* As the kidney is mostly placed below the cecum and ascending, the right side is favored for the surgical ease of doing vascular anastomoses of the renal vessels maybe to the aorta and vena cava due to the size of the kidney.
- *Simultaneous pancreas and KT:* With the vertical midline transperitoneal method, complications such as twisting of the renal pedicle with KT thrombosis have been reported.[9] Procedures such as nephropexy or retroperitoneal implantation of the kidney graft can be done to such avoid torsion. The iliac fossa can be found by inserting an index finger into the prevesical region immediately lateral to the midline.

Incision

An oblique Rutherford Morison[10] or curvilinear incision is made in the right or left lower quadrant of the abdomen beginning in the midline and curving upward parallel to the inguinal ligament and approximately 2 cm above it and ending just above the anterior superior iliac spine of the iliac crest. In a child or small adult, this incision can be carried up to the costal margin to increase exposure.[11] **Figure 2** shows the technique of incision for adults and children.

Along the incision line, the external oblique muscle and fascia are divided and split to the wound's lateral extent. This incision is carried medially onto the rectus sheath to allow a piece of the rectus muscle to be retracted or divided, allowing the bladder to be exposed later. The internal oblique and transverse muscles are divided to expose the peritoneum. To avoid division of the internal oblique and transverse muscles, the confluence of the oblique muscles and the rectus sheath can also be divided medially, lateral to the rectus muscle as a pararectus incision.

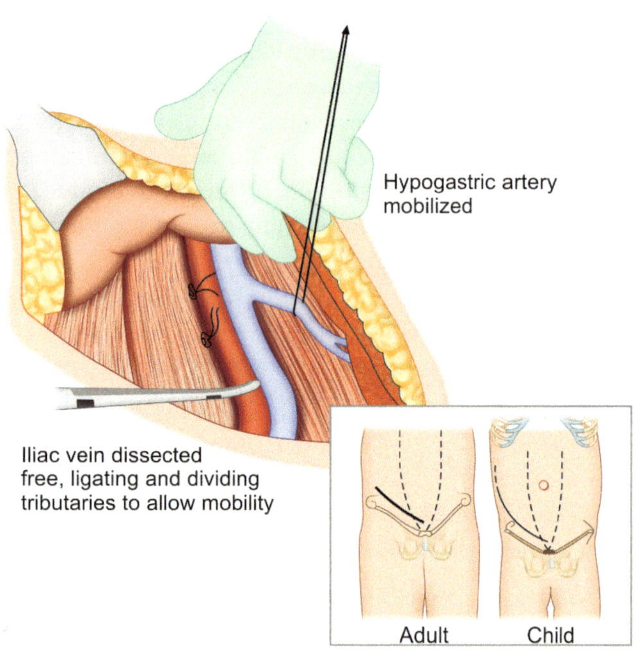

Fig. 2: Preparation of the bed in the renal recipient. Inset—incision for adult and child.
Source: Lee HM. Surgical techniques of renal transplantation. In: Morris PJ (Ed). Kidney Transplantation. London: Academic Press/Grune & Stratton; 1979. p. 146.

Note: In case there is the presence of multiple renal arteries, it is important that the inferior epigastric vessels should be preserved first.

Operative Bed Preparation

After exposing the transversalis fascia and peritoneum, the psoas muscle and iliac vessels are shown by separating the transversalis fascia and reflecting the peritoneum upward and medially. Now, a self-retaining retractor can be inserted.

Depending on whether the internal iliac artery (IIA) is to be anastomosed to the transplant kidney's renal artery or the renal artery with a cuff of aorta is to be anastomosed to the exterior iliac artery, dissection is performed first to expose the external, common, and IIA.

Ligation of Lymphatics

Ligation of lymphatics (rather than cauterizing) them that runs along and across the vessels with a nonabsorbable suture such as silk helps to avoid the development of lymphocele later.

In scenarios where the IIA is to be utilized, it is important to mobilize a section of the common and external iliac arteries (EIA) in a certain way that the IIA can be twisted laterally with no kink happening at its origin and common and EIA can be clamped if needed, for example, when the IIA is short.

After exposing the correct iliac arteries, dissection of the external iliac vein is done. If a long left renal vein is available, dissection of the external iliac vein by itself usually results in a strain-free anastomosis. If a kidney with a short renal vein is to be utilized, or if the patient is fat, the internal iliac vein and usually one or two gluteal veins can be ligated and divided with silk. The peritoneum is needed to be reflected higher up laterally to create the final pocket for the kidney in the parapsoas gutter.

Once the kidney has been prepped and is ready for implantation, the vessels are ready to be clamped. Heparin is commonly administered at a low dose of 30 IU/kg. If an end-to-side anastomosis is to be performed, vascular clamps are applied to the EIA proximally and distally, and a vascular clamp is applied to the IIA at its origin or to the common and EIA if the IIA is to be used.

After the IIA has been split distally, the lumen is flushed with heparinized saline. If the external or common iliac arteries are to be used, an arteriotomy of the proper size is made, which is then enlarged with a vascular punch and the lumen is washed out with heparinized saline. Similarly, the venotomy is flushed out with heparinized saline, and any valves present should be carefully removed. To ensure that the anastomoses are established in the best possible position, the surgeon should mentally envision the kidney in its parapsoas gutter, as well as the route that the renal artery and vein would follow, before conducting an arteriotomy or venotomy.

Kidney Preparation

In the case of a deceased donor: The kidney must be dissected to various degrees when it is received in ice. Because the kidneys are generally removed as part of an en bloc procedure, significant dissection is required in the case of a cadaver kidney. On a back table, with the kidney in a bowl of ice slush, this should be done carefully and under good lighting. Before the transplant, the cadaver kidney is dissected in case there is a defect that would prevent the surgery from going through. During the dissection, the blood supply to the ureter must be safeguarded, and the so-called golden triangle must not be crossed.

In a living donor kidney: Mostly, there is only one renal artery. In the situation of multiple renal arteries, a common trunk is formed by joining the arteries at their orifices or an end-to-side anastomosis is done between the smaller artery and a bigger renal artery on the back table. Revascularizing a lower polar artery is crucial since it is inevitably the source of ureteric blood flow. Although one can use the epigastric artery to revascularize the lower polar artery, the common practice is to do anastomosis of a lower polar artery to the major renal artery, which can be either an end-to-side anastomosis or a common trunk.

A renal artery or arteries should be cut to size and used for anastomosis to the EIA in case of an aortic patch from the deceased donor. If the two renal arteries on the aortic patch are far apart, the patch can be divided and inserted into EIA separately, or one end-to-side and the other into a branch of the IIA.

In the presence of more than one renal vein, ligation of smaller veins is done, assuming that there is only one large renal vein. There are concerns for recurrent venous infarction in case ligation of two similar renal veins not starting from a Carrel patch is done; hence, it is advised to connect the veins to establish a common trunk for the anastomosis.

The anastomoses are conducted while the kidney is still cool when it is finally ready for implantation.

This method not only keeps the kidney cool throughout the anastomosis, but also makes it easier to handle the kidney because an artery clamp may be used to hold the kidney in position on the glove itself. After the anastomoses are finished, the glove is removed and the kidney is reperfused.

Revascularization

- After preparing the implantation site, the surgeon should shift the graft to its final location transiently so that the anastomosis sites can be examined more thoroughly. The goal is to reduce the time it takes for the arterial and venous systems to clamp together.
- First, the site of each anastomosis and the position of the graft should be accurately identified based on the size and length of the arteries, the length of the ureter, the position of the recipient bladder or ureter, and the eventual position of the implanted kidney.
- The IIA and external iliac vein are used for vascular anastomoses.
- We do the arterial anastomosis first (the risk of deep vein thrombosis is involved).
  Note: The venous anastomosis should be performed first if (1) the vein is short, (2) the left iliac fossa is to be utilized for graft implantation, and (3) the abdominal cavity, inferior vena cava (IVC), aorta, or EIA are to be utilized.
- Vascular anastomosis follows the same principles as any other vascular surgery. For venous and arterial anastomosis, the optimal suture sizes are commonly 5-0 and 6-0 Prolene® sutures.
- The needle size is dictated by the anastomosis location, although taper-point or taper-cutting-tip round-bodied 3/8 circle needles with 11–13 mm length are recommended for optimal results. Smaller arteries may benefit from 7-0 or 8-0, 1/2 circle, 7–9.3 mm needles.
- Application of vascular clamps, at the starting vessel, prevents kinking or rotation. This is to be done after determining the correct length and position of the anastomosis region.
- Bulldog clamps are used on the IIA and veins, while Satinsky clamps are used on the EIA and common iliac arteries, as well as the aorta and IVC. During anastomosis, the vessels can be irrigated with heparinized saline.

ARTERIAL ANASTOMOSIS

The IIA is anastomosed end-to-end to the renal artery with a 5-0 or 6-0 monofilament vascular suture using a three-point anastomosis technique **(Fig. 3)**. If the renal artery and the IIA have a large diameter difference, the renal artery should be spatulated along one side to widen the anastomosis.

An end-to-side anastomosis of the renal artery to the EIA is frequently performed using an aortic cuff attached to the renal artery that has been properly trimmed.

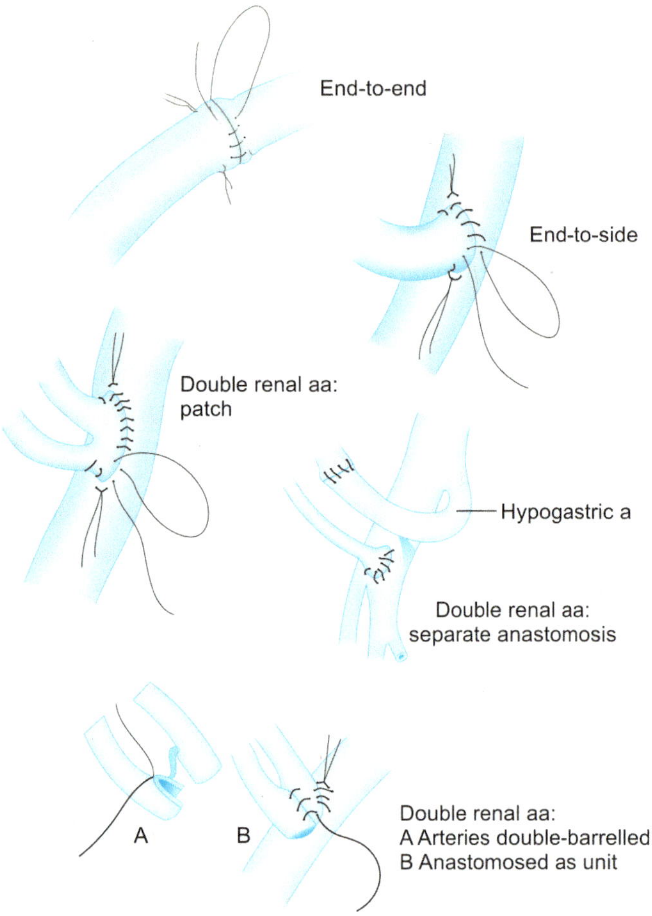

Fig. 3: Variations of the renal artery anastomoses (aa).

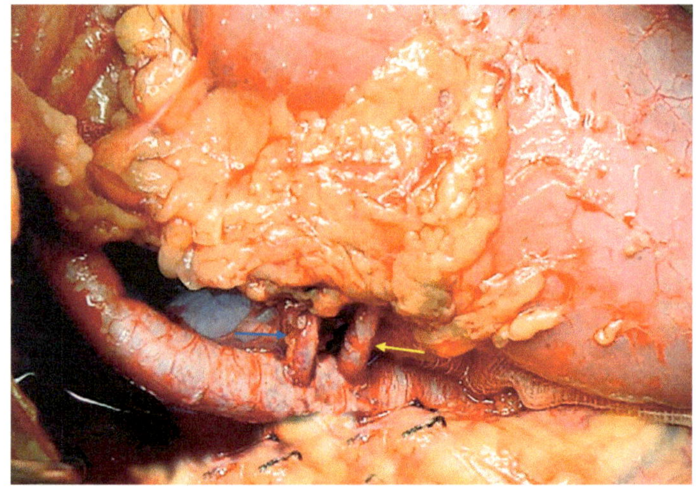

Fig. 4: Two renal arteries in a donor being anastomosed sequentially. The two arteries (yellow and blue arrows) are frequently implanted individually to the external or common iliac artery.
Source: Humar A, Matas AJ. Atlas of Organ Transplantation; 2018.

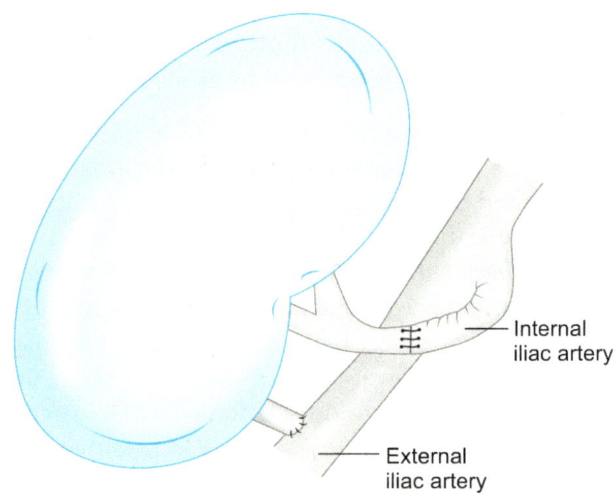

Fig. 5: Two renal arteries being joined on the bench and then being anastomosed in the recipient.

If necessary, an arteriotomy is performed in the EIA, and the anastomosis is finished with a continuous 5-0 or 6-0 monofilament vascular suture **(Figs. 4 to 7)**.

Anastomosis of the renal artery to hypogastric artery: At least one-third of the anastomosis should have interrupted sutures to allow for growth if both arteries are small.

VENOUS ANASTOMOSIS

An end-to-side anastomosis is usually done between the renal vein and the external iliac vein with a continuous 5-0 monofilament vascular suture. The initial sutures are placed at either end of the venotomy **(Fig. 8)**.

A crucial component of this method is the placement of an anchor suture at the midpoint of the lateral wall, which allows the EIV and renal vein on the lateral side of the anastomosis to be brought clear of the medial wall of the anastomosis. While the medial wall is being sutured, this approach reduces the chance of the rear wall becoming entangled in the suture. The anastomosis can connect the renal vein to the external iliac vein lateral or medial to the EIA.

If the external and common iliac veins have been mobilized, the venous anastomosis can usually be done medial to the artery, even if the vein is short. Regardless of where the anastomosis is made, it is vital to verify that the renal vein is not twisted or under tension before initiating the anastomosis.

Note: When an adult kidney is being transplanted into a small child receives, the renal vein is needed to be shortened to avoid kinking, especially if the vein is anastomosed to the IVC.

We tie the last suture loosely and leave a "growth factor" or "expansion factor" in all other continuous anastomoses (artery or vein) to avoid the purse-string effect of the continuous suture on constricting the anastomosis, as first described by Starzl in the portal anastomosis of liver transplantation.

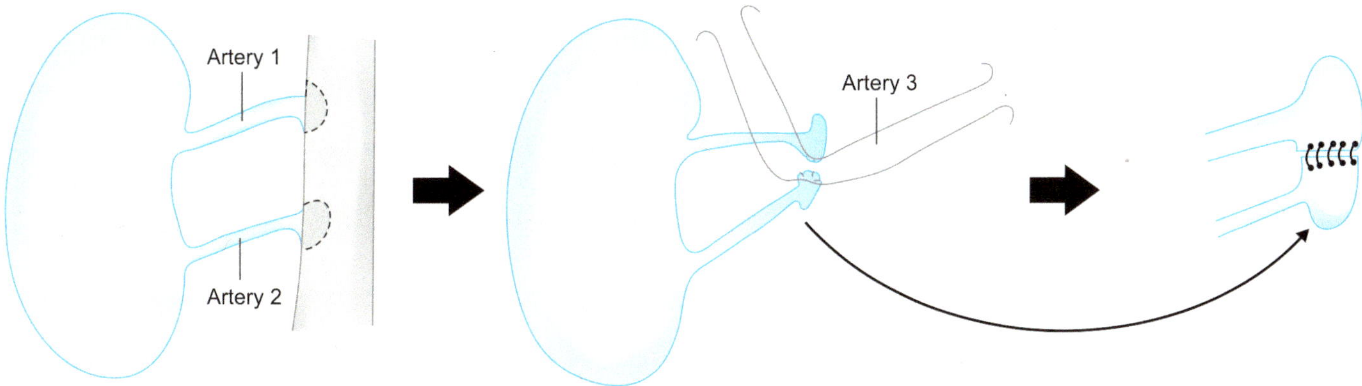

Fig. 6: Three renal arteries in a donor. Artery 1 and 2 have been joined on a common patch whereas artery 3 has been joined end to side to artery 1.

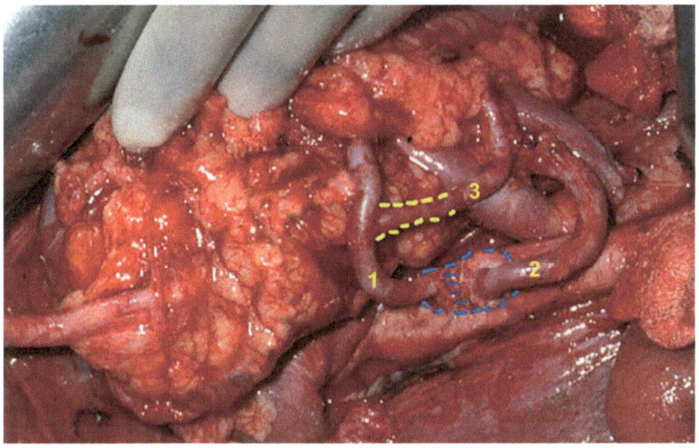

Fig. 7: Connecting one vessel to the other in an end-to-side arrangement is another option. Arteries 1 and 2 have been sewed together with a common patch (broken blue line) in this example with three renal arteries, whereas artery 3 has been anastomosed to artery 1 in an end-to-side method (broken yellow line).
Source: Humar A, Matas AJ. Atlas of Organ Transplantation; 2018.

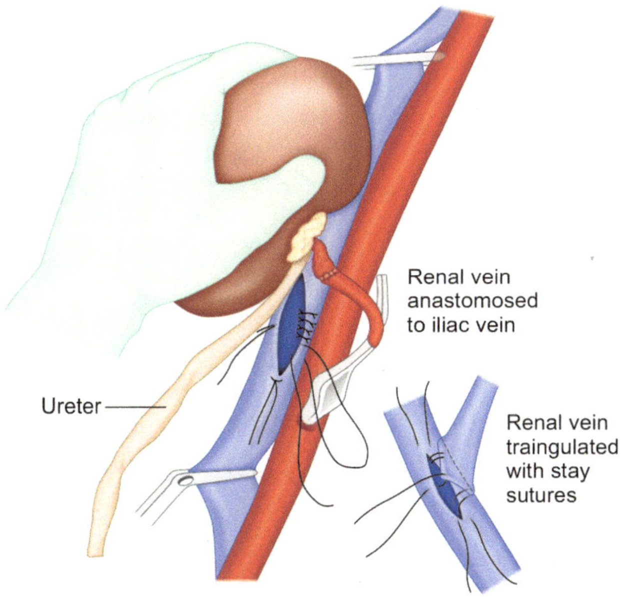

Fig. 8: Vein anastomosis with triangular stay sutures in place.

RECONSTRUCTION OF THE URINARY TRACT

The graft kidney is positioned at its ultimate surgical location after renal revascularization followed by restoration of urinary tract continuity. When the left kidney is transplanted into the right iliac fossa and the right kidney is transplanted into the left iliac fossa, the normal anterior-to-posterior relationship of the vein, artery, and collecting system is reversed, and the renal pelvis and ureter of the KT are the most medial and superficial of the hilar structures.[6]

Note: Common factors on which the approach to urinary tract reconstruction depends upon are:
- Length and condition of the donor ureter
- Status of the recipient's bladder or bladder substitute
- Condition of the recipient's ureter
- Surgeon's familiarity with the technique.

The suture material is a matter of personal choice. Synthetic absorbable sutures are now available and have features that are beneficial to immunocompromised KT recipients who may have delayed wound healing.[12] We use 3-0 for bladder closure and 4-0 or 5-0 for ureteric or renal pelvic anastomoses, and polydioxanone has proven to be sufficient.

Ureteroneocystostomy

The most common type of urinary tract restoration is ureteroneocystostomy. Its benefits are as follows:
- It can be done regardless of the recipient ureter's quality or existence.
- The vascular anastomoses are several centimeters away.
- The original ureter can still be used to treat ureteric problems.
- A native nephrectomy is not required.

The most common approach used for ureter reimplantation into the bladder is by using the Lich-Gregoir technique, in which the ureter is reimplanted extravesically. The goal is to make a 2–3 cm submucosal tunnel with ureter muscle backing, so that when the bladder contracts, a valve prevents urine from refluxing up the ureter.[13-16]

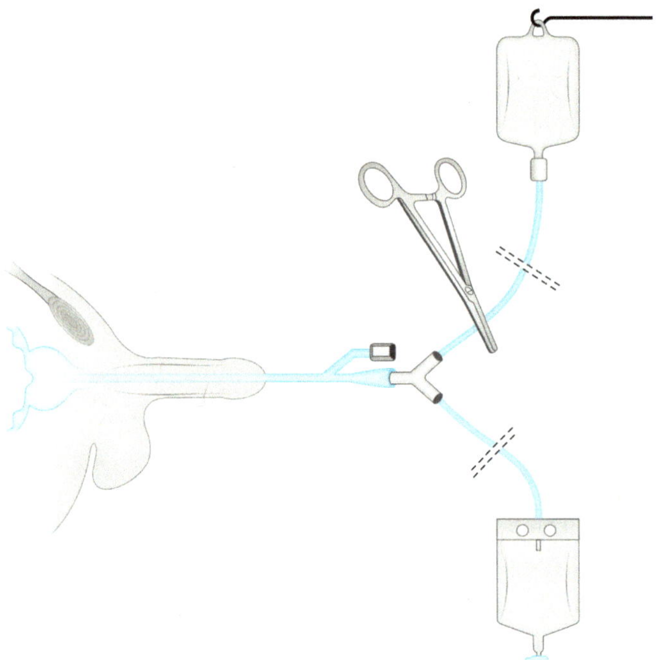

Fig. 9: Y-tube system for rinsing, filling, and draining bladder or bladder substitute.

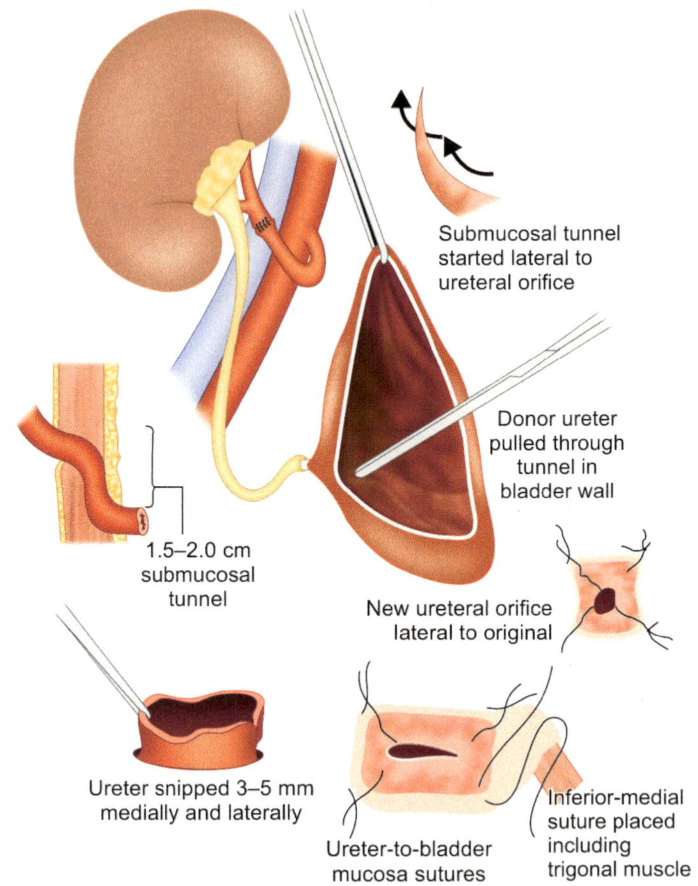

Fig. 10: Steps of transvesical ureteroneocystostomy.
Source: Lee DM. Surgical techniques of renal transplantation. In: Morris PJ (Ed). Kidney Transplantation. London: Academic Press/ Grune & Stratton; 1979. p. 153.

A few examples of other less frequently used approaches are:

- Barry technique
- The single-stitch Taguchi technique
- Intravesical Leadbetter–Politano technique.

A sterile Y-tube system connects the lubricated balloon retention catheter to the Y-tube system.[17] **Figure 9** shows the Y-tube system for rinsing, filling, and draining bladder or bladder substitute.

On one line there is an antibiotic solution bag and on the other a collection bag. This approach allows the bladder to be filled, irrigated, drained, and refilled during the operation. This technique is particularly beneficial when the urinary bladder is hard to locate due to scar tissue in the pelvis, an obese recipient, or diminished capacity.[18]

Steps of transvesical ureteroneocystostomy are shown in **Figure 10**.

Extravesical Ureteroneocystostomy

Extravesical techniques are speedier than transvesical operations because they do not require a separate cystotomy and require less ureteric length. These parameters should cut down on operating time, bladder spasms, and hematuria, as well as increase the chances of a good distal ureteric blood supply **(Figs. 11 and 12)**.[19]

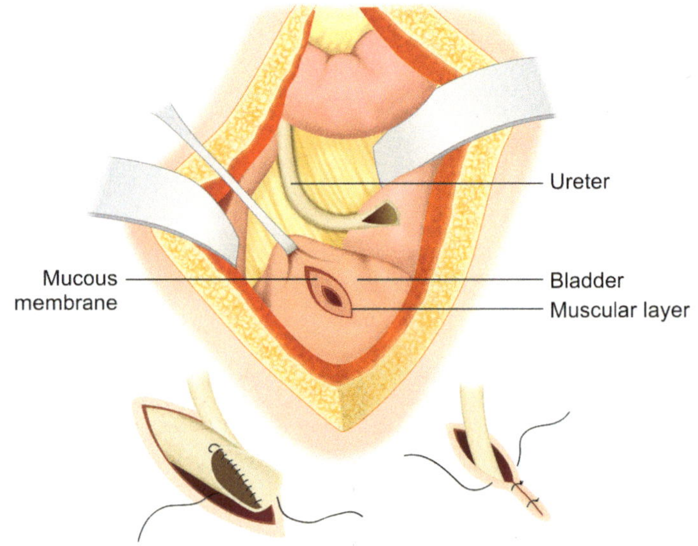

Fig. 11: Extravesical ureteroneocystostomy.

Catheter and Stent Management

During ureteral anastomosis, an indwelling stent is placed in most cases. In the majority of transplant centers, the urinary bladder or reservoir catheter is removed after 3–5 days following the transplant surgery. The stent is usually removed in an outpatient clinic 6–12 weeks later.

CLOSURE

Closure methods may vary, but the commonly used procedure is:

Skin closure with subcuticular nylon or polyglactin, as well as loop nylon in two layers—internal oblique and transverse muscles followed by external oblique muscles.

Drainage is a debatable topic since it has the potential to allow microorganisms to enter. If drainage is required, it should be a suction-only system with drains removed as quickly as practicable. Every day, the drain's exit point is cleaned with an antibiotic solution and dressed until it is no longer visible.

The excess perirenal fat is removed, and the graft is placed in a retroperitoneally created pouch parallel to the psoas muscle. This approach prevents compression of the graft between the abdominal wall and the pelvic bones.

Note: Inability to recover abdominal muscles adequately can lead to "compartment syndrome" if the kidney's capacity surpasses this gap or the renal vasculature or ureter is shorter than normal. Such a situation results in good renal artery input but disturbed outflow due to abdominal wall strain on the renal vein. Eventually, blockage of the graft leads to decreased urinary flow with elevated renal venous pressure. The final result would be reduced renal artery flow followed by thrombosis, and subsequently, transplant failure.

In case repositioning the graft in the supravesical location and anchoring it to the abdominal wall is not possible without causing vascular kinking, the following options can be considered.

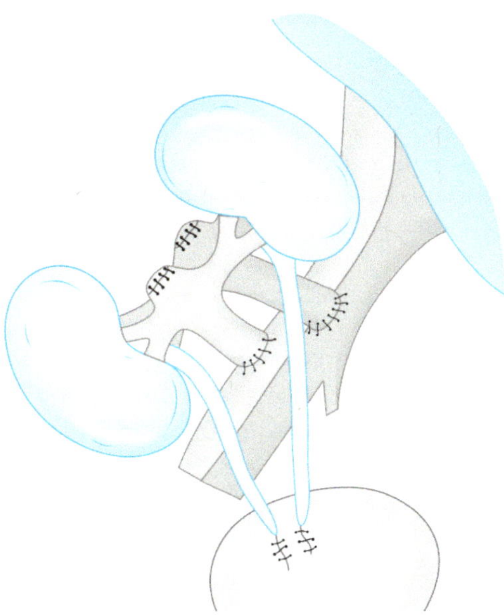

Fig. 12: Transplantation of pediatric kidneys into an adult. The anastomoses are conducted on the recipient's iliac vessels. The two ureters can be anastomosed into the recipient's bladder independently.

- Incise the rectus sheath after the muscles have been closed.
- Close the abdominal wall from the distal to the proximal end, and the area covering the kidney can be left open or closed with a hernia repair mesh.
- Expose the abdominal musculature completely, with only the skin protecting it. The resultant incisional hernia can be repaired later, usually 3 months after the transplant.

Such complications can be avoided by matching the size of donor and recipient, carefully examining the lengths of the graft's vasculature and ureter, and constructing the pouch at earlier stages (preferably the first step).

SURGICAL VARIATIONS

Pediatric Recipient Kidney Transplant

The surgical techniques for kidney transplantation in children, particularly in older children, are fairly similar to those described for adult recipients.

We favor an intraperitoneal method with a kidney from an adult-sized living donor for individuals weighing <20 kg. The kidney is located behind the right colon on the right side **(Figs. 13 to 17)**. The distal aorta and cava are usually anastomosed.

Pediatric Donor En Bloc Kidneys

Adult receivers can get kidneys from small pediatric donors (weighing <15 kg). However, in this case, both kidneys should be transplanted together into the same recipient.

Multiple Renal Arteries

In 10–15% of instances, several renal arteries are present. Reconstruction possibilities vary on the basis of the size

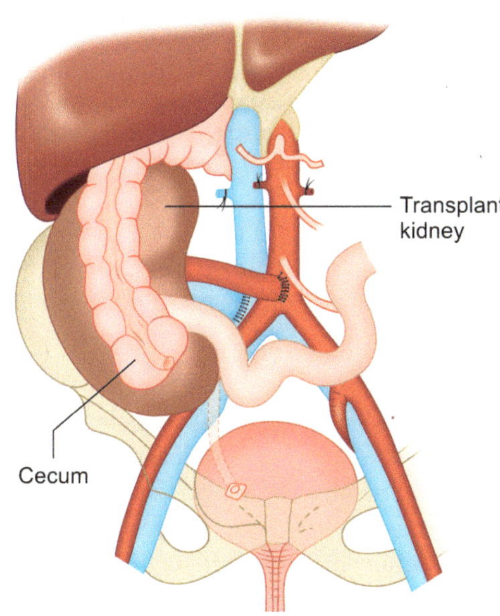

Fig. 13: Pediatric recipient kidney transplant.

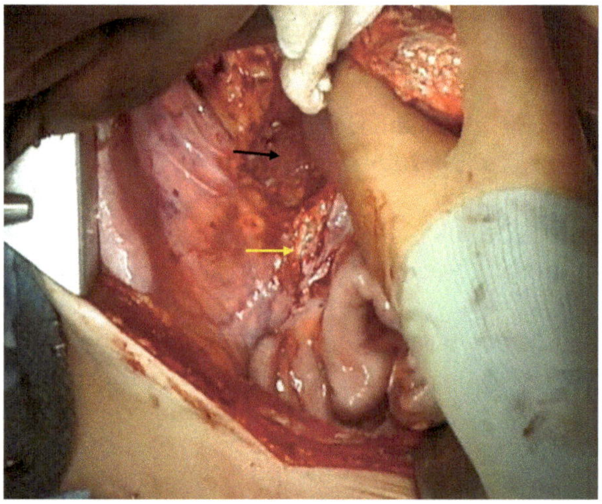

Fig. 14: Transplantation in children. To enter the peritoneal cavity, the surgery begins with a large midline incision. The right colon is mobilized and reflected medially to reveal the right retroperitoneal region, which includes the psoas muscle (black arrow) and the distal aorta/proximal iliac arteries (yellow arrow).
Source: Humar A, Matas AJ. Atlas of Organ Transplantation; 2018.

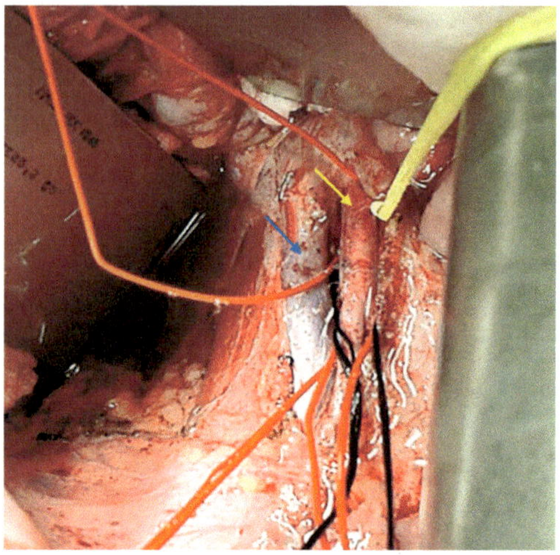

Fig. 15: Preparation of the vessels in a child. Isolate and encircle the infrarenal cava (blue arrow), infrarenal aorta (yellow arrow), and proximal iliac arteries.
Source: Humar A, Matas AJ. Atlas of Organ Transplantation; 2018.

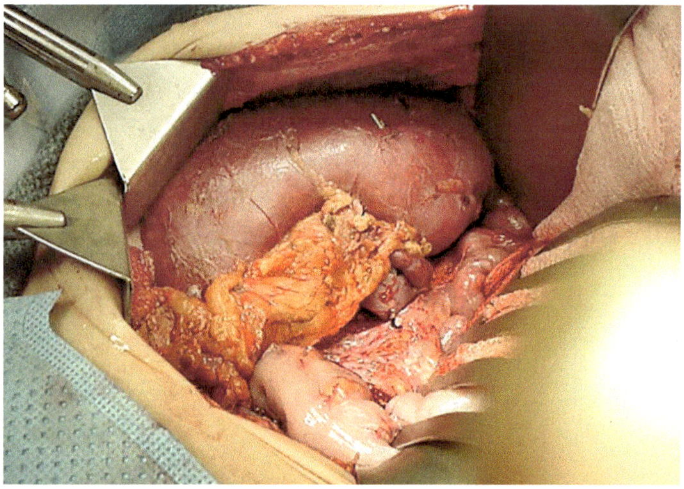

Fig. 16: Renal transplantation in a child. The renal artery is anastomosed to the distal aorta and the renal vein is anastomosed to the distal cava in the same way that it is for adult patients. Adult bladder anastomoses, as previously indicated, can also be performed. After that, the colon is placed in front of the transplanted kidney in its proper location. The incision is then stitched up.
Source: Humar A, Matas AJ. Atlas of Organ Transplantation; 2018.

of the vessels, their location, the donor source (alive vs. deceased), and the quality of the recipient's vessels.

Horseshoe Kidney

In these circumstances, abnormal vasculature is the norm. Ectopic kidneys that are crossed-fused or non-fused have the same issue. One way to deal with such a situation is to incise the isthmus between the two conjoined kidneys and then use each kidney in a separate recipient.

In this condition, two grafts with complicated vascular anatomy and short and numerous ureters are the key issues. Most centers prefer this strategy due to the scarcity of donor organs. However, separating the horseshoe kidney might be difficult at times and can harm both kidneys. In these circumstances, it is preferable to treat the aberrant kidney as a separate graft, with the aorta and IVC serving as the graft's arterial inflow and venous outflow, respectively.

Because such massive grafts cannot be inserted retroperitoneally, they must be implanted in the intraperitoneal area. Other vascular abnormalities that complicate the transplantation operation include circumaortic or retroaortic

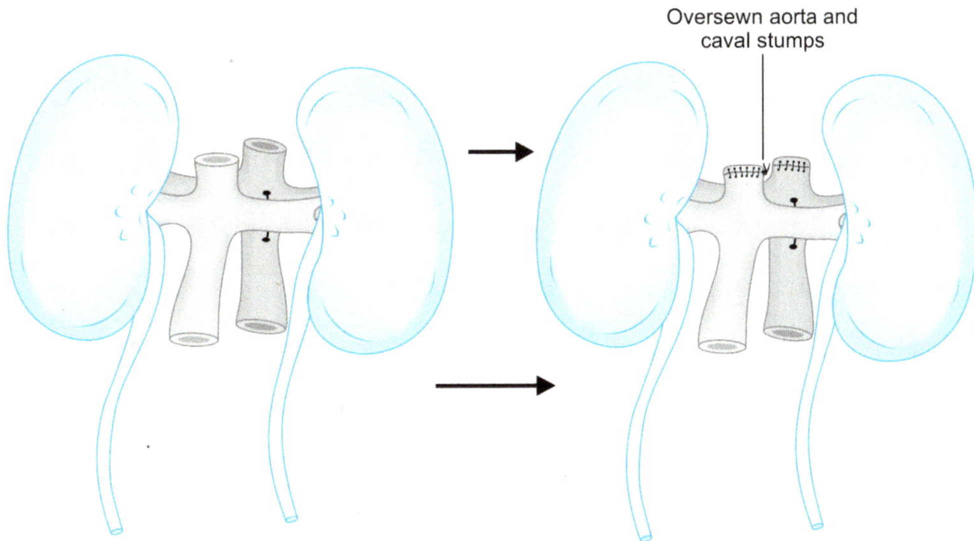

Fig. 17: Preparation of pediatric donor kidneys for use in an adult. On the back table, the kidneys are being prepared. The aorta and cava, as well as the two kidneys, are left intact. The cava and aorta's proximal ends are oversewn. The anastomoses to the recipient's vessels can then be performed using the distal ends.

renal veins. Even from a living donor, these anomalies are not a contraindication for donation in the hands of skilled hands. Because huge grafts cannot be introduced retroperitoneally, they have to be placed intraperitoneally.

REFERENCES

1. Kakaei F, Nikeghbalian S, Malekhosseini SA. Kidney transplantation techniques. In: Rath T (Ed). Current Issues and Future Direction in Kidney Transplantation. London: IntechOpen; 2013.
2. Humar A, Matas AJ. Atlas of Organ Transplantation. Springer; 2018.
3. Brazilian Society of Urology, Silvinato A, Bernardo WM, Santos LS. Guidelines in focus. Rev Assoc Med Bras. 2018; 64(12).
4. Mandal AK, Cohen C, Montgomery RA, Kavoussi LR, Ratner LE. Should the indications for laparascopic live donor nephrectomy of the right kidney be the same as for the open procedure? Anomalous left renal vasculature is not a contraindication to laparoscopic left donor nephrectomy. Transplantation. 2001;71(5):660-4.
5. IntechOpen. (2013). Current issues and future direction in kidney transplantation. [online] Available from https://www.intechopen.com/books/3257 [Last accessed September, 2022].
6. Hameed AM, Yao J, Allen RDM, Hawthorne WJ, Pleass HC, Lau H. The evolution of kidney transplantation surgery into the robotic era and its prospects for obese recipients. Transplantation. 2018;102:1650-65.
7. Hume DM, Magee JH, Kauffman HM, Rittenbury MS, Prout Jr GR. Renal homotransplantation in man in modified recipients. Ann Surg. 1963;158:608-41.
8. Kuss R, Tsenturier J, Milliez P. Quelgues essais de greffos du rein chez l'homme. Med Acad Chir. 1951;77:755.
9. Merrill JP, Murray JE, Harrison JH. Successful homotransplantation of the human kidney between two identical twins. JAMA. 1956;160:277.
10. Michon L, Hamburger J, Oeconomos N, Delinotte P, Richet G, Vaysse J, et al. Une tentative de transplantation renale chez l'homme aspects medicaux et abiologiques. Presse Med. 1953;61:1419.
11. Starzl TE, Marchioro TL. Technique of renal homotransplantation: experience with 42 cases. Arch Surg. 1964; 89:87.
12. West MS, Stevens RB, Metrakos P, Foshager MC, Jessurun J, Sutherland DE, et al. Renal pedicle torsion after simultaneous kidney-pancreas transplantation. J Am Coll Surg. 1998; 187:80.
13. Lawrie R. Surgery of access to the abdomen. In: Rob C, Smith R, Morgan CN (Eds). Operative Surgery, 2nd edition. Philadelphia: JB Lippincott; 1969. p. 16.
14. Lee HM. Surgical techniques of renal transplantation. In: Morris PJ (Ed). Kidney Transplantation. London: Academic Press/Grune & Stratton; 1979. p. 145.
15. Rosen NA, McAninch JW. Wound closures and suture techniques in reconstructive procedures. In: McAninch JW (Ed). Traumatic and Reconstructive Urology. Philadelphia: WB Saunders; 1996. p. 49.
16. Lich R, Howerton LW, David LA. Recurrent urosepsis in children. J Urol. 1961;86:554.
17. Paquin Jr AJ. Ureterovesical anastomosis: the description and evaluation of a technique. J Urol. 1959;82:573.
18. Politano VA, Leadbetter WF. An operative technique for the correction of vesicoureteral reflux. J Urol. 1958;79:932.
19. Stevens AR, Marshall VF. Reimplantation of the ureter into the bladder. Surg Gynecol Obstet. 1943;77:585.
20. Kootstra G. Kidney transplantation. In: Kremer B, Broelsch CE, Henne-Bruns D (Eds). Atlas of Liver, Pancreas, and Kidney Transplantation. Stuttgart: Georg Thieme Verlag; 1994. p. 128.
21. Barry JM, Lemmers MJ, Meyer MM, De Mattos A, Bennett WM, Norman DJ. Cadaver kidney transplantation in patients more than 65 years old. World J Urol. 1996; 14:243.

CHAPTER 5

Surgical and Vascular Complications After Kidney Transplantation

Aneesh Srivastava, Akshay Kriplani

INTRODUCTION

Complications after renal transplant form an important part of the natural course of post-transplant events and can have a significant bearing on the graft outcome. With improved understanding of pre- and post-transplant workup, surgical techniques, and immunosuppression protocols, surgical complications have reduced significantly, with the current incidence of 2.9–12.5%.[1,2] Surgical complications can be classified into urological, vascular, or lymphatic complications.[3,4] Ureteric obstruction and urinary leak are major urological complications. Common post-transplant vascular complications include renal artery thrombosis, renal vein thrombosis, and renal artery stenosis. Lymphatic complications can have a wide clinical spectrum from lymphorrhea to the formation of lymphoceles. In the clinical setting of graft dysfunction, these complications should be ruled out based on their specific clinical features and the timeline of presentation. In this chapter, the common surgical complications have been classified and summarized as per their usual timeline of presentation **(Table 1)** to provide a clear guidance to the transplant surgeons for a targeted follow-up care.

INTRAOPERATIVE COMPLICATIONS

EXTERNAL ILIAC ARTERY DISSECTION

External iliac artery dissection is a rare complication of renal transplantation, mostly occurring intraoperatively but can even present in the immediate or early postoperative period. Dissection can be either at the site of anastomosis **(Fig. 1)** or at the site of vascular clamping. Plaque rupture in atherosclerotic vessels at the site of vascular clamping or improper suturing during anastomosis leads to endothelial injury, intimal flap, and medial dissection. Other risk factors include male gender, diabetes, hypertension, collagen vascular disorder, and polycystic kidney disease.[5] Improper graft perfusion after declamping with no palpable pulse or flow on Doppler ultrasound in the distal external iliac artery is usually diagnostic.[6] Urgent intervention, i.e., graft explantation and reperfusion with thrombus evacuation from the iliac artery, is required to restore graft and lower limb perfusion. Modalities of repair include excision of the pathological segment with reconstruction using a synthetic or autologous vascular graft or endovascular stenting. Endarterectomy with intimal tacking has also been reported.[6] Preventive measures include the selection of soft segments free of plaques for anastomosis, application of soft clamps, and ensuring inclusion of intimal layer during suturing **(Fig. 2)**.

RENAL ARTERY KINK

Long donor renal artery (such as right kidney with short renal vein and longer renal artery), end-to-end anastomosis with long internal iliac artery stump **(Figs. 3A and B)**, end-to-side anastomosis on the too lateral or too medial wall of the external iliac artery, malalignment of vessels in recipients

TABLE 1: Common post-transplant surgical complications with the expected timeline of presentation.

Intraoperative complications	*0–6 hours*	*6 hours–7 days*	*1 week–2 months*	*2 months onward*
External iliac artery dissection	Renal allograft compartment syndrome	Perigraft hematoma	Ureteral leak	Ureteric obstruction
Renal artery kink	Graft torsion	Renal vein thrombosis	Lymphocele	Renal artery stenosis
Venous outflow obstruction		Renal artery thrombosis	Pseudoaneurysm	Vesicoureteral reflux
			Paratransplant hernia	Incisional hernia
			Wound complications	

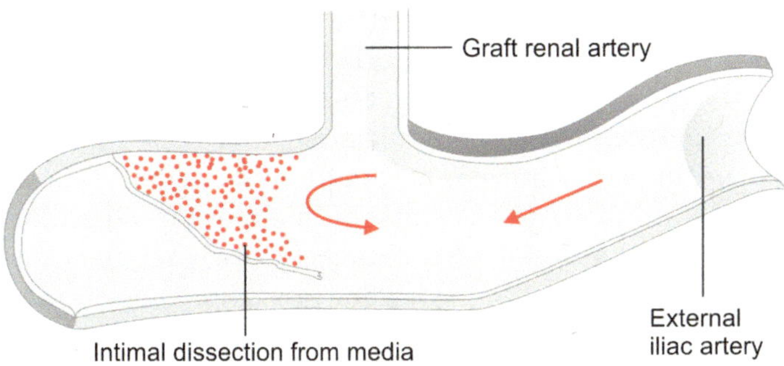

Fig. 1: Dissection of intima from media at the anastomotic site of renal artery with external iliac artery.

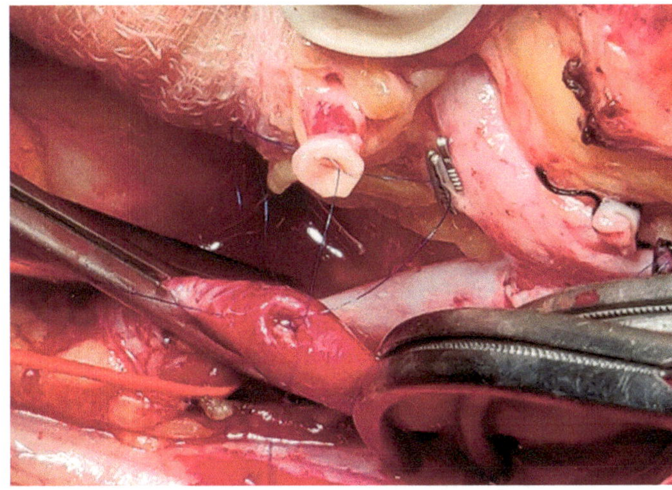

Fig. 2: Deep bites including the intima in atherosclerotic donor and recipient artery to avoid dissection.

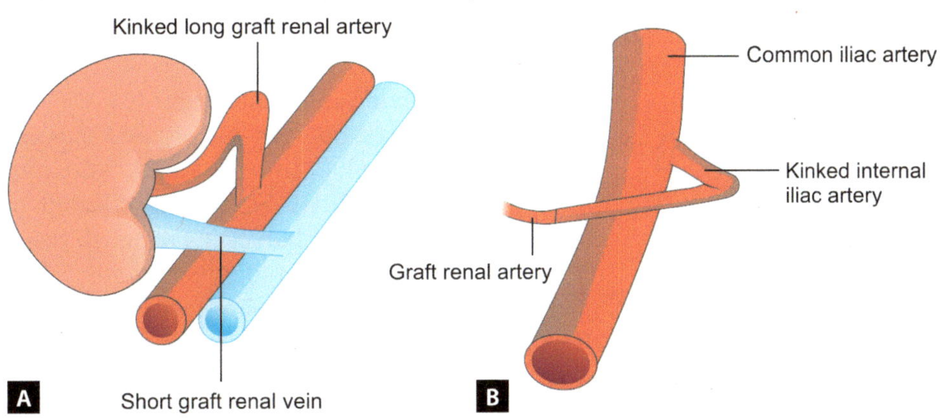

Figs. 3A and B: (A) Kink of long right renal artery after end-to-side anastomosis with external iliac artery; (B) Kink of long internal iliac artery after end-to-end anastomosis with graft renal artery.

with narrow pelvis, thin/short recipients receiving large kidneys, and too distal vascular anastomosis are common predisposing factors for renal artery kink.[7] In most cases, the kink is mild and seldom causes graft hypoperfusion, but rarely acute kink, especially during abdominal closure to accommodate the graft, leads to sudden decreased urine output. Uncorrected kinks cause turbulence potentially leading to artery thrombosis or stenosis.[8,9] Arterial bruit over the graft can raise the clinical suspicion, but Doppler ultrasound [elevated kinked artery peak systolic velocity (PSV) >3.5 times than iliac artery and post-stenotic parvus et tardus pattern],[9] computed tomography (CT) or magnetic resonance (MR) angiography or digital subtraction angiography (DSA) is usually diagnostic. Percutaneous transluminal renal angioplasty (PTEA) with intra-arterial stenting reestablishes graft perfusion.[10] Rarely surgical graft repositioning and nephropexy are required.

VENOUS OUTFLOW OBSTRUCTION

Kinking or rotation of a long left donor renal vein, compressed short right renal vein, apposition of walls during suturing, inclusion of valve cusps in the anastomosis, or ligation of significant caliber second renal vein can lead to poor venous outflow and graft congestion and necessitates anastomotic revision.

CHAPTER HIGHLIGHTS

- Surgical (urological, vascular, or lymphatic) complications can have a significant bearing on the graft outcome
- During graft dysfunction evaluation, surgical complications should be ruled out based on their specific clinical features and the timeline of presentation **(Table 1)**
- Lack of awareness and standard diagnostic protocol precludes early identification and prompt management of renal allograft compartment syndrome (RACS)
- Renal artery stenosis is the most common vascular complication after renal transplantation (1–23%)

POSTOPERATIVE COMPLICATIONS

0–6 HOURS

Renal Allograft Compartment Syndrome

Early graft dysfunction due to ischemic injury and extrinsic compression on the graft has a reported incidence of 1–2%.[11,12] Lack of awareness of this entity leads to underreporting and, therefore, forms an important cause of delayed graft function. Lack of standard diagnostic protocol precludes early identification and prompt management. Size mismatch between graft and recipient fossa leads to a cascade of events during the closure of abdominal layers **(Flowchart 1)**[12] resulting in graft dysfunction. Classical presentation is a sudden fall in urine output after abdominal wall closure under tension to accommodate a large-for-space graft (adult kidney in a pediatric patient). Immediate decompression is needed to restore graft perfusion, and tension-free abdominal closure can be achieved by mesh repair, fasciotomy, anterior rectus sheath flap closure **(Figs. 4A to C)**, or intraperitonealization of graft.[13-15]

6 HOURS TO 7 DAYS

Perigraft Hematoma

Bleeding after renal transplantation is common (0.2–14%)[16] and multifactorial with common sites being bleeding from anastomotic sites, graft perihilar vessels, retroperitoneal veins, drain insertion site, and slipped ligature of deep circumflex iliac vein.[16] In case of anastomosis of the second renal artery with inferior epigastric artery, small missed branches of the inferior epigastric artery may be in spasm initially and bleed postoperatively.

Postoperative persistent tachycardia, hypotension requiring ionotropic support, high drain output, falling urine output, serial drop in hemoglobin level, and perigraft pain are clinical indicators of an ongoing hemorrhage causing a compressing perigraft hematoma. These indicators are enough to necessitate immediate surgical reexploration, but Doppler ultrasound and plain CT scan can be supportive imaging to identify the hematoma **(Fig. 5)**. On the other hand, a clinically inapparent expanding hematoma in a closed extraperitoneal space is another cause of compartment syndrome leading to a fall in urine output.

Sometimes diffuse oozing, probably due to various medical factors, obviate any specific major bleeding point but mere clot evacuation relieves the pressure in the extraperitoneal space improving the output immediately.

Flowchart 1: Cascade of events during renal allograft compartment syndrome (RACS) leading to ischemic injury.

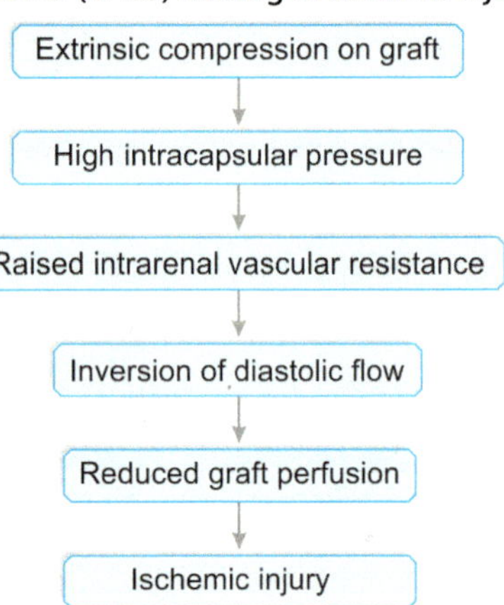

Vascular Thrombosis

Thrombotic complications (0.5–6%)[17,18] have a multifactorial etiology but can be broadly classified by being due to endothelial injury, stasis, and hypercoagulable state (Virchow's triad). Technical errors such as graft intimal injury during harvesting or bench preparation, inappropriate recipient arteriotomy or venotomy, recipient intimal injury or flaps, inadequate inclusion of intima during suturing, suturing of the opposite vessel wall, plaque rupture in atherosclerotic vessels, vascular kinking or graft torsion, and wide disparity in vessel size commonly predispose to activate the Virchow's triad. External compression by hematoma or lymphocele can also be contributory. Vascular complications are comparatively more in right-sided graft kidneys probably due to short renal vein and/or lengthening procedures for a tension-free anastomosis.[18,19] Intravascular hypovolemia, acute tubular necrosis (ATN), and early vascular rejection are important predisposing factors; therefore, adequate fluid resuscitation, reducing ischemia time, and early diagnosis and management of rejection should be ensured. Recipients with a history

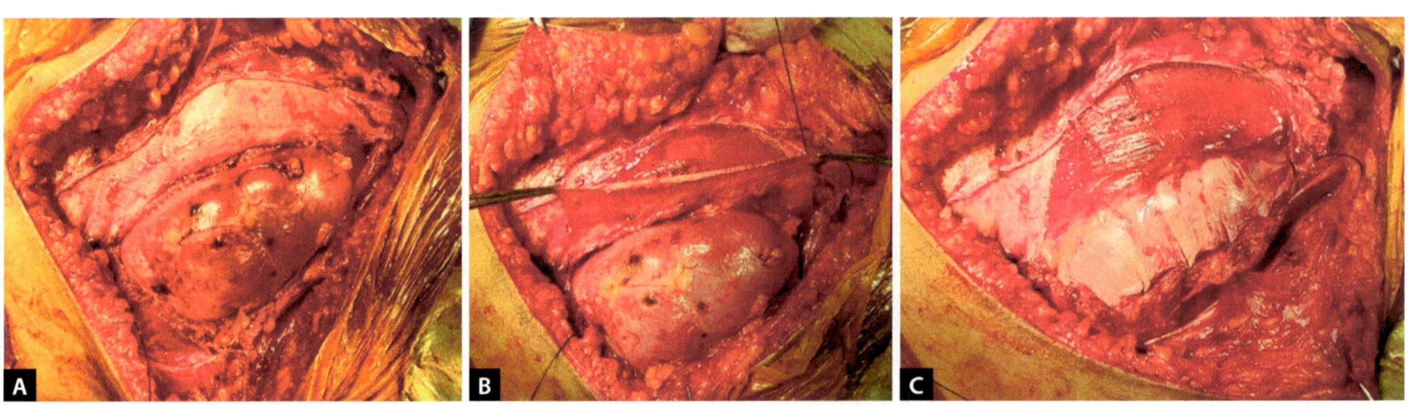

Figs. 4A to C: (A) Difficult abdominal wall closure for a large-for-space graft; (B) Anterior rectus sheath flap raised to cover the graft; (C) Tension-free closure of anterior rectus sheath flap and internal oblique and transversus abdominus muscle.

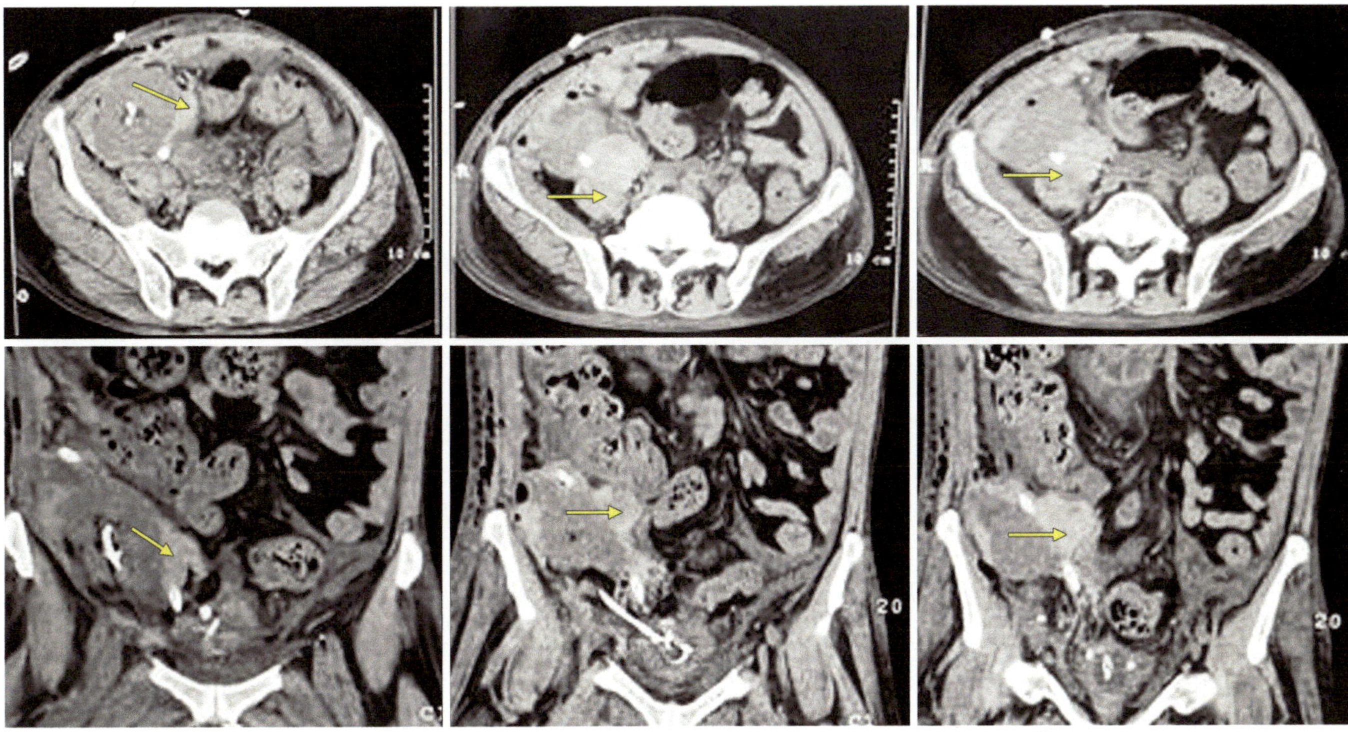

Fig. 5: A 50-year-old male post-ABO-incompatible (ABOi) transplant developed tachycardia, hypotension, increasing ionotropic requirement, and fall in urine output. Plain computed tomography (CT) at 7 hours post-transplant showing perigraft hematoma (arrows).

of multiple failed arteriovenous fistulas, thrombosed central venous dialysis catheters, deep vein thrombosis, or family history of thrombotic events should be screened for hypercoagulable states such as protein C, protein S, antithrombin III deficiency, factor V Leiden mutation, acquired antiphospholipid antibody (APLA), anticardiolipin, and lupus antibody. Calcineurin inhibitors, especially cyclosporin, are prothrombotic and should be switched to mammalian target of rapamycin (mTOR) inhibitors in case of thrombotic events.[20]

Renal Vein Thrombosis

With a prevalence of 0.1–4.2%[3,17,21] renal vein thrombosis can be a dramatic early vascular complication. Extreme graft site pain, rapid onset oliguria, and hematuria are classical signs. Ultrasound shows an enlarged graft with a perigraft hematoma due to venous congestion and graft rupture. Color Doppler findings include absence of venous flow and plateau-like reversed diastolic flow waveform in the renal artery.[20] Magnetic resonance venography is accurate but seldom used.[22] Immediate surgical reexploration is mandated, venotomy and thrombectomy to salvage the graft are not always successful thereby requiring graft nephrectomy.[23] Percutaneous transluminal angioplasty (PTA) with or without thrombolysis for early and partial thrombosis has been reported.[22,24]

Renal Artery Thrombosis

Commonly considered as a "silent" cause of early graft loss with a prevalence of 0.5–3.5%.[17,22] Sudden fall in urine output, rise in serum creatinine, and worsening hypertension in an otherwise asymptomatic recipient with no or low flow in renal artery or intrarenal branches on color Doppler are diagnostic.[23] Digital subtraction angiography or MR angiography can be confirmatory. Immediate surgical exploration is a rule. Arteriotomy, thrombectomy, and in situ graft reperfusion should be attempted. Rarely the graft is salvageable if reperfused successfully, but commonly allograft nephrectomy is inevitable. Catheter-directed thrombolysis has been attempted,[25,26] but unclear success rate and bleeding complications make it less favorable. High index of suspicion for early diagnosis based on clinical and radiological assessment is paramount.

1 WEEK TO 2 MONTHS

Ureteral Leak

Ureteral complications after renal transplant are common (2.9–21%)[27,28] and include ureteral leak or ureteral obstruction. Ureteral leak (0–9.3%)[29,30] can be due to technical or nontechnical etiology. Leak due to surgical errors usually presents early (first 24 hours) while those due to ureteric ischemia or necrosis occur within the first 14 days.[31,32] Surgical errors such as completely skeletonizing the ureter, ureteric injury during graft retrieval, faulty ureteroneocystostomy suturing, and inadvertent bladder injury are usually responsible. The most common site of leak is vesicoureteric anastomotic site, and rarely bladder injury. Proximal ureter/pelvis injury, or calyceal leak due to localized renal infarction due to ligated accessory artery may also contribute.[32] Laparoscopic donor nephrectomy does not

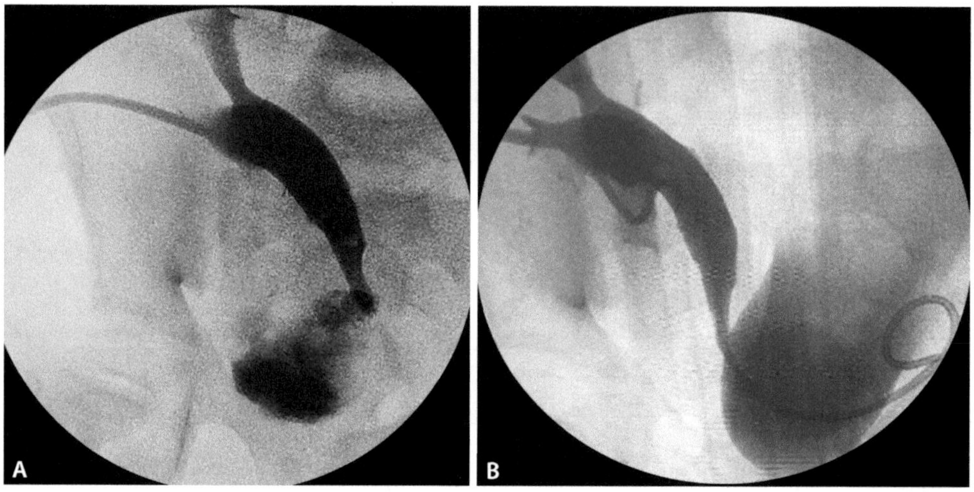

Figs. 6A and B: A 12-year-old girl on postoperative day (POD) 14 developed graft site pain and sudden fall in urine output after double-J (DJ) stent removal. Ultrasound and plain computed tomography (CT) showed perigraft collection. (A) Percutaneous nephrostomy and antegrade nephrostogram demonstrating leak and its (B) resolution after prolonged DJ stenting and indwelling Foley catheter.

increase the risk of ureteral complications.[33,34] Preservation of the periureteric fat (golden triangle) and lower pole accessory renal artery during donor nephrectomy and keeping the ureter short and tension-free before ureterovesical stented anastomosis, with pink bleeding lower margins, ensure proper vascularity. Extravesical (Lich–Gregoir) stented anastomosis has a comparatively lower incidence of ischemic ureteral complications compared to intravesical Politano–Leadbetter anastomosis.[35,36] Nontechnical risk factors include older donors, pediatric or elderly recipients, high immunosuppression in ABOi or 6/6 human leukocyte antigen (HLA) mismatch transplants, post-transplant anemia, hypoalbuminemia, or hyperglycemia.[37-40] A sudden increase in drain output with a fall in urine output is the classical presentation. High drain fluid creatinine level confirms the diagnosis. Leak can be demonstrated on CT cystogram, single-photon emission CT (SPECT) or CT fusion, isotope renogram, or antegrade nephrostogram **(Figs. 6A and B)**.[32,41] Small leaks usually respond to conservative management by decompression (percutaneous nephrostomy) and urinary diversion (prolonged catheterization) and long indwelling stent (4–6 weeks), whereas larger ureteric defects due to necrosis require surgical reimplantation or ureteroureterostomy with the native ureter.[42-44]

Lymphocele

A pseudocystic perigraft collection of lymph lined by a nonepithelized fibrous capsule[45-47] is one of the common complications occurring after 2 weeks to 6 months post-transplant.[48] Its incidence ranges between 5 and 50%.[46,48,49] The source of lymphorrhagia is both recipient lymphatics along the iliac vessels and donor lymphatics at the renal hilum. The risk factors can be divided into surgical and medical causes.[45] Surgical causes include incomplete ligation of lymphatic channels along the iliac vessels during bed preparation and around the donor renal hilum or perinephric fat. Medical causes include use of mTOR inhibitors, steroids, anticoagulants, diuretics, ABOi transplants, immunocompromised state, hypoalbuminemia, obesity, or delayed graft function/acute rejection.[45,46,48,50,51] Majority are asymptomatic collections diagnosed on routine ultrasound. Large anteromedial lymphoceles compressing on the ureter may cause graft hydroureteronephrosis and graft dysfunction **(Figs. 7A and B)**. Compression on iliac vessels can cause limb or external genitalia edema. Bladder compression can cause increased frequency or rarely bladder outlet obstruction.[46] Lymph can tract through the abdominal layers to cause a subcutaneous collection or a lymphocutaneous fistula through the surgical wound or drain site **(Fig. 8)**. Ultrasound and plain CT scans define the extent, number, and character of the collection. Asymptomatic small lymphoceles (<100 mL) or even large posterolateral lymphoceles should be managed conservatively. Aspiration for biochemical confirmation (fluid creatine level) rules out urine leak. Aspiration of small symptomatic collections can be curative. Ultrasound-guided percutaneous drain placement in recurrent or large collections followed by sclerosant (povidone-iodine) instillation has a failure rate of <11%.[49,52,53] Laparoscopic or open fenestration/deroofing or marsupialization into peritoneal cavity is the modality of choice in persistent high output (>300 mL/day) lymphocele or recurrent collections.

Pseudoaneurysm

Juxta-anastomotic pseudoaneurysm is an uncommon but dangerous complication occurring in <1% renal transplants.[54-57] These can be classified into infective and noninfective pseudoaneurysms. Noninfective pseudoaneurysms occur early and can be due to intimal injury during harvesting or anastomosis or faulty suturing technique.[58] Immunological injury after vascular rejection

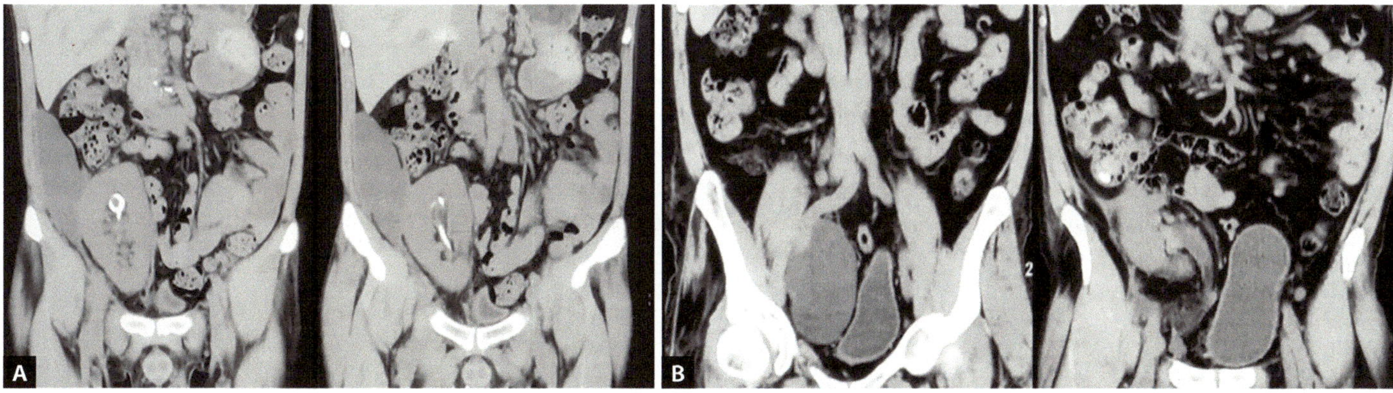

Figs. 7A and B: (A) Silent posterolateral lymphocele with no signs of graft obstruction; (B) Large obstructive anteromedial lymphocele causing graft hydroureteronephrosis.

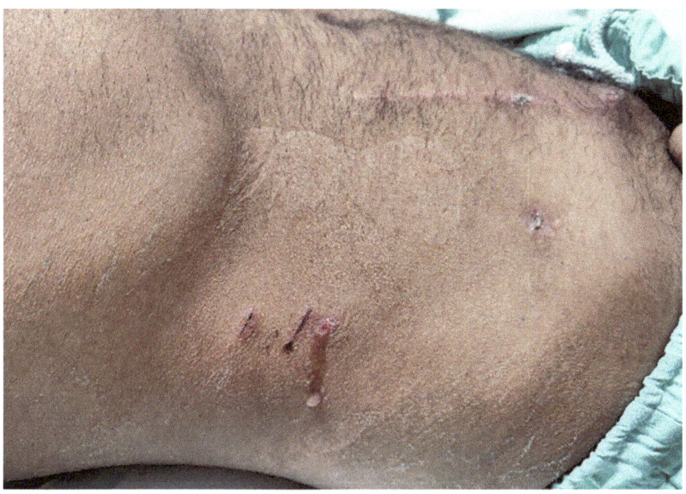

Fig. 8: Lymphocutaneous fistula from the drain site with an underlying lymphocele.

can also lead to endothelial damage. Infective/mycotic pseudoaneurysm is present in the second or third week post-transplant and is mostly of fungal (*Candida* and *Aspergillus*) or bacterial (*Staphylococcus, Pseudomonas,* and *Klebsiella*) origin.[55] The infective source can be the donor aortic patch, infected irrigation fluid, or any distant septic foci in an immunocompromised recipient. Clinical presentation can be varied ranging from being silent **(Figs. 9A to D)** or causing asymptomatic graft dysfunction to cause graft site pain, fever, lower limb swelling or ischemia or hemorrhagic shock secondary to ruptured pseudoaneurysm. Intervention is indicated in patients with symptoms, size >2.5 cm, rapidly increasing in size, impending rupture, compressive features, or graft dysfunction.[54,56,59]

Graft nephrectomy with excision of a large infected pseudoaneurysm with vascular reconstruction is mostly inevitable. Exclusion of small noninfected pseudoaneurysms by covered endovascular stents has been attempted but is seldom successful. Endovascular coiling or ultrasound-guided thrombin/glue injection has been described for small narrow-necked pseudoaneurysms.[54,56] Long-term antibiotic and antifungal therapy as per blood and tissue (excised pseudoaneurysm) culture is required.

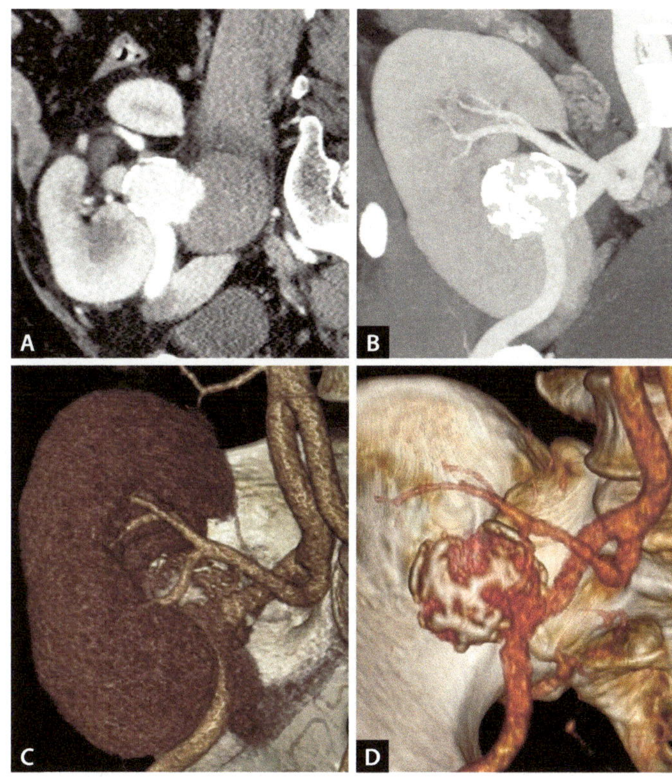

Figs. 9A to D: Computed tomography (CT) angiogram with three-dimensional (3D) reconstruction of a 55-year-old male, 11 years post-transplant with an incidentally detected 65 x 47 mm calcified juxta-anastomotic pseudoaneurysm at the inferior renal artery to right external iliac artery anastomotic site. The graft was well perfused by superior renal artery anastomosed to right internal iliac artery.

Wound-related Complications

Subcutaneous seroma, wound infection, and wound dehiscence **(Fig. 10)** are common wound-related complications post-transplant. Common risk factors include obesity, old age, diabetes, and immunosuppression, especially mTOR inhibitors.[60,61] Placement of subcutaneous drain in obese patients reduces the incidence of subcutaneous seromas.[62] The incidence of surgical site infection (SSI) after kidney transplant is 5–27%.[63,64] Wound complications do not impair graft function but add to the treatment cost, prolong hospitalization, and impair quality of life.

2 MONTHS ONWARD

Ureteric Obstruction

Ureteric obstruction has an incidence of 0.6–10.5%[65] and can be due to intrinsic or extrinsic factors. Ureteric kink, blood clots, tight-tunneled anastomosis, native graft calculi, or faulty suturing cause early ureteric obstruction (<3 months). Perigraft collections can cause extrinsic compression. Late stenosis (>6 months) occurs due to fibrosis, ischemia, healed ureteric leaks, BK virus nephropathy, rejection, or high immunosuppression.[31,44,66] Significant obstruction causes hydronephrosis and graft dysfunction and should be intervened early by prompt decompression by percutaneous nephrostomy.[44] Short strictures (<1 cm) on antegrade nephrostogram can be considered for balloon dilatation and antegrade stenting **(Fig. 11)**.[31,67] Failed intervention and long strictures (>3 cm) require ureteral reimplantation or ureteroureterostomy or pyeloureterostomy.[44]

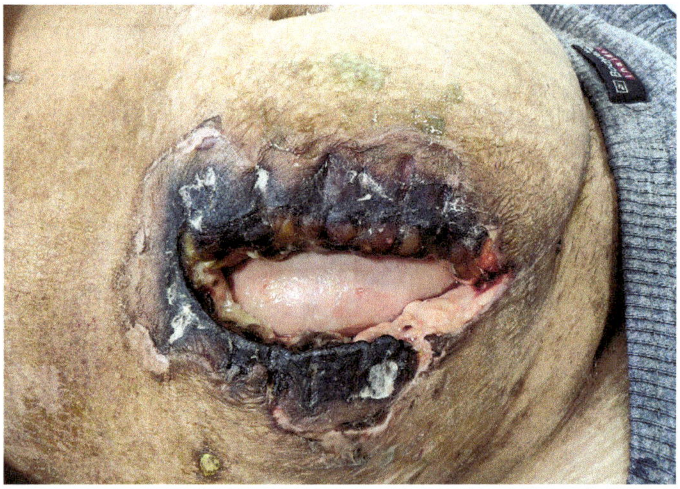

Fig. 10: A 34-year-old obese female developed wound gaping and ischemic necrosis of subcutaneous fat due to thrombotic microangiopathy secondary to tacrolimus toxicity.

Renal Artery Stenosis

Renal artery stenosis is the most common vascular complication after renal transplantation (1–23%)[68] mostly presenting between 2 months and 2 years.[69] Stenosis is multifactorial and can be either significant (>50% occlusion) to cause refractory hypertension and graft dysfunction[22] or be silent and detected incidentally on routine Doppler ultrasound.

Stenosis presenting early is usually at the anastomotic site and mostly due to technical reasons. Not achieving a wide-open anastomosis or intimal injury/flap during graft harvesting, anastomosis or traumatic clamping is usually responsible.[70] Atherosclerotic donor artery commonly predisposes to delayed and proximal stenosis.[17] The most common cause of delayed stenosis is juxta-anastomotic intimal hyperplasia and fibrosis.[70] Vascular rejection or cytomegalovirus (CMV) infection is also known to cause endothelial injury and distal stenosis or diffuse multiple stenosis.[71,72] Long-standing arterial kink may also eventually stenose.

Ultrasound Doppler is the first investigation with a sensitivity of 63–100%.[73] High PSV of >2.5 m/s (specificity 67–100%) suggests a significantly stenosed renal artery at the hilum. High acceleration time at renal and intrarenal artery ≥0.1 seconds and renal artery to iliac artery PSV >1.8. Intrarenal parvus et tardus pattern with resistive index (RI) <0.5 has a sensitivity of 90–100% and a specificity of 87–100%.[74-76]

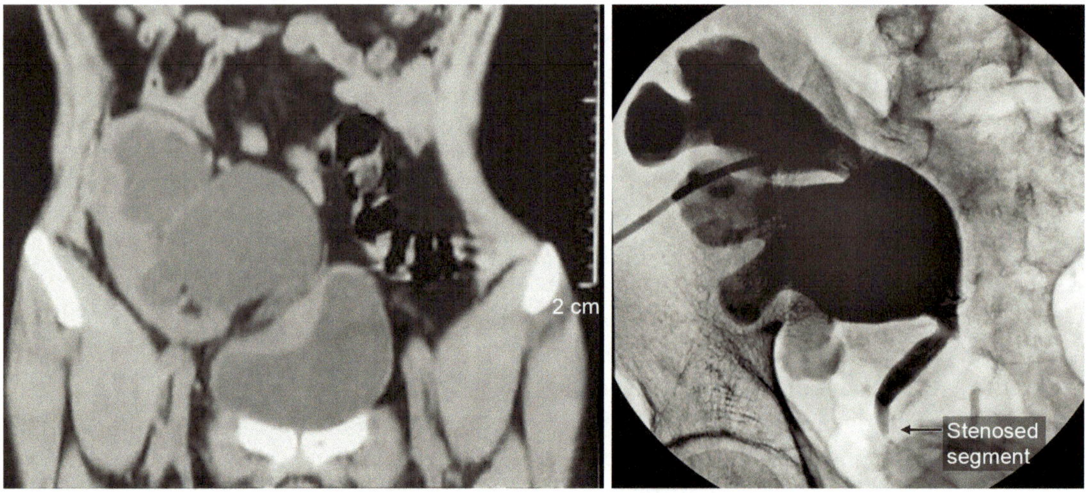

Fig. 11: A 56-year-old male, 10 years postrenal transplant, developed graft dysfunction with hydroureteronephrosis. Percutaneous nephrostomy and antegrade nephrostogram showing narrowing at vesicoureteric junction.

Computed tomography or MR angiography carries the risk of contrast-induced nephropathy. Carbon dioxide (CO_2) angiography is a non-nephrotoxic alternative.[77] Digital subtraction angiography is the gold standard with the inherent advantage of accurate diagnosis and intervention in the same sitting. Pressure gradient >10 mm Hg across the stenosed segment is an indication for intervention. Percutaneous transluminal angioplasty is the current standard treatment with a technical success rate of 85–93% and clinical success rate of 75–86%.[78,79] It has the best results for a short segment, linear, and nonostial stenosis.[74] Potential complications include restenosis, arterial dissection, aneurysm, and hematoma formation. Reintervention rate in PTA only versus PTA with stenting is 16–62% versus <10%,[79,80] although the long-term outcomes are comparable.[81] Surgical reexploration and revision of anastomosis with or without vascular grafts are reserved for complex nonostial stenosis or failed angioplasty.[82]

Vesicoureteric Reflux

With a reported incidence of 3–12.4%,[83,84] graft vesicoureteric reflux (VUR) occurs due to the inability to achieve an effective nonrefluxing vesicoureteric anastomosis. It is diagnosed on micturating cystourethrogram (MCU) **(Fig. 12)** in patients with recurrent urinary tract infection (UTI) and commonly managed by long-term antibiotics. Breakthrough UTI or recurrent graft pyelonephritis requires Deflux injection or ureteric reimplantation.[29]

Hernia

Post-transplant hernia can be incisional hernia or paratransplant hernia **(Fig. 13)**.

- Incisional hernia is due to the loss of integrity of the musculofascial layer at the surgical site. Although common with midline abdominal incisions (10–20%),[85] its incidence with transverse abdominal incisions for abdominal surgeries is 1.1–18%.[86] The incidence is 4–5-fold lower with oblique (Rutherford Morison) incision than hockey stick (modified Gibson) incision.[87-89] Risk factors include old age, obesity, diabetes, smoking, immunosuppression, large lymphocele, delayed graft function, surgical reexploration, and dual kidney transplantation apart from SSI or faulty suturing technique.[90,91] The incidence of incisional hernia increases from 3.7 to 18.1% with sirolimus-based regimen.[89] Although it does not affect the graft function, it adds to the morbidity and adversely affects the patient's well-being. Treatment options include primary repair, synthetic or biological mesh repair or grafts or flap repair.[90,92]
- Paratransplant hernia is the extrusion of bowel loops from a defect in peritoneum, into the perigraft space. It is a rare variant of internal hernia with an incidence of 0.18–0.45%.[93,94] Missed peritoneal rent during bed preparation or accidental bites through it during abdominal wall closure is the postulated cause. It is a potentially

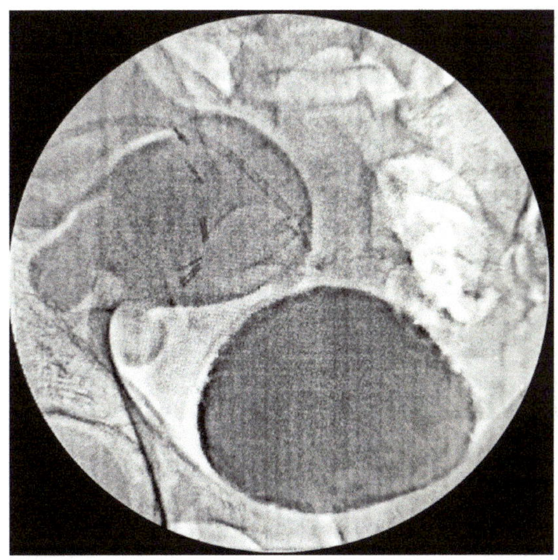

Fig. 12: Cystogram of a 45-year-old male with recurrent urinary tract infection (UTI) 2 years after transplant showing reflux into the transplanted kidney.

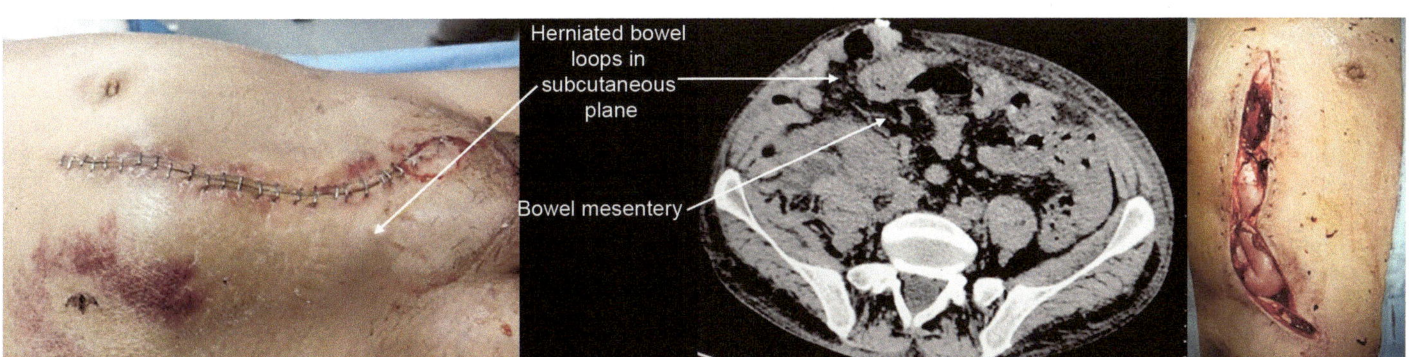

Fig. 13: A 68-year-old diabetic male on postoperative day 18 of an ABOi transplant developed slowly progressive subcutaneous swelling and constipation. Plain computed tomography (CT) scan showed components of both paratransplant and incisional hernia with bowel loops in subcutaneous plane. Emergency exploration ensured viable bowel segments, and peritoneal and fascial defects were repaired.

serious complication due to the risk of bowel obstruction and strangulation.[95] Plain CT scan confirms the diagnosis once clinically suspected, and emergent surgical reexploration is warranted.[96]

REFERENCES

1. Deininger S, Nadalin S, Amend B, Guthoff M, Heyne N, Königsrainer A, et al. Minimal-invasive management of urological complications after kidney transplantation. Int Urol Nephrol. 2021;53(7):1267-77.
2. Inci MF, Ozkan F, See TC, Tatli S. Renal transplant complications: diagnostic and therapeutic role of radiology. Can Assoc Radiol J. 2014;65(3):242-52.
3. Pillot P, Bardonnaud N, Lillaz J, Delorme G, Chabannes É, Bernardini S, et al. Risk factors for surgical complications after renal transplantation and impact on patient and graft survival. Transplant Proc. 2012;44(9):2803-8.
4. Lempinen M, Stenman J, Kyllönen L, Salmela K. Surgical complications following 1670 consecutive adult renal transplantations: a single center study. Scand J Surg. 2015; 104(4):254-9.
5. Kırnap M, Özçelik Ü, Akdur A, Soy EHA, Işıklar İ, Karakayalı FY, et al. Reconstruction of traumatic external iliac artery dissection due to vascular clamping. Exp Clin Transplant. 2017;4.
6. Lushina N, Lee A, Cuadra S, Whang M, Sun H. External iliac artery dissection during renal transplantation: a case report and literature review. Transplant Proc. 2019;51(2):538-40.
7. Guleria S, Abdullah S, Bansal R, Reddy VS. A kink in transplantation: a rare cause of early graft dysfunction. Saudi J Kidney Dis Transplant. 2013;24(5):965.
8. Meier R, Fournier I, Toso C, Berney T, Bednarkiewicz M. Surgical repair of a living-donor kidney graft artery kink by a postanastomotic external iliac artery rotation and reanastomosis. Ann Vasc Surg. 2017;44:414.e5-9.
9. Frauchiger B, Bock A, Spoendlin M, Eichlisberger R, Vogelbach P, Landmann J, et al. Early renal transplant dysfunction due to arterial kinking stenosis. Nephrol Dial Transplant. 1994;9(1):76-9.
10. Miah M, Madaan S, Kessel DJ, Newstead CG, Guleria S. Transplant renal artery kinking: a rare cause of early graft dysfunction. Nephrol Dial Transplant. 2004;19(7):1930-1.
11. Damiano G, Maione C, Maffongelli A, Ficarella S, Carmina L, Buscemi S, et al. Renal allograft compartment syndrome: is it possible to prevent? Transplant Proc. 2016;48(2):340-3.
12. El-Bandar N, Lerchbaumer M, Hubatsch M, Lichy IM, Schulz MRG, Friedersdorff F. Renal allograft compartment syndrome: a case report and review of the literature. Urol Int. 2020;104(7-8):646-50.
13. Beasley KA, McAlister VC, Luke PPW. Mesh hood fascial closure in renal allograft compartment syndrome. Transplant Proc. 2003;35(7):2418-9.
14. Heer MK, Trevillian PR, Hardy DB, Hibberd AD. Salvaging kidneys with renal allograft compartment syndrome. Transpl Int. 2012;25(4):e47-9.
15. Tang L, Lee T, Yuen L, Pleass H. Renal allograft compartment syndrome: a review. ANZ J Surg. 2021;91(12):2606-9.
16. Hachem LD, Ghanekar A, Selzner M, Famure O, Li Y, Kim SJ. Postoperative surgical-site hemorrhage after kidney transplantation: incidence, risk factors, and outcomes. Transpl Int. 2017;30(5):474-83.
17. Poli D, Antonucci E, Zanazzi M. Hemostatic complications in renal transplantation. Semin Thromb Hemost. 2017;43(7): 742-9.
18. Ammi M, Daligault M, Sayegh J, Abraham P, Papon X, Enon B, et al. Evaluation of the vascular surgical complications of renal transplantation. Ann Vasc Surg. 2016;33:23-30.
19. Amézquita Y, Méndez C, Fernández A, Caldes S, Pascual J, Muriel A, et al. Risk factors for early renal graft thrombosis: a case-controlled study in grafts from the same donor. Transplant Proc. 2008;40(9):2891-3.
20. El Zorkany K, Bridson JM, Sharma A, Halawa A. Transplant renal vein thrombosis. Exp Clin Transplant. 2017;15(2): 123-9.
21. Szabo-Pap M, Zadori G, Fedor R, Illesy L, Toth F, Kanyari Z, et al. Surgical complications following kidney transplantations: a single-center study in Hungary. Transplant Proc. 2016; 48(7):2548-51.
22. Dimitroulis D, Bokos J, Zavos G, Nikiteas N, Karidis NP, Katsaronis P, et al. Vascular complications in renal transplantation: a single-center experience in 1367 renal transplantations and review of the literature. Transplant Proc. 2009;41(5):1609-14.
23. Tavakkoli M, Zafarghandi RM, Taghavi R, Ghoreifi A, Zafarghandi MM. Immediate vascular complications after kidney transplant: experience from 2100 recipients. Exp Clin Transplant. 2017;15(5):504-8.
24. Santos JE, Gaspar A, Querido S, Jorge C, Weigert A, Gabriel HM, et al. Unexpected success in early post-transplantation renal vein thrombosis: a case report and literature review. Clin Nephrol Case Stud. 2021;9:19-25.
25. Rouvière O, Berger P, Béziat C, Garnier JL, Lefrançois N, Martin X, et al. Acute thrombosis of renal transplant artery: graft salvage by means of intra-arterial fibrinolysis. Transplantation. 2002;73(3):403-9.
26. Ayvazoglu Soy EH, Akdur A, Kirnap M, Boyvat F, Moray G, Haberal M. Vascular complications after renal transplant: a single-center experience. Exp Clin Transplant. 2017; 15(Suppl. 1):79-83.
27. Choi YS, Kim KS, Choi SW, Bae WJ, Hong SH, Lee JY, et al. Ureteral complications in kidney transplantation: analysis and management of 853 consecutive laparoscopic living-donor nephrectomies in a single center. Transplant Proc. 2016;48(8):2684-8.
28. Zavos G, Pappas P, Karatzas T, Karidis NP, Bokos J, Stravodimos K, et al. Urological complications: analysis and management of 1525 consecutive renal transplantations. Transplant Proc. 2008;40(5):1386-90.
29. Sui W, Lipsky MJ, Matulay JT, Robins DJ, Onyeji IC, James MB, et al. Timing and predictors of early urologic and infectious complications after renal transplant: an analysis of a New York statewide database. Exp Clin Transplant. 2018;16(6):665-70.
30. Kayler L, Kang D, Molmenti E, Howard R. Kidney transplant ureteroneocystostomy techniques and complications: review of the literature. Transplant Proc. 2010;42(5):1413-20.
31. Englesbe MJ, Dubay DA, Gillespie BW, Moyer AS, Pelletier SJ, Sung RS, et al. Risk factors for urinary complications after renal transplantation. Am J Transplant. 2007;7(6):1536-41.
32. Hamouda M, Sharma A, Halawa A. Urine leak after kidney transplant: a review of the literature. Exp Clin Transplant. 2018;16(1):90-5.

33. Fuller TF, Deger S, Büchler A, Roigas J, Schönberger B, Schnorr D, et al. Ureteral complications in the renal transplant recipient after laparoscopic living donor nephrectomy. Eur Urol. 2006;50(3):535-40; discussion 540-1.
34. El-Galley R, Hood N, Young CJ, Deierhoi M, Urban DA. Donor nephrectomy: a comparison of techniques and results of open, hand assisted and full laparoscopic nephrectomy. J Urol. 2004;171(1):40-3.
35. Akoh JA, Opaluwa AS, Weller D. Urological complications of renal transplantation: reducing the risk. Saudi J Kidney Dis Transplant. 2009;20(6):1005-9.
36. Friedersdorff F, Weinberger S, Biernath N, Plage H, Cash H, El-Bandar N. The ureter in the kidney transplant setting: ureteroneocystostomy surgical options, double-J stent considerations and management of related complications. Curr Urol Rep. 2020;21(1):3.
37. Neri F, Tsivian M, Coccolini F, Bertelli R, Cavallari G, Nardo B, et al. Urological complications after kidney transplantation: experience of more than 1,000 transplantations. Transplant Proc. 2009;41(4):1224-6.
38. French CG, Acott PD, Crocker JF, Bitter-Suermann H, Lawen JG. Extravesical ureteroneocystostomy with and without internalized ureteric stents in pediatric renal transplantation. Pediatr Transplant. 2001;5(1):21-6.
39. Karam G, Maillet F, Parant S, Soulillou JP, Giral-Classe M. Ureteral necrosis after kidney transplantation: risk factors and impact on graft and patient survival. Transplantation. 2004;78(5):725-9.
40. Faenza A, Spolaore R, Selleri S, Rocca M, Corbucci Vitolo G, Gozzetti G, et al. Late ureteric stenosis after kidney transplantation: a possible consequence of rejection. Contrib Nephrol. 1989;70:75-80.
41. Minnee RC, Surachno S, Kox C, ten Berge IJM, Aronson DC, Idu MM. Is a selective splinted ureterocystostomy protocol feasible in renal transplantation? An analysis of 475 renal transplantations. Transpl Int. 2006;19(7):558-62.
42. Mazzucchi E, Souza GL, Hisano M, Antonopoulos IM, Piovesan AC, Nahas WC, et al. Primary reconstruction is a good option in the treatment of urinary fistula after kidney transplantation. Int Braz J Urol. 2006;32(4):398-403; discussion 403-4.
43. El-Mekresh M, Osman Y, Ali-El-Dein B, El-Diasty T, Ghoneim MA. Urological complications after living-donor renal transplantation. BJU Int. 2001;87(4):295-306.
44. Manassero F, Vistoli F, Mogorovich A, DE Maria M, Boggi U, Selli C. Early and late ureteral complications after renal transplant. Minerva Urol Nefrol. 2017;69(6):613-8.
45. Lucan CV, Jurchis I, Suciu M, Selicean SE, Buttice S. Modern lymphatic dissection techniques for preventing post renal transplant lymphocele. Clujul Med. 2017;90(4):416-9.
46. Singh AG, Jai SJ, Ganpule AP, VijayKumar M, Sabnis RB, Desai MR. Critical appraisal of consecutive 36 cases of post renal transplant lymphocele: a proposed algorithm. World J Urol. 2017;35(9):1443-50.
47. Pacovsky J, Hyspler R, Husek P, Navratil P, Brodak M. Colloid osmotic pressure participates on the post-transplant lymphocele pathogenesis. Transplant Proc. 2018;50(10):3422-5.
48. Heer MK, Clark D, Trevillian PR, Sprott P, Palazzi K, Hibberd AD. Functional significance and risk factors for lymphocele formation after renal transplantation: functional significance of lymphocele. ANZ J Surg. 2018;88(6):597-602.
49. Golriz M, Klauss M, Zeier M, Mehrabi A. Prevention and management of lymphocele formation following kidney transplantation. Transplant Rev. 2017;31(2):100-5.
50. Jänigen BM, Salabè C, Glatz T, Thomusch O, Lässle C, Fichtner-Feigl S, et al. Single cohort study: ABO-incompatible kidney transplant recipients have a higher risk of lymphocele formation. Langenbecks Arch Surg. 2019;404(8):999-1007.
51. Sayilar E, Ersoy A, Ayar Y, Aydin MF, Sahin AB, Coskun B, et al. Factors influencing lymphocele development after kidney transplant: single center experience. Exp Clin Transplant. 2019. [online] Available from http://www.ectrx.org/detail/epub/1/1/1/0/830/0 [Last accessed June, 2022].
52. Baboudjian M, Tadrist A, Gondran-Tellier B, McManus R, Akiki A, Gaillet S, et al. Povidone-iodine sclerotherapy of primary symptomatic lymphocele after kidney transplantation. Int Urol Nephrol. 2021;53(4):685-90.
53. Sureka SK, Yadav P, Singh UP, Lal H, Kapoor R, Ansari MS, et al. Role of early povidone iodine instillation in post-renal transplant lymphorrhea: a prospective randomized study. Turk J Urol. 2019;45(6):461-6.
54. Bracale UM, Santangelo M, Carbone F, del Guercio L, Maurea S, Porcellini M, et al. Anastomotic pseudoaneurysm complicating renal transplantation: treatment options. Eur J Vasc Endovasc Surg. 2010;39(5):565-8.
55. Chung MT, Chan YC, Law Y, Cheng SW. Infectious anastomotic pseudoaneurysm complicating renal allograft: case report and review of literature. Int J Nephrol Renovasc Dis. 2017;10:55-60.
56. Vijayvergiya R, Kasinadhuni G, Sharma A, Lal A. Endovascular repair of a post-renal transplant internal iliac artery pseudoaneurysm. Vasc Endovascular Surg. 2021;55(6):651-3.
57. Marcu CB, Nijveldt R, Van Rossum AC. Unsuspected chronic traumatic aortic pseudoaneurysm—what to do about it. Late post-traumatic aortic pseudoaneurysm. Can J Cardiol. 2008;24(2):143-4.
58. Sharma N, Bidnur S, Caldas M, McNally D, Murray A, Turnbull R, et al. Renal transplant anastomotic pseudoaneurysms: case report of open repair and endovascular management. IJU Case Rep. 2019;2(2):86-9.
59. Che H, Men C, Yang M, Zhang J, Chen P, Yong J. Endovascular repair of a transplant renal artery anastomotic pseudoaneurysm using the snorkel technique. J Vasc Surg. 2014;60(4):1052-5.
60. Fockens MM, Alberts VP, Bemelman FJ, van der Pant KAMI, Idu MM. Wound morbidity after kidney transplant. Prog Transplant. 2015;25(1):45-8.
61. Tay HWM, Sim PY, Teo YA, Rahman L, Tiong HY. Review of stentless, tubeless, apposed renal (STAR) transplant wound management programme. Singapore Med J. 2021;62(10):529-34.
62. Fujii T, Tabe Y, Yajima R, Yamaguchi S, Tsutsumi S, Asao T, et al. Effects of subcutaneous drain for the prevention of incisional SSI in high-risk patients undergoing colorectal surgery. Int J Colorectal Dis. 2011;26(9):1151-5.
63. Humar A, Ramcharan T, Denny R, Gillingham KJ, Payne WD, Matas AJ. Are wound complications after a kidney transplant more common with modern immunosuppression? Transplantation. 2001;72(12):1920-3.
64. Menezes FG, Wey SB, Peres CA, Medina-Pestana JO, Camargo LFA. Risk factors for surgical site infection in kidney transplant recipients. Infect Control Hosp Epidemiol. 2008;29(8):771-3.

65. Breda A, Bui MH, Liao JC, Gritsch HA, Schulam PG. Incidence of ureteral strictures after laparoscopic donor nephrectomy. J Urol. 2006;176(3):1065-8.
66. Dinckan A, Tekin A, Turkyilmaz S, Kocak H, Gurkan A, Erdogan O, et al. Early and late urological complications corrected surgically following renal transplantation. Transpl Int. 2007;20(8):702-7.
67. Kaskarelis I, Koukoulaki M, Georgantas T, Bairamidis E, Kokkinos C, Ieronymou M, et al. Ureteral complications in renal transplant recipients successfully treated with interventional radiology. Transplant Proc. 2008;40(9):3170-2.
68. Li X, Zhang J, Meng Y, Yang L, Wang F, Li B, et al. Transplant renal artery stenosis caused by the stretch of an artey branch: a case report and literature review. BMC Nephrol. 2018;19(1):56.
69. Baird DP, Williams J, Petrie MC, Smith JR. Transplant renal artery stenosis. Kidney Int Rep. 2020;5(12):2399-402.
70. Nicholson ML, Yong C, Trotter PB, Grant L, Hosgood SA. Risk factors for transplant renal artery stenosis after live donor transplantation. Br J Surg. 2019;106(3):199-205.
71. Patel NH, Jindal RM, Wilkin T, Rose S, Johnson MS, Shah H, et al. Renal arterial stenosis in renal allografts: retrospective study of predisposing factors and outcome after percutaneous transluminal angioplasty. Radiology. 2001;219(3):663-7.
72. Wong W, Fynn SP, Higgins RM, Walters H, Evans S, Deane C, et al. Transplant renal artery stenosis in 77 patients—does it have an immunological cause? Transplantation. 1996; 61(2):215-9.
73. Pedersen EB. New tools in diagnosing renal artery stenosis. Kidney Int. 2000;57(6):2657-77.
74. Chen W, Kayler LK, Zand MS, Muttana R, Chernyak V, DeBoccardo GO. Transplant renal artery stenosis: clinical manifestations, diagnosis and therapy. Clin Kidney J. 2015; 8(1):71-8.
75. Bruno S, Ferrari S, Remuzzi G, Ruggenenti P. Doppler ultrasonography in posttransplant renal artery stenosis: a reliable tool for assessing effectiveness of revascularization? Transplantation. 2003;76(1):147-53.
76. Ardalan MR, Tarzamani MK, Shoja MM. A correlation between direct and indirect Doppler ultrasonographic measures in transplant renal artery stenosis. Transplant Proc. 2007;39(5):1436-8.
77. Elmously A, Stern JR, Greenberg J, Agrusa CJ, Schneider DB, Ellozy SH, et al. Carbon dioxide angiography in the treatment of transplant renal artery stenosis. Ann Vasc Surg. 2020; 63:198-203.
78. Ghazanfar A, Tavakoli A, Augustine T, Pararajasingam R, Riad H, Chalmers N. Management of transplant renal artery stenosis and its impact on long-term allograft survival: a single-centre experience. Nephrol Dial Transplant. 2011; 26(1):336-43.
79. Ngo AT, Markar SR, De Lijster MS, Duncan N, Taube D, Hamady MS. A systematic review of outcomes following percutaneous transluminal angioplasty and stenting in the treatment of transplant renal artery stenosis. Cardiovasc Intervent Radiol. 2015;38(6):1573-88.
80. Hagen G, Wadström J, Magnusson M, Magnusson A. Outcome after percutaneous transluminal angioplasty of arterial stenosis in renal transplant patients. Acta Radiol. 2009;50(3):270-5.
81. Wongpraparut N, Chaipruckmalakarn T, Tongdee T, Jaspttananon A, Vongwiwatana A, Premasathian N, et al. Long-term outcome of percutaneous transluminal renal angioplasty (PTRA) versus PTRA with stenting (PTRAS) in transplant renal artery stenosis. BMC Cardiovasc Disord. 2021;21(1):212.
82. Shames BD, Odorico JS, D'Alessandro AM, Pirsch JD, Sollinger HW. Surgical repair of transplant renal artery stenosis with preserved cadaveric iliac artery grafts. Ann Surg. 2003;237(1):116-22.
83. Torricelli FCM, Watanabe A, Piovesan AC, Antonopoulos IM, David-Neto E, Nahas WC. Urological complications, vesicoureteral reflux, and long-term graft survival rate after pediatric kidney transplantation. Pediatr Transplant. 2015;19(8):844-8.
84. Routh JC, Yu RN, Kozinn SI, Nguyen HT, Borer JG. Urological complications and vesicoureteral reflux following pediatric kidney transplantation. J Urol. 2013;189(3):1071-6.
85. Denys A, Monbailliu T, Allaeys M, Berrevoet F, van Ramshorst GH. Management of abdominal wound dehiscence: update of the literature and meta-analysis. Hernia. 2021;25(2): 449-62.
86. Røine E, Bjørk IT, Oyen O. Targeting risk factors for impaired wound healing and wound complications after kidney transplantation. Transplant Proc. 2010;42(7):2542-6.
87. Nanni G, Tondolo V, Citterio F, Romagnoli J, Borgetti M, Boldrini G, et al. Comparison of oblique versus hockey-stick surgical incision for kidney transplantation. Transplant Proc. 2005;37(6):2479-81.
88. Smietański M, Bury K, Tomaszewska A, Lubowiecka I, Szymczak C. Biomechanics of the front abdominal wall as a potential factor leading to recurrence with laparoscopic ventral hernia repair. Surg Endosc. 2012;26(5):1461-7.
89. Shahrestani S, Tran HM, Pleass HC, Hawthorne WJ. Optimal surgical management in kidney and pancreas transplantation to minimise wound complications: a systematic review and meta-analysis. Ann Med Surg. 2018;33:24-31.
90. Gioco R, Sanfilippo C, Veroux P, Corona D, Privitera F, Brolese A, et al. Abdominal wall complications after kidney transplantation: a clinical review. Clin Transplant. 2021; 35(12):e14506.
91. Durinka JB, Parsikia A, Karipineni F, Campos S, Khanmoradi K, Zaki R, et al. Association between delayed graft function and incisional hernia after renal transplant. Exp Clin Transplant. 2017;15(1):27-33.
92. Vennarecci G, Mascianà G, De Werra E, Sandri GBL, Ferraro D, Burocchi M, et al. Effectiveness and versatility of biological prosthesis in transplanted patients. World J Transplant. 2017;7(1):43-8.
93. Moris D, Vernadakis S. Renal paratransplant hernia. An uncommon variant of internal hernia. Are we aware of it? Transplantation. 2014;97(11):e65-6.
94. Igarashi Y, Miyake K, Yamano M, Shimoyama R, Kashiwagi H, Kawachi J. Laparoscopic treatment for renal paratransplant hernia: a case report. Int J Surg Case Rep. 2021;82:105849.
95. Di Cocco P, Kandilis A, Rajagopal P, Hakim N. Paratransplant hernia: a true emergency after renal transplant. Exp Clin Transplant. 2015;13(4):363-4.
96. Moris D, Bokos J, Vailas M, Kakavia K, Spartalis E, Athanasiou A, et al. Renal paratransplant hernia revealed: a review of the literature. Hernia. 2017;21(3):363-7.

CHAPTER 6

Perioperative Care of Kidney Transplant Recipient

Ratan Jha, Rakesh Kumar Ambati, Aman Jha

INTRODUCTION

Kidney transplant (KTx) is an elective (live transplant) or semi-elective emergency surgery (cadaveric transplant) in dialysis-dependent renal failure patients who have undergone detailed evaluation preoperatively. Most of the chronic dialysis patients will be in optimal health condition with a consequent good outcome post-transplant, unlike patients awaiting heart, liver, or lung transplant who are generally sick. An uncomplicated KTx recipient usually leaves the hospital in 1–2 weeks. Preoperative care should be focused on the initiation of immunosuppression, avoiding fluid overload and hyperkalemia prior to surgery. Intraoperative care includes maintaining hemodynamics, reducing cold ischemia time, and ensuring good surgical anastomosis of the artery, vein, and ureter. Postoperative care should focus on surgical and medical issues to ensure a safe outcome. This perioperative care is usually done as a fixed protocol based on the center's experience and preference which spans 2 weeks approximately from admission to discharge that impacts the successful long-term renal outcome. We will divide the perioperative care into three phases for discussion: (1) preoperative care (usually 1–2 days), (2) intraoperative care (usually 4–6 hours), and (3) postoperative care (0–14 days).

The three phases of perioperative care are a multidisciplinary team approach. Preoperative care involves revisiting last minute no missed issues of concern. Intraoperative care includes reducing cold ischemia and timely use of cold perfusion fluid in live KTx, monitoring hemodynamic stability, immunosuppression coverage, meticulous surgical, and anesthetic care. Postoperative care entails focused care with early diagnosis of complications, including diagnosis of graft dysfunctions.[1,2]

IMMUNOSUPPRESSION AND REGIMEN

Once the patient is found fit to undergo a renal transplant, an initial immunosuppression regimen is chosen based on immunological risk **(Box 1 and Table 1)** and centers protocol.

BOX 1: Immunological risk assessment for kidney transplantation.

- *Very low risk:* Identical twin donor
- *Low risk:* HLA-identical sibling donor, no DSA
- *Average risk:* HLA-mismatched donor, no DSA
- *High risk:* HLA-mismatched donor, detectable DSA, negative crossmatch, or ABO-incompatible donor following desensitization
- *Very high risk:* HLA-mismatched donor, detectable DSA, positive crossmatch

(DSA: donorspecific antibody; HLA: human leukocyte antigen)
Source: Kronish K, Olmos A, Niemann CU. Perioperative care of patients undergoing kidney transplantation. In: Knechtle S, Marson L, Morris P (Eds). Kidney Transplantation—Principles and Practice, 8th edition. Philadelphia: Elsevier Inc; 2020. pp. 184-97 [Chapter 13].

TABLE 1: Immunological risk assessment for antibody-mediated rejection based on crossmatch.

Immunological risk category	*CDC-XM (IgG)*	*FC-XM*	*Luminex-SAB DSA*
High	Positive	Positive	Positive (MFI > 5,000)
Intermediate	Negative	Positive	Positive (MFI > 2,000)
Low	Negative	Negative	Positive (MFI 500–2,000)
Standard	Negative	Negative	Negative (MFI < 500)

(CDC: complement-dependent cytotoxicity; DSA: donor-specific antibody; FC: flow crossmatch; IgG: immunoglobulin G; MFI: mean fluorescent intensity; SAB: single antigen bead; XM: crossmatch)
Source: Fuggle SV, Taylor CJ. Histocompatibility in renal transplantation. In: Knechtle S, Marson L, Morris P (Eds). Kidney Transplantation—Principles and Practice, 8th edition. Elsevier Inc; 2020. pp. 139-56 [Chapter 10].

BOX 2: Perioperative prophylaxis.

- Gastroprotection with PPI while on high dose steroids
- *Bacterial prophylaxis:* Perioperative antibiotic therapy prescribed based on local guidelines and adapted for recipient multiresistant organism colonization or potential donor infection
- *PJP prophylaxis:* 6-12 months co-trimoxazole. May consider lifelong therapy
- *UTI prophylaxis:* 6 months co-trimoxazole
- *Oropharyngeal candidiasis prophylaxis:* Oral nystatin suspension or clotrimazole troches, systemic medications such as fluconazole, rarely used
- *Systemic fungal prophylaxis:* Not generally prescribed due to low incidence of invasive fungal infection
- *CMV prophylaxis:* Oral valganciclovir. Duration depending on donor and recipient serostatus
- Unfractionated heparin and mechanical calf compressors unless contraindicated till the patient is mobile

(CMV: cytomegalovirus; PJP: *Pneumocystis jirovecii* pneumonia; PPI: proton pump inhibitor; UTI: urinary tract infection; VTE: venous thromboembolism)

Source: Kronish K, Olmos A, Niemann CU. Perioperative care of patients undergoing kidney transplantation. In: Knechtle S, Marson L, Morris P (Eds). Kidney Transplantation—Principles and Practice, 8th edition. Elsevier Inc; 2020. pp. 184-97 [Chapter 13].

Initial immunosuppression regimen and induction protocol have been discussed in detail in separate chapters.[1-3]

Most patients receiving KTx get some form of induction immunosuppression, such as basiliximab or thymoglobulin which is followed by triple drug immunosuppression, namely tacrolimus, mycophenolate, and prednisolone. The choice of regimen in highly sensitized recipient with donor-specific antibody (DSA) and ABO-incompatible transplant, though somewhat similar, is center specific and incorporates plasmapheresis as routine. Other regimens such as steroid-free protocols are usually considered in the pediatric age group to support catch-up growth and height **(Box 2)**.

PREOPERATIVE FACTORS

The standard evaluation of KTx patients consists of medical fitness, cardiac and vascular status, absence of infection, status of the immune system, absence of malignancy, or obstructive uropathy, which may risk the individual undergoing transplant.[3]

At the admission time in the transplanting hospital, blood is collected for routine investigations, immunological crossmatch (lymphocytic and Luminex assay) along with chest radiograph, and electrocardiogram (ECG). One needs to relook carefully at the recent medical problems with focused clinical examination and do appropriate medical counseling based on recent assessments (clinical/lab) about the risk, if any. These are the following medical history of relevance **(Box 3)**:

- Any new medical comorbidities (angina, peripheral foot ulceration)
- Any active infection (fever, constitutional symptoms, lymphadenopathy), occult sepsis (diabetic foot ulcers) or chronic untreated viral infections (hepatitis B/hepatitis C/human immunodeficiency virus) or pulmonary tuberculosis, unexplained weight loss
- Signs or symptoms of fluid overload, electrolyte and hematocrit—to decide the need for preoperative

BOX 3: Protocol for preoperative check at admission of the recipient before transplantation.

Preoperative assessment on the most recent items:

1. Preoperative need for dialysis
2. Any evidence of current infection?
3. Preoperative requirement of IV fluids
4. Current diuresis (mL/day)
5. Physical examination of heart and lungs, record blood pressure
6. Examination of pulse—femoral arteries, foot ulcers in diabetics
7. Current list of medication
8. Consent forms checked

Order preoperative immunosuppression:

1. Tacrolimus and mycophenolate mofetil given orally in the ward preoperatively
2. Induction therapy (basiliximab or ATG) can be given in the ward or in the operating room
3. Methylprednisolone 500 mg IV given before the start of the operation
4. Availability of cold perfusion fluid

Order antibiotic prophylaxis: Cefuroxime 1.5 g IV preoperatively/cefoperazone/sulbactum 1.5 g as a one/two dose treatment

Order co-medication: Antihypertensives, pantoprazole, and hypnotics to continue:

Operative assessment:

1. Anesthetists evaluation of patient records
2. Check the preoperative blood sample and chest X-ray
3. Final check that the crossmatch was negative—Luminex/CDC
4. Transplant surgeon decision of site preference—left or right side of the patient's abdomen for transplantation and part preparation
5. Blood crossmatch—two units leukocyte depleted/one unit for live donor
6. Preparation for surgery—shower, shaving, clothing
7. Check and note weight preoperative
8. CAPD catheter—should empty the abdomen before going to the operating room (preferably off PD and one HD preoperative)

(ATG: antithymocyte globulin; CAPD: continuous ambulatory peritoneal dialysis; CDC: Centers for Disease Control and Prevention; HD: hemodialysis; IV: intravenous; PD: peritoneal dialysis)

TABLE 2: Intraoperative management protocol.

CVC	***CVC is inserted in the operating room by anesthesiologist***
Intravenous fluids	Depending on hydration status—around 1.5–2.5 L of fluid is given intraoperatively
Antibiotics	Cefuroxime/cefoperazone sulbactam preoperatively as a one dose treatment
Urine output	Urine output is to be recorded intra- and postoperatively, and hourly records should be maintained
Blood transfusion	Avoid transfusions and if it becomes necessary CMV negative blood (leukocyte depleted) given
Peritoneal dialysis/hemodialysis catheter	If the patient has a PD/HD catheter, it should be removed at the end of the transplant surgery

(CMV: cytomegalovirus; CVC: central venous catheter; PD: peritoneal dialysis; HD: hemodialysis)

hemodialysis (HD) and blood transfusion. Usually, HD is done 24 hours prior to surgery, and if needed, a short heparin-free HD 2 hours prior to surgery for hyperkalemia or fluid overload.

The diagnosis of potential new medical problems, such as angina or heart failure and active or smoldering infection would mean postponing the decision for renal transplant till such factors are dealt with. Recipient factors that may affect perioperative course, such as high-grade vesicoureteral reflux (VUR), large polycystic kidney, neurogenic bladder, cardiac diseases on antiplatelets, obesity, or latent obstructive uropathies, need detailed work up for urological disorders. Donor factors known to be associated with delayed graft function (DGF) (prolonged cold ischemia time, donation from nonheart beating donor) may need supplemental dialysis. DGF discussed in Chapter 10.1 in deatail.

BOX 4: Intraoperative documentation.

- Donor graft—graft anatomy, backbench surgery, renal capsule tear
- Graft perfusion—appearance on cross-clamp release. Cold and warm ischemia time
- Hemodynamics—blood pressure profile, CVP, need for inotropic support, blood loss volume
- Fluid charting—volume of intravenous fluid administration during the procedure, urine output
- Biochemistry—intraoperative insulin dextrose. Postoperative renal chemistry panel including urea, creatinine, and potassium
- Assessment of the above factors helps guide and predict perioperative management

(CVP: central venous pressure)

Source: Kronish K, Olmos A, Niemann CU. Perioperative care of patients undergoing kidney transplantation. In: Knechtle S, Marson L, Morris P (Eds). Kidney Transplantation—Principles and Practice, 8th edition. Philadelphia: Elsevier Inc; 2020. pp. 184-97 [Chapter 13].

Management of Continuing Comorbidity Medication

Dialysis-dependent patients are usually receiving many medications and supplements, some of which can be stopped abruptly, such as phosphate binders, cinacalcet, erythropoietin, oral antidiabetics, and statins. Antihypertensive drugs such as amlodipine, metoprolol, and clonidine are continued unless blood pressure (BP) is on the lower side.

Preoperative Care of Hyperglycemia

Severe hyperglycemia may develop in nondiabetics or controlled diabetics before actual transplant due to steroid and calcineurin inhibitor (CNI), which usually needs IV insulin infusion to control glucose quickly and safely. Hypoglycemia, if occurs, is treated, as usual, with IV dextrose.

INTRAOPERATIVE PERIOD

Transplant kidney is usually placed in the iliac fossa extraperitoneally, and the anastomosis of artery, vein, and ureter is established (renal artery end to end with internal iliac artery or end to side with external iliac artery, renal vein end to side external iliac vein, ureter drained to bladder near trigone through submucosal tunnel). Proper perfusion of the donor's kidney is done with appropriate cold saline with heparin (live KTx) or histidine-tryptophan-ketoglutarate (HTK) perfusion fluid in cadaver KTx. Usually, blood loss during surgery is <300 mL, but occasionally can be around 500 mL, which requires replacement. Induction therapy during operation and methylprednisolone before the release of renal arterial clamp postanastomosis are routine.[4]

Intraoperative Fluid Therapy

There is no fixed or universally accepted fluid strategy practiced or promoted. It needs individualization. It is believed that fluid loading maintains cardiac output and optimize renal perfusion, but one needs to tread carefully to avoid volume overload. Hence, repeated clinical assessment based on heart rate, BP, central venous pressure (CVP), basal lung rales, O_2 saturation, and the trend of such parameters are utilized to assess fluid balance intraoperative. Diuretics such as furosemide and occasionally mannitol is administered following vascular anastomosis and vascular clamp release to precipitate diuresis, thereby reducing the need for early or frequent HD **(Table 2 and Box 4)**.

POSTOPERATIVE PERIOD

In the early postoperative period, management of KTx involves a rapid diagnosis of surgical and medical complications, which are complex and need the highest vigilance to avoid graft loss and patient death. The course is largely determined by the degree of renal function recovery. Three types of response are seen—good and progressive recovery with diuresis, nonoliguric status postsurgery with slow recovery, and oliguric or DGF with a prolonged phase of dialysis needing close watch for complications. In this period, the focus is on electrolytes, immunosuppression, labs, and diagnosis of any complication **(Boxes 5 and 6)**.

Postoperative Medical Issues

- *Hematological:* Anemia, leukopenia, thrombocytopenia
- *BP:* High or low and volume status

BOX 5: Postoperative orders—first week (nursing care).

- Vital signs are to be checked every hour for 24 hours, then every 4 hours once the patient is stable
- Intake and output every hour for 24 hours, then every four hours once the patient is stable
- Daily weight
- Intravenous fluids as directed by the physician
- To encourage incentive spirometry, turning in the bed, deep breathing, cough every hour
- To ambulate from the first postoperative day
- Head end of the bed is to be elevated to 30°
- No blood pressure monitoring, IV cannula in the extremity of AV access
- Check dialysis access for function every day
- Dressing is to be changed every day and more frequently if soaked
- Irrigate Foley's catheter with 30 mL of normal saline for removing blood clots if poor flow
- Alert if urine output drops to <50 mL/h
- Notify if systolic blood pressure is <110 mm Hg or >180 mm Hg
- Electrocardiogram sos
- NPO until told otherwise by transplant surgeon on day 1 and then introduction oral fluid and food as per comfort

(AV: arteriovenous; IV: intravenous)

Source: Amend W, Vincenti F, Tomlanovich S. The first three post-transplantation months. In: Danovitch G (Ed). Handbook of Kidney Transplantation, 4th edition. Philadelphia: Lippincott William & Wilkins; 2005. pp. 212-35.

BOX 6: Common postoperative laboratory tests.

- *Blood tests:* Complete blood count with platelet, electrolytes, creatinine, glucose and blood urea nitrogen twice a day: LFT, calcium, phosphorus after 7 days
- Calcineurin inhibitor level twice a week
- Urine culture and sensitivity after catheter removal or sos
- Postoperative chest radiograph
- Duplex ultrasound imaging, usually at days 2–4 post-transplant
- DTPA renogram as indicated by clinical progress

(DTPA: diethylenetriaminepentaacetic acid; LFT: liver function test)

Source: Kronish K, Olmos A, Niemann CU. Perioperative care of patients undergoing kidney transplantation. In: Knechtle S, Marson L, Morris P (Eds). Kidney Transplantation—Principles and Practice, 8th edition. Philadelphia: Elsevier Inc; 2020. pp. 184-97 [Chapter 13].

- *Metabolic issues:* Electrolytes (potassium, magnesium), hyperglycemia
- Infections and prophylaxis
- Need for dialysis
- *Fluid balance:* Proper intake/output chart, IV fluid as 0.45% saline, or Ringer's lactate (as per blood electrolytes)
- Fluid intake should be output plus 50 mL if urine output is below 250 mL/h, equal to output if urine is 250–500 mL/h, minus 100 if output is 500–1,000, and minus 200 if above 1 L/h (on the first postoperative day)
- Immunosuppression regimen and monitoring are done as per local protocol.

Postoperative Surgical Issues

- *Catheter care:* Urinary, drains, incision site care, removal of catheter (7 days and ureteric stent by 3–4 weeks)
- Allowing oral feed and fluids.

Postoperative Anesthetic Issues

Pain management/epidural anesthesia/ventilator care/IV lines—central and peripheral—are looked at.

GENERAL ISSUES

The general issues are psychological support/ambulation, chest physiotherapy, and deep venous thrombosis (DVT) prophylaxis.

INVESTIGATION PROTOCOLS

Investigation protocols include labs, radiology [ultrasound abdomen, diethylenetriamine pentaacetate (DTPA) nuclear scan of kidneys, X-ray chest], and drug levels **(Box 6)**.

Early Postoperative Complications

Diverse complications could be seen postoperatively **(Table 3 and Box 6)**. Usually, a set protocol of labs and

TABLE 3: Early surgical and medical complications after surgery.

Surgical	*Medical*
Ureteral obstruction	Prerenal/volume factors AKI
Urinary leak	Acute rejection
Hematuria	*Drug toxicity:* Acute calcineurin inhibitor-induced nephrotoxicity
Arterial thrombosis/kinking	Infection—graft/systemic
Renal vein thrombosis	Delayed graft function—ATN
Postoperative hemorrhage	Recurrent disease
Lymphocele	Systemic complication—PTE/ACS

(ACS: acute coronary syndrome; AKI: acute kidney injury; ATN: acute tubular necrosis; PTE: pulmonary thromboembolism)

Source: Schroder PM, Marson LP, Knechtle SJ. Early course of the patient with a kidney transplant. In: Knechtle S, Marson L, Morris P (Eds). Kidney Transplantation—Principles and Practice, 8th edition. Philadelphia: Elsevier Inc; 2020. pp. 198-211 [Chapter 14].

radiological investigations are employed by all centers for timely diagnosis of complications.[5-7]

Allograft Dysfunction

Postoperative oligoanuria is commonly seen in cadaveric KTx but is unusual in live transplant and needs appropriate evaluation of possible causes. When the kidney fails to recover, and the patient needs HD in the first postoperative week, it is referred to as DGF. Such delay in graft function predisposes to a higher incidence of acute rejection and is associated with poorer graft survival.

An early renal transplant duplex ultrasound is a useful noninvasive bedside first radiological investigation that can readily identify vascular anastomotic complications such as renal artery or venous thrombosis or compression of vessel from hematoma/other collections. Even the ureteric dilatation due to compression from blood, urine, or lymph collection can be picked up easily. In the absence of vascular or ureteric complications in oligoanuric patients, abnormality of parenchymal echo texture, size of kidney allograft, and resistive index (RI) can suggest the need for renal biopsy to exclude rejection. The RI (measured as peak systolic velocity–end-diastolic velocity/peak systolic velocity) normally lies between 0.60 and 0.80 levels and has its own limitations of etiological diagnosis. Even the nuclear medicine imaging with isotope DTPA or ethylene cysteine (EC) or sulfur colloid scan can help in the assessment of allograft perfusion, early graft dysfunction, possibility of superimposed rejection based on pattern recognition, if done on a serial basis. Nuclear imaging can identify a ureteric anastomotic leak in a functioning graft easily.

Biochemical, Metabolic, and Hematological Abnormality

Dyselectrolytemia is frequent in the early postoperative period. Perioperative initial hyperkalemia is followed by hypokalemia once diuresis starts. Hypomagnesemia is not infrequent and gets exacerbated by CNI therapy. Use of CNI is associated with an increased risk of post-transplant diabetes mellitus, which can worsen dyselectrolytemia. A low inorganic phosphorus level (hypophosphatemia) is universal but usually needs no treatment. To reduce the risk of arrhythmias, choosing appropriate fluid as IV electrolyte replacement is important. One should aim to target serum potassium and magnesium in the normal range. The stress of surgery combined with steroid and CNI (mostly tacrolimus) leads to severe perioperative hyperglycemia in both diabetics and nondiabetics (post-transplant diabetes).

Hematological abnormalities are common, such as anemia, thrombocytopenia, and leukopenia, and have to be analyzed for appropriate action. Leukopenia due to myelosuppression in post-transplant patients may need drug dose modification of mycophenolate mofetil (MMF)/azathioprine, or discontinuation of cotrimoxazole or dose adjustment of valganciclovir. Severe and persistent thrombocytopenia, if observed post-transplant, one needs to look for any thrombotic microangiopathy **(Box 7)**. Any acute drop of hematocrit needs evaluation for transfusion need and source of blood loss.[5]

BOX 7: Lab tests for diagnosis of thrombotic microangiopathy (TMA).

- Thrombocytopenia—platelet count <150,000/mL[3]
- Microangiopathic hemolytic anemia (MAHA)—hemoglobin <10 g/dL with evidence of red cell fragments on blood film (schistocytes), elevated reticulocyte count
- Elevated lactate dehydrogenase
- Elevated bilirubin

Source: Kronish K, Olmos A, Niemann CU. Perioperative care of patients undergoing kidney transplantation. In: Knechtle S, Marson L, Morris P (Eds). Kidney Transplantation—Principles and Practice, 8th edition. Philadelphia: Elsevier Inc; 2020. pp. 184-97 [Chapter 13].

Hypotension

Hypotension in the postoperative period is not uncommon. It may be due to hypovolemia or due to vasoplegia from drugs used as an anesthetic or narcotic analgesics, or occasionally from the anaphylactoid reaction of monoclonal or polyclonal induction agents or can be due to acute coronary syndrome. Initial management involves fluid boluses to optimize fluid status and to exclude other causes, such as blood loss, sepsis, and cardiac dysfunction. Renal transplant recipient who continues to remain hypotensive despite fluid boluses can be supported with vasopressors and inotropes as per center-specific protocol, but ruling out acute coronary syndrome (ACS) by ECG, 2D echo, and the cardiac enzyme is essential in such situation.

Cardiovascular Complications

Hypertension is common and not considered as a complication. It is seen to occur in nearly 50–70% of recipients and well tolerated. It is caused or contributed by multiple factors (prior hypertension, stoppage of oral antihypertensive drugs due to surgery, IV fluid administration, steroid, and CNI use). The dihydropyridine agents may be used along with clonidine, beta blockers, and alpha blockers. Renin-angiotensin system (RAS) blockers and diltiazem are usually avoided.

Despite pretransplant cardiac screening, ACS still is a perioperative risk. ACS in this setting is a serious and challenging complication to manage. The risk of bleeding from antiplatelet and anticoagulant therapy needs to be balanced against the benefit of usual care and needs a multidisciplinary approach for decision-making in this difficult situation.

Vascular Complications

In transplant recipients with a good urine output postoperatively, the sudden development of oliguria or anuria should prompt exclusion of urinary catheter block as well as the possibility of renal artery or venous thrombosis. Duplex ultrasound imaging and knowledge of donor vessel status at the time of surgery known well to transplant surgeons can give the diagnosis early for emergency reexploration.

Ureteric Complications and Perinephric Collection

Urine leak-producing urinoma is an uncommon urological complication these days and gets prevented by routine stenting by certain urologist. Perinephric collection could be urinoma, lymphocele, or hematoma, which can be aspirated and analyzed biochemically for clarity.

Infection (Local, Graft, or Systemic)

Immunosuppressed transplant patients are particularly prone to acquire infections in the perioperative phase which are usually bacterial. However, sepsis can be challenging to diagnose. In general, any change in physiological vital parameters (such as BP, pulse, respiration, sensorium, or temperature) or unexplained clinical deterioration, even if afebrile, should alert to the possibility of sepsis and appropriate samples be sent.

Rejection

In recent times, developing hyperacute rejection has become extremely rare, consequent to better immunological assays that detect the presence of preformed anti-human leukocyte antigen (HLA) antibodies. However, early acute rejection continues to be common, with a reported incidence of 10–25% depending on immunological risk, choice of induction agent, and immunosuppression.

CONCLUSION

Kidney transplantation is considered to be the best treatment option for all eligible patients with end-stage kidney disease. This successful evolution of transplant care has seen many milestones and developments in the surgical field (laparoscopic donor nephrectomy) as well as in the medical field (highly effective immunosuppressives and monoclonals), which has improved patient and graft survival together with tools that aid immunological monitoring.

Protocol-driven multidisciplinary care in the perioperative period is achieving excellent allograft outcomes. Early optimized postrenal transplant care has decreased the risk of mortality (due to infections, cardiovascular issues, and rarely surgical complications) to <1–2% in the immediate perioperative period in most centers. So, the adage of "well begun is half done" needs reinforcement in all transplant care centers to get the desired result.

REFERENCES

1. Kidney Disease: Improving Global Outcomes (KDIGO) Transplant Work Group. KDIGO clinical practice guideline for the care of kidney transplant recipients. Am J Transplant. 2009;9(Suppl. 3):S1-155.
2. Chadban SJ, Ahn C, Axelrod DA, Foster BJ, Kasiske BL, Kher V, et al. KDIGO clinical practice guideline on the evaluation and management of candidates for kidney transplantation. Transplantation. 2020;104(4S1 Suppl 1):S11-103.
3. Fuggle SV, Taylor CJ. Histocompatibility in kidney transplantation. In: Knechtle S, Marson L, Morris P (Eds). Kidney Transplantation—Principles and Practice, 8th edition. Philadelphia: Elsevier Inc; 2020. pp. 139-56 [Chapter 10].
4. Kronishk, Olmos A, Niemann CU. Perioperative care of patients undergoing kidney transplantation. In: Knechtle S, Marson L, Morris P (Eds). Kidney Transplantation—Principles and Practice, 8th edition. Philadelphia: Elsevier Inc; 2020. pp. 185-97 [Chapter 13].
5. Hultin S, Hawley CM, Johnson DW, Francis RS. In: Vitin A (Ed). Perioperative Care for Organ Transplant Recipient. London: Intech Open; 2019. p. 160.
6. Schroder PM, Marson LP, Knechtle SJ. Early course of the patient with a kidney transplant. In: Knechtle S, Marson L, Morris P (Eds). Kidney Transplantation—Principles and Practice, 8th edition. Elsevier Inc; 2020. pp. 198-211 [Chapter 14].
7. Amend W, Vincenti F, Tomlanovich S. The first three post-transplantation months. In: Danovitch G (Ed). Handbook of Kidney Transplantation, 4th edition. Philadelphia: Lippincott William & Wilkins; 2005. pp. 212-35.

CHAPTER 7

Kidney Transplantation in Abnormal Urinary Bladder

PP Varma, Prateek Kumar

CASE VIGNETTE

A 15-year-old male developed end-stage kidney disease and is awaiting renal transplantation. He is suffering from neurogenic bladder and has a history of recurrent urinary tract infections (UTIs) and pyelonephritis. He is on hemodialysis for the last 2 years.

a. How would you evaluate this patient for renal transplantation?
b. What are graft outcomes in a renal transplant patient with abnormal bladder?

INTRODUCTION

Workup to transplantation shows that 10% of adults and 25–30% of pediatric end-stage renal failure patients have abnormal bladder. Advances in medical and surgical therapeutics have improved the outcome of transplantation, and abnormal bladder is no longer considered a contraindication to transplantation.[1-3]

NORMAL AND ABNORMAL BLADDER

Normal adults and children over the age of 12 years have bladder capacity of 300–500 mL. It is supplied by sympathetic, parasympathetic, and somatic nerves. Bladder emptying is a coordinated mechanism. When the bladder gets filled, afferent fibers carry sensations to the spinal cord. These sensations are conveyed to upper centers in pons and cerebrum and by interneurons to the efferents. In very young children, the micturition center in pons is not developed, so efferents contract the bladder whenever sensation of fullness arrives. Parasympathetics contract the detrusor muscle and relax the internal sphincter. Upper centers exert inhibitory control over the bladder. Only when the surroundings are comfortable, the upper centers relax the external sphincter and cause contraction of the detrusor. Normal bladder is compliant, low-pressure reservoir, nonleaky, and empties fully on natural voiding. When a person starts micturition, intravesical pressure is around 10 cmH_2O. If intravesical pressure exceeds 40 cmH_2O (due to obstruction or noncompliant bladder), urine ceases to come from the ureters with resultant damage to the upper tract.[1,4] An abnormal bladder maybe of small or large capacity, maybe noncompliant, maybe leaky, has high intravesical pressure, and does not empty fully. So, all efforts are made to make the bladder a low-pressure reservoir prior to transplantation.

Bladder capacity in children can be calculated by either of these two formulae:[4-6]

- Age <2 years = 2 × age in years + 2 = capacity (ounces)
  Age >2 years = age in years (divided by) 2 + 6 = capacity (ounces)
- (Age + 1) × 30 mL (with 400 mL for those older than 12 years)

Causes of Abnormal Bladder

- *Neurogenic bladder:* Diabetes, cauda equina syndrome, spinal cord injury—bladder maybe large and sensationless. It has high pressure and does not empty fully.
- *Obstruction:* Posterior urethral valves, urethral stricture, a prostatic enlargement where the bladder is working against resistance (urine bladder has high pressure, is thick-walled, and trabeculated).
- *Dysplasia:* Prune belly syndrome
- *Voiding dysfunction:* Hinman–Allen syndrome
- Postradiation, postchemotherapy, interstitial fibrosis, post-tuberculosis, schistosomiasis, etc.—bladder becomes small, low capacity, and noncompliant.

PRETRANSPLANT WORKUP OF BLADDER

The foundation of evaluation is a detailed history, especially focusing on a diary, recording voided volumes, frequency of urination, incontinence episodes, presence of nocturia, and UTI episodes over several days or months.

In patients without any symptoms suggestive of bladder abnormality, the absence of residual urine on ultrasonography and a normal uroflow study is sufficient to rule out significant bladder dysfunction. Residual urine estimation using ultrasonography is a simple and quick test without any radiation exposure. Uroflowmetry is a noninvasive urodynamic test which gives important information in the form of pattern of urine flow, and the maximal and average flow rate. Patients with a urine flow rate of >15 mL/s and postvoid volume of <100 mL can go ahead with transplant. A voiding cystourethrogram provides an estimate of bladder capacity, evaluates urethral anatomy, and determines the presence of vesicoureteral reflux. Invasive urodynamic studies, like cystomanometry, and electromyography of the pelvic floor maybe needed in select cases.[6] Videourodynamics is the simultaneous performance of a voiding cystourethrogram and cystomanometry.

Cystoscopy is indicated in cases in which the urinary flow is abnormal, residual urine volume is significant, or there is difficulty in urethral catheterization. The absence of obstruction in these cases warrants neurological investigation, including magnetic resonance imaging of the spinal cord, to exclude neuropathic voiding dysfunction.[7,8]

Algorithms for evaluation and approach are shown in **Flowcharts 1 and 2**.

Flowchart 1: Approach to management of bladder dysfunction.

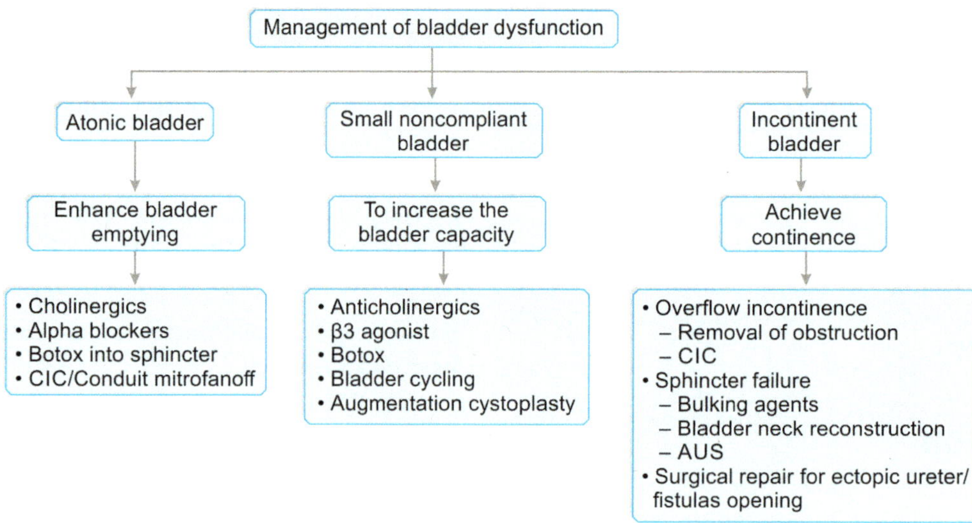

(AUS: artificial urinary sphincter; CIC: clean intermittent catheterization)

Flowchart 2: Approach to a patient with bladder abnormality.

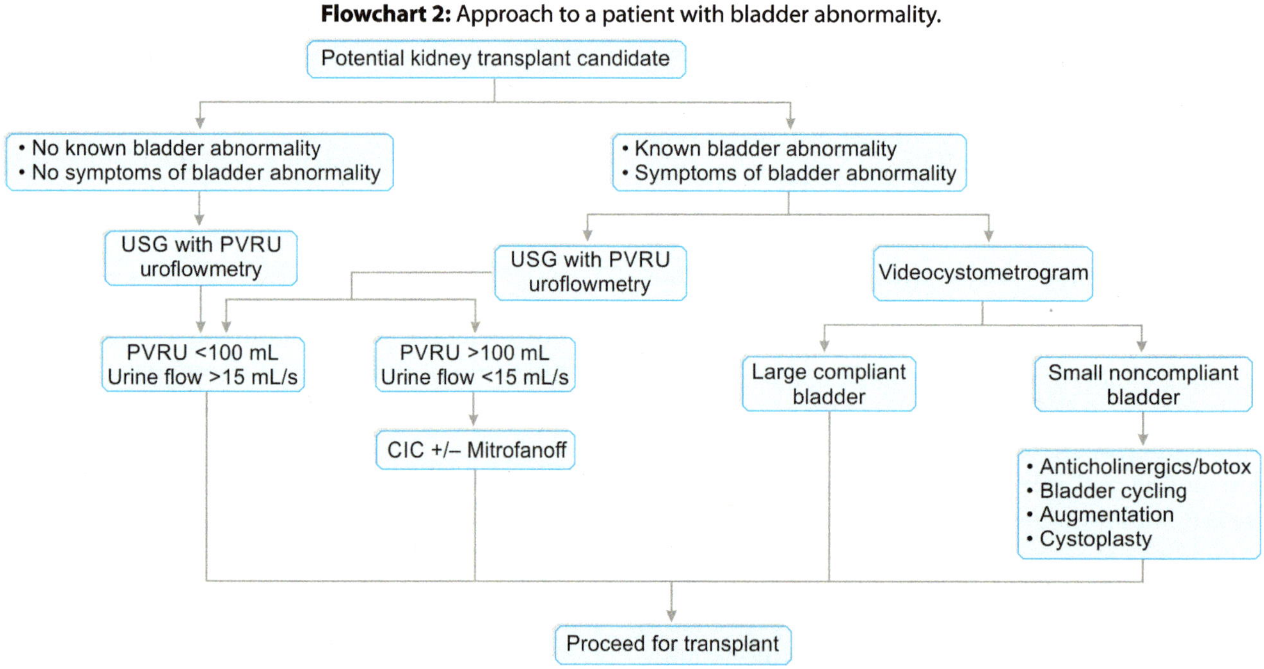

(PVRU: postvoid residual urine; USG: ultrasonography)

CHAPTER HIGHLIGHTS

- Up to 10% of adults and 25–30% of pediatric end-stage renal failure patients have abnormal bladder during their workup to transplantation.
- The incidence of UTI in renal transplant recipients with abnormal bladder ranges from 6 to 86%.
- The best timing of bladder reconstruction surgery in renal transplant candidates is controversial.
- There is a higher chance of UTI in patients who undergo surgery such as reconstruction or rehabilitation of bladder.
- Recurrent UTIs can affect graft survival in such patients.

GOAL FOR INTERVENTION

The goal is to make the bladder compliant and low-pressure reservoir with adequate capacity.

MANAGEMENT STRATEGIES

- Clean intermittent catheterization (CIC)
- Medical management-anticholinergics, muscle relaxants, botulinum toxin A, neuromodulation (NM)
- Augmentation cystoplasty (AC) and conduit for catheterization.

Clean Intermittent Catheterization

Clean intermittent catheterization has revolutionized the management of abnormal high-pressure bladder. In CIC, a patient has to do self-catheterization every 4–6 hours by passing catheter in the native urethra. Hand washing and catheter cleaning with soap are the only requirement. Lapides et al. in 1972[9] used this technique for the first time in 218 of his patients with obstructive uropathy, neurogenic bladder, and decompensated detrusor. There was a significant improvement in urinary incontinence, bladder emptying, upper tract infection, and importantly improvement in emotional status of the patients. CIC reduces the intravesical pressure and prevents upper tract damage. Today, CIC is the backbone in the management of abnormal bladder. If it is not possible to catheterize from native urethra because of structural reasons or embarrassment of doing CIC in public places, especially in ladies, then a conduit can be made from the bladder to the outside by Mitrofanoff or Monti's procedure.[1] The commonly used Mitrofanoff procedure uses appendix vermiformis as a conduit. If appendix is not available, then small intestine (Monti's procedure) is used for making conduit. One end of the appendix or intestinal conduit is in the bladder and the other end is brought out through an opening (stoma), which is made in the umbilicus or little below that on the right side. Bladder end is passed through detrusor in such a way that it acts like a valve, so that urine does not leak out in-between catheterizations.[1,10] There has been debate about reuse of catheters. A prospective multicentric study comparing single-use hydrophilic-coated catheters with reuse catheter found that single-use catheter improved the quality of life ($p = 0.01$). The reused catheters were full of debris and biofilm (74%) and were contaminated with microorganisms.[11] The only problem with CIC is the increase in the incidence of UTI and noncompliance by some patients.

Medical Management (Anticholinergics, Botulinum Toxin A, Neuromodulation)

Propantheline bromide is an anticholinergic, antimuscarinic drug which relaxes the bladder muscle and reduces the pressure. It has been used in bladder overactivity with a success rate of 50%. However, poor absorption and side effects such as dry mouth, palpitations, and blurring of vision have made it unpopular.

Oxybutynin: It has less side effects and a negligible discontinuation rate (1%). Long-acting oxybutynin is to be taken once a day. It relaxes bladder, lowers intravesical pressure, and prevents upper tract damage. It reduces incontinence episodes by 80–90%, and the continence rate is reported between 40 and 50%. Tolterodine and solifenacin are also antimuscarinic and muscle relaxants and are useful. Tolterodine is as effective as oxybutynin. OBJECT (Overactive Bladder: Judging Effective Control and Treatment) trial, a multicentric trial with 315 women and 63 men, compared sustained-release oxybutynin with tolterodine over 12 weeks' period. Extended-release oxybutynin 10 mg OD (once a day) was more effective than tolterodine 2 mg BD (twice daily), as measured by end-of-study urge incontinence, total incontinence, and micturition frequency episodes ($p < 0.01$) with similar side effects.[1,4,12] Mirabegron, a β-3 adrenergic receptor agonist, causes relaxation of the detrusor muscle and increases bladder capacity. It is indicated for an overactive bladder (OAB) with symptoms of urge urinary incontinence and urinary frequency. The American Urological Association recommends β-3 adrenergic receptor agonists as second-line therapy in patients with an inadequate response to behavioral therapy.[13]

In case medical modality is not satisfactory, then botulinum toxin A can be used. It has been approved by the Food and Drug Administration (FDA) for urinary incontinence and bladder overactivity, where anticholinergics have failed. Its effect lasts for 6–9 months. Onabotulinum toxin A 100–200 units are injected at 20–30 sites around trigone during cystoscopy, the only drawback being repeated injections with increased risk of UTI. Its effectiveness has reduced the need for AC. Cost comparison studies find that over a 5-year follow-up, botulinum works out cheaper than AC.[14] Other studies comparing NM with botulinum find both to be equally effective.

Neuromodulation: Neuromodulation is again an effective strategy, especially in those with OAB having poor response to medical therapy. A stimulator stimulates the sacral nerve fibers or post-tibial nerve. In OAB afferents from bladder go the spinal cord and stimulate the efferent and bladder contracts. In NM, impulses travel from stimulator to spinal cord and they block the afferents coming from the bladder. One can change the frequency/timing and intensity of stimulus. For sacral stimulation, the stimulator is placed near S3 foramina and for post-tibial little above the medial malleolus. Stimulation is tried for up to 12 weeks. If there is over 50% benefit in incontinence, then in the second surgery, a sitting stimulator is implanted under the skin. The results of this modality are very rewarding.[1,4,10]

Bladder Augmentation: Augmentation Cystoplasty

With availability of effective medical management, the need for AC has gone down. But for patients who have refractory OAB or those having small bladder need AC. Mikulicz initially described augmentation ileocystoplasty in humans in 1889. The technique gained acceptance in the 1950s for the management of tuberculous bladders and was further popularized by Bramble in the 1980s in conjunction with CIC. For the last two decades, newer modalities such as laparoscopic and robotic surgery have gained popularity.

In AC, a flap is made from ileum or colon or stomach or megaureter (if available) and stitched to the bladder. Ileum is the most common organ used **(Figs. 1A to C)**. There are certain inherent problems with use of ileum for AC. Intestinal epithelium secretes mucus which can block the catheter, especially in children who have thin catheters. So daily irrigation is required. Second, there is a loss of bicarbonate from the epithelium so patients universally have metabolic acidosis. A megaureter if available is free from both these major problems. The resection of ileum is complicated by intestinal obstruction in up to 5% of patients. The attached ileum does not contract synergistically with detrusor and therefore patients need to use pressure/strain to empty the bladder. Therefore, CIC use along with augmented bladder is common (20–100%). Constant exposure of intestinal epithelium to urine, the accumulation of nitrosamines and infections can lead to premalignant and malignant degeneration in the long term with incidences of 1.2–10.3%. Because of urinary stasis and acidosis-induced calcium release from bones, stone formation is reported in 15–40% patients. Those with urethral CIC are 5 times and those with Mitrofanoff technique 10 times prone to stone formation. Bladder rupture due to ischemia at the anastomotic site is also reported. Over 80% patients feel satisfied after AC. Because of the stasis and repeated catheterizations, UTI is common. Some of the studies suggest that bacteriuria is seen in 75% patients, but infections occur only in 20%.[4,5,10,15]

To obviate problems associated with ileocystoplasty, a lot of research is going on to make bioengineered bladder augmentation. With the help of tissue engineering technology, efforts have been made to (1) grow urothelial cells (UC) and smooth muscle cells (SMC) taken from the bladder biopsy, in the artificial media. Then these are put on (2) the scaffold. Cellular and acellular scaffolds have been tried. However, the results have not been very encouraging because of fibrosis, inflammatory reaction, and shrinkage of scaffold. Another challenge is the blood and nerve supply to this scaffold.

Ideal timing of reconstruction surgeries of the urinary tract in transplant candidates is controversial. It depends on practices of different transplant centers. Such surgeries are not usually performed along with transplant because of higher incidence of infective complications and impaired wound healing. There is lack of studies comparing the outcomes in patients in whom bladder reconstruction is done prior, at the time or after the transplantation.

Now bioprinting technology is being tried in vivo. In this, bioink is made up of UC and SMC. A Biopen is mounted on an endoscope, which is advanced in bladder, and bioprinting is done. Even capillary bioprinting can be done **(Figs. 2A to D)**. Though in preliminary stages, bioprinting is offering hope for bladder augmentation in near future.[10,16]

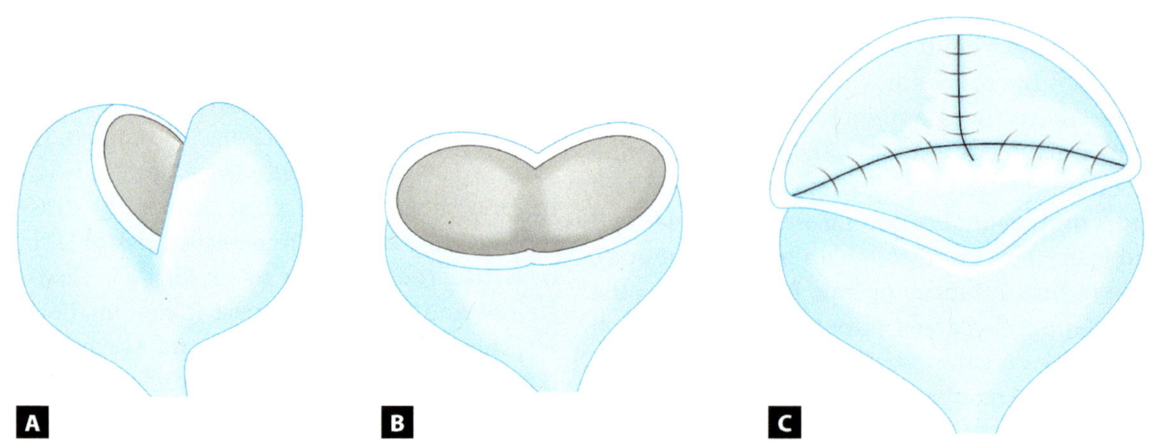

Figs. 1A to C: Bladder augmentation. (A) Bladder incision; (B) Bladder cut open; (C) U-shaped flap anastomoses to bladder.

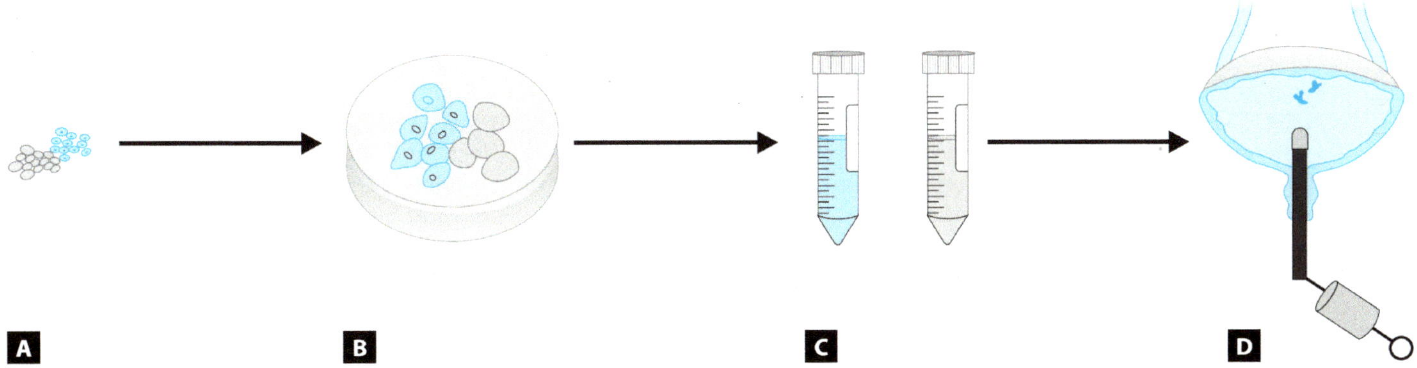

Figs. 2A to D: Bioprinting: (A) UCs and SMCs cells; (B) UCs and SMCs propagation; (C) Bioink; (D) In situ in vivo bioprinting inside a bladder. (SMC: smooth muscle cells; UC: urothelial cells)

GRAFT OUTCOME

Indian and international data suggest that graft outcome in patients with abnormal bladder is almost similar to the ones with normal bladder, though episodes of UTI are common. Salman et al. compared 30 transplants in abnormal bladder patients with an equal number in normal bladders. Graft survival was not significantly different between the study and the control groups at 1 year (90% vs. 97%; $p = 0.30$), 3 years (88% vs. 91%; $p = 0.67$), and 5 years (82% vs. 87%; $p = 0.68$). Desai et al. reported outcome of 14 patients with rehabilitated bladder and found short-term outcome to be not much different. After 3 years, all grafts were functioning but they had significant episodes of UTI and pyelonephritis. A 20-year data of patients transplanted for congenital anomalies of kidney and urinary tract (CAKUT) in New Zealand and Australia (with diagnosis of PUV, renal dysplasia, and reflux nephropathy) reported a 10-year graft survival of 70%, 76%, and 70% and 20-year graft survival as 30%, 53%, and 49%, respectively. After adjusting for age at transplant, graft source and human leukocyte antigen (HLA) matching, there was evidence for poorer graft survival in PUV [hazard ratio (HR), 1.65; 95% confidence interval (CI), 1.15–2.38] after 10 years. A similar observation was reported by McKay et al., who found no difference in graft survival till 10 years; however, after 10 years, the graft outcome was inferior in these patients.[17-20]

CONCLUSION

The target of all therapies, medical or surgical, is to make abnormal bladder a low-pressure reservoir. Anticholinergics, botulinum toxin, NM, and CIC, alone or in combination, have brought relief to majority. A minority with refractory OAB or small bladder needs AC. Bioengineering techniques are likely to reduce the inherent complications associated with AC. For the initial 10 years, the graft outcome in patients transplanted with abnormal bladder is similar to those with normal bladder but is inferior thereafter.

REFERENCES

1. Barry JM. Kidney transplantation into patients with abnormal bladder. Transplantation. 2004;77:1120-23.
2. Desai P, Yadav R, Chaturvedi S, Maheshwari R, Gulia A, Kumar A. Kidney transplant in patients with abnormal bladder: experience of tertiary care center in developing country-is the outcome same? Ind J Transpl. 2018;12:136-42.
3. Mishra SK, Muthu V, Rajapurkar MM, Desai MR. Kidney transplantation in abnormal bladder. Indian J Urol. 2007;23(3):299-304.
4. Fontaine C, Papworth E, Pascoe J, Hashim H. Update on the management of overactive bladder. Ther Adv Urol. 2021;13:17562872211039034.
5. Nankivell G, Caldwell PH. Paediatric urinary incontinence. Aust Prescr. 2014;37:192-5.
6. Kaefer M, Zurakowski D, Bauer SB, Retik AB, Peters CA, Atala A, et al. Estimating normal bladder capacity in children. J Urol. 1997;158(6):2261-4.
7. Hijalmas K. Urodynamics in normal infants and children. Scand J Urol Nephrol Suppl. 1988;114:20-7.
8. Winters JC, Dmochowski RR, Goldman HB, Herndon CDA, Kobashi KC, Kraus SR, et al. Urodynamic studies in adults: AUA/SUFU guidelines. J Urol. 2012;188:2464-72.
9. Lapides J, Diokno AC, Gould FR, Lowe BS. Further observations on self-catheterization. J Urol. 1976;116:169-71.
10. Langer S, Radtke C, Györi E, Springer A, Metzelder ML. Bladder augmentation in children: current problems and experimental strategies for reconstruction. Wien Med Wochenschr. 2019;169:61-70.
11. Newman DK, New PW, Heriseanu R, Petronis S, Håkansson J, Håkansson MÅ, et al. Intermittent catheterization with single- or multiple-reuse catheters: clinical study on safety and impact on quality of life. Int Urol Nephrol. 2020;52(8):1443-51.
12. Appell RA, Sand P, Dmochowski R, Anderson R, Zinner N, Lama D, et al. Prospective randomized controlled trial of extended-release oxybutynin chloride and tolterodine tartrate in the treatment of overactive bladder: results of the OBJECT study. Mayo Clin Proc. 2001;76(4):358-63.
13. Vaughan CP, Markland AD. Urinary incontinence in women. Ann Intern Med. 2020;172(3):ITC17-32.

14. Padmanabhan P, Scarpero HM, Milam DF, Dmochowski RR, Penson DF. Five-year cost analysis of intra-detrusor injection of botulinum toxin type A and augmentation cystoplasty for refractory neurogenic detrusor overactivity. World J Urol. 2011;29(1):51-7.
15. Veeratterapillay R, Thorpe AC, Harding C. Augmentation cystoplasty: contemporary indications, techniques and complications. Indian J Urol. 2013;29(4):322-7.
16. Wang X, Zhang F, Liao L. Current applications and future directions of bioengineering approaches for bladder augmentation and reconstruction. Front Surg. 2021;8: 664404.
17. Amesty MV, García-Vaz C, Espinosa L, Martínez-Urrutia MJ, López-Pereira P. Long-term renal transplant outcome in patients with posterior urethral valves. Prognostic factors related to bladder dysfunction management. Front Pediatr. 2021;9:646923.
18. López Pereira P, Ortiz R, Espinosa L, Martínez Urrutia MJ, Lobato R, Alonso A, et al. Does bladder augmentation negatively affect renal transplant outcome in posterior urethral valve patients? J Pediatr Urol. 2014;10(5):892-7.
19. Salman B, Hassan A, Sultan S, Tophill P, Halawa A. Renal transplant in the abnormal bladder: long-term follow-up. Exp Clin Transplant. 2018;16(1):10-5.
20. McKay AM, Kim S, Kennedy SE. Long-term outcome of kidney transplantation in patients with congenital anomalies of the kidney and urinary tract. Pediatr Nephrol. 2019;34:2409-15.

CHAPTER

8

Evaluation of Acute Allograft Dysfunction

Joyita Bharati, Harbir S Kohli

CASE VIGNETTE 1

A case of graft dysfunction presenting at 1-week post-transplant.

A 34-year-old male was evaluated for reduced urine output (500 mL/day) and absence of fall in serum creatinine (5 mg/dL) after 5 days of first kidney transplant with his wife as the donor. He had received 2 units of blood transfusion 6 months prior to transplant, and there were no chronic or bloodstream infections in the past. Recent donor specific antibodies (DSAs) [by single antigen bead (SAB)] were done 3 months back which were negative, and complement-dependent lymphocytotoxicity crossmatch was negative. Human leukocyte antigen (HLA) match was only one sixth with the donor. He underwent a standard risk living donor transplant with his spouse as the donor, with antithymocyte globulin as induction therapy followed by tacrolimus, mycophenolate mofetil (MMF), and steroids maintenance therapy. There were no adverse events during the intraoperative and immediate postoperative periods. Calcineurin inhibitor (CNI) trough levels were difficult to be maintained within the expected range between 10 and 15 ng/mL, likely due to individual metabolism differences. There was no evidence of infection. His urine output did not return to normal despite 5 days post-transplant and serum creatinine was stuck at 5 mg/dL. Ultrasound/Doppler of the graft showed normal blood flow and no urinary obstruction. Urine protein was 1+ (by dipstick) without any cells/casts. Kidney allograft biopsy was done and was reported as glomerulitis (g1), peritubular capillaritis (ptc2), and minimal interstitial inflammation (i1) suggestive of active antibody-mediated rejection. C4d staining along peritubular capillaries was positive by immunofluorescence. Repeat DSA titers were negative. He was diagnosed with antibody-mediated rejection (ABMR) despite lack of DSAs based on C4d staining and evidence of microvascular inflammation.[1] He responded to treatment of ABMR (plasmapheresis and rituximab) with serum creatinine falling down to 1.7 mg/dL over the subsequent week. The reason for having a negative DSA despite active histological and clinical ABMR is not clear. There is a school of thought that HLA incompatibility in the form of HLA mismatches and reduced doses of tacrolimus (probably due to genetic difference in metabolism of CNIs) in the early post-transplant period led to development of DSAs (to HLA antigens) causing ABMR. The negative DSAs could be due to methodological flaws or possible fleeting DSAs or due to the presence of HLA-specific memory B cells.[2] Similar to previous studies,[2] this patient with ABMR (histological) without donor-specific anti-HLA antibodies responded favorably to treatment in a short time.

CASE VIGNETTE 2

A case of acute graft dysfunction presenting at 3 months post-transplant.

A 55-year-old male presented with complaints of reduced urine output on and off for 2 weeks after undergoing kidney allograft biopsy for acute graft dysfunction elsewhere. He was 3 months postkidney transplant with his wife as the donor with no immediate complications after transplant. 2 weeks back, he presented to the previous hospital with complaints of increasing serum creatinine from a baseline of 1.3 to 2.7 mg/dL over a 2-week period for which he was treated with steroid pulses and plasmapheresis for a diagnosis of ABMR. After treatment, his serum creatinine fell to 1.7 mg/dL over 5 days; however, he started developing reduced urine output. The urine volume fluctuated between 100 and 500 mL/day initially to become completely absent over the last 24 hours. Physical examination revealed minimal graft site tenderness, but no obvious swelling or redness or warmth. His serum creatinine was 2.4 mg/dL at presentation to our hospital and an urgent ultrasonography (USG) of the graft showed moderate hydronephrosis and a cystic mass outside the ureter almost compressing the lower part of the ureter. Per urethral catheter was placed immediately and a single time aspiration of the cyst was attempted. Urine output improved to 1,000 mL/day on the per-urethral catheter. Fluid from the cyst showed creatinine of 3.5 mg/dL (not significantly high as compared to serum creatinine) and predominant lymphocytes on differential count. Later, a pigtail drainage catheter was placed in the cyst which drained clear fluid, not suggestive of urine. Computed tomography (CT) urography was then done which was not suggestive of urinoma as the cause of the cyst, and the volume of the cyst was ~50 mL without any septations inside the cyst. After 3–4 days of pigtail drainage and then removal of the catheter, the cyst started to shrink in size along with sustained good urine output. Serum creatinine also fell back to 1.6 mg/dL on follow-up. Therefore, a definitive treatment was not done. The diagnosis of lymphocele was made on the basis of imaging and laboratory findings in this case. Precedence of an episode of acute ABMR and its treatment in this case is similar to other reports[3,4] showing acute rejection (and treatment agents) as a risk factor for lymphocele. Our patient presented with acute urinary retention after a treated episode of acute rejection. Alternative diagnosis of urinoma/leak and hematoma was excluded using laboratory findings (drain fluid creatinine/plasma creatinine ratio of >1.5–6 times[5,6] is considered suggestive of urine leak) and imaging, respectively. This case highlights the importance of clinical history, urgent imaging, and systematic approach to evaluation of differential diagnoses in kidney transplant recipients presenting with acute graft dysfunction. One has to be vigilant as more than one factor may be playing a role in graft dysfunction. A sound and updated knowledge of the different conditions that could present as graft dysfunction in kidney transplant recipients is crucial to appropriately managing such patients and avoiding graft failure.

INTRODUCTION

Acute allograft dysfunction is a common complication after kidney transplant and has varied risk factors depending on timing of presentation after transplant. Acute graft dysfunction is usually defined as a rise in serum creatinine of ≥25% from the baseline within days to weeks. The incidence of acute graft dysfunction within the 1st year after transplant varies between centers with an average between 5 and 30%. Acute graft dysfunction, if recognized promptly, is usually reversible; however, if unmanaged, acute graft dysfunction ends in graft failure.

CLINICAL PRESENTATION OF ACUTE GRAFT DYSFUNCTION

Patients are typically diagnosed on routine monitoring when serum creatinine is noted to increase on serial testing. Others present with full-blown symptoms of severe acute kidney injury in the form of reduced urine output and uremic complications. Those with acute graft dysfunction immediately after transplant (delayed graft function) generally present with lack of reduction of serum creatinine and an increase in urine output, respectively, leading to dialysis in most. Patients with significant residual kidney function would mostly continue to have urine output immediately after kidney transplant despite allograft dysfunction; therefore, information about urine output just prior to kidney transplant must be sought.

CHAPTER HIGHLIGHTS

- Acute graft dysfunction is caused by different etiologies, mostly based on the timing of presentation after transplant.
- Urgent evaluation using bedside imaging tools, laboratory markers, and allograft biopsy help in promptly diagnosing the cause of acute graft dysfunction.
- Although the incidence rates of acute rejection have fallen to 10% after kidney transplant, other causes of acute graft dysfunction occur commonly based on center skills and protocols.
- Lymphocele can present with acute urinary retention and graft dysfunction, and acute rejection is reported as a risk factor of lymphocele.
- Urinary leak/urinoma can have overlapping features as lymphocele; however, advanced imaging and fluid chemistry help in distinguishing them.
- DSA negative but histopathological ABMR are reported; however, the exact cause of negative DSA is unclear.

CAUSES OF ACUTE ALLOGRAFT DYSFUNCTION

Causes of acute graft dysfunction vary based on the timing of presentation after transplant—less than 1 week and after 1 week, respectively. The common causes are as follows.

Within 1 Week of Transplant

- *Acute tubular necrosis:* Ischemic (either from long cold ischemia time or intraoperative vasodilation from anesthetic agents/other drug reaction/cardiac event or hypovolemia)
- *Acute rejection:* Acute cellular rejection (ACR) or ABMR
- Acute CNI nephrotoxicity
- *Vascular thrombosis:* Due to surgical issues such as arterial dissection, kinking, or compression from hematoma or anastomotic leak, multiple renal arteries and due to thrombophilic state, hyperacute rejection or severe vascular rejection or hypovolemia
- Vascular obstruction
- Urinary leak
- *Recurrence of basic disease:* For example, focal segmental glomerulosclerosis (FSGS), thrombotic microangiopathy (TMA), primary hyperoxaluria
- Graft pyelonephritis.

After 1 Week of Transplant

- Acute rejection
- Acute CNI nephrotoxicity
- Recurrence of basic disease
- Transplant renal artery stenosis
- BK virus (BKV) nephropathy
- Graft pyelonephritis
- Lymphocele
- Acute tubular necrosis—hypovolemia related.

EVALUATION OF ACUTE GRAFT DYSFUNCTION PRESENTING WITHIN 1 WEEK OF TRANSPLANT

On suspicion of acute graft dysfunction in a patient within 1 week after transplant, the approach to evaluation is depicted in **Flowchart 1**.

- *Prerenal causes:* Information about fluid loss, blood loss, intraoperative cardiac event, intraoperative hypotension, drug reaction, surgical difficulties, or inadvertent vascular injuries is sought to exclude *prerenal* causes of acute graft dysfunction.
- *Surgical causes:* Urine output is quantified every hourly and *reversible postrenal* causes of urinary retention such as obstructed Foley's catheter should be relieved. An urgent USG of the allograft and native kidneys and urinary bladder (KUB) is performed bedside to check for *surgical causes of urinary tract obstruction*, and Doppler of renal vessels is done bedside for checking blood flow to the allograft kidney and exclude *vascular thromboses*.
- *Acute rejection or CNI toxicity:* In patients without any abnormality in the USG, kidney allograft biopsy is performed immediately to evaluate for other causes of acute graft dysfunction such as *acute rejection and acute CNI nephrotoxicity*. Hyperacute rejection usually occurs within minutes or hours of the transplant, especially in the background of either HLA or ABO incompatibility. DSAs to HLA antigens are tested using the SAB method in patients with acute rejection. Routine monitoring of DSAs is not practiced widely due to financial restraints and therefore, only patients with ABMR are evaluated for DSAs. However, sensitized patients who undergo desensitization and then transplant are serially monitored for DSAs and increasing DSAs in them is an indication for kidney biopsy and/or prompt treatment irrespective of clinical graft dysfunction. A high trough level of CNI indicates acute *CNI toxicity*; however, it might be normal in patients with acute CNI nephrotoxicity, particularly TMA.
- *Recurrence of basic disease:* Urine protein in nephrotic range (dipstick 3+ or more and/or spot/24 hour-urine protein-creatinine ratio >2–3) points toward the recurrence of FSGS (and rarely other glomerular diseases such as C3 glomerulopathy and membranous nephropathy) in the immediate post-transplant period; however, a biopsy with electron microscopy (light microscopy is likely to miss FSGS lesions as sclerosis develops over months) is must to confirm the diagnosis.[7]
- *Unusual causes:* In some cases, unusual causes of acute graft dysfunction such as recurrence of primary hyperoxaluria in the background of unknown basic kidney disease or unevaluated kidney stones prior to kidney transplant and invasive fungal infection of the allograft are also diagnosed. Although rare, these diagnoses are worthy of note due to the ominous course that follows.

Fluid challenge (300–500 mL crystalloid) is given in patients without volume overload to take care of a possibility of hypovolemia-induced hemodynamic acute graft dysfunction. In case of a failed fluid challenge, intravenous frusemide at 1–1.5 mg/kg/dose (may require higher doses in patients with advanced kidney dysfunction, such as those with delayed graft function after deceased donor transplant) is administered and urine output (expected 200 mL over 2 hours) is observed. Negative frusemide challenge is used to predict future progression of acute graft dysfunction.[8] In cases with abnormal USG graft and KUB, surgical exploration is undertaken for relieving obstruction of the urinary tract and vascular thromboses.

It is important to keep in mind that it is the course of illness which decides the next line of evaluation. Even after managing obstruction if the patient is not improving, the patient may need a graft biopsy to uncover ongoing rejection.

Flowchart 1: Algorithm to evaluate acute graft dysfunction presenting within 1 week of transplant.

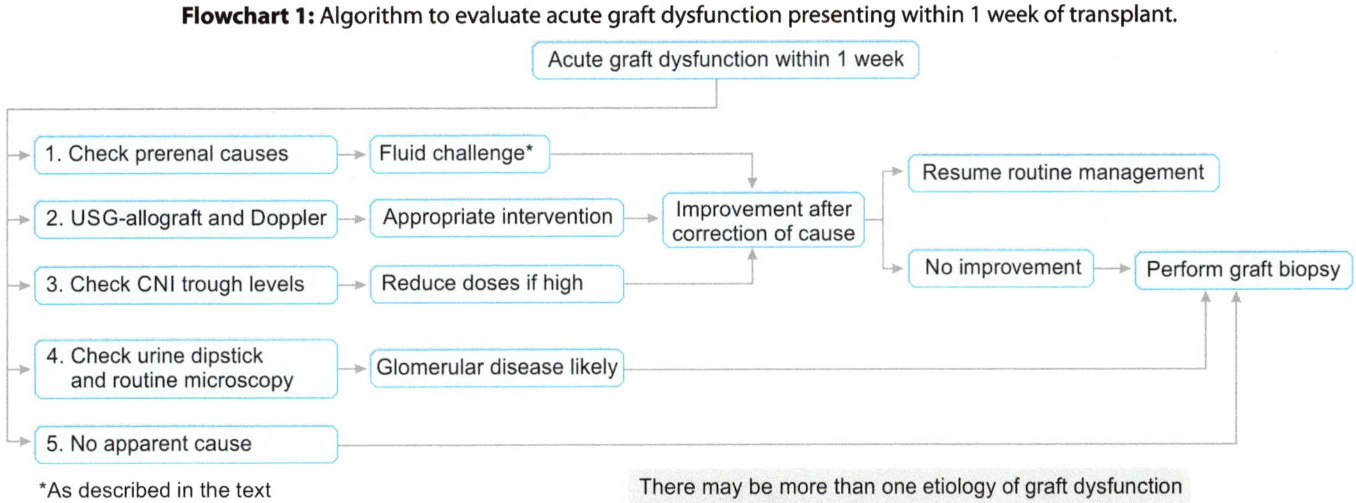

(CNI: calcineurin inhibitor; USG: ultrasonography)

EVALUATION OF ACUTE GRAFT DYSFUNCTION PRESENTING AFTER 1 WEEK OF TRANSPLANT

On suspicion of acute graft dysfunction in a patient after 1 week of transplant, based on "how many months after transplant has the patient presented," etiologies vary and, therefore, the approach to evaluation **(Flowchart 2)** varies. The etiologies of acute graft dysfunction among those presenting early versus those presenting late, in fact, vary in the order of common occurrence, rather than them being truly varying conditions. Patients with acute graft dysfunction (as defined above) after 1 week of kidney transplant are also evaluated with clinical history, physical examination, and basic investigations like those presenting within 1 week of transplant; however, postsurgical complications and acute/hyperacute rejection become less common after the 1st week. Basic investigations of patients with acute graft dysfunction after 1 week of transplant include: (1) USG graft and KUB and Doppler, (2) urine microscopy and dipstick, (3) CNI trough level, and (4) BKV deoxyribonucleic acid (DNA) polymerase chain reaction (PCR) and cytomegalovirus (CMV) DNA PCR.

Although *acute rejection* remains the most supreme cause of acute graft dysfunction that must be ruled out, allograft biopsy is not always performed promptly at the first presentation in patients with acute graft dysfunction later (>1 week) after transplant as other causes of graft dysfunction, such as CNI toxicity, opportunistic infections related-graft dysfunction, recurrence of basic disease, and late surgical complications, also start manifesting. Plasma levels of donor-derived cell-free DNA (>1%) have been shown to reliably distinguish rejection (either ACR or ABMR) from nonrejection causes of acute graft dysfunction. In patients with high CNI trough levels and acute graft dysfunction suggestive of *acute CNI nephrotoxicity*, the dose of CNI is down-titrated first and serum creatinine monitored before performing a kidney allograft biopsy. It is crucial to look for newly added drugs which could interfere with the metabolism and absorption of CNIs. In patients with fever and graft site pain/tenderness, *graft pyelonephritis* must be excluded before performing allograft biopsy. Those with evidence of *hypovolemia-related acute tubular necrosis* are treated with oral (for mild dehydration) or intravenous (for severe or hypotensive) fluids, and serum creatinine is monitored. Patients with nephrotic range proteinuria (with or without hypoalbuminemia) and acute graft dysfunction due to *recurrence of basic disease*, especially if known to have FSGS (as the basic disease), are considered for plasmapheresis and high-dose steroids while awaiting kidney biopsy report. In patients with evidence of *surgical cause* of acute graft dysfunction, if even after treatment of the cause, serum creatinine does not fall to baseline,

Flowchart 2: Algorithm to evaluate acute graft dysfunction presenting after 1 week of transplant.

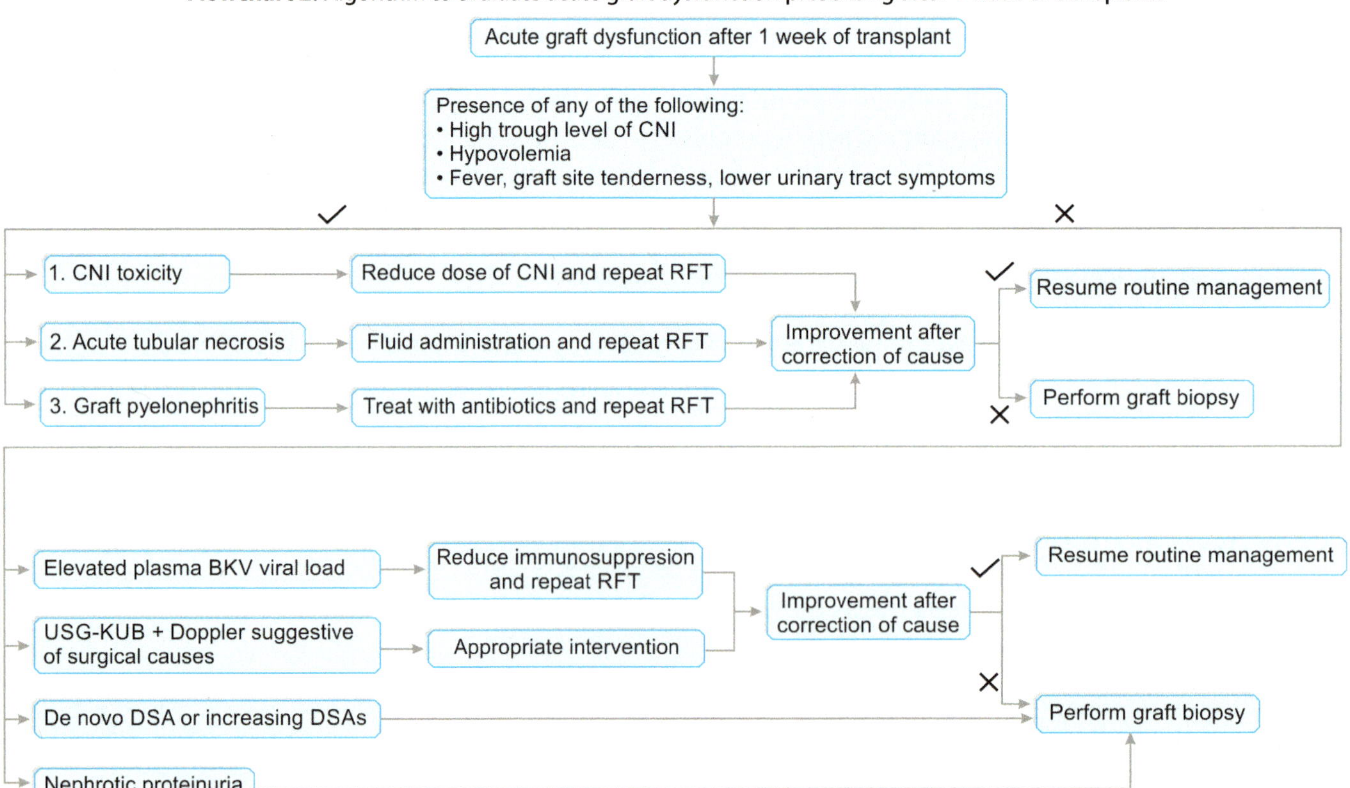

(BKV: BK virus; CNI: calcineurin inhibitor; DSA: donor-specific antibodies; KUB: kidneys and urinary bladder; RFT: renal function tests; USG: ultrasonography)

a kidney allograft biopsy is done to evaluate for coexisting pathologies. In patients with high plasma BKPyV viral load ($>10^4$ copies/mL) and acute graft dysfunction, a presumptive diagnosis of *BKPyV-associated nephropathy* is made in some centers, whereas others routinely perform kidney biopsy to diagnose BKPyV nephropathy. In patients with no obvious cause of acute graft dysfunction from clinical history and basic investigations, prompt kidney allograft biopsy would be absolutely necessary to identify the pathology and control the cause.

REFERENCES

1. Haas M, Loupy A, Lefaucheur C, Roufosse C, Glotz D, Seron D, et al. The Banff 2017 Kidney Meeting Report: revised diagnostic criteria for chronic active T cell-mediated rejection, antibody-mediated rejection, and prospects for integrative endpoints for next-generation clinical trials. Am J Transplant. 2018;18(2):293-307.
2. Senev A, Coemans M, Lerut E, Sandt VV, Daniëls L, Kuypers D, et al. Histological picture of antibody-mediated rejection without donor-specific anti-HLA antibodies: clinical presentation and implications for outcome. Am J Transplant. 2019;19(3):763-80.
3. Schweizer RT, Cho S, Koutz KS, Belzer FO. Lymphoceles following renal transplantation. Arch Surg. 1972;104:42-5.
4. Choudhrie AV, Kumar S, Gnanaraj L, Devasia A, Chacko N, Kekre NS. Symptomatic lymphocoeles post renal transplant. Saudi J Kidney Dis Transpl. 2012;23:1162-8.
5. Flores-Gama F, Bochicchio-Riccardelli T, Mondragon-Ramirez G. Determination of creatinine in drained liquid. Urinary leak of lymphocele? Cir Cir. 2010;78(4):327-32.
6. Regmi SK, Bearrick EN, Hannah PTF, Sathianathen N, Kalapara A, Konety BR. Drain fluid creatinine-to-serum creatinine ratio as an initial test to detect urine leakage following cystectomy: a retrospective study. Indian J Urol. 2021;37(2):153-8.
7. Shoji J, Mii A, Terasaki M, Shimizu A. Update on recurrent focal segmental glomerulosclerosis in kidney transplantation. Nephron. 2020;144(Suppl 1):65-70.
8. Powell TC, Warnock DG. The furosemide stress test and predicting AKI outcomes. J Am Soc Nephrol. 2015;26(8): 1762-4.

CHAPTER

9 Immunosuppressive Drugs

9.1 Induction Therapy in Kidney Transplantation

Arunkumar S, D Bhaumik

CASE VIGNETTE

A 32-year-old female patient with chronic glomerulonephritis related end-stage-renal-disease on maintenance hemodialysis for 6 months was planned for live related renal transplantation with mother as a donor. She has a history of 2 units PRBC transfusion at the time of initiation of hemodialysis and one-unit PRBC was transfused during delivery of her second child (P2L2A1) three years back. An immunological workup for renal transplantation revealed haplotype HLA match in the donor-recipient pair with a negative complement-dependent cytotoxicity (CDC) test. Flow cytometry crossmatch was negative and patient had 25% panel reactive antibody (PRA) to HLA class I and 11% PRA to HLA class II. The patient was then assessed for donor-specific antibody by flow single antigen beads which detected DSA to A2 (MFI:1321) and B5 (578) with CREG antibody detected to HLA-A69 (1800). As the patient was having a high immunological risk (DSA positivity), rabbit antithymocyte globulin (rATG) induction at a dose of 1 mg/kg/day was administered for three consecutive days, starting peri-operatively. The DSA titers were not very high, and hence pre-transplant desensitization therapy with plasma exchange ± IvIg was not considered. She was treated with standard triple drug immunosuppression and had an uneventful postoperative course with a stable serum creatinine of 0.9–1.1 mg/dL. DSA was repeated at the end of first month post-transplantation and DSA was detected to HLA A2 (430) alone. Patient is planned for sequential DSA monitoring and titration of maintenance immunosuppressive therapy on follow-up.

INTRODUCTION

The success of kidney transplantation is largely dependent on the use of optimal immunosuppressive drugs. Considerable progress in the understanding of transplant immunology has resulted in the development of drugs with specific mechanisms of action targeting a particular component of the immune system (T lymphocytes, B lymphocytes, plasma cells, complement components, costimulatory signals, etc.). Immunosuppressive therapies are categorized into induction therapy, maintenance therapy, or antirejection therapy (rescue therapy). Induction therapies are potent and powerful drugs used in higher doses at the time of transplant surgery to prevent acute rejection. Over the last couple of decades, the use of induction therapy has been increasing consistently across the world. However, their role in improving graft and patient survival needs to be counterbalanced with the risks of infections, malignancy, and other complications. In addition to risk-benefit analysis, clinician preference and center-specific practices cause wide variability in the usage of these agents. This chapter summarizes the various induction agents and their utility in different clinical scenarios.

INDUCTION THERAPY—TIMELINE OF DEVELOPMENT AND CLASSIFICATION

The goal of immunosuppressive therapy is to prevent allograft rejection. Till 1980, azathioprine and steroids were the only available immunosuppressive drugs, and no separate induction therapy was available. Major advances in transplant immunosuppression were in the 1980s when antilymphocyte globulin (ALG) and muromonab-CD3 were developed as induction agents. In one of the first controlled trials on ALG, Sansom et al. reported a significantly better graft survival with a reduced risk of rejection in the ALG group.[1] This period also saw the introduction of calcineurin inhibitors (CNI) as part of maintenance therapy. This was followed by the replacement of ALG by rabbit antithymocyte globulin (rATG) and, thereafter, the development of rituximab, basiliximab, and alemtuzumab in the last two decades.[2] The Food and Drug Administration (FDA) approval for interleukin-2 receptor antagonists (IL2RA) increased the use of these drugs significantly. The timeline of the development of the various immunosuppressive drugs is given in **Figure 1**. The induction agents can be classified as depleting or nondepleting agents based on their T-cell depleting capacity or into monoclonal or polyclonal agents based on their origin and binding specificity **(Table 1)**. Of all the available agents, rATG and basiliximab continue to be the most widely used induction agents worldwide.

Muromonab-CD3 (OKT3): Murine monoclonal antibody (mAb) against CD3 of T-cell receptor complex is the first mAb used clinically. It was used earlier as part of induction therapy (FDA off-label use) and also for treatment of rejection but is now discontinued. A common adverse effect was the cytokine release syndrome with febrile reaction, nausea, vomiting, and in severe cases pulmonary edema and hemodynamic instability. Patients can develop antimouse antibodies, which can limit its efficacy.

Interlukin-2 receptor antagonists (IL2RA): Basiliximab (chimeric) and daclizumab (humanized) are mAbs targeting CD25 (α subunit) of interleukin-2 (IL-2) receptor. Activated T cells release IL-2, which in turn promotes further differentiation and proliferation of T cells. This is prevented by IL-2 inhibitors. Basiliximab is administered intraoperatively (during transplant surgery) at a dose of 20 mg and repeated on day 4. This saturates the IL-2 receptor for 4–6 weeks. It is well tolerated with no particular adverse effects. Hypersensitivity reactions are rare (<1%). Though daclizumab has a similar mechanism of action, its cumbersome dosing schedule and high costs have led to its discontinuation from clinical use.

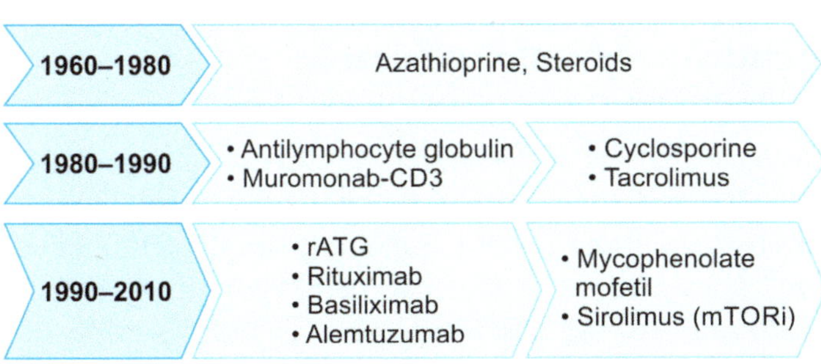

Fig. 1: Timeline of development of various immunosuppressive agents in kidney transplantation. (mTORi: mammalian target of rapamycin inhibitors; rATG: rabbit antithymocyte globulin)

TABLE 1: Classification of induction immunosuppressive therapy used in kidney transplantation.

Depleting capacity	***Binding specificity and origin***
• *Depleting antibodies:* rATG, ATGAM, OKT3, alemtuzumab • *Nondepleting antibodies:* Basiliximab, daclizumab	• *Polyclonal:* rATG, ATGAM, rATG-Fresenius • *Monoclonal:* Basiliximab, daclizumab, alemtuzumab, OKT3

(ATGAM: antithymocyte globulin; OKT3: muromonab-CD3; rATG: rabbit antithymocyte globulin)

Antithymocyte globulin (ATG): Polyclonal immunoglobulins are obtained by injecting human thymus-derived lymphoid cells into animals (rabbit or horse) and obtaining their sera with immunoglobulins. The initial ALG was obtained by injecting human lymphocytes obtained from the thoracic duct. ATG induces T-cell depletion through both antibody and complement-mediated cytotoxicity, opsonization, and phagocytosis of antibody-recovered T lymphocytes. It also affects leukocyte adhesion and T-cell activation. ATG interferes with T cell-dependent activation of B cells, mediates complement-mediated lysis, induces apoptosis of B cells, and thereby affects B cells too.[3]

Rabbit antithymocyte globulin (thymoglobulin) is more potent and has fewer infusion-related adverse effects compared to equine ATG and is used in kidney transplantation as an induction agent (off-label use). The recommended dosage regimen is 1–6 mg/kg divided over 3–7 days. Most centers use 1–1.5 mg/kg/day for 3–5 days for induction. rATG is also used in the management of cellular rejection. Common adverse effects include cytokine release syndrome, and premedication with hydrocortisone and antihistaminic is needed. Thrombophlebitis and thrombosis can occur when administered from the peripheral line; hence, rATG has to be administered via the central venous route. Cytopenias are common and often necessitate dose adjustment. Thymoglobulin dose has to be reduced to one half if the white blood cell (WBC) count is between 2,000 and 3,000 cells/mm^3 and/or platelet count is between 50,000 and 75,000 cells/mm^3 and should be stopped with further cytopenia (WBC <2,000 cells/mm^3 or platelet <50,000 cells/mm^3). CD3 count monitoring helps to optimize rATG

CHAPTER HIGHLIGHTS

- Induction therapies are potent and powerful drugs used in higher doses at the time of transplant surgery to prevent acute rejection.
- The induction agents can be classified as depleting or nondepleting agents based on their T-cell depleting capacity or into monoclonal or polyclonal agents based on their origin and binding specificity.
- Basiliximab and rATG are the commonly used induction agents both in India and worldwide.
- The choice of induction agent depends on immunologic risk assessment of the recipient and also on the clinician/center's preference.
- Basiliximab is preferred for low-risk transplantation, while rATG is preferred for high-risk recipients. rATG or alemtuzumab can be used for patients planned for steroid-free maintenance.

TABLE 2: Polyclonal globulins used in kidney transplantation.

	Thymoglobulin	***ATG-Fresenius***	***Grafalon***	***ATGAM***
Species source	Rabbit	Rabbit	Rabbit	Horse
Immunogen	Thymocyte	Jurkat cell line	Jurkat cell line	Thymocyte
Dose/day	1–2.5 mg/kg	5 mg/kg	2–5 mg/kg	10–20 mg/kg
Manufacturer	Genzyme-Sanofi	Fresenius	Zydus	Pfizer

(ATG: antithymocyte globulin)

dose. The different types of polyclonal globulins available for kidney transplantation are given in **Table 2**. The long-lasting immunosuppressive effects of ATG increase the risk of infectious complications and malignancies in the kidney transplant recipient.

Alemtuzumab (Campath): It is a humanized mAb targeting CD52 present on both T and B lymphocytes (and also on macrophages, natural killer cells, and granulocytes). Hence, it acts as a pan-lymphocyte-depleting agent. Campath is FDA approved for chronic lymphocytic leukemia and has been tried as an induction agent in kidney transplantation. It is administered as a 30-mg single intraoperative dose. Alemtuzumab use results in prolonged lymphocyte depletion and cytopenias (neutropenia, lymphopenia, thrombocytopenia, etc.) and increases the risk of infections.

Rituximab: It is a chimeric mAb directed against CD20 on B cells. Rituximab is commonly used in hemato-oncology for use in non-Hodgkin's lymphoma and as a part of many chemotherapy regimens. In kidney transplantation, rituximab is part of the induction therapy of ABO-incompatible (ABOi) transplantation and desensitization of human leukocyte antigen (HLA) incompatible transplantation. Infusion reactions are common and are usually mild.

EFFICACY OF INDUCTION AGENTS

The efficacy of various induction agents is usually evaluated by their potential to prevent acute rejections. The lack of adequately powered controlled trials is a limiting factor for generating evidence on induction therapy in kidney transplantation. Moreover, the role of induction agents in improving graft and patient survival has not been reliably demonstrated. This is because most are retrospective studies, have focused more on short-term outcomes and are not adequately powered to detect adverse outcomes such as post-transplant lymphoproliferative diseases (PTLD). The lack of standardized criteria to stratify "high-risk" and "low-risk" transplant recipients also affect our interpretation of most studies. The use of different combinations of maintenance therapies is a confounding factor.

Basiliximab versus no Induction

In the United States Simulect Renal Study, basiliximab was shown to reduce the number of acute rejection episodes (35.3% vs. 49.1%) and was well tolerated.[4] Even after the routine use of mycophenolate-based maintenance regimen, basiliximab had a reduced rate of rejection episodes (15.3% vs. 26.6%, no induction).[5] A retrospective analysis of the Scientific Renal Transplant Registry (SRTR) also confirmed the reduction in acute rejection episodes with basiliximab (11.6% vs. 13%).[6] None of the trials, however, could show a survival benefit with basiliximab. The Cochrane systematic review in 2010 suggested a beneficial effect of using IL2RA to reduce the risk of rejections.[7] However, it should be remembered that the standard triple-drug maintenance was not used in most of the trials conducted prior to the year 2000.

A recent propensity score analysis of the Organ Procurement and Transplantation (OPTR) registry of patients on maintenance with tacrolimus and mycophenolate failed to show any benefit for IL2RA induction over no induction for standard-risk patients.[8] With the present triple-drug maintenance therapy, the small additional benefit (1–4%) offered by IL2RA raises questions about the justification for its use in low-risk patients.[9]

Antithymocyte Globulin versus no Induction

Registry analysis of the United Network for Organ Sharing (UNOS) database concluded that induction therapies improve graft and patient outcomes, and depleting agents are more effective.[2] The use of rATG with tacrolimus maintenance had the least risk of acute rejection in a European study.[10] Though similar results have been obtained in other studies, there is a significantly increased incidence of cytomegalovirus (CMV) infections with use of rATG.[11] One added advantage of rATG is the possibility of implementing steroid avoidance or CNI sparing immunosuppression protocols.[12] Though the risk of malignancies is reported to be higher with rATG, the study by Hall et al. failed to show an increased risk of any solid malignancy or lymphoma with rATG use. The risk of melanoma was the only significant risk with rATG use.[13] A recent Cochrane systematic review on induction therapy in kidney transplantation showed that rATG reduced the risk of rejection with or without calcineurin therapy.[14] The incidence of CMV infection and cytopenias was increased with rATG use.

Antithymocyte Globulin versus Basiliximab

In immunologically low-risk patients, rATG did not show any superiority over basiliximab, even after rapid steroid withdrawal in the Harmony study. This suggests that low-risk patients may benefit from a lesser degree of immunosuppression and rATG induction is not a prerequisite for steroid avoidance.[15] In an earlier meta-analysis by Liu et al. with six randomized controlled trials (RCTs), there was no difference with regard to acute rejections, patient, and graft survival between basiliximab and rATG.[16] Another study, however, showed the benefit of rATG therapy with reduced incidence of delayed graft function and no incremental risk of infection.[17] An economic analysis supports the use of basiliximab as it is associated with a lower first post-transplant year cost as compared to rATG irrespective of the degree of immunologic risk.[18] The use of rATG in moderate to high-risk deceased donor transplantation results in a significantly reduced risk of rejection (14.2% vs. 25% basiliximab) with better graft survival on follow-up.[19,20] Even with kidneys of donors after circulatory death (DCD), rATG is more advantageous than both basiliximab and alemtuzumab.[21]

ALEMTUZUMAB

Alemtuzumab reduces the risk of acute rejection in both low-risk and high-risk transplant recipients. There is a significant advantage when compared to IL2RA for low-risk patients. However, the graft and patient survival are similar with an increased incidence of late rejection.[22] Alemtuzumab relatively spares regulatory T cells; hence, in spite of the lymphopenia, patients can develop donor-specific antibody (DSA), which may be one of the reasons for late rejections. The 3C study reported a significant acute rejection risk reduction with alemtuzumab and allowed for successful steroid avoidance but with similar graft and patient survival rates.[23] A recent Cochrane systematic review showed a positive result for alemtuzumab with comparable rates of acute rejection (vs. rATG), even with early steroid withdrawal.[14]

INDIAN STUDIES

Indian data on induction therapy in kidney transplantation is mostly from retrospective studies **(Table 3)**. Studies on basiliximab in standard-risk patients have shown some reduction in the risk of acute rejection but no extra benefit

TABLE 3: Indian studies on induction therapy in kidney transplantation.

Author	*Center*	*Induction therapy*	*Outcomes*
IL2R versus no induction			
Atlani et al.[25]	SGPGIMS, Lucknow	• IL2R ($n = 57$) • No induction ($n = 312$)	• *IL2R:* Significantly better prevention of acute rejection (14% vs. 25%) • Graft survival at 5 years similar in both groups
Gundlapalli et al.[26]	PGIMER, Chandigarh	• IL2R ($n = 46$) • No induction ($n = 56$)	• Similar acute rejection rates, graft survival • No extra advantage of IL2R in intermediate risk live donor transplants
Bansal et al.[27]	Medanta, Gurgaon	• IL2R ($n = 202$) • No Induction ($n = 58$)	• Similar graft rejection rates, graft survival, and patient survival • No advantage of IL2R in first kidney recipients of living donors
Gosain et al.[28]	SCB, Cuttack	• IL2R ($n = 52$) • No induction ($n = 52$)	• *IL2R:* Lower rejection and lower patient death risk
IL2R versus ATG			
Kesiraju et al.[29]	KIIMS and Mahavir hospitals, Hyderabad	• IL2R ($n = 44$) • ATG ($n = 42$)	• *ATG:* Lesser acute rejection (14.2% vs. 18.1%); better graft survival (83.4% vs. 77.3%)
Radhakrishnan et al.[30]	CMC Vellore	• IL2R ($n = 403$) • ATG ($n = 42$) • No Induction ($n = 160$)	• No extra benefit of induction therapy in low immunologic risk • Increased risk of BK viremia with rATG • Benefit of induction lost with TAC-MPA regimen
Thymoglobulin versus Grafalon			
Singh et al.[31]	SGRH, New Delhi	• Thymoglobulin ($n = 25$) • Grafalon ($n = 22$) • ABOi Tx patients	• Higher rejection rate with Grafalon (32% vs. 20%): Not statistically significant • Overall outcomes similar between groups
Jha et al.[32]	Medanta, Gurgaon	• Thymoglobulin ($n = 355$) • Grafalon ($n = 78$)	• Higher acute rejection rate with Grafalon (12.8% vs. 5.1%) • Similar short-term patient and graft survival; infection rates comparable

(ABOi: ABO incompatible; ATG: antithymocyte globulin; CMC: Christian Medical College; IL2R: interleukin-2 receptor antagonists; MPA: mycophenolic acid; TAC: tacrolimus)

with regard to long-term outcomes. rATG has shown to reduce the risk of acute rejection with better graft survival with an increased risk of infections (BK viremia). In a study from India, Ray et al. reported a lower rejection rate, better survival, and renal function at 6 months and 1 year with rATG in Indian patients.[24] 17.7% of the patients reported infections on follow-up. Grafalon is a type of rATG available in India. Studies with Grafalon have shown an increased incidence of rejection with similar overall patient outcomes.

APPROACH TO INDUCTION THERAPY

Personalized immunosuppressive therapy is the need of the hour. Every patient should be assessed individually, and immunosuppressive regimens need to be decided accordingly. The first step in this regard will be to assess the immunologic risk of the patient.[33] The various patient-related factors deciding the immunologic risks are as follows:

- *Low-risk:* Zero HLA mismatch, live donors, absence of DSA, the first transplant
- *High-risk:* HLA mismatch, younger recipient/old donor age, blood group incompatibility, presence of DSA, high panel reactive antibody, second/retransplant, delayed graft function.

A simplified protocol for induction immunosuppression suitable for clinical practice is shown in **Flowchart 1**. Induction therapy in haploidentical live-related renal transplantation (LRRT) does not add any benefit to standard maintenance therapy and can be avoided if there are no other risk factors. A recent analysis of the data from the United States Organ Procurement and Transplant Network revealed that in well-matched kidney transplant recipients, the use of any type of induction therapy does not improve outcomes.[34] The Kidney Disease: Improving Global Outcomes (KDIGO) guidelines for transplant recipients recommend IL2RA as the first-line induction therapy (grade 1B), while lymphocyte-depleting agents should be used in those with high immunologic risk (grade 2B).[35] rATG and alemtuzumab induction therapy may be preferred in patients planned for steroid-free maintenance therapy. All patients of deceased donor transplantation should preferably receive rATG induction therapy.

Flowchart 1: Approach to induction immunosuppression therapy in living donor kidney transplantation.

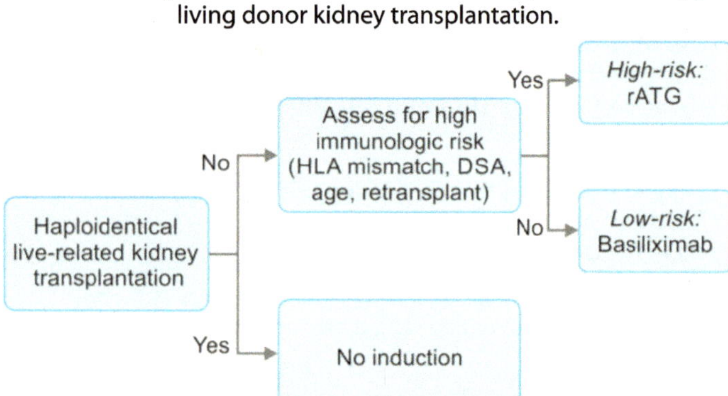

(DSA: donor-specific antibody; HLA: human leukocyte antigen)

CONCLUSION

Induction therapy is an integral part of kidney transplantation. Advances in immunosuppressive therapy have improved the rejection rates and short-term graft survival substantially. Induction therapy is used in over 80% of kidney transplant recipients. Both rATG and basiliximab have proven efficacy and safety data in kidney transplantation, and a choice of agent will have to be done based on an individualized risk–benefit analysis. Though the choice of an induction agent is still debatable, low-risk patients may go with basiliximab and high-risk patients will need rATG induction for transplantation. Well-matched haploidentical donors with no other risk factors may not require any induction therapy. The lack of appropriately powered controlled trials is still an issue for generating evidence on induction therapy in kidney transplantation. Newer well-planned controlled trials are the need of the hour to address these shortcomings.

REFERENCES

1. Sansom JR, Barnes AD, Hall CL. A randomized prospective clinical trial of antilymphocyte globulin in 100 cadaveric renal transplants. Postgrad Med J. 1976;52(Suppl. 5):75-8.
2. Cai J, Terasaki PI. Induction immunosuppression improves long-term graft and patient outcome in organ transplantation: an analysis of United Network for Organ Sharing registry data. Transplantation. 2010;90(12):1511-5.
3. Bamoulid J, Staeck O, Crépin T, Halleck F, Saas P, Brakemeier S, et al. Anti-thymocyte globulins in kidney transplantation: focus on current indications and long-term immunological side effects. Nephrol Dial Transplant. 2017;32(10): 1601-8.
4. Kahan BD, Rajagopalan PR, Hall M. Reduction of the occurrence of acute cellular rejection among renal allograft recipients treated with basiliximab, a chimeric anti-interleukin-2-receptor monoclonal antibody. United States Simulect Renal Study Group. Transplantation. 1999; 67(2):276-84.
5. Lawen JG, Davies EA, Mourad G, Oppenheimer F, Molina MG, Rostaing L, et al. Randomized double-blind study of immunoprophylaxis with basiliximab, a chimeric anti-interleukin-2 receptor monoclonal antibody, in combination with mycophenolate mofetil-containing triple therapy in renal transplantation. Transplantation. 2003;75(1):37-43.
6. Gralla J, Wiseman AC. The impact of IL2ra induction therapy in kidney transplantation using tacrolimus- and mycophenolate-based immunosuppression. Transplantation. 2010;90(6):639-44.
7. Webster AC, Ruster LP, McGee RG, Matheson SL, Higgins GY, Willis NS, et al. Interleukin 2 receptor antagonists for kidney transplant recipients. Cochrane Database Syst Rev. 2010;2010(1):CD003897.
8. Tanriover B, Zhang S, MacConmara M, Gao A, Sandikci B, Ayvaci MUS, et al. Induction therapies in live donor kidney transplantation on tacrolimus and mycophenolate with

or without steroid maintenance. Clin J Am Soc Nephrol. 2015;10(6):1041-9.

9. Hellemans R, Bosmans JL, Abramowicz D. Induction therapy for kidney transplant recipients: do we still need anti-IL2 receptor monoclonal antibodies? Am J Transplant. 2017;17(1):22-7.
10. Charpentier B, Rostaing L, Berthoux F, Lang P, Civati G, Touraine JL, et al. A three-arm study comparing immediate tacrolimus therapy with antithymocyte globulin induction therapy followed by tacrolimus or cyclosporine A in adult renal transplant recipients. Transplantation. 2003;75(6):844-51.
11. Mourad G, Garrigue V, Squifflet JP, Besse T, Berthoux F, Alamartine E, et al. Induction versus noninduction in renal transplant recipients with tacrolimus-based immunosuppression. Transplantation. 2001;72(6):1050-5.
12. Malvezzi P, Jouve T, Rostaing L. Induction by anti-thymocyte globulins in kidney transplantation: a review of the literature and current usage. J Nephropathol. 2015;4(4):110-5.
13. Hall EC, Engels EA, Pfeiffer RM, Segev DL. Association of antibody induction immunosuppression with cancer after kidney transplantation. Transplantation. 2015;99(5): 1051-7.
14. Hill P, Cross NB, Barnett ANR, Palmer SC, Webster AC. Polyclonal and monoclonal antibodies for induction therapy in kidney transplant recipients. Cochrane Database Syst Rev. 2017;1(1):CD004759.
15. Thomusch O, Wiesener M, Opgenoorth M, Pascher A, Woitas RP, Witzke O, et al. Rabbit-ATG or basiliximab induction for rapid steroid withdrawal after renal transplantation (Harmony): an open-label, multicentre, randomised controlled trial. Lancet. 2016;388(10063):3006-16.
16. Liu Y, Zhou P, Han M, Xue CB, Hu XP, Li C. Basiliximab or antithymocyte globulin for induction therapy in kidney transplantation: a meta-analysis. Transplant Proc. 2010;42(5):1667-70.
17. Dedinská I, Graňák K, Vnučák M, Skálová P, Laca Ĺ, Krivuš J, et al. Induction therapy with ATG compared with anti-IL2 basiliximab in low-immunologic risk kidney transplant recipients. Transplant Proc. 2019;51(10):3259-64.
18. Polsky D, Weinfurt KP, Kaplan B, Kim J, Fastenau J, Schulman KA. An economic and quality-of-life assessment of basiliximab vs antithymocyte globulin immunoprophylaxis in renal transplantation. Nephrol Dial Transplant. 2001;16(5): 1028-33.
19. Brennan DC, Daller JA, Lake KD, Cibrik D, Castillo DD, Thymoglobulin Induction Study Group. Rabbit antithymocyte globulin versus basiliximab in renal transplantation. N Engl J Med. 2006;355(19):1967-77.
20. Brennan DC, Schnitzler MA. Long-term results of rabbit antithymocyte globulin and basiliximab induction. N Engl J Med. 2008;359(16):1736-8.
21. Asderakis A, Sabah TK, Watkins WJ, Khalid U, Szabo L, Stephens MR, et al. Thymoglobulin versus alemtuzumab versus basiliximab kidney transplantation from donors after circulatory death. Kidney Int Rep. 2022;7(4):732-40.
22. Hanaway MJ, Woodle ES, Mulgaonkar S, Peddi VR, Kaufman DB, First MR, et al. Alemtuzumab induction in renal transplantation. N Engl J Med. 2011;364(20):1909-19.
23. 3C Study Collaborative Group, Haynes R, Harden P, Judge P, Blackwell L, Emberson J, et al. Alemtuzumab-based induction treatment versus basiliximab-based induction treatment in kidney transplantation (the 3C study): a randomised trial. Lancet. 2014;384(9955):1684-90.
24. Ray DS, Gang S, Mandrekar A. Rabbit antithymocyte globulin (rATG) as induction therapy in Indian patients undergoing renal transplantation: clinical experience from rise registry. Nephrol Dial Transplant. 2021;36(Suppl. 1).
25. Atlani M, Sharma RK, Gupta A. Basiliximab induction in renal transplantation: long-term outcome. Saudi J Kidney Dis Transpl. 2013;24(3):473.
26. Gundlapalli S, Rathi M, Kohli HS, Jha V, Sharma A, Minz M, et al. Efficacy of basiliximab induction in poorly matched living donor renal transplantation. Indian J Nephrol. 2013;23(6):409-12.
27. Bansal SB, Pathania D, Sethi SK, Jha PK, Nandwani A, Jain M, et al. Basiliximab induction in living donor kidney transplant with tacrolimus-based triple immunosuppression. Indian J Transplant. 2019;13(2):104.
28. Gosain V, Kar C, Rout S. SAT-338 the dilemma of induction immunosuppression in low immunological risk kidney transplant recipients- a prospective randomised study from eastern India comparing basiliximab versus no induction immunosuppression. Kidney Int Rep. 2020;5(3):S141-2.
29. Kesiraju S, Paritala P, Rao Ch UM, Athmakuri SM, Reddy VS, Sahaiah S. Anti-thymocyte globulin versus basiliximab induction in renal transplant recipients: long-term outcome. Saudi J Kidney Dis Transpl. 2014;25(1):9-15.
30. Radhakrishnan RC, Basu G, Mohapatra A, Alexander S, Valson AT, Jacob S, et al. Utility of induction agents in living donor kidney transplantation. Indian J Transplant. 2019;13(3):202.
31. Singh R, Bhalla A, Gupta A, Malik M, Gupta A, Bhargava V, et al. Comparative study of ATG vs ATG-F (Grafalon) as an induction agent in ABO incompatible kidney transplantation. Transplantation. 2020;104(S3):S340.
32. Jha PK, Rana A, Kher A, Bansal SB, Sethi S, Nandwani A, et al. Grafalon® vs. Thymoglobulin® as an induction agent in renal transplantation – a retrospective study. Indian J Nephrol. 2021;31(4):336.
33. Pratschke J, Dragun D, Hauser IA, Horn S, Mueller TF, Schemmer P, et al. Immunological risk assessment: the key to individualized immunosuppression after kidney transplantation. Transplant Rev (Orlando). 2016;30(2):77-84.
34. Evans RDR, Lan JH, Kadatz M, Brar S, Chang DT, McMichael L, et al. Use and outcomes of induction therapy in well-matched kidney transplant recipients. Clin J Am Soc Nephrol. 2022;17(2):271-9.
35. Kidney Disease: Improving Global Outcomes (KDIGO) Transplant Work Group. KDIGO clinical practice guideline for the care of kidney transplant recipients. Am J Transplant. 2009;9(Suppl. 3):S1-155.

9.2 Steroid

Kapil N Sejpal, PS Priyamvada

CASE VIGNETTE

A 50-year-old lady is seeking a second kidney transplant. Her native kidney disease was IgA nephropathy. Her first transplantation was done at the age of 35 years, from an HLA identical sibling. She did not receive any induction and was maintained on cyclosporine, MMF and low dose steroids. She had no biopsy proven acute rejections any time following the first kidney transplant. She had developed post-transplant diabetes mellitus (PTDM). Seven years after transplant, she sustained a fracture of the femoral neck and was found to have severe osteoporosis. She had a gradual increase in serum creatinine levels noticed around the 9th year of transplantation. A graft biopsy showed glomerular sclerosis, interstitial fibrosis and tubular atrophy. Eventually she was reinitiated on dialysis and registered for a cadaveric donor.

Considering her background history of bone disease and PTDM, what would be the best management option regarding steroids, in the event of a second transplant?

a. Is it possible to avoid steroids completely?
b. Can steroids be given and withdrawn at a later date? If so, what is the optimal time for steroid withdrawal?

INTRODUCTION

In the early 1960s, corticosteroids were initially used to reverse acute rejections in the renal allograft.[1] Administering a single dose of prednisolone resulted in a rapid reduction in the fever associated with rejections, followed by improved kidney function. Subsequently, steroids became an integral part of kidney transplantation and became part of the immunosuppressive regimen. However, steroids come with many short-term and long-term adverse effects. Along with the advent of induction agents and potent immunosuppressants, the concerns on steroid toxicity gained considerable attention and resulted in steroid minimization and avoidance protocols.

MECHANISM OF ACTION

Steroids induce anti-inflammatory and immunosuppressive properties via genomic (direct and indirect mechanisms) and nongenomic pathways, or both **(Fig. 1)**. Steroids bind to the intracellular glucocorticoid receptor (GR) complex leading to transactivation on transrepression of downstream genes.[2]

Genomic Effects

Following steroid binding, the GR translocates to the nucleus and undergoes homodimerization. The GR homodimers interact with the palindromic glucocorticoid responsive elements (GRE), leading to the transactivation of multiple genes, resulting in the downregulation of pro-inflammatory and upregulation of anti-inflammatory cytokines.

- Steroids upregulate the anti-inflammatory cytokine interleukin (IL)-10 production from mononuclear cells.
- Steroids upregulate the anti-inflammatory dual-specificity phosphatase 1 (DUSP1), also known as mitogen-activated protein kinase phosphatase 1 (MKP-1). DUSP1 dephosphorylates the mitogen-activated protein kinases (MAPK), thus reducing inflammatory cell signaling.

Direct upregulation of I-kappa-B-alpha (IκBα), an inhibitor of nuclear factor kappa B (NF-κB) inhibitor, in specific tissues. Steroids also cause upregulation of glucocorticoid-induced leucine zipper (GILZ), which can bind to NF-κB. GILZ also increases Treg cell production, which is essential for immunologic tolerance.[3]

After steroid binding, the GR monomer can lead to a "direct transrepression." The GR monomer directly tethers with other transcription factors, such as NF-κB, interferon regulatory factor 3 (IRF3), and activator protein 1 (AP-1).[4,5]

Nongenomic Effects[6,7]

- The nongenomic effects occur much more rapidly. At high concentrations (≥30 mg prednisolone equivalents), steroid directly intercalates into the plasma membranes of inflammatory cells. The resultant decrease in calcium trafficking leads to the suppression of inflammatory cytokine production. Steroids also inhibit oxidative phosphorylation by increasing the mitochondrial proton leak.
- Steroid-binding with the cytosolic GR complex may cause some kinases like Src to dissociate from the GR complex. Src inhibits various inflammatory mediators.
- Steroids upregulate annexin-1 expression by genomic as well as nongenomic mechanisms. Annexin-1 reduces phospholipase A2 activity, enhances mononuclear cell phagocytosis and neutrophil apoptosis, and reduces T-cell proliferation and activation.
- Steroids cause reduced phospholipase A2 activity, thus inhibiting the arachidonic acid metabolism, with subsequent reductions in levels of various inflammatory mediators.

PHARMACOKINETICS

Most protocols start with a fixed-dose methylprednisolone pulse (5 to 10 mg/kg) followed by a transition to oral prednisolone by days 3–5. A bolus administration of

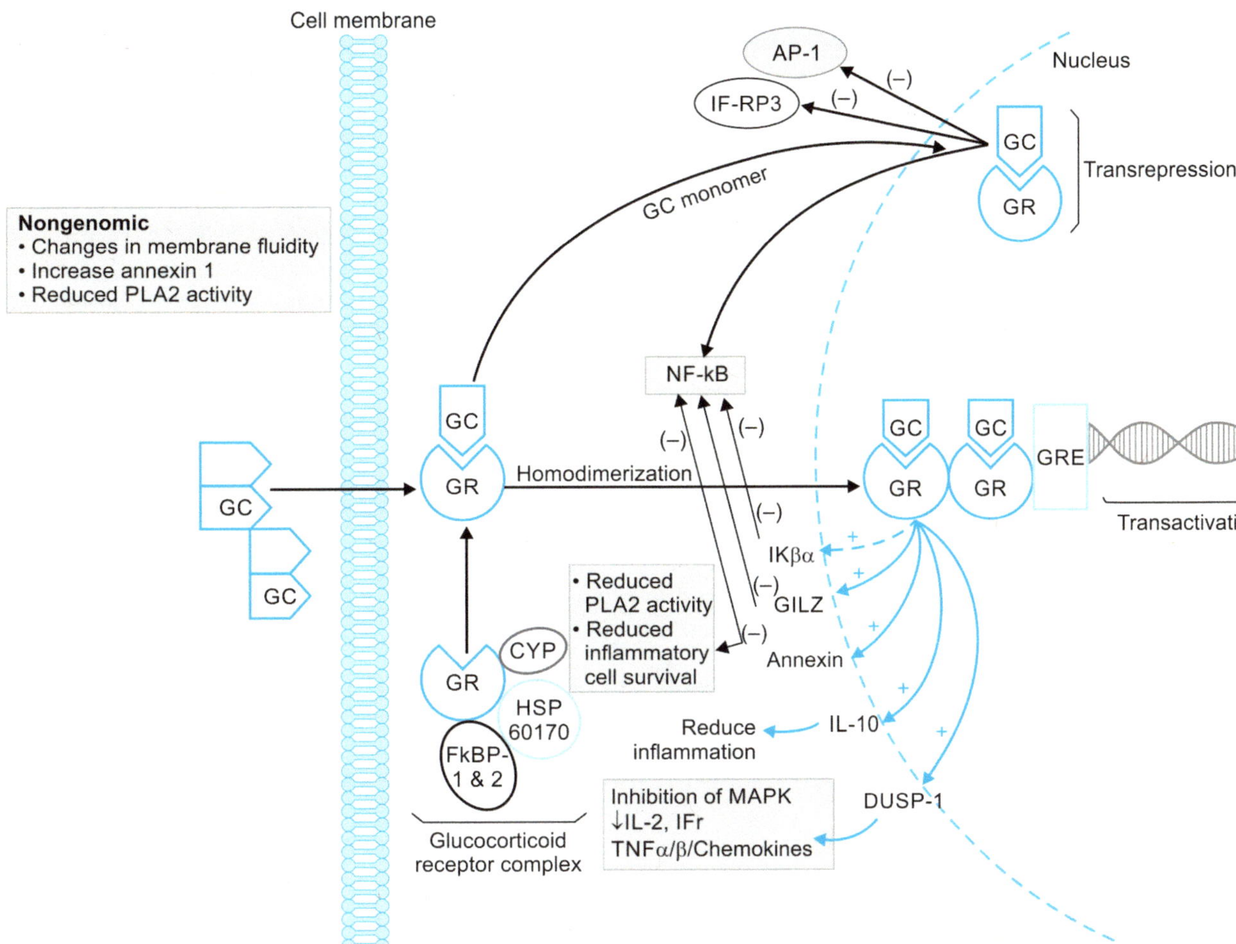

Fig. 1: Mechanism of action of steroids.
Nongenomic effects include changes in membrane fluidity and altered expression of phospholipase A2 (PLA2).
Genomic pathways: Steroids (GC) bound to glucocorticoid receptor (GR) can undergo homodimerization. The homodimers interact with glucocorticoid response elements (GRE) and cause transactivation and regulation of downstream inflammatory mediators. Glucocorticoid monomers can directly tether to many multiple cytokine genes, inducing a state of transrepression. (AP-1: activator protein 1; CYP: cytochrome P; DUSP-1: dual specificity phosphatase 1; FkBP: Fk binding protein; GC: glucocorticoid; GILZ: glucocorticoid-induced leucine zipper; GR: glucocorticoid receptor; GRE: glucocorticoid responsive element; HSP: heat shock protein; IL-10: interleukin 10; IL-2: interleukin 2; IF-RP3: interferon regulatory factor 3; IκBα: I-kappa-B-alpha; MAPK: mitogen-activated protein kinases; NF-κB: nuclear factor Kb; PLA2: phospholipase A2; TNF: tumor necrosis factor)
Courtesy: Illustration by Dr Vidhya K Zachariah.

methylprednisolone (maximum 500 mg) during the transplant operation is a common practice at various centers. Oral prednisolone is tapered to the physiologic dose or 5 mg over a few weeks following the transplant. The evidence for the optimal steroid dosing in kidney transplantation is sparse.

Prednisolone is an active drug, whereas prednisone is a prodrug. Both drugs are interconvertible by the liver. Prednisolone is approximately 77% plasma protein-bound; only the free drug contributes to the drug activity. At doses varying from 1 to 5 mg/kg body weight (KBW) of methylprednisolone, the free drug levels exhibit linear pharmacokinetics; however, this becomes nonlinear at dosages >15 mg/KBW.[8] Following steroid ingestion, the peak blood levels are reached in about 2–3 hours, with no measurable drug level detected at 24 hours. The kidney clears the majority of the drug. Drug clearance is delayed by kidney failure; faster elimination occurs in pediatric patients, especially those under 5 years.[9]

Sizeable interindividual variability is noticed among the transplant population. Time since transplantation, organ dysfunction, sex, body weight, serum albumin concentration, other medications' exposure, and genetic polymorphisms in metabolic enzymes and drug transporters contribute to the pharmacokinetic variability.[10] Those who exhibit higher drug clearances are reported to be vulnerable to early rejections.[11] In theory, individualized dosages with therapeutic drug monitoring (TDM) may help avoid rejections and reduce the adverse effects. However, TDM for steroids is seldom done in clinical practice. The variable metabolism, drug interactions, lack of standardized tests for the "steroid effect," and absence of data on TDM are significant hindrances in formulating evidence-based guidelines.

CHAPTER HIGHLIGHTS

- Steroids reduce the expression of multiple inflammatory mediators via genomic and nongenomic mechanisms.
- Steroids enhance the elimination of CNI and Sirolimus and possibly increase drug clearance of mycophenolate mofetil (MMF).
- The use of low dose steroids for maintenance immunosuppression is relatively safe and widely practiced.
- The potential benefits of steroid withdrawal include lower post-transplant diabetes mellitus, bone disease and better patient and graft survival.
- Factors like the type of induction agents and concomitant immunosuppression and patients immunologic risk influence the graft outcomes following steroid withdrawal.
- Late steroid withdrawal without induction may be possible in selected patients with low immunologic risk.
- Early steroid withdrawal in six months post-transplant might increase the risk of rejections.
- Steroid withdrawal within the first two weeks post-transplant, with usage of induction agents, does not increase death and graft loss. Even though there might be increased in acute rejections, this does not appear to affect long-term graft outcome.
- The data on steroid-free immunosuppression remains sparse and inadequate to come to a conclusion.

INTERACTIONS WITH OTHER IMMUNOSUPPRESSANTS

Steroids are substrates as well as inducers of CYP3A and P glycoprotein. This would enhance the metabolism and the transmembrane efflux of calcineurin inhibitors (CNIs) and sirolimus.[12] Clinically relevant elevations in CNI levels may occur on steroid cessation. Glucocorticoid (GC) induces the activity of uridine diphosphate-glucuronosyltransferase enzymes and multidrug resistance-associated protein 2, presumably increasing metabolism and drug clearance of mycophenolate mofetil (MMF).[13,14]

ADVERSE EFFECTS

Steroid therapy is associated with multiple long-term adverse effects **(Table 1)**. Some adverse effects may show a linear relationship with dosage (ecchymosis, cushingoid appearance, skin changes, edema, and sleep disturbance). Some other changes appear above a threshold dose (e.g., weight gain at prednisolone >5 mg daily, glaucoma, depression, hypertension at >7.5 mg daily).[15] Initially, the use of steroids can be associated with elevation in mood, rarely psychosis and disruption of sleep. Longer duration use might cause sleep disruption, restlessness and depression (including increased risk of suicidality), and cognitive impairment.

Cushingoid appearance is a poor marker of steroid toxicities in the transplant population. Long-term steroid therapy is an independent predictor of cardiovascular morbidity and death in renal allograft recipients; also, steroids increase the economic burden in the post-transplant setting.[16,17] These adverse effects might be considerably lower with the current low-dose regimens (usually around 5 mg).

TABLE 1: Adverse effects with long-term steroids exposure relevant to kidney transplantation.

Adverse effects	***Proposed mechanisms***
Hypertension	• Increased sensitivity of vessels to adrenergic agonist • Activation of renal mineralocorticoid receptors
Post-transplant diabetes mellitus (PTDM)	• Increased insulin resistance • Increased hepatic glucose production through proteolysis and lipolysis
Cataracts/ glaucoma	• Changes in transmembrane transport • Increased reactive oxygen species • Increased extracellular matrix deposition in the trabecular meshwork, increasing the aqueous fluid outflow resistance
Osteoporosis	• Apoptosis of osteoblasts • Increased activation of osteoclasts • Osteocyte apoptosis • Altered intestinal and renal calcium handling
Dyslipidemia	• Reduced lipoprotein lipase • Increased activity of HMG-CoA reductase
Growth retardation	• Impaired release of growth hormone • Decreased activity of insulin-like growth factor (IGF-1)

(HMG-CoA: 3-hydroxy-3-methyl-glutaryl-coenzyme A)

Steroids and Post-transplant Diabetes Mellitus

The recipient age, steroid dose, duration of therapy, use of CNI—especially tacrolimus (TAC)—and type of steroid used can affect the prevalence of post-transplant diabetes mellitus (PTDM). In addition to increased glucose output from the liver, steroids induce apoptosis of the beta cells and also enhance insulin resistance. The mechanisms of reduced glucose entry to the cell include direct down-regulation of GLUT 4, enhanced lipolysis, leading to tissue accumulation of acetyl CoA and increased cellular glucose production mediated by the peroxisomal proliferator-activated receptor α.[18] The available data from India on PTDM is limited—single center studies have reported the prevalence varying from 15 to 23% with triple-drug immunosuppression.[19-22] An Indian study using an early withdrawal of corticosteroids reported a lower cumulative prevalence of PTDM (6.9%).[23]

Late unscheduled steroid withdrawal at physicians' discretion is associated with reductions/cessation of hypoglycemic agents used in the long term.[16] A blinded randomized controlled trial (RCT) demonstrated a similar prevalence of PTDM after steroid withdrawal on day 7 (21.5 vs. 20.9%); however, fewer steroid withdrawal subjects required insulin at 5 years (3.7 vs. 11.6%).[24] Similar results were reported from another RCT with steroid withdrawal at day 7. The prevalence of PTDM was identical (39.3 vs. 39.4%), but with lower requirements of insulin therapy in the steroid withdrawal group after a 5-year follow-up.[25] Both studies have used only 5 mg of prednisolone—much lower than the physiologic replacement doses—in the maintenance arm, which might explain the similar prevalence of PTDM. Steroid withdrawal reduces PTDM to a greater extent with cyclosporine A (CsA)-based therapy compared TAC.[26]

Steroids and Post-transplant Bone Disease

Long term use of even small doses of steroids (7.5 mg/day) is reported to accelerate the loss of cortical bone, leading to osteoporosis, fractures, or even avascular necrosis. The use of CNI compounds the loss in bone mineral density (BMD). Steroids interfere with the normal bone remodeling by inducing apoptosis of bone cells and enhancing the secretion of sclerostin and Dickkopf-related protein 1 (DKK1) by osteocytes, leading to inhibition of the osteoblast. Other mechanisms include a higher NF-κB ligand (RANKL)/osteoprotegerin (a decoy receptor for RANKL) ratio facilitating osteoclastic bone reabsorption. Also, steroids suppress the insulin-like growth factor 1, growth hormone, and gonadal hormones, which may contribute to bone mineral loss.[27] Factors such as age, comorbidities, patient, disease-related factors, and CNIs also contribute.

An Indian study reported that despite having good BMD, at baseline, a 16% decline in BMD was observed in the initial 6 months after transplant.[28] Another study from South India also reported a significant decrease in the spinal BMD in the initial 3 months following transplantation.[29] Data from the United States Renal Data System (USRDS) reported that early corticosteroid withdrawal is associated with a 31% reduction in fracture risk.[30] The HARMONY trial has shown that rapid withdrawal of GC is associated with significant decreases in the prevalence of osteoporosis at 12 months (12% with steroid continuation vs. 5% and 6% with rapid withdrawal).[31,32]

STEROID WITHDRAWAL AND AVOIDANCE

There has been a gradual tendency to minimize steroids even before the advent of CSA in the 1980s.[33] The introduction of CNI and induction agents has facilitated steroid withdrawal and avoidance. As per the USRDS data, 23% of renal allograft recipients were discharged without steroids.[34] Steroid reductions are associated with a lower incidence of steroid-induced adverse effects, but the lingering question is whether it negatively affects long-term graft survival. Kidney Disease Improving Global Outcomes (KDIGO) 2009 guidelines recommend steroid withdrawal during the 1st week following transplant in low-risk patients.[35] However, there has been accumulating evidence on steroid withdrawal and avoidance since the publication of these guidelines. There are no uniform definitions on what constitutes early versus late steroid withdrawal. The ensuing discussion covers various aspects of steroid withdrawal in the adult transplant setting.

Late Steroid Withdrawal

In the CSA era without induction agents, randomized trials reported that steroids could be withdrawn in around two-third of patients with stable kidney function after 1 year.[34,35] Even though many of the steroid effects were reversed, the withdrawal arm showed increased rejections (with CSA alone as maintenance)[36] or a reduced kidney function in the long-term despite the absence of rejections [with CSA + Azathioprine (AZA)].[37] The introduction of MMF was postulated to facilitate steroid withdrawal in CSA-treated patients without increasing rejections.[38]

Long-term prospective studies with steroid withdrawal after 6 months transplant have reported better patient survival, graft survival (81.9 vs. 75.3%), and death-censored graft survival (91.8 vs. 87.9%) after a follow-up period of 7 years.[39] A retrospective study from Spain, with data dating to the 1990s, showed that late steroid withdrawal after a mean of 3.7 ± 2.8 years post-transplant had no harmful effects on graft function, irrespective of the type of immunosuppression used. It was found that steroid continuation was associated with a 1.5-fold increase in death-censored graft loss.[16] A meta-analysis reported a 77% higher chance of rejections following steroid withdrawal in the first year of transplant.[40] However, no differences in the patient mortality, graft loss, PTDM, or cytomegalovirus (CMV) infection prevalence were noticed at the end of 5 years. More rejections were detected with CSA use [risk ratio (RR) 2.08, 95% confidence interval (CI) 1.29–3.35] and absence of induction treatment (RR 1.93, 95% CI 1.26–2.94). The use of MMF in addition to CNI reduced the risk for rejections.[40] The patient profile appears to be the most important determinant of outcomes for steroid withdrawal. It might be possible to withdraw steroids in individuals with low immunologic risk and stable graft function.

Steroid Withdrawal after 2 Weeks and within 6 Months of Surgery

A meta-analysis published in the preinduction era reported that early steroid withdrawal in 6 months might increase rejections.[41] Of the seven studies included, six withdrew steroids before 3 months of transplant; four studies used CSA alone for immunosuppression and the remaining used CSA + Aza. The use of induction agents and TAC and MMF might impact the outcomes of steroid withdrawal. Steroid withdrawal within 3–6 months of CSA-based regimens is associated with a 42% higher incidence of rejections. In contrast, TAC allowed steroid withdrawal without inducing rejections.[42] A retrospective analysis of the Austrian Dialysis and Transplant Registry data reported a higher incidence of biopsy-proven rejections with steroid withdrawal the first 18 months following transplant despite induction with IL-2 blockers. The risk for rejection was most increased in the initial 6 months following transplant, decreasing in a time-bound manner.[43] Steroid withdrawal increases rejections in early months; however, it does not appear to affect the short-term graft outcomes and possibly offers a survival advantage. However, whether the high incidence of rejections may reduce graft survival in the long term remains unresolved.

Steroid Withdrawal in High-risk Populations

Steroid withdrawal in populations with high immunologic risk is even more contentious. There is a lack of well-performed clinical trials addressing this issue. A propensity score-matched analysis of United Network for Organ Sharing (UNOS) data showed that early steroid withdrawal is associated with a similar risk of graft loss and a 9% lower risk of death in Afro-Americans.[44] The mortality advantage was more apparent later (>4 years post-transplant). Around 67% received cytolytic induction therapy, which had a modifying effect on the long-term outcomes. Acute rejections were slightly higher in the corticosteroid continuation group but without impacting long-term graft function. Another retrospective study showed that steroid withdrawal could be safely made in subjects who receive a kidney from expanded criteria donors.[45] Among those who received rabbit antithymocyte globulin (rATG) for induction, steroid continuation led to a 32% higher chance of graft failure and 46% higher mortality. However, the outcomes were similar in patients who withdrew steroids with alemtuzumab and IL-2 blocking agents. Similarly, withdrawal of steroids does not affect the graft outcomes in retransplantation with rATG induction; however, steroid continuation was associated with a 44% higher chance of graft survival with alemtuzumab.[46] Observational studies with small sample sizes have reported that successful early steroid withdrawal is possible in ABO-incompatible transplant.[47,48]

Steroid-free Maintenance (Withdrawal within the First 2 Weeks)

Steroid-free maintenance includes using steroids for <2 weeks—most often a bolus with or without oral tapering—along with induction therapy. Steroid-free maintenance is often preferred over steroid withdrawal at a later date. In 2008, the FREEDOM trial showed that steroid-free immunosuppression with basiliximab induction/CSA/MMF regimen did not compromise graft function at 1 year.[49] Another RCT published in the same year looked at the effect of steroid withdrawal on day 7 versus very low-dose maintenance steroids (5 mg/day after 6 months). Biopsy-proven acute rejection was higher in the withdrawal group (17.8 vs. 10.8%) at the end of 5 years but did not attain statistical significance. Most rejections were mild—Banff 1A responsive to steroid therapy. There were no differences in the graft loss, death, or moderate-to-severe rejections at 5 years.[24]

A meta-analysis in 2011 (9 studies, all with antibody induction) reported that steroid withdrawal in the first 2 weeks did not increase death and graft loss.[26] However, acute rejections were 1.6-fold higher when the CSA-based regimen was used.[26] Another meta-analysis comprising 11 studies published in 2016 reported steroid withdrawal within 14 days of transplantation is associated with a 58% higher incidence for acute rejection compared to steroid withdrawal at a later time point. The 5-year patient mortality and graft loss remained similar.[40] The HARMONY trial tested steroid withdrawal on day 8 with two induction agents (rATG vs. basiliximab) versus low-dose steroid maintenance. At 1 year, the graft function was comparable, and there was no difference in the number of rejections.[31] The ADVANCE trial tested the impact of two steroid withdrawal regimens—one arm with bolus steroids and the other arm with bolus and oral steroid withdrawal. The bolus-only arm had higher rejections, but graft and patient survival and mean estimated glomerular filtration rate were comparable at 6 months.[50] An interim analysis from the ALLEGRO trial has shown that steroid-free maintenance with IL-2 induction is associated with similar kidney function compared to steroid maintenance.[51] There was a higher prevalence of biopsy-proven rejections in the steroids withdrawal arm; however, this was insignificant.

A retrospective study from India reported an increased incidence of rejections (20.5 vs. 7.5%) on steroid withdrawal in TAC/MMF + basiliximab induction; the graft function was comparable at 6 months.[52] Another retrospective from India employing low-dose rituximab + antithymocyte globulin (ATG) induction with TAC/MMF-based immunosuppression has reported 86% graft survival at 12 years following steroid withdrawal at day 5; biopsy-proven acute rejections were noted in 6.56%.[23]

The optimal immunosuppressive regimen in steroid avoidance remains unknown. One RCT compared the efficiency of the sirolimus/MMF versus TAC/MMF regimen in patients who had withdrawn steroids on day 4. Sirolimus did not improve GFR at 1 year; by the end of 2 years, 63% had withdrawn sirolimus owing to adverse effects or rejections.[53] The current evidence suggests the possibility of steroid-free maintenance regimens. However, it should be remembered that most of the trials had short follow-up periods. The impact of steroid withdrawal on long-term graft function remains unknown. The results from the major trials are summarized in **Table 2**. It was reported that steroid withdrawal might predispose to recurrent immunoglobulin A (IgA) nephropathy; however, the relationship

TABLE 2: Major trials on steroid-free maintenance.

Trial name	Study details	Immunosuppression regimen	eGFR at endpoint (mL/min/1.73 m^2)	Graft outcomes	Patient outcomes	Rejections
FREEDOM[49]	12 months Three arms Steroid withdrawal on day 7	Basiliximab, CsA, and MMF complete steroid avoidance ($n = 112$) Basiliximab, CsA, and MMF and steroid withdrawal by day 7 ($n = 115$) Basiliximab, CsA, MMF, and standard steroids ($n = 109$)	58.6 in steroid avoidance versus 59.1 in steroid-free maintenance versus 60.8 in the standard steroid group	Graft loss 2.4 versus 1.1 versus 2.3% (p = NS)	Death 3.5 versus 1.1 versus 0 (p = NS)	28.2 versus 23.6 versus 14.0% ($p = 0.004$ for steroid-free versus steroid maintenance)
HARMONY[31]	12 months Three arms Steroid withdrawal on day 8	Basiliximab/TAC/MMF and steroids ($n = 206$) Basiliximab/TAC/MMF and steroid withdrawal day 8 ($n = 189$) rATG/TAC/MMF and steroid withdrawal day 8 ($n = 192$)	46.3 in standard steroid arm versus 47.4 in basiliximab group versus 50.2 in rATG group ($p = 0.25$)	(Death censored graft survival) 96.1 versus 96.8 versus 95.8% ($p = 0.87$)	Survival 94.7 versus 94.7 versus 96.9% (p = NS)	11.2 versus 10.6 versus 9.9% (p = NS)
ADVANCE[50]	6 months Two arms	Basiliximab/TAC/MMF and steroids till day 10 ($n = 528$) Basiliximab/TAC/MMF and only bolus steroids ($n = 553$)	47.1 in steroid-free maintenance versus 47.3 in the steroid avoidance group ($p = 0.875$)	Graft survival 95.2 versus 95% ($p = 0.90$)	Survival 98.4% versus 99% ($p = 0.334$)	18.2% versus 25.9% ($p = 0.001$) BPAR—8.7% versus 13.6%
ALLEGRO[51] (interim analysis)	6 months Two arms	Basiliximab/TAC/MMF and steroids for 6 months Basiliximab/TAC/MMF and methylprednisolone day 0–2	45.0 in the standard steroid versus 43.2 in the steroid-free maintenance ($p = 0.408$)	Graft survival 98% versus 96.9% ($p = 0.370$)	Survival 98% versus 99% ($p = 0.737$)	13.6% versus 18.6% ($p = 0.289$)

(ADVANCE: Advagraf-based immunosuppression regimen examining new onset diabetes mellitus in kidney transplant recipients; ALLEGRO: Amsterdam, LEiden, GROningen; BPAR: biopsy proved acute rejections; CsA: cyclosporine A; FREEDOM: A Randomized, Multicenter Study of Steroid Avoidance, Early Steroid Withdrawal or Standard Steroid Therapy in Kidney Transplant Recipients by FREEDOM study group; HARMONY: Rabbit-ATG or basiliximab induction for rapid steroid withdrawal after renal transplantation (Harmony): an open-label, multicentre, randomised controlled trial; MMF: mycophenolate mofetil; NS: non significant; rATG: rabbit antithymocyte globulin; TAC: tacrolimus)

disappeared after matching for immunosuppression and induction protocols.[54,55]

Complete Steroid Avoidance

The data on steroid-free immunosuppression remains sparse. The FREEDOM trial tested the efficacy of steroid avoidance and steroids-free maintenance strategies against steroid maintenance. At the end of 1 year, the kidney function was comparable among all groups; however, the steroid avoidance arm showed a significantly higher incidence of biopsy-proven rejections (26.1%) than the steroid maintenance arm (14.7%).[49] The *SAILOR* (steroid-free immunosuppressive protocol, based on ATG induction and low dose tacrolimus) study compared steroid avoidance with ATG induction/TAC/MMF versus maintenance steroids/TAC/MMF, and basiliximab induction in low immunologic risk patients. At 1 year, the incidence of biopsy-proven rejections was similar (15% in steroid avoidance vs. 13.8% in maintenance). Also, graft and patient outcomes were comparable at the end of 2 years.[56]

CONCLUSION

Even though beneficial in reducing inflammation, steroids are associated with significant adverse effects. The use of low-dose steroids for maintenance is relatively safe and widely practiced. It is unclear whether late steroid withdrawal is secure. The use of induction agents, especially ATG and alemtuzumab, facilitates steroid withdrawal. A few well-designed clinical trials have provided critical evidence on steroid withdrawal early in the course of transplant. However, the risk of rejections following early withdrawal is higher and whether this affects the long-term graft function is unknown.

REFERENCES

1. Starzl TE, Marchioro TL, Waddell WR. The reversal of rejection in human renal homografts with subsequent development of homograft tolerance. Surg Gynecol Obstet. 1963;117:385-95.
2. Libert C, Dejager L. How steroids steer T cells. Cell Rep. 2014;7(4):938-9.

3. Chakraborty S, Pramanik J, Mahata B. Revisiting steroidogenesis and its role in immune regulation with the advanced tools and technologies. Genes Immun. 2021; 22(3):125-40.
4. Coutinho AE, Chapman KE. The anti-inflammatory and immunosuppressive effects of glucocorticoids, recent developments and mechanistic insights. Mol Cell Endocrinol. 2011;335(1):2-13.
5. Vandevyver S, Dejager L, Tuckermann J, Libert C. New insights into the anti-inflammatory mechanisms of glucocorticoids: an emerging role for glucocorticoid-receptor-mediated transactivation. Endocrinology. 2013;154(3): 993-1007.
6. Stahn C, Buttgereit F. Genomic and nongenomic effects of glucocorticoids. Nat Clin Pract Rheumatol. 2008;4(10): 525-33.
7. Perretti M, D'Acquisto F. Annexin A1 and glucocorticoids as effectors of the resolution of inflammation. Nat Rev Immunol. 2009;9(1):62-70.
8. Steiner RW, Awdishu L. Steroids in kidney transplant patients. Semin Immunopathol. 2011;33(2):157.
9. del Mar Fernández de Gatta M, Santos-Buelga D, Domínguez-Gil A, García MJ. Immunosuppressive therapy for paediatric transplant patients: pharmacokinetic considerations. Clin Pharmacokinet. 2002;41(2):115-35.
10. Bergmann TK, Barraclough KA, Lee KJ, Staatz CE. Clinical pharmacokinetics and pharmacodynamics of prednisolone and prednisone in solid organ transplantation. Clin Pharmacokinet. 2012;51(11):711-41.
11. Keller F, Hemmen T, Schöneshöfer M, Schwarz A, Offermann G. Pharmacokinetics of methylprednisolone and rejection episodes in kidney transplant patients. Transplantation. 1995;60(4):330-3.
12. Anglicheau D, Flamant M, Schlageter MH, Martínez F, Cassinat B, Beaune P, et al. Pharmacokinetic interaction between corticosteroids and tacrolimus after renal transplantation. Nephrol Dial Transplant. 2003;18(11): 2409-14.
13. Lam S, Partovi N, Ting LSL, Ensom MHH. Corticosteroid interactions with cyclosporine, tacrolimus, mycophenolate, and sirolimus: fact or fiction? Ann Pharmacother. 2008; 42(7):1037-47.
14. Cattaneo D, Perico N, Gaspari F, Gotti E, Remuzzi G. Glucocorticoids interfere with mycophenolate mofetil bioavailability in kidney transplantation. Kidney Int. 2002; 62(3):1060-7.
15. Yasir M, Goyal A, Bansal P, Sonthalia S. (2021). Corticosteroid Adverse Effects. StatPearls. [online] Available from https://www.ncbi.nlm.nih.gov/books/NBK531462/. [Last accessed January, 2022].
16. Gonzalez-Molina M, Gentil MA, Burgos D, Cabello M, Cobelo C, Bustamante J, et al. Effect of long-term steroid withdrawal in renal transplant recipients: a retrospective cohort study. NDT Plus. 2010;3(Suppl. 2):ii32-6.
17. Augustine JJ, Hricik DE. Steroid sparing in kidney transplantation: changing paradigms, improving outcomes, and remaining questions. Clin J Am Soc Nephrol. 2006;1(5):1080-9.
18. Tamez-Pérez HE. Steroid hyperglycemia: prevalence, early detection and therapeutic recommendations: a narrative review. World J Diabetes. 2015;6(8):1073.
19. Jayam J, Balakrishnan MA, Srinivasaprasad N, Fernando ME. Prevalence and risk factors for posttransplant diabetes mellitus: data from government tertiary care center. Indian J Transplant. 2018;12(2):119.
20. Choudhury PS, Mukhopadhyay P, Roychowdhary A, Chowdhury S, Ghosh S. Prevalence and predictors of "new-onset diabetes after transplantation" (NODAT) in renal transplant recipients: an observational study. Indian J Endocrinol Metab. 2019;23(3):273.
21. Prakash J, Rathore SS, Singh TB, Choudhury TA, Prabhakar U. New onset diabetes after transplantation (NODAT): analysis of pre-transplant risk factors in renal allograft recipients. Indian J Transplant. 2022;6(3):77.
22. Saxena S, Dash SC, Guleria S, Mittal R, Agarwal SK, Tiwari SC, et al. Post transplant diabetes mellitus in live related renal allograft recipients: a single centre experience. J Assoc Physicians India. 1996;44(7):472, 477-9.
23. Pathak V, Madhavan D, Narayanasamy K, Kumar S, Ramalingam V, Sengodagounder B, et al. Low-dose rituximab and thymoglobulin induction with steroid-free maintenance immunosuppression and protocol biopsies improves long-term patient and graft survival after kidney transplantation: survival and safety outcomes in more than 1100 patients from a single center. Transplant Direct. 2019;5(8): e475.
24. Woodle ES, First MR, Pirsch J, Shihab F, Gaber AO, Van Veldhuisen P. A prospective, randomised, double-blind, placebo-controlled multicenter trial comparing early (7 day) corticosteroid cessation versus long-term, low-dose corticosteroid therapy. Ann Surg. 2008;248(4):564-77.
25. Pirsch JD, Henning AK, First MR, Fitzsimmons W, Gaber AO, Reisfield R, et al. New-onset diabetes after transplantation: results from a double-blind early corticosteroid withdrawal trial. Am J Transplant. 2015;15(7):1982-90.
26. Pascual J, Royuela A, Galeano C, Crespo M, Zamora J. Very early steroid withdrawal or complete avoidance for kidney transplant recipients: a systematic review. Nephrol Dial Transplant. 2012;27(2):825-32.
27. Buckley L, Humphrey MB. Glucocorticoid-induced osteoporosis. N Engl J Med. 2018;379(26):2547-56.
28. Govindarajan S, Khandelwal N, Sakhuja V, Jha V. Bone mineral density in patients with end-stage renal disease and its evolution after kidney transplantation. Indian J Nephrol. 2011;21(2):85.
29. Ramakrishna M, Arun C, Sreedharan S, Pavithran PV, Bhavani N, Bhaskaran R, et al. Changes in bone mineral density in patients undergoing kidney transplantation. Indian J Transplant. 2021;15(3):199.
30. Nikkel LE, Mohan S, Zhang A, McMahon DJ, Boutroy S, Dube G, et al. Reduced fracture risk with early corticosteroid withdrawal after kidney transplant. Am J Transplant. 2012;12(3):649-59.
31. Thomusch O, Wiesener M, Opgenoorth M, Pascher A, Woitas RP, Witzke O, et al. Rabbit-ATG or basiliximab induction for rapid steroid withdrawal after renal transplantation (harmony): an open-label, multicentre, randomised controlled trial. Lancet. 2016;388:3006-16.
32. Thomusch O, Hugo C. Steroid withdrawal and bone disease after kidney transplantation—authors' reply. Lancet. 2017; 389(10081):1796.

33. Siegel RR, Luke RG, Hellebusch AA. Reduction of toxicity of corticosteroid therapy after renal transplantation. Am J Med. 1972;53(2):159-69.
34. Andreoni KA, Brayman KL, Guidinger MK, Sommers CM, Sung RS. Kidney and pancreas transplantation in the United States, 1996–2005. Am J Transplant. 2007;7(Suppl. 1): 1359-75.
35. Transplant recipient—KDIGO. [online] Available from https://kdigo.org/guidelines/transplant-recipient/. [Last accessed January, 2022].
36. Hollander AAMJ, Hene RJ, Hermans JO, Van Es LA, Van Der Woudee FJ. Late prednisone withdrawal in cyclosporine-treated kidney transplant patients: a randomised study. J Am Soc Nephrol. 1997;8(2):294-301.
37. Ratcliffe PJ, Dudley CRK, Higgins RM, Firth JD, Smith B, Morris PJ. Randomised controlled trial of steroid withdrawal in renal transplant recipients receiving triple immunosuppression. Lancet. 1996;348(9028):643-8.
38. Grinyo JM, Gil-Vernet S, Serón D, Cruzado JM, Moreso F, Fulladosa X, et al. Steroid withdrawal in mycophenolate mofetil-treated renal allograft recipients. Transplantation. 1997;63(11):1688-90.
39. Opelz G, Döhler B, Laux G. Long-term prospective study of steroid withdrawal in kidney and heart transplant recipients. Am J Transplant. 2005;5(4 Pt. 1):720-8.
40. Haller MC, Royuela A, Nagler EV, Pascual J, Webster AC. Steroid avoidance or withdrawal for kidney transplant recipients. Cochrane Database Syst Rev. 2016;2016(8): CD005632.
41. Hricik DE, O'Toole MA, Schulak JA, Herson J. Steroid-free immunosuppression in cyclosporine-treated renal transplant recipients: a meta-analysis. J Am Soc Nephrol. 1993;4(6):1300-5.
42. Pascual J, Galeano C, Royuela A, Zamora J. A systematic review on steroid withdrawal between 3 and 6 months after kidney transplantation. Transplantation. 2010;90(4): 343-9.
43. Haller MC, Kammer M, Kainz A, Baer HJ, Heinze G, Oberbauer R. Steroid withdrawal after renal transplantation: a retrospective cohort study. BMC Med. 2017;15(1):8.
44. Taber DJ, Hunt KJ, Gebregziabher M, Srinivas T, Chavin KD, Baliga PK, et al. A comparative effectiveness analysis of early steroid withdrawal in black kidney transplant recipients. Clin J Am Soc Nephrol. 2017;12(1):131-9.
45. Hussain SM, Marcus RJ, Ko TY, Nashar K, Thai NL, Sureshkumar KK. Outcomes of early steroid withdrawal in recipients of deceased-donor expanded criteria kidney transplants in the era of induction therapy. Exp Clin Transplant. 2016;14(3):287-93.
46. Sureshkumar KK, Hussain SM, Nashar K, Marcus RJ. Steroid maintenance in repeat kidney transplantation: influence of induction agents on outcomes. Saudi J Kidney Dis Transpl. 2014;25(4):741-9.
47. Nanmoku K, Shinzato T, Kubo T, Shimizu T, Kimura T, Yagisawa T. Steroid withdrawal using everolimus in ABO-incompatible kidney transplant recipients with post-transplant diabetes mellitus. Transplant Proc. 2018;50(4):1050-5.
48. Tojimbara T, Yashima J, Shirai H, Yamazaki T, Koyama I, Nakajima I. Early steroid withdrawal protocol with basiliximab and rituximab in ABO-incompatible kidney transplant recipients. Transplant Proc. 2020;52(6):1705-8.
49. Vincenti F, Schena FP, Paraskevas S, Hauser IA, Walker RG, Grinyo J. A randomised, multicenter study of steroid avoidance, early steroid withdrawal or standard steroid therapy in kidney transplant recipients. Am J Transplant. 2008;8(2):307-16.
50. Mourad G, Glyda M, Albano L, Viklický O, Merville P, Tydén G, et al. Incidence of posttransplantation diabetes mellitus in de novo kidney transplant recipients receiving prolonged-release tacrolimus-based immunosuppression with 2 different corticosteroid minimization strategies: ADVANCE, a randomized controlled trial. Transplantation. 2017;101(8):1924-34.
51. van Sandwijk MS, de Vries APJ, Bakker SJL, ten Berge IJM, Berger SP, Bouatou YR, et al. Early steroid withdrawal compared with standard immunosuppression in kidney transplantation—interim analysis of the Amsterdam-Leiden-Groningen randomized controlled trial. Transplant Direct. 2018;4(6):e354.
52. Bansal SB, Sethi S, Sharma R, Jain M, Jha P, Ahlawat R, et al. Early corticosteroid withdrawal regimen in a living donor kidney transplantation program. Indian J Nephrol. 2014;24(4):232.
53. Heilman RL, Younan K, Wadei HM, Mai ML, Reddy KS, Chakkera HA, et al. Results of a prospective randomised trial of sirolimus conversion in kidney transplant recipients on early corticosteroid withdrawal. Transplantation. 2011; 92(7):767-73.
54. Leeaphorn N, Garg N, Khankin EV, Cardarelli F, Pavlakis M. Recurrence of IgA nephropathy after kidney transplantation in steroid continuation versus early steroid-withdrawal regimens: a retrospective analysis of the UNOS/OPTN database. Transpl Int. 2018;31(2):175-86.
55. Kurian SM, Bagsic SRS, Case J, Barrick BL, Schaffer R, Rice JC, et al. UNOS/OPTN data guided assessment of IgA nephropathy recurrence after kidney transplantation and evaluation of immunosuppressive protocols in a steroid free center. Transplant Rep. 2020;5(4):100063.
56. Ekberg J, Baid-Agrawal S, Jespersen B, Källén R, Rafael E, Skov K, et al. A randomized controlled trial on safety of steroid avoidance in immunologically low-risk kidney transplant recipients. Kidney Int Rep. 2021;7(2):259-69.

9.3 Calcineurin Inhibitors

Abhijit Taraphder, Padmini Sirkanungo, Govardhan Gupta

CASE VIGNETTE 1

Mrs. A.M., a 38-year-old housewife with biopsy-proven focal and segmental glomerulosclerosis (FSGS) diagnosed 16 years ago, developed end-stage renal disease and underwent live-related renal transplantation, her sister being the donor with no induction therapy. She was keeping well with triple immunosuppression [tacrolimus (TAC)/mycophenolate mofetil (MMF)/steroid] with a stable graft function. In view of her financial constraint, her TAC dose was reduced and her anti-hypertensive drug was substituted with diltiazem. Though urine output remained steady, her serum creatinine started to rise. A graft biopsy was performed. Likely findings in the histology suggest the following:

a. Acute cellular rejection
b. Recurrent FSGS
c. TAC toxicity
d. Acute tubular necrosis

CASE VIGNETTE 2

A 36-year-old male executive underwent renal transplantation with the donor being his wife. He was on triple immuno-suppression, namely TAC, MMF, and steroid. Though he was maintaining a good graft function, 6 months post-transplant, he developed post-transplant diabetes mellitus (PTDM) and TAC was substituted with cyclosporine A (CsA). Recently, his renal function deteriorated and investigation revealed a low trough level of MMF. The possible explanation could be:

a. Diabetes-induced abnormal gut motility hindering MMF absorption
b. Inhibition of excretion of mycophenolic acid glucuronide in bile by CsA
c. Chronic diarrhea induced by MMF leading to impaired MMF absorption

INTRODUCTION

Although the era of chemical immunosuppression in solid organ transplantation began more than 60 years ago, the scenario had observed a sea change since the advent of calcineurin inhibitors (CNIs). CsA was the first to be introduced followed by TAC, both being of fungal origin. CsA was first used clinically in the late 1970s, whereas TAC was introduced in liver transplantation (1994) followed by renal transplantation (1997). The widespread use of CNIs has improved 1-year graft survival to >90%.[1] Of the two, TAC has largely replaced CsA over the past 20 years.[2,3]

Cyclosporine A is a cyclic polypeptide consisting of 11 amino acids, whereas TAC is a 23-membered macrolide lactone. Both are insoluble in water and neither is significantly dialyzed.

MECHANISM OF ACTION

Both of these compounds inhibit calcineurin, which in normal situations acts as a phosphatase enzyme that dephosphorylates certain nuclear regulatory proteins, thereby facilitating their passage through the nuclear membrane. At the initial step, they form a complex with their cytoplasmic receptor protein, namely cyclophilin for CsA and TAC-binding protein for TAC. These complexes bind with calcineurin, and inhibition of calcineurin impairs the expression of cytokines. The net effect is a quantitative reduction of cytokine production and lymphocyte proliferation **(Flowchart 1)**.

Hence, CNIs cause a selective inhibition of the immune response, in the sense that they do not inhibit neutrophilic phagocyte activity nor suppress the bone marrow. Patients receiving CNIs maintain a certain degree of immune responsiveness in spite of an adequate CNI-based immuno-suppressive regimen.

Flowchart 1: Mechanism of action of calcineurin inhibitor.

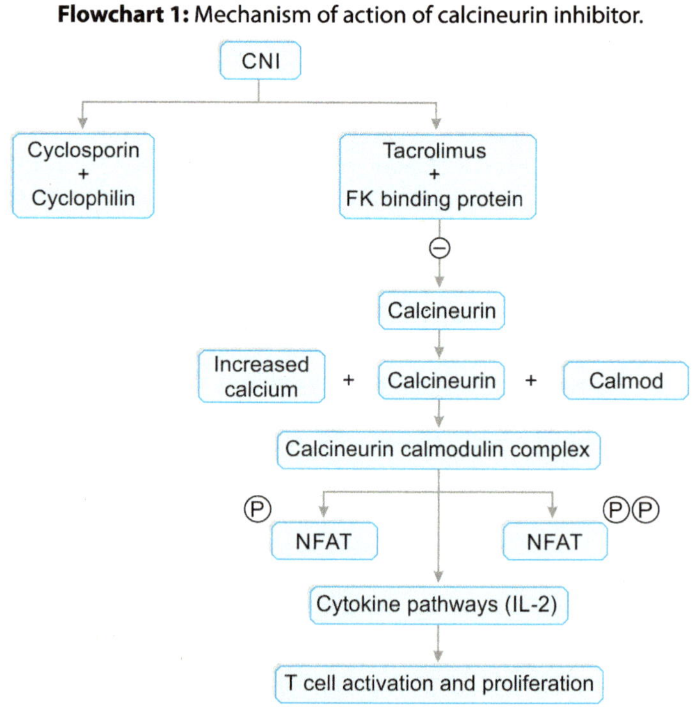

(CNI: calcineurin inhibitor; IL-2: interleukin 2; NFAT: nuclear factor of activated T cell)

CHAPTER HIGHLIGHTS

- Calcineurin inhibitors (CNIs), namely cyclosporine A (CsA) or tacrolimus (TAC) in combination with corticosteroids and azathioprine (Aza) or mycophenolate mofetil (MMF), constitute the cornerstone of maintenance immunosuppressive regimen in >90% of the renal transplantation cases.
- These agents have a narrow therapeutic window and need constant monitoring of therapeutic blood levels to avoid toxicity.
- They also interact with a number of drugs in a way that some drugs tend to raise the blood levels of CNIs, while others tend to reduce them, requiring a constant vigil on important drug interactions.

CLINICAL PHARMACOKINETICS

Cyclosporine A is available as an oil-based and as a microemulsion form. Both are available as 100 mg/mL solution and soft gelatin capsules (25 and 100 mg). Mixing with grapefruit juice should be avoided. Gelatin capsules that are exposed to heat or has been kept out of the blister package for >2 weeks may show decreased efficacy. TAC is available as 0.5-, 1-, and 5-mg immediate-release capsules and in an intravenous formulation. The immediate-release products are administered twice daily. Long-acting once-daily formulations are also available which are marketed as 0.5-, 1-, and 5-mg capsules and 0.75-, 1-, and 4-mg prolonged-release tablets. Intravenous dose is approximately one third of the total oral dose and administered via 24-hour continuous infusion. Sublingual dose is usually one half of the oral dose.

After a dose of CNI is taken, the blood concentration reaches a peak level referred to as C_{max}, declining thereafter owing to distribution and elimination, until it reaches the trough level, referred to as C_0, the timing of which corresponds to that of the immediate next dose. Both the CNI's, cyclosporine A and TAC share similar profile **(Box 1)** with some differences **(Box 2)**.

BOX 1: Comparison between cyclosporine A and tacrolimus.

Similarities
- Both are calcineurin inhibitors
- Both have oral and intravenous preparations
- Drug interactions are more or less identical
- Hyperuricemia develops with both, but clinical gout is more common with CsA
- Acute and chronic nephrotoxicity develop with both
- Sodium retention and hypertension in both, but more with CsA
- Pancreatic islet cell toxicity and PTDM develop with both, but more common with TAC
- Neurotoxicity may develop in both, but more severe with TAC treatment
- Hypomagnesemia may develop with both

(CsA: cyclosporine A; PTDM: post-transplant diabetes mellitus; TAC: tacrolimus)

BOX 2: Comparison between cyclosporine A and tacrolimus.

Differences
- Sublingual preparation and prolonged-release formulation are available only with TAC
- Gingival hyperplasia is found with CsA
- CsA treatment may give rise to hypertrichosis
- Alopecia is typically found in patients receiving TAC
- Hypercholesterolemia is a characteristic feature of CsA
- Gastrointestinal motility disorders, specially diarrhea, are more common with TAC
- Combination of TAC and MMF has an edge over the combination of CsA and MMF because of favorable effect on enterohepatic circulation in the former

(CsA: cyclosporine A; MMF: mycophenolate mofetil; TAC: tacrolimus)

Absorption and Distribution

The absorption of CsA depends on the presence of food, bile acids, certain other drugs, time of the day, and gastrointestinal motility. The bioavailability of the microemulsion formulation is better than the original form. The bioavailability of the orally administered formulation is around 30–45% of the intravenous infusion and the conversion ratio is 3:1. Bioavailability increases with time and reaches a steady state 4–8 weeks after transplantation. The microemulsion form reaches maximum blood concentration in 2 hours, of which one third is bound to lipoproteins and the remaining to erythrocytes. The toxic effects of CsA may be exaggerated in low-cholesterol states when a large amount of unbound CsA is in circulation.

The absorption of TAC is bile independent. Immediate-release TAC is absorbed primarily from the proximal small intestine. TAC has a mean bioavailability of around 25% (31% in pediatric population). TAC also has an affinity for erythrocytes.

Both CsA and TAC cross the placenta and enter breast milk at a very low level.

Metabolism and Elimination

Cyclosporine A is metabolized almost entirely in the liver and excreted through bile. TAC, in addition, has intestinal metabolism, though to a lesser extent. Both are excreted primarily in the bile; hence, renal dysfunction does not necessitate dose adjustment. Pediatric patients require larger doses, whereas a larger dosage interval is indicated in the elderly. Severe liver dysfunction with mean Pugh score >10 affects the drug clearance.

Both CsA and TAC require the cytochrome P450 (CYP) 3A enzymes, specially CYP3A4 and CYP3A5 for their metabolism. This takes place primarily in the liver, small intestine, and, to a lesser extent, in the kidney. P-glycoprotein (P-gp) efflux pumps also have a role. These adenosine triphosphate (ATP)-dependent pumps are located at hepatocytes, intestinal epithelial cells, renal tubular cells, and in the capillary endothelial cells of the brain. P-gp is encoded in the *ABCB1* gene. Genetic polymorphism in the expression of ABCB1 and CYP3A4/5 may affect the metabolism of CNIs which will modify the drug concentration at target sites and influence the efficacy vis-à-vis toxicity of the drugs.

Genetic variations in CYP3A5 can affect the metabolism of TAC. Individuals homozygous for the G allele at the single nucleotide polymorphism (SNP) rs776746 (CYP3A5*3/*3) have a nonfunctional CYP3A5 protein, are slow metabolizers, and are called "non expressors." They require a reduced dosing to achieve therapeutic drug concentration. Those having a genotype CYP3A5*1/*3 are called "expressors," requiring a higher dose.

Unlike TAC, CYP3A4 plays a more dominant role in the metabolism of CsA. The intrinsic clearance of CsA is approximately two- to threefold higher for CYP3A4 than for CYP3A5. Only CsA has inhibitory properties on organic anion transporter protein B1 (OATP1B1) in the liver and P-gp inhibitor in enterocytes.

Higher TAC dose requirement in expressors and higher TAC drug toxicity in nonexpressors have been observed in two studies published in the North Indian[4] and South Indian[5] transplant populations recently.

Tacrolimus is preferentially absorbed in the proximal small intestine and metabolized by the CYP3A4 and CYP3A5 isoforms located in the liver and intestine. The concentration of CYP3A congeners is the highest in the duodenum and jejunum and relatively less in stomach and distal intestinal mucosa. TAC is also a substrate for P-gp pump, which operates by actively transporting TAC from the mucosal cell back into the intestinal lumen. The P-gp system predominantly operates in the colon.

In severe diarrhea (more than three loose stools a day), the metabolism of TAC by CYP3A is affected. Also is affected the back transport of TAC by the P-gp system in the colonic mucosa due to reduced enzymatic activity of the CYP3A and P-gp system. Moreover, due to a shortened ileal transit time, a higher amount of TAC is being delivered to the colon, which is not prepared to handle it. The other reasons which are thought to raise TAC concentration in blood during acute diarrhea are hemoconcentration due to fluid loss, reduced hepatic metabolism, and fasting. It has been observed that diarrhea precedes the rise in TAC blood levels suggesting that diarrhea is the cause and not a consequence of TAC toxicity.

Mycophenolate mofetil is known to cause mild diarrhea. It is reported that MMF-induced diarrhea may be associated with a loss of the normal villous structure of the small bowel. This might affect intestinal metabolism of TAC resulting in an elevated trough level of TAC. Ongoing mild diarrhea may give rise to unnoticed chronic TAC overexposure leading to irreversible CNI nephrotoxicity.

THERAPEUTIC DRUG-LEVEL MONITORING AND DOSING

The therapeutic window is narrow. That makes measurement of blood level an integral part of management. There is a large interpatient and intrapatient variability of CNI metabolism. The relationship between blood levels and episodes of rejection vis-à-vis toxicity is not linear.

As the absorption of CsA Neoral is consistent, its peak level (2 hours after dosing) has been found to correlate better with drug exposure and clinical events. Hence, C_2 monitoring is applied. For TAC, the trough levels are normally considered for adequate approximation of drug response.

For CsA, a whole-blood ethylenediaminetetraacetic acid (EDTA) anticoagulated sample is the recommended specimen type. High-performance liquid chromatography (HPLC) is the gold standard. Because it is expensive and not available universally, immunoassays are the usual practice. TAC levels are measured using microparticle enzyme immunoassays (MEIA).

Calcineurin inhibitors are generally started 2 days prior to transplantation except in ABO-incompatible transplants where it is to be started 10–14 days prior. The target trough level of TAC is 7–10 ng/mL for the first month, which comes down to 3–7 ng/mL subsequently. The C_2 level for CsA is between 800 and 1,000 ng/mL to start with, gradually tapered to between 200 and 300 ng/mL.

RELEVANT DRUG INTERACTIONS

Drugs that have an impact on CYP3A 4/5 or P-gp activity have the potential to interact with the CNIs. It is CsA that has been incriminated more often.

Calcium channel blockers, notably verapamil and diltiazem and antifungals, e.g., ketoconazole, tend to increase CNI levels and permit reduction of CNI dose.

Sometimes, they are intentionally added to reduce the dose of CNI to curtail the cost of therapy. Antibiotics such as erythromycin and antiretroviral agents such as ritonavir can raise CNI levels.

Corticosteroids are inducers of CYP3A. Hence, when the dose of corticosteroid is suddenly reduced as after steroid pulse therapy for acute rejection, or corticosteroids are withdrawn as a part of steroid-avoidance therapy, the TAC level may suddenly increase. This may give rise to raised serum creatinine levels producing therapeutic confusion.

Of the drugs which reduce CNI levels, anticonvulsants such as phenytoin and barbiturates, and rifampicin, an antitubercular agent, are few examples. Cholestyramine and sevelamer reduce gastrointestinal absorption of CNIs.

Cyclosporine A inhibits enterohepatic circulation of MMF, which TAC does not. Coadministration of TAC and sirolimus results in decreased trough levels of sirolimus

TABLE 1: Drugs increasing calcineurin inhibitor levels.

Class of drugs	*Drugs*
Calcium channel blockers	Verapamil, amlodipine, nicardipine
Antifungal agents	Fluconazole, itraconazole, voriconazole
Antibiotics	Erythromycin, chloramphenicol
Hormones	Steroids, somatostatin, testosterone
Others	• Metoclopramide • Statins • Protease inhibitors • Allopurinol • Amiodarone • Ranitidine

Note: See text for mechanism of action.

TABLE 2: Drugs decreasing calcineurin inhibitor (CNI) levels.

Class of drugs	*Drugs*
Antitubercular drugs	Rifampicin, rifabutin, isoniazid
Anticonvulsants	Phenytoin, carbamazepine, barbiturates
Antibiotics	Nafcillin, imipenem, cephalosporins
Antidepressive herbals	St John's wort
Others	Ticlopidine, sevelamer, steroids

Note: See text for mechanism of action.

(Details of drug interactions of CNIs are given in **Tables 1 and 2.**)

ADVERSE EFFECTS

Calcineurin Inhibitor Nephrotoxicity

The spectrum of CNI nephrotoxicity may be acute or chronic/progressive. Some of them improve with dose reduction, and few require CNI withdrawal. The spectrum also includes electrolyte abnormalities.

Acute

- *Functional decrease in renal blood flow:* CNIs tend to produce a dose-dependent reversible vasoconstriction predominantly affecting the afferent arteriole, clinically manifested as a transient reversible blood level-dependent elevation of serum creatinine or a delayed recovery of a malfunctioning graft. It is more pronounced with CsA.
- *Tubulopathy:* Both TAC and CsA cause isometric vacuolization of tubular cells, mainly in the proximal straight tubules.
- *Vasculopathy:* It is present as afferent arteriolopathy characterized by endothelial swelling, vacuolation necrosis, and hyaline replacements of myocytes.

TABLE 3: Mechanism of hypertension, acidosis, and dyselectrolytemia caused by calcineurin inhibitor (CNI).

Disorders	*Possible explanations*
Hypertension	• Impaired sodium excretion secondary to CNI-mediated vasoconstriction • Activation of renin–angiotensin–aldosterone system (RAAS) • Decreased production of nitric oxide
Renal tubular acidosis • Early and late forms • Early tend to develop dyselectrolytemia • Late tend to cause CNI nephrotoxicity	• Impaired mineralocorticoid transcriptional activity in distal tubular cells leading to aldosterone resistance manifesting as hyperkalemia and acidosis • Dysregulation of acid–base transporters such as H+V-ATPase, sodium bicarbonate cotransporter, and anion exchanger (AE) • Inhibition of prolyl-cis-trans isomerase activity of cyclophilin by cyclosporine, thereby interrupting the remodeling of intercalated cell • From bicarbonate-secreting beta form to acid-secreting alpha form in cortical collecting duct
Hyperkalemia	• Impaired renal response to aldosterone • Inhibition of cortical collecting duct potassium secretory channels
Hypomagnesemia	• Downregulation of epidermal growth factor and distal collecting tubule TRPM6 channel • Volume expansion • Metabolic acidosis • Insulin resistance • *Net effect:* Tubular magnesium wasting

- *Thrombotic microangiopathy (TMA):* The mean time from transplantation to the onset of microangiopathy is 9.3 ± 7.9 months. Pronounced arterial intimal changes are not typical of CNI-induced TMA. Plasmapheresis, plasma exchange, and anticoagulation are tried with mixed results.

Chronic

Interstitial fibrosis, which is typically patchy or striped, associated with arteriolar lesions is the usual feature. Hyaline arteriolopathy tends to affect the distal interlobular arteries and afferent arterioles. On staining, it appears as a pearl necklace pattern.

Dyselectrolytemias

The spectrum includes sodium retention leading to hypertension, hyperkalemia, hyperchloremic acidosis, hypomagnesemia, and hypercalciuria. Hyperuricemia occurs in both, but clinical gout is more common with CsA therapy. (Details are mentioned in **Table 3.**)

NONRENAL SIDE EFFECTS OF CALCINEURIN INHIBITORS

Post-transplant Diabetes Mellitus

Post-transplant diabetes mellitus is encountered more with TAC therapy. In the ELITE-Symphony trial, the TAC arm had shown higher incidence of PTDM. CNIs are said to be directly toxic to pancreatic islet cells. The effect is dose related and exaggerated by concomitant use of corticosteroid, obesity, old age, hepatitis C infection, and a family history of diabetes.

Hypertension

Incidence of elevated blood pressure (BP) is more common with CsA compared to TAC.

Hyperlipidemia

Occupation of low-density lipoprotein (LDL) receptor by CsA or abnormal LDL feedback control by the liver is the possible mechanism.

Cosmetic

Cyclosporine A therapy is associated with hypertrichosis, whereas TAC produces alopecia. Gingival hyperplasia may develop with CsA therapy. It is exacerbated by poor dental hygiene and concomitant use of calcium channel blockers. Azithromycin is said to reduce it.

Gastrointestinal

Asymptomatic elevation of liver enzymes, cholelithiasis, and mild hyperbilirubinemia is more common with CsA and reflects disturbed bile secretion. Gastrointestinal motility disorders are common with TAC.

Neurological

Headache, insomnia, paresthesia, and coarse tremor may develop with both, being more common with TAC. Administration of higher evening dose compared to the morning dose and switch to prolonged-release formulation of TAC may reduce it. Discrete cognitive impairments are uncommon and isolated seizures are occasional. Full-blown leukoencephalopathy is a rare complication.

Malignancy

The most common malignancies reported are those of skin and lymphoid tissue. Post-transplant lymphoproliferative disorder (PTLD) has a higher risk in children and its incidence is marginally higher with TAC therapy.

TABLE 4: Landmark clinical trials.

Study name/purpose	*Authors/year of publication*	*Study design*	*Outcome*
TAC versus CsA in combination with azathioprine	Vincenti et al., 2002[1]	An open-label phase 3 randomized multicenter study in 19 US centers in 412 patients after cadaveric renal transplantation	• Incidence of biopsy-proven acute rejection at 1 year was 30.7% in the TAC group compared with 46.4% in the CsA group ($p = 0.001$) • A significant number of patients in the CsA group crossed over to TAC secondary to refractory rejection with CsA at 3- and 5-year follow-up
ELITE-Symphony Study: TAC versus CsA in combination with MMF Importance of low-dose TAC	Ekberg et al., 2007[6]	A combination of low-dose TAC (target level aimed between 3 and 7 ng/mL), fixed daily dose of 2 g MMF, corticosteroids and daclizumab was compared with standard-dose CsA, low-dose CsA, and low-dose sirolimus with identical combination	• After 3 years follow-up, the low-dose TAC group remained superior in terms of cumulative acute rejection episodes, graft function, and survival • However, though the target TAC trough level was between 3 and 7 ng/mL, actual achieved level averaged 6.4 ng/mL at 12 months and 6.5 ng/mL at 36 months
CNI conversion/ avoidance protocol	Rostaing et al., 2011[7]	Switching from CNI-based regimens to a belatacept-based regimen at 6–36 months post-transplant	At 1-year GFR increased by 7 ± 11.99 mL/min in belatacept group, while it was 2.1 ± 10.34 mL/min in the CNI group
TRANSFORM trial: Low-dose TAC in combination with m-TOR inhibitors	Pascual et al., 2018[8]	2,037 subjects were randomized to low-dose TAC (target trough level between 2 and 4 ng/mL) in combination with everolimus or standard MMF/TAC-based regimen having a target trough level between 6 and 10 ng/mL	• At 1-year post-transplant, there was no difference in terms of biopsy-proven acute rejection graft loss or death • There were fewer CMV or BKV infections in the everolimus arm

(BKV: BK virus; CMV: cytomegalovirus; CsA: cyclosporine A; CNI: calcineurin inhibitor; GFR: glomerular filtration rate; MMF: mycophenolate mofetil; m-TOR: mammalian target of rapamycin; TAC: tacrolimus)

Pregnancy and Lactation

Calcineurin inhibitors are extensively metabolized by the placenta; hence, dose requirement increases during gestation. They can cause transient hyperkalemia and an elevated creatinine level in neonates.

THERAPEUTIC USE AND CALCINEURIN INHIBITOR-BASED PROTOCOLS

Though CNIs have been used as part of rescue therapy[9] and induction immunosuppression,[10,11] their main role lies in maintenance immunosuppression. The important trials in this respect are mentioned in **Table 4**.

WAY FORWARD

New Formulations and New Agents

Once-daily dosing of TAC is gradually becoming the new practice. Newer CNIs are in the horizon. Voclosporin is such an agent, which, in the PROMISE study, has shown to be as efficacious as TAC in preventing acute rejection.[12] It has already been approved in the treatment of lupus nephritis.

Balancing between Chronic Alloimmunity and Chronic Nephrotoxicity

It was long being held that alloimmunity as evidenced by antibody-mediated injury is the major cause of long-term graft loss. But a recent study performed 10 years post-transplant in 145 surveillance biopsies has shown arteriolar hyalinosis, mesangial sclerosis, and global glomerulosclerosis in 50–70% biopsies which are nonimmunologic in nature suggesting chronic CNI toxicity.[13]

REFERENCES

1. Vincenti F, Jensik SC, Filo RS, Miller J, Pirsch J. A long-term comparison of Tacrolimus (FK506) and cyclosporine in kidney transplantation: evidence for improved allograft survival at five years. Transplantation. 2002;73(5):775-82.
2. Matas AJ, Smith JM, Skeans MA, Thompson B, Gustafson SK, Stewart DE, et al. OPTN/SRTR 2013 annual data report: kidney. Am J Transplant. 2015;15(Suppl. 2):1-34.
3. Patel DD, Modi KP, Patel AK. Prescription trends of immunosuppressant drugs in Indian renal transplant patients. Int J Ph Sc Dr Res. 2015;7(4):334-9.
4. Prasad N, Jaiswal A, Behera MR, Agarwal V, Kushwaha R, Bhadauria D, et al. Melding pharmacogenomic effect of MDR1 and CYP3A5 gene polymorphism on tacrolimus dosing in renal transplant recipients in Northern India. Kidney Int Rep. 2019;5(1):28-38.
5. Fernando ME, Sellappan M, Srinivasa Prasad ND, Suren S, Thirumalvalavan K. Influence of CYP3A5 and ABCB1 polymorphism on tacrolimus drug dosing in South Indian renal allograft recipients. Indian J Nephrol. 2019;29(4):261-6.
6. Ekberg H, Tedesco-Silva H, Demirbas A, Vítko S, Nashan B, Gürkan A, et al. Reduced exposure to calcineurin inhibitors in renal transplantation. N Engl J Med. 2007;357(25):2562-75.
7. Rostaing L, Massari P, Garcia VD, Mancilla-Urrea E, Nainan G, del Carmen Rial M, et al. Switching from calcineurin inhibitor-based regimens to a belatacept-based regimen in renal transplant recipients: a randomized phase II study. Clin J Am Soc Nephrol. 2011;6:430-9.
8. Pascual J, Berger SP, Witzke O, Tedesco H, Mulgaonkar S, Qazi Y, et al. Everolimus with reduced calcineurin inhibitor exposure in renal transplantation. J Am Soc Nephrol. 2018;29(7):1979-91.
9. Jordan ML, Shapiro R, Vivas C, Scantlebury V, McCauley J, McMichael J, et al. Outcome of tacrolimus conversion therapy for renal allograft rejection: 5-year follow-up. Transplant Proc. 1999;31(7A):S81-3.
10. Davis S, Gralla J, Klem P, Tong S, Wedermyer G, Freed B, et al. Lower tacrolimus exposure and time in therapeutic range increase the risk of de novo donor-specific antibodies in the first year of kidney transplantation. Am J Transplant. 2018;18(4):907-15.
11. Wojciechowski D, Wiseman A. Long-term immunosuppression management opportunities and uncertainties. Clin J Am Soc Nephrol. 2021;16:1264-71.
12. Busque S, Cantarovich M, Mulgaonkar S, Gaston R, Gaber AO, Mayo PR, et al. The PROMISE study: a phase 2b multicenter study of voclosporin (ISA247) versus tacrolimus in de novo kidney transplantation. Am J Transplant. 2011;11(12):2675-84.
13. Stegall MD, Cornell LD, Park WD, Smith BH, Cosio FG. Renal allograft histology at 10 years after transplantation in the tacrolimus era: evidence of pervasive chronic injury. Am J Transplant. 2018;18:180-8.

9.4 Mycophenolate Mofetil

Kristin George, Soumita Bagchi

CASE VIGNETTE

Mr A, case of diabetic kidney disease with end-stage renal disease, underwent renal transplantation with mother as donor, blood group compatible. He did not receive any induction immunosuppression and is on stable dose of tacrolimus, mycophenolate mofetil (MMF), and steroid. 2 months post-transplant, he comes with loose stools, 5–6 episodes per day, watery nonbloody, nonmucoid, not associated with pain in the abdomen. Stool examination is negative for common bacterial and parasitic pathogens. The symptoms are recurrent and persistent despite short course of antibacterial agents. Which of the following medications could be causing his symptoms?

a. Steroid
b. MMF
c. Tacrolimus
d. None of the above

Ans. b

INTRODUCTION

Mycophenolate mofetil is one of the most frequently used immunosuppressive drugs in solid organ transplant recipients including kidney transplant. While CNIs, cyclosporine, and tacrolimus block early signals in cytokine production and T-cell activation, the antiproliferatives which include azathioprine and MMF exert effects downstream in the cell cycle, interfering with cytokine-dependent signals and lymphocyte proliferation.[1]

Mycophenolate mofetil is an inhibitor of inosine-5′-monophosphate and is able to preferentially inhibit B-cell and T-cell function. The effective immunosuppressive properties have made MMF one of the most successful antirejection drugs in kidney transplant patients.

DRUG DEVELOPMENT

Azathioprine, along with corticosteroids, was used as the primary maintenance immunosuppression in renal transplantation till the early 1980s, when cyclosporine A (CsA) was introduced. The "triple" therapy, with CsA, azathioprine, and steroids, then became the widely practiced immunosuppressive protocol. MMF was developed in the early 1990s as an alternative to azathioprine and soon became the standard therapy along with CNIs and steroids.

Mycophenolic acid (MPA) is a fermentation product of *Penicillium brevicompactum* and related fungi. It was initially considered as a potential antitumor agent, but soon scientists began to study the in vitro effect of MPA on lymphocyte function. This was followed by animal studies on graft outcomes, wherein they observed that optimal kidney graft outcomes in dogs occurred when MPA was combined with low-dose CsA and prednisone.

Three large multicenter double-blinded trials rigorously conducted studies involving large numbers of patients in solid-organ transplantation. The European Study Group compared two doses of MMF with placebo in patients receiving CsA and prednisone but no induction therapy. The incidence of acute rejection at 6 months was reduced from 46.4% in the placebo group to 17.0% and 13.8% in the 2 g MMF and 3 g MMF groups, respectively ($p = 0.001$).[2]

The US Renal Transplant Mycophenolate Mofetil Study Group compared the same two doses of MMF to azathioprine (AZA) in patients receiving CsA, steroids, and antithymocyte globulin induction therapy. The incidence of acute rejection at 6 months was reduced from 38.0% in the Aza group to 19.8% and 17.5% in the 2 g MMF and 3 g MMF groups, respectively ($p = 0.002$).[3] The Tricontinental Study Group trial patients also received either MMF (2 or 3 g) or AZA with CsA and steroids, but induction therapy was not given. Biopsy-proven rejection or treatment failure within the first 6 months was 38.2%, 34.8%, and 50.0% for patients receiving MMF 2 g, MMF 3 g, or AZA, respectively.[4]

To summarize, the findings of all the three trials were similar: A 50% reduction in rates of acute rejection with MMF within the first 6 months after transplantation, with identical graft and patient survival among treatment arms at 1 and 3 years.[2-4] **Table 1** summarizes the important clinical trials.

An important development in the subsequent years was the development of enteric-coated formulation, mycophenolate sodium (EC-MPS, Myfortic). While MMF administration releases MPA in the stomach, mycophenolate sodium (MPS) releases it in the small intestine.

MECHANISM OF ACTION

Mycophenolate mofetil is a morpholinoethyl ester and a prodrug of MPA, a potent inhibitor of IMPDH.[5]

The observations in children with two genetic disorders prompted the development of MMF as an immunosuppressive drug. Children with an absence of adenosine deaminase, an enzyme responsible for the de novo production of guanosine monophosphate, had a combined immunodeficiency involving deficiencies in both T and B lymphocytes.[6] Children born with deficiency of hypoxanthine-guanine phosphoribosyltransferase (Lesch-Nyhan syndrome), an enzyme for salvage production of guanosine monophosphate, suffered from neurologic

TABLE 1: Important clinical trials of mycophenolate mofetil (MMF).

Study	Year	Study design	Drugs	Primary outcome	Results/remarks
European Mycophenolate Mofetil Cooperative Study Group[2]	1995	RCT	• MMF 2 g versus 3 g versus placebo • All patients on CsA + steroid, no induction	BPAR or treatment failure at 6 months	30.3%, 38.8%, and 56.0% for patients receiving MMF 2 g, MMF 3 g, or placebo, respectively ($p = 0.001$)
Sollinger[3]	1995	RCT	• MMF 2 g versus 3 g versus AZA • All patients on CsA + steroid, ATG induction	Biopsy-proven rejection or treatment failure 6 months	31.1%, 31.3%, and 47.6% for MMF 2 g, MMF 3 g, and AZA, respectively. $p = 0.002$ for either MMF group versus AZA
Tricontinental Mycophenolate Mofetil Renal Transplantation Study Group[4]	1996	RCT	• MMF 2 g versus 3 g versus AZA • All patients on CsA + steroid, no induction	BPAR or treatment failure at 6 months	38.2%, 34.8%, and 50.0% for patients receiving MMF 2 g, MMF 3 g, or AZA, respectively $p = 0.03$ for either MMF group versus AZA
Ojo et al.[7]	2000	Retrospective registry-based study	MMF versus AZA		4-year patient survival (91.4% vs. 89.9%; $p = 0.002$) and graft survival (85.6% vs. 81.9%; $p = 0.0001$) were significantly better for those patients receiving MMF than for those receiving AZA
Miller et al.[8]	2000	Multicenter RCT	TAC/AZA, TAC/MMF 1 g/day, or TAC/MMF 2 g/day		The incidence of acute rejection at 1 year was 32.2%, 32.2%, and 8.6% for the TAC/AZA, TAC/MMF 1 g/day, and TAC/MMF 2 g/day groups, respectively ($p = 0.01$ for the TAC/MMF 2 g/day group vs. the other arms)
Johnson et al.[9]	2000	RCT	TAC/AZA, TAC/MMF, or CsA/MMF	Acute rejection, graft survival, or patient survival at 1 year	All regimens yielded similar acute rejection rates and graft survival, but the TAC + MMF regimen was associated with the lowest rate of steroid resistant rejection requiring antilymphocyte therapy

(ATG: antithymocyte globulin; AZA: azathioprine; BPAR: biopsy proven acute rejection; CsA: cyclosporine A; MMF: mycophenolate mofetil; RCT: randomized controlled trial; TAC: tacrolimus)

abnormalities and gout, but had normal immune function.[10] These observations led to the search for an inhibitor specific for de novo guanosine monophosphate synthesis.

Mycophenolic acid is an inhibitor of IMPDH and preferentially inhibits de novo guanosine synthesis. Depletion of de novo guanosine causes a lack of deoxyguanosine triphosphate, suppressing DNA synthesis, and proliferation of T and B lymphocytes.[1] MPA is a selective inhibitor of the type II isoform of IMPDH which is expressed almost exclusively in activated T and B lymphocytes, while the type I isoform is expressed in most other cells. Therefore, the activity of MPA is specifically targeted toward T and B lymphocytes.[11] **Flowchart 1** illustrates the mechanism of action of MMF.

DOSING

In adult kidney transplant patients, MMF is most commonly administered orally at a dose of 1 g twice daily. In pediatric patients, the recommended dose of MMF oral suspension is 600 mg/m^2 at 12-hour intervals up to a maximum of 2 g daily. EC-MPS is administered orally at a dose of 720 mg twice daily in adults.

CHAPTER HIGHLIGHTS

- Mycophenolate mofetil (MMF) along with corticosteroids and calcineurin inhibitors (CNIs) form the backbone of modern immunosuppressive protocols in kidney transplantation.
- Mycophenolic acid (MPA), the active form of MMF, is a reversible, noncompetitive inhibitor of inosine-5′-monophosphate dehydrogenase (IMPDH). It acts by suppressing deoxyribonucleic acid (DNA) synthesis and proliferation of T and B lymphocytes.
- The prominent adverse effects include gastrointestinal symptoms, bone marrow suppression, and an increased risk of infections.

ABSORPTION

Mycophenolate mofetil, when orally administered, is hydrolyzed to MPA and almost completely absorbed from the stomach and upper small intestine. The time to maximal concentration (T_{max}) of MMF is <1 hour and is independent of hepatic or renal function.

The EC-MPS does not release MPA under acidic conditions (pH < 5) as in the stomach but does so in a neutral pH environment like the intestine.[12] Hence, it has a T_{max} of 1.5–2.75 hours. Food intake affects MPA absorption with

Flowchart 1: Mechanism of action of mycophenolate mofetil by inhibition of de novo purine synthesis.

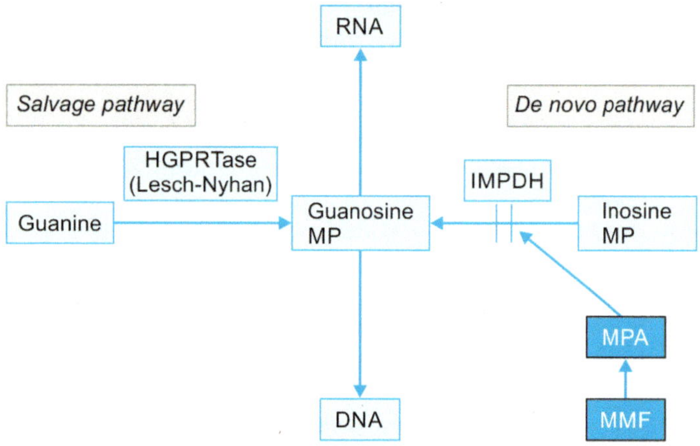

(DNA: deoxyribonucleic acid; HGPRTase: hypoxanthine guanine phosphoribosyltransferase; IMPDH: inosine monophosphate dehydrogenase; MMF: mycophenolate mofetil; MP: monophosphate; MPA: mycophenolic acid; RNA: ribonucleic acid)

EC-MPS and to avoid variability, it should be taken on an empty stomach.

DISTRIBUTION

In the whole blood, 99.99% of MPA is found in the plasma fraction with 97–99% bound to albumin. Significant renal dysfunction, liver disease, and hypoalbuminemia can alter MPA serum albumin binding, changing the fraction of free MPA available.

METABOLISM AND EXCRETION

Mycophenolic acid is rapidly metabolized to an inactive glucuronide mycophenolic acid glucuronide (MPAG) (7-0-glucuronide metabolite) in the gastrointestinal tract and liver with elimination half-life of 17.9 hours in healthy volunteers.[13] Another minor metabolite is mycophenolic acyl-glucuronide (AcMPAG), which has been shown to inhibit IMPDH in vitro and may contribute to hypersensitivity, drug toxicity, and immune response in patients on MMF.[14] Following oral administration, 93% of the drug is excreted in urine as MPAG and AcMPAG while 6% is excreted in the feces.[15]

ENTEROHEPATIC RECIRCULATION

The glucuronide metabolites are excreted into bile [mediated by multidrug resistance-related protein 2 (MRPR2)] and subsequently undergo deglucuronidation by intestinal bacteria followed by reabsorption of MPA. This results in a secondary peak in plasma MPA concentrations 8–12 hours after oral drug administration. This enterohepatic recirculation has a significant contribution to the overall MPA exposure, such that the interruption of the same leads to a decrease in area under the curve (AUC) of about 40%.[16] **Figure 1** shows the clinical pharmacokinetics of MMF.

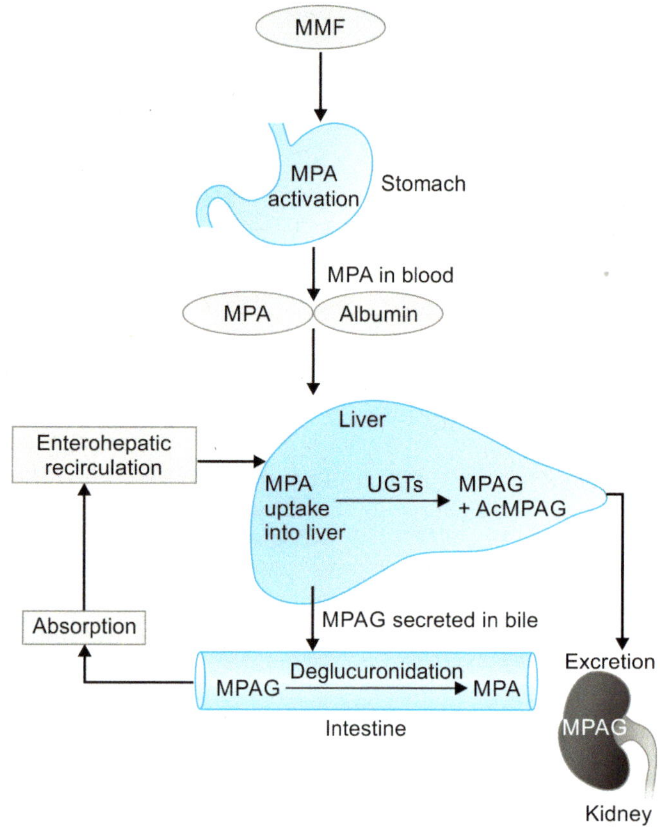

Fig. 1: Clinical pharmacokinetics of mycophenolate mofetil (MMF). (AcMPAG: mycophenolic acyl-glucuronide; MPA: mycophenolic acid; MPAG: mycophenolic acid glucuronide; UGTs: uridine 5′-diphosphoglucuronosyltransferase)

Drugs that block the MRPR2 like cyclosporine (not tacrolimus) impair the enterohepatic circulation leading to lower plasma levels of MPA. Both MMF and EC-MPS show this interaction with cyclosporine. Antibiotic therapy disrupting the gastrointestinal flora may also interfere with deglucuronidation and enterohepatic recirculation, decreasing drug levels.

Clinical Implications of the Drug-drug Interaction

Lower plasma levels of MPA, indicated by MPA-AUC, have been associated with an increased risk of acute rejection. Although MMF was introduced as a fixed-dose drug, the 40% difference in MPA-AUC between cyclosporine and noncyclosporine-based regimens suggests that 1 g bid may not be the appropriate dose in all the cases.[17] It has been shown that MMF dose escalations up to 2 g bid in cyclosporine-treated patients are required to reach the target MPA-AUC and result in decreased incidence of rejection.[18]

Another important clinical application of this drug interaction is that, on discontinuation of cyclosporine, the MPA concentration increases and can result in adverse effects like leukopenia while the patient is on the same dose of MMF.

ADVERSE EFFECTS

Gastrointestinal Adverse Reactions

Gastrointestinal symptoms including nausea, vomiting, diarrhea, indigestion, bloating, and abdominal pain are the most commonly reported adverse effects with MMF therapy. These adverse effects improve with MMF dose reduction or in some cases by splitting the dose into more frequent smaller doses (e.g., 500 mg four times daily rather than 1,000 mg twice daily). As gastric and early small-bowel exposure is believed to cause symptoms of gastrointestinal toxicity, EC-MPS, by delaying MPA release and absorption in the gut, leads to fewer adverse gastrointestinal events.

One of the most common and bothersome side effects is diarrhea, which has been reported by about 35% of study participants.[19] MMF has been associated with erosive enterocolitis characterized by crypt distortion, focal inflammation, and faster colonic transit. This is believed to be mediated by the action of the acyl-MPAG metabolite on absorptive cells, leading to a predominance of goblet cells.[20]

In the post-transplant setting, other causes of diarrhea need to be ruled out like cytomegalovirus (CMV), *Campylobacter*, *Giardia*, microsporidiosis, or antibiotic-related diarrhea. This often requires colonoscopy and biopsy besides stool examinations and may show apoptosis of intestinal gland epithelial cells and atrophy of the intestinal villi. Though nonspecific, these changes have been observed to normalize after stoppage of MMF.[21]

Diarrhea as a side effect is more common in patients receiving MMF along with tacrolimus as compared to cyclosporine.[22]

Bone Marrow Suppression

Bone marrow suppression is a dose-dependent adverse effect of MMF. Leukopenia defined as total leukocyte count less than 3,000 leukocyte/mm^3 is reported in 14–23% of kidney transplant recipients.[23] Other causes of leukopenia like infections, especially CMV infections, need to be ruled out in a transplant recipient presenting with leukopenia.

Concurrent medications like valganciclovir and cotrimoxazole are also associated with leukopenia and may require dose reduction or withdrawal. Reducing the dose of MMF and in some cases recombinant granulocyte-colony stimulating factors (G-CSF), such as filgrastim (Neupogen) administration, may be required if leukopenia is severe and persistent.

Infections

Mycophenolate mofetil increases the risk of infections, especially viral infections such as herpes simplex, herpes zoster, and tissue-invasive CMV disease. It was observed that while MMF was successful in reducing early acute rejection and prolonging graft survival, there was a significantly higher rate of CMV disease in patients receiving MMF at the standard dose of 2 g/day versus azathioprine.[24]

BK virus (BKV) infection has emerged as an important infection in the transplant recipient and can lead to allograft dysfunction and graft failure in severe cases. BKV viremia has been associated with the use of higher dose immunosuppressive regimens. Several studies have shown that regimens that include MMF with tacrolimus increase the incidence of BKV viremia.[25]

Mycophenolate mofetil use has been associated with lesser incidence of *Pneumocystis jiroveci* pneumonia in few retrospective studies.[26] But there are other studies which showed an increased risk of infection.[27]

The approach to modify immunosuppressive drugs depends on the severity of infection. In severe infections such as CMV, varicella, and pneumonia, the first step is to stop the antimetabolite which in most cases is MMF. In less severe cases, MMF dose is reduced.

Vaccination

Live attenuated vaccines have a significant risk of unchecked vaccine strain proliferation and vaccine-induced disease in kidney transplant recipients and hence should be avoided in patients taking MMF. Inactivated and subunit vaccines, though safe, have decreased efficacy especially in the initial 3–6 months of intensive immunosuppression after kidney transplantation.[28]

A suboptimal response to COVID-19 messenger ribonucleic acid (mRNA) vaccines in kidney transplant recipients has been observed. MMF, by blocking the proliferation of follicular helper $CD4^+$ T (T_{FH} cells) which are instrumental for the differentiation of spike-specific B cells into antibody-producing plasma cells, especially results in a dampened immune response in these patients. Additional third or fourth booster doses and MMF dose reduction in selected cases have been suggested to improve vaccine efficacy.[29]

Neoplastic Diseases

Though early data indicated a possible increase in malignancies like lymphoma in patients on MMF as compared to azathioprine, large case-control studies and registry data showed little or no additional increase in the risk of lymphoma.[30,31]

Pregnancy

Mycophenolate mofetil use in pregnant women has been associated with fetal malformations and hence is a US Food and Drug Administration (FDA) Category D drug for pregnancy. The patients are also advised to continue contraception for at least 6 weeks after stopping MMF to minimize any residual drug effect.[32]

MYCOPHENOLIC ACID DRUG LEVEL MONITORING

Mycophenolate mofetil, though commonly given as a fixed dose drug, has wide pharmacokinetic variability between patients resulting in difference in drug exposure.

Two randomized controlled trials (RCT) of concentration controlled dosing (CCD) in kidney transplantation (RCCT and APOMYGRE) showed substantially reduced kidney rejection when doses were individualized to a target MPA-AUC in the 12 hours post dose (AUC_{0-12}).[18,33,34]

But the two largest RCTs, "fixed-dose concentration-controlled trial (FDCC)" and "Opticept," failed to significantly differentiate MPA exposure between the treatment arms. The proportion of patients achieving MPA-AUC values within the therapeutic range of 30–60 mg/L.h was similar in the therapeutic drug monitoring (TDM) and fixed dosing (FD) groups. Outcomes such as treatment failure and biopsy-proven acute rejection (BPAR) were also similar in the two groups.[35,36]

Possible role of TDM could be in patients with high immunological risk, those on reduced-dose CNI, CNI withdrawal or avoidance protocols, and steroid withdrawal or avoidance regimens.[17]

Although some experts advocate for MPA-$AUCt_{0-12}$ target of 40 mg/L.h in the initial post-transplant period,[37] the benefit of CCD in comparison to FD still remains contentious.

To summarize, MMF remains the backbone of current immunosuppressive protocol in kidney transplantation along with CNIs (tacrolimus) and steroid. A thorough understanding of the mechanism of action, pharmacokinetics, and the adverse effects of this drug is essential for optimal management of the renal transplant recipient.

REFERENCES

1. Allison AC, Eugui EM. Mechanisms of action of mycophenolate mofetil in preventing acute and chronic allograft rejection. Transplantation. 2005;80(Suppl. 2):S181-90.
2. European Mycophenolate Mofetil Cooperative Study Group. Placebo-controlled study of mycophenolate mofetil combined with cyclosporin and corticosteroids for prevention of acute rejection. Lancet. 1995;345(8961):1321-5.
3. Sollinger HW. Mycophenolate mofetil for the prevention of acute rejection in primary cadaveric renal allograft recipients. U.S. Renal Transplant Mycophenolate Mofetil Study Group. Transplantation. 1995;60(3):225-32.
4. Tricontinental Mycophenolate Mofetil Renal Transplantation Study Group. A blinded, randomized clinical trial of mycophenolate mofetil for the prevention of acute rejection in cadaveric renal transplantation. Transplantation. 1996;61(7): 1029-37.
5. Allison AC, Eugui EM. Mycophenolate mofetil and its mechanism of action. Immunopharmacology. 2000;47: 85-118.
6. Giblett ER, Anderson JE, Cohen F, Pollara B, Meuwissen HJ. Adenosine-deaminase deficiency in two patients with severely impaired cellular immunity. Lancet. 1972;2:1067-9.
7. Ojo AO, Meier-Kriesche H-U, Hanson JA, Leichtman AB, Cibrik D, Magee JC, et al. Mycophenolate mofetil reduces late renal allograft loss independent of acute rejection. Transplantation. 2000;69:2405.
8. Miller J, Mendez R, Pirsch JD, Jensik SC. Safety and efficacy of tacrolimus in combination with mycophenolate mofetil (MMF) in cadaveric renal transplant recipients. FK506/ MMF Dose-Ranging Kidney Transplant Study Group. Transplantation. 2000;69:875.
9. Johnson C, Ahsan N, Gonwa T, Halloran P, Stegall M, Hardy M, et al. Randomized trial of tacrolimus (Prograf) in combination with azathioprine or mycophenolate mofetil versus cyclosporine (Neoral) with mycophenolate mofetil after cadaveric kidney transplantation. Transplantation. 2000;69:834.
10. Allison AC, Hovi T, Watts RW, Webster AD. Immunological observations on patients with Lesch–Nyhan syndrome, and on the role of de-novo purine synthesis in lymphocyte transformation. Lancet. 1975;2:1179-83.
11. Carr SF, Papp E, Wu JC, Natsumeda Y. Characterization of human type I and type II IMP dehydrogenases. J Biol Chem. 1993;268:27286-90.
12. Arns W, Breuer S, Choudhury S, Taccard G, Lee J, Binder V, et al. Enteric-coated mycophenolate sodium delivers bioequivalent MPA exposure compared with mycophenolate mofetil. Clin Transplant. 2005;19(2):199-206.
13. Atcheson BA, Taylor PJ, Mudge DW, Johnson DW, Hawley CM, Campbell SB, et al. Mycophenolic acid pharmacokinetics and related outcomes early after renal transplant. Br J Clin Pharmacol. 2005;59(3):271-80.
14. Shipkova M, Armstrong VW, Oellerich M, Wieland E. Acyl glucuronide drug metabolites: toxicological and analytical implications. Ther Drug Monit. 2003;25(1):1-16.
15. Bullingham RE, Nicholls AJ, Kamm BR. Clinical pharmacokinetics of mycophenolate mofetil. Clin Pharmacokinet. 1998;34(6):429-55.
16. Cremers S, Schoemaker R, Scholten E, den Hartigh J, König-Quartel J, van Kan E, et al. Characterizing the role of enterohepatic recycling in the interactions between mycophenolate mofetil and calcineurin inhibitors in renal transplant patients by pharmacokinetic modelling. Br J Clin Pharmacol. 2005;60:249-56.
17. Kuypers DR, Le Meur Y, Cantarovich M, Tredger MJ, Tett SE, Cattaneo D, et al. Consensus report on therapeutic drug monitoring of mycophenolic acid in solid organ transplantation. Clin J Am Soc Nephrol. 2010;5:341-58.
18. Le Meur Y, Büchler M, Thierry A, Caillard S, Villemain F, Lavaud S, et al. Individualized mycophenolate mofetil dosing based on drug exposure significantly improves patient outcomes after renal transplantation. Am J Transplant. 2007; 7:2496-503.
19. Halloran P, Mathew T, Tomlanovich S, Groth C, Hooftman L, Barker C. Mycophenolate mofetil in renal allograft recipients: a pooled efficacy analysis of three randomized, double-blind, clinical studies in prevention of rejection. The International

Mycophenolate Mofetil Renal Transplant Study Groups. Transplantation. 1997;63(1):39-47.
20. Shapiro R, Jordan ML, Scantlebury VP, Vivas C, Marsh JW, McCauley J, et al. A prospective, randomized trial of tacrolimus/prednisone versus tacrolimus/prednisone/mycophenolate mofetil in renal transplant recipients. Transplantation. 1999;67(3):411-5.
21. Ducloux D, Ottignon Y, Semhoun-Ducloux S, Labbé S, Saint-Hillier Y, Miguet J-P, et al. Mycophenolate mofetil-induced villous atrophy. Transplantation. 1998;66(8):1115-6.
22. Silva HT, Yang HC, Abouljoud M, Kuo PC, Wisemandle K, Bhattacharya P, et al. One-year results with extended-release tacrolimus/MMF, tacrolimus/MMF and cyclosporine/MMF in de novo kidney transplant recipients. Am J Transplant. 2007;7(3):595-608.
23. Bouamar R, Elens L, Shuker N, van Schaik RHN, Weimar W, Hesselink DA, et al. Mycophenolic acid-related anemia and leucopenia in renal transplant recipients are related to genetic polymorphisms in CYP2C8. Transplantation. 2012;93(10):e39-40.
24. Jorge S, Guerra J, Santana A, Mil-Homens C, Prata MM. Mycophenolate mofetil: ten years' experience of a renal transplant unit. Transplant Proc. 2008;40:700-4.
25. Mengel M, Marwedel M, Radermacher J, Eden G, Schwarz A, Haller H, et al. Incidence of polyomavirus-nephropathy in renal allografts: influence of modern immunosuppressive drugs. Nephrol Dial Transplant. 2003;18:1190-6.
26. Neff RT, Jindal RM, Yoo DY, Hurst FP, Agodoa LY, Abbott KC. Analysis of USRDS: incidence and risk factors for *Pneumocystis jiroveci* pneumonia. Transplantation. 2009;88:135-41.
27. Eitner F, Hauser IA, Rettkowski O, Rath T, Lopau K, Pliquett RU, et al. Risk factors for *Pneumocystis jiroveci* pneumonia (PcP) in renal transplant recipients. Nephrol Dial Transplant. 2011;26(6):2013-7.
28. Danziger-Isakov L, Kumar D. AST infectious diseases community of practice. Vaccination in solid organ transplantation. Am J Transplant. 2013;13(Suppl. 4):311-7.
29. Caillard S, Thaunat O. COVID-19 vaccination in kidney transplant recipients. Nat Rev Nephrol. 2021;17:785-7.
30. Funch DP, Ko HH, Travasso J, Brady J, Kew 2nd CE, Nalesnik MA, et al. Posttransplant lymphoproliferative disorder among renal transplant patients in relation to the use of mycophenolate mofetil. Transplantation. 2005;80(9):1174-80.
31. Robson R, Cecka JM, Opelz G, Budde M, Sacks S. Prospective registry-based observational cohort study of the long-term risk of malignancies in renal transplant patients treated with mycophenolate mofetil. Am J Transplant. 2005;5(12):2954-60.
32. McKay DB, Josephson MA. Pregnancy after kidney transplantation. Clin J Am Soc Nephrol. 2008;3(Suppl. 2):S117-25.
33. Hale MD, Nicholls AJ, Bullingham RE, Hené R, Hoitsma A, Squifflet JP, et al. The pharmacokinetic-pharmacodynamic relationship for mycophenolate mofetil in renal transplantation. Clin Pharmacol Ther. 1998;64:672-83.
34. van Gelder T, Hilbrands LB, Vanrenterghem Y, Weimar W, de Fijter JW, Squifflet JP, et al. A randomized double-blind, multicenter plasma concentration controlled study of the safety and efficacy of oral mycophenolate mofetil for the prevention of acute rejection after kidney transplantation. Transplantation. 1999;68:261-6.
35. van Gelder T, Silva HT, de Fijter JW, Budde K, Kuypers D, Tyden G, et al. Comparing mycophenolate mofetil regimens for de novo renal transplant recipients: the fixed-dose concentration-controlled trial. Transplantation. 2008;86:1043-51.
36. Gaston RS, Kaplan B, Shah T, Cibrik D, Shaw LM, Angelis M, et al. Fixed- or controlled-dose mycophenolate mofetil with standard- or reduced-dose calcineurin inhibitors: the Opticept trial. Am J Transplant. 2009;9:1607-19.
37. Metz DK, Holford N, Kausman JY, Walker A, Cranswick N, Staatz CE, et al. Optimizing mycophenolic acid exposure in kidney transplant recipients: time for target concentration intervention. Transplantation. 2019;103:2012-30.

9.5 mTOR Inhibitors

Pallavi Prasad, Dinesh Khullar

CASE VIGNETTE

A 36-year-old male patient, 1-month postrenal transplant, presented with a rise in serum creatinine to 1.4 mg/dL. Urine protein-creatinine ratio (PCR) was 200 mg/g creatinine. The patient was on tacrolimus (TAC), mycophenolate mofetil (MMF), and steroid. The TAC level was 10 ng/mL. A kidney biopsy was suggestive of TAC toxicity with tubular cytoplasmic vacuolation. The TAC dose was decreased to maintain a trough level between 7 and 9 ng/mL. He comes 15 days later with a further rise in serum creatinine, and you consider shifting him to everolimus. In which of the following scenarios would it be safe to shift the patient to everolimus?

a. Serum creatinine 2.3 mg/dL, urine PCR 1 g/g creatinine
b. Serum creatinine 1.6 mg/dL, urine PCR 1 g/g creatinine
c. Serum creatinine 2.3 mg/dL, urine PCR 0.4 g/g creatinine
d. Serum creatinine 1.6 mg/dL, urine PCR 0.4 g/g creatinine

INTRODUCTION

Mammalian target of rapamycin (mTOR) inhibitors are a class of drugs which block the cell cycle and prevent T-cell proliferation. Although, they have been studied in a wide variety of diseases including cancer chemotherapy, cystic kidney diseases, and psoriasis, the first field in which they were used in a clinical setting and where they were approved for use was transplantation. Sirolimus and everolimus are used in kidney transplantation.

MECHANISM OF ACTION

There are two mTOR complexes (mTORC): mTORC1 and mTORC2. mTORC1 promotes cell proliferation, lipid synthesis, and messenger ribonucleic acid (mRNA) translation, in response to growth factors, stress, and toll-like receptor stimulation. mTORC2 maintains cytoskeletal integrity. mTOR inhibitors enter the cell and bind to immunophilin FK binding protein which inhibits mTOR complexes (mTORC1 > mTORC2).

The immunosuppressive effect of mTOR inhibitors has been attributed to their inhibitory effect on T-cell proliferation **(Fig. 1)**, causing cell cycle arrest in activated lymphocytes in the late G1 phase. They also have a differential action on various T-cell subsets, paradoxically causing a proliferative action on T regulatory cells.

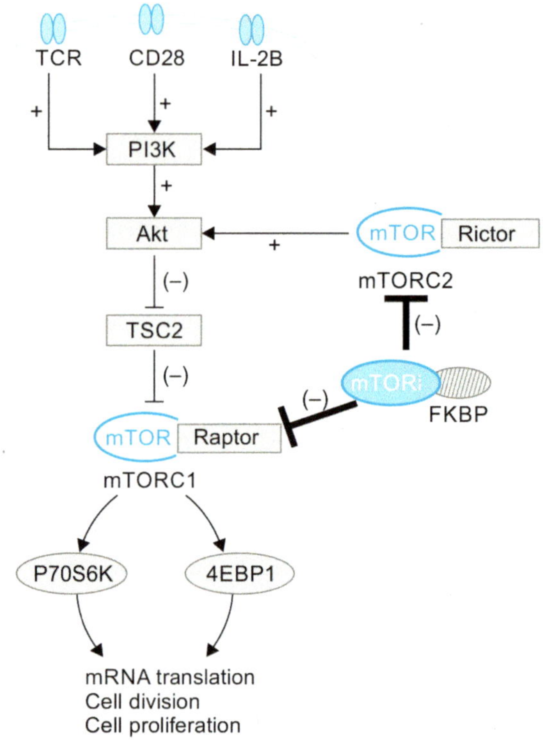

Fig. 1: Mechanism of action of mTORi. PI3K pathway is stimulated after antigen presentation via T cell receptor-CD28 costimulation and after binding of IL-2 to its receptor. This leads to stimulation of mTOR pathway via Akt. mTORi binds to FKBP after entering the cell and inhibits mTORC1 > mTORC2. This prevents mRNA translation, protein synthesis, and cell cycle arrest at G1 phase. (IL-2B: interleukin-2B; mRNA: messenger ribonucleic acid; mTOR: mammalian target of rapamycin; mTORC1: mammalian target of rapamycin complex 1; mTORC2: mammalian target of rapamycin complex 2; P13K: phosphoinositide 3-kinase; Raptor: rapamycin associated TOR complex; Rictor: rapamycin insensitive companion of mTOR)
Source: McMahon G, Weir MR, Li XC, Mandelbrot DA. The evolving role of mTOR inhibition in transplantation tolerance. J Am Soc Nephrol. 2011;22(3):408-15.

CLINICAL PHARMACOKINETICS INCLUDING METABOLISM AND EXCRETION

Absorption is from the small intestine. Both drugs are metabolized by CYP3A4/CYP3A5 (3A4 > 3A5) in the intestinal wall and liver. Large interindividual variability in everolimus is caused by different activities of cytochrome P (CYP) enzymes (3A4, 3A5, and 2C8), and the efflux pump P-glycoprotein. Sirolimus has a longer half-life (60 hours) and requires a loading dose, as against everolimus ($t_{1/2}$ = 16 hours, no loading dose).

It reaches peak concentration after 1.3–1.8 hours and a steady state is reached within 7 days. The steady state peak and trough concentrations and area under the concentration-time curve are proportional to the dose. Primary excretion (about 98%) of everolimus is in the bile in the form of metabolites and only 2% of everolimus is eliminated in the urine. In patients with hepatic impairment, the apparent clearance of everolimus decreased and thus dose reduction is required.

CHAPTER HIGHLIGHTS

- mTOR inhibitors act on T lymphocytes and prevent their proliferation.
- Use of mTOR inhibitors in kidney transplantation without calcineurin inhibitors (CNIs) leads to a high rate of biopsy-proven acute rejection (BPAR). They may be used along with CNIs to reduce CNI related toxicity in low-risk renal transplant candidates.
- mTOR inhibitors may be useful agents in post-transplant malignancies, CNI-related toxicity including thrombotic microangiopathy (TMA), and BK virus (BKV)-associated nephropathy.
- Adverse effects include impaired wound healing, oral ulcers, lymphedema, proteinuria, and dyslipidemia.

DRUG LEVEL MONITORING

Therapeutic drug level monitoring can be done by high-performance liquid chromatography (HPLC) or enzyme-linked immunosorbent assay (ELISA) techniques. Area under curve (AUC) correlates with trough concentrations. Trough levels should be measured just before dosing the drug after 3–5 days of change in drug dosage or if CYP inhibitors/inducers are introduced.

DOSING

Sirolimus is available as an oral tablet and solution, whereas everolimus comes in a capsule form.

For sirolimus when used in combination with CNI, a one-time loading dose of 6 or 15 mg (three times the maintenance dose), followed by a maintenance dose of either 2 or 5 mg/day, is used to maintain trough level of 5–15 ng/mL.

An initial everolimus dose of 0.75 mg given orally twice daily is recommended when used with CNI. The target trough concentration is 3–8 ng/mL.

RELEVANT DRUG INTERACTIONS

- Mammalian target of rapamycin (mTOR) inhibitors increase cyclosporine levels and vice versa. The time gap between cyclosporine and mTOR inhibitor dose affects the concentration which should be kept constant in an individual patient (concomitant with everolimus and 4 hours gap with sirolimus).
- mTOR inhibitors decrease TAC levels.
- mTOR inhibitors (particularly sirolimus) increase mycophenolic acid levels as compared to patients on cyclosporine.
- mTOR inhibitors lead to reduced AUC for prednisolone as compared to cyclosporine.

ADVERSE EFFECTS

Adverse effects of mammalian target of rapamycin inhibitor (mTORi) are summarized in **Table 1**. Sirolimus has more propensity to cause adverse effects compared to everolimus.

TRIALS

Landmark trials of mTORi use in kidney transplantation are summarized in **Table 2**.

TABLE 1: Adverse effects of mammalian target of rapamycin (mTOR) inhibitors.

Adverse effects	***Comments***
Infections	Bacterial, fungal, viral infections; less risk of CMV and BKV compared to CNIs
Interstitial pneumonia	• Noninfectious pneumonitis with peripheral and basal lung involvement; maybe early or late manifestation[1,2] • Changes reverse with drug withdrawal
Oral and nasal ulcers/mucositis	Aphthous like ulcers in 1st week of therapy,[3] often improve on their own
Delayed wound healing	• Sirolimus > everolimus • Incisional hernia, wound dehiscence, and lymphoceles may occur • *Risk factors:* Early post-transplant, obesity, malnourishment, corticosteroid use
Post-transplant diabetes mellitus	• Incidence lower than with CNIs • Induce insulin resistance, increase gluconeogenesis and decrease β-cell function
Dyslipidemia	• Increased in triglycerides and cholesterol • May require lipid-lowering therapy
Hematological side effects	Microcytic hypochromic anemia, leukopenia, and thrombocytopenia may occur
Gonadal toxicity	In men, azoospermia, low sperm count, and decreased ejaculate volume have been reported with mTORi therapy. Oligomenorrhea, amenorrhea, and ovarian cysts may occur in women
Proteinuria	• Occurs due to loss of vasoconstrictive effect of CNI on the afferent arteriole, decreased VEGF causing podocyte loss or injury (FSGS), alteration of podocyte slit diaphragm proteins • Avoid mTORi when proteinuria > 500 mg/day[4] • ACEI/ARB may help decrease proteinuria[5] • Reversible with drug discontinuation

Contd...

Contd...

Adverse effects	***Comments***
Electrolyte abnormalities	Hypokalemia and hypophosphatemia may occur
Delayed graft function	Seen with sirolimus not everolimus. Antiproliferative effect may prevent recovery from ischemia-reperfusion injury
Thrombotic microangiopathy (TMA)	• Sirolimus > everolimus. Combination with CNIs may increase the risk of TMA • Drug discontinuation mandatory if mTORi is an implicated cause[6]

(ACEI: angiotensin-converting enzyme inhibitor; ARB: angiotensin-receptor blockers; BKV: BK virus; CMV: cytomegalovirus; CNIs: calcineurin inhibitors; mTORi: mammalian target of rapamycin inhibitor; VEGF: vascular endothelial growth factor)

TABLE 2: Landmark trials of mammalian target of rapamycin inhibitor (mTORi) use in kidney transplantation.

Trial name and year	***Trial arms***	***Primary outcome***	***Other significant results***
Sirolimus			
ELITE-symphony[7] (*N* = 1,645)	Four arms (low-dose sirolimus, low-dose cyclosporine, standard dose cyclosporine, low-dose TAC) with mycophenolate mofetil (MMF) + steroids	eGFR at 12 months significantly lower in the sirolimus arm compared to the low-dose TAC arm (56.7 mL/min vs. 65.4 mL/min)	• Higher rate of biopsy-proven acute rejection (BPAR) at 6 months, lower allograft survival at 12 months • Higher incidence of serious adverse events
CONVERT trial[8] (*N* = 830)	Calcineurin inhibitor (CNI) continuation versus switch to sirolimus (SRL) at 6–120 months after transplantation	Nankivell GFR and composite endpoint of BPAR, death, graft loss at 12 months: No difference in endpoint in GFR > 40 mL/min	• Study in 20–40 mL/min GFR group discontinued early in view of higher incidence of safety end points in SRL group • Lower rate of post-transplant malignancies
Spare the nephron[9] (*N* = 299)	CNI continuation versus switch to SRL 30–180 days after transplantation	Mean percentage change in renal function (GFR) from baseline to 12 months higher in SRL group as compared to CNI group	• Lesser number of BPAR and deaths in SRL arm (*p* = NS)
ORION study[10] (*N* = 469)	Three arms: Group 1 SRL + TAC with TAC withdrawal at week 13, Sirolimus + MMF, TAC + MMF	Nankivell GFR at 1 year in the groups (59.1, 59.3, and 62.2 mL/min for groups 1, 2, and 3)—no difference	• Group 2 discontinued early due to high rate of BPAR • Higher BPAR in CNI free groups
Everolimus			
ZEUS[11] (*N* = 503)	Cyclosporine continuation versus switch to everolimus (EVR) at 4.5 months	*GFR at 12 months:* Significant improvement in EVR arm (71.8 mL/min vs. 61.9 mL/min)	• Higher rates of BPAR in EVR arm after randomization but incidence not different for the entire study duration
SOCRATES[12] (*N* = 126)	• De novo kidney transplants on CNI + MMF + steroid randomized to three arms at day 15 • Everolimus + steroid (CNI—withdrawal) • Everolimus (EVR) + CNI (steroid withdrawal) • Control arm (continuation of CNI + MMF + steroid)	Mean eGFR (Nankivell) at month 12 for CNI-WD versus control was 65.1 mL/min/1.73 m^2 versus 67.1 mL/min/1.73 m^2 by intention to treat (ITT), which met predefined noninferiority criteria (*p* = 0.026)	• The steroid withdrawal arm was terminated prematurely because of excess discontinuations • Higher rate of BPAR in CNI-withdrawal group and a trend toward higher composite treatment failure (BPAR, graft loss, death, loss to follow-up)
ELEVATE[13] (*N* = 715)	• CNI + MMF + steroid versus EVR + MMF + steroid • CNI to everolimus switch at week 10–14	No difference in the primary endpoint (change in eGFR from randomization to month 12)	• Higher rate of BPAR in EVR versus TAC (no difference vs. cyclosporine) • Higher rate of de novo donor-specific antibody (DSA) formation and more drug discontinuation in EVR arm
TRANSFORM[14] (*N* = 2,037)	• EVR with low-dose CNI versus MPA + standard dose CNI	• No difference in composite endpoint of treated BPAR or eGFR <50 mL/min/1.73 m^2	• No difference in BPAR or de novo DSA • Lower incidence of CMV and BKV infections

Contd...

Contd...

Trial name and year	*Trial arms*	*Primary outcome*	*Other significant results*
ATHENA study[15] (*N* = 338)	De novo KTR were randomized to everolimus with TAC, everolimus with CsA or MPA with TAC, with similar TAC exposure in both groups	Noninferiority of primary end point (eGFR Nankivell at 12 months) was not shown for the EVR/TAC or EVR/CsA groups versus the MPA/TAC group	• The incidence of treatment failure (BPAR, graft loss or death) was not significant for EVR/TAC but significant for EVR/CsA versus MPA/TAC • Cytomegalovirus and BK virus infections were significantly more frequent with MPA/TAC

(CsA: cyclosporine A; eGFR: estimated glomerular filtration rate; GFR: glomerular filtration rate; KTR: kidney transplant recipient; MPA: mycophenolic acid; TAC: tacrolimus)

Lessons learned from these trials include the following:

- Sirolimus is associated with a higher incidence of adverse effects as compared to everolimus, including wound healing complications, lymphoceles, and hyperlipidemia.
- The use of mTORi can decrease CNI-related nephrotoxicity and epithelial mesenchymal transition linked to interstitial fibrosis but at the cost of higher BPAR and de novo donor specific antibodies (DSAs).
- A pre-emptive approach with the use of mTORi (at 1 month from transplantation or de novo use) may limit the development of chronic allograft nephropathy (CAN)/interstitial fibrosis and tubular atrophy (IFTA) and preserve renal function.
- De novo use of mTORi with reduced dose CNI limits the increased rate of BPAR associated with complete CNI withdrawal (switch to mTORi) in kidney transplantation. The TRANSFORM trial, which had the strength of recruiting the largest population of de novo kidney transplant recipients randomized in a trial till date, demonstrated that low-dose CNI–everolimus combination was noninferior to MPA (mycophenolic acid)-standard dose CNI regimen for a novel composite primary endpoint of treated BPAR and estimated glomerular filtration rate (eGFR) < 50 mL/min/1.73 m^2.
- mTOR inhibitor use may be associated with reduced incidence of viral infections [cytomegalovirus (CMV), BKV] as compared to CNI use.

INDICATIONS WHERE mTOR INHIBITORS MAY BE USED IN KIDNEY TRANSPLANTATION

- As a de novo maintenance immunosuppressive agent in combination with CNI in low immunological risk transplants: In view of high risk of BPAR in CNI-free regimes, mTOR inhibitors are best used in combination with CNIs.
- *Chronic CNI toxicity:* CNI minimization with mTOR inhibitor leads to decreased nephrotoxicity.
- TMA (CNI related)
- *Post-transplant malignancies:* The mTOR pathway is constitutively active in malignant cells and promotes tumor proliferation and angiogenesis. Stemming from this, mTOR inhibitors tend to have a protective effect in post-transplant malignancies, especially in comparison to CNIs. Switching to mTOR inhibitors may induce remission in patients of cutaneous Kaposi's sarcoma[16] and decrease in recurrence of other cutaneous malignancies including squamous cell carcinoma of skin.[17] Although mTOR inhibitors have been shown to in vitro suppress Epstein–Barr virus (EBV) related transformed lymphocytes, there is not enough evidence to prove that they protect from post-transplant lymphoproliferative disorder (PTLD) or are efficacious in its treatment.[17,18]
- *BKV nephropathy:* There is some evidence that BKV nephropathy may be less frequent in patients on mTOR inhibitors compared to CNI-based regime.[14] mTOR inhibitors may have some effect on the protein kinase pathways of the virus which may explain the protective role in BKV nephropathy.

CONCLUSION

mTOR inhibitors are proliferation signal inhibitors which can be used in low-risk transplant patients in cases of CNI toxicity, viral infections, or post-transplant malignancies. They are best used in combination with CNIs before onset of significant proteinuria or glomerular filtration rate (GFR) decline.

REFERENCES

1. Weiner SM, Sellin L, Vonend O, Schenker P, Buchner NJ, Flecken M, et al. Pneumonitis associated with sirolimus: clinical characteristics, risk factors and outcome—a single-centre experience and review of the literature. Nephrol Dial Transplant. 2007;22(12):3631-7.
2. Champion L, Stern M, Israël-Biet D, Mamzer-Bruneel MF, Peraldi MN, Kreis H, et al. Brief communication: sirolimus-associated pneumonitis: 24 cases in renal transplant recipients. Ann Intern Med. 2006;144(7):505-9.
3. Kaplan B, Qazi Y, Wellen JR. Strategies for the management of adverse events associated with mTOR inhibitors. Transplant Rev (Orlando). 2014;28(3):126-33.

4. Kidney Disease: Improving Global Outcomes (KDIGO) Transplant Work Group. KDIGO clinical practice guideline for the care of kidney transplant recipients. Am J Transplant. 2009;9(Suppl. 3):S1-155.
5. Diekmann F, Andrés A, Oppenheimer F. mTOR inhibitor-associated proteinuria in kidney transplant recipients. Transplant Rev (Orlando). 2012;26(1):27-9.
6. Noris M, Remuzzi G. Thrombotic microangiopathy after kidney transplantation. Am J Transplant. 2010;10(7): 1517-23.
7. Ekberg H, Tedesco-Silva H, Demirbas A, Vítko S, Nashan B, Gürkan A, et al. Reduced exposure to calcineurin inhibitors in renal transplantation. N Engl J Med. 2007;357(25):2562-75.
8. Schena FP, Pascoe MD, Alberu J, del Carmen Rial M, Oberbauer R, Brennan DC, et al. Conversion from calcineurin inhibitors to sirolimus maintenance therapy in renal allograft recipients: 24-month efficacy and safety results from the CONVERT trial. Transplantation. 2009;87(2):233-42.
9. Weir MR, Mulgaonkar S, Chan L, Shidban H, Waid TH, Preston D, et al. Mycophenolate mofetil-based immunosuppression with sirolimus in renal transplantation: a randomized, controlled Spare-the-Nephron trial. Kidney Int. 2011;79(8):897-907.
10. Flechner SM, Glyda M, Cockfield S, Grinyó J, Legendre Ch, Russ G, et al. The ORION study: comparison of two sirolimus-based regimens versus tacrolimus and mycophenolate mofetil in renal allograft recipients. Am J Transplant. 2011; 11(8):1633-44. [Erratum in: Am J Transplant. 2012;12(1): 268].
11. Budde K, Becker T, Arns W, Sommerer C, Reinke P, Eisenberger U, et al. Everolimus-based, calcineurin-inhibitor-free regimen in recipients of de-novo kidney transplants: an open-label, randomised, controlled trial. Lancet. 2011; 377(9768):837-47.
12. Chadban SJ, Eris JM, Kanellis J, Pilmore H, Lee PC, Lim SK, et al. A randomized, controlled trial of everolimus-based dual immunosuppression versus standard of care in de novo kidney transplant recipients. Transpl Int. 2014;27(3): 302-11.
13. de Fijter JW, Holdaas H, Øyen O, Sanders JS, Sundar S, Bemelman FJ, et al. Early conversion from calcineurin inhibitor- to everolimus-based therapy following kidney transplantation: results of the randomized ELEVATE trial. Am J Transplant. 2017;17(7):1853-67.
14. Pascual J, Berger SP, Witzke O, Tedesco H, Mulgaonkar S, Qazi Y, et al. Everolimus with reduced calcineurin inhibitor exposure in renal transplantation. J Am Soc Nephrol. 2018; 29(7):1979-91.
15. Sommerer C, Suwelack B, Dragun D, Schenker P, Hauser IA, Witzke O, et al. An open-label, randomized trial indicates that everolimus with tacrolimus or cyclosporine is comparable to standard immunosuppression in de novo kidney transplant patients. Kidney Int. 2019;96(1):231-44.
16. Stallone G, Schena A, Infante B, Di Paolo S, Loverre A, Maggio G, et al. Sirolimus for Kaposi's sarcoma in renal-transplant recipients. N Engl J Med. 2005;352(13):1317-23.
17. Euvrard S, Morelon E, Rostaing L, Goffin E, Brocard A, Tromme I, et al. Sirolimus and secondary skin-cancer prevention in kidney transplantation. N Engl J Med. 2012; 367:329-39.
18. Caillard S, Dharnidharka V, Agodoa L, Bohen E, Abbott K. Posttransplant lymphoproliferative disorders after renal transplantation in the United States in era of modern immunosuppression. Transplantation. 2005;80(9):1233-43.

9.6 Azathioprine

Umapati Hegde

CASE VIGNETTE

Mr X, a case of end-stage renal disease, underwent ABO-compatible renal transplantation with his father as donor. He was on a stable dose of tacrolimus and azathioprine (AZA) steroid. 6 months post-transplant, he was found to have hyperuricemia and the physician prescribed allopurinol to reduce the uric acid. He was evaluated and found to have anemia and severe leukopenia. What is the reason for severe leukopenia?

a. Idiosyncratic reaction to allopurinol
b. Allopurinol reducing the metabolism of AZA
c. Reducing the metabolism of tacrolimus
d. None of the above

INTRODUCTION

Renal transplant is the best form of renal replacement available for end-stage renal failure. AZA is one of the oldest immunosuppressive agents used today.[1] Triple-drug immunosuppression consisting of prednisolone, calcineurin inhibitors [tacrolimus or cyclosporine (CsA)], and antiproliferative agents [AZA or mycophenolate mofetil (MMF)] which exert effects downstream in the cell cycle to reduce lymphocyte proliferation.

HISTORY OF AZATHIOPRINE

Azathioprine is an imidazolyl derivative of 6-mercaptopurine (6-MP). It was synthesized in 1957 by George Herbert Hitchings and Gertrude Elion.[2] The immunosuppressive effect of 6-MP in rabbits was investigated by Robert Schwartz in 1958 and showed that it significantly suppresses the formation of antibodies.[3] In animal experiments of kidney and heart transplants, 6-MP was used as an immunosuppressant by Sir Roy Calne[3] which was shown to be effective, and the bone marrow toxicity was within acceptable limits; AZA and prednisone became the effective combination immunosuppression in 1962 for kidney transplantation. AZA is being replaced by MMF for organ transplantation because of a lower incidence of acute rejection, its less bone marrow toxicity, and fewer opportunistic infections. AZA is being used in the treatment of hematologic malignancies, prevention of rejection in solid organ transplantation, rheumatologic diseases, and inflammatory bowel disease to suppress immune activity.

MECHANISM OF ACTION

Azathioprine is an imidazolyl derivative of 6-MP and it inhibits purine synthesis.[4] It is converted within tissues to 6-MP or 6-thioguanine. Both 6-thioguanine and 6-MP are first conjugated with ribose and then phosphorylated to inhibit glutamine phosphoribosylpyrophosphate amidotransferase (GPAT), the enzyme involved in purine biosynthesis. By blocking the de novo pathway of purine synthesis, deoxyribonucleic acid (DNA) and ribonucleic acid (RNA) synthesis is reduced in actively replicating cells such as T and B lymphocytes causing immunosuppression. Triphosphate form bind to GTP-binding protein Rac1 and blocks the synthesis of Bcl-xL causing susceptibility to apoptosis of activated T cells and mononuclear cells.[5] Tiede et al. reported that AZA resulted in increased apoptosis, the most likely mechanism being CD28 costimulation blockade, leading to either apoptosis or T-cell anergy[6] by inhibition of signal transducer and activator of transcription 3 (STAT3) and nuclear factor kappa B (NF-κB).

DOSING, METABOLISM, AND MONITORING

Dose

Azathioprine is used at 2.5 mg/kg/day with steroid alone and 1.5 mg/kg when used with CsA with careful monitoring of leukocyte counts[7] as once daily or in divided doses.

Pharmacokinetics

Azathioprine is well absorbed (88%) with variable bioavailability (30 and 90%) between the individuals because of first-pass metabolism by the liver.[8] Plasma peak concentration is achieved by 1–2 hours. The average plasma half-life of AZA is 26–80 minutes and the half-life for the drug plus metabolites is 3–5 hours. Only 20–30% of the drug is protein bound. AZA undergoes metabolism in the liver and is excreted via the kidneys, which increases its toxicity in renal failure. It usually requires 6–8 weeks for AZA to work.

Metabolism

Azathioprine is reduced to 6-MP by glutathione and other sulfhydryl-containing compounds. 6-MP is then enzymatically converted into 6-thiouric acid, 6-methyl-MP, and 6-thioguanine. 6-MP undergoes two major inactivation routes as shown in **Flowchart 1**. (1) Thiol methylation is catalyzed by the enzyme thiopurine *S*-methyltransferase (TPMT) to form the inactive metabolite methyl-6-MP (6-MeMP). (2) The catabolism of 6-MP to 6-thiouric acid is mediated by xanthine oxidase. The cytotoxicity of AZA is partly due to the incorporation of 6-thioguanine nucleotide (6-TGN) into DNA.

Monitoring

Complete blood count (CBC) and liver function test (LFT) need to be monitored weekly in the initial first 4–8 weeks

Flowchart 1: Azathioprine metabolism.

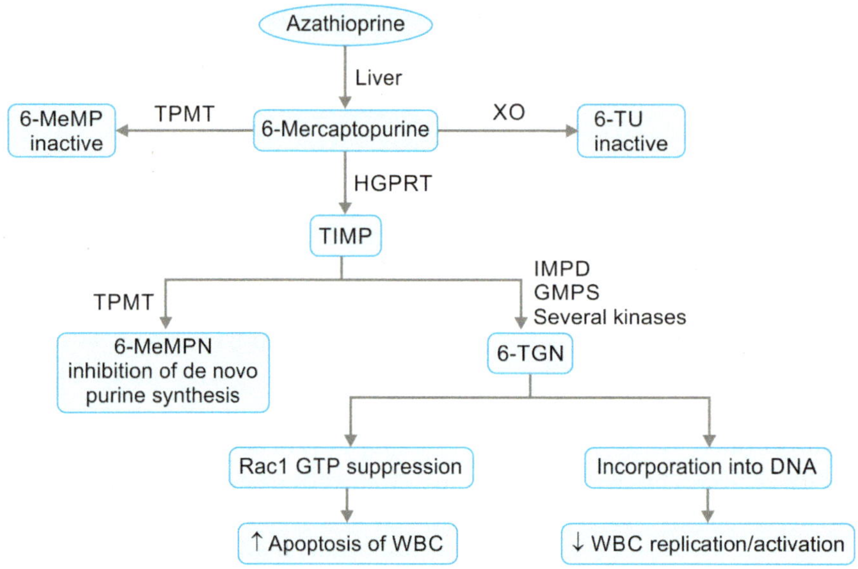

(DNA: deoxyribonucleic acid; GMPS: guanosine monophosphate synthetase; GTP: guanosine triphosphate; HGPRT: hypoxanthine-guanine phosphoribosyltransferase; IMPD: inosine monophosphate dehydrogenase; MeMP: methylmercaptopurine; MeMPN: methyl-mercaptopurine nucleotide; TGN: thioguanine nucleotide; TIMP: thioinosine monophosphate; TPMT: thiopurine S-methyltransferase; TU: thiouric acid; WBC: white blood cell; XO: xanthine oxidase; Rac1: Ras-related C3 botulinum toxin substrate 1)

and then every 3 monthly. Leukopenia is the most common; therefore, the dose needs to be reduced if the white blood cell (WBC) count is <3,000/mm^3. Polymorphisms in the TPMT enzyme,[9] which catalyzes the *S*-methylation of 6-MP, may be associated with an increased likelihood of myelotoxicity. TPMT activity is usually measured in erythrocytes, with erythrocyte activity reflecting what is found in other tissues. Although approximately 89% of whites and blacks have high TPMT activity and 11% have intermediate activity. TPMT activity correlates inversely with 6-TGN levels in erythrocytes/hemopoietic tissues since these cells have negligible xanthine oxidase activities. Erythrocyte 6-thioguanine nucleotide levels may be a better indicator of AZA activity.

CHAPTER HIGHLIGHTS

- Azathioprine (AZA) is an antiproliferative agent used since 1962 for the prevention of renal transplant rejection.
- AZA blocks the de novo pathway of purine synthesis leading to reduced deoxyribonucleic acid (DNA) and ribonucleic acid (RNA) synthesis and proliferation of T and B lymphocytes.
- The prominent adverse effects include hematological, gastro-intestinal symptoms, and an increased risk of infections.

SIDE EFFECTS AND OVERDOSE

Bone marrow suppression most commonly manifests as leukopenia. In severe cases, it may cause megaloblastic anemia and thrombocytopenia. Dose reduction or temporary withdrawal of the medication improves leukopenia. Patients with low or absent TPMT activity may have more bone marrow suppression. Due to the consequences of its bone-marrow suppression in severe cases, it may cause spontaneous bleeding and oral ulcers.

Nausea, vomiting, and diarrhea are more common (10–15%) in the initial few months, which may improve with reducing the dose or taking post meal. Hepatotoxicity manifesting as mild elevation in bilirubin and liver enzymes is seen in some transplant recipients, especially in the first 6 months. It reverses with dose reduction.

With increasing dose and duration of AZA, there may be increased risk of infection and malignancy, especially nonmelanoma skin cancers in transplant recipients.

Very rarely, a serious allergic interaction to this drug may manifest as rash, itching, swelling, severe dizziness, or trouble in breathing needing emergency medical care. AZA is dialyzable, and 45% of the drug is eliminated by 8 hours of hemodialysis.

Vaccination

The vaccine may not work as well and may not fully protect you from the disease. Live vaccines including measles, mumps, rubella (MMR), polio, rotavirus, typhoid, yellow fever, varicella (chickenpox), and zoster (shingles) are contraindicated with AZA.

DRUG INTERACTIONS AND CONTRAINDICATIONS

Purine analogs inhibit xanthine oxidase, the enzyme that metabolizes AZA, increase the drug level, and cause toxicity of AZA[10] as shown in **Table 1**. AZA interferes with niacin metabolism and causes pellagra and medullary aplasia. It decreases the anticoagulation effects of the warfarin.

Contraindications to the use of AZA are hypersensitivity to AZA/6-MP, severe infections, severely impaired hepatic or bone marrow function, and pancreatitis.

TABLE 1: Drug interactions of azathioprine.	
Drug class	***Drug effect or interaction***
Aminosalicylates • Sulfasalazine • 5-Aminosalicylic acid	Inhibits thiopurine methyltransferase pathway of azathioprine metabolism
Angiotensin-converting-enzyme inhibitors	Induces anemia and leukopenia when used concurrently
Carbamazepine, clozapine, co-trimoxazole	Exacerbate hematological toxicity
Warfarin	Azathioprine may inhibit the anticoagulant effect of warfarin
Xanthine oxidase inhibitors • Allopurinol • Febuxostat	Inhibit the xanthine oxidase pathway of azathioprine metabolism
Ribavirin	Induces severe pancytopenia and may increase the risk of azathioprine-related myelotoxicity

PLACE OF AZATHIOPRINE IN RENAL TRANSPLANT AND TRIALS

Three landmark randomized controlled trials conducted during the 1990s compared MMF with AZA as a component of initial immunosuppression in deceased donor kidney transplantation. A comparison of major trials is shown in **Table 2.**

- *Mycophenolate steroids sparing (MYSS) study:* A multicenter randomized controlled trial by Remuzzi et al.[11,12] involving 336 patients undergoing a deceased donor renal transplant was randomly assigned to MMF or AZA along with CsA microemulsion and corticosteroids. Corticosteroids were continued for the first 6 months (phase A), after which they were slowly withdrawn, and patients were followed for another 15 or more months (phase B). The incidence of clinical rejection was the same in both groups. Considering the high cost of MMF and comparable efficacy among patients with or without steroid therapy, standard immunosuppression regimens for kidney transplantation should perhaps include AZA rather than MMF.
- *US MMF study group:* A double-blind randomized, multicenter study to evaluate the safety and efficacy of MMF[13,14] enrolled 499 patients undergoing first transplant and randomized to MMF 2 g, 3 g, or AZA. Quadruple sequential immunosuppression consisted of antithymocyte globulin (ATGAM) induction and maintenance therapy with CsA, AZA/MMF, and corticosteroids. Treatment failure or biopsy-proven acute rejection episode occurred in 47.6% of patients with AZA as compared to 31.1% ($p = 0.0015$) and 31.3% ($p = 0.0021$) of patients with MMF 2- and 3-g dose, respectively.
- *Tricontinental study:* This large randomized study involved 503 patients[15] to receive AZA, 2 or 3 g of MMF per day, along with CsA and prednisone. The incidence of biopsy-proven acute graft rejection (BPR) in the first 6 months was reduced by ~50%. The major cause of graft loss was rejection in all groups: AZA (9.9%), MMF 2 g (5.8%), and MMF 3 g (3.0%). Gastrointestinal toxicity, cytomegalovirus (CMV) disease, and leukopenia were more common in the MMF 3 g group in the first year of transplantation. The study concluded that MMF significantly reduced the incidence of early rejections.
- Miller et al.[16] reported reduced rejection rates with 2 g at 1 year [AZA (32.2%), MMF 1 g (32%), and 2 g (8.6%) ($p < 0.01$)].
- *UK database:* 238 deceased donors who donated one kidney to a patient treated with MMF and the other kidney to AZA, transplanted between 1999 and 2002, were identified by Shah et al.[17] Three-year unadjusted graft survival was inferior in MMF (90 vs. 96%). The increased cost above AZA with the use of MMF is approximately £2,500.00 per patient per year.
- In a retrospective analysis of adult solitary renal transplant recipients from 1998 to 2006 with the national SRTR database consisting of 98,580 patients, MMF (n = 94,747) and AZA (n = 3,833) were analyzed.[18] 1-year acute rejection rates were reduced for MMF (10 vs. 13%, $p < 0.01$); AZA was associated with a lower risk for graft loss with concomitant tacrolimus. A similar study by Bansal et al. also showed tacrolimus-based immunosuppression, AZA may be as good as MMF as maintenance immunosuppressive drug in living donor kidney transplantation.[19]
- *ATHENA trial: AZA is considered safe and cost-effective option for kidney transplant recipients.* Ruggenenti et al.[20] designed ATHENA trial to test the safety and efficacy of AZA compared to MMF. At 3 years, of follow-up chronic allograft nephropathy, biopsy-proven acute cellular rejection, graft failure, and estimated glomerular filtration rate (eGFR) were similar with AZA and MMF.

SYSTEMATIC ANALYSIS

A systematic review by Knight et al.,[21] including a total of 3,143 patients from 19 relevant studies, showed that MMF significantly reduced the risk of acute rejection in combination with calcineurin inhibitor (relative risk 0.62, 0.55–0.87, $p < 0.00001$). The hazard for graft loss, including death with a functioning graft, was significantly reduced with MMF therapy (hazard ratio 0.76, 0.59–0.98, $p = 0.037$). There was an increased risk of diarrhea in MMF-treated patients.

A Cochrane review consisting of 23 studies involving 3,301 patients treated with MPA or AZA showed that MMF is more effective than AZA for reducing the risk of graft loss by 20% and acute rejection by 30%.[22] There was no difference in mortality or graft function.

TABLE 2: Comparison of major trials of azathioprine in renal transplant.

Author and year of publication	*Study design*	*Immunosuppressive medications*	*Results*
Sang Cho 1999 *US MMF study group*	*n* = 499 (MMF 2 g; *n* = 165), (MMF 3 g; *n* = 166), or (AZA: 164) Randomized, double-blind, multicenter study	MMF or AZA in addition CsA, corticosteroids, and ATGAM induction	• First BPAR occurred in 38.0%: AZA compared with 19.8% (MMF 2 g) and 17.5% (MMF 3 g) • BPAR or treatment failure was significantly higher in 47.6% (AZA) compared with 31.1% (MMF 2 g) and 31.3% (MMF 3 g) ($p = 0.0021$) • Increased incidence of infection (invasive CMV, *Aspergillus*, and mucormycosis) was seen in the MMF • The long-term data shows MMF is a safe and valuable alternative to azathioprine
Mathew 1998[15] *Tricontinental study*	*n* = 503 (Randomized AZA: 166), (MMF 2 g; *n* = 173), or (MMF 3 g; *n* = 164)	Azathioprine: 100–150 mg/day was compared to MMF 2 g/3 g along with cyclosporine and steroid in de novo renal transplants	• BPAR was 50% lower with MMF [19.7% (MMF 2 g); 15.9 (MMF 3 g) vs. 35.5% (AZA)] • The incidence of treatment failure was significantly less in MMF • Graft function was comparable in all groups 3 years after cadaver kidney transplantation
Remuzzi et al. 2004[11] *MYSS study*	*n* = 336 (MMF: 122)/(AZA: 121) Multicenter randomized controlled trial	MMF or AZA in addition to cyclosporine microemulsion and corticosteroids	• Phase A: ACR in MMF versus AZA was 34 and 35%, respectively • Rates of allograft loss, serum creatinine concentration, graft loss (6.8 vs. 6.1%), and proteinuria (25.0 vs. 27.4%) were the same in both groups • MMF has no advantages over azathioprine in preventing acute rejections and is about 15 times more expensive
Shah et al. 2006[17]	*n* = 238; UK database A paired kidney analysis was undertaken to account for all donor effects and era effects	MMF-treated recipients were taking more often tacrolimus (47 vs. 26%) as compared to CsA (43 vs. 64%). 53% of patients at 3 months were receiving <2 g/days MMF	• 3-year unadjusted graft survival was inferior in MMF (90 vs. 96%, $p = 0.03$) • Patient survival was similar in both groups (92 vs. 95%, $p = 0.16$) • AR rates (45 vs. 30%) and DGF (10 vs. 12%) were not significantly different • There were increased rejection rates in patients receiving MMF; however, there was no difference in patient or graft outcome
Bansal et al. 2011[19]	*n* = 205 (AZA: 113 and MMF: 921) Retrospective analysis	MMF or AZA along with tacrolimus and steroid	• AR was 13% in MMF and 17.6% in the AZA ($p = 0.36$) • Patient and graft survival were not different between MMF and AZA • The incidence of infections was also not different
Ruggenenti et al.[20] *ATHENA study 2020*	Prospective, multicentered trial 233 (MMF: 119 and AZA: 114)	Low-dose thymoglobulin/basiliximab MMF 750 mg BD and azathioprine 75–125 mg/day	• 33% (MMF) and 35.2 (AZA) patients developed CAN • 16.8% in MMF and 29.8% in AZA had biopsy-proven AR • Patient and graft survival, DGF, 3-year GFR [53.8 (40.6; 65.7) vs. 49.8 (36.8; 62.5) mL/min/1.73 m^2] were not different • CsA and no steroids, MMF had no significant benefits over AZA

(ACR: acute cellular rejection; AR: acute rejection; ATGAM: antithymocyte globulin [equine]; AZA: azathioprine; BPAR: biopsy proven acute rejection; CAN: chronic allograft nephropathy; CMV: cytomegalovirus; CsA: cyclosporine; DGF: delayed graft function; GFR: glomerular filtration rate; MMF: mycophenolate mofetil; MYSS: mycophenolate steroids sparing)

Conversion from Mycophenolate Mofetil to Azathioprine

Study by Wüthrich RP et al. showed replacing MMF with AZA at 6 months postrenal transplant in low immunologic risk recipients is safe and is not associated with the altered graft function in the short-term.[23]

Conversion from Azathioprine to Mycophenolate Mofetil

A retrospective study by Chu et al.[24] enrolled 36 chronic allograft nephropathy, 20 changed to MMF and 16 continued on AZA. The serum creatinine decreased initially in the group on MMF, but renal function deteriorated progressively after 6 months.

PREGNANCY AND BREASTFEEDING

Azathioprine crosses the placenta, but the immature fetal liver lacks the enzyme inosinate pyrophosphorylase needed to convert AZA to mercaptopurine; hence, it protects the fetus from toxic drug exposure.[25] A population-based study using AZA from Denmark showed that it has resulted in a sevenfold increase in fetal abnormalities.[26] Teratogenesis was observed when given to animals; however, no significant abnormalities were documented in humans. Therefore, the transplant patients planning to become pregnant should not discontinue AZA.

Azathioprine and its metabolites are either absent or present in negligible amounts in breast milk. Mercaptopurine content in breast milk within the first 4 hours after drug intake and the estimated maximum exposure of drug to the infant was <0.008 mg mercaptopurine/kg/day, representing <1% of maternal which is considered to be safe.[25]

SUMMARY

Azathioprine antiproliferative agent is an important drug, a part of triple-drug immunosuppressive agent, in renal transplantation. It being cheap saves a lot of money. The trials and systematic analysis showed good graft and patient survival despite increased early rejections.

REFERENCES

1. Hartono C, Muthukumar T, Suthanthiran M. Immunosuppressive drug therapy. Cold Spring Harb Perspect Med. 2013;3(9):a015487.
2. Goel RM, Blaker P, Mentzer A, Fong SCM, Marinaki AM, Sanderson JD. Optimizing the use of thiopurines in inflammatory bowel disease. Ther Adv Chronic Dis. 2015;6(3):138-46.
3. Hurst J. A modern Cosmas and Damian: Sir Roy Calne and Thomas Starzl receive the 2012 Lasker~Debakey Clinical Medical Research Award. J Clin Invest. 2012;122(10):3378-82.
4. Morris PJ. Azathioprine. In: Morris PJ, Knechtle SJ (Eds). Kidney Transplantation—Principles and Practice, 7th edition. Philadelphia, PA: W.B. Saunders; 2014. pp. 216-20 [chapter 15].
5. Maltzman JS, Koretzky GA. Azathioprine: old drug, new actions. J Clin Invest. 2003;111(8):1122-4.
6. Tiede I, Fritz G, Strand S, Poppe D, Dvorsky R, Strand D, et al. CD28-dependent Rac1 activation is the molecular target of azathioprine in primary human CD4+ T lymphocytes. J Clin Invest. 2003;111(8):1133-45.
7. IMURAN® (azathioprine). [online] Available from https://www.accessdata.fda.gov/drugsatfda_docs/label/2011/017391s015lbl.pdf. [Last accessed June, 2022].
8. Patel AA, Swerlick RA, McCall CO. Azathioprine in dermatology: the past, the present, and the future. J Am Acad Dermatol. 2006;55(3):369-89.
9. McLeod HL, Siva C. The thiopurine S-methyltransferase gene locus—implications for clinical pharmacogenomics. Pharmacogenomics. 2002;3(1):89-98.
10. Madrazo L, Jones E, Hsia CC. Azathioprine-induced severe anemia potentiated by the concurrent use of allopurinol. Can Med Assoc J. 2021;193(3):E94-7.
11. Remuzzi G, Cravedi P, Costantini M, Lesti M, Ganeva M, Gherardi G, et al. Mycophenolate mofetil versus azathioprine for prevention of chronic allograft dysfunction in renal transplantation: the MYSS follow-up randomized, controlled clinical trial. J Am Soc Nephrol JASN. 2007;18(6):1973-85.
12. Remuzzi G, Lesti M, Gotti E, Ganeva M, Dimitrov BD, Ene-Iordache B, et al. Mycophenolate mofetil versus azathioprine for prevention of acute rejection in renal transplantation (MYSS): a randomised trial. Lancet. 2004; 364(9433):503-12.
13. Sollinger HW. Mycophenolate mofetil for the prevention of acute rejection in primary cadaveric renal allograft recipients. U.S. Renal Transplant Mycophenolate Mofetil Study Group. Transplantation. 1995;60(3):225-32.
14. Mycophenolate mofetil in cadaveric renal transplantation. US Renal Transplant Mycophenolate Mofetil Study Group. Am J Kidney Dis. 1999;34(2):296-303.
15. Mathew TH. A blinded, long-term, randomized multicenter study of mycophenolate mofetil in cadaveric renal transplantation: results at three years. Tricontinental Mycophenolate Mofetil Renal Transplantation Study Group. Transplantation. 1998;65(11):1450-4.
16. Miller J, Mendez R, Pirsch JD, Jensik SC. Safety and efficacy of tacrolimus in combination with mycophenolate mofetil (MMF) in cadaveric renal transplant recipients. FK506/MMF Dose-Ranging Kidney Transplant Study Group. Transplantation. 2000;69(5):875-80.
17. Shah S, Collett D, Johnson R, Thuraisingham R, Raftery M, Rudge C, et al. Long-term graft outcome with mycophenolate mofetil and azathioprine: a paired kidney analysis. Transplantation. 2007;82:1634-9.
18. Schold JD, Kaplan B. AZA/tacrolimus is associated with similar outcomes as MMF/tacrolimus among renal transplant recipients. Am J Transplant. 2009;9(9):2067-74.
19. Bansal SB, Saxena V, Pokhariyal S, Gupta P, Kher V, Ahlawat R, et al. Comparison of azathioprine with mycophenolate mofetil in a living donor kidney transplant programme. Indian J Nephrol. 2011;21(4):258-63.
20. Ruggenenti P, Cravedi P, Gotti E, Plati A, Marasà M, Sandrini S, et al. Mycophenolate mofetil versus azathioprine in kidney transplant recipients on steroid-free, low-dose cyclosporine immunosuppression (ATHENA): a pragmatic randomized trial. PLoS Med. 2021;18(6):e1003668.
21. Knight SR, Russell NK, Barcena L, Morris PJ. Mycophenolate mofetil decreases acute rejection and may improve graft survival in renal transplant recipients when compared with azathioprine: a systematic review. Transplantation. 2009;87(6):785-94.
22. Wagner M, Earley AK, Webster AC, Schmid CH, Balk EM, Uhlig K. Mycophenolic acid versus azathioprine as primary immunosuppression for kidney transplant recipients. Cochrane Database Syst Rev. 2015;(12):CD007746.
23. Wüthrich RP, Cicvara S, Ambühl PM, Binswanger U. Randomized trial of conversion from mycophenolate mofetil to azathioprine 6 months after renal allograft transplantation. Nephrol Dial Transplant. 2000;15(8):1228-31.
24. Chu S-H, Wu C-T, Chou C-C, Chen Y, Liu K-L, Chiang Y-J. Clinical experience of mycophenolate mofetil in the treatment of chronic allograft nephropathy in kidney transplantation: three-year follow-up. Transplant Proc. 2004; 36(7):2073-5.
25. Gisbert JP. Safety of immunomodulators and biologics for the treatment of inflammatory bowel disease during pregnancy and breast-feeding. Inflamm Bowel Dis. 2010;16(5):881-95.
26. Nørgård B, Pedersen L, Fonager K, Rasmussen SN, Sørensen H. Azathioprine, mercaptopurine and birth outcome: a population-based cohort study. Aliment Pharmacol Ther. 2003;17:827-34.

9.7 Belatacept

Anshul Bhalla, Divyanshu Malhotra

CASE VIGNETTE 1

A 60-year-old man with history of end-stage kidney disease or end-stage renal disease (ESRD) secondary to diabetic kidney disease undergoes a deceased donor kidney transplant. Donor is a young Caucasian male with kidney donor profile index (KDPI) of 10%. Recipient calculated panel reactive antibody (cPRA) is 0%. Patient receives basiliximab induction. His diabetes has been poorly controlled with a recent hemoglobin A1c (HbA1c) of 8.5%. He also has a history of seizures related to prior costovertebral angle (CVA) and is currently on antiepileptic medications. You are concerned about tacrolimus exacerbating his underlying seizure disorder and worsening his hyperglycemia. Which medication can be used to minimize the tacrolimus exposure for this patient?

a. Cyclosporine A (CsA)
b. Belatacept
c. Thymoglobulin
d. Eculizumab

CASE VIGNETTE 2

A 65-year-old male, a case renal allograft recipient (deceased renal allograft recipient), basic disease of CKD. Hypertension presents for his regular follow-up after 3 years. He received Thymoglobulin induction and is currently on maintenance immunosuppression (IS) with tacrolimus, mycophenolate, and prednisone. He has been adherent to his IS medications. He has had difficulty controlling his blood pressure (BP) despite being on two antihypertensive medications. His serum creatinine has gradually increased from nadir of 1 mg/dL 1-month post-transplant to 1.6 mg/dL over the past 3 years. His urine protein/creatinine ratio is 0.4 g/g. Antihuman leukocyte antigens (HLA) donor-specific antibody (DSA) is negative. Allograft biopsy shows vacuolization of tubules, 40% interstitial fibrosis, and tubular atrophy, and moderate arteriolar hyalinosis along with moderate vascular fibrosis without acute or chronic rejection. Which medication is best suited to minimize the tacrolimus exposure for this patient?

a. CsA
b. Belatacept
c. Rituximab
d. Eculizumab

INTRODUCTION

The key cellular mediator of rejection in kidney transplantation is the T lymphocyte. T cells can either cause direct injury or facilitate the activation and maturation of B lymphocytes into antibody-producing plasma cells, which can then elaborate DSA and mediate humoral rejection of the allograft.

T-cell activation by antigen-presenting cells (APC) and subsequent cellular proliferation constitute three signaling pathways. Signal 2 or costimulation is an essential part of the alloimmune response. It is nonantigen specific, and targeting this pathway can lead to T-cell anergy and trigger apoptosis. Conventional IS protocols do not target the costimulatory pathway.

Belatacept is a human fusion protein containing cytotoxic T-lymphocyte-associated antigen 4 (CTLA-4) fused with Fc fragment of human IgG1. It binds to CD80 and CD86 on APCs and prevents their binding with CD28 on the T-cell membrane, preventing the subsequent intracellular release of calcineurin and other antiapoptotic proteins. It was Food and Drug Administration (FDA) approved in 2011 for use in kidney transplantation **(Fig. 1)**.[1,2]

Calcineurin inhibitors (CNI) have reduced the risk of acute rejection (AR) and improved short-term kidney allograft survival but are associated with chronic allograft dysfunction, long-term risk of diabetes, hypertension, and hyperlipidemia. Belatacept can serve as an alternative, minimizing side effects and improving long-term patient, and graft outcomes. It can also be used in cases where CNIs

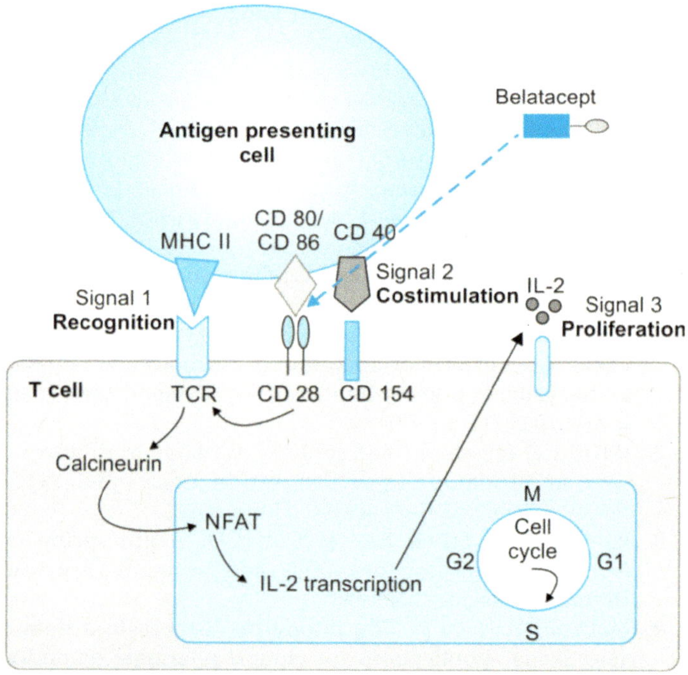

Fig. 1: Mechanism of action of belatacept. Belatacept inhibits the signal 2 and, in turn, inhibits antigen presenting cell mediated T-cell activation via the calcineurin pathway. (CD: cluster of differentiation; stages of cell cycle: G1: gap 1, G2: gap 2, S: synthesis, M: mitosis; IL: interleukin; MHC: major histocompatibility complex; NFAT: nuclear factor of activated T cell; TCR: T-cell receptor)

are contraindicated or avoided (such as history of seizures, thrombotic microangiopathy).

CHAPTER HIGHLIGHTS

- As part of the Immunosuppression armamentarium, belatacept can be used as an adjunct or substitute to CNI to minimize side effects and prolong the allograft survival.
- Belatacept can slow eGFR decline, lower risk of hyperlipidemia, hypertension, and diabetes mellitus.
- Risk of acute rejection is higher with belatacept. This can be minimized by either utilizing it in low immunological risk patients or combining with low dose CNI.
- Belatacept has a favorable effect on DSA and is increasingly being used for highly sensitized patients or patients with chronic AMR.
- Its use should be avoided in EBV seronegative patients. Higher risks of PTLD and viral infections and lower response to vaccination with belatacept should be accounted for inpatient selection and monitoring.

DE NOVO USE OF BELATACEPT

De novo use of belatacept in kidney transplantation is based on two landmark trials—BENEFIT (Belatacept Evaluation of Nephroprotection and Efficacy as First-line Immunosuppression) and BENEFIT-EXT (Belatacept Evaluation of Nephroprotection and Efficacy as First-line Immunosuppression-EXTended criteria donors). Both trials had a similar study design and compared the use of more-intensity (MI) or low-intensity (LI) belatacept with CsA for maintenance IS. Induction agent used was predominantly basiliximab, though Thymoglobulin was used for patients in CsA arm who were at risk of delayed graft function (DGF).[3,4] All recipients were at low immunological risk. Whereas the BENEFIT trial included transplants with standard criteria donors, BENEFIT-EXT trial included expanded criteria donors. These included older donors with history of stroke, hypertension or Cr > 1.5 mg/dL; donors with increased cold ischemia time or donation after circulatory death (DCD).

At 1 year follow-up, belatacept regimens had similar patient and graft survival, better kidney function (percent with measured glomerular filtration rate (GFR) < 60 mL/min/1.73 m^2 at 12 months or a decrease in measured GFR (mGFR) ≥10 mL/min/1.73 m^2 between months 3 and 12), and a higher mGFR. Incidence of AR was significantly higher in the belatacept groups in the BENEFIT study but similar across all groups in the BENEFIT-EXT study. Majority of AR episodes occurred early (within 6 months) and responded to corticosteroids. Belatacept-treated patients also had better BP and lipid control compared with CsA controls.

Long term follow-up data over 7 years from these studies further supported the beneficial effects of belatacept.[5,6] Risk of death or graft loss was reduced by 43% in the MI and the LI belatacept regimens as compared with the CsA regimen. Belatacept groups had higher estimated GFR (eGFR). Cumulative rate of formation of de novo DSA was significantly lower with the belatacept regimens. Adverse events were generally similar in the different groups, but post-transplant lymphoproliferative disorder (PTLD) was more common in the belatacept groups, especially in the recipients with negative Epstein–Barr virus (EBV) serology.

Although, these studies were celebrated as a success in development and introduction of newer non-CNI-based IS protocols, the lack of comparison with standard of care tacrolimus-based IS, and the higher incidence of AR prevented its adoption as a mainstream agent.

Adams et al. developed a belatacept dosing strategy to mitigate some of these limitations. In their analysis of patients treated with belatacept compared to a historical cohort receiving tacrolimus-based IS protocol, introducing a tacrolimus course early post-transplant and tapered over 11 months lead to similar rates and grades of AR within 1 year when compared to the tacrolimus only cohort and significantly less rejection than either the belatacept alone or belatacept plus short tacrolimus cohorts (16% vs. 20.5% vs. 50.5% vs. 33.3%, respectively) and was associated with superior eGFR at 4 years.[7]

A Cochrane database review from 2014 summarized that there was no evidence of any difference in the effectiveness of belatacept and CNI in preventing AR, graft loss, and death, but treatment with belatacept was associated with reduced chronic kidney scarring [risk ratio (RR) 0.72] and improved kidney allograft function [eGFR: Mean difference 9.96 mL/min/1.73 m^2, 95% confidence intervals (CI) 3.28–16.64]. Belatacept also improved the cardiovascular and metabolic outcomes with lower BP, better lipid profile, and reduced incidence of new onset diabetes after transplantation (NODAT) (RR 0.61).[8]

The efficacy of belatacept in reducing anti-HLA antibodies was investigated in 60 highly sensitized patients with cPRA 98–100% treated with belatacept plus tacrolimus taper. HLA class 1 antibodies and cPRA reduced significantly in the belatacept group.[9] In another prospective clinical trial of 49 patients with preformed DSA [mean-fluorescence intensity (MFI) 500–3,000], participants treated with a de novo belatacept-based IS, significantly higher number of patients displayed complete disappearance of class II DSAs in the belatacept group ($p = 0.001$). No patient experienced antibody-mediated rejection (AMR) in the belatacept group with excellent patient and allograft survival at 1 year. However, the 12-month incidence of acute T cell-mediated rejection was 25%, significantly higher than the control group on CNI ($p = 0.003$).[10]

CONVERSION TO BELATACEPT FOR CALCINEURIN INHIBITOR TOXICITY

Long-term exposure to CNI can lead to allograft dysfunction. CNI minimization or avoidance strategies have been attempted by conversion to a belatacept-based regimen. Rostaing et al. in a phase 2 randomized controlled trial (RCT) of low immunological risk kidney transplants who were 6–36 months post-transplant, randomized patients to continue CNI-based IS or switch to belatacept. Mean change from baseline in eGFR was higher in the belatacept group at 1 year follow-up (7 vs. 2.1 mL/min/1.73 m^2, $p = 0.0058$). The improved renal function benefit persisted in 2 and 3 years follow-up studies. Incidence of serious infections and malignancies was similar in the two groups, albeit higher incidence of AR was seen in the belatacept group.[11-13]

In patients with established allograft dysfunction, multiple studies have shown a benefit of switching to belatacept. In a retrospective study of 53 patients with a median of 2.5 year follow-up, Gupta et al. showed an improvement of mean eGFR from baseline of 31 to 40.2 mL/min/1.73 m^2 ($p < 0.001$) by 6 months postconversion and stabilization thereafter.[14] Budde et al. published a randomized phase 3b trial of 446 patients of which half switched to belatacept and rest continued CNI (90% of which were on tacrolimus). BPAR was higher in the belatacept group [hazard ratio (HR) 2.09] but de novo DSA formation was lower (1% vs. 7%). 24-month eGFR was higher with belatacept (55.5 vs. 48.5 mL/min/1.73 m^2). Both groups had similar rates of serious adverse events, infections, and discontinuations, with no unexpected adverse events. One patient in the belatacept group had PTLD.[15]

CONVERSION TO BELATACEPT IN HIGH IMMUNOLOGICAL RISK RECIPIENTS

Gupta et al. presented their initial experience of conversion from tacrolimus to belatacept in six sensitized kidney transplant recipients for presumed CNI toxicity and/or interstitial fibrosis/tubular atrophy. Five patients had more than one transplant and four had a positive DSA at the time of transplant with median cPRA of 88%. There was a significant increase in peak mean eGFR at a mean follow-up of 16.5 months without rejection episodes or subclinical rejection on surveillance biopsies. No development of DSA was noted.[16] In another retrospective analysis of 29 highly sensitized patients, out of which 16 had anti-HLA DSA, and were switched to belatacept, pre-existing DSA decreased or stabilized after a median follow-up of 308 days and no patient developed de novo DSA in the DSA-positive group. One patient had AMR after conversion to belatacept.[17]

Sethi et al. followed 108 patients after conversion from CNI to belatacept, out of which 29 were HLA sensitized (HS) and 79 were not sensitized (non-HS). There was no difference in rejection-free survival at 5 years follow-up; however, rejection-free survival was lower among sensitized recipients converted within the 1st-year post-transplant compared to non-HS recipients (HS: 55.6%; non-HS: 75.0%, $p = 0.03$). There was no difference in patient survival or graft survival. eGFR rate slope improved in nonsensitized recipients but declined in sensitized recipients.[18]

CONVERSION TO BELATACEPT FOR CHRONIC ANTIBODY-MEDIATED REJECTION

The lower rate of development of DSA in RCT and retrospective cohort studies was used as a rationale for conversion of patients with findings of chronic active AMR and high degree of chronicity on biopsy in a prospective cohort of 19 patients at 44 months postkidney transplant. When compared to a 1:2 propensity-matched control cohort maintained on CNI, the belatacept group had progressive improvement in eGFR and a higher eGFR at 12 months. The preconversion and postconversion paired biopsies showed no worsening in microvascular inflammation or chronicity. The paired tissue gene expression analysis showed improved mean total rejection score ($p = 0.02$) and a trend toward improved AMR score ($p = 0.06$).[19]

BELATACEPT AND VIRAL INFECTIONS

The BENEFIT and the BENEFIT-EXT trials did not find a significant difference in the rates of viral infections between the CsA and the belatacept cohorts. Some subsequent follow-up studies which looked at conversion of CNI to belatacept have shown a trend toward higher incidence of viral infections including CMV in the belatacept groups, especially in older patients, lower eGFR at conversion and early conversion (<6 months) after transplant.[20-22] One needs to be cautious in the timing and carefully choose the candidates for conversion from CNI to belatacept. When infected by severe acute respiratory syndrome coronavirus 2 (SARS-CoV-2), there is a trend for more hospitalizations overall and cases in intensive care units (ICUs), and more deaths of belatacept-treated kidney transplant recipients compared to a CNI-based treatment. However, without prospective, controlled trials, it is difficult to ascertain that this increased risk is related to the belatacept treatment.[23]

Belatacept adversely affects the response to COVID vaccines in kidney transplant recipients. In a cohort of 101 patients who received the vaccine on the same day as belatacept, antispike antibody response was only 2% after the first dose of Pfizer vaccine and 5.7% after the second dose.[24] The response remained poor even after the third dose.[25] Another study comparing immune response to Pfizer in patients on tacrolimus-based IS, belatacept-based IS response remained low.[26] In another study, timing the vaccine 21 days after the infusion helped to improve the vaccine response.[27]

BELATACEPT USE IN SPECIAL POPULATIONS

Pediatric Patients

Data on belatacept use in pediatric population is limited. Blew et al. demonstrated that a de novo belatacept-based regimen in three adolescent renal transplant patients resulted in comparable short-term eGFR and side effects observed with pediatric CNI regimens.[28] When considering CNI to belatacept switch, Lerch et al. showed that six patients converted from a CNI-based regimen primarily due to nonadherence and rejection, showed better adherence, stabilization, or improvement in eGFR, and no unexpected adverse effects were encountered.[29] A tailored approach to the use of belatacept in the pediatric population can be used especially in adolescence to improve adherence and ensure regular follow-up, while we await studies with larger cohorts and longer-term follow-up.

Post-transplant Pregnant Patients

Safety of belatacept in pregnant post-transplant patients has not been completely established and the manufacturer recommends using it only if potential benefit to mother outweighs the risk to fetus. The drug was not found to be teratogenic in pregnant rats and rabbits who received 16–19 times the maximum recommended human dose and it has not been studied in humans.[30] Two case reports from the Transplant Pregnancy Registry International described live births with no adverse effects in both cases with exposure to belatacept throughout the pregnancy.[31] One of the women had previously experienced two miscarriages, one of which occurred during belatacept therapy but could not be attributed to belatacept as she was on mycophenolic acid (MPA) as well. Another case report of successful pregnancy in a liver transplant on belatacept further supports its safety.[32]

Although belatacept labeling requires its use with prednisone and MPA, we recommend switching mycophenolate to alternate IS before and during the pregnancy. More experience with abatacept, a fusion protein such as belatacept that binds CD80 and CD86 and is used in autoimmune disease such as rheumatoid arthritis, did not show teratogenicity in animals and human studies of maternal or paternal exposure to abatacept did not show a pattern of congenital anomalies.[33]

Multiorgan Transplants

Belatacept has been used as an alternate to CNI for patients with simultaneous pancreas-kidney (SPK) to reduce the adverse kidney effects of CNI. In a case report of two patients (one with SPK and other with pancreas alone), switching to belatacept leads to stabilization of kidney function without any episode of rejection even after a year of discontinuing CNI.[34] However, a more recent phase 2 multicenter open-label randomized trial of SPK recipients randomized to CNI-based IS versus a low dose CNI plus belatacept with intended CNI withdrawal arm was stopped mid-enrollment due to increased pancreas rejection after CNI withdrawal. Rate of kidney allograft rejection was similar in both arms. Pancreas allograft survival at 52 weeks was 100% in CNI group and 86% in the belatacept arm.[35] In the authors' experience, off label use of belatacept in SPK recipients can allow for CNI minimization in patients with nonadherence but the risk of pancreas rejection outweighs the benefits of complete CNI discontinuation. Successful reports of using belatacept in kidney after liver or heart transplants suggests its increasing acceptability as a CNI avoiding agent in these cases, although more data is needed for mainstream application.[36-38]

BELATACEPT-RESISTANT REJECTIONS

Multiple mechanisms have been studied to explain the increased risk of AR with belatacept-based IS. T cells of the effector-memory phenotype develop an escape mechanism against belatacept to mediate allogeneic response. T-cell inhibition by belatacept is dose-dependent and despite higher doses, the inhibition of T-cell proliferation is <70%. Hence, a residual T-cell proliferation of ~30% can still occur and mediate cell injury. Additionally, CD28 positive T cells can either differentiate into CD28 null T cells (loss of CD28 expression) which makes them resistant to the effect of belatacept or down-regulate CD28 expression on surface cell membrane after allogeneic stimulation.[39] The belatacept induced CD28 downregulation promotes effector memory cells proliferation as well as cellular infiltration into the renal allograft, causing more cytotoxic injury. Other mechanisms including CD57 expression on the membranes of CD28 negative T cells and effector memory CD8+CD28++ EMRA cells could play a role in driving the escape mechanism of T cells.[40]

Upstream action of belatacept at the level of TCR versus a downstream action of CNI in the process of T-cell activation also accounts for the lack of complete T-cell inhibition. Immunomic analysis of biopsies with rejection in tacrolimus versus belatacept patients showed no difference in the intragraft gene expression and immunohistochemistry of markers that are involved in rejection, implying a final common pathway.[41]

Further studies to understand the mechanism of belatacept-resistant rejections will help in recognition of biomarkers that could identify patients most likely to benefit and ones most at risk of rejection.

ADVERSE REACTIONS

Most common adverse reactions (≥20%) are anemia, diarrhea, urinary tract infection, peripheral edema, constipation, hypertension, pyrexia, graft dysfunction, cough, nausea, vomiting, headache, hypokalemia, hyperkalemia, and leukopenia. Infusion reactions are uncommon and decreased with premedication.

Contraindications

Absolute: Transplant patients who are EBV seronegative or with unknown EBV serostatus due to increased risk for PTLD.

One should avoid belatacept conversions in the setting of active infection.

DOSING/PHARMACOKINETICS

Belatacept is dosed based on actual body weight at the time of transplantation, and dose is modified if there is a change in body weight of >10% during the therapy.[42] It is administered as an IV infusion over 30 minutes. Although premedication is not necessary, many centers use acetaminophen and diphenhydramine prior to the administration. The elimination half-life is around 10 days. No dose adjustment is needed for CYP450 substrates. Volume of distribution is 0.11 L/kg and higher clearance of the drug might be seen with increasing body weight.

Dose for de novo Use

- *Initial phase:* 10 mg/kg on day 1 (day of transplant, prior to implantation) and on day 5 (~96 hours after day 1 dose), followed by 10 mg/kg at week 2, 4, 8, and 12 following transplantation
- *Maintenance phase:* 5 mg/kg every 4 weeks (±3 days) beginning at the end of week 16 following transplantation

Dose for Conversion: Off Label Dosing

- *Initial phase:* 5 mg/kg on transition days 1, 15, 29, 43, and 57
- *Maintenance phase:* 5 mg/kg every 4 weeks beginning 4 weeks after completion of the initial phase

Monitoring

All patients should be monitored closely for infusion reactions including anaphylaxis which has been very rarely described. Given the findings of higher rates of AR on belatacept within the first 6 months,[3] we recommend close monitoring of allograft function with labs with every induction. Subsequently, labs including serum creatinine, urinalysis with every 4-week maintenance infusion within the first 6–12 months is reasonable. Novel biomarkers including donor-derived cell-free deoxyribonucleic acid (DNA) or gene expression profiling can be used for non-invasive monitoring for rejection in this setting. If these are utilized, we recommend checking them at the time of initiation of belatacept and every 3–6 months thereafter. While no drug levels need to be monitored, careful attention should be paid toward the appearance of side effects as described earlier.

CONCLUSION

Belatacept is a first-in-class costimulation blocker that selectively blocks T-cell activation. It was approved by the FDA in 2011 for use in kidney transplant recipients to prevent rejection and prolong graft survival. It has significant benefits including improved long-term graft function, better cardiovascular, and metabolic profile when compared to CNI-based regimens. Its use has expanded from low immunological risk patients to high immunological risk as well as patients with chronic AMR. Belatacept allows the transplant community to individualize IS and improve long-term outcomes. However, it does come with logistical challenges including cost and the need for IV access and increased risk of certain complications, and thus should be chosen in a thoughtful manner.

REFERENCES

1. Larsen CP, Pearson TC, Adams AB, Tso P, Shirasugi N, Strobert E, et al. Rational development of LEA29Y (belatacept), a high-affinity variant of CTLA4-Ig with potent immunosuppressive properties. Am J Transplant. 2005;5(3):443-53.
2. Archdeacon P, Dixon C, Belen O, Albrecht R, Meyer J. Summary of the US FDA approval of belatacept. Am J Transplant. 2012;12(3):554-62.
3. Vincenti F, Charpentier B, Vanrenterghem Y, Rostaing L, Bresnahan B, Darji P, et al. A phase III study of belatacept-based immunosuppression regimens versus cyclosporine in renal transplant recipients (BENEFIT study). Am J Transplant. 2010;10(3):535-46.
4. Durrbach A, Pestana JM, Pearson T, Vincenti F, Garcia VD, Campistol J, et al. A phase III study of belatacept versus cyclosporine in kidney transplants from extended criteria donors (BENEFIT-EXT study). Am J Transplant. 2010;10(3):547-57.
5. Vincenti F, Rostaing L, Grinyo J, Rice K, Steinberg S, Gaite L, et al. Belatacept and long-term outcomes in kidney transplantation. N Engl J Med. 2016;374(4):333-43.
6. Durrbach A, Pestana JM, Florman S, Del Carmen Rial M, Rostaing L, Kuypers D, et al. Long-term outcomes in belatacept-versus cyclosporine-treated recipients of extended criteria donor kidneys: final results from BENEFIT-EXT, a phase III randomized study. Am J Transplant. 2016;16(11):3192-201.
7. Adams AB, Goldstein J, Garrett C, Zhang R, Patzer RE, Newell KA, et al. Belatacept combined with transient calcineurin inhibitor therapy prevents rejection and promotes improved long-term renal allograft function. Am J Transplant. 2017;17(11):2922-36.
8. Masson P, Henderson L, Chapman JR, Craig JC, Webster AC. Belatacept for kidney transplant recipients. Cochrane Database Syst Rev. 2014(11):CD010699.
9. Parsons RF, Zahid A, Bumb S, Decker H, Sullivan HC, Eun-Hyung Lee F, et al. The impact of belatacept on third-party HLA alloantibodies in highly sensitized kidney transplant recipients. Am J Transplant. 2020;20(2):573-81.
10. Leibler C, Matignon M, Moktefi A, Samson C, Zarour A, Malard S, et al. Belatacept in renal transplant recipient with mild immunologic risk factor: a pilot prospective study (BELACOR). Am J Transplant. 2019;19(3):894-906.
11. Rostaing L, Massari P, Garcia VD, Mancilla-Urrea E, Nainan G, del Carmen Rial M, et al. Switching from calcineurin inhibitor-based regimens to a belatacept-based regimen in renal transplant recipients: a randomized phase II study. Clin J Am Soc Nephrol. 2011;6(2):430-9.
12. Grinyo J, Alberu J, Contieri FL, Manfro RC, Mondragon G, Nainan G, et al. Improvement in renal function in kidney transplant recipients switched from cyclosporine or tacrolimus to belatacept: 2-year results from the long-term extension of a phase II study. Transpl Int. 2012;25(10):1059-64.
13. Grinyo JM, Del Carmen Rial M, Alberu J, Steinberg SM, Manfro RC, Nainan G, et al. Safety and efficacy outcomes

3 years after switching to belatacept from a calcineurin inhibitor in kidney transplant recipients: results from a phase 2 randomized trial. Am J Kidney Dis. 2017;69(5):587-94.
14. Gupta G, Raynaud M, Kumar D, Sanghi P, Chang J, Kimball P, et al. Impact of belatacept conversion on kidney transplant function, histology, and gene expression—a single-center study. Transpl Int. 2020;33(11):1458-71.
15. Budde K, Prashar R, Haller H, Rial M, Kamar N, Agarwal A, et al. Conversion from calcineurin inhibitor to belatacept-based maintenance immunosuppression in renal transplant recipients: a randomized phase 3b trial. J Am Soc Nephrol. 2021;32(12):3252-64.
16. Gupta G, Regmi A, Kumar D, Posner S, Posner MP, Sharma A, et al. Safe conversion from tacrolimus to belatacept in high immunologic risk kidney transplant recipients with allograft dysfunction. Am J Transplant. 2015;15(10):2726-31.
17. Ulloa CE, Anglicheau D, Snanoudj R, Scemla A, Martinez F, Timsit MO, et al. Conversion from calcineurin inhibitors to belatacept in HLA-sensitized kidney transplant recipients with low-level donor-specific antibodies. Transplantation. 2019;103(10):2150-6.
18. Sethi S, Najjar R, Peng A, Choi J, Lim K, Vo A, et al. Outcomes of conversion from calcineurin inhibitor to belatacept-based immunosuppression in HLA-sensitized kidney transplant recipients. Transplantation. 2020;104(7):1500-7.
19. Kumar D, Raynaud M, Chang J, Reeve J, Yakubu I, Kamal L, et al. Impact of belatacept conversion on renal function, histology, and gene expression in kidney transplant patients with chronic active antibody-mediated rejection. Transplantation. 2021;105(3):660-7.
20. Bertrand D, Chavarot N, Gatault P, Garrouste C, Bouvier N, Grall-Jezequel A, et al. Opportunistic infections after conversion to belatacept in kidney transplantation. Nephrol Dial Transplant. 2020;35(2):336-45.
21. Bertrand D, Terrec F, Etienne I, Chavarot N, Sberro R, Gatault P, et al. Opportunistic infections and efficacy following conversion to belatacept-based therapy after kidney transplantation: a French multicenter cohort. J Clin Med. 2020; 9(11):3479.
22. Chavarot N, Divard G, Scemla A, Amrouche L, Aubert O, Leruez-Ville M, et al. Increased incidence and unusual presentations of CMV disease in kidney transplant recipients after conversion to belatacept. Am J Transplant. 2021;21(7):2448-58.
23. Terrec F, Jouve T, Malvezzi P, Janbon B, Naciri Bennani H, Rostaing L, et al. Belatacept use after kidney transplantation and its effects on risk of infection and COVID-19 vaccine response. J Clin Med. 2021;10(21):5159.
24. Chavarot N, Ouedrani A, Marion O, Leruez-Ville M, Vilain E, Baaziz M, et al. Poor anti-SARS-CoV-2 humoral and T-cell responses after 2 injections of mRNA vaccine in kidney transplant recipients treated with belatacept. Transplantation. 2021;105(9):e94-5.
25. Chavarot N, Morel A, Leruez-Ville M, Vilain E, Divard G, Burger C, et al. Weak antibody response to three doses of mRNA vaccine in kidney transplant recipients treated with belatacept. Am J Transplant. 2021;21(12):4043-51.
26. Bertrand D, Hamzaoui M, Lemee V, Lamulle J, Hanoy M, Laurent C, et al. Antibody and T cell response to SARS-CoV-2 messenger RNA BNT162b2 vaccine in kidney transplant recipients and hemodialysis patients. J Am Soc Nephrol. 2021;32(9):2147-52.
27. Noble J, Langello A, Bouchut W, Lupo J, Lombardo D, Rostaing L. Immune response post-SARS-CoV-2 mRNA vaccination in kidney transplant recipients receiving belatacept. Transplantation. 2021;105(11):e259-60.
28. Blew KH, Chua A, Foreman J, Gbadegesin R, Jackson A, Nagaraj S, et al. Tailored use of belatacept in adolescent kidney transplantation. Am J Transplant. 2020;20(3):884-8.
29. Lerch C, Kanzelmeyer NK, Ahlenstiel-Grunow T, Froede K, Kreuzer M, Drube J, et al. Belatacept after kidney transplantation in adolescents: a retrospective study. Transpl Int. 2017;30(5):494-501.
30. Bristol-Myers Squibb Company. NULOJIX Prescribing Information. [online] Available from https://www.accessdata.fda.gov/drugsatfda_docs/label/2017/125288s070lbl.pdf [Last accessed May, 2022].
31. Combs J, Kagan A, Boelkins M, Coscia L, Moritz M, Hofmann RM. Belatacept during pregnancy in renal transplant recipients: two case reports. Am J Transplant. 2018;18(8):2079-82.
32. Klintmalm GB, Gunby Jr RT. Successful pregnancy in a liver transplant recipient on belatacept. Liver Transpl. 2020; 26(9):1193-4.
33. Kumar M, Ray L, Vemuri S, Simon TA. Pregnancy outcomes following exposure to abatacept during pregnancy. Semin Arthritis Rheum. 2015;45(3):351-6.
34. Mujtaba MA, Sharfuddin AA, Taber T, Chen J, Phillips CL, Goble M, et al. Conversion from tacrolimus to belatacept to prevent the progression of chronic kidney disease in pancreas transplantation: case report of two patients. Am J Transplant. 2014;14(11):2657-61.
35. Stock PG, Mannon RB, Armstrong B, Watson N, Ikle D, Robien MA, et al. Challenges of calcineurin inhibitor withdrawal following combined pancreas and kidney transplantation: results of a prospective, randomized clinical trial. Am J Transplant. 2020;20(6):1668-78.
36. Schenk AD, Anderson DJ, Cole RT, Badell IR, Larsen CP. De novo belatacept in a kidney-after-heart transplant recipient. Transplant Direct. 2020;6(1):e515.
37. Kumar D, Yakubu I, Cooke RH, Halloran PF, Gupta G. Belatacept rescue for delayed kidney allograft function in a patient with previous combined heart-liver transplant. Am J Transplant. 2018;18(10):2613-4.
38. Cristea O, Karadkhele G, Kitchens WH, Vasanth P, Larsen CP, Badell IR. Belatacept conversion in kidney after liver transplantation. Transplant Direct. 2021;7(11):e780.
39. de Graav GN, Hesselink DA, Dieterich M, Kraaijeveld R, Weimar W, Baan CC. Down-regulation of surface CD28 under belatacept treatment: an escape mechanism for antigen-reactive T-cells. PLoS One. 2016;11(2):e0148604.
40. Kumar J, Reccia I, Virdis F, Podda M, Sharma AK, Halawa A. Belatacept in renal transplantation in comparison to tacrolimus and molecular understanding of resistance pattern: meta-analysis and systematic review. World J Transplant. 2021;11(3):70-86.
41. van der Zwan M, Baan CC, Colvin RB, Smith RN, White RA, Ndishabandi D, et al. Immunomics of renal allograft acute T cell-mediated rejection biopsies of tacrolimus- and belatacept-treated patients. Transplant Direct. 2019;5(1):e418.
42. NULOJIX. [online] Available from https://www.accessdata.fda.gov/drugsatfda_docs/label/2017/125288s070lbl.pdf [Last accessed May, 2022].

CHAPTER 10

Allograft Rejection

10.1 Acute Allograft Rejection

Anna Gupta, Mehakinder Singh, Raja Ramachandran

CASE VIGNETTE

A 29-year-old female, a case of end-stage kidney disease (ESKD) with chronic glomerulonephritis as the primary disease and a dialysis vintage of 5 months, underwent kidney transplantation with an unrelated donor (kidney-pair donation) in December of 2020, elsewhere. The sensitization history includes one pregnancy in the past. The induction included rabbit anti-thymocyte globulin (rATG), and triple immunosuppression. The patient developed acute graft dysfunction in the immediate operative period with biopsy suggestive of mixed rejection antibody-mediated rejection (ABMR) (peritubular capillaritis-2 and glomerulitis-2 and acute tubular necrosis) + T-cell-mediated rejection (TCMR) (1a). The treatment included pulse methylprednisolone, followed by plasma exchange (PLEX) (seven sessions) with intravenous immunoglobulin (IVIG). Pre-PLEX donor-specific antibody (DSA) was 19,594 mean fluorescence intensity (MFI) to human leukocyte antigen (HLA)-A and the DSA reduced to 1,434 MFI post-treatment. Presently, she is on triple immunosuppression with creatinine being 1.4 mg/dL.

a. What is allograft rejection?
b. When to suspect rejection?
c. What are the types of rejection?
d. What is the gold standard test to diagnose rejection?
e. What are the noninvasive biomarkers to diagnose rejection?
f. What are the treatment options?

INTRODUCTION

Kidney transplantation is unarguably the best treatment for ESKD. As the donor's kidney acts as an alloantigen for the recipient, it is critical to consider various factors for matching the donor's kidney with the recipient. The donor kidney (antigen) stimulates the induction of immune response in a genetically diverse recipient. This alloimmune response, if not controlled, can elicit both acute and chronic damage to the allograft. This whole process is called "allograft rejection."[1] Several years of research continue to shed light on these response mechanisms. The aforementioned subsequently led to an evolution of highly effective immunosuppressive medications which restrain the recipient's immune response. Currently, triple immunosuppressive therapy has led to a consistent decline in acute rejection rates from nearly 100% in the pre-azathioprine era to approximately 10–15% with the current regimens.[2] However, it is vital to diagnose acute rejection, as it is the most significant factor determining long-term allograft survival.

DEFINITIONS[1]

Based on the time frame, the rejection can be:

- *Hyperacute:* Occurring within minutes, maybe up to a day. However, its existence in the current era of immunosuppression is scarce.
- *Acute:* Occurring within days to weeks. It is classified into:
  - *ABMR:* Characterized by the presence of circulating DSA and histologically by evidence of tissue injury.
  - *TCMR:* Characterized by infiltration of the tubules, interstitium, and sometimes the arterial intima by lymphocytes. Mostly, acute rejection episodes are T-cell mediated, whereas an ABMR component accounts for only 12–37% of cases.[3]
- *Chronic:* It can be either TCMR or ABMR. It usually occurs 6 months to years after transplantation.
- *Chronic active:* It is an ongoing acute rejection superimposed on chronic rejection.

We may also classify them according to:

- Pathophysiological changes (cellular—interstitial, vascular, antibody—endothelial)
- Severity (extent of histologic inflammation and injury, as scored and graded by the Banff schema)
- Response to treatment (presence or absence of glucocorticoid resistance)
- Absence or presence of kidney injury (clinical or subclinical rejection, respectively)
- Immune-related mechanisms (innate or adaptive immune system response).

ETIOLOGY AND RISK FACTORS

Factors associated with an increased risk of rejection after the transplantation are:[4,5]

- Previous sensitization (blood transfusion, pregnancy, or organ transplantation)
- Presence of panel reactive antibodies
- *Nature of transplant:* Higher rejection with deceased donor than with a live donor
- ABO incompatibility
- HLA mismatch and incompatibility
- *Race (recipient):* Black race more than White race
- *Age (recipient):* Younger recipients have more rejection than older ones
- Old age donors
- Delayed graft function
- Prolonged cold ischemia time (CIT)
- Previous episodes of rejections
- Therapy noncompliance or inadequate immunosuppression
- Cytomegalovirus (CMV) infection.

PATHOPHYSIOLOGY

Allograft Rejection

The immunological response of the patient (recipient) against the nonself (foreign) antigen in the allograft leads to inflammation with specific pathological changes, with or without allograft dysfunction.

Depending upon the type of rejection, various pathophysiological mechanisms are postulated. These are:

- *Hyperacute rejection:* It occurs due to the presence of preexisting antibodies, usually against donor HLA or ABO antigen. These antibodies are present in the recipient's blood at the time of transplantation which bind to and damage the transplanted kidney either immediately or within a few hours after the surgery.
- *Acute TCMR:* The recipient's lymphocytes recognize donor antigens in the transplanted kidney either through direct pathway or through indirect pathway with the contribution of antigen-presenting cells (APCs), thereby leading to T-cell activation and infiltration and kidney damage.
- *Acute ABMR:* Here, antibodies (mostly HLA-related and rarely non-HLA-related) act against donor antigens, leading to allograft injury by activating the complement-dependent and -independent mechanisms with the recruitment of natural killer (NK) cells, polymorphonuclear cells, and macrophages. These antibodies can be preexisting, i.e., present before the transplant at a low level or synthesized de novo after transplant.
- *Chronic rejection:* Noncompliance and subtherapeutic immunosuppressive medication are the main factors responsible for chronic rejection. As discussed above, it can be either ABMR (due to DSA formed against donor HLA) or TCMR.

CLINICAL MANIFESTATIONS

Most patients are asymptomatic who have acute graft dysfunction. Occasionally, patients can present with fever, oliguria, weight gain, and graft tenderness. These clinical findings are commonly nonspecific, and we should work the patient up for other etiologies of graft dysfunction. Since most patients are clinically asymptomatic, an increase in serum creatinine, proteinuria, or hypertension should lead to suspicion of acute rejection. A rise in the serum creatinine level usually suggests significant histologic damage and hence develops relatively late in the course of a rejection episode.

DIAGNOSIS

When to suspect acute rejection?

We should suspect acute kidney allograft rejection in patients with one or more of the following:

- New rise in serum creatinine of ≥25% from baseline values or a serum creatinine that is greater than expected (such as in recently transplanted patients who have a nonresolving kidney injury as suggested by the elevated serum creatinine or a slower decline in the serum creatinine, than the usual trajectory post-transplant)
- Proteinuria >1 g/day
- Worsening hypertension.

HISTOPATHOLOGY

The allograft biopsy is the best modality to differentiate between different rejections for grading and guiding the subsequent therapy. It is the gold standard for diagnosing rejection.

The initial (also major) classification system for the pathological diagnosis of kidney allograft included the Cooperative Clinical Trials in Transplantation (CCTT) and Banff classification system. Later, to standardize the diagnosis of kidney allograft biopsy, both aforementioned classification systems were incorporated into the Banff 1997 classification. Subsequently, the Banff classification is constantly updated; the latest one was in 2019.

TABLE 1: Summary of studies for management of antibody-mediated rejection (ABMR).

PLEX	Rapidly removes preformed antibodies and is considered a standard part of therapy	• PLEX was found to be beneficial in a study done by Bonomini et al.[8] and Pascual et al.[9] (80% patients, i.e., four out of five patients) had improved kidney function and decreased DSAs to their pretransplant levels after 4–7 treatment of PLEX • However, a study done by Blake et al.[10] and Allen et al.[11] found PLEX had no added advantage. Allen et al. included 27 patients, out of which 13 received daily PLEX for 6 consecutive days whereas 14 had received standard immunosuppression. However, these results could not be generalized due to variable patient population, small sample size, and different maintenance immunosuppression protocols
IVIG	As a monotherapy, IVIG has a limited use	• Jordan et al. in 2004 included 98 sensitized patients, out of which 48 received IVIG and 50 were in placebo arm. Patients in the IVIG arm received monthly IVIG for 4 months and then at 12 and 24 months. Mean serum creatinine at 2 years was 1.68 ± 0.28 mg/dL in the IVIG arm and 1.28 ± 0.13 mg/dL in the placebo arm[12] • There are better allograft outcomes with combination therapy with rituximab and PLEX
PLEX and IVIG	Standard of care according to international guidelines (FDA 2017 Public workshop and KDIGO 2010)	Combination therapy with PLEX and IVIG was superior to PLEX alone, according to the study done by Slatinska et al. in 2009.[13] It included 24 patients out of which 13 received PLEX and 11 patients received combination therapy of PLEX and IVIG (0.5 g/kg). At 1-year PLEX plus IVIG group had higher graft and patient survival as compared to PLEX alone, i.e., 90.9 versus 46.2% and 100 versus 76.9%, respectively
Rituximab	It is an optional treatment according to KDIGO	• Evidence is low despite its frequent use, and two small randomized trials conducted by Zarkhin et al.[14] and Sautenet et al.[15] did not show any benefit • In contrast, several retrospective studies demonstrate some positive effects of rituximab in patients with ABMR, Roberts et al.,[16] Wan et al.,[17] and Faguer et al.,[18] especially with vascular lesions in combination with steroids, intravenous immunoglobulin, and PLEX
Bortezomib	Proteosome inhibitor (rationale being removing antibody-producing plasma cells) as a rescue therapy for treatment of ABMR in combination with plasma exchange, IVIG, or rituximab with some encouraging result	• There is limited data (case series) supporting the use of bortezomib with some beneficial effects when used in a multimodal treatment regimen of steroids, PLEX, intravenous immunoglobulin, and rituximab • However, prospective RCT done by Eskandary et al. in "late" ABMR did not show any benefit of bortezomib alone[19]

(ABMR: antibody-mediated rejection; DSA: donor-specific antibody; FDA: Food and Drug Administration; IVIG: intravenous immunoglobulin; KDIGO: Kidney Disease: Improving Global Outcomes; PLEX: plasma exchange; RCT: randomized controlled trial)

It is crucial to ensure kidney biopsy tissue adequacy for a decisive interpretation. Kidney biopsy maybe classified as:

- *Adequate:* Having thickness of 3–4 μm, containing 10 glomeruli and 2 arteries
- *Marginal:* Containing 7–10 glomeruli and 1 artery
- *Unsatisfactory:* If there are less than seven glomeruli or no arteries.[6]

As the rejection findings are often patchy and focal in the early stages, transplant physicians should obtain at least two separate cores to decrease sampling errors. The Banff classification of rejection is shown in **Table 1**.[7]

NONINVASIVE BIOMARKERS OF KIDNEY ALLOGRAFT REJECTION

- Functional cell-based immune monitoring—interferon (IFN)-gamma enzyme-linked immunospot (ELISPOT) assay
- Molecular blood biomarkers
- Kidney Solid Organ Response Test (kSORT)
- TruGraf v1 assay
- Donor-derived cell-free deoxyribonucleic acid (dd-cfDNA)—the injured allograft releases dd-cfDNA into the blood during allograft rejection. There are various methods for measuring dd-cfDNA which include:
    - Quantitative reverse transcription polymerase chain reaction (RT-PCR)
    - Droplet digital PCR (dd-PCR)
    - Targeted next-generation sequencing

A dd-cfDNA level of over 1% could differentiate between biopsy specimens showing rejection (TCMR or ABMR) and those without rejection with a positive predictive value and negative predictive value for active rejection being 61 and 84%, respectively.[20]

- Quantification of micro-ribonucleic acids (miRNAs) in peripheral blood
- Urinary messenger RNA (mRNA), miRNA, and proteomics.

DIFFERENTIAL DIAGNOSIS

Besides rejection in patients with fever, malaise, oliguria, or graft pain/tenderness, other diagnoses include infection, urinary leak, and ureteric obstruction. In addition, other diseases, such as CMV disease, post-transplant lymphoproliferative disease (PTLD), interstitial nephritis, BK (polyomavirus) nephropathy, and acute pyelonephritis, may mimic histologic findings of allograft rejection.

PROPHYLAXIS AND PREVENTION

Major risk factors for recipient sensitization and ABMR are pregnancy or abortions, blood transfusions, and previous organ transplantation. Therefore, prevention of ABMR depends upon the detection of DSA which can be preexisting, i.e., prior to, or de novo, i.e., after transplant. Registry data suggest an association between HLA mismatch and adverse transplant outcomes. In addition, several studies demonstrate that mismatches at individual HLA loci do not have equal weight regarding transplant outcomes. In particular, there is a strong association between HLA matching at the HLA-A, -B, -DR, and -DQ loci and patient and graft outcomes compared to HLA-C and -DP.

TREATMENT

The management of acute rejection depends on reliably diagnosing the type of rejection. The management strategies of both acute TCMR and ABMR depend on the severity of lesions **(Flowchart 1)**.

Flowchart 1: Algorithm for treatment of acute kidney allograft rejection.

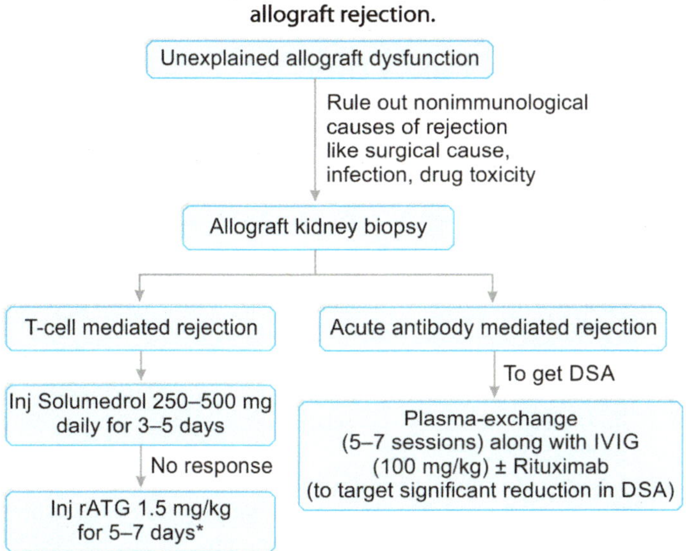

Banff category Iia, IIb, and III-rATG upfront
(DSA: donor specific antibodies; Inj: Injection; IVIG: intravenous immunoglobulin; rATG: rabbit anti-thymocyte globulin)

ACUTE T CELL-MEDIATED REJECTION

The class of the lesion guides the treatment of TCMR. Majority of Banff class 1a lesions respond to pulse corticosteroids (commonly, methylprednisolone 250–500 mg daily for 3–5 days).[21] However, experts suggest rATG for class 1b lesions besides pulse steroids. Similarly, TCMR with higher Banff grades, i.e., grade II and above lesions, mandate T-cell depleting therapy, most commonly rATG (1–1.5 mg/kg/day for five to seven doses, in limited-resource setting; clinicians also use a CD3-targeted therapy). ATG is superior to steroid therapy in reversing TCMR with no effect on patient survival or on subsequent acute rejection incidence, according to an updated Cochrane Database.

ACUTE ANTIBODY-MEDIATED REJECTION

The principles of ABMR management include depleting antibody-producing B cells (rituximab) or plasma cells (bortezomib) and removal of antibodies (DSA) (PLEX), and/or inhibiting the subsequent complement-mediated allograft damage (eculizumab). Evidence supporting antibody removal therapies (PLEX and immunoadsorption) is of low quality, and very low quality for all other treatments according to recent meta-analysis. PLEX and IVIG, with or without rituximab, remained the standard of care for the treatment of ABMR.[17] The most commonly used regimen is PLEX daily or on alternate days (1.5 volume removal per session) followed by IVIG at 100–200 mg/kg, with or without a single dose of rituximab at 375 mg/m^2.[21]

The study (observational) by Slatinska et al. reported superior results with combination therapy of PLEX and IVIG to PLEX alone.[13] The other therapies include bortezomib and eculizumab. Bortezomib, a proteasome inhibitor to treat multiple myeloma, has been shown in a case series to reduce plasma cell infiltrate in patients with ABMR and stabilize graft function. Historically, plasma cell–rich acute rejection, which is a rare histologic finding, is associated with poor outcomes despite aggressive treatment. In ABMR, various case series support additive bortezomib treatment with a positive effect within a combination therapy of steroids, PLEX, IVIG, and depleting antibodies. However, a randomized, double-blind placebo-controlled trial of bortezomib therapy does not suggest any benefit in late ABMR. The humanized monoclonal antibody eculizumab, because of its complement component C5 inhibition mechanism, has been targeted to prevent and treat antibody-mediated injury. A summary of studies on the management of ABMR is shown in **Table 1**.

PROGNOSIS AND OUTCOME

Acute T cell-mediated Rejection

It is common during the first year after transplantation and infrequent after wards, unless complicated by reduced immunosuppression. We attribute each acute rejection episode with a potential to reduce the longevity of allograft survival. A higher histologic severity [acute TCMR (i.e., Banff grade greater than IA), especially vascular rejection] and later onset of rejection (>3 months post-transplant) are associated with adverse outcomes.[22,23]

Antibody-mediated Rejection

Active and chronic ABMR are both associated with inferior outcomes. Transplant recipients with active ABMR are at increased risk for chronic ABMR and allograft loss. Similarly, chronic ABMR has a higher risk for adverse outcomes, including graft loss and patient death. Risk factors for graft loss in patients with ABMR depend on the degree of kidney injury biopsy findings [mixed rejection, presence of thrombotic microangiopathy (TMA), C4d positivity] and DSA [presence of complement-fixing (C1q) antibodies and persistent antibodies, despite treatment].

CONCLUSION

An increasingly effective immunosuppressive protocols translate to low acute rejection rates nonetheless. Acute rejection episodes continue to affect the allograft survival; hence, it is very important to detect graft dysfunction early and prompt treatment should be initiated. It is advised to obtain tissue biopsy in a patient who has unexplained acute allograft dysfunction. In addition, latest Banff criteria update 2019 for diagnosing ABMR no longer requires the combination of DSA and C4d deposition. Corticosteroids are the mainstay of TCMR-1a; however, higher grades mandate rATG. Currently, PLEX with IVIG is the mainstay of acute ABMR. For chronic rejection (TCMR or ABMR), continuing triple immunosuppressive therapy is the cornerstone of therapy.

REFERENCES

1. Nankivell BJ, Alexander SI. Rejection of the kidney allograft. N Engl J Med. 2010;363(15):1451-62.
2. Hart A, Smith JM, Skeans MA, Gustafson SK, Stewart DE, Cherikh WS, et al. OPTN/SRTR 2015 Annual Data Report: kidney. Am J Transplant. 2017;17(Suppl. 1):21-116.
3. Mauiyyedi S, Colvin RB. Humoral rejection in kidney transplantation: new concepts in diagnosis and treatment. Curr Opin Nephrol Hypertens. 2002;11(6):609-18.
4. Pallardó Mateu LM, Sancho Calabuig A, Capdevila Plaza L, Franco Esteve A. Acute rejection and late renal transplant failure: risk factors and prognosis. Nephrol Dial Transplant. 2004;19(Suppl. 3):iii38-42.
5. Joosten SA, Sijpkens YWJ, van Kooten C, Paul LC. Chronic renal allograft rejection: pathophysiologic considerations. Kidney Int. 2005;68(1):1-13.
6. Colvin RB, Cohen AH, Saiontz C, Bonsib S, Buick M, Burke B, et al. Evaluation of pathologic criteria for acute renal allograft rejection: reproducibility, sensitivity, and clinical correlation. J Am Soc Nephrol. 1997;8(12):1930-41.
7. Loupy A, Haas M, Roufosse C, Naesens M, Adam B, Afrouzian M, et al. The Banff 2019 Kidney Meeting Report (I): updates on and clarification of criteria for T cell- and antibody-mediated rejection. Am J Transplant. 2020;20(9): 2318-31.
8. Bonomini V, Vangelista A, Frascà GM, Di Felice A, Liviano D'Arcangelo G. Effects of plasmapheresis in renal transplant rejection. A controlled study. Trans Am Soc Artif Intern Organs. 1985;31:698-703.
9. Pascual M, Saidman S, Tolkoff-Rubin N, Williams WW, Mauiyyedi S, Duan JM, et al. Plasma exchange and tacrolimus-mycophenolate rescue for acute humoral rejection in kidney transplantation. Transplantation. 1998;66(11):1460-4.
10. Blake P, Sutton D, Cardella CJ. Plasma exchange in acute renal transplant rejection. Prog Clin Biol Res. 1990;337:249-52.
11. Allen NH, Dyer P, Geoghegan T, Harris K, Lee HA, Slapak M. Plasma exchange in acute renal allograft rejection. A controlled trial. Transplantation. 1983;35(5):425-8.
12. Jordan SC, Tyan D, Stablein D, McIntosh M, Rose S, Vo A, et al. Evaluation of intravenous immunoglobulin as an agent to lower allosensitization and improve transplantation in highly sensitized adult patients with end-stage renal disease: report of the NIH IG02 trial. J Am Soc Nephrol. 2004;15(12): 3256-62.
13. Slatinska J, Honsova E, Burgelova M, Slavcev A, Viklicky O. Plasmapheresis and intravenous immunoglobulin in early antibody-mediated rejection of the renal allograft: a single-center experience. Ther Apher Dial. 2009;13(2):108-12.
14. Zarkhin V, Li L, Kambham N, Sigdel T, Salvatierra O, Sarwal MM. A randomized, prospective trial of rituximab for acute rejection in pediatric renal transplantation. Am J Transplant. 2008;8:2607-17.
15. Sautenet B, Blancho G, Büchler M, Morelon E, Toupance O, Barrou B, et al. One-year results of the effects of rituximab on acute antibody-mediated rejection in renal transplantation: RITUX ERAH, a multicenter double-blind randomized placebo-controlled trial. Transplantation. 2016;100:391-9.
16. Roberts DM, Jiang SH, Chadban SJ. The treatment of acute antibody-mediated rejection in kidney transplant recipients—a systematic review. Transplantation. 2012;94:775-83.
17. Wan SS, Ying TD, Wyburn K, Roberts DM, Wyld M, Chadban SJ. The treatment of antibody-mediated rejection in kidney transplantation: an updated systematic review and meta-analysis. Transplantation. 2018;102:557-68.
18. Faguer S, Kamar N, Guilbeaud-Frugier C, Fort M, Modesto A, Mari A, et al. Rituximab therapy for acute humoral rejection after kidney transplantation. Transplantation. 2007;83(9): 1277-80.
19. Eskandary F, Regele H, Baumann L, Bond G, Kozakowski N, Wahrmann M, et al. A randomized trial of bortezomib in late antibody-mediated kidney transplant rejection. J Am Soc Nephrol. 2018;29:591-605.
20. Bloom RD, Bromberg JS, Poggio ED, Bunnapradist S, Langone AJ, Sood P, et al. Cell-free DNA and active rejection in kidney allografts. J Am Soc Nephrol. 2017;28(7):2221-32.
21. Kidney Disease: Improving Global Outcomes (KDIGO) Transplant Work Group. KDIGO clinical practice guideline for the care of kidney transplant recipients. Am J Transplant. 2009;9(Suppl. 3):S1-155.
22. Naesens M, Kuypers DR, De Vusser K, Evenepoel P, Claes K, Bammens B, et al. The histology of kidney transplant failure: a long-term follow-up study. Transplantation. 2014;98:427.
23. Wu K, Budde K, Schmidt D, Neumayer HH, Rudolph B. The relationship of the severity and category of acute rejection with intimal arteritis defined in Banff classification to clinical outcomes. Transplantation. 2015;99:e105.

10.2 Chronic Allograft Rejection

Praveen Kumar Etta, Arpita Ray Chaudhury

CASE VIGNETTE

A 56-year-old kidney transplant (KT) recipient presented at 6 years after transplant, with gradually progressive graft dysfunction, hypertension, and proteinuria with edema from 6 months. His native kidney disease was presumed as chronic glomerulonephritis. Dialysis vintage before transplant was 5 months. Human leukocyte antigen (HLA) mismatch was 2/6 (donor was brother). He did not receive induction and was prescribed the standard triple-drug immunosuppression with near-normal graft function till 6 months ago. However, the patient was noncompliant and missed drug doses due to financial constraints. There was no tenderness at graft site. His laboratory investigations revealed a creeping rise in creatinine level over 6 months (2.1, 3.7, and then to 4.6 mg/dL) with significant proteinuria. Complete urine examination showed 3+ albumin with—six to eight red blood cells per high-power field. Spot urine protein to creatinine ratio was 3.2 g/g. Serum albumin was 3.0 g/dL. Tacrolimus trough level was 3.1 ng/mL. HLA donor-specific antibody (DSA) assay was positive for class II antigens. Ultrasound and Doppler showed increased echogenicity of the graft with raised resistive index. Allograft biopsy confirmed the diagnosis of chronic active antibody-mediated rejection (ABMR) with transplant glomerulopathy (TG) and C4d positivity. The patient and was unable to afford plasma for plasma exchange and intravenous immunoglobulin (IVIg). Hence, he was treated with bortezomib, and his maintenance drug doses were increased with a targeted tacrolimus trough level of 6–8 ng/mL. At 6 months follow-up, his graft function remains stable with serum creatinine of 4.3 mg/dL.

Observation: Chronic allograft injury with significant proteinuria most commonly results from chronic active ABMR.

INTRODUCTION

Kidney transplantation (KT) is the best choice of kidney replacement therapy (KRT) for majority of patients with end-stage kidney disease (ESKD), especially due to progress in immunosuppressive regimens and post-transplant management. With the advances in KT protocols, short-term graft survival has improved, but long-term survival of transplants is still unsatisfactory and it remains to be improved. Late allograft loss can be due to both immunologic and nonimmunologic factors. Chronic allograft rejection is a broad category of late immunological graft injury characterized by progressive reduction in graft function that usually starts to manifest after the first year of transplantation and is usually associated with proteinuria and hypertension. It plays a very important role in chronic allograft injury leading to graft failure, which results in significant morbidity and mortality as KT recipients return to dialysis. The current 10-year death-censored graft survival is about 40–50% in deceased donor and 60–65% in living donor KTs. Optimizing immunosuppression to both prevent rejection and minimize drug toxicity remains a challenge. The two major phenotypes of chronic rejection are chronic T-cell-mediated (cellular) rejection (TCMR) and chronic ABMR. In this chapter, we plan to elaborate the recent knowledge of etiopathogenesis, pathology, management of chronic rejection, and chronic active ABMR in particular, it being the Achilles heel of long-term allograft function.

EPIDEMIOLOGY

The overall incidence and prevalence of chronic rejection depend on the timing and indication of graft biopsies, with higher incidence observed with protocol biopsies. Chronic rejection, especially due to ABMR, is one of the most common causes of late graft loss after KT. The incidence of acute rejection within the first year is around 8%. Overall, the rate of acute rejection is lower in living-donor than deceased-donor KTs; this is likely related to better matching and shorter cold ischemia time. The incidence of subclinical rejection with protocol biopsies at 1 year is about 25%. Graft outcomes have improved in the past few decades, and the 1-year graft survival rate is over 95%. In spite of the improvement, the long-term graft failure rate is still high. For deceased donor recipients, 10-year graft failure is around 50% and for living donor recipients, it is around 35%. An algorithm has been developed and validated to predict the long-term risk of allograft failure among KT recipients. This algorithm incorporates functional, histologic, and immunological parameters to calculate a prognostic score (named the iBox) for an individual patient. The incidence of chronic ABMR increased over time in recent years, and it is the most common cause of long-term graft failure caused by chronic rejection. This is especially due to advances in histopathological characterization. In a prospective study, 64% of long-term graft failure among indication biopsies was due to ABMR, of which 50% were chronic active ABMR.

RISK FACTORS

The primary risk factor for chronic rejection is noncompliance with immunosuppressive medication. The other common risk factors for the development of rejection include the presence of DSAs, HLA mismatches, pediatric recipient, elderly donor, African-American ethnicity, blood group incompatibility, prolonged cold ischemia time, delayed graft function, medication nonadherence and prior

CHAPTER HIGHLIGHTS

- Late allograft loss can be due to both immunologic and non-immunologic factors.
- Chronic allograft rejection is a broad category of late immunological graft injury characterized by progressive reduction in graft function that usually starts to manifest after the first year of transplantation.
- It plays a very important role in chronic allograft injury leading to graft failure, which results in significant morbidity and mortality.
- Optimizing immunosuppression to both prevent rejection and minimize drug toxicity remains a challenge.
- In this chapter, we summarized the recent knowledge of etiopathogenesis, pathology, and management of chronic allograft rejection.

sensitization identified with high panel reactive antibody (PRA), prior transplant, multiple pregnancies, and blood transfusions. Acute rejection episodes are one of the important predisposing factors for late graft loss and chronic rejection. Others like ischemia-reperfusion injury with delayed graft function and post-transplant infectious diseases also play a role in chronic rejection.

PATHOGENESIS AND MECHANISMS

The fundamental component of graft rejection is the detection of antigens on the donor's tissues as "foreign entities" by the recipient's immune system. However, the degree of immune reaction, and thereby degree and speed of graft rejection, depends on the histocompatibility between donor and recipient.

Alloimmune Injury

Rejection of graft is primarily mediated by activation of antigen-presenting cells (APCs) such as dendritic cells, macrophages and B lymphocytes, and alloreactive T cells. Following KT, the recipient immune system reacts to the donor alloantigens (HLA and others) and leads to stimulation of adaptive immune response mediated by T cells or antibodies resulting in TCMR or ABMR, respectively. This process leads to the release of proinflammatory mediators with subsequent recruitment of the effector cells and allograft injury.[1]

Human Leukocyte Antigen and Epitope Matching

The degree of HLA mismatch influences risk of rejection and long-term graft survival. HLA typing and matching in relation to transplant immunology mainly consider only antigens in HLA-A, B, and DR loci. However, the majority of de novo DSAs (dnDSAs) after KT is class 2 antibodies, especially HLA-DQ. During antigen–antibody binding, the DSA binds to a limited area of the HLA molecule comprising a 15–25 amino acid sequence. This specific binding area of the HLA is called an "epitope." While some of these epitopes are unique to a single HLA (private epitopes), others are shared among numerous antigens (public epitopes). Epitope-based matching has been shown to be more predictive of alloimmune injury and subsequent graft outcome compared to HLA-based matching. Use of epitopes and eplets may also help in determining permissible HLA mismatches. HLA Matchmaker is a computer algorithm developed to evaluate donor/receptor compatibility by comparing sequences of polymorphic amino acids (eplets) present in HLA molecules.

Phenotypes of Rejection

The major phenotypes of rejection are hyperacute, accelerated, acute, subacute, subclinical rejection, and chronic rejection. The two major distinct types of chronic rejection are chronic active TCMR and chronic active ABMR. Sometimes, both TCMR and ABMR can coexist and predispose to abrupt graft loss.

T cell-mediated (cellular) rejection can involve both the tubulointerstitial and the vascular compartments. APCs present donor-derived antigens to recipient T cells, which then get access to allograft interstitium and produce several cytokines such as interferon-gamma (IFN-γ) and transforming growth factor-beta (TGF-β). This process triggers an inflammatory cascade leading to tubulitis and interstitial inflammation, the characteristic features of TCMR. Type 2 helper (Th2) lymphocytes and their cytokines such as interleukin (IL)-4, -5, -6, -10, and -13, are responsible for interstitial fibrosis and other features of chronic rejection. TCMR can also involve the vascular compartment manifesting as arteritis and arterial intimal fibrosis. Eventually, progressive interstitial fibrosis/tubular atrophy (IF/TA) may be a late consequence of chronic active TCMR. Most cases of chronic rejection are due to chronic active ABMR which is characterized by TG, peritubular capillary basement membrane multilayering and arterial intimal fibrosis. This results from a repetitive pattern of thrombotic events and inflammatory changes that lead to endothelial cell injury and allograft matrix remodeling. Preceding TCMR is a risk factor for development of dnDSA and chronic active ABMR. Memory B and T cells are generated from exposure to environmental antigens or prior rejection episodes and once activated, they enter into the graft interstitium and secrete many cytokines such as IFN-γ and TGF-β, and ultimately trigger an inflammatory cascade.

Pathogenesis of T Cell-mediated (Cellular) Rejection

T cell-mediated (cellular) rejection is characterized by immune cell infiltration into the graft mainly composed of CD8 T cells, CD4 T cells, monocytes, macrophages, and B cells. This is associated with interstitial inflammation and may involve epithelial cells (tubulitis) and vessels (arteritis).

Within local draining lymph nodes, dendritic cells (APCs)–T cell interaction in the presence of alloantigen results in recipient T-cell activation through direct antigen presentation, indirect antigen presentation, or via semidirect antigen presentation. The indirect activation can stimulate the activity of activated B cells, which then leads to the production of antibodies against the graft tissues. Hence, the indirect pathway is the main predictor for chronic rejection.

The cytotoxicity of CD8$^+$ T cells plays a key role in allograft injury by the production of lytic molecules such as perforin and granzyme. Perforin forms pores in target cell membranes, allowing delivery of granzymes to the cytosol, where granzymes induce apoptosis through activation of caspases and the mitochondrial pathway. Binding of Fas and tumor necrosis factor-related apoptosis-inducing ligand (TRAIL) on the CD8$^+$ T cell to their receptors Fas ligand (FasL) and tumor necrosis factor-related apoptosis-inducing ligand receptor (TRAILR) on the target cells also induce caspase activation **(Fig. 1)**.

Type 2 helper lymphocyte cells and their cytokines such as IL-4, -5, -6, -10, and -13 play a major role in the pathogenesis of chronic rejection and tissue fibrosis.[2] This fact has been further validated in clinical studies. Immune-deficient recipients injected with Th2 cells showed features of chronic rejection and blocking the effect of their cytokines after injection of anti-IL-4 antibodies prevented fibrosis in skin grafts. IL-4 released by Th2 cells stimulates the activity of fibroblasts that increase the production of extracellular matrix and precipitate the process of fibrosis. In a similar way, a high level of IL-10 inhibits macrophages and the production of metalloproteinases which digest the excessive extracellular matrix. In addition, Th2 cytokines also potentiate the production of antibodies. The production of IFN-γ and IL-2 by Th1 lymphocytes also promotes this process. Alloreactive CD8$^+$ effector memory T cells (T_{EM}) are also implicated in the development of TCMR. Unlike naïve T cells, T_{EM} cells are known for their low activation threshold, robust effector functions, and resistance to conventional immunosuppression and costimulation blockade. Memory T cells are originated from environmental antigens or generated from previous rejection episodes, and once activated, they enter into the renal interstitium and secrete several cytokines such as IFN-γ and TGF-β and subsequently trigger a cascade of inflammation. Chronic active TCMR occurs as a persistent or recurrent form of acute TCMR. Due to inadequate immunosuppression during acute TCMR, persistent immune activation may result in T-cell invasion of renal fibrotic parenchyma and initiation of i-IF/TA and tubulitis, the pathological components of chronic active TCMR.

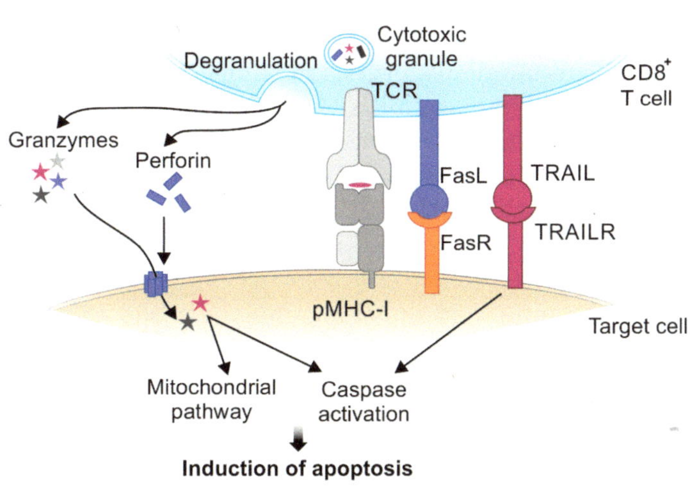

Fig. 1: Mechanisms of CD8$^+$ T-cell cytotoxicity. (FasL: Fas ligand; FasR: Fas receptor; pMHC: peptide major histocompatibility complex; TCR: T-cell receptor; TRAIL: tumor necrosis factor-related apoptosis-inducing ligand)

Pathogenesis of Antibody-mediated Rejection

B cells are immune cells of the lymphoid lineage that develop in the bone marrow. They are characterized by the expression of antibody as their surface antigen receptor, i.e., the B-cell receptor (BCR), and other markers such as CD20 and CD19. Once activated, alloreactive T cells differentiate into T follicular helper (Tfh) cells, which help B cells to transform into plasma cells producing high-affinity class switch antibodies.[3] When B cells encounter an antigen that binds their surface BCR, they may either develop into short-lived plasmablasts that produce early, germ-line encoded antibody or alternatively migrate to a B-cell follicle with the Tfh cells and develop a germinal center (GC). Memory B cells and long-lived plasma cells (LLPCs) are produced in GC. Here, they divide and mutate their variable region genes (somatic hypermutation) in an attempt to produce antibody with a higher affinity for antigen. They also undergo class switching, so that the heavy chain present in antibody changes from μ to one of the other isotypes. During many rounds of division and hypermutation, B cells with a high-affinity BCR are positively selected and differentiate into either memory B cells or plasma cells. The LLPCs are devoid of CD20 receptor, but they are capable of secreting a large number of antibodies and offer long-lasting humoral immunity via IL-6 and a proliferation-inducing ligand in bone marrow.[4] On the other hand, memory B cells can hypermutate and express CD19, CD20, and B lymphocyte stimulator [BLyS or B-cell activating factor (BAFF)] receptors. On re-exposure to target antigens, these can proliferate rapidly and transform into short-lived plasma cells which secrete antibodies. The hypermutations occurring at antigen-binding sites of memory B cells may lead to formation of several forms of dnDSA with multiple unpredicted HLA specificities. The persistent low-grade activation and transformation of memory B cells to plasma cells may trigger accumulation of DSA, resulting in slowly progressive and long-term graft dysfunction.

The pathogenicity of DSA is dynamic and varies according to the immunoglobulin G (IgG) subclass profile.[5] Over the course of immune response and antibody production, there is a sequential IgG subclass switching, typically from IgG3 to IgG1 to IgG2 to IgG4. IgG1 and IgG3 are usually complement-binding subclasses. IgG1 is the most abundant subclass and mirrors the total IgG level, but IgG3 has the greater binding efficiency to C1q and activate complement cascade.[6] Although IgG2 can activate complement weakly, IgG4 does not activate complement at all, but both can recruit effector cells through the Fc receptor. IL-6 is found to have a prominent role in the function and differentiation of Th cells, and IL-6 antagonist can arrest or prevent the differentiation of B cells into plasma cells or memory B cells, and decrease long-term survival of plasma cells. The BAFF molecule is a critical survival factor in the function and replication of B cells.

Antibody-mediated rejection results due to alloantibodies against foreign (nonself) donor antigens, mainly HLA, which leads to damage to the allograft through activation of the complement-dependent pathway as well as independent mechanisms recruiting natural killer (NK) cells, polymorphonuclear cells, platelets, and macrophages to attack the allograft.[7] These antibodies can be either preexisting at a low level before the transplant or synthesized de novo post-transplant. Chronic active ABMR usually shares a different phenotype than acute ABMR, namely dnDSA against class 2 HLA, antibodies of IgG2 and IgG4 subclasses, and activation of the complement-independent pathways (C4d negative), and may generally have a poor and incomplete response to currently available therapies.

Donor-specific antibodies binding to allograft endothelium expressing alloantigens can activate a variety of inflammatory mechanisms: (1) *Complement-dependent cytotoxicity:* Activation complement via the classical pathway. The anaphylatoxins are released with recruitment of inflammatory cells and finally lead to generation of the membrane attack complex, ultimately causing microvascular inflammation (MVI) in the graft and tissue injury. Additionally, C4d, a degradation product of the classical complement pathway, covalently binds to the endothelial basement membrane surface and persists there as an in situ marker of complement activation. (2) *Antibody-dependent cellular toxicity:* Innate immune cells such as NK cells and macrophages having Fc receptor bind to the Fc region of DSAs leading to activation of these cells which triggers degranulation, phagocytosis, and cell lysis. (3) *Direct endothelial injury:* The binding of DSA to alloantigens expressed on endothelial cells can also lead to activation and proliferation of endothelial cells, upregulating fibroblast growth factor receptor, and increasing its ligand binding as well as other signaling pathways for cellular recruitment **(Fig. 2)**. The absence of C4d staining in more than half of biopsies with late ABMR highlights the importance of complement independent mechanisms in mediating the deleterious effects of DSAs. Some IgG isotypes (IgG4) cannot fix complement, whereas IgG2 has a limited complement-activating capacity compared with IgG1 and IgG3.[8]

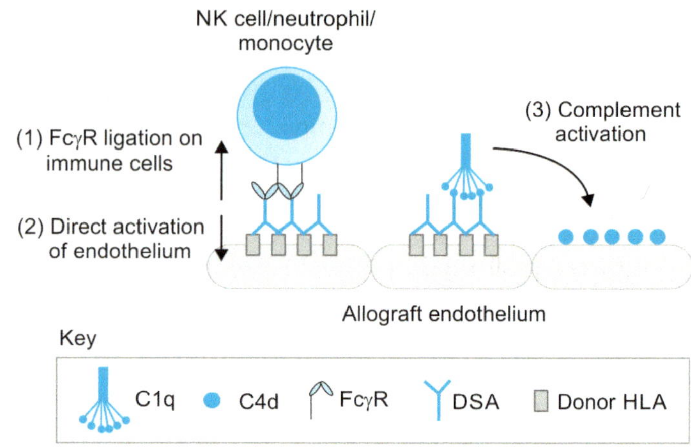

Fig. 2: Pathogenetic mechanisms of DSAs leading to allograft injury: (1) Engagement of Fcγ receptors on local and circulating immune cells; (2) Direct activation of allograft endothelium; (3) Activation of complement via the classical pathway. (DSA: donor-specific antibody; HLA: human leukocyte antigen; NK: natural killer)

The interaction of DSAs with graft HLA, especially class II antigens expressed by vascular endothelial cells, leads to a cascade of molecular events, including complement pathway activation that may contribute to endothelial injury, cellular dysfunction, MVI, and remodeling, and ultimately results in irreversible graft injury characteristic of chronic ABMR.

In addition to activation of alloimmune response due to inadequate immunosuppression or medication nonadherence, inflammatory events in the early post-transplant period such as ischemia-reperfusion injury, acute rejection episodes, and viral infections are suggested to be risk factors for production of dnDSA. In general, dnDSA is a new DSA detected after >3 months post-transplant in the context of inadequate immunosuppression which is either due to patient nonadherence, physician directed, or genetically determined variability in metabolism of immunosuppressive drugs. The development of dnDSA after KT was reported in 13–30% of previously nonsensitized patients. The risk factors for dnDSA include the following: (1) High HLA mismatches (especially DQ mismatches); (2) inadequate immunosuppression and nonadherence; and (3) graft inflammation, such as viral infection, cellular rejection, or ischemic injury, which can increase graft immunogenicity. The majority of dnDSAs after KT are class 2 antibodies, especially DQ, and are commonly noncomplement binding IgG2 or IgG4 subclass. They tend to be persistent and are associated with chronic ABMR and TG.[9]

Natural killer cells via their CD16a Fc receptors are also involved in ABMR pathogenesis. After exposure to alloantigens, they increase IFN-γ production through antibody-dependent cellular cytotoxicity-like mechanisms. NK cell infiltration in graft biopsy is a poor prognostic factor. The absence of self HLA class I ligands on the allograft is recognized by inhibitory killer cell immunoglobulin-like receptors (KIRs) expressed on NK cells; this leads to mitigation of inhibitory signals and finally eliminates the target. This missing-self-induced NK-cell activation may be one mechanism of immunological graft injury leading to chronic rejection. In C4d-negative ABMR, endothelial activation and NK cells were suggested as the primary causes of chronic rejection.

As discussed above, the activation of complement-dependent and -independent mechanisms that recruit NK cells, polymorphonuclear neutrophils, platelets, and macrophages, contributes to peritubular capillaritis, glomerulitis, cellular necrosis, and thrombotic microangiopathy (TMA). In chronic active ABMR, the sustained MVI over a longer period leads to microvascular remodeling of the glomerular and peritubular capillaries (PTCs) and arterial intimal fibrous thickening.

In transplanted kidneys, the magnitude of microvascular involution during the first 3 months following transplantation is a major negative predictor of long-term renal allograft function. Recent studies using in vivo imaging and electron microscopy demonstrated a tight correlation between peritubular capillary dysfunction/rarefaction and renal fibrosis in both murine models of acute kidney injury and human kidney biopsy samples.

PATHOLOGY

Histologic evaluation of the allograft remains the gold standard for the diagnosis of rejection. Chronic rejection is characterized by changes affecting all compartment parts of the kidneys, including the glomeruli, tubules, interstitium, and arteries. Chronic active TCMR involves mainly the renal tubules, interstitium, and arteries, leading to tubulitis, interstitial inflammation, and chronic allograft arteriopathy, respectively. Variable degrees of IF/TA are common. Arterial intimal fibrosis is the characteristic of chronic allograft arteriopathy. Chronic active ABMR leads to microzvascular remodeling in both the glomerular and the PTCs. At the glomerular level, this manifests as TG, which is characterized by double contouring of glomerular capillary walls **(Figs. 3A to D)**. Other features of chronic

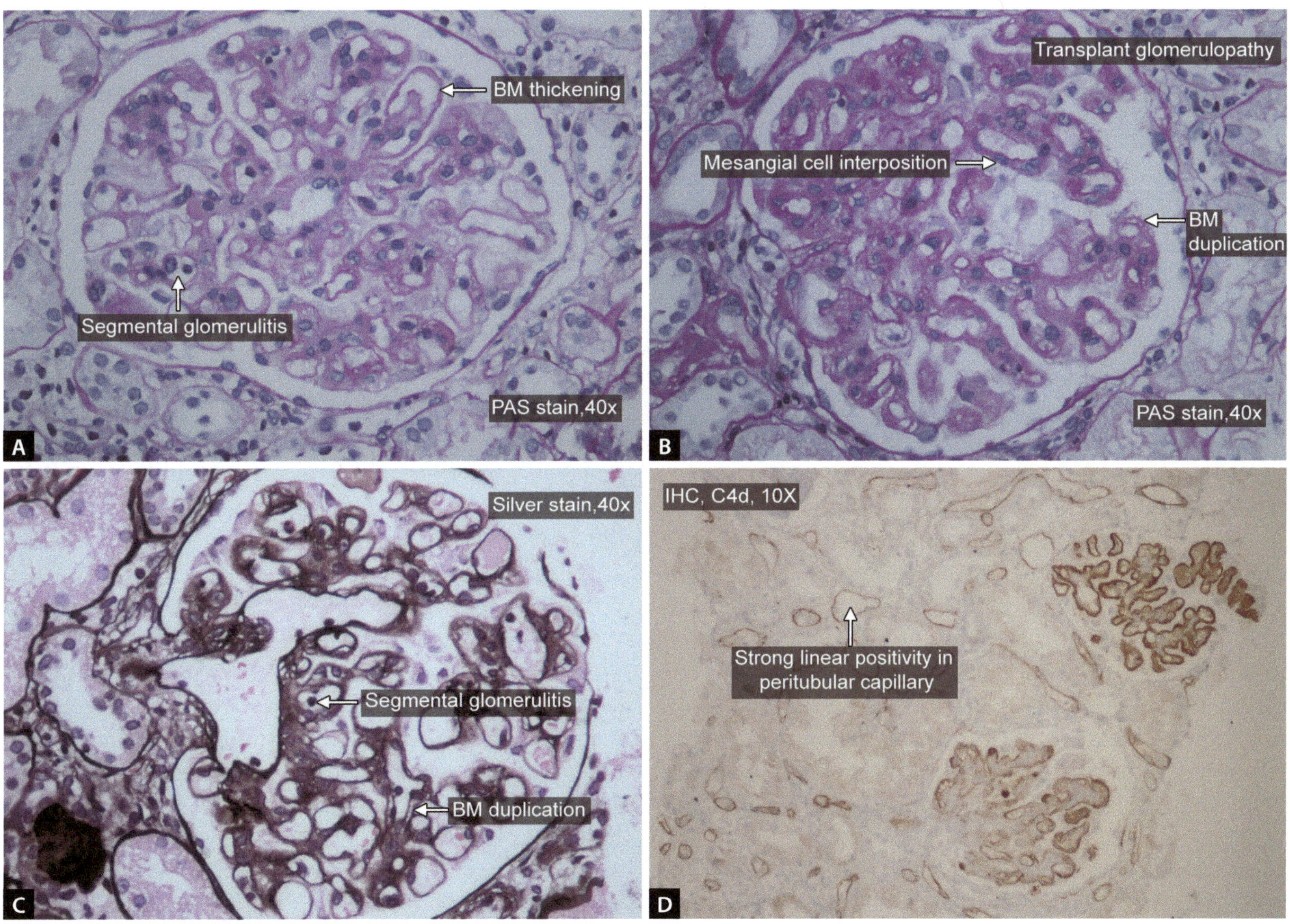

Figs. 3A to D: Composite picture of kidney allograft biopsy showing features of C4d positive chronic active antibody-mediated rejection (ABMR).

BOX 1: Conditions associated with C4d positivity.

- Hyperacute rejection
- Active ABMR (previously termed acute/active ABMR)
- Chronic active ABMR
- Chronic ABMR
- Smoldering and indolent ABMR
- C4d staining without evidence of rejection

(ABMR: antibody-mediated rejection)

active ABMR include peritubular capillary basement membrane multilayering and arterial intimal fibrosis.[10] (Read detailed pathology in Chapter 10.1.)

C4d is a degradation product of the complement pathway and binds covalently to the endothelium. It serves as an immunologic footprint of complement activation and ABMR **(Box 1)**.[11] Its prevalence in PTCs varies from 36 to 91% with TG, 12 to 61% diagnosed with chronic rejection and renal dysfunction, and 2% of protocol specimens. ABMR without C4d occurs in 20–30% of cases (termed "C4d-negative"). ABO-incompatible allografts commonly display harmless C4d staining. C4d staining in at least 10% of PTCs (C4d2 or C4d3) by IF on frozen sections or in any PTCs by immunoperoxidase on paraffin sections (C4d score > 0) is regarded as sufficient for the diagnosis of ABMR in the presence of tissue injury and DSAs. Some patients have morphologic evidence of ABMR with little or no C4d staining. Diagnostic criteria for C4d-negative ABMR were incorporated into the 2013 Banff update.[12]

CLINICAL FEATURES

Chronic rejection is manifested by slowly progressive loss of graft function that usually starts to manifest after the first year following KT and usually accompanied by proteinuria and hypertension. It usually occurs in patients with insufficient or inadequate immunosuppression, or drug noncompliance. Diagnosis is suggested only by an increase in the serum creatinine, worsening of hypertension, or proteinuria and is confirmed by allograft biopsy. A rising serum creatinine level, however, is a relatively late phenomenon and usually indicates the presence of significant histologic damage. Sometimes, rejection (especially acute) may present with fever, pain at the graft site, graft tenderness, hematuria, dysuria, fluid retention, and decreased urine output. Many of these symptoms are typically absent in chronic rejection. As most patients are asymptomatic, delay in diagnosis is common. Late stages of chronic rejection can manifest with azotemia, including nausea, vomiting, metallic taste, oliguria, pericardial friction rub, and asterixis.

Important points to note in history in a patient with chronic allograft injury are history of medication nonadherence and drug toxicity, basic kidney disease and its recurrence rate, previous transplantation, prior rejection episodes and viral infections, and baseline HLA sensitization. Unexplained decrease in drug levels in blood can point toward drug noncompliance as a cause for chronic rejection. Medication history is also essential, as many commonly used drugs affect the metabolism of immunosuppressive drugs, decreasing or increasing their blood levels leading to rejection and drug toxicity, respectively. Examination findings are usually noncontributory and nonspecific but may reveal edema and hypertension.

EVALUATION AND DIAGNOSIS

Testing for Donor-specific Antibodies

Testing for DSAs is crucial as post-transplant generation of dnDSA has been implicated as one of the most common causes of chronic graft loss, and these can be detected before significant graft dysfunction ensues.[13]

Testing for anti-HLA DSA is negative in 10–15% of chronic active ABMR cases (usually false negative). Cases in which C4d staining is positive but DSA cannot be detected may result from DSA being below the level of detection due to immunoadsorption by the graft (sink effect) or it can also be due to the presence of non-HLA antibodies. This issue has been particularly discussed in the 2017 Banff conference. Though molecular diagnostics were first introduced in 2013 Banff, its 2017 update has recommended indications for use of these tests in the diagnosis of ABMR.[14] C4d as well as molecular classifiers were recognized as surrogate markers for DSA.[15] (Detailed discussion on DSA is given in Chapter 1.3.)

Nonhuman Leukocyte Antigen Donor-specific Antibodies

Nonhuman leukocyte antigen donor-specific antibodies can also result in rejection and C4d deposition.[16] In cases where there are no detectable HLA DSAs but a biopsy specimen meeting criterion for ABMR (MVI score ≥ 1 and C4d positive; MVI score ≥ 2 and C4d negative), testing for non-HLA antibodies is strongly advised.[17] (Detailed discussion on non-HLA DSAs is given in Chapter 1.4.)

NOVEL DIAGNOSTIC MARKERS

Although histological examination through allograft biopsy remains the gold standard diagnostic criterion, it cannot be carried out frequently due to its invasiveness and risk of complications. A variety of promising noninvasive biomarkers have been detected that can be used to monitor the alloimmune response in a particular KT recipient. Some of these include estimating the plasma level of donor-derived cell-free deoxyribonucleic acid (DNA) (dd-cfDNA testing by AlloSure), microribonucleic acids (microRNAs), chemokines, and microarray-based assay of the mRNA expression level of genes associated with rejection or leukocyte trafficking [kidney solid organ response test (kSORT) and molecular microscope diagnostic system (MMDx)].[18] Molecular methods require a graft biopsy specimen for analysis of microarray data. Sellarés et al.[19,20] looked at transplant biopsy histology and tried to match is with microarray data to develop classifiers that assigned ABMR scores to each biopsy. They concluded that microarray assessment of gene expression can assign a probability of ABMR along with chronic changes such as TG to transplant biopsies without knowledge of HLA antibody status, histology, or C4d staining and predicts future failure. The microarray data-derived MMDx also improved the uncertainty for ABMR diagnosis in graft biopsy.

In India at present, dd-cfDNA testing is available. The test was validated in the Diagnosing Acute Rejection in Kidney Transplant Recipients (DART) study which included patients with active ABMR, chronic active ABMR, or TCMR. At 1% threshold of dd-cfDNA, it had 81% positive predictive value (PPV) and 83% negative predictive value (NPV) for active ABMR. Identification of DSA was complementary and the combined use of dd-cfDNA and DSA improved the prediction of active ABMR, including chronic active ABMR noninvasively. The elevation of dd-cfDNA was associated with the development of dnDSA and estimated glomerular filtration rate (eGFR) decline. dd-cfDNA can be monitored sequentially in patients with a higher risk of allograft rejection. However, urinary tract infection or BK virus nephropathy may increase dd-cfDNA of ABMR. The use of routine monitoring of dd-cfDNA after KT may allow clinicians to identify subclinical immunological graft injury and intervene prior to development of clinically significant graft injury.[21] In a recently published ADMIRAL (Assessing AlloSure Dd-cfDNA Monitoring Insights of Renal Allografts with Longitudinal Surveillance) study, authors evaluated data from more than one thousand KT recipients monitored for dd-cfDNA over a 3-year period and was analyzed to assess the association of dd-cfDNA with histologic evidence of allograft rejection. Elevation of dd-cfDNA (0.5% or more) was significantly correlated with clinical and subclinical allograft rejection. dd-cfDNA values of 0.5% or more were associated with a nearly threefold increase in risk development of dnDSA [hazard ratio (HR) 2.71] and were determined to be elevated a median of 91 days (interquartile range of 30–125 days) ahead of DSA identification. Persistently elevated dd-cfDNA (more than one result above the 0.5% threshold) predicted over a 25% decline in the eGFR over 3 years (HR 1.97).[22] Thus, persistently low dd-cfDNA levels may accurately identify allograft quiescence or absence of immunological injury, paving the way for personalization of immunosuppression trials.

Other novel tests include IFN-γ enzyme-linked immunosorbent spot assay evaluating circulating antidonor T-cell alloreactivity, gene expression analysis including AlloMap score, urine gene analysis panel, urinary chemokines including CXCL9 and CXCL10, and microRNAs.[23] All these tests may act complementary to the current standard and help in the identification of graft rejection in combination with pathological data on biopsy. These tests can be positive even before the actual rise in serum creatinine, enabling early detection of possible rejection.

MANAGEMENT

The management of chronic rejection remains a difficult task, mainly due to irreversibility of the disease in most of the patients at the time of diagnosis. Hence, management should focus on the acute rejection, its prevention, early detection, and prompt management rather than treating chronic rejection. The goals of therapy should be to stabilize or reduce the rate of decline in GFR, proteinuria, histological injury score, and titer of DSA while minimizing drug toxicity. Currently, no immunotherapies are clinically proven to be significantly effective in preventing and treating chronic rejection.

Tailoring of immunosuppression based on individual patient characteristics is actually needed. Risks (infections and cost) versus benefit (minimizing graft injury) should be analyzed before intensifying immunosuppression in chronic rejection.[24] Nonimmunological interventions include controlling several risk factors such as managing hypertension, hyperglycemia, and dyslipidemia. Renin–angiotensin–aldosterone system (RAAS) blockers should be used cautiously with calcineurin inhibitors (CNIs) due to a greater risk of hyperkalemia and azotemia.

T Cell-mediated (Cellular) Rejection

Chronic active TCMR is variably responsive to immunosuppressive therapy, and it is often associated with insufficient immunosuppression. Intensification of immunosuppression with steroid pulse therapy ± ATG, and escalating doses and types of oral maintenance immunosuppressives might improve graft survival in chronic active TCMR. Few authors suggested using a strategy of combining the four immunosuppressive agents from different classes [including mammalian target of rapamycin (mTOR) inhibitors] which might enhance immunosuppression and reduce toxicity by reducing the dosage of individual drugs. The response to therapy is variable and depends mainly on the timing of diagnosis, severity of graft dysfunction, and histological grading, especially the extent of chronicity in biopsy.

Antibody-mediated Rejection

In 2019, The Transplantation Society Working Group developed an expert consensus on the appropriate treatment for active and chronic active ABMR. There is no conclusive evidence to support any specific therapy. Aggressive immunosuppression may severely compromise the safety of the patient with high treatmentrelated mortality and morbidity. In one study on management of ABMR comparing supportive therapy with aggressive treatment (with double filtration plasmapheresis, pulse corticosteroids, IVIg, rituximab, and bortezomib) showed that the graft survival was better in the later group but with high therapy emergent adverse effects.

Most of the studies on ABMR therapy were small, heterogeneous, and retrospective as shown in **Table 1**. Chronic ABMR pathogenesis is distinct from active (acute) ABMR and mainly relies on LLPCs producing high-affinity multispecificity anti-HLA DSAs and abundance of Tfh cells and hypermutated B cells in GC reaction.[38] GC is relatively resistant to therapeutic armamentarium currently available. In chronic tissue injury cases (evidence of TG, PTC multilayering, and chronic vasculopathy), it is important to recognize for evidence of acute injury, i.e., MVI (g + PTC > 2), C4d positivity in immunofluorescence (IF) or immunohistochemistry (IHC) staining, raised DSA or upregulated molecular or genetic transcripts in C4d negative patients, because in this clinical scenario, addition of other immunosuppressants should be considered. In the Indian scenario, where molecular or genetic transcripts are not available for C4d negative chronic ABMR patients presenting with proteinuria, excluding basic disease recurrence with TG-like picture is important. While interpreting MVI, glomerular or tubular neutrophilic infiltration, infection or infection-related glomerulonephritis should be kept in mind.

The treatment strategies are directed mainly toward depleting DSAs. These include therapeutic plasma exchange (TPE), IVIg, CD20 antibody (rituximab), proteasome inhibitor (bortezomib), and anticomplement monoclonal antibody (eculizumab), either single or in combination. Early treatment will reduce the risk of further graft injury and chronic graft loss. These therapies have limited success either alone or in combination in chronic active ABMR in spite of their effectiveness in treating active (acute) ABMR. The use of IVIg and TPE, with or without rituximab, has not been shown to improve outcomes in patients with chronic active ABMR (as distinct from active ABMR). Splenectomy can be considered in patients refractory to other therapies. Important studies using immunomodulatory therapies in chronic ABMR are mentioned in **Table 1**.

TABLE 1: Studies for therapy of chronic antibody-mediated rejection (ABMR).

Intervention	*Study design*	*Diagnosis*	*Therapy*	*Follow-up*	*Outcome*	*Graft function*	*Reference*
TPE + IVIg	Retrospective	Chronic active ABMR	Steroids, IVIg, TPE, RTX, or ATG versus no intervention; all received CNIs	4.3 years	Steroids + IVIg hazard ratio 0.38 for graft loss. No additional benefit of RTX or ATG	NR	Redfield et al.[25] (2016)
TPE + IVIg	Retrospective	Chronic active ABMR	IVIg + steroids	6.3 years	Graft survival at 1, 3, and 5 years after chronic active ABMR diagnosis. Responders: 100, 75, and 59%; non-responders: 89, 57, and 20%	ΔeGFR −9.8/year prior to tx; −6.3/year after tx ($p < 0.05$)	Sablik et al.[26] (2019)
RTX	Prospective (20 pediatric patients)	Chronic ABMR	All received IVIg + RTX along with steroids + MMF + CNIs	2 years	20% graft loss	ΔeGFR from −7.6 during 6 months prior to tx to −2.1 during 6 months after tx ($p < 0.05$)	Billing et al.[27] (2012)
RTX	Retrospective	Chronic ABMR	IVIg + RTX + steroids versus steroids. All received CNIs	>2 years	HR for graft loss 0.24	ΔeGFR 0.2/month in RTX group ($p < 0.05$ compared to the pre-6 months ΔeGFR); ΔeGFR −1.4/month in control group (p = NS compared to the pre-6 months ΔeGFR)	Chung et al.[28] (2014)

Contd...

Contd…

Intervention	Study design	Diagnosis	Therapy	Follow-up	Outcome	Graft function	Reference
RTX	Retrospective	Chronic ABMR with TG	IVIg + steroids + RTX versus no IVIg + RTX; 95% on CNIs in RTX group, 80% on CNIs in control group	2 years	53% graft loss in RTX group, 60% in control group	NR	Bachelet et al.[29] (2015)
RTX	Retrospective	Chronic active ABMR with TG	IVIg + TPE + RTX versus no intervention	27 months	No difference in graft loss	No difference	Piñeiro et al.[30] (2018)
RTX	RCT	Chronic ABMR + TG ± C4d in PTC; anti-HLA DSA	RTX + IVIg versus placebo; all patients received CNIs + MMF	1 year	8% graft loss in both groups	ΔeGFR −4.2 in RTX group, −6.6 in placebo group (p = NS)	Moreso et al.[31]
Bortezomib	Prospective cohort study	Early acute ABMR (13) and late acute ABMR (17)	All received TPE + RTX + bortezomib along with TAC + MMF	7 months	10% graft loss in early ABMR, 20% in late ABMR	eGFR from 40 prior to tx to 66 after tx in early ABMR ($p < 0.05$); eGFR from 27 prior to tx to 37 after tx in late ABMR ($p < 0.05$)	Walsh et al. (2011)[32]
Bortezomib	RCT	44 with late ABMR (28 chronic active ABMR)	Bortezomib versus placebo. All received steroids + MMF + CNIs	2 years	19% graft loss in bortezomib group, 4% in placebo group (p = NS)	eGFR slope −4.7/year in bortezomib group, −5.2/year in placebo group (p = NS)	Eskandary et al.[33]
Eculizumab	Nonblinded RCT	Chronic ABMR: DSA MFI >1,100; 20% reduction in eGFR; no severe fibrosis	Eculizumab versus placebo. All received CNIs or rapamycin	1 year	Graft loss was not reported	No difference in graft function	Kulkarni et al.[34] (2017)
C1 inhibitor	Prospective phase 1 study (10)	Late ABMR (9 with chronic active ABMR)	All received C1 INH along with steroids + MMF + CNIs	50 days	Graft loss was not reported	Stable graft function	Eskandary et al.[35]
Tocilizumab	Prospective cohort study (36)	Chronic ABMR with TG	All received tocilizumab along with steroids + MMF + TAC	3.3 years	11.1%	Stable graft function	Choi et al.[36]
Clazakizumab	Randomized, placebo controlled, parallel-group phase 2 trial (20)	Late active or chronic active ABMR, ≥365 days post-transplantation with a molecular pattern of ABMR	Clazakizumab versus placebo. 18 received CNIs or mTOR inhibitor-based triple therapy, two received dual therapy without steroids	52 weeks	Graft loss in one at 3 months after last visit	eGFR slope −0.96/month in clazakizumab group, −2.43/month in placebo group ($p < 0.05$) Improvement of eGFR slope in PTS switched from placebo to clazakizumab ($p < 0.05$)	Doberer et al.[37]

(ABMR: antibody-mediated rejection; ATG: antithymocyte globulin; C1-INH: C1 esterase inhibitor CNIs: calcineurin inhibitors; DSA: donor-specific antibody; eGFR: estimated glomerular filtration rate; HR: hazard ratio; IVIg: intravenous immunoglobulin; MFI: mean fluorescence intensity; MMF: mycophenolate mofetil; mTOR: mammalian target of rapamycin; NR: not reported; PTC: peritubular capillary; RCT: randomized controlled trial; RTX: rituximab; TAC: tacrolimus; TG: transplant glomerulopathy; TPE: therapeutic plasma exchange)

Plasmapheresis (Therapeutic Plasma Exchange) and Intravenous Immunoglobulin

These two therapies are the mainstay to treat active ABMR and for pretransplant desensitization, however, their use in chronic ABMR is yet to get strong evidence of benefit. Usually, five to six sessions of TPE are used, tailored to non-detection of DSA level. Though TPE can reduce levels of circulating antibodies and graft injury, it has a transient effect in most of the cases. Several studies looked at the efficacy of TPE in reduction of DSA depending on their types and graft life as well, where they found better clearance of type 1 DSAs compared to type 2 DSAs, and older grafts were likely to have more type 2 DSAs particularly to DQ and DR, which showed lesser clearance than DSAs against class 1, while younger grafts showed creatinine improvement better than the older grafts. TPE is also associated with a rebound in DSAs, which may be explained by the fact that the graft antigens are persistent to stimulate DSA production constantly. TPE does not affect LLPCs, who are a key player for chronic ABMR by producing dnDSA, and the negative feedback on DSA production by high DSA titer is also diminished by transient DSA clearance. So, there is a rebound of DSA post-TPE which has to be taken care of by IVIg and other immunosuppressive medications. Hence, the combination of treatments that inhibit the formation and favor removal of DSA is crucial.

Anti-CD20 Monoclonal Antibody—Rituximab

Long-lived plasma cells, which produce alloantibodies in chronic ABMR do not have CD20 receptor and are therefore resistant to rituximab. Therefore, rituximab may not effectively improve the outcome of ABMR, although it may have some beneficial effects in active ABMR. Earlier studies reported that rituximab would be beneficial in chronic active ABMR patients by increasing their graft survival. But later studies published failed to show any improvement in short or long term; they rather documented an increase in infective complications and GI side effects. Obinutuzumab is another anti-CD20 molecule which can deplete B cells more effectively and had been used in sensitized KT patients with IVIg as desensitization protocol but did not cause any effective reduction of DSA.

Proteasome Inhibitors

Bortezomib is a selective inhibitor of the 26S proteasome and leads to accumulation of unfolded proteins, thereby inducing apoptosis of short- and long-lived plasma cells. It was initially thought to lead to the inhibition of the production of dnDSA. Two trials raised this hope: One from Mayo clinic, where it eliminated DSA effectively from sensitized transplant patients, and in another study, where acute ABMR patients, early or late, had shown improvement of eGFR when treated with a combination of rituximab, bortezomib, and TPE. The cause of failure was explored by various researcher groups where they opined that bortezomib-induced plasma cell depletion is associated with rebound plasma cell formation from bone marrow resident cells, generation of new plasma cells from GC, and memory B cells, where bortezomib fails to inhibit B cell–Tfh cell interaction and proliferation of high-affinity antibody-producing B cells.

Carfilzomib is an irreversible proteasome inhibitor. Studies performed in highly sensitized KT patients, it reduced anti-HLA DSA, only to rebound after a few months. This resistance to carfilzomib in plasma cells may be due to structural changes of proteasome and immune proteasome formation.

Complement-based Therapy

Eculizumab is a humanized monoclonal antibody that blocks the cleavage of C5 into C5a and C5b. As shown by Marks et al.[39] and other studies, eculizumab showed the potential to improve graft function in early active ABMR. Schinstock et al.[40] have also showed this early ABMR incidence reduction benefit in highly sensitized KT patients but over a period of 6-year follow-up, it did not reduce the chronic ABMR incidence or outcome. Other studies used this molecule in KT recipients with DSA >1,100 mean fluorescence intensity (MFI) where renal function was stabilized but the expression of endothelial-associated transcripts (ENDATs) predicting acute humoral injury was not reduced.[41] As an attempt to explain relative ineffectiveness, the likelihood of involvement of complement-independent pathways in chronic ABMR pathogenesis seems important, as well as activation of upstream complement factors, like the anaphylatoxin C3a, triggering chronic injury and inflammation and sublytic levels of the membrane attack complex causing endothelial cell injury and activation can be other probabilities.

Novel Therapies

Certain novel therapeutic agents which are in pipeline for management of the ABMR include IL-6/IL-6R blockade [tocilizumab (TCZ), an anti-IL-6 receptor monoclonal antibody], C1 esterase inhibitor (C1 INH), and BLyS or BAFF inhibitor (belimumab).

C1 Esterase Inhibitor

The C1 INH inhibits complement proteases C1r and C1s. These complement inhibitors have the potential to prevent and treat ABMR.[42] Studies by Montgomery et al.[43] and others had shown beneficial effect of C1 INH in improving graft function and preventing TG in acute ABMR. Eskandary et al.[35] tried this molecule in a small number of patients with late ABMR, with no improved outcomes.

Anti-C1s monoclonal antibody BIVV009 inhibited the complement pathway, but there was no change in MVI, gene expression patterns, DSA levels, or graft function in 5-week follow-up biopsies. As the studies are few with heterogeneous design and participants are small, it is difficult to comment upon the future utility of this molecule.

Interleukin-6 Blockade: Tocilizumab

Interleukin 6 is a pleiotropic, proinflammatory cytokine that plays an integral role in the development of acute and chronic rejection after KT. It plays a role in the differentiation of a mature B cell into a cell capable of secreting antibodies. TCZ is being evaluated in many prospective trials and randomized controlled trials (RCTs) either alone or in combination with other molecules. Shin et al.[44] had shown that it reduced total IgG and IgG 1–3 anti-HLA DSA levels. Choi et al.[36] treated 36 patients of chronic ABMR with TCZ and 86% with high type 2 DSA who failed standard of care therapy with steroids + IVIg + rituximab ± TPE; they had significant reduction of DSAs with stabilized renal function.

Clazakizumab, a humanized monoclonal antibody directed against the IL-6 molecule (rather than the IL-6 receptor), is undergoing evaluation currently. In a recent phase 2 randomized clinical trial by Doberer et al.,[37] clazakizumab was associated with an early decrease in DSA levels, modulated ABMR activity, and slowed the decline of renal function.

Anti-CD38 Molecule: Daratumumab

Daratumumab, a human IgG1 monoclonal antibody targeting CD38, has become an established therapy in plasma cell neoplasia and is being tried in ABMR too. In a nonhuman primate model, the molecule was used to treat rejection, where it reduced anti-HLA DSA and NK cells, but there was subsequent rebound in DSA with TCMR.[45]

Immunoglobulin G Endopeptidase

Imlifidase is an IgG-degrading enzyme derived from *Streptococcus pyogenes* (IdeS) that cleaves human IgG into F(ab′)2 and Fc fragments, thereby protecting against complement-dependent cytotoxicity and antibody-dependent cellular cytotoxicity. Favorable outcomes with its use for desensitization in HLA-incompatible KT have engendered interest in its use for ABMR. It is a novel agent that cleaves all four human subclasses of IgG. Data from clinical trials in KT demonstrated rapid degradation of anti-HLA DSA facilitating HLA-incompatible transplantation, which led to conditional approval of imlifidase by the European Medicines Agency for desensitization in KT recipients of a deceased donor with a positive crossmatch. Imlifidase is currently being evaluated in comparison to plasmapheresis in clinical trials and is a potential therapy for ABMR.

Costimulation Blockade: Belatacept

Belatacept could bind to CD80 and CD86 and prevent the costimulation at CD28 in Tfh cells and decrease plasmablast differentiation, production of antibody, especially IgG2 and IgG4, and prevent activation of Tfh cells in KT recipients.[46] In a series by Jain et al.,[47] who combined belatacept and bortezomib in his six KT patients with ABMR, DSAs showed reduced and ABMR reversed.

Other Therapies

Banham et al.[48] studied the combination of belimumab to standard of care immunosuppression in adult KT recipients and concluded that belimumab might be a useful adjunct in KT, with no major increased risk of infection and potential beneficial effects on humoral alloimmunity. Blocking the IL21 receptor with antiIL21 receptor monoclonal antibody may change the Tfh/Tfr balance and inhibit DSA generation.

PREVENTION

Optimizing HLA matching reduces the chances of immunological graft injury. The selection of a most appropriate, immune-compatible donor is needed. Avoiding unrelated living kidney donation, and organ allocation for deceased donor using HLAMatchmaker software may be appropriate suggestions in Indian scenario. The crucial step is the usage of different immunosuppressive drugs in ideal combination that can inhibit the proliferation and action of immune cells to decrease the chances of graft rejection in the longer run. The prevention of ABMR depends upon the early detection of DSAs prior to (preexisting DSA) or after (dnDSA) transplant. A higher level of DSA predicts higher risk of ABMR and graft loss. Monitoring for dnDSA is recommended in high-risk situations such as reduced immunosuppression, drug noncompliance, medication nonadherence, or rejection. DSA analysis may predict the risk of developing ABMR, but the diagnostic value for ABMR is likely to be low. In a recent study, 21.4% of grafts with simultaneous dnDSA and ABMR failed during a mean follow-up period of 4.2 years, and no graft failure occurred in patients with only dnDSA. The incidence of chronic AMBR was not correlating with the MFI values. These findings may indicate that not all DSAs are pathological and cause graft injury. Adequacy of immunosuppression, medication adherence, and drug compliance is pivotal to preventing rejection. Minimizing individual nonadherence and iatrogenic drug lowering, particularly CNIs, may help. Whenever CNI dose is decreased, drug levels and creatinine are to be monitored closely and if required, dnDSA monitoring may be done. Early diagnosis of ABMR and TCMR and treating them adequately can prevent progression to chronic forms. Minimizing surgery related ischemia-reperfusion injury and prevention of delayed graft function may also affect long-term outcome.

PROGNOSIS AND OUTCOME

The prognosis and outcome of chronic rejection depend on several factors such as the type and timing of rejection, severity, previous acute rejections, degree of chronicity (IF/TA) on biopsy, graft dysfunction at the time of diagnosis and reversibility after treatment. Serum creatinine >3 mg/dL and proteinuria >1 g/day were identified as poor prognostic markers. Rejections occurring after 3 months, vascular rejections, higher histologic scores (e.g., i: Interstitial inflammation, t: Tubulitis, v: Intimal arteritis) and the rejections not responding to therapy (serum creatinine not reaching 75% of baseline value) are associated with poor graft survival. Certain characteristics of DSAs such as their strength, subclass, complement-binding capacity, type (dnDSA > preexisting DSA), and response to treatment can affect outcomes among patients with ABMR.

REFERENCES

1. Becker LE, Morath C, Suesal C. Immune mechanisms of acute and chronic rejection. Clin Biochem. 2016;49(4-5):320-3.
2. Siu JHY, Surendrakumar V, Richards JA, Pettigrew GJ. T cell allorecognition pathways in solid organ transplantation. Front Immunol. 2018;9:2548.
3. Laguna-Goya R, Suàrez-Fernández P, Paz-Artal E. Follicular helper T cells and humoral response in organ transplantation. Transplant Rev (Orlando). 2019;33(4):183-90.
4. Ionescu L, Urschel S. Memory B cells and long-lived plasma cells. Transplantation. 2019;103(5):890-8.
5. Zhang R. Donor-specific antibodies in kidney transplant recipients. Clin J Am Soc Nephrol. 2018;13:182-92.
6. Lefaucheur C, Viglietti D, Bentlejewski C, Duong van Huyen JP, Vernerey D, Aubert O, et al. IgG donor-specific anti-human HLA antibody subclasses and kidney allograft antibody-mediated injury. J Am Soc Nephrol. 2016;27(1):293-304.
7. Leibler C, Thiolat A, Elsner RA, El Karoui K, Samson C, Grimbert P. Costimulatory blockade molecules and B-cellmediated immune response: current knowledge and perspectives. Kidney Int. 2019;95(4):774-86.
8. Etta PK, Rao MV. Renal allograft dysfunction: an update on immunological graft injury. Indian J Transplant. 2019; 13:69-77.
9. Aubert O, Loupy A, Hidalgo L, Duong van Huyen JP, Higgins S, Viglietti D, et al. Antibody-mediated rejection due to preexisting versus de novo donor-specific antibodies in kidney allograft recipients. J Am Soc Nephrol. 2017;28(6): 1912-23.
10. Haas M. The relationship between pathologic lesions of active and chronic antibody-mediated rejection in renal allografts. Am J Transplant. 2018;18(12):2849-56.
11. Roufosse C, Simmonds N, Clahsen-van Groningen M, Haas M, Henriksen KJ, Horsfield C, et al. A 2018 reference guide to the Banff classification of renal allograft pathology. Transplantation. 2018;102:1795-814.
12. Etta PK. C4d staining and antibody-mediated rejection in renal transplantation: current status. Indian J Transplant. 2020;14:197-201.
13. Etta PK. Testing for donor-specific antibodies in renal transplantation: Indian perspective. Indian J Transplant. 2020;14:90-3.
14. Loupy A, Haas M, Roufosse C, Naesens M, Adam B, Afrouzian M, et al. The Banff 2019 Kidney Meeting Report (I): updates on and clarification of criteria for T cell- and antibody-mediated rejection. Am J Transplant. 2020;20(9):2318-31.
15. Haas M. Evolving criteria for the diagnosis of antibody-mediated rejection in renal allografts. Curr Opin Nephrol Hypertens. 2018;27(3):137-43.
16. Zhang Q, Reed EF. The importance of non-HLA antibodies in transplantation. Nat Rev Nephrol. 2016;12(8):484-95.
17. Etta PK, Madhavi T, Parikh N. Pathobiology of non-HLA immunity in renal transplantation. Indian J Transplant. 2021;15:147-56.
18. Erpicum P, Hanssen O, Weekers L, Lovinfosse P, Meunier P, Tshibanda L, et al. Non-invasive approaches in the diagnosis of acute rejection in kidney transplant recipients, part II: omics analyses of urine and blood samples. Clin Kidney J. 2017;10:106-15.
19. Sellarés J, Reeve J, Loupy A, Mengel M, Sis B, Skene A, et al. Molecular diagnosis of antibody-mediated rejection in human kidney transplants. Am J Transplant. 2013;13(4): 971-83.
20. Sellarés J, de Freitas DG, Mengel M, Reeve J, Einecke G, Sis B, et al. Understanding the causes of kidney transplant failure: the dominant role of antibody-mediated rejection and nonadherence. Am J Transplant. 2012;12(2):388-99.
21. Puliyanda DP, Swinford R, Pizzo H, Garrison J, De Golovine AM, Jordan SC. Donor-derived cell-free DNA (dd-cfDNA) for detection of allograft rejection in pediatric kidney transplants. Pediatr Transplant. 2021;25(2):e13850.
22. Bu L, Gupta G, Pai A, Anand S, Stites E, Moinuddin I, et al. Clinical outcomes from the assessing donor-derived cell-free DNA monitoring insights of kidney allografts with longitudinal surveillance (ADMIRAL) study. Kidney Int. 2022;101(4):793-803.
23. Salvadori M, Tsalouchos A. Biomarkers in renal transplantation: an updated review. World J Transplant. 2017;7: 161-78.
24. Kim MY, Brennan DC. Therapies for chronic allograft rejection. Front Pharmacol. 2021;12:651222.
25. Redfield RR, Ellis TM, Zhong W, Scalea JR, Zens TJ, Mandelbrot D, et al. Current outcomes of chronic active antibody mediated rejection—A large single center retrospective review using the updated BANFF 2013 criteria. Hum Immunol. 2016;77(4):346-52.
26. Sablik KA, Clahsen-van Groningen MC, Looman CWN, Damman J, van Agteren M, Betjes MGH. Treatment with intravenous immunoglobulins and methylprednisolone may significantly decrease loss of renal function in chronic-active antibody-mediated rejection. BMC Nephrol. 2019;20(1):218.
27. Billing H, Rieger S, Süsal C, Waldherr R, Opelz G, Wühl E, et al. IVIG and rituximab for treatment of chronic antibody-mediated rejection: a prospective study in paediatric renal transplantation with a 2-year follow-up. Transpl Int. 2012;25(11):1165-73.
28. Chung BH, Kim Y, Jeong HS, Hong YA, Choi BS, Park CW, et al. Clinical outcome in patients with chronic antibody-mediated rejection treated with and without rituximab and intravenous

immunoglobulin combination therapy. Transpl Immunol. 2014;31(3):140-4.
29. Bachelet T, Nodimar C, Taupin JL, Lepreux S, Moreau K, Morel D, et al. Intravenous immunoglobulins and rituximab therapy for severe transplant glomerulopathy in chronic antibody-mediated rejection: a pilot study. Clin Transplant. 2015;29(5):439-46.
30. Piñeiro GJ, De Sousa-Amorim E, Solé M, Ríos J, Lozano M, Cofán F, et al.. Rituximab, plasma exchange and immunoglobulins: an ineffective treatment for chronic active antibody-mediated rejection. BMC Nephrol. 2018;19(1):261.
31. Moreso F, Crespo M, Ruiz JC, Torres A, Gutierrez-Dalmau A, Osuna A, et al. Treatment of chronic antibody mediated rejection with intravenous immunoglobulins and rituximab: a multicenter, prospective, randomized, double-blind clinical trial. Am J Transplant. 2018;18(4):927-35.
32. Walsh RC, Brailey P, Girnita A, Alloway RR, Shields AR, Wall GE, et al. Early and late acute antibody-mediated rejection differ immunologically and in response to proteasome inhibition. Transplantation. 2011;91(11):1218-26.
33. Eskandary F, Regele H, Baumann L, Bond G, Kozakowski N, Wahrmann M, et al. A randomized trial of bortezomib in late antibody-mediated kidney transplant rejection. J Am Soc Nephrol. 2018;29(2):591-605.
34. Kulkarni S, Kirkiles-Smith NC, Deng YH, Formica RN, Moeckel G, Broecker V, et al. Eculizumab therapy for chronic antibody-mediated iInjury in kidney transplant recipients: a pilot randomized controlled trial. Am J Transplant. 2017;17(3):682-91.
35. Eskandary F, Jilma B, Mühlbacher J, Wahrmann M, Regele H, Kozakowski N, et al. Anti-C1s monoclonal antibody BIVV009 in late antibody-mediated kidney allograft rejection-results from a first-in-patient phase 1 trial. Am J Transplant. 2018;18(4):916-926.
36. Choi J, Aubert O, Vo A, Loupy A, Haas M, Puliyanda D, et al. Assessment of tocilizumab (anti-interleukin-6 receptor monoclonal) as a potential treatment for chronic antibodymediated rejection and transplant glomerulopathy in HLA-sensitized renal allograft recipients. Am J Transplant. 2017;17(9):2381-9.
37. Doberer K, Duerr M, Halloran PF, Eskandary F, Budde K, Regele H, et al. A randomized clinical trial of anti-IL-6 antibody clazakizumab in late antibody-mediated kidney transplant rejection. J Am Soc Nephrol. 2021;32(3):708-22.
38. Yan L, de Leur K, Hendriks RW, van der Laan LJW, Shi Y, Wang L, et al. T follicular helper cells as a new target for immunosuppressive therapies. Front Immunol. 2017;8:1510.
39. Marks WH, Mamode N, Montgomery RA, Stegall MD, Ratner LE, Cornell LD, et al. Safety and efficacy of eculizumab in the prevention of antibody-mediated rejection in livingdonor kidney transplant recipients requiring desensitization therapy: a randomized trial. Am J Transplant. 2019; 19(10):2876-88.
40. Schinstock CA, Mannon RB, Budde K, Chong AS, Haas M, Knechtle S, et al. Recommended treatment for antibodymediated rejection after kidney transplantation: the 2019 expert consensus from the Transplantation Society Working Group. Transplantation. 2020;104:911-22.
41. Tatapudi VS, Montgomery RA. Therapeutic modulation of the complement system in kidney transplantation: clinical indications and emerging drug leads. Front Immunol. 2019;10:2306.
42. Viglietti D, Gosset C, Loupy A, Deville L, Verine J, Zeevi A, et al. C1 inhibitor in acute antibody-mediated rejection nonresponsive to conventional therapy in kidney transplant recipients: a pilot study. Am J Transplant. 2016;16: 1596-603.
43. Montgomery RA, Orandi BJ, Racusen L, Jackson AM, Garonzik-Wang JM, Shah T, et al. Plasma-derived C1 esterase inhibitor for acute antibody mediated rejection following kidney transplantation: results of a randomized doubleblind placebo-controlled pilot study. Am J Transplant. 2016;16:3468-78.
44. Shin BH, Everly MJ, Zhang H, Choi J, Vo A, Zhang X, et al. Impact of tocilizumab (anti-IL-6R) treatment on immunoglobulins and anti-HLA antibodies in kidney transplant patients with chronic antibody-mediated rejection. Transplantation. 2020;104(4):856-63.
45. Doberer K, Kläger J, Gualdoni GA, Mayer KA, Eskandary F, Farkash EA, et al. CD38 antibody daratumumab for the treatment of chronic active antibody-mediated kidney allograft rejection. Transplantation. 2021;105(2):451-7.
46. Burghuber CK, Manook M, Ezekian B, Gibby AC, Leopardi FV, Song M, et al. Dual targeting: combining costimulation blockade and bortezomib to permit kidney transplantation in sensitized recipients. Am J Transplant. 2019;19(3):724-36.
47. Jain D, Rajab A, Young JS, Yin D, Nadasdy T, Chong AS, et al. Reversing donor-specific antibody responses and antibodymediated rejection with bortezomib and belatacept in mice and kidney transplant recipients. Am J Transplant. 2020;20(10):2675-85.
48. Banham GD, Flint SM, Torpey N, Lyons PA, Shanahan DN, Gibson A, et al. Belimumab in kidney transplantation: an experimental medicine, randomised, placebo-controlled phase 2 trial. Lancet. 2018;391(10140):2619-30.

CHAPTER 11

Histopathology of Kidney Transplantation

Swarnalata Gowrishankar, Pallav Gupta

INTRODUCTION

Renal transplantation pathology is complex as the allograft biopsy is prone to immune reactions, notably rejections and nonimmune reactions, which are peculiar to the graft such as infections, drug toxicity, and donor and recurrent disease. Besides, all conditions which affect the native kidney can theoretically affect the graft. It is for all the above reasons that the interpretation of a graft biopsy needs to be systematic and a correlation with all the clinical findings and investigations is necessary to come to a right diagnosis and for the management to maintain renal function.

BANFF SCHEMA

The first international meeting was held in 1991 at Banff in Canada to standardize the nomenclature for reporting renal allograft biopsies. These meetings have been christened the Banff meetings and have subsequently held every 2 years across the world, and our understanding of graft pathology in general and rejections in particular has evolved with discussions and publications arising out of these meetings.[1] The schema is unique in that the criteria are based on consensual discussion, scientific studies, and continues to remain modern and updated.[1,2]

APPROACH TO ALLOGRAFT BIOPSY INTERPRETATION

The Banff criteria for adequacy are 10 glomeruli and two arteries. However, valuable information can be obtained from even smaller biopsies. While the cortical tissue is essential for diagnosing rejections confidently, the renal medulla is useful in the diagnosis of polyomavirus nephropathy (PVN), granulomatous inflammation, recurrent/de novo disease such as crystalline nephropathy, amyloid, monoclonal deposition disease, medullary angiitis, and SV40 and C4d immunohistochemistry (IHC) can be reported confidently even in medullary tissue.

The changes in the four compartments which are of particular importance in renal allograft biopsies are listed below:

1. *Glomeruli:* Glomerulitis, fibrin thrombi, and basement membrane duplication or transplant glomerulopathy **(Figs. 1A to C)**.
2. *Tubules:* Tubular injury including cytoplasmic vacuolation, viral cytopathic changes, tubulitis **(Fig. 1D)**, crystals within lumina, and tubular atrophy.
3. *Interstitium:* Interstitial edema, inflammation including the type of inflammatory cells, granuloma, any unusual or atypical lymphoid infiltrate, interstitial fibrosis, and striped fibrosis.
4. *Vessels:* Arteriolar hyalinosis in particular, whether it is peripheral and nodular, thrombotic microangiopathy (TMA), endarteritis **(Fig. 1E)**, peritubular capillaritis **(Fig. 1F)**, and arteriosclerosis.

The above morphologic changes are graded 1 to 3 using objective criteria and these are listed in **Table 1**.

ANCILLARY TESTS ON A RENAL BIOPSY

- C4d staining by immunofluorescence (IF) or IHC is mandatory in all allograft biopsies, even if the biopsy includes only medullary tissue.
- Direct IF with the full battery of antibodies is mandated in cases with proteinuria or suspected recurrent disease.
- *Electron microscopy (EM):* Ideally, this is recommended in all 'for cause' biopsies ≥3 months post-transplant and all biopsies ≥6 months post-transplant, to detect early transplant glomerulopathy, a manifestation of an antibody-mediated rejection (ABMR). Biopsies in which the light microscopy (LM) and IF study suspect a glomerular disease are again benefitted by an EM study. The guidelines and the recommendations for reporting are tabled in the Banff 2019 paper.[3]
- *Banff scores:* The scores are semiquantitatively graded from 0 to 3 according to the severity and are enlisted in **Table 2**. They lend an objectivity to the analysis and these

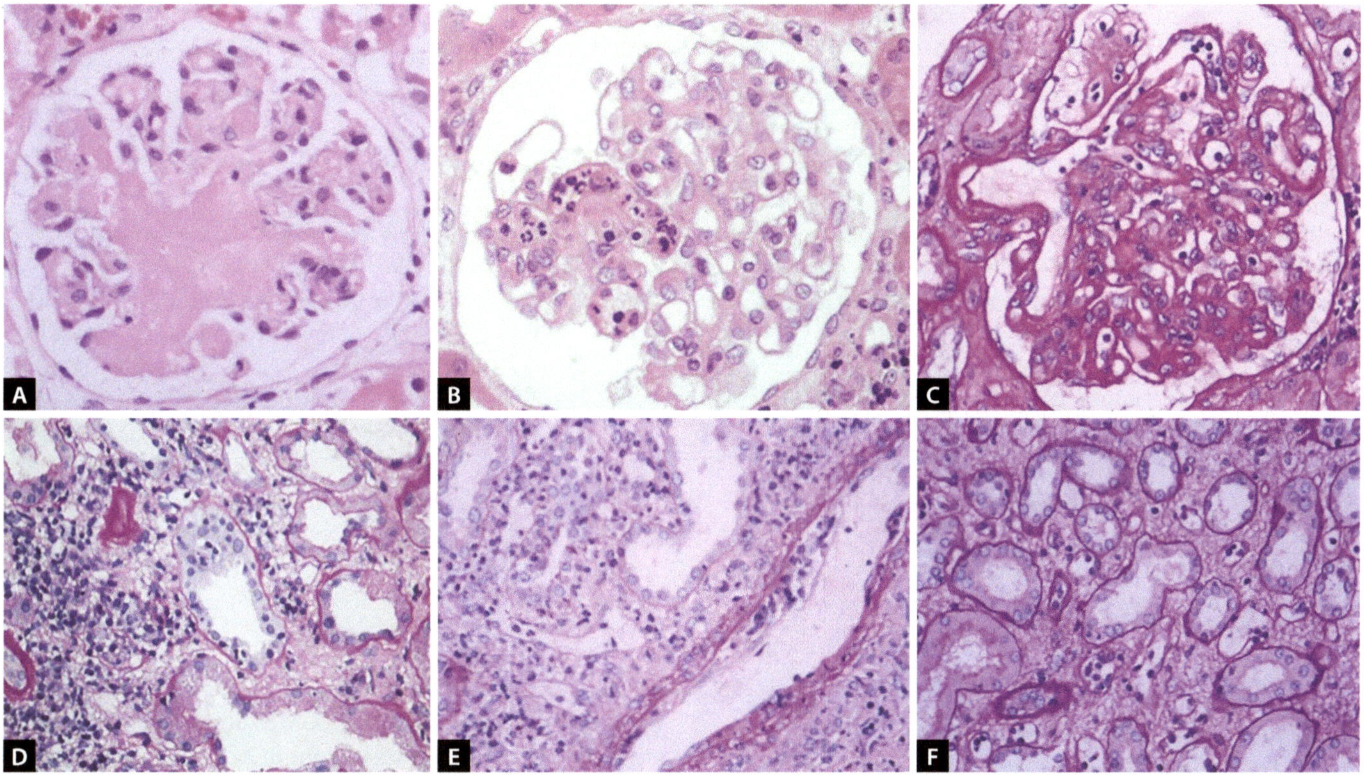

Figs. 1A to F: Changes seen in rejection. (A) [Hematoxylin and eosin (H&E) 400×] Glomerulus with a creeping thrombus obliterating the capillary lumina; (B) (H&E 400×) Segmental glomerulitis with swelling of the endothelium and an infiltrate of neutrophils and lymphomononuclear cells obliterating the capillary lumen; (C) [Periodic acid–Schiff (PAS) 400×] Transplant glomerulopathy with glomerulitis and a thickening and duplication of the capillary basement membrane; (D) (PAS 200×) Tubulitis with lymphocytes infiltrating the tubular epithelium: (E) (PAS 200×) Endarteritis with a subendothelial infiltrate of lymphomononuclear cells, protruding into the vascular lumen; (F) (PAS 200×) Peritubular capillary (PTC) dilatation and cells within the capillaries indicating peritubular capillaritis.

TABLE 1: Description of Banff scores.

Lesion	*Definition*	*Short form*	*Score 0*	*Score 1*	*Score 2*	*Score 3*
Glomerulitis (number of glomeruli involved)	Endothelial swelling with an infiltration of mononuclear cells and/or neutrophils within a capillary lumen of the tuft	g	None	≤25%	26–50%	>50%
Interstitial inflammation	Percentage of the nonscarred area of cortex with inflammatory cells	i	<10%	10–25%	26–50%	>50%
Tubulitis	No of lymphocytes between tubular epithelial cells or between the tubular lining and basement membrane. Very atrophic tubules to be excluded	t	None	1–4	5–10	>10
Endarteritis	Percentage of lumen occluded by subendothelial inflammation	v	None	<25%	≥25%	Transmural necrosis
Transplant glomerulopathy	GBM double contours in the maximally involved glomerulus	cg	None	<25% (LM)*	26–50%	>50%
Interstitial fibrosis	Percentage of atrophic tubules in the cortex	ci	≤5%	6–25%	26–50%	>50%
Tubular atrophy	Percentage of atrophic cortical tubules	ct	None	≤25%	26–50%	>50%
Fibrous intimal thickening	Percentage of narrowing of luminal area by intimal fibrosis without elastosis, may have inflammatory cells away from the intima	cv	None	<25%	26–50%	>50%
Mesangial matrix widening	Intercapillary width is more than two-cell diameter in at least two lobules; graded according to the percentage of nonsclerosed glomeruli involved	mm	None	<25%	26–50%	>50%

Contd...

Contd...

Lesion	Definition	Short form	Score 0	Score 1	Score 2	Score 3
Total inflammation	Percentage of entire cortex, scarred and nonscarred occupied by inflammatory cells	ti	<10%	11–25%	26–50%	>50%
Inflammation in atrophic areas	Percentage of scarred area occupied by inflammatory cells	i-IFTA	<10%	11–25%	26–50%	>50%
Peritubular capillaritis	Maximum leukocytes in a capillary with >10% of PTC having at least one leukocyte	ptc	<3	3–4	5–10	>10
Arteriolar hyalinosis	PAS positive arteriolar hyaline thickening	ah	None	Mild to moderate in ≥1	Moderate to severe in >1	Severe in many
Hyaline arteriolar thickening	Peripheral nodular hyalinosis	aah	None	Noncircum-ferential in one vessel	Noncircum-ferential in many vessels	Circum-ferential in one vessel
C4d (by IHC)	Percentage of PTCs with circumferential linear staining, cortex, and medulla	C4d	None	<10%	10–50%	>50%

*By electron microscopy (EM), duplication observed in more than one loop is scored 1a.
(GBM: glomerular basement membrane; IHC: immunohistochemistry; LM: light microscopy; PAS: periodic acid–Schiff; PTC: peritubular capillary)

TABLE 2: Banff categories.[2]

Category 1	When the biopsy is normal or the changes are nonspecific and do not fit into any of the categories below
Category 2	Antibody-mediated rejection (ABMR)
Category 3	Suspicious (borderline) for acute rejection
Category 4	T-cell-mediated rejection (TCMR)
Category 5	IFTA (interstitial fibrosis and tubular atrophy) This is divided into mild (ci1 and/or ct1), moderate (ci2 and/or ct2), and severe (ci3 and/or ct3). *Note:* An underlying cause for the IFTA needs to be always searched for by correlating with the other histologic, IF, and EM findings; clinical details and other investigations including imaging before a case is diagnosed as IFTA of no special type
Category 6	All other changes which are considered not rejected are in this category. The important conditions include acute tubular injury, infections including polyomavirus nephropathy (PVN), drug toxicity including that due to CNI, and recurrent and de novo renal disease

(CNI: calcineurin inhibitor; EM: electron microscopy; IF: immunofluorescence)

scores in turn determine the types and grades of rejection. They can also be used to objectively analyze the response to therapy and progress of the lesions in repeat biopsies.[2-4]

DIAGNOSIS AND CLASSIFICATION OF REJECTIONS

The renal biopsy remains the gold standard for diagnosing rejections. The criteria for diagnosing and typing rejections have been laid out in the Banff schema:[2-4]

- *T cell-mediated rejections (TCMR):*[5,6] These can be borderline, suspicious of TCMR, acute or chronic active.
- *Borderline changes suspicious of TCMR:* This is diagnosed when the criteria for TCMR mentioned below are not met.
- *Acute TCMR:* This is graded into type I (A and B) and type II. The presence of endarteritis will upgrade the rejection to type II irrespective of the grade of interstitial inflammation and tubulitis.
  - *IA:* Interstitial inflammation (i2 or i3) and moderate tubulitis (t2)
  - *IB:* Interstitial inflammation (i2 or i3) and severe tubulitis (t3)
  - *IIA:* Any grade of interstitial inflammation and tubulitis with mild endarteritis (v1)
  - *IIB:* Any grade of interstitial inflammation and tubulitis with moderate endarteritis (v2)
  - *III:* Any grade of interstitial inflammation and tubulitis with severe transmural arteritis (v3)
- *Isolated "v" lesions:* This refers to the presence of endarteritis without tubulointerstitial inflammation. This can be considered as ABMR when C4d positive and TCMR when the diagnostic criteria for ABMR are not met.

Chronic Active T Cell-mediated Rejection

- *Grade IA:* Total inflammation at least moderate (ti ≥ 2), moderate inflammation in atrophic areas (i-IFTA ≥ 2) and moderate tubulitis (t2)
- *Grade IB:* Total inflammation at least moderate (ti ≥ 2), moderate inflammation in atrophic areas (i-IFTA ≥ 2) and severe tubulitis (t3)
- *Grade II:* Presence of transplant arteriopathy (arterial intimal thickening and fibrosis with or without leukocytes occluding the lumina).

Antibody-mediated Rejection[5,6]

This can be active, chronic active, or chronic. For each of the above, there are three sets of criteria and at least one criterion from each set needs to be fulfilled to give a definitive diagnosis.

Active Antibody-mediated Rejection

Note: The terminology in ABMR is active while that in TCMR is acute for the reason that ABMR is not always acute in presentation.

Criterion 1: Evidence of injury mediated by antibody, which can be in the form of:

- Microvascular inflammation, namely glomerulitis and/or peritubular capillaritis
- Endarteritis (*Note:* Endarteritis can also be seen in TCMR.)
- TMA, in the absence of other causes
- Tubular injury, in the absence of other causes.

Criterion 2: Evidence that the injury was indeed mediated by antibody

- C4d positivity by IF or IHC (*Note:* As IF is more sensitive, a score of >0 is considered positive on IHC and a score >1 for IF.)
- Moderate microvascular inflammation (g + ptc score ≥ 2 with none being 0). (*Note:* This criterion can be used when C4d is negative, but there should be no evidence of recurrent or de novo disease, borderline or acute TCMR, or infection.)
- Increased expression of genes which are upregulated in ABMR. This should be a validated assay. [*Note:* These assays are ribonucleic acid (RNA)-based assays on renal biopsies and for practical purposes, there is no laboratory in India which offers a validated assay at present.]

Criterion 3: Demonstration of the antibody

- *Donor-specific antibody (DSA):* This can be anti-human leukocyte antigen (HLA) or non-HLA antibodies directed against the graft.
- *C4d positivity:* As C4d positivity is a very strong indicator of the presence of antibody at the site of reaction, the requirement for checking for DSA has been dispensed with, when C4d is positive.
- Increased expression of validated gene transcripts (if this test is available and increased expression of a set of validated genes is demonstrated, then ABMR can be diagnosed even if C4d and DSA are negative).

Chronic Active Antibody-mediated Rejection

Here, the injury is presumed to be due to persistent antibodies and the pattern of injury is chronic and different from that in active ABMR. Criteria 2 and 3 remain the same as above.

Criterion 1: Evidence of chronic injury mediated by antibodies, which can be in the form of:

- Transplant glomerulopathy by LM or EM. Cases of chronic TMA due to other causes are excluded.
- PTC basement membrane multilayering, demonstrated on EM (seven or more layers in one capillary and five or more layers in two more)
- Arterial intimal fibrosis of new onset

Criterion 2: Same as above

Criterion 3: Same as above

Note: In practice, a C4d-negative ABMR (active or chronic active) diagnosis is made when the histologic changes are present, but C4d is negative and DSA is positive at the time of biopsy.

A diagnosis of chronic active ABMR can be confusing as it gives treating physicians limited information on appropriate treatment options. The diagnostic line could therefore read "chronic active ABMR with (mild/moderate/severe) activity and (mild/moderate/severe) chronicity" and include the Banff lesion scores in the text of the diagnostic line.

Chronic ABMR (no active in the name): This diagnosis can be made when there is evidence of chronic injury (criterion 1 of chronic active ABMR above), negative C4d, with a prior documented diagnosis of active/chronic active ABMR, or a prior DSA positivity.

The findings in the various forms of rejection, CNI toxicity and polyoma virus nephropathy are summarized in **Table 3**.

MOLECULAR DIAGNOSTICS[7,8]

Conventional pathology with IF and EM is a pattern-based diagnosis and, while helpful and forming the backbone for diagnosis of rejections presently, does not always meet the demand for precise and mechanism-based diagnosis. As in the field of oncopathology, molecular techniques are rapidly evolving.

Molecular classifier systems have been developed for TCMR where the molecular phenotype involves T-cell effector mechanisms, namely granzymes, perforin, γ-interferon, etc., and the inflammatory molecules CXCL9, 10, 11, etc., and for the ABMR phenotype, where molecular transcripts involving endothelial and natural killer (NK) cell activation predominate. The molecular analysis will find a special use in borderline rejections (TCMR vs. no TCMR), isolated "v" lesions (ABMR vs. TCMR vs. no rejection), PVN (with/without TCMR), ABMR with absent C4d or absent C4d and DSA (ABMR vs. no ABMR), and C4d positivity without any changes (ABMR vs. no ABMR).

These molecular tests are expensive, sophisticated, and require an elaborate validation before they can be in routine use. But a combination of these and the conventional tests offers a promise of improved diagnostics with personalized therapy regimens and improved long-term outcome for transplant recipients.

TABLE 3: Summary of the changes seen in the four compartments of the kidney in various conditions.

Compartment	*A-TCMR*	*CA-TCMR*	*A-AMR*	*CA-AMR*	*PVN*	*CNI toxicity*
Glomeruli	Glomerulitis±	Glomerulitis±	Glomerulitis thrombi	Glomerulitis thrombi Transplant glomerulopathy	*	Thrombi, mesangial widening, segmental sclerosis, collapsing GN
Tubules	Tubulitis (≥t2)	Tubulitis (≥t2)	*	*	Viral cytopathic changes, tubulitis, calcification	Isometric vacuoles
Interstitium	Inflammation (≥i2)	Fibrosis inflammation In atrophic areas (≥i-IFTA ≥ 2)	*	*	Plasma cell-rich inflammation, fibrosis	Striped fibrosis
Vessels	Endarteritis	Endarteritis, transplant arteriopathy	Endarteritis, thrombotic microangiopathy	Endarteritis, thrombotic microangiopathy, transplant arteriopathy	*	Thrombotic microangiopathy, smooth muscle vacuoles, peripheral nodular hyalinosis

*Changes can occur but are not specific.

(A-AMR: active antibody-mediated rejection; A-TCMR: acute T cell-mediated rejection; CA-AMR: chronic active antibody-mediated rejection; CA-TCMR: chronic active T cell-mediated rejection; CNI: calcineurin inhibitor; GN: glomerulonephritis; i-IFTA: inflammation in areas of interstitial fibrosis and tubular atrophy; PVN: polyomavirus nephropathy)

ABO-INCOMPATIBLE GRAFT[9,10]

Diagnosis of rejection in the ABO-incompatible (ABOi) graft: ABO antigens are present in the endothelium and distal tubules of the kidneys. ABO antibodies occur "naturally" and are of the immunoglobulin G (IgG) and immunoglobulin M (IgM) isotypes. Pretransplant removal of circulating ABO antibodies has made ABOi transplants possible. A minority of patients develop ABMR due to anti-ABO-Ab (4–30%), with the risk being greatest in the first 3 weeks. A2 blood group allografts are less vulnerable to rejection. The pathologic features are similar to anti-HLA ABMR. Simultaneous development of ABMR due to anti-HLA Ab is rare. 94% of ABOi grafts continue to be C4d positive even at the end of 1 year, without inflammation and are considered to be a form of accommodation and occurs due to a lack of Fc receptors for the dominant IgM isotype of blood group antigens. Hence, donor-specific antibodies need to be demonstrated in an ABOi graft for the diagnosis of ABMR.

Nonhuman Leukocyte Antigen Antibodies[11-13]

Human leukocyte antigen incompatibility is the major driver of alloantibody response. Presence of HLA–DSA is a key diagnostic criterion. ABMR can, however, occur in the absence of detectable HLA–DSA in 30–45% and can even occur in HLA-identical twins. Non-HLA antibodies are directed against polymorphic antigens expressed on endothelial cells, basement membrane, and extracellular matrix which are expressed in allograft injury and which differ between the donor and the recipient. Of these, antibodies to angiotensin type I receptor expressed on multiple cell types including endothelial cells are the best studied. These antibodies have also been shown to directly stimulate peripheral mononuclear cells to release proinflammatory cytokines and chemokines. What this means is that these reactions while akin to anti-HLA antibody-mediated ABMR morphologically can be C4d negative. They are believed to also act in synergy with the anti-HLA antibodies. In the future, we can expect commercially available solid-phase assays to detect non-HLA antibodies, especially where the usual donor-specific HLA antibodies are negative, and they would also influence the type of treatment including specific targeted therapies.

CASE VIGNETTE 1

*A 40-year-old male with native kidney disease of immunoglobulin A (IgA) nephropathy, and a spousal donor, presented with a raised serum creatinine of 1.6 mg/dL, 4.5 months post-transplant. There was a history of decrease in mycophenolate dosage due to leukopenia **(Figs. 2A to D)**.*

CASE VIGNETTE 2

*A 45-year-old woman, 2 years post-live related transplant presented with fluctuating s. creatinine between 1.4 and 1.8 mg/dL. She had a history of biopsy proven ABMR 6 months post-transplant and COVID-19 infection 3 weeks prior to this biopsy **(Figs. 3A to F)**.*

CALCINEURIN INHIBITOR TOXICITY[14-17]

Calcineurin inhibitor (CNI) toxicity includes toxicity due to cyclosporin and tacrolimus and can produce characteristic changes due to epithelial, endothelial, and smooth muscle injury. The toxicity can be functional due to afferent arteriolar

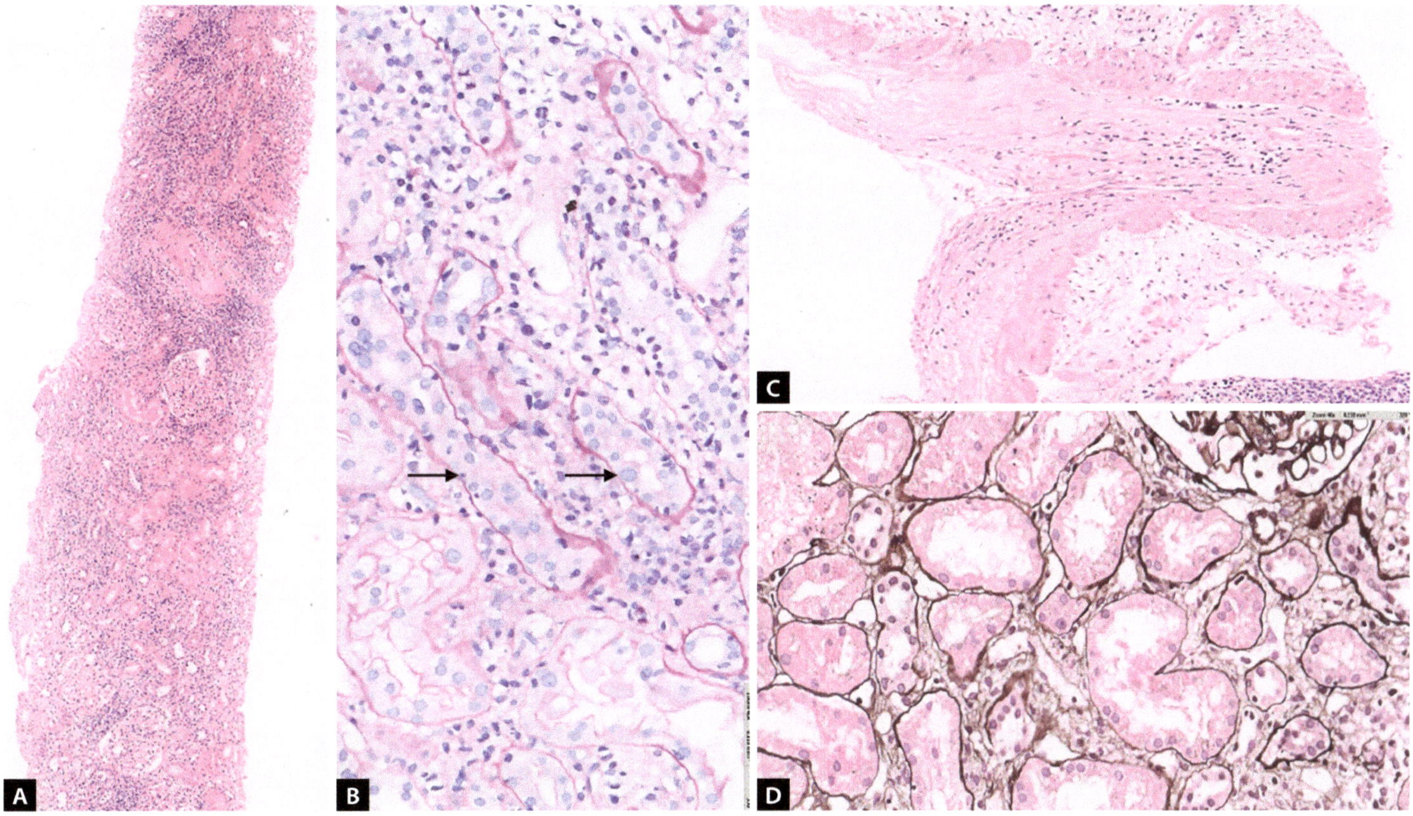

Figs. 2A to D: (A) A significant interstitial inflammation exceeding 25%. Moderate tubulitis is indicated by arrows in (B), significant endarteritis partially occluding the vascular lumen in (C), and there no peritubular capillaritis in (D). C4d was negative. The diagnosis in this case is acute TCMR, type IB.

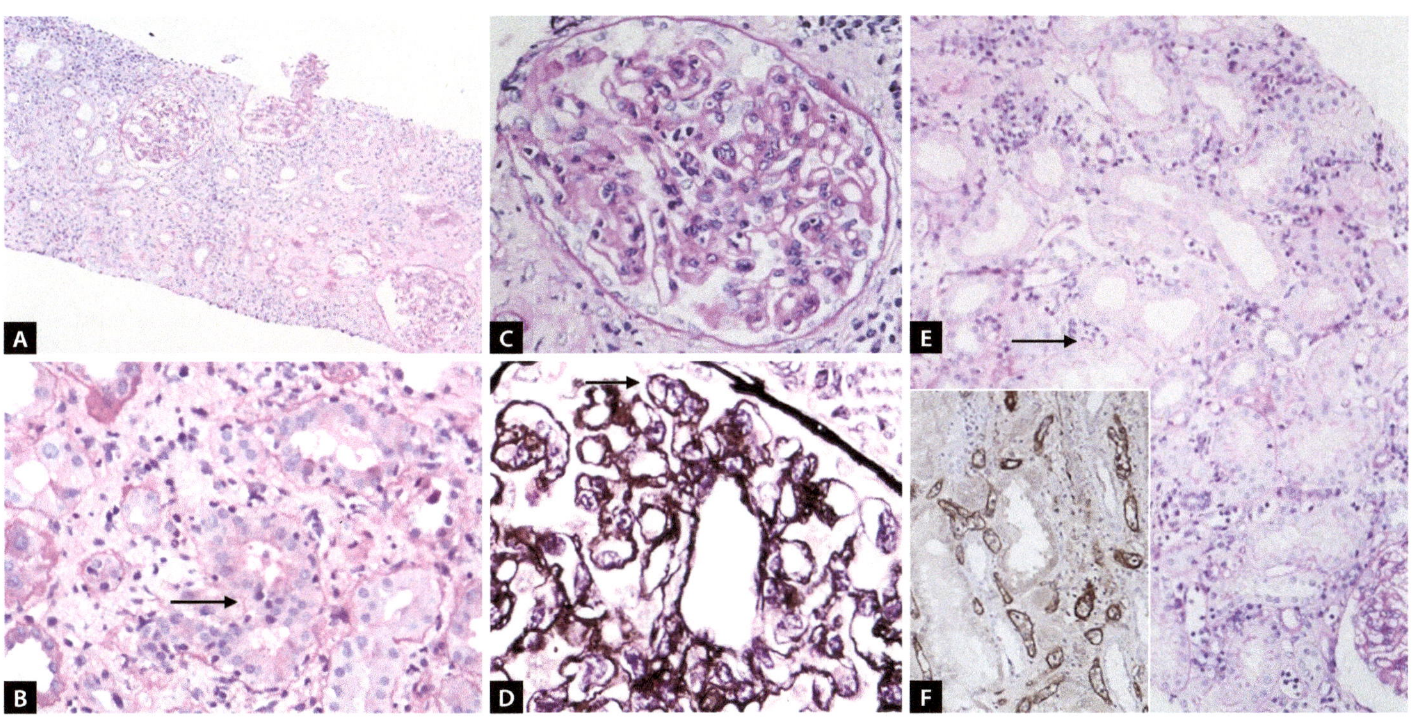

Figs. 3A to F: (A) Significant interstitial inflammation and (B) moderate tubulitis fulfilling the criteria for TCMR IA. However, there is also microvascular inflammation as the glomeruli show glomerulitis (C) and early transplant glomerulopathy as evinced by basement membrane duplication (D), and peritubular capillaritis (E). C4d is strongly positive (F) and so this is a case of combined chronic active TCMR, type IA, and chronic active ABMR.

vasoconstriction, and this produces no changes or it can be structural which can be acute or chronic.

Acute toxicity in the tubules manifests as isometric proximal tubular vacuolization, intratubular microcalcification, and acute tubular injury. In the vessels, changes of a TMA [fibrin thrombi, fragmented red blood cells (RBCs), intimal myxoid change, and onion-skinning or myointimal hyperplasia], smooth muscle dropout, and vacuolization in the arteriolar wall with separation of the myocytes are manifestations.

Chronic toxicity is seen as striped fibrosis, namely radial fibrosis of the corticomedullary rays interspersed with nonscarred areas. In the vessels, the necrosed outer media is replaced by hyaline forming peripheral nodular hyalinosis or the "chain of pearls" appearance. Glomerular changes include double contours of the basement membrane due to chronic TMA, ischemic change, global and segmental glomerulosclerosis, and collapsing glomerulopathy (***See* Table 1**).

While none of the above changes is pathognomonic of CNI toxicity, combined tubular and vascular changes on a biopsy increase the probability of CNI toxicity. These changes are also often focal, and hence a study of step sections is important. As some of the chronic changes are attributed to immunologic injury, some authors have questioned the existence of a chronic CNI toxicity **(Figs. 4A to E)**.

CASE VIGNETTE 3

A 32-year-old female, native kidney disease being IgA nephropathy, with donor being sister with a full-house HLA match, on tacrolimus, mycophenolate mofetil (MMF), and steroids had a rise in serum creatinine from 1.2 to 1.6 on third post-transplant day ***(Figs. 5A to D)****.*

GLOMERULONEPHRITIS FOLLOWING RENAL TRANSPLANTATION

Glomerulonephritis following renal transplantation can be

- Recurrent glomerulonephritis
- De novo glomerulonephritis.

Recurrent Glomerulonephritis

- Both primary and secondary glomerulonephritis can reoccur.
- Clinical manifestations of recurrent glomerulonephritis are the same as those of native disease.
- Recurrence can be seen in between 10 and 20% of the renal transplant recipients.
- Allograft failure due to recurrent glomerular diseases can be seen in ~20% patients.

De Novo Glomerulonephritis

- De novo glomerulonephritis usually develops several years after the transplantation.

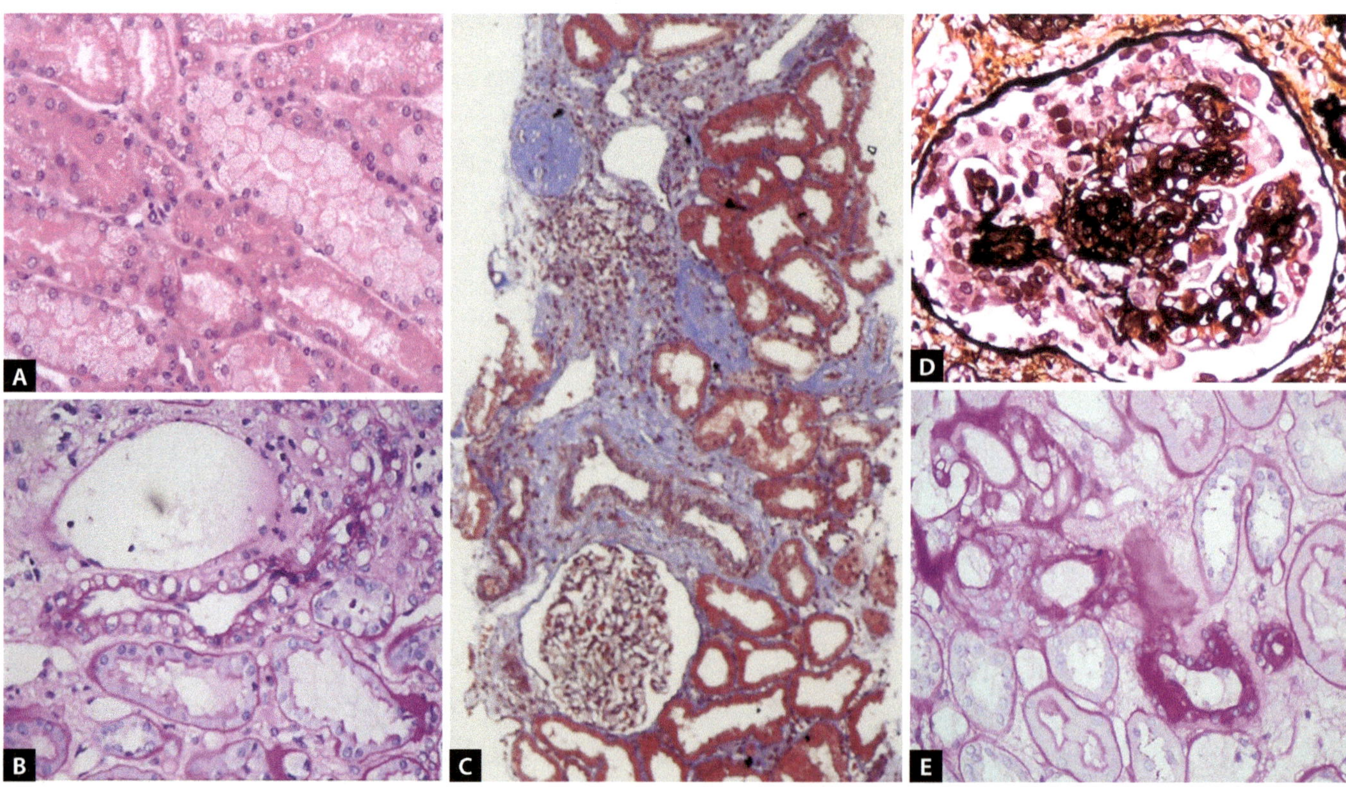

Figs. 4A to E: Spectrum of calcineurin inhibitor toxicity. (A) [Hematoxylin and eosin (H&E) 100×] Fine isometric vacuolation in proximal tubules; (B) (H&E 100×) Vacuolation of the myocytes in an arteriole; (C) (Mason trichrome 100×) A zone of "striped" fibrosis with nonscarred cortex on either side; (D) (Jones silver 400×) Collapsing glomerulopathy with collapse of the tuft and hyperplasia of the overlying podocytes; (E) [Periodic acid–Schiff (PAS) 100×] Peripheral nodular hyalinosis in an arteriole.

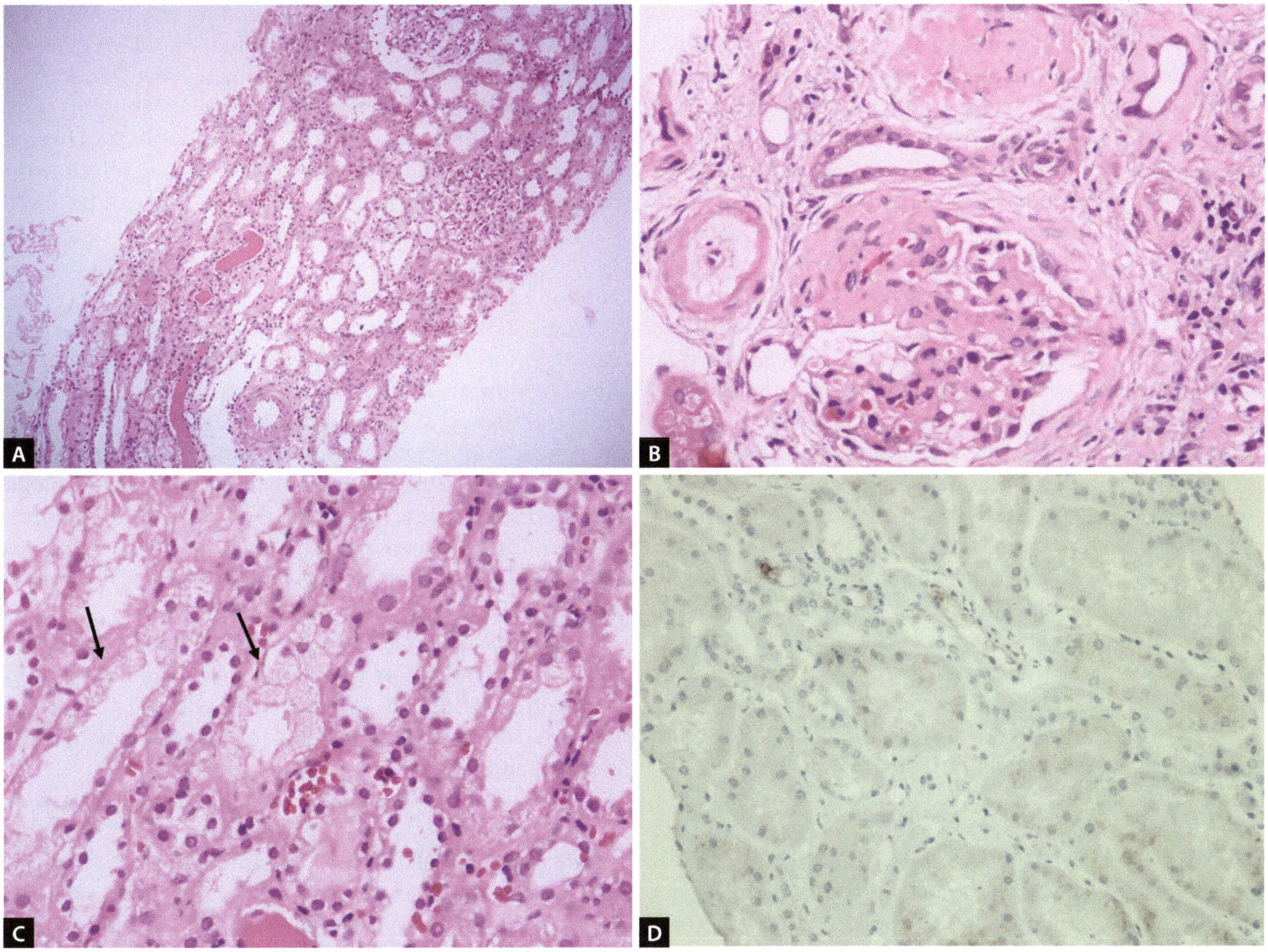

Figs. 5A to D: (A) Tubular dilatation and injury with no significant interstitial inflammation are shown; (B) One glomerulus with an intraglomerular thrombus and the small vessel to the left prominent intimal myxoid change with partial luminal occlusion; (C) Fine isometric tubular vacuolization of the proximal tubules is noted. C4d immune stain in (D) is negative. This combination of tubular changes and endothelial injury with negative C4d makes it likely to be an acute CNI toxicity. With a decrease in tacrolimus dosage, there was a reversion of renal function to normal.

- It is unrelated to disease in native kidney biopsy.
- Glomerular hyperfiltration, nephron loss, and exposure of cryptic podocyte antigens contribute to the development of de novo glomerulonephritis.

All forms of glomerulonephritis can reoccur after renal transplantation.[18] The rate of recurrence of glomerulonephritis following transplantation ranges from 10 to 20% in various studies.[19-21] It can account for 8–20% of graft failures on long-term follow-up and is the third most common cause of graft loss after chronic rejections and death.[22-24] In one study, incidence of allograft glomerulonephritis was 5.2% at 1 year, 21.7% at 5 years, and 42.3% at 10 years post-transplantation.[25] Centers performing protocol biopsies pick up recurrent glomerulonephritis early as it may remain clinically silent for many years. Also, histology of early recurrent glomerulonephritis can be different from more advanced form of disease diagnosed on native biopsies.[25]

Immunoglobulin A nephropathy is the most common recurrent glomerulonephritis in renal transplant recipients followed by focal segmental glomerulosclerosis (FSGS) and immune complex-mediated membranoproliferative glomerulonephritis (MPGN), and membranous nephropathy.[22,25] Patients with a diagnosis of C3 glomerulopathy (formerly MPGN type II) undergoing renal transplants can show recurrence in 50–70% cases with evidence of early graft loss.[22,26] Time to reoccurrence is shorter for patients with FSGS as compared to patients with IgA nephropathy.[26] FSGS recurrence can be seen in 30–40% of the patients post-transplantation, recurrence being higher in patients younger in age and those with higher levels of proteinuria prior to transplantation. It is also higher among those in whom time to progression of FSGS to end-stage renal disease (ESRD) is shorter in the pretransplant period, biopsies with diffuse mesangial hypercellularity, and those with collapsing variant of FSGS.[27,28] The IgA nephropathy recurrence rate ranges from 8 to 50% with a higher number of recurrences reported by centers performing protocol biopsies. Similar to risk factors for recurrent FSGS, IgA nephropathy recurrence is more common in patients with younger age at transplantation, those with higher levels of proteinuria, and rapid progression of native disease in the pretransplant period. Other factors which are thought to play a role in recurrence include type of donor (recurrence in living donor being higher as compared to deceased donor).[29] Some studies also claim reduced recurrence rates in ABOi renal transplants.[30] Patients with recurrent IgA nephropathy can have no to minimal mesangial hypercellularity with infrequent presence of crescents. IF will show typical mesangial IgA deposits as seen in native biopsies.[31,32] MEST scores can be applied to recurrent IgA nephropathy cases as in native biopsies and would provide useful prognostic information.[33]

In early post-transplant period, cases of recurrent primary FSGS may not have demonstrable segmental sclerosis and shall have minimal change nephropathy like morphologic appearance.[34,35] Some studies have shown recurrences to be more common in collapsing and cellular variants, whereas others show similar recurrences for all histological variants of FSGS.[34-36] At the ultrastructural level, evolution of changes observed in recurrent FSGS is in the form of diffuse effacement of visceral epithelial cell foot process along with marked villous transformation followed by podocyte detachment, dropout, segmental sclerosis, and presence of glomerular capillary foam cells.[37]

In the spectrum of C3 glomerular diseases, dense deposit disease recurrence is more common in patients with presence of crescents in native biopsies. On IF, exclusive C3 deposits without significant immunoglobulin deposits can be seen in an intramembranous and mesangial pattern. Patients with dense deposit disease having crescent in recurrent disease have been shown to have early graft loss.[38,39] Recurrent C3 glomerulonephritis can present with a mesangioproliferative or membranoproliferative pattern with C3 deposits without immunoglobulin or minimal immunoglobulin deposit (trace to 1+). In one study, an average of 16% globally sclerosed glomeruli were present in biopsy at the time of recurrence.[26]

Membranoproliferative glomerulonephritis type I recurrence will show a membranoproliferative pattern as seen in native biopsies with some cases showing the presence of crescents. On IF, C3-dominant deposits are seen along the glomerular basement membrane (GBM) and mesangium accompanied by IgG deposits. It is important to differentiate MPGN type I from transplant glomerulopathy due to chronic antibody-mediated and cellular rejection and also from chronic CNI toxicity. In latter cases, no or minimum immune deposits will be seen and GBM can have multilayering on EM.[40]

Among the secondary glomerular diseases, lupus nephritis, TMA, anti-GBM nephritis, and rarely pauci-immune crescentic glomerulonephritis can show recurrence. Metabolic diseases including diabetic nephropathy, amyloidosis, oxalosis, and Fabry's disease have been shown to reoccur in grafts.[41,42]

De novo membranous nephropathy will have minimal morphological changes of glomerular capillary basement membranes and may show infrequent argyrophilic spikes but can have some increase in mesangial cellularity. On IF and EM, immune deposits (IgG) can be smaller and irregular in distribution and will show lack of phospholipase A2 receptor (PLA2r) expression, although C4d can be seen in deposits.[43-45] Some studies have documented the association with chronic active ABMR and presence of donor-specific antibodies in these patients.[43,45]

Anti-GBM necrotizing and crescentic glomerulonephritis can develop in post-transplant setting in patients with Alport syndrome. The morphological features are similar to what is observed in native anti-GBM disease.[46,47]

Autosomal recessive congenital nephrotic syndrome of Finnish type (*NPHS1* mutant) can lead to post-transplant nephrotic syndrome. Glomeruli may appear normal on LM with endothelial cell swelling evident on ultrastructural studies in the absence of any basement membrane abnormality.[48]

De novo FSGS can be seen late in the post-transplant period as a result of glomerular hyperfiltration injury and nephron loss or secondary to chronic CNI toxicity with perihilar variant being the common morphologic manifestation.[49]

De novo collapsing glomerulopathy has been described in association with cytomegalovirus (CMV) infections, parvovirus, and CNI toxicity.[50] De novo diabetic nephropathy has been seen in renal allograft several years after renal transplantation following the development of new-onset diabetes after renal transplantation (NODAT).[51] All the diseases occurring in native biopsies can also be seen in the form of de novo glomerular diseases post-transplant and can be associated with impaired graft function and long-term graft survival.[52]

CASE VIGNETTE 4

A 35-year-old male renal allograft recipient in 2014 on triple-drug immunosuppression came with complaints of rise in serum creatinine from 1.1 to 1.3 mg/dL and numerous RBCs on urine routine examination. Urine protein (P):creatinine (C) ratio was 0.53. Patient had biopsy-proven IgA nephropathy prior to renal transplantation. Renal biopsy was done ***(Figs. 6A and B)****.*

RENAL BIOPSY SUMMARY

- Minimal increase in mesangial cellularity in few glomeruli (MO), no endocapillary hyperplasia (E), no segmental sclerosis (S0), no tubular atrophy (T0), no crescents (C0)
- No tubulitis (t0), no interstitial inflammation (i0), no glomerulitis (g0), no peritubular capillaritis (ptc0), no arteritis (v0), no GBM double contour (cg0), no significant interstitial fibrosis and tubular atrophy (IFTA), no viral cytopathic changes

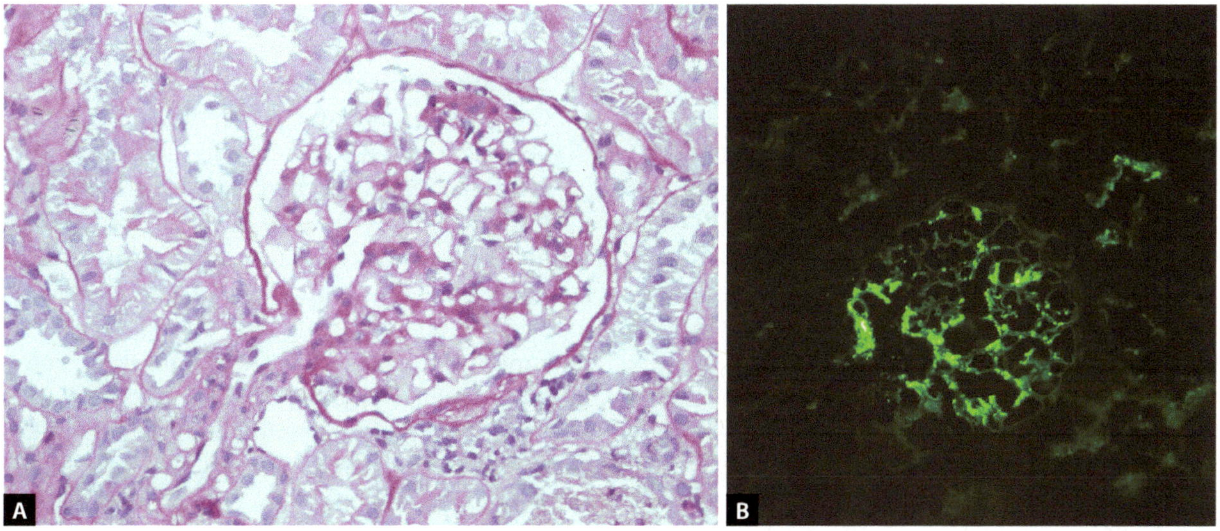

Figs. 6A and B: (A) Glomerulus showing minimal segmental increase in mesangial cellularity [periodic acid–Schiff (PAS), ×200 original magnification]; (B) Immunofluorescence showing mesangial granular immunoglobulin A (IgA) deposits [IgA, fluorescein isothiocyanate (FITC)].

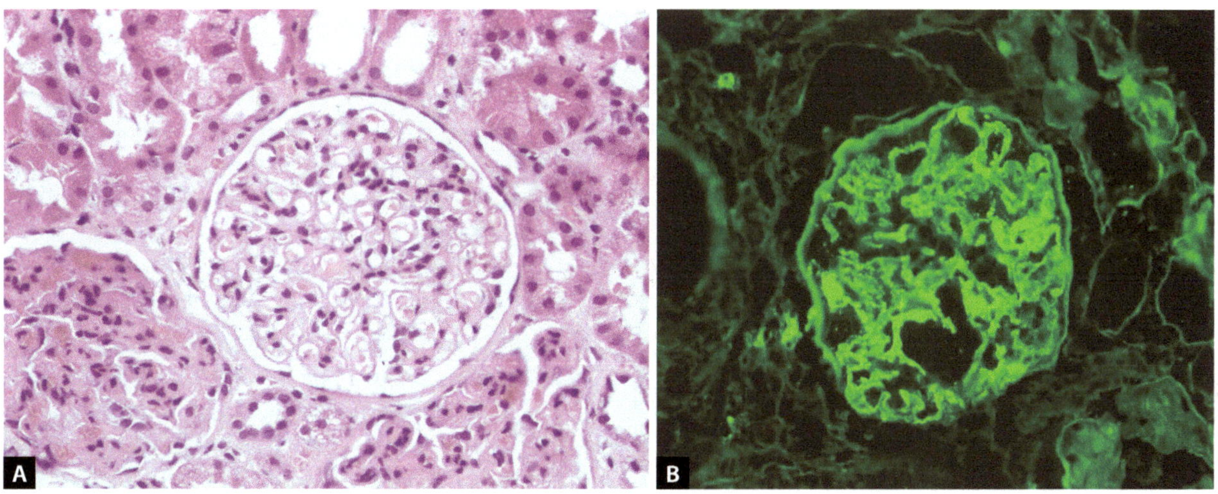

Figs. 7A and B: (A) Glomerulus showing thickening of glomerular capillary basement membrane [hematoxylin and eosin (H&E) stain, ×200 original magnification]; (B) Immunofluorescence showing discontinuous capillary wall granular IgG deposits [immunoglobulin G (IgG), fluorescein isothiocyanate (FITC)].

- C4d was negative in PTCs
- *On IF:* IgA (3+), C3 (1+), kappa (2+), lambda (3+) mesangial granular deposits. No capillary wall deposits were seen
- *Final diagnosis:* Recurrent IgA nephropathy

CASE VIGNETTE 5

A 28-year-male renal allograft recipient 8 years post-transplant presented with proteinuria (24-hour urine protein 3.2 g/day) with normal renal function (serum creatinine 0.9 mg/dL). Basic disease before renal transplantation was biopsy-proven FSGS. Renal biopsy was done ***(Figs. 7A and B)****.*

RENAL BIOPSY SUMMARY

- Mild thickening of glomerular capillary basement membrane, no definite argyrophilic spikes, no segmental sclerosis seen
- No glomerulitis (go), GBM double contour (cg0), tubulitis (to), interstitial inflammation (i0), peritubular capillaritis (ptc0), or arteritis (v0)
- C4d was negative in PTCs
- IF showed IgG (3+) granular deposits along GBM along with C3 (1+), kappa (3+), and lambda (3+)
- *Final diagnosis:* De novo membranous nephropathy

THROMBOTIC MICROANGIOPATHY AFTER RENAL TRANSPLANTATION

See Chapter 13.8.

POST-TRANSPLANT INFECTIONS OF THE RENAL ALLOGRAFT

Post-transplant infections of the renal allograft are important causes of graft dysfunction.

Most common infections affecting the renal allograft include:

- BK PVN
- CMV nephritis
- Adenoviral infections
- Acute pyelonephritis
- Fungal infections of renal allograft

BK PVN is the most common infection affecting the renal allograft post-transplantation affecting <1–20% of the allograft.[53-56] It is caused by reactivation of latent infection in donor kidneys. In majority of cases, it is confines to renal allograft, although urothelium can also be affected.[53,54]

Cytomegalovirus infections usually affect the renal allograft during the first 3 months post-transplantation and causes viral-induced tissue injury.[57]

Adenovirus infections are also seen in the early post-transplant period usually within the first 3 months post-transplantation.[58]

For acute pyelonephritis, most common causative pathogens implicated are *Escherichia coli* and *Klebsiella pneumoniae.*[59]

The most common invasive fungal infections affecting the renal allograft include mucormycosis, aspergillosis, and candidiasis. Other rare fungi infecting the renal allograft include cryptococcus and histoplasmosis.[60,61]

Renal Biopsy in Viral-induced Nephropathy Affecting Renal Allograft

BK Virus Nephropathy

Renal biopsy is diagnostic of BK virus (BKV) nephropathy. The viral cytopathic changes affect the tubular epithelial cell. In addition, they can also rarely affect the parietal epithelial cells of the glomeruli. The characteristic changes include the intranuclear inclusions which can be of four types:[53,54]

1. Ground-glass amorphous appearance of intranuclear inclusions is the most common type
2. Central inclusion surrounded by halo
3. Granular inclusions without a halo
4. Vesicular nuclei with irregular clumping of viral inclusions.

Based on the degree of viral replication and the extent of tubular injury induced by BK polyomavirus, it has been divided into three grades based on the Banff Working Group classification of definitive BK PVN.[1] Instead of the following grades, you could consider giving details of Banff PVN classes I, II, and III according to polyomavirus load (pvl) scores and the ci score:

- *Grade 1:* Minimal tubular injury and only a few intranuclear inclusions and no significant interstitial changes. Chiefly identified by performing IHC against SV40 large T-antigen.
- *Grade 2:* There are marked tubulointerstitial changes in the form of acute tubular injury, denudation of basement membrane of tubules, foci of tubulitis, interstitial lymphoplasmacytic infiltrate, and marked intranuclear inclusions.
- *Grade 3:* Chronic tubulointerstitial changes in the form of tubular atrophy and interstitial fibrosis are seen with focal viral replication and minimal inflammation.

Viral cytopathic changes can affect both renal cortical tubules and collecting ducts. In case of focal infections, medullary collecting ducts should be observed carefully for viral cytopathic changes. Varying degrees of cortical and medullary interstitial inflammation can be seen. Infiltrate is chiefly composed of lymphocytes, plasma cells, and macrophages and can be dominated by plasma cells. Nonnecrotizing granulomas can also be seen. Unlike the CMV infection, inflammatory cells, mesenchymal cells, and endothelial cells will not show viral cytopathic changes.[53-55]

Immunohistochemistry for antibody against SV40 large T-antigen helps in confirmation. Crisp intranuclear positivity (≥2 out of 4) indicates significant viral replication. An in situ hybridization technique can also be used. Another method is to employ antibodies directed against viral capsid antigens although it is less often used.[53,55]

In some cases, focal tubular basement membrane staining can be seen against immunoglobulins, complement C4d, and light chains, although the clinical significance of these is not well established.[62]

On EM, 30–40-nm viral particles are seen in the intranuclear location. These may sometimes be seen as crystalloid structures. The noninvasive method of detection of BK polyomavirus is by detecting three-dimensional viral aggregates (Haufen) on voided urine samples by EM.[63]

Cytomegalovirus Nephritis

Renal biopsy is important to identify viral cytopathic changes induced by CMV and thereby to confirm CMV nephritis. Proximal tubules, collecting ducts, and endothelial cells are primarily affected in the kidney. Both intranuclear and intracytoplasmic viral inclusions can be seen. The viral-induced changes can be patchy and focal in distribution. Nucleomegaly is seen with typical owl's eye appearance of intranuclear inclusion characterized by central round inclusion body surrounded by halo. Smudgy intranuclear homogeneous inclusions can be seen rarely. Cytoplasmic basophilic viral inclusions can be often seen in viral infected cells. Endothelial cells of the PTCs, blood vessels, and glomerular capillary endothelial cells can also show inclusions. Interstitium can show the presence of plasma cells, mononuclear cells, or granulomas and sometimes even microabscess.[64,65] TMA can be associated with CMV infection of the graft.[66]

Immunohistochemistry against early antigen of CMV helps in confirmation of diagnosis. EM will show enveloped virion with a central electron-dense core measuring around 150 nm.[64]

Adenoviral Nephritis

Tubulointerstitial compartment of kidney is primarily involved in adenovirus infection. Severe destruction of tubules with rupture of tubular basement membranes, polymorphonuclear infiltrate, and necrotizing tubulointerstitial inflammation is seen and gives a clue for diagnosis. Interstitium shows the presence of polymorphs, plasma cells, and often granulomas. Interstitial hemorrhage can also be seen. Smudge cells (adenovirus-infected tubular cells) are characterized by basophilic intranuclear central viral inclusions surrounded by halo or amorphous ground-glass inclusions.[67,68] Parietal epithelial cells of glomeruli can rarely show viral cytopathic changes. Blood vessels are not affected. IHC directed against the adenovirus antigens and EM will help in confirming the diagnosis. 70–80-nm virions can be seen in the inclusion-bearing tubular epithelial cells within the nuclei or the cytoplasm. EM done on urine samples of patients with adenovirus nephritis can show the presence of free viral particles. Hemorrhagic cystitis due to adenoviral infections is an important manifestation.[58,67-69]

ACUTE PYELONEPHRITIS

Morphology is the same as seen on the native kidneys. Intratubular neutrophils and neutrophilic casts can be seen along with interstitial polymorphonuclear infiltrate and edema. Medullary interstitium is commonly involved and should be carefully examined in cases of patchy diseases.[59,70,71]

Fungal Infections

Mucormycosis is characterized by broad ribbon-like aseptate hyphae. Angioinvasion is common in these fungi resulting in large areas of ischemic necrosis. *Aspergillus* infections have septate hyphae with parallel walls and acute angle branching. *Candida* is seen as budding yeast forms (3–8 μm) and pseudohyphae. Neutrophilic infiltration and formation of microabscesses are common in *Candida pyelonephritis*.[61]

CASE VIGNETTE 6

A 59-year-old female received live-related renal transplant in 2012. The patients disease was suspected to be chronic tubulo-interstitial nephritis. She received induction therapy with three doses of thymoglobulin at 0.9 mg/kg and triple-drug immunosuppression in the form of tacrolimus, MMF, and prednisolone. She received CMV prophylaxis with valganciclovir for 3 months and trimethoprim–sulfamethoxazole for 1 year. 2 years later, she developed rising serum creatinine (2.3 mg/dL) without any associated fever, dysuria, or decreased urine output. Renal biopsy was performed **(Figs. 8A and B).** BKV deoxyribonucleic acid (DNA) was identified in the serum—2,784,000 copies/mL.

RENAL BIOPSY SUMMARY

- No glomerulitis (g0), tubulitis (t0), peritubular capillaritis (ptc0), or intimal arteritis (v0)
- Mild interstitial lymphoplasmacytic infiltrate was seen (i1).
- Tubular epithelial cells showed nuclear enlargement with ground-glass intranuclear inclusions.

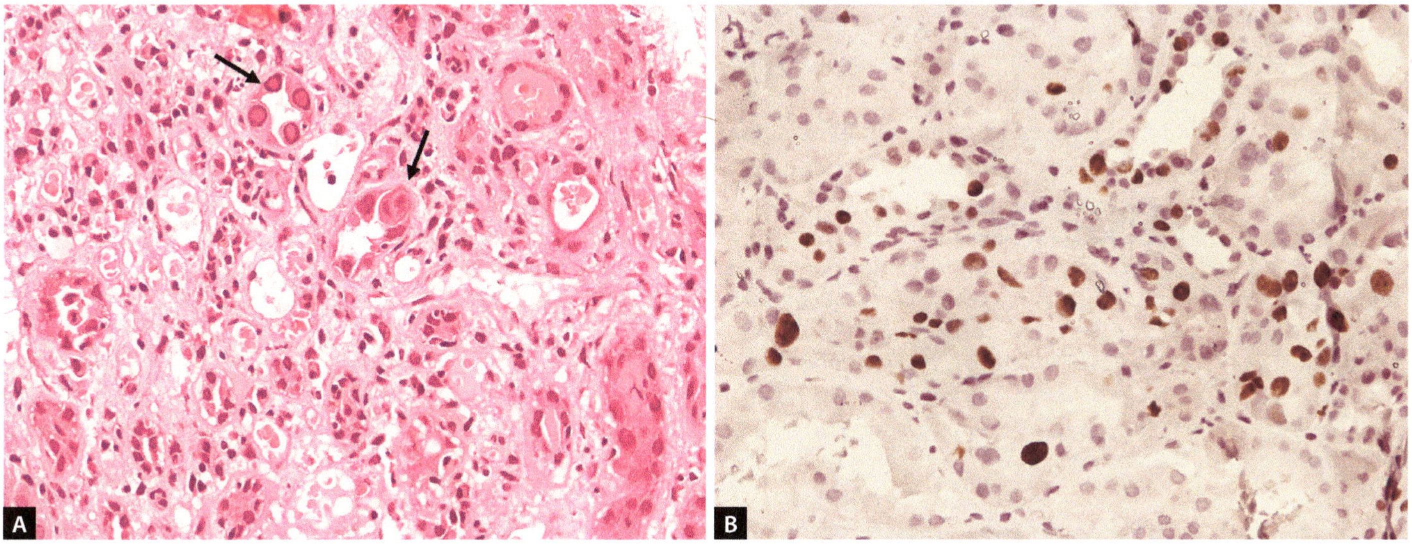

Figs. 8A and B: (A) Tubular epithelial cells showing nuclear enlargement with many ground-glass eosinophilic inclusions (hematoxylin and eosin stain ×200); (B) Immunohistochemistry shows positive staining for SV40 large T-antigen in many nuclei of tubular epithelial cells [immunohistochemistry (IHC) ×200].

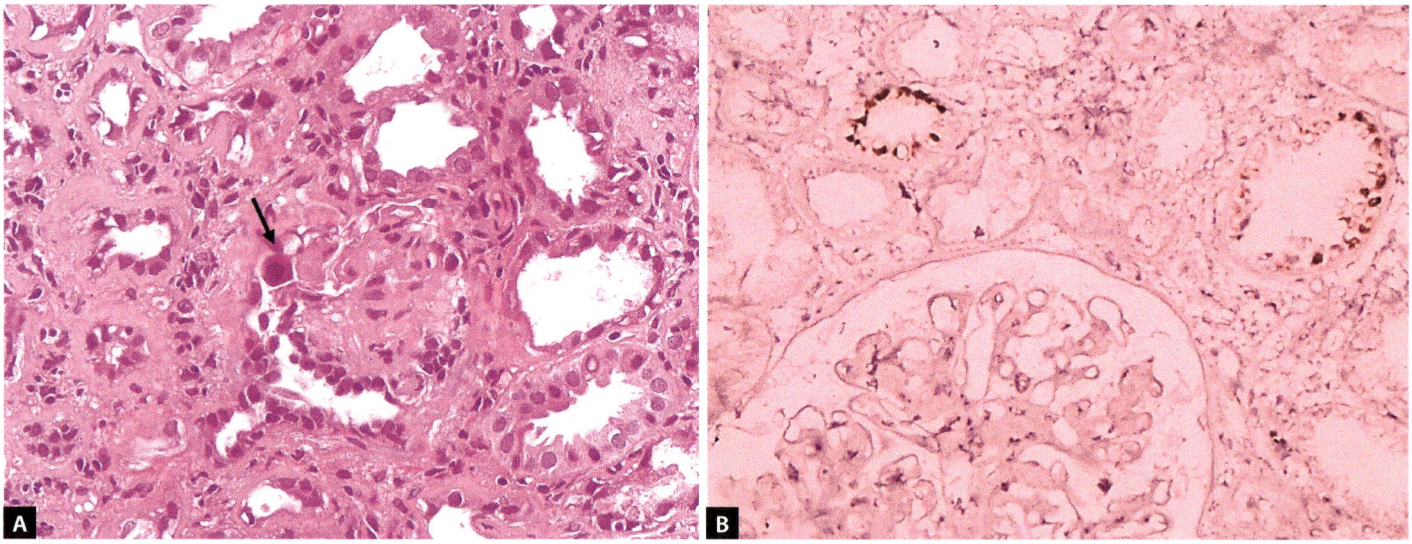

Figs. 9A and B: (A) Tubular epithelial cell showing nucleomegaly and cytomegaly with characteristic intranuclear inclusion (hematoxylin and eosin stain ×200); (B) Immunohistochemistry shows positive staining for cytomegalovirus (CMV) in many nuclei of tubular epithelial cells [immunohistochemistry (IHC) ×200].

- IHC for SV40 large T-antigen confirmed the diagnosis of BKV nephropathy.

CASE VIGNETTE 7

A 48-year-old female received live-related renal transplant in 2013 outside our hospital. The patient's basic disease was chronic glomerulonephritis. She was on triple-drug immunosuppression in the form of tacrolimus, MMF, and prednisolone. She had not received CMV prophylaxis. She presented with rising serum creatinine (2.1 mg/dL) 5 months post-transplant. Renal biopsy was performed ***(Figs. 9A and B).***

RENAL BIOPSY SUMMARY

- No glomerulitis (g0), peritubular capillaritis (ptc0), or intimal arteritis (v0)
- Mild interstitial lymphocytic infiltrate was seen (i1) and occasional focus of tubulitis was seen.
- Tubular epithelial cells showed intranuclear inclusions.
- IHC for CMV confirmed the diagnosis of CMV nephritis.

CASE VIGNETTE 8

A 50-year-old male, live-related renal transplant recipient on triple-drug immunosuppression presented with fever and nonfunctioning graft with raised total leukocyte count. Ultrasonography (USG) showed enlarged kidney with perigraft collection. Computed tomography (CT) showed enlarged kidney with multiple low-density areas. The patient underwent graft nephrectomy ***(Figs. 10A and B).***

GRAFT NEPHRECTOMY SUMMARY

- Large areas of ischemic coagulative necrosis involving cortex and medulla
- Ghost outlines of renal tubules and glomeruli were seen.
- Ribbon-like nonseptate hyphae with nonparallel walls were seen within glomerulus, tubules, and within vessel wall (angioinvasion).
- Chromic silver methenamine stain highlighted fungal hyphae of mucormycosis.

POST-TRANSPLANT LYMPHOPROLIFERATIVE DISORDER

Lymphoid or plasmacytic proliferation as a consequence of immunosuppression in a recipient of a solid organ/bone marrow/stem cell allograft.

Categories (2017 World Health Organization Classification)[72]

- Nondestructive post-transplant lymphoproliferative disorder (PTLD)
  - Plasmacytic hyperplasia
  - Infectious mononucleosis
  - Florid follicular hyperplasia
- Polymorphic PTLD
- Monomorphic PTLD (classify according to the lymphoma they resemble)
  - B-cell neoplasms
    - Diffuse large B-cell lymphoma
    - Burkitt lymphoma
    - Plasma cell myeloma
    - Plasmacytoma
    - Others
  - T-cell neoplasms
    - Peripheral T-cell lymphoma, not otherwise specified

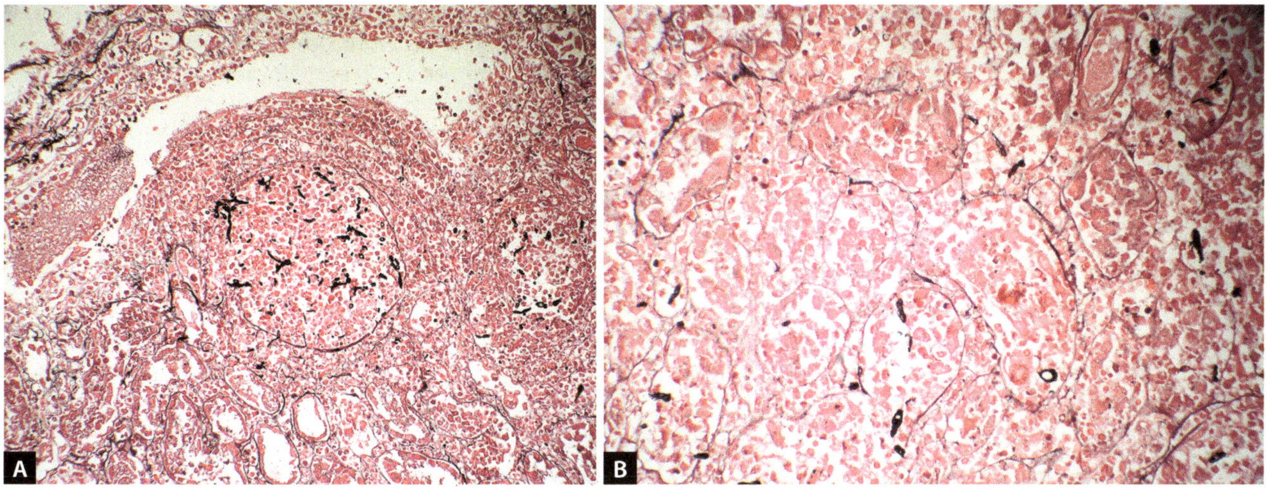

Figs. 10A and B: (A) Ischemic necrosis of glomeruli with infiltrating ribbon-like nonseptate fungal hyphae of mucor (CSM, ×100); (B) Ischemic necrosis with ghost outline of renal tubules along with ribbon-like nonseptate fungal hyphae of mucor (CSM, ×200).

    - Hepatosplenic T-cell lymphoma
    - Others
- Classical Hodgkin lymphoma PTLD

Note: Indolent small B-cell lymphomas not included with the exception of Epstein–Barr virus (EBV)-positive marginal zone lymphoma (MZL).

Etiology

Majority are due to EBV A infection (30% EBV negative) and are of host origin. Human herpesvirus-8 (HHV8) can also be a causative agent. Lymph nodes, lungs, gastrointestinal tract, and liver are the common sites of involvement. Allograft involvement is more common in early onset EBV-positive disease, but among the solid organ allografts, renal involvement is rare (<1%).

Risk factors for PTLD include EBV seronegative at the time of transplant, intensity of immunosuppression, pediatric allografts, unrelated/HLA mismatch donors, and use of antithymocyte globulin (ATG)/CD3 antibodies.[73]

The differential diagnoses of lymphoid infiltrates in the graft include TCMR; infections, notably polyomavirus; pyelonephritis when neutrophil rich with neutrophilic casts; allergic tubulointerstitial nephritis when eosinophil rich with the clinical triad of fever, rash, and eosinophiluria; and PTLD.[74]

Post-transplant lymphoproliferative disorder in the allograft biopsy is rare and needs to be suspected in grafts with lymphoid infiltration in resistant rejections (polymorphic <1 year, monomorphic >1 year) and when the infiltrates are expansile, with geographic necrosis, polymorphic, atypical, and with sparing of arteries. On immune staining, the cells would be a mixture of T and B cells with absent lymphoid follicles and positivity on Epstein–Barr encoding region-in situ hybridization (EBER-ISH) stains.

REFERENCES

1. Loupy A, Mengel M, Haas M. 30 years of the international Banff classification for allograft pathology: the past, present and future of kidney transplant diagnostics. Kidney Int. 2022;101(4):678-91.
2. Roufosse C, Simmonds N, Clahsen-van Groningen M, Haas M, Henriksen KJ, Horsfield C, et al. A 2018 reference guide to the Banff classification of renal allograft pathology. Transplantation. 2018;102(11):1795-814.
3. Mengel M, Loupy A, Haas M, Roufosse C, Naesens M, Akalin E, et al. Banff 2019 Meeting Report: molecular diagnostics in solid organ transplantation—consensus for the Banff Human Organ Transplant (B-HOT) gene panel and open source multicenter validation. Am J Transplant. 2020;20(9):2305-17.
4. Racusen LC, Solez K, Colvin RB, Bonsib SM, Castro MC, Cavallo T, et al. The Banff 97 working classification of renal allograft pathology. Kidney Int. 1999;55(2):713-23.
5. Loupy A, Haas M, Roufosse C, Naesens M, Adam B, Afrouzian M, et al. The Banff 2019 Kidney Meeting Report (I): updates on and clarification of criteria for T cell- and antibody-mediated rejection. Am J Transplant. 2020;20(9): 2318-31.
6. Haas M, Loupy A, Lefaucheur C, Roufosse C, Glotz D, Seron D, et al. The Banff 2017 Kidney Meeting Report: revised diagnostic criteria for chronic active T cell-mediated rejection, antibody-mediated rejection, and prospects for integrative endpoints for next-generation clinical trials. Am J Transplant. 2018;18(2):293-307.
7. Adam B, Mengel M. Transplant biopsy beyond light microscopy. BMC Nephrol. 2015;16:132.
8. Snijders MLH, Varol H, van der Zwan M, Becker JU, Hesselink DA, Baan CC, et al. Molecular analysis of renal allograft biopsies: where do we stand and where are we going? Transplantation. 2020;104(12):2478-86.
9. Fehr T, Stussi G. ABO-incompatible kidney transplantation. Curr Opin Organ Transplant. 2012;17(4):376-85.
10. Crew RJ, Ratner LE. ABO-incompatible kidney transplantation: current practice and the decade ahead. Curr Opin Organ Transplant. 2010;15(4):526-30.

11. Lefaucheur C, Louis K, Philippe A, Loupy A, Coates PT. The emerging field of non-human leukocyte antigen antibodies in transplant medicine and beyond. Kidney Int. 2021; 100(4):787-98.
12. Lefaucheur C, Viglietti D, Bouatou Y, Philippe A, Pievani D, Aubert O, et al. Non-HLA agonistic anti-angiotensin II type 1 receptor antibodies induce a distinctive phenotype of antibody-mediated rejection in kidney transplant recipients. Kidney Int. 2019;96(1):189-201.
13. Dragun D, Catar R, Philippe A. Non-HLA antibodies against endothelial targets bridging allo- and autoimmunity. Kidney Int. 2016;90(2):280-8.
14. Leal R, Tsapepas D, Crew RJ, Dube GK, Ratner L, Batal I. Pathology of calcineurin and mammalian target of rapamycin inhibitors in kidney transplantation. Kidney Int Rep. 2017; 3(2):281-90.
15. Liptak P, Ivanyi B. Primer: histopathology of calcineurin-inhibitor toxicity in renal allografts. Nat Clin Pract Nephrol. 2006;2(7):398-404.
16. Sharma A, Jain S, Gupta R, Guleria S, Agarwal S, Dinda A. Calcineurin inhibitor toxicity in renal allografts: morphologic clues from protocol biopsies. Indian J Pathol Microbiol. 2010;53(4):651-7.
17. Matas AJ. Chronic progressive calcineurin nephrotoxicity: an overstated concept. Am J Transplant. 2011;11(4):687-92.
18. Mathew TH. Recurrence of disease following renal transplantation. Am J Kidney Dis. 1988;12:85-9.
19. Jiang SH, Kennard AL, Walters GD. Recurrent glomerulonephritis following renal transplantation and impact on graft survival. BMC Nephrol. 2018;19(1):344.
20. Infante B, Rossini M, Leo S, Troise D, Netti GS, Ranieri E, et al. Recurrent glomerulonephritis after renal transplantation: the clinical problem. Int J Mol Sci. 2020;21(17):5954.
21. Choy BY, Chan TM, Lai KN. Recurrent glomerulonephritis after kidney transplantation. Am J Transplant. 2006;6(11): 2535-42.
22. Blosser CD, Bloom RD. Recurrent glomerular disease after kidney transplantation. Curr Opin Nephrol Hypertens. 2017;26(6):501-8.
23. Morozumi K, Takeda A, Otsuka Y, Horike K, Gotoh N, Watarai Y. Recurrent glomerular disease after kidney transplantation: an update of selected areas and the impact of protocol biopsy. Nephrology (Carlton). 2014;19(Suppl. 3):6-10.
24. Sprangers B, Kuypers DR. Recurrence of glomerulonephritis after renal transplantation. Transplant Rev (Orlando). 2013;27(4):126-34.
25. Cosio FG, Cattran DC. Recent advances in our understanding of recurrent primary glomerulonephritis after kidney transplantation. Kidney Int. 2017;19:302-14.
26. Zand L, Lorenz EC, Cosio FG, Fervenza FC, Nasr SH, Gandhi MJ, et al. Clinical findings, pathology, and outcomes of C3GN after kidney transplantation. J Am Soc Nephrol. 2014;25:1110-7.
27. Pinto J, Lacerda G, Cameron JS, Turner DR, Bewick M, Ogg CS. Recurrence of focal segmental glomerulosclerosis in renal allografts. Transplantation. 1981;32:83-9.
28. Shoji J, Mii A, Terasaki M, Shimizu A. Update on recurrent focal segmental glomerulosclerosis in kidney transplantation. Nephron. 2020;144(Suppl. 1):65-70.
29. Wyld ML, Chadban SJ. Recurrent IgA nephropathy after kidney transplantation. Transplantation. 2016;100(9):1827-32.
30. Sato Y, Ishida H, Shimizu T, Tanabe K. Evaluation of tonsillectomy before kidney transplantation in patients with IgA nephropathy. Transpl Immunol. 2014;30(1):12-7.
31. Ortiz F, Gelpi R, Koskinen P, Manonelles A, Räisänen-Sokolowski A, Carrera M, et al. IgA nephropathy recurs early in the graft when assessed by protocol biopsy. Nephrol Dial Transplant. 2012;27(6):2553-8.
32. Tang Z, Ji SM, Chen DR, Wen JQ, Chen JS, Liu ZH, et al. Recurrent or de novo IgA nephropathy with crescent formation after renal transplantation. Ren Fail. 2008;30: 611-6.
33. Moroni G, Longhi S, Quaglini S, Gallelli B, Banfi G, Montagnino G, et al. The long-term outcome of renal transplantation of IgA nephropathy and the impact of recurrence on graft survival. Nephrol Dial Transplant. 2013;28:1305-14.
34. IJpelaar DH, Farris AB, Goemaere N, Amann K, Goldschmeding R, Nguyen TQ, et al. Fidelity and evolution of recurrent FSGS in renal allografts. J Am Soc Nephrol. 2008;19(11):2219-24.
35. Canaud G, Dion D, Zuber J, Gubler MC, Sberro R, Thervet E, et al. Recurrence of nephrotic syndrome after transplantation in a mixed population of children and adults: course of glomerular lesions and value of the Columbia classification of histological variants of focal and segmental glomerulosclerosis (FSGS). Nephrol Dial Transplant. 2010;25(4):1321-8.
36. Tejani A, Stablein DH. Recurrence of focal segmental glomerulosclerosis posttransplantation: a special report of the North American Pediatric Renal Transplant Cooperative Study. J Am Soc Nephrol. 1992;2(12 Suppl):S258-63.
37. Verani RR, Hawkins EP. Recurrent focal segmental glomerulosclerosis. A pathological study of the early lesion. Am J Nephrol. 1986;6(4):263-70.
38. Braun MC, Stablein DM, Hamiwka LA, Bell L, Bartosh SM, Strife CF. Recurrence of membranoproliferative glomerulonephritis type II in renal allografts: The North American Pediatric Renal Transplant Cooperative Study experience. J Am Soc Nephrol. 2005;16(7):2225-33.
39. Appel GB, Cook HT, Hageman G, Jennette JC, Kashgarian M, Kirschfink M, et al. Membranoproliferative glomerulonephritis type II (dense deposit disease): an update. J Am Soc Nephrol. 2005;16(5):1392-403.
40. Lorenz EC, Sethi S, Leung N, Dispenzieri A, Fervenza FC, Cosio FG. Recurrent membranoproliferative glomerulonephritis after kidney transplantation. Kidney Int. 2010; 77(8):721-8.
41. Golgert WA, Appel GB, Hariharan S. Recurrent glomerulonephritis after renal transplantation: an unsolved problem. Clin J Am Soc Nephrol. 2008;3:800-7.
42. Ponticelli C, Moroni G, Glassock RJ. De novo glomerular diseases after renal transplantation. Clin J Am Soc Nephrol. 2014;9(8):1479-87.
43. Honda K, Horita S, Toki D, Taneda S, Nitta K, Hattori M, et al. De novo membranous nephropathy and antibody-mediated rejection in transplanted kidney. Clin Transplant. 2011;25(2):191-200.
44. Collins AB, Beck Jr LH, Satoskar AA, Saidman SL, Karel DL, Farkash EA, et al. De novo MGN is immunologically distinct from idiopathic MGN and associated with C4d deposition. J Am Soc Nephrol. 2010;(Abstract).
45. Patel K, Hirsch J, Beck L, Herlitz L, Radhakrishnan J. De novo membranous nephropathy in renal allograft associated with

antibody-mediated rejection and review of the literature. Transplant Proc. 2013;45(9):3424-8.
46. Kalluri R, Torre A, Shield 3rd CF, Zamborsky ED, Werner MC, Suchin E, et al. Identification of alpha3, alpha4, and alpha5 chains of type IV collagen as alloantigens for Alport posttransplant anti-glomerular basement membrane antibodies. Transplantation. 2000;69(4):679-83.
47. Browne G, Brown PAJ, Tomson CRV, Fleming S, Allen A, Herriot R, et al. Retransplantation in Alport post-transplant anti-GBM disease. Kidney Int. 2004;65(2):675-81.
48. Patrakka J, Ruotsalainen V, Reponen P, Qvist E, Laine J, Holmberg C, et al. Recurrence of nephrotic syndrome in kidney grafts of patients with congenital nephrotic syndrome of the Finnish type: role of nephrin. Transplantation. 2002; 73(3):394-403.
49. Nadasdy T, Allen C, Zand MS. Zonal distribution of glomerular collapse in renal allografts: possible role of vascular changes. Hum Pathol. 2002;33(4):437-41.
50. Patel AM, Zenenberg RD, Goldberg RJ. De novo CMV-associated collapsing focal segmental glomerulosclerosis in a kidney transplant recipient. Transpl Infect Dis. 2018; 20(3):e12884.
51. Prasad N, Gupta P, Jain M, Bhadauria D, Gupta A, Sharma RK, et al. Outcomes of de novo allograft diabetic nephropathy in renal allograft recipients. Exp Clin Transplant. 2013;11:215-21.
52. Lim WH, Shingde M, Wong G. Recurrent and de novo glomerulonephritis after kidney transplantation. Front Immunol. 2019;10:1944.
53. Nickeleit V, Singh HK, Dadhania D, Cornea V, El-Husseini A, Castellanos A, et al. The 2018 Banff Working Group classification of definitive polyomavirus nephropathy: a multicenter validation study in the modern era. Am J Transplant. 2021;21(2):669-80.
54. Gupta P, Gupta A, Bhalla AK, Malik M, Gupta A, Bhargava V, et al. BK virus nephropathy in living donor renal allograft recipients: an observational study from a large transplant center in India. Saudi J Kidney Dis Transpl. 2018;29(6): 1366-70.
55. Mengel M, Marwedel M, Radermacher J, Eden G, Schwarz A, Haller H, et al. Incidence of polyomavirus-nephropathy in renal allografts: influence of modern immunosuppressive drugs. Nephrol Dial Transplant. 2003;18(6):1190-6.
56. Gabardi S, Townsend K, Martin ST, Chandraker A. Evaluating the impact of pre-transplant desensitization utilizing a plasmapheresis and low-dose intravenous immunoglobulin protocol on BK viremia in renal transplant recipients. Transpl Infect Dis. 2013;15(4):361-8.
57. Giakoustidis D, Antoniadis A, Fouzas I, Sklavos A, Giakoustidis A, Ouzounidis N, et al. Prevalence and clinical impact of cytomegalovirus infection and disease in renal transplantation: ten years of experience in a single center. Transplant Proc. 2012;44(9):2715-7.
58. Rady K, Walters G, Brown M, Talaulikar G. Allograft adenovirus nephritis. Clin Kidney J. 2014;7(3):289-92.
59. Kamath NS, John GT, Neelakantan N, Kirubakaran MG, Jacob CK. Acute graft pyelonephritis following renal transplantation. Transpl Infect Dis. 2006;8(3):140-7.
60. Gupta KL, Bagai S, Ramachandran R, Kumar V, Rathi M, Kohli HS, et al. Fungal infection in post-renal transplant patient: single-center experience. Indian J Pathol Microbiol. 2020;63(4):587-92.
61. Gupta RK, Gupta P (Eds). Pathology of Opportunistic Infections: An Illustrative Atlas. Singapore: Springer; 2016.
62. Bracamonte E, Leca N, Smith KD, Nicosia RF, Nickeleit V, Kendrick E, et al. Tubular basement membrane immune deposits in association with BK polyomavirus nephropathy. Am J Transplant. 2007;7(6):1552-60.
63. Singh HK, Donna Thompson B, Nickeleit V. Viral Haufen are urinary biomarkers of polyomavirus nephropathy: new diagnostic strategies utilizing negative staining electron microscopy. Ultrastruct Pathol. 2009;33(5):222-35.
64. Battegay EJ, Mihatsch MJ, Mazzucchelli L, Zollinger HU, Gudat F, Thiel G, et al. Cytomegalovirus and kidney. Clin Nephrol. 1988;30(5):239-47.
65. Rane S, Nada R, Minz M, Sakhuja V, Joshi K. Spectrum of cytomegalovirus-induced renal pathology in renal allograft recipients. Transplant Proc. 2012;44(3):713-6.
66. Liapis H, Storch GA, Hill DA, Rueda J, Brennan DC. CMV infection of the renal allograft is much more common than the pathology indicates: a retrospective analysis of qualitative and quantitative buffy coat CMV-PCR, renal biopsy pathology and tissue CMV-PCR. Nephrol Dial Transplant. 2003; 18(2):397-402.
67. Florescu DF, Schaenman JM, AST Infectious Diseases Community of Practice. Adenovirus in solid organ transplant recipients: guidelines from the American Society of Transplantation Infectious Diseases Community of Practice. Clin Transplant. 2019;33(9):e13527.
68. Friedrichs N, Eis-Hubinger AM, Heim A, Platen E, Zhou H, Buettner R. Acute adenoviral infection of a graft by serotype 35 following renal transplantation. Pathol Res Pract. 2003; 199(8):565-70.
69. Bruno B, Zager RA, Boeckh MJ, Gooley TA, Myerson DH, Huang ML, et al. Adenovirus nephritis in hematopoietic stem-cell transplantation. Transplantation. 2004;77(7): 1049-57.
70. Gołębiewska J, Dębska-Ślizień A, Zadrożny D, Rutkowski B. Acute graft pyelonephritis during the first year after renal transplantation. Transplant Proc. 2014;46:2743-7.
71. Jennette JC, D'Agati VD, Olson JL, Silva FG. Heptinstall's Pathology of the Kidney, 7th edition. Philadelphia, PA: Wolter Kluwer; 2014.
72. Swerdlow SH, Campo E, Harris NL, Jaffe ES, Pileri SA, Stein H, Thiele J (Eds). WHO Classification of Tumours of Haematopoietic and Lymphoid Tissues. Lyon: IARC; 2017.
73. Dharnidharka VR, Webster AC, Martinez OM, Preiksaitis JK, Leblond V, Choquet S. Post-transplant lymphoproliferative disorders. Nat Rev Dis Primers. 2016;2:15088.
74. Randhawa PS, Magnone M, Jordan M, Shapiro R, Demetris AJ, Nalesnik M. Renal allograft involvement by Epstein-Barr virus associated post-transplant lymphoproliferative disease. Am J Surg Pathol. 1996;20(5):563.

CHAPTER 12

Infections in Kidney Transplantation

12.1 Overview of Infections in Kidney Transplantation

Vaibhav Tiwari, AK Bhalla, Ashwani Gupta

CASE VIGNETTE

48-year-old, renal allograft recipient (9 months back), donor-father, ABO compatible, presented with slowly rising creatinine from 0.9 mg/dL to 2.7 mg/dL over a period of 2 months. The patient denied any history of nephrotoxic drugs or missing his immunosuppression medications. His Lab parameters were unremarkable with urine showing bland sediments with few pus cells. Tacrolimus level was maintained within 7 µg/L range. His USG graft Doppler showed mildly resistive flows (Resistive Index = 0.81). Plasma BK viral load was positive with 5 log copies. A kidney biopsy was performed which showed focal inflammation and tubular epithelial cell nuclear positivity for simian virus-40 immunostain, confirming BK nephropathy without rejection. His immunosuppression medications were modified with Mycophenolate mofetil being stopped, tacrolimus level was lowered to 4 µg/L and prednisolone was reduced to 5 mg/kg. A month later his serum creatinine was decreased to 1.4 mg/dL. His plasma BK viral load decreased to 3.2 log copies. After 2 months, creatinine further decreased to 1.2 mg/dL and viral load decreased to 1.3 log copies. One year after the diagnosis, his creatinine is stable at 1.4 mg/dL with plasma BK viral load being undetectable. He was maintained on dual immunosuppression with DSA being monitored 6 monthly.

INTRODUCTION

Transplantation is considered successful when the recipient's immunological barrier has been adequately suppressed so that the donor's kidney persists in the hostile environment. However, it is a continuous battle between the recipient immunological forces and donor graft antigens which are aided by immunosuppressive medications. Not so infrequently, this battle results in collateral damage in the form of infections by community-acquired as well as opportunistic infections. Infections are the second most common cause of mortality and morbidity among transplant patients.

Infection in kidney transplant recipients (KTRs) can be categorized according to the type of pathogens, source of infection, and site of infection, although the most common and useful way to classify infection is to categorize them according to a particular timetable in which they occur in the post-transplant period **(Table 1)**.[1,2]

EARLY TRANSPLANT PERIOD (FIRST MONTH POST-TRANSPLANTATION)

During the initial period, most infections arise from:

- *Donor derived:* Especially in cadaveric donation when there is a shortage of time to completely evaluate the donor
- During the organ procurement
- During the transplant surgery
- The perioperative period associated with indwelling catheters, central lines, etc.
- Surgical site infections
- Activation of latent infection in the recipient.

Donor-derived and recipient-origin infections are rare and generally manifest within the first 30 days. Donor-derived infection can be further classified as follows:[1]

- *Expected:* When the pathogens are known to present in donors and may not be possible to eradicate before the transplantation [e.g., cytomegalovirus (CMV), Epstein–Barr virus (EBV)]
- *Unexpected:* When the infection is initially not recognized and simultaneously occurs in other recipients.

TABLE 1: Timeline of common infections in transplant patients.

<1 Month	1–6 Months	>6 Months
Bacterial infection: • Urinary tract infection • Respiratory tract infection • Catheter infection • Wound infection • Intra-abdominal infection • Multidrug-resistant infection • *Clostridium difficile* colitis *Fungal: Candida*, azole-resistant *Candida* species (recipient pre-Tx colonization or donor derived) *Donor-derived infection (uncommon):* HSV, CMV, HIV *Recipient-derived infection (colonization): Aspergillus, Pseudomonas*	*Opportunistic or unconventional infections:* • *Viral:* CMV, EBV, VZV Influenza, BK infection • *Fungal: Aspergillus* species, *Cryptococcus* • *Bacterial: Nocardia, Mycobacterium* species, tuberculosis • *Parasitic: Pneumocystis jiroveci, Toxoplasma* and *Strongyloides* species, leishmaniasis	Community-acquired pneumonia, urinary tract infection Infection with aspergillus, atypical moulds, *Mucor* species Infection with *Nocardia, Rhodococcus* species • *Late viral infections:* CMV infection (colitis and retinitis) • Hepatitis (HBV, HCV) • HSV encephalitis • Community-acquired (SARS, West Nile virus infection) • JC polyomavirus infection (PML) • Shin cancer, lymphoma (PTLD)

(CMV: cytomegalovirus; EBV: Epstein–Barr virus; HBV: hepatitis B virus; HCV: hepatitis C virus; HSV: herpes simplex virus; PML: progressive multifocal leukoencephalopathy; PTLD: post-transplant lymphoproliferative disorder; VZV: varicella-zoster virus)
Source: Morton L, Landgren O, Chatterjee N. Hepatitis C virus infection and risk of post-transplant lymphoproliferative disorder among solid organ transplant recipients. Blood. 2007;110:4599-605.

CHAPTER HIGHLIGHTS

- Infections in transplant are a major cause of morbidity and mortality.
- Etiological spectrum of infection varies according to the time period and immune status of the patient.
- During the initial first month bacterial infection deriving from urinary catheter, surgical sites, central line predominate.
- In the next 6 months, opportunistic infections account for the majority of infections.
- After the initial 6 months, community acquired infections especially lower tract infections and urinary tract infections (UTIs) become more common.
- UTI has been by far the most common infections especially in India subcontinent.
- Reactivation of Tuberculosis is common in the initial few years owing to immunosuppressed state.
- BK virus infection is an exclusive infection seen in solid organ transplant patients commonly in first year and presents a challenging situation of treatment by reduction of immunosuppression along with risk of concurrent rejection.
- Gastroenteritis is common among transplant recipient, mostly due to immunosuppression medication as well as common enteropathogens like Norovirus, Girdia, E. coli etc.

Majority of infections in the early transplant period are due to urinary tract infection (UTI), surgical site infection, infected collections, pneumonia, and catheter-related bloodstream infection (CRBSI). Most of the common community-acquired and opportunistic infections are conspicuously absent in this period.

SECOND PERIOD (1–6 MONTHS POST-TRANSPLANTATION)

This is the period when cumulative dose immunosuppression is at the peak and similar is reflected in the spectrum of microorganisms. The opportunistic and latent infections take the center stage. BK virus (BKV), CMV, hepatitis B, hepatitis C, tuberculosis (TB), herpes simplex virus (HSV), and varicella-zoster become predominant infections. This is also the period when rejections frequently occur, resulting in more immunosuppression exposure and a net state of excessive immunosuppression. Due to this reason, prophylaxis with valganciclovir and co-trimoxazole is recommended during this period.

THIRD PERIOD (>6 MONTHS POST-TRANSPLANTATION)

From 6 to 12 months onwards, the spectrum of pathogens changes and community-acquired infectious predominate albeit with more frequency and severity than the general population. However, few patients (20–30%) deviate from this standard path. These are the patients who have experienced rejections and high-risk patients who have had greater exposure to immunosuppression. These patients continue to experience opportunistic infections as well as community-acquired infections with a much more frequency than the rest of the transplant recipients. Patients with chronic infections such as hepatitis B and C, BKV, and CMV may experience flare and progressive organ damage.

The most important steps in reducing infections in KTRs are pretransplant screening, vaccination, and optimal antibacterial and antiviral prophylaxis.

CHALLENGES IN DIAGNOSIS

Classic signs and symptoms of infections in KTRs may be absent or mitigated owing to the effect of immunosuppression. Even the laboratory markers of infection such as leukocytosis may not be as pronounced as in the general population due to the influence of drugs such as azathioprine and mycophenolate mofetil (MMF). Other markers such as C-reactive protein (CRP) may also not be a distinctive marker as it can also be elevated in cases of acute rejections. The rise in procalcitonin levels can also be seen in noninfective conditions such as following the administration of antithymocyte globulin (ATG) or after a major surgery.[3] Presence of atypical clinical features and reduced immune response to a pathogen can conceal a severe infection. Not only the typical common pathogens of community and nosocomial infections but also atypical, opportunistic, and very rare pathogens can complicate the course of transplantation.

PRETRANSPLANT SCREENING

Thorough screening of donors and recipients for the infections is essential prior to the transplantation, especially for the infections that can be transmitted via organ donation or at high risk of reactivation in the recipient in the suppressed state by virtue of immunosuppressive agents. Refer to Chapter 2 for recommended screening protocol for infections in recipient and donors.

VACCINATIONS

Waiting list candidates for kidney transplantation (KT) should be assessed for their vaccination status. For a better response, it is advised to vaccinate the patients prior to the transplantation than after. Vaccination for pneumococcus, influenza, and hepatitis B virus (HBV) should be given special consideration. Refer to Chapter 25 for a detailed discussion on vaccination in KTRs.

DATA FROM INDIA

In a retrospective study of 510 post-KTRs, around 75% of the patients suffered from the infections. The most common infection was UTI (53%) followed by chest infection and bacteremia. The common isolates were *Escherichia coli* (160), *Staphylococcus aureus*, *Enterococcus*, and *Pseudomonas*.[4]

In another retrospective study, out of 144 KTRs, 73 patients developed infections. UTIs were the most common infections (34.5%), followed by viral (31.2%), sepsis, mycobacterial, fungal, and parasitic infections (1.4%). CMV and BKV accounted for 14.5 and 5.5% of the total infections, respectively. Majority of the infection occurred in the first 6 months of KT.[5]

In an analysis by Gupta et al. on opportunistic infections in KTRs, the spectrum of infections was bacterial infection (5.9%) followed by TB (4.9%), viral (3.8%), and fungal (2.1%). The most common site was the lung, followed by the urinary tract. Higher infection rates were found in the first 6 months of KT.[6]

RISK FACTORS

Risk of complications in KTRs is determined by multiple factors such as epidemiological exposure, net state of immunosuppression, vaccination and chemoprophylaxis status. The net immunosuppressed status of the KTR is based on factors such as age, gender, underlying clinical condition, and the ongoing immunosuppressive medications. Other conditions such as leukopenia, post-transplant diabetes mellitus, poor graft function and malnutrition also play a role in determining the overall immunity of the patient.[7]

Data from the United States Renal Data System (USRDS) medicare on primary KTR showed a higher adjusted hazard ratio for infections in recipients aged <18 years, donors with positive CMV IgG, delayed graft function, primary renal diagnosis, chronic pyelonephritis, associated pretransplant diabetes, and female sex.[8]

A study from Korea reported a higher incidence of early post-transplant infection in older recipients. Older KTRs had more mycobacterial infections, coinfections, and multiple site infections compared with younger recipients. Female gender, longer hospitalization after KT, and occurrence of acute rejection were the independent risk factors for the development of infections during the post-transplantation period.[9]

Some other variables such as lupus erythematosus, malignancy, cancer, prior KT, history of antirejection therapy, and a basal serum albumin concentration < 3.5 mg/dL have also been recognized as risk factors for infection in KTRs in other studies.[10]

NOTABLE INFECTIONS

Urinary Tract Infection

Urinary tract infection is the most common infection in transplant patients.[11] It is difficult to estimate the true incidence of UTI in the post-transplant period as almost half of the infections are asymptomatic. In a study of 100 patients, asymptomatic bacteriuria (ASB), uncomplicated UTI, complicated UTI, and recurrent UTI were found in 44, 32, 23, and 14%, respectively.[12] Extending the pattern from the general population, *E. coli* is the most frequent organism in transplantation patients followed by *Klebsiella pneumoniae*.[13] Trimethoprim-sulfamethoxazole (TMP-SMX) is preferred for prophylaxis against UTI in the post-transplant period. ASB is common in the post-transplant period, but its treatment is controversial and still a matter of debate.[14] (Read details in Chapter 12.6.)

Cytomegalovirus

Cytomegalovirus is the most common opportunistic infection among transplant recipients. The seroprevalence is variable; however, it is reported between 20 and 97%.[15] The incidence of CMV in the renal transplant population is estimated to be between 8 and 32%. The most important risk factor in the development of symptomatic CMV disease is transplantation between the seronegative recipient and seropositive donor.[15] Other factors include induction with ATG, concomitant other viral infections, older donors (>60 years), simultaneous kidney-pancreas transplantation, and acute rejection episodes. In view of the significant effect of CMV infection on patient and graft survival, especially during the early period, standard prophylaxis is recommended in D+/R–, D+/R+, and D–/R+ using valganciclovir for a minimum of 3 months after transplantation and 1–3 months after ATG treatment.[16] (Read details in Chapter 12.2.1.)

BK Virus

BK virus is a human polyomavirus that is ubiquitous. Infection occurs during childhood and the virus lies dormant in the uroepithelial cells of 80–90% of adults. Initially, asymptomatic viruria is seen in 25–40% of patients in the first year. Subsequently, in patients with persistent viruria and high urinary viral loads, 10–20% develop viremia after a few weeks. BK polyomavirus-associated nephropathy occurs in 1–10% of all patients.[17] BVN has the highest incidence during the first year of transplant. No specific treatment has been approved against the BKV. Early detection by screening, monitoring, and modification of immunosuppression is still the mainstay of the management of BKV. Certain medications which have shown in vivo efficacy and are offered in resistant cases including IVIg, leflunomide, cidofovir, and fluoroquinolones.[18-20] (Read details in Chapter 12.2.2.)

Tuberculosis

Tuberculosis is one of the leading infectious complications in renal transplant patients. Its incidence is highly variable with developing countries like India reporting 12.3%. Around 45–60% of TB occur in the first year after transplantation.[21] Reactivation is the most common mode of infection. Clinical presentation of TB in immunocompromised patients differs with around 30% of all cases of active infection involving disseminated disease or extrapulmonary sites, compared with approximately less than one-fifth of cases in normal hosts. Mantoux and interferon gamma (IFN-γ) are not recommended for diagnosing the active disease. High clinical suspicion is required to diagnose the disease with the occult site. Treatment of active disease as in the general population should contain a four-drug regimen of isoniazid, rifampin, pyrazinamide, and ethambutol for 2 months followed by rifampin and isoniazid alone for 4 additional months is recommended for active TB, although bone, joint, and central nervous system infection may require longer treatment.[22] (Read details in Chapter 12.7.)

Gastroenteritis

Acute gastroenteritis is a cause of significant morbidity and mortality among renal transplant patients. The etiology of diarrhea is most difficult to establish as immunosuppressive agents, especially MMF, are also a known cause of significant diarrhea. However, it's of paramount importance to distinguish between infective and noninfective etiology as dose modification or withholding immunosuppressive agents invariably increase the risk of rejection. The most common pathogens involved are *Norovirus, E. coli, Giardia cryptosporidium*, CMV, *Clostridium, Shigella, Salmonella, Cyclospora*, and *Microsporidia*.[23] Diagnosis is usually established by microbiological confirmation; however, the yield of routine tests including microscopy and culture is usually low. Multiplex polymerase chain reaction (PCR) kits are now available, which can diagnose more than 20 pathogens in a short span of time with high sensitivity and specificity.[23]

Fungal Infection

Pneumocystis jirovecii is the most important fungal infection in the initial post-transplant period. It is known to cause fulminant pneumonia with a mortality of 29–50%. Its incidence has drastically reduced with the introduction of universal prophylaxis of co-trimoxazole.[24] Other common fungal infections include candidiasis, aspergillosis, cryptococcosis, and zygomycosis. The main sites of fungal infections in admitted patients are esophageal candidiasis, pneumonia, and urogenital candidiasis. Risk factors for fungal infections in transplant recipients include the use of high immunosuppression, especially corticosteroids, multiple or recent rejection episodes, poorly controlled blood sugars, reduced graft function, leukopenia, and advanced age.[25] Treatment of fungal infections especially with azoles should be carefully reviewed because of the potentially drug interaction with calcineurin inhibitors (CNIs). A pre-emptive CNI dose reduction of 50% should be done empirically while initiating the azoles.[26] (Read details in Chapter 12.3.)

REFERENCES

1. Agrawal A, Ison MG, Danziger-Isakov L. Long-term infectious complications of kidney transplantation. Clin J Am Soc Nephrol. 2022;17(2):286-95.
2. Karuthu S, Blumberg EA. Common infections in kidney transplant recipients. Clin J Am Soc Nephrol. 2012;7(12): 2058-70.
3. Dasdelen S, Grebe S-O. Infections after renal transplantation. Laboratoriums Medizin. 2017;41(s1):20170094.
4. Sharma KK, Ayyagiri A, Dhole TN, Prasad KN, Kishore J. Prevalence of infections in renal transplant recipients of north India. Indian J Pathol Microbiol. 2007;50(2):453-7.

5. Sriperumbuduri S, Kalidindi K, Guditi S, Taduri G. Declining trend of infections in renal transplant recipients in a tertiary care hospital from India. Indian J Transplant. 2017;11:143-8.
6. Gupta KL, Bagai S, Joshi K, Rathi M, Kohli HS, Jha V, et al. Opportunistic infections occurring in renal transplant recipients in tropical countries. Indian J Transplant. 2019; 13:110-4.
7. Jha V. Post-transplant infections: an ounce of prevention. Indian J Nephrol. 2010;20:171-8.
8. Dharnidharka VR, Agodoa LY, Abbott KC. Risk factors for hospitalization for bacterial or viral infection in renal transplant recipients—an analysis of USRDS data. Am J Transplant. 2007;7(3):653-61.
9. Kim JS, Jeong KH, Lee DW, Lee SY, Lee SH, Yang J, et al. Epidemiology, risk factors, and clinical impact of early post-transplant infection in older kidney transplant recipients: the Korean organ transplantation registry study. BMC Geriatr. 2020;20(1):519.
10. Valdez-Ortiz R, Sifuentes-Osornio J, Morales-Buenrostro LE, Ayala-Palma H, Dehesa-López E, Alberú J, et al. Risk factors for infections requiring hospitalization in renal transplant recipients: a cohort study. Int J Infect Dis. 2011;15(3):e188-96.
11. De Souza RM, Olsburgh J. Urinary tract infection in the renal transplant patient. Nat Clin Pract Nephrol. 2008;4(5):252-64.
12. Ariza-Heredia EJ, Beam EN, Lesnick TG, Cosio FG, Kremers WK, Razonable RR. Impact of urinary tract infection on allograft function after kidney transplantation. Clin Transplant. 2014;28(6):683-90.
13. Hollyer I, Ison MG. The challenge of urinary tract infections in renal transplant recipients. Transpl Infect Dis. 2018;20(2):e12828.
14. Coussement J, Kaminski H, Scemla A, Manuel O. Asymptomatic bacteriuria and urinary tract infections in kidney transplant recipients. Curr Opin Infect Dis. 2020; 33(6):419-25.
15. de Matos SB, Meyer R, de Mendonça Lima FW. Cytomegalovirus infection after renal transplantation: occurrence, clinical features, and the cutoff for antigenemia in a university hospital in Brazil. Infect Chemother. 2017;49(4):255-61.
16. Luscalov S, Loga L, Dican L, Junie LM. Cytomegalovirus infection in immunosuppressed patients after kidney transplantation. Clujul Med. 2016;89(3):343-6.
17. Schwarz A, Linnenweber-Held S, Heim A, Framke T, Haller H, Schmitt C. Viral origin, clinical course, and renal outcomes in patients with BK virus infection after living-donor renal transplantation. Transplantation. 2016;100(4):844-53.
18. Sood P, Senanayake S, Sujeet K, Medipalli R, Van-Why SK, Cronin DC, et al. Donor, and recipient BKV-specific IgG antibody and posttransplantation BKV infection: a prospective single-center study. Transplantation. 2013;95(6):896-902.
19. Sener A, House AA, Jevnikar AM, Boudville N, McAlister VC, Muirhead N, et al. Intravenous immunoglobulin as a treatment for BK virus associated nephropathy: one-year follow-up of renal allograft recipients. Transplantation. 2006;81(1):117-20.
20. Josephson MA, Gillen D, Javaid B, Kadambi P, Meehan S, Foster P, et al. Treatment of renal allograft polyoma BK virus infection with leflunomide. Transplantation. 2006; 81(5):704-10.
21. John GT. Infections after renal transplantation in India. Indian J Nephrol. 2022;13(1):14.
22. Singh N, Paterson DL. Mycobacterium tuberculosis infection in solid-organ transplant recipients: impact and implications for management. Clin Infect Dis. 1998;27(5):1266-77.
23. Tiwari V, Anand Y, Gupta A, Divyaveer S, Bhargava V, Malik M, et al. Etiological spectrum of infective diarrhea in renal transplant patient by stool PCR: an Indian perspective. Indian J Nephrol. 2021;31(3):245-53.
24. Martin SI, Fishman JA. Pneumocystis pneumonia in solid organ transplantation. Am J Transplant. 2013;13(Suppl. 4): 272-79.
25. Abbott KC, Hypolite I, Poropatich RK, Hshieh P, Cruess D, Hawkes CA, et al. Hospitalizations for fungal infections after renal transplantation in the United States. Transpl Infect Dis. 2001;3(4):203-11.
26. Thomas LD, Miller GG. Interactions between antiinfective agents and immunosuppressants. Am J Transplant. 2009; 9(Suppl. 4):S263-6.

12.2 Viral Infections

12.2.1 Cytomegalovirus

K Sampathkumar

CASE VIGNETTE

A 38-year-old female underwent living-related renal transplantation after being on hemodialysis for 2 years. She received antithymocyte globulin (ATG) for induction, followed by triple-drug immunosuppression with tacrolimus, mycophenolate mofetil, and prednisolone. The pretransplant cytomegalovirus (CMV) serostatus was D–/R+. She received CMV prophylaxis of oral valganciclovir (VGCV) for 6 months. 11 months post-transplant, she was admitted with fever, malaise, headache, and dysphagia. Her laboratory investigations were suggestive of anemia with leukopenia. She had serum creatinine of 1.4 mg/dL.

a. How do you evaluate her further?
b. What do you find in renal histopathology in cases of CMV nephritis?

Ans. Read text for the answers.

BACKGROUND AND EPIDEMIOLOGY

The lives of kidney transplant recipients (KTRs) patients who undergo renal transplantation show a transformative change for the better. More potent immunosuppressive agents have pushed the first-year patient and graft survival rates close to 100%. But infections continue to play spoilsport which still remain the most common cause of morbidity and mortality. The reasons are not far to seek. Post-transplant immunosuppressives are predicated on intentional T-lymphocyte inhibition, which creates ideal conditions for a variety of viral infections to set in.

Human Cytomegalovirus (CMV) is a ubiquitous double-stranded double-deoxyribonucleic acid (DNA) bearing β-herpesvirus. It is the most common opportunistic viral infection among KTRs occurring in 15–50% of patients not on prophylaxis during the first year of transplantation. Multiple risk factors such as donor positive and recipient negative serostatus (D+/R–), induction therapy with antilymphocyte globulins, acute rejection episodes, and net state of immunosuppression underlie post-transplant CMV disease.

A serological mismatch between the donor and the recipient (D+/R–) poses the highest risk for development of CMV disease; CMV D–/R+ transplantations are at intermediate risk whereas CMV D–/R– transplantations are at low risk (<5% incidence).

We seem to be conquering this menace in recent years due to enhanced surveillance and universal prophylaxis. Nevertheless, CMV can still pose a diagnostic and therapeutic challenge. In the absence of a National Renal Transplant Registry in India, single-center publications are the alternative sources of data that show a 14% incidence of CMV disease in the setting of renal transplantation.[1]

DEFINITIONS

Cytomegalovirus latent infection is a term used when the presence of virus is identified only by serology [immunoglobulin G (IgG) anti-CMV antibodies positive]. Active infection is identified by replication of CMV in blood; the patient may or may not be symptomatic. CMV disease requires both its active replication and clinical manifestations, which can be CMV syndrome (fever, malaise, leukopenia, thrombocytopenia) or tissue-invasive disease where end-organ disease develops (enterocolitis, hepatitis, pneumonitis, nephritis, meningoencephalitis, retinitis).[2]

There are two clinical patterns of infection in KTR:

1. *Reactivation:* Most common pattern. The patient carries the virus in latent form as evidenced by positive IgG reactivity. T-cell depletion therapy results in 50% reactivation status in the absence of chemoprophylaxis. The incidence, however, is reduced to <10% with adequate preventive therapy.
2. *Primary infection:* This is rare in Indian context. It is precipitated by D+/R– CMV serostatus resulting in illness within the first months of renal transplant. The source of the virus is renal allograft where it resides and proliferates under the niche provided by human leukocyte antigen (HLA) mismatch between the donor and the host. Life-threatening CMV syndromes can develop.

PATHOGENESIS

Indians have near-universal exposure to the virus during the childhood and adolescence in contrast to the Western population. Primary infection is contained by the host's robust immune response and is passed off as a minor illness. It is followed by prolonged persistence of CMV in undifferentiated cells of the myeloid lineage ($CD34^+$ and $CD14^+$ monocytes). These cells periodically exit the bone marrow and differentiate to macrophages and/or dendritic cells in various tissue compartments. A prolonged latency period of many years follows, which is broken with the advent of host immunosuppression. During the reactivation, intracellular CMV activation in the endothelial and the epithelial cells is promoted by inflammatory cytokines with sequential activation of transforming growth factor alpha (TGF-α) and nuclear factor kappa B (NF-κB). The latter moves into the nucleus to activate CMV enhancer/replicative sequences. A vicious cycle is propagated wherein the CMV itself immunomodulates the T-cell reactivity leading to multiple superinfections with bacteria, tuberculosis (TB), and fungi.

IMMUNOMODULATORY EFFECTS

The virus inhibits the T helper type 1 (Th1) pathway which results in diminished production of interferon gamma (INF-γ) from lymphocytes. There is also enhanced secretion of interleukin-6 (IL-6) and interleukin-10 (IL-10). Immunomodulation by CMV is suspected on diverse conditions such as chronic allograft dysfunction, cardiovascular disease, post-transplant diabetes mellitus, risk of coinfections, vascular thrombosis, and malignancy.

CLINICAL FEATURES

Cytomegalovirus infection commonly presents as nonspecific malaise, body ache, and low-grade irregular fever. Lower gastrointestinal manifestations include abdominal pain and diarrhea. Rectal involvement with bloody stools and tenesmus may develop. Upper gastrointestinal symptoms such as nausea, vomiting, and abdominal pain can also be seen. Ulcerative lesions of esophagus, stomach, and colon reveal the extent of tissue invasion. To add to the diagnostic confusion, quantitative nucleic acid testing (QNAT) tests may return negative in gastrointestinal involvement.[3] Mucosal biopsies with immunohistochemistry provide the final diagnosis. The dreaded pulmonary complications are ushered in by cough, tachypnea, and hypoxemia. Lower lung peripheral interstitial shadows mimicking COVID-19 pneumonia develop, which is followed by more widespread lung involvement. Rare manifestations include adrenal necrosis, retinitis, and hemophagocytic syndrome. **Table 1** shows the clinical laboratory features of active CMV disease.

CHAPTER HIGHLIGHTS

- CMV is a DNA virus of the herpesvirus family and is a common complication in KTRs.
- CMV disease has been associated with atherosclerosis, acute, and chronic rejection along with decreased patient and graft survival.
- Risk of CMV infection is highest in KTRs with CMV seropositive donor/CMV seronegative recipient (D+/R–).
- Commonly involved organs are gastrointestinal tract, liver, lung, kidneys, and central nervous system.
- VGCV is currently the most commonly used drug for prophylaxis.

HISTOPATHOLOGY

The cytomegalic cells are two to four times enlarged than the surrounding cells. They contain intranuclear inclusions which are eccentrically placed and surrounded by a clear halo, causing an "owl's eye" appearance. The predominant form of involvement in the renal allograft is tubulointerstitial nephritis.[4] Rarely isolated glomerular involvement in the form of cytopathic changes in the podocytes and endothelial cells with minimal inflammation can be seen **(Figs. 1 to 3)**.

Pattern 1: Predominant tubulopathy with interstitial inflammation. The tubular epithelial cell shows prominent nuclear inclusions. There is mononuclear and plasma cell interstitial infiltration.

Pattern 2: Endothelial cells of glomeruli and/or peritubular capillaries show viral cytopathic changes. The interstitium is relatively spared.

Pattern 3: Glomerular involvement is characterized by diffuse proliferation. This is the least common manifestation.

DIAGNOSTIC TESTING

A high index of suspicion should be entertained in a patient who presents in the post-transplant period with symptoms and signs suggestive of CMV infection. Quantitative polymerase chain reaction (PCR) is the gold standard for diagnosis. PCR has a broad linear range with

TABLE 1: Clinical and laboratory features of Cytomegalovirus (CMV) disease.

Common manifestations	***Symptoms***	***Signs (uncommon)***	***Laboratory features***
Pneumonitis, gastrointestinal illness, hepatitis, retinitis, nephritis	• Fever • Nonspecific malaise Body ache • Diarrhea • Bloody stools • Cough, tachypnea • Altered sensorium • Seizures • Oliguria • Diminished visual acuity	• Hepatomegaly • Splenomegaly • Rash • Neck stiffness • Lung crackles • Edema • Retinal exudates	• Leukopenia • Thrombocytopenia • Transaminitis • Proteinuria • Raised serum creatinine • Raised serum amylase, lipase

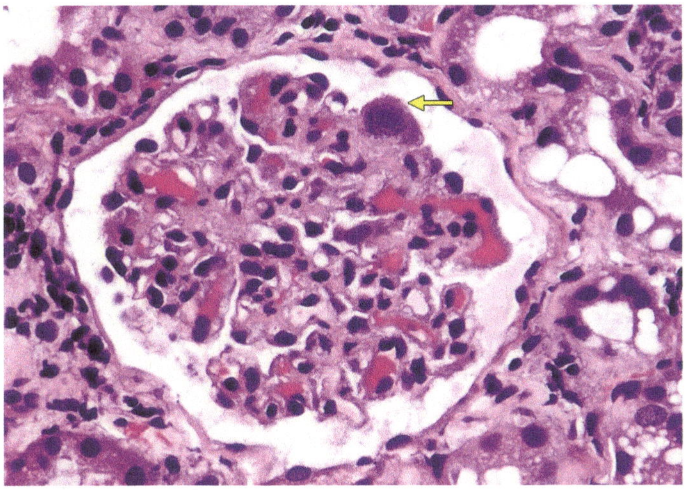

Fig. 1: Cytomegalovirus (CMV) infected podocyte (arrow).

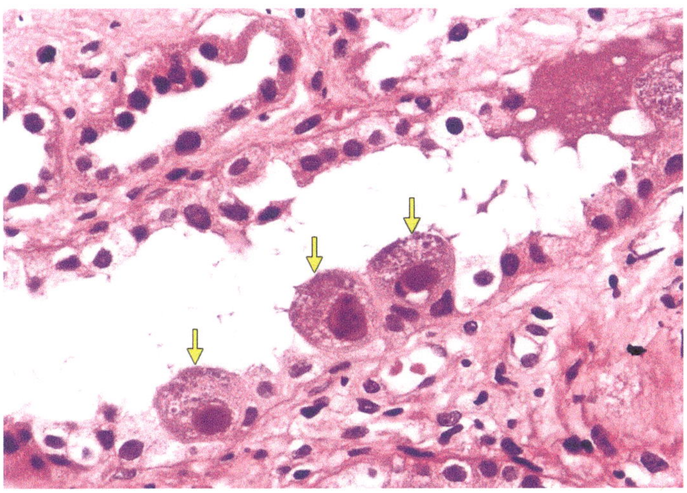

Fig. 2: Cytomegalovirus (CMV) infected tubular epithelial cells (arrows).

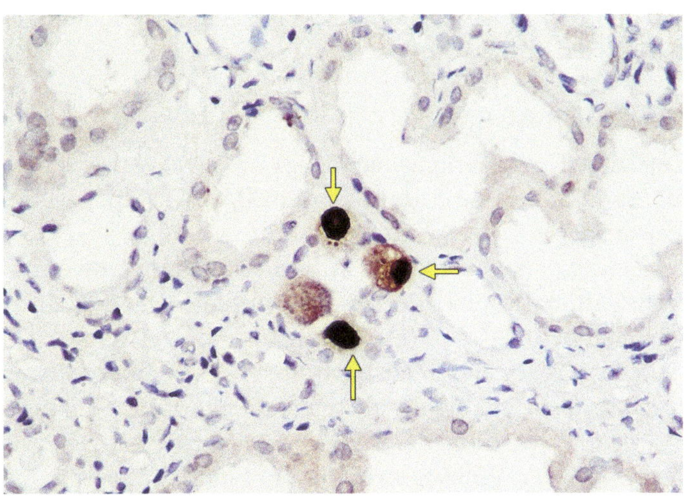

Fig. 3: Immunohistochemistry for cytomegalovirus (CMV) antigens (arrows).
Courtesy: Dr. Anila Abraham, Renopath Lab, Chennai.

excellent sensitivity. Variations in tests mandate that the same laboratory is utilized in serial testing of samples for uniformity in reporting. Because of variability in CMV viral load testing when measured in copies/mL, the World Health Organization (WHO) approved an international standard for the CMV PCR test with results reported in international units (IU) per milliliter. CMV DNA is detected earlier and in greater amounts in whole blood as compared to plasma.

There are no widely accepted PCR thresholds that differentiate among latent, low-level active infection, and CMV disease. Clinical judgment must be used when evaluating QNAT results. In many centers, immunofluorescence assay that detects CMV antigens (pp65) in the peripheral blood leukocytes is also used. Though it costs less, results are operator dependent with standardization issues. Anti-CMV immunoglobulin M (IgM) seropositivity has poor sensitivity and should not be relied upon to make a diagnosis of CMV disease.

PREVENTION

The strategy of preemptive therapy relies on weekly PCR testing and close follow-up which is challenging to implement in the Indian context due to logistics and cost. On the other hand, universal prophylaxis is popular with the advent of generics with reduced cost of therapy. Oral VGCV is started within the first post-transplant week at a renal adjusted dose of 900 mg [450 mg if the estimated glomerular filtration rate (eGFR) is <60 mL/min]. The duration of universal prophylaxis varies depending on the perceived risk. A minimum of 6 months for D+/R– serostatus which is followed by active surveillance in the form of QNAT testing on a monthly basis is recommended. In R+/D± status, 3 months of prophylaxis is indicated. In the rare D–/R– status, the risk of primary infection should be reduced by stricter policies on blood transfusions and environmental exposures. Late reactivation has to be guarded against. This is partly due to the virostatic nature of ganciclovir (GCV) and partly because these antivirals do not target latently infected cells. One additional benefit of universal prophylaxis is the protection against herpes simplex and varicella zoster viruses. It is recommended to reinitiate prophylaxis or preemptive therapy when antilymphocyte antibodies and high doses of steroids are used for treatment of rejections.

IMMUNE MONITORING ASSAYS

Several immune monitoring tools which depend on the release of IFN-γ from peripheral blood mononuclear cells are currently available in the West. These include CMV-specific QuantiFERON, enzyme-linked immune absorbent spot (ELISPOT), and intracellular cytokine staining (ICS) platforms. If the virus-specific $CD4^+$ and $CD8^+$ responses are negative, a higher risk for CMV disease is predicted. **Table 2** shows how these can help in decision-making when used along with viral nucleic acid testing (NAT) assays. However, these are not yet widely available in India. The table shows the utility of these tests.

TABLE 2: Cytomegalovirus (CMV)-specific immune monitoring assays—guidelines.

Clinical setting	*Interferon assay*	*Interpretation*	*Decision*
Pretransplant monitoring	Negative	High risk	Prophylaxis indicated
Post-transplant 3–6 months for end of prophylaxis	+	Protection	Stop prophylaxis
	–	Risk	Continue prophylaxis

TREATMENT

Ganciclovir is a nucleoside analog which is phosphorylated to form GCV triphosphate inside body; the active drug preferentially inhibits the viral DNA polymerase UL54. Phosphorylation of GCV by CMV-encoded UL97 kinase is the first step which is followed by host cellular kinases-driven phosphorylation. Thus, tissue selectivity of infected cells is ensured by the initial viral kinase encoded phosphorylation step. Intravenous GCV therapy is indicated in those with life-threatening CMV disease and gastrointestinal illness and in pediatric patients.

The dose is 5 mg/kg which is adjusted for the renal function. It is crucial to use renal dose adjustment to prevent both underdosing and drug toxicity. The duration of therapy is usually 14–21 days. Therapy can be complicated by leukopenia, which is treated by injections of granulocyte-macrophage colony stimulating factor (GM-CSF) without dose reduction. Other side effects are thrombocytopenia, diarrhea, and intravenous catheter-related infections. Regular QNAT tests to monitor the progress are required since effective therapy leads to progressive reduction in viral load.[5] Parenteral therapy is followed by 3 months of secondary prophylaxis with oral VGCV therapy. Preemptive therapy is continued until two negative plasma CMV PCR DNA (quantitative) tests results are done within a gap of 1 week.

This is indicated due to the virostatic nature of GCV in addition to the fact that the drug is ineffective in latent infection of cells. When the situation is life-threatening with multi-organ involvement, CMV immunoglobulins or intravenous immunoglobulin (IVIG) (with passive antibody transfer from multiple donors) therapy is instituted with variable results.

Reduction of immunosuppression is advised if there is presence of CMV disease, inadequate clinical response, high viral loads, or cytopenia. Mainly, antimetabolite immunosuppressants are stopped.

Mild manifestations of CMV infection can be treated by 900 mg twice daily of oral VGCV therapy. This is a prodrug which is rapidly metabolized to active GCV in the GI mucosa and liver; a corollary is to use parenteral GCV when GI involvement is prominent. Oral VGCV and intravenous GCV treatment have been found to be associated with similar long-term outcomes in CMV syndrome and tissue-invasive CMV disease based on the VICTOR study.[6]

DRUG RESISTANCE

Ganciclovir-resistant CMV infection is rare seen in 1–2% of KTR. It is suspected when viral counts do not show a downward trend after the 1–2 weeks of adequate antiviral therapy or if there is clinical progression.

Alterations in the *UL97* gene are more common and appear first in about 90% of cases, resulting in impairment in the processing of GCV to its triphosphorylated form. Mostly GCV-resistant CMV strains are susceptible to foscarnet (FOS), as it does not require activation and blocks the viral DNA polymerase by a noncompetitive mechanism. An inadequately dosed prophylactic regimen is an important risk factor. Testing for gene mutations (*UL54*, *UL97*) is not widely available. If suspected, intravenous GCV dose is prolonged by a few more weeks or sometimes these cases respond to increased dose of GCV. *UL54* DNA polymerase gene mutations confer increased GCV resistance and likely cross-resistance to cidofovir (CDV) and/or FOS.

Alternative agents have increased side-effect profile and toxicity. Intravenous FOS in a dose of 90 mg/kg twice a day for 2 weeks is used in drug-resistant forms. The drug is nephrotoxic and can lead to renal magnesium and potassium wasting. Cardiac arrhythmias and genital ulcerations are other side effects. Another alternative is intravenous CDV therapy at a dose of 5 mg/kg weekly for 2 weeks followed by 3 mg/kg every 2 weeks. CDV is again nephrotoxic (excreted by kidneys) in addition to tendency for neutropenia and metabolic acidosis. Leflunomide is used as off label drug with mixed results.

NEWER AGENTS

Letermovir and maribavir are drugs which recently received US Food and Drug Administration (USFDA) approval as newer agents.

Letermovir is available in both oral and intravenous formulations, inhibits the viral terminase enzyme complex encoded by UL56, and does not share cross-resistance with GCV. Its efficacy and safety have already been demonstrated in a hematopoietic stem cell transplantation (HSCT) patient.

Maribavir inhibits CMV UL97, available in oral formulation. It inhibits viral maturation and egress. It has not been found to be associated with myelosuppression or nephrotoxicity.

Brincidofovir is a lipid conjugated derivative of CDV with improved intracellular active drug delivery. It is an inhibitor of viral DNA polymerase. It has better safety profile than CDV.

Cytomegalovirus vaccines are in the early phases of development. They aim to prevent or modulate CMV replication and/or CMV disease. As of now, no recommendations have been made.

INDIAN EXPERIENCE

A recent publication from the Postgraduate Institute of Medical Education and Research (PGIMER), Chandigarh, highlights their 18-year experience of managing post-transplant CMV disease with an incidence of 14%. Diagnostic testing with both pp65 antigenemia assay and QNAT were employed with excellent agreement between them. A protocolized regimen of initial parenteral GCV for 3 weeks followed by oral VGCV therapy for 3 months resulted in remarkable results of zero graft failure or mortality. Another publication from the same center showed the renal histopathologic changes of CMV infection in the form of tubulointerstitial involvement (most common) followed by isolated glomerular involvement without proliferation and thrombotic microangiopathy.

CONCLUSION

Cytomegalovirus infection is an important viral infection in the postrenal transplantation period which tests the clinician's diagnostic and decision-making skills. In recent years, universal chemoprophylaxis during the initial months of the post-transplant period has shifted the timeline to late reactivation which should be recognized and treated without delay.

REFERENCES

1. Minz RW, Kumar M, Kanwar DB, Sharma A, Singh P, Singh J, et al. Cytomegalovirus infection in postrenal transplant recipients: 18 years' experience from a tertiary referral center. Transplant Proc. 2020;52:3173-8.
2. Knechtle SJ, Marson LP, Morris PJ. Kidney Transplantation: Principles and Practice, 8th edition. Philadelphia: Elsevier; 2020.
3. Kotton CN, Kumar D, Caliendo AM, Huprikar S, Chou S, Danziger-Isakov L, et al. The Third International Consensus Guidelines on the management of cytomegalovirus in solid-organ transplantation. Transplantation. 2018;102:900-31.
4. Rane S, Nada R, Minz M, Sakhuja V, Joshi K. Spectrum of cytomegalovirus-induced renal pathology in renal allograft recipients. Transplant Proc. 2012;44:713-6.
5. Santos CAQ, Vella J, Brennan DC. Clinical manifestations, diagnosis, and management of cytomegalovirus disease in kidney transplant patients. UpToDate, Version—30.38.0. Waltham, MA: Wolters aKluwer; 2022.
6. Asberg A, Humar A, Jardine AG, Rollag H, Pescovitz MD, Mouas H, et al. Long-term outcomes of CMV disease treatment with valganciclovir versus IV ganciclovir in solid organ transplant recipients. Am J Transplant. 2009;9:1205-13.

12.2.2 BK Virus Nephropathy

Raj Kumar Sharma, Sonia Mehrotra

INTRODUCTION

BK virus (BKV) was first reported in 1971. It is a small, nonenveloped deoxyribonucleic acid (DNA) virus that belongs to the Polyomaviridae family and is present globally. BKV infects the majority of the population in their childhood and usually is asymptomatic or associated with fever and mild upper respiratory symptoms.[1] At the time of secondary infection, BKV enters a resting state and gets located into the renal tubular and uroepithelial cells and causes asymptomatic viruria in 7–15% of healthy subjects.[2] Polyomavirus infection in kidney transplant recipients is difficult to manage due to lack of effective antiviral therapy. BKV nephropathy could be a serious complication early after kidney transplantation when recipients are on heavy immunosuppression.[3,4] There are no specific medications or effective antiviral therapies for BKV infection. Insufficient immunosuppression usage can influence the development of acute or chronic rejection, leading to graft dysfunction and graft loss.[5]

EPIDEMIOLOGY

Many publications have suggested that BKV has high prevalence and low morbidity in healthy individuals. In newborns, maternal antibodies protect infants from BKV infection, and after the disappearance of maternal antibodies, BKV infection starts to manifest, with 10–30% seropositivity in infants and 65–>90% seropositivity during childhood. Primary BKV infection in immunocompetent patients is usually a subclinical event and is associated with mild nonspecific symptoms, after which BKV can persist in many organs of the body such as renal tubules, uroepithelium, and peripheral blood leukocytes.[2,6]

PREVALENCE

BK virus as a primary infection establishes as lifelong infection in renal tubular and uroepithelial cells. Both primary infection and persistent infection could be clinically silent and not associated with any known adverse effects for most individuals.

BK virus nephropathy (BKVN) can occur in kidney transplant recipients through reactivation of hidden infection or transmission of new infection via the donor kidney resulting in allograft nephropathy. During the first year after transplantation when cellular immunity is most suppressed and when recipients are on heavy immunosuppression, viral replication most commonly occurs. Viruria can occur in 30–40% of the patients, and viremia may follow viruria in a few weeks.

Approximately 1–10% of kidney transplant recipients will develop BKVN. Historically, BKVN is associated with graft loss rates that could exceed 50%. With the implementation of standardized screening protocols and reduction of immunosuppression rates, short-term graft loss due to BKVN has dropped significantly.[7,8]

RISK FACTORS

Risk factors for BKVN after renal transplantation include deceased donors transplant and episodes of acute and chronic rejection.

Other risk factors for BKVN in clinical studies reported are as follows:

- *Donor factors:* Deceased donor, high BKV antibody titers, female gender of donor, degree of human leukocyte antigen (HLA) mismatches, positivity of HLA A9, and negativity of HLA C7.
- *Recipient factors:* Older age, male gender, ABO incompatibility, history of hemodialysis, low BKV antibody titers, race, diabetes, positivity of HLA A2, negativity of HLA C7, and HLA B51.
- *Post-transplant factors:* Cold ischemia time, delayed graft function, acute rejection and antirejection treatment, steroid exposure, tacrolimus and/or mycophenolate mofetil (MMF)-based maintenance immunosuppression, lower total lymphocyte percentage, and ureteral stent insertion.

A single-center report noted that the absence of the HLA C7 allele in the donor or recipient increases the risk for sustained BKV in the recipient at least threefold. Other studies have reported that a lower proportion of Black race Americans develop BKV, independent of other confounding risk factors **(Table 1)**.[9-15]

TABLE 1: Summary of proposed risk factors for BK virus infection.[4]

Donor risk factors	• BK virus seropositive donor • Degree of HLA mismatching • HLA C7
Recipient risk factors	• Older recipient age • Male recipient • Recipient race (non-African American) • Diabetes
Transplant risk factors	• Acute rejection episodes • Cold ischemia time • Delayed graft function • Ureteral stent placement • Antithymocyte globulin induction • Tacrolimus and/or MMF-based maintenance immunosuppression

(HLA: human leukocyte antigens; MMF: mycophenolate mofetil)

CHAPTER HIGHLIGHTS

- BKV is a small, nonenveloped deoxyribonucleic acid (DNA) virus that belongs to the Polyomaviridae family.
- Early diagnosis and management need to differentiate rejection from BKV nephropathy and intervention to prevent allograft failure.
- BK virus nephropathy (BKVN) in adult renal transplant recipients initially presents with graft dysfunction and later can result in graft loss.
- Factors associated with BKVN are immunosuppressive drugs, allograft rejection, donor's previous BKV infection, autoimmunity, gender, race, human leukocyte antigen (HLA) mismatch, and cold ischemia time.
- The role of a transplant nephrologist is to reduce immunosuppression through early diagnosis of BKVN.
- The American Society of Transplantation guidelines and Banff grading of BKV nephritis suggest allograft biopsy and estimation of BKV viral load for all kidney transplant recipients with BKVN.
- After allograft loss due to BK nephropathy, retransplantation can be done. Many studies suggest that before retransplantation nephrectomy is not required, but BK viral load should not be detectable prior to retransplant.

VIROLOGY

BK viruses are small, nonenveloped viruses with a core of circular double-stranded DNA that replicates bidirectionally. The chief proteins are divided into three regions: (1) early encoding region, (2) late encoding region, and (3) noncoding control region. The transcription of early and late coding regions proceeds in a bidirectional way. The early coding regions encode for the early regulatory proteins, nonstructural polypeptides, and two tumors antigens (small-T and large-T antigens). Antibody against T antigens is useful to detect BKV infection by polymerase chain reaction (PCR). The base-pair genome encodes three capsid proteins on viral proteins and late structural proteins [viral capsid protein 1 (VP1), VP2, and VP3 and also agnoprotein]. The genome also contains a noncoding control region that contains the replication and transcription factor binding sites. The agnoprotein and its protein products help regulate virus replication and disrupt host cell processes. After attachment, BKV is internalized via caveolae-mediated endocytosis (bulb-shaped plasma membrane called caveolae). Once inside the cell, the virus transports to the nucleus and establishes a suppressed or lytic infection.[5]

PATHOGENESIS

BK virus viruria can occur in pregnancy, cancer, human immunodeficiency virus (HIV) infection, diabetes, and after organ transplantation. Replication of BKV occurs in recipients on immunosuppression.[13]

The primary BKV infection is prevented by the innate immune system of the body, while adaptive humoral response prevents or limits BKV reactivation.

BK virus replication typically progresses through three stages. Asymptomatic viruria occurs in approximately one-quarter to one-third of patients during the first post-transplant year. Viremia follows viruria in approximately one-half of patients. In a subset of viremic patients, viral replication progresses leading to damage to renal tubular epithelium and BKVN. Like viruria and viremia, BKVN is typically asymptomatic, and a rise in serum creatinine maybe the sole presenting sign. Without control of viral replication, allograft loss can ensue within a period of months.

The BKV multiplies in the interstitium and crosses into the peritubular capillaries, causing viremia and finally attacking the allograft, resulting in various tubulointerstitial lesions. The infected renal tubular epithelial cells detach from the basement membrane and appear in urine as decoy cells. The renal tubulointerstitium with profound inflammation (BKV-associated nephropathy) in kidney transplant recipients is the result of continued intragraft inflammation, tubular injury, and upregulation of profibrotic mediators. Damage to the bladder's transitional epithelium and blood vessels can result in hemorrhagic cystitis in transplant recipients.

BK virus nephropathy could progress in 1–10% of recipients showing viral infection in urine (viruria) and could result in BK viremia. The pathogenesis of BKVN includes recipient allograft immune activation and ineffective immune response by the infected T lymphocytes. If humoral immunity dose does not trigger an effective anti-BKV immune response, BKVN can result.

CLINICAL MANIFESTATIONS

Tubulointerstitial nephritis is the most common manifestation of BKVN. In asymptomatic recipients, urine analysis shows white blood cells (WBCs), red blood cells (RBCs) and cellular casts. There is an associated increase in serum creatinine levels. BKV infection generally occurs 10–13 months post-transplant. BKVN may occur early at week 1 post-transplant or as late as 5 years post-transplant as acute or chronic graft dysfunction. Primary BKV infection transmission occurs via vertical transmission from mother to baby during the period immediately before and after childbirth with gastrointestinal or respiratory transmission.[16,17]

BK Virus and Renal Disease

The virus starts replication in the uroepithelial cells and shows findings in urine as uroepithelial cells (viruria) in few days and later in the blood (viremia) and causes BKVN. BKV-associated nephropathy could be asymptomatic with viruria, hematuria, and subclinical chronic allograft injury. Severe renal dysfunction, ureteric stenosis, and hemorrhagic cystitis can occur in renal transplant patients due to BKV infection.

BK nephropathy can also occur in hematopoietic stem cell transplantation, in heart and lung transplant recipients, and in immunocompromised HIV-infected patients and can also present as acute kidney injury (AKI).

Other clinical manifestations due to BKV infection can occur in other parts of the body including ophthalmologic, hepatic, autoimmune, pulmonary, neurological manifestation, and malignancy.

Kidney Disease Improving Global Outcomes (KDIGO) and American Transplant Society guidelines suggest that screening of BKVN should start immediately after transplantation and to be continued for up to 2 years (monthly for 6 months, then every 3 monthly for 2 years post-transplant).[5,18]

Screening Technique (Table 2)

Decoy cells do not occur in every renal allograft recipient with BKVN. This marker is generally available at all labs. It is a useful marker in the identification of BKV infection but cannot replace viral load.

Urine Electron Microscopy

Presence of Haufen bodies in urine smear of transplant patients corresponds to high levels of BK viremia. Haufen bodies are three-dimensional cast-like polyomavirus aggregates (termed "Haufen" after the German word for "cluster or stack"). They can be observed in voided urine samples by negative staining electron microscopy (EM), but its interpretation is difficult and needs expertise for EM. Urinary EM examination is not practical for routine practice.

Quantitative Polymerase Chain Reaction on Plasma for BK Virus

Plasma can be tested in renal transplant patients to assess the risk for BKV nephropathy. BKV PCR viral load of $>5 \times 10^3$ copies/mL plasma suggests risk for BKV disease. In the plasma, BKV load of ≥10,000 copies/mL or (greater than or equal to 4 log copies/mL) correlates highly with nephropathy and is considered "presumed nephropathy." Some patients may not develop renal disease despite high viral loads in the plasma sample. They should be monitored at intervals. Graft renal biopsy maybe required to differentiate the graft rejection from BKVN.

TABLE 2: BK virus screening methods.[20,22,24,26]

Screening method	Positive predictive value (%)	Negative predictive value (%)	Sensitivity (%)	Specificity (%)
BK serum PCR	50–60	100	100	88
BK urine PCR	40	100	100	78
Decoy cells	29	100	25	84
Haufen	97	100	100	99
VP1 urinary mRNA	95	100	93.8	93.9

(mRNA: messenger ribonucleic acid; PCR: polymerase chain reaction)

Benefits of quantitative polymerase chain reaction: Polymerase chain reaction technique has faster results, ability to monitor viral load for BKV disease, and response to therapy (real-time TaqMan PCR targeting BKV large T-antigen gene).

Quantitative BK Virus Polymerase Chain Reaction in Urine for BK Virus

Urine should not be tested alone but should be tested in parallel with plasma BKV PCR. Standardization is required for different markers to diagnose hemorrhagic cystitis. Viral loads of $>10^7$ copies/mL in urine are associated with BKV disease. The negative predictive value of a negative BKV PCR in urine is high. Rapid BKV culture provides qualitative results in 2–3 days. It detects only high titers of BKV in urine ($>10^7$ copies/mL). High titers correlate fairly well with clinical BKV disease.[19]

Difficulties in Standardization of Quantitative BK Virus Polymerase Chain Reaction

Higher BK viral load values in plasma and urine have a positive predictive value for BKV disease. There are no exact viral load cutoff levels to diagnose BKVN.

Sample types, PCR quantitative standards, gene targets, and test protocols can make associations of viral loads among different laboratories difficult to interpret. Mutations in primer or probe-binding sites can lead to low viral load quantification and can result in false-negative results.[20-25]

Urinary BK-messenger ribonucleic acid (mRNA) in the urinary cells detects BK VP1-mRNA replication; this method is considered highly specific and sensitive for BKV disease but would require validation to report.[26]

Histology of Renal Allograft Biopsy

This is the "gold standard" to diagnose rejection, chronic allograft nephropathy, and acute tubular necrosis. Renal allograft dysfunction due to viral infection (BKVN) can be missed sometime in biopsy. BKVN on histology needs to be correlated with other laboratory findings. The allograft involvement is usually focal; thus there is a possibility of sampling error. Therefore, two cores containing medulla are required for an adequate biopsy sample.

The Banff classification of BKVN is divided into three stages:[27] Of the various factors associated with the clinical presentation of BKVN, two independent histological variables (the intrarenal viral load and the extent of interstitial fibrosis) show strong association with BKVN.

- *Stage 1:* No or minimal number of injuries to tubular epithelial cells in some of the virus-infected cells.
- *Stage 2:* More than two cells show tubular epithelial cell necrosis or lysis with denudation of the basement membrane.
- *Stage 3:* Interstitial fibrosis affecting >50% of the cortex as with any degree of tubular injury.

American Society of Transplantation Classification of BKVN: The American Society of Transplantation (AST) classification semiquantifies the histological findings into patterns (stages A, B, and C). Staging of BKV-associated nephropathy (BKVAN) is based on viral cytopathic changes, interstitial inflammation, tubular atrophy, and interstitial fibrosis.[28] It especially focuses on the presence of interstitial inflammation and pattern percentage in stage B.

- *Stage A:* Cytopathic effects in <25% of biopsy with BKV infection and no inflammation specified >10%.
- *Stage B:* Degree of tubular injury and significant inflammation affecting virus-infected cells in a number of cells less than 25% (B1), between 25 and 50% (B2), and >50% (B3) in biopsy.
- *Stage C:* Any degree of tubular injury and tubular atrophy/fibrosis affecting >50% of biopsy with virus-infected cells.

SUMMARIZED LABORATORY FINDINGS OF VARIOUS TEST RESULTS TO DIAGNOSE BK VIRUS NEPHROPATHY

- Increase in serum creatinine levels, urine decoy cells with an enlarged nucleus containing single basophilic intranuclear inclusion, tubular casts, and inflammatory cells.
- Blood BK PCR can detect BK viremia suggesting BKVN, hemorrhagic cystitis or ureteral stenosis, increased detection of RBC, and protein in urine.
- Urine BK PCR with counts $>10^7$ copies/mL, renal biopsy histology (BKVN) showing enlarged intranuclear inclusions and cell detachments, cytopathic changes starting at medulla and distal tubules, and progressing to proximal tubules.

TREATMENT (TABLE 3)

There is no specific antiviral therapy to treat BKVN. Recommended guidelines by the AST is to start treatment for BKVN at a high level of viral load in the blood, which should be detected by routine screening. The management includes mainly reduction in immunosuppression.

Overview of Treatment for BK Virus Nephropathy

Recipients going for transplantation should have prior screening for BKV viral load by reverse transcription-PCR (RT-PCR) (plasma and urine) in both recipient and donor. Post-transplantation urine and plasma viral loads and urine cytology should be done every month up to 6 months and every 3 months up to 5 years. If BKV viral load is detected, then closely monitor renal function. If creatinine increases from baseline, the recipient should undergo an allograft biopsy (with histology grading). If there is any rejection, then the recipient should be treated for antirejection therapy. Monitor for donor-specific antibodies or drug toxicity. Reduction in immunosuppression should be done if BKV viral load in blood is positive. Reduction in calcineurin inhibitors (CNI), antiproliferative drug, and corticosteroids would be required in stages. First, MMF dose should be reduced by 50% or stopped if indicated by the persistence of viremia. CNI reduction would be required in the second stage. Switching immunosuppression may include, from tacrolimus to cyclosporine, mycophenolic acid (MPA) to leflunomide (active metabolite inhibits viral replication via pyrimidine depletion), switch from MPA to mammalian target of rapamycin (mTOR) inhibitors (inhibits the proliferation of specific T-cell BKV and controls the differentiation of memory $CD8^+$ responses), addition of intravenous immunoglobulin (IVIG) to neutralize antibodies to BKV, and close monitoring of BKV viremia until BKV viral load becomes negative with follow-up of serum creatinine levels and BKV viral load to show that antiviral response is cornerstone of BKVN management strategy. BK PCR monitoring should be done every 2–4 weeks for 3–12 months after any immunosuppression increase.[29-35]

Cidofovir is a nucleotide analog of cytosine. It acts against DNA viruses and is approved for topical treatments and for cytomegalovirus (CMV) retinitis (inflammation of the retina), adenovirus infection, and BKV disease. BKV replication is inhibited by fluoroquinolones as an antiviral effect (BKV) in both hematopoietic stem cell and kidney transplant recipients. Fluoroquinolones show in vitro inhibition of BKV replication. IVIG can be used with reduced immunosuppression to neutralizing antibodies of BKV. Leflunomide, an immunosuppressive drug, is approved for use in rheumatoid arthritis. It can be used for BKVN following the discontinuation of MMF. Everolimus inhibits mTOR kinase activity and can be used to replace MMF **(Flowchart 1)**.[36-40]

None of these therapies has demonstrated clear benefit.

For established BKVN, ciprofloxacin 500 mg twice daily for 60 days, low-dose cidofovir (0.1–1.0 mg/kg every 2 weeks with probenecid for four doses), elimination or substitution

TABLE 3: Summary of treatment strategies for BK virus and BK virus nephropathy.[4,41-50]

Treatment	Reference	Immunosuppression adjustment strategy	Patients with BKV or BKVN	Outcome	Adverse events
Immunosuppression reduction	Hirsch et al.[11]	Varied; CNI minimization or switch of agent	5	4/5 cleared BKV	• Three episodes of rejection • No allograft losses to BKVN
	Alméras et al.[41]	CNI and MMF dose reduction simultaneously	11	8/11 cleared BKV	• Three episodes of rejection • No allograft losses to BKVN
	Weiss et al.[42]	Withdrawal of CNI or MMF versus dose reduction of both CNI and MMF	35	19/35 retain allograft function	CNI withdrawal is associated with superior allograft survival compared with dose reduction strategy
	Schaub et al.[43]	CNI minimization followed by discontinuation of MMF	38	35/38 cleared BKV	• Three episodes of acute rejection • No graft losses due to BK • No difference in patient or kidney survival with BK
	Hardinger et al.[44]	MMF discontinuation followed by minimization of the CNI	23	12/23 cleared BKV	• Five episodes of acute rejection • No graft losses due to BK • Patient survival was inferior in the BK group, but allograft survival was similar
Leflunomide	Faguer et al.[45]	MMF replaced with leflunomide	11	5/11 cleared BKV	• One episode of acute rejection • One graft lost to BKVN
	Leca et al.[46]	MMF replaced with "low-dose" or "high-dose" leflunomide	21	11/21 cleared BKV	Four graft losses
Cidofovir	Kuypers et al.[47]	MMF/CNI reduction with/without "adjuvant" cidofovir	21	6/8 cidofovir patients cleared BKV	• Two acute rejections in the cidofovir group • No graft losses in the cidofovir group
Intravenous immunoglobulin (IVIG) *Dose:* IV: 0.25–2.0 g/kg	Vu et al.[48]	Treatment with IVIG was given only to patients who did not respond to 8 weeks of the adjustment of immunosuppression and leflunomide	30	90% had a positive response in clearing viremia	No serious adverse events reported
	Moon et al.[48]	IVIG (1.0 g/kg) given if high viral load persisted for 4 weeks, even after treatment with a combination of leflunomide therapy and immunosuppression reduction	52	BK DNA viral load significantly lowered in patients with persistent BKVN	No significant side effects noted

(BKV: BK virus; BKVN: BK virus nephropathy; CNI: calcineurin inhibitors; DNA: deoxyribonucleic acid; MMF: mycophenolate mofetil)

of MMF with leflunomide, loading dose of 100 mg daily for 5 days followed by 40 mg daily to attain blood level 50–100 µg/mL when MMF is discontinued (all these are weak antiviral agents) or azathioprine, IVIG therapy, and IVIG dose 100 mg/kg weekly for 10 weeks (total dose 1 g/kg) (for BKVN with rejection) are all potential treatments, which have shown some benefits in small studies.

Late rejection after reduction in immunosuppression can occur in 15% of BKVN kidneys. After sustained viral clearance, immunosuppression maybe increased modestly. Regular monitoring for relapse of BKVN viremia should be done.

SOME CLINICAL SCENARIOS

CASE VIGNETTE 1

Urinary Chemokine as Biomarker

BKV replication in different stages can be detected using urinary C-X-C motif chemokine-10 (uCXCL10) as a diagnostic biomarker. Studies suggest that urinary chemokines levels are increased in patients with BKV infection. In kidney transplant recipients, uCXCL10 increases with BKV viral load but not with increased BKV in urine. uCXCL10 could be used as a prognostic biomarker of estimated glomerular filtration rate (eGFR) decrease, and it also predicts higher inflammatory burden and poor renal outcomes.[51-53]

Flowchart 1: Proposed algorithm for the management of kidney transplant recipient with BK viremia or BK nephropathy.

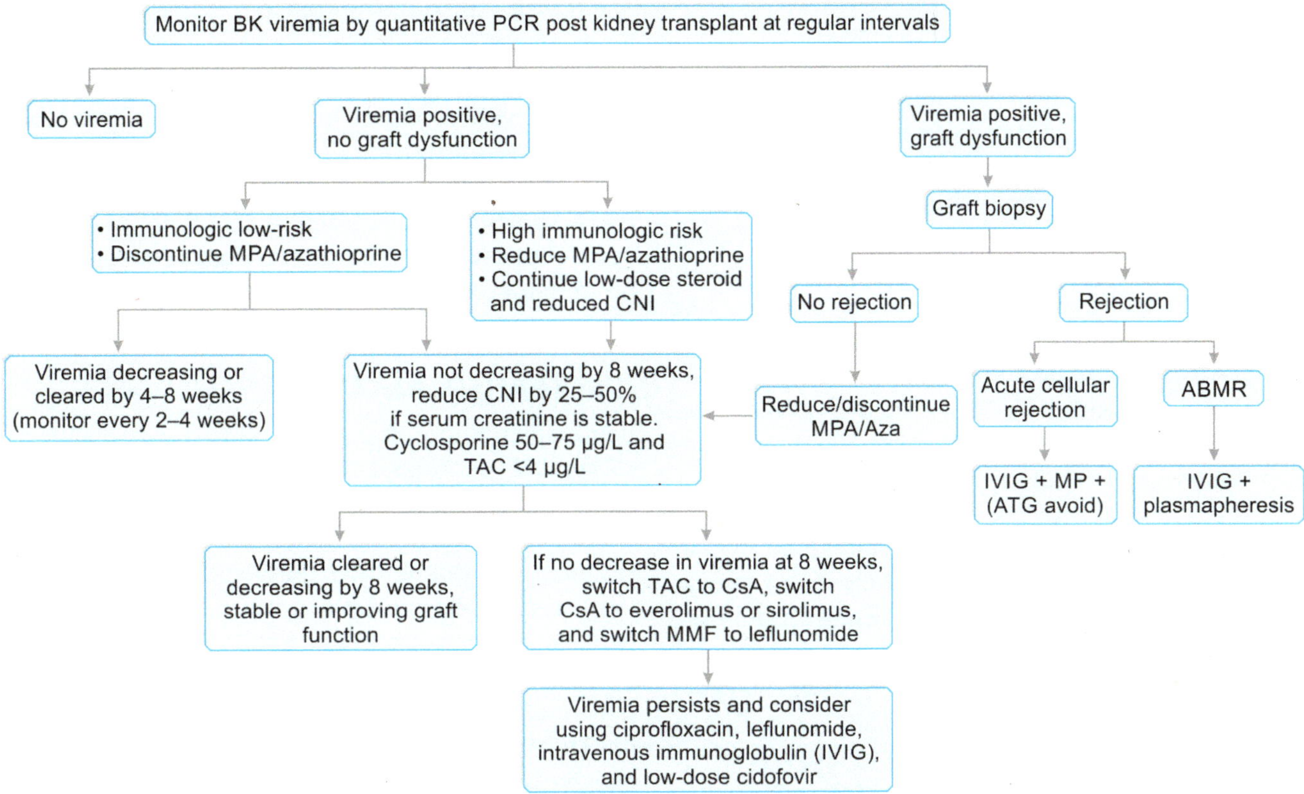

Note: Monitor digital subtraction angiography (DSA), acute rejection, and viral load for relapse of viremia.
(ABMR: antibody-mediated rejection; ATG: antithymocyte globulin; Aza: azathioprine; CNI: calcineurin inhibitors; CsA: cyclosporine A; MMF: mycophenolate mofetil; MP: methylprednisolone; MPA: mycophenolic acid; PCR: polymerase chain reaction; TAC: tacrolimus)

CASE VIGNETTE 2

Concomitant COVID-19 Infection

COVID-19 infection can stimulate viral replication in kidney transplant recipients on immunosuppressive drugs with recurrence of BKVN. COVID-19 infection is associated with weak cytotoxic T-cell (CD8+) response, which triggers BKV replication and development of BKVN.[54]

CASE VIGNETTE 3

Absence of BK Virus Viremia and BK Virus Nephropathy

A renal transplant patient from a living related donor had biopsy-proven acute antibody-mediated and cellular rejection after 1 year and was treated with methylprednisolone, plasmapheresis, and IVIG. Serum creatinine came down to baseline, but the patient developed CMV infection with pancytopenia and transaminitis treated with ganciclovir. Ultrasound showed partial obstruction of the proximal ureter with moderate hydronephrosis, and quantitative PCR assay for BKV DNA was negative in plasma. Graft kidney biopsy showed viral cytopathic changes in the tubular epithelium with interstitial inflammation. BKV infection was confirmed by in situ hybridization. BKVN was confirmed by graft biopsy with no viremia. This was treated with immunosuppression reduction.[55]

CASE VIGNETTE 4

BK Virus Nephropathy in Native Kidney in Nonrenal Transplant

Case report of BKVN in a patient who underwent heart transplantation. Kidney biopsy showed active chronic tubulointerstitial nephritis associated with late-stage polyomavirus nephritis, and the blood viral load for BKV was positive. The immunosuppressive treatment was reduced. After 2 years of follow-up, the patient had a stable renal function. A high index of suspicion, kidney biopsy, and BK viremia and viruria can diagnose BKV infection and BKVN, in nonrenal solid organ transplantation.[56]

CASE VIGNETTE 5

BK Virus Nephropathy in Pediatric Transplant

Case reports of treatment with IVIG in pediatric renal transplant recipients with BKV infection and allograft dysfunction. BKVN can occur even at low plasma viral loads. Treatment with IVIG is successful in persistent BK viremia and BKVN, although the reduction in immunosuppression is the main treatment. Other therapies such as cidofovir, leflunomide, and fluoroquinolones have also been used to treat BKVN in pediatric renal transplants.[57] *But the benefit of these therapies has not been shown.*

INDIAN CLINICAL STUDIES AND CASE REPORTS

In renal transplant recipients, BKV causes allograft dysfunction in 2–5% due to tubulointerstitial nephritis. Sachdeva et al. in the first report of BKV infection among Indian renal transplant recipients used routine histologic examination, immunohistochemistry, and EM to retrospectively screen for BK polyomavirus in 414 renal allograft biopsy specimens from 321 transplant recipients presenting with allograft dysfunction. All patients had received a combination of cyclosporine, azathioprine, and prednisolone. A total of 30 biopsy specimens (9.3%) were positive for BK polyomavirus. They concluded that a high incidence of BKV infection in Indian transplant recipients coexisted with acute rejection in a majority of patients.[58]

Reports of BKVN with the features of acute cellular rejection in a patient with ureteric stenosis caused by BKV infection, which was managed successfully with stepwise modification of immunosuppression along with double-J stenting, leading to stabilization of graft function. Etta et al. concluded in their case study that BKV infection can occur with acute rejection. Immunosuppression reduction is required. Timely management can help in recovery of the graft function and better long-term graft outcome. Rejection with vasculitis maybe associated with BKV infection. Both can cause ureteric stenosis and would require urologic intervention.[59]

Gupta et al. conclude in their study that immunosuppression activates BKVN and manifests as tubulointerstitial nephritis causing renal allograft dysfunction. A total of 402 patients who underwent renal allograft biopsy from 2013 to 2016 were included in this study. Six patients were diagnosed to have BKVN. Histopathology showed ground-glass intranuclear inclusions accompanied by acute tubular injury, interstitial inflammation, and varying degrees of interstitial fibrosis and tubular atrophy. Patients were managed with a reduction in the overall immunosuppression. Only one patient progressed to graft failure on follow-up. The overall prevalence of polyomavirus infection in this report is 1.49%.[60]

Thakur et al. studied prospectively the activation of BKV in renal transplant. 32 renal allograft recipients were prospectively monitored with protocol biopsies of allografts, BKV DNA load in plasma, and viral particles in urine by EM on day 1, and at 1, 3, and 6 months. The baseline BKV DNA load in plasma was quantitated in 21 corresponding donors. The study showed a total of 15.7% and 25% urine, and plasma samples were positive for BKV at any time during a 6-month follow-up. The highest incidence of BK viruria and viremia occurred at 1 month. In protocol biopsies, focal positivity of SV-40 T Ag was seen in 8% biopsies.[61]

Shah et al. reported BKVN in nonrenal transplant patients who developed biopsy-proven BKVN in native kidneys.

In the first case of a heart transplant patient on maintenance immunosuppression, 3 years post-transplant, the patient developed AKI and underwent a kidney biopsy, which showed acute tubular injury and tubulointerstitial nephritis with moderate interstitial fibrosis and serum BK virus PCR was positive.

A systematic review of the literature on biopsy-proven BKVN in native kidney showed that there are 65 reported cases of BKVN in native kidneys. Evaluation for BKN should be considered in immunocompromised patients who exhibit unexplained renal failure.[62]

RETRANSPLANTATION

Retransplantation after graft failure due to BKVN can be successfully performed. Kidney transplant loss due to BKVN should not be a barrier to retransplantation. Pretransplant clearance of plasma BK viral load is necessary for both recipient and donor. After retransplantation, it was found that graft nephrectomy did not protect from BKVN in patients with loss of graft due to BKVN. BKV may persist and relapse of previous BKV or new infection could emerge again after retransplant. Close monitoring through recommended investigations is required to manage BKVN in retransplant recipients **(Table 3)**.[63]

REFERENCES

1. Helle F, Brochot E, Handala L, Martin E, Castelain S, Francois C, et al. Biology of the BKPyV: an update. Viruses. 2017;9(11):327.
2. De Gascun CF, Carr MJ. Human polyomavirus reactivation: disease pathogenesis and treatment approaches. Clin Dev Immunol. 2013;2013:373579.
3. Dall A, Hariharan S. BK virus nephritis after renal transplantation. Clin J Am Soc Nephrol. 2008;3(Suppl. 2):S68-75.
4. Sawinski D, Goral S. BK virus infection: an update on diagnosis and treatment. Nephrol Dial Transplant. 2015;30:209-17.
5. Shen CL, Wu BS, Lien TJ, Yang AH, Yang CY. BK polyomavirus nephropathy in kidney transplantation: balancing rejection and infection. Viruses. 2021;13(3):487.
6. Stolt A, Sasnauskas K, Koskela P, Lehtinen M, Dillner J. Seroepidemiology of the human polyomaviruses. J Gen Virol. 2003;84:1499-504.
7. Bohl DL, Brennan DC. BK virus nephropathy and kidney transplantation. Clin J Am Soc Nephrol. 2007;2(Suppl. 1): S36-46.
8. Schwarz A, Held SL, Heim A, Framke T, Haller H, Schmitt C. Viral origin, clinical course, and renal outcomes in patients with BK virus infection after living-donor renal transplantation. Transplantation. 2016;100(4):844-53.
9. Lamarche C, Orio J, Collette S, Senécal L, Hébert MJ, Renoult E, et al. BK polyomavirus and the transplanted kidney: immunopathology and therapeutic approaches. Transplantation. 2016;100(11):2276-87.
10. Sánchez DM, García LJ, Sánchez DM, Jiménez IL, Luján IMS, Soriano MJG, et al. Renal function impairment in kidney transplantation: importance of early BK virus detection. Transplant Proc. 2019;51(2):350-2.

11. Hirsch HH, Knowles W, Dickenmann M, Passweg J, Klimkait T, Mihatsch MJ, et al. Prospective study of polyomavirus type BK replication and nephropathy in renal transplant recipients. N Engl J Med. 2002;347:488-96.
12. Hirsch HH, Randhawa PS, AST Infectious Diseases Community of Practice. BK polyomavirus in solid organ transplantation. Am J Transplant. 2013;13:179-88.
13. Schold JD, Rehman S, Kayle LK, Magliocca J, Srinivas TR, Meier-Kriesche HU. Treatment for BK virus: incidence, risk factors and outcomes for kidney transplant recipients in the United States. Transplant Int. 2009;22:626-34.
14. Steubl D, Baumann M, Schuster T, Fischereder M, Krämer BK, Heemann U, et al. Risk factors and interventional strategies for BK polyomavirus infection after renal transplantation. Scand J Urol Nephrol. 2012;46:466-74.
15. Bohl DL, Storch GA, Ryschkewitsch C, Gaudreault-Keener M, Schnitzler MA, Major EO, et al. Donor origin of BK virus in renal transplantation and role of HLA C7 in susceptibility to sustained BK viremia. Am J Transplant. 2005;5:2213-21.
16. Hirsch HH, Babel N, Comoli P, Friman V, Ginevri F, Jardine A, et al. European perspective on human polyomavirus infection, replication and disease in solid organ transplantation. Clin Microbiol Infect. 2014;20:74-88.
17. Drachenberg CB, Papadimitriou JC, Chaudhry MR, Ugarte R, Mavanur M, Thomas B, et al. Histological evolution of BK virus-associated nephropathy: importance of integrating clinical and pathological findings. Am J Transplant. 2017; 17:2078-91.
18. Kidney Disease: Improving Global Outcomes Transplant Work Group. KDIGO clinical practice guideline for the care of kidney transplant recipients. Am J Transplant. 2009; 9(Suppl. 3):S1-155.
19. Balba GP, Javaid B, Timpone Jr JG. BK polyomavirus infection in the renal transplant recipient. Infect Dis Clin North Am. 2013;27:271-83.
20. Chung BH, Hong YA, Kim HG, Sun IO, Choi SR, Park HS, et al. Clinical usefulness of BK virus plasma quantitative PCR to prevent BK virus associated nephropathy. Transpl Int. 2012;25:687-95.
21. Viscount HB, Eid AJ, Espy MJ, Griffin MD, Thomsen KM, Harmsen WS, et al. Polyomavirus polymerase chain reaction as a surrogate marker of polyomavirus-associated nephropathy. Transplantation. 2007;84:340-5.
22. Chan GCW, Leung AY, Wong AS, Chan KW, Kwong YL, Lai KN, et al. Quantification of BK viral load in asymptomatic renal allograft recipients. Ren Fail. 2012;34(5):550-4.
23. Ma MKM, Leung AYH, Lo KY, Lio WI, Chan HW, Wong I, et al. Screening algorithm for BK virus-associated nephropathy using sequential testing of urinary cytology: a probabilistic model analysis. Am J Nephrol. 2015;42(6):410-7.
24. Zakaria ZE, Elokely AM, Ghorab AA, Bakr AI, Halim MA, Gheith OA, et al. Screening for BK viremia/viruria and the impact of management of BK virus nephropathy in renal transplant recipients. Exp Clin Transplant. 2019;17(Suppl. 1): 83-91.
25. Varella RB, Almeida JR, de Fátima Lopes P, Matos JP, Menezes P, Lugon JR. BK polyomavirus in kidney transplant recipients: screening, monitoring and clinical management. J Bras Nefrol. 2014;36(4):529-34.
26. Ding R, Medeiros M, Dadhania D, Muthukumar T, Kracker D, Kong JM, et al. Noninvasive diagnosis of BK virus nephritis by measurement of messenger RNA for BK virus VP1 in urine. Transplantation. 2002;74(7):987-94.
27. Nickeleit V, Singh HK, Randhawa P, Drachenberg CB, Bhatnagar R, Bracamonte E, et al. The Banff Working Group classification of definitive polyomavirus nephropathy: morphologic definitions and clinical correlations. J Am Soc Nephrol. 2018;29(2):680.
28. Hirsch HH, Randhawa PS, AST Infectious Diseases Community of Practice. BK polyomavirus in solid organ transplantation-guidelines from the American Society of Transplantation Infectious Diseases Community of Practice. Clin Transplant. 2019;33:e13528.
29. Demey B, Tinez C, François C, Helle F, Choukroun G, Duverlie G, et al. Risk factors for BK virus viremia and nephropathy after kidney transplantation: a systematic review. J Clin Virol. 2018;109:6-12.
30. van Aalderen MC, Heutinck KM, Huisman C, ten Berge IJM. BK virus infection in transplant recipients: clinical manifestations, treatment options and the immune response. Neth J Med. 2012;70(4):172-83.
31. Cohen-Bucay A, Ramirez-Andrade SE, Gordon CE, Francis JM, Chitalia VC. Advances in BK virus complications in organ transplantation and beyond. Kidney Med. 2020;2(6):771-86.
32. Saleh A, El Din Khedr MS, Ezzat A, Takou A, Halawa A. Update on the management of BK virus infection. Exp Clin Transplant. 2020;18(6):659-70.
33. Celik B, Shapiro R, Vats A, Randhawa PS. Polyomavirus allograft nephropathy: sequential assessment of histologic viral load, tubulitis, and graft function following changes in immunosuppression. Am J Transplant. 2003;3:1378-82.
34. Saad ER, Bresnahan BA, Cohen EP, Lu N, Orentas RJ, Vasudev B, et al. Successful treatment of BK viremia using reduction in immunosuppression without antiviral therapy. Transplantation. 2008;85:850-4.
35. Peinemann F, de Villiers EM, Dörries K, Adams O, Vögeli TA, Burdach S. Clinical course and treatment of haemorrhagic cystitis associated with BK type of human polyomavirus in nine paediatric recipients of allogeneic bone marrow transplants. Eur J Pediatr. 2000;159:182-8.
36. Zaman RA, Ettenger RB, Cheam H, Malekzadeh MH, Tsai EW. A novel treatment regimen for BK viremia. Transplantation. 2014;97:1166-71.
37. Polanco N, Monte EG, Folgueira MD, Morales E, Martínez EG, Bengoa I, et al. Everolimus-based immunosuppression therapy for BK virus nephropathy. Transplant Proc. 2015;47: 57-61.
38. Patel SJ, Knight RJ, Kuten SA, Graviss EA, Nguyen DT, Moore LW, et al. Ciprofloxacin for BK viremia prophylaxis in kidney transplant recipients: results of a prospective, double-blind, randomized, placebo-controlled trial. Am J Transplant. 2019;19(6):1831-7.
39. Lopez V, Sola E, Gutierrez C, Burgos D, Cabello M, García I, et al. Anterior uveitis associated with treatment with intravenous cidofovir in kidney transplant patients with BK virus nephropathy. Transplant Proc. 2006;38:2412-3.
40. Lee BT, Gabardi S, Grafals M, Hofmann RM, Akalin E, Aljanabi A, et al. Efficacy of levofloxacin in the treatment

of BK viremia: a multicenter, double-blinded, randomized, placebo-controlled trial. Clin J Am Soc Nephrol. 2014;9: 583-9.

41. Alméras C, Foulongne V, Garrigue V, Szwarc I, Vetromile F, Segondy M, et al. Does reduction in immunosuppression in viremic patients prevent BK virus nephropathy in de novo renal transplant recipients? A prospective study. Transplantation. 2008;85:1099-104.
42. Weiss AS, Gralla J, Chan L, Klem P, Wiseman AC. Aggressive immunosuppression minimization reduces graft loss following diagnosis of BK virus-associated nephropathy: a comparison of two reduction strategies. Clin J Am Soc Nephrol. 2008;3:1812-9.
43. Schaub S, Hirsch HH, Dickenmann M, Steiger J, Mihatsch MJ, Hopfer H, et al. Reducing immunosuppression preserves allograft function in presumptive and definitive polyomavirus-associated nephropathy. Am J Transplant. 2010;10:2615-23.
44. Hardinger KL, Koch MJ, Bohl DJ, Storch GA, Brennan DC. BK virus and the impact of pre-emptive immunosuppression reduction: 5 year results. Am J Transplant. 2010;10:407-15.
45. Faguer S, Hirsch HH, Kamar N, Guilbeau-Frugier C, Ribes D, Guitard J, et al. Leflunomide treatment for polyomavirus BK associated nephropathy after kidney transplantation. Transplant Int. 2007;20:962-9.
46. Leca N, Muczynski KA, Jefferson JA, de Boer IH, Kowalewska J, Kendrik EA, et al. Higher levels of leflunomide are associated with hemolysis and are not superior to lower levels for BK virus clearance in renal transplant patients. Clin J Am Soc Nephrol. 2008;3:829-35.
47. Kuypers DR, Vandooren AK, Lerut E, Evenepoel P, Claes K, Snoeck R, et al. Adjuvant low-dose cidofovir therapy for BK polyomavirus interstitial nephritis in renal transplant recipients. Am J Transplant. 2005;5:1997-2004.
48. Vu D, Shah T, Ansari J, Naraghi R, Min D. Efficacy of intravenous immunoglobulin in the treatment of persistent BK viremia and BK virus nephropathy in renal transplant recipients. Transplant Proc. 2015;47(2):394-8.
49. Moon J, Chang Y, Shah T, Min DI. Effects of intravenous immunoglobulin therapy and Fc gamma receptor polymorphisms on BK virus nephropathy in kidney transplant recipients. Transpl Infect Dis. 2020;22(4):e13300.
50. Sawinski D, Trofe-Clark J. BK virus nephropathy. Clin J Am Soc Nephrol. 2018;13(12):1893-6.
51. Tinel C, Vermorel A, Picciotto D, Morin L, Devresse A, Sauvaget V, et al. Deciphering the prognostic and predictive value of urinary CXCL10 in kidney recipients with BK virus reactivation. Front Immunol. 2020;11:604353.
52. Hricik DE, Nickerson P, Formica RN, Poggio ED, Rush D, Newell KA, et al. Multicenter validation of urinary CXCL9 as a risk-stratifying biomarker for kidney transplant injury. Am J Transpl. 2013;13(10):2634-44.
53. Hirt-Minkowski P, Amico P, Ho J, Gao A, Bestland J, Hopfer H, et al. Detection of clinical and subclinical tubulo-interstitial inflammation by the urinary CXCL10 chemokine in a real-life setting. Am J Transpl. 2012;12(7):1811-23.
54. Masset C, Ville S, Halary F, Gaborit B, Bressolette-Bodin C, Deltombe C, et al. Resurgence of BK virus following Covid-19 in kidney transplant recipients. Transpl Infect Dis. 2021;23:e13465.
55. Ruangkanchanasetr P, Pumchandh N, Satirapoj B, Termmathurapoj S, Pongthanapisith V. Biopsy-proven BK virus nephropathy without detectable BK viremia in a one-year post-kidney transplant recipient. Southeast Asian J Trop Med Public Health. 2015;46(4):657-61.
56. Nieto-Ríos JF, Benavides-Henao DA, Aristizabal-Alzate A, Morales-Contreras C, Chacón-Jaimes DC, Zuluaga-Valencia G, et al. BK virus nephropathy in a heart transplant recipient. J Bras Nefrol. 2021;43(3):434-9.
57. Anyaegbu EI, Hmiel SP. Intravenous immunoglobulin in BK virus nephropathy. Open Urolo Nephrol J. 2014;7(2):129-32.
58. Sachdeva MS, Nada R, Jha V, Sakhuja V, Joshi K. The high incidence of BK polyoma virus infection among renal transplant recipients in India. Transplantation. 2004;77(3):429-31.
59. Etta PK, Madhavi T, Gowrishankar S. Coexistent BK-virus-associated nephropathy and ureteric stenosis in a patient with acute cellular rejection after renal transplantation: a case report and review of literature. Indian J Transplant. 2020;14:147-51.
60. Gupta P, Gupta A, Bhalla AK, Malik M, Gupta A, Bhargava V, et al. BK virus nephropathy in living donor renal allograft recipients: an observational study from a large transplant center in India. Saudi J Kidney Dis Transpl. 2018;29:1366-70.
61. Thakur R, Arora S, Nada R, Minz M, Joshi K. Prospective monitoring of BK virus reactivation in renal transplant recipients in North India. Transpl Infect Dis. 2011;13:575-83.
62. Shah A, Kumar V, Palmer MB, Trofe-Clark J, Laskin B, Sawinski D, et al. Native kidney BK virus nephropathy, a systematic review. Transpl Infect Dis. 2019;21(4):e13083.
63. Funahashi Y. BK virus-associated nephropathy after renal transplantation. Pathogens. 2021;10(2):150.

12.2.3 Hepatitis C Virus

Ruju Gala, Narayan Prasad

CASE VIGNETTE

A 45-year-old male patient with end-stage kidney disease (ESKD) is awaiting living donor renal transplant. He is positive for anti-hepatitis C virus (HCV) antibodies.

a. How would you evaluate this patient further?
b. When would you like him to start on direct antiviral agents (DAA)?

Ans. Refer to text

INTRODUCTION

The hepatitis C virus (HCV), a member of the Flaviviridae family, is a single-stranded, enveloped, positive-sense ribonucleic acid (RNA) virus. Choo et al. first described it in 1989.[1] HCV virus has seven genotypes with several distinct subtypes distributed worldwide, with genotype-1 being the most common. Genotype 3 is predominant in India.[2]

Hepatitis C virus causes a chronic infection 80–85% of the time, with mild symptoms of fatigue and nonspecific arthralgias. In 20–35% of these patients, the liver disease progresses to cirrhosis over 20–30 years, causing significant morbidity and mortality.[3] While 180 million people are infected with HCV worldwide, anti-HCV seroprevalence in the Indian population is estimated to be 5.2 and 13 million (0.4–1%). Of these, 3–9 million people are estimated to have an active HCV infection.[4]

Hepatitis C virus prevalence is higher in high-risk groups such as the chronic kidney disease population on maintenance hemodialysis. The Dialysis Outcomes and Practices Patterns Study showed a mean HCV prevalence of 13.5% in hemodialysis units across seven countries, ranging from 2.6% to as high as 22.9%.[5] As per the Organ Procurement and Transplantation Network database, 1,470 (4.4%) of the 33,357 adult primary kidney transplant recipients were HCV positive.[6]

HEPATITIS C VIRUS EVALUATION OF TRANSPLANT CANDIDATES

A significant number of prospective transplant candidates on dialysis, awaiting a renal transplant, are infected with HCV, given the high HCV prevalence of patients on hemodialysis. Risk factors for HCV among transplant candidates include dialysis vintage period, exposure to blood products before the universal screening, and the prevalence of HCV infection in the hemodialysis unit.

SCREENING RECOMMENDATIONS

Screening for HCV infection is recommended for all prospective transplant recipients. Moreover, prospective transplant candidates receiving hemodialysis at a center should be subjected to periodic screening at an interval of 6 months.[5]

Serological assays for detecting anti-HCV antibodies are based on enzyme immunoassays or chemiluminescence immunoassays. If immunoassay is positive, HCV viremia is ascertained by Nucleic Acid Amplification Testing (NAT) for HCV RNA.[5]

In areas with a high prevalence of HCV, transplant candidates should be screened by HCV RNA testing because false-negativity rates for HCV antibody tests can be as high as 17.9% in dialysis units in such areas.[7] NAT is also needed to screen transplant candidates with a history of HCV infection to screen for reinfection, as anti-HCV antibody remains positive.

Hepatitis C virus infection in a transplant candidate is not a contraindication to renal transplantation. In HCV-infected persons, kidney transplantation offers a survival benefit over maintenance hemodialysis. A meta-analysis inferred that HCV-infected end-stage renal disease (ESRD) patients, even in the absence of cirrhosis, had 2.19 times higher relative risk of death, higher risk of cardiovascular disease, and a similar risk of liver disease than HCV-infected patients who received a kidney transplant.[8]

STAGING OF LIVER DISEASE

- *Noninvasive:* Ascertaining the stage of liver disease is a standard procedure in the routine evaluation of HCV-infected patients, including transplant candidates. Initially, noninvasive methods of assessment such as transient elastography (TE) or strain elastography are performed.[9] TE is a radiological diagnostic modality that uses shear wave imaging to estimate liver stiffness and thus provide a reasonably accurate evaluation of liver fibrosis in patients with ESKD. However, its use is unreliable in patients with ascites and obesity. The ideal time to perform TE should be after a dialysis session since liver stiffness measurements have been shown to decrease significantly after hemodialysis.[10,11]
- *Invasive:* Liver biopsy is considered to be the gold standard for the evaluation of HCV-infected transplant candidates for the presence of cirrhosis but is reserved in cases when noninvasive test results are discordant or when liver comorbidities are suspected.[5] Results of staging test help assess the degree of liver compromise

and initiate appropriate anti-HCV therapy. Patients with cirrhosis detected clinically or on liver biopsy or patients with suspected advanced fibrosis should undergo evaluation for portal hypertension to decide on the type of transplantation for these patients.

CHAPTER HIGHLIGHTS

- Anti-HCV seroprevalence in the Indian population is estimated to be 5.2 and 13 million (0.4–1%).
- Screening for HCV infection is recommended for all prospective transplant recipients and donors.
- In HCV-infected persons, kidney transplantation offers a survival benefit over maintenance hemodialysis.
- The advent of safe pangenotypic regimens after 2018 allows safe institution of DAAs in transplant recipients and waiting list candidates.

TYPES OF TRANSPLANTATION: LIVER–KIDNEY COMBINED VERSUS KIDNEY ALONE

- The presence of decompensated liver cirrhosis in patients with ESKD prompts the decision of a combined liver–kidney transplant over a single kidney transplant. Liver cirrhosis is considered to be decompensated if ascites, hepatic encephalopathy, coagulopathy (deranged prothrombin time), hypoalbuminemia, and/or hyperbilirubinemia are evidently present.[5] Patients with severe portal hypertension [defined as a hepatic venous pressure gradient (HVPG) ≥ 10 mm Hg], even with compensated cirrhosis, are an indication for a combined liver–kidney transplant. HVPG is a good predictor of clinical decompensation even in compensated cirrhosis and increases mortality risk.[12]
- HCV-infected patients with compensated liver cirrhosis without portal hypertension (HVPG < 10 mm Hg), may receive kidney transplantation alone with acceptable outcomes. Two case series showed similar 3-year patient and graft survival rates in HCV-infected patients with biopsy-proven cirrhosis with HVPG < 10 mm Hg when compared with recipients without cirrhosis.[13,14]

EFFECT OF HEPATITIS C VIRUS POSITIVITY ON POST-TRANSPLANT OUTCOMES

Studies have shown HCV-positive renal transplant recipients have a decreased patient and graft survival. Hanafusa et al. found a significant decline in the 20-year survival rates (64 vs. 88%) in HCV-positive patients. The relative risk for liver disease was five times higher, twice the risk of graft loss and three times higher risk of mortality when compared with HCV-negative transplant recipients.[15,16] The higher mortality risk in HCV-positive transplant recipients is attributed to increased diabetes, cardiovascular disease, infections, and malignancy.[17] The need for treatment of HCV serostatus in HCV-positive transplant recipients, due to the aforementioned reasons, cannot be stressed enough.

COMPLICATIONS OF HEPATITIS C VIRUS IN TRANSPLANT RECIPIENTS

Kidney Disease Improving Global Outcomes (KDIGO) 2018 guidelines recommend that kidney transplant recipients with chronic HCV infection should be assessed for proteinuria estimation by spot urine protein–creatinine ratio or 24-hour urine protein every 6 months. The new-onset proteinuria, with quantification that exceeds >1 g/day, or urine protein to creatinine ratio (UPCR) >1 g/g on two or more occasions, or microscopic hematuria is an indication of allograft biopsy. The histological examination should include light microscopy, immunofluorescence, and electron microscopy. Supportive care with renin-angiotensin-aldosterone system (RAAS) blockade should be commenced.[5] The kidney diseases seen in transplant recipients with HCV infection are as follows:

- Membranoproliferative glomerulonephritis (MPGN), the most common immune-mediated glomerulonephritis (GN) in HCV-positive transplant recipients, may be a de novo or recurrent disease. MPGN was reported in 45% of the graft biopsies in HCV-positive transplant recipients, done for worsening renal function, of which 18% had a de novo disease.[18] De novo variant progresses to ESKD more rapidly.
- *Cryoglobulinemic MPGN:* This histological diagnosis warrants the use of specific immunosuppressive treatment in addition to DAA.[18]
- *Membranous nephropathy:* A relatively uncommon association, more commonly seen in HCV-positive renal transplant recipients than the normal adult population. The post-transplant outcomes are similar to post-transplant idiopathic de novo membranous GN, with persistent massive proteinuria and gradual worsening of graft functions.[19]
- *Renal thrombotic microangiopathy:* More common in HCV-infected transplant recipients, associated with anticardiolipin antibodies.[20]
- Transplant glomerulopathy (TG) is the glomerular manifestation of chronic rejection. The occurrence of TG in HCV-infected transplant recipients is as high as 36%, while merely 5% of the overall kidney transplant population develops TG. Also, the progression to allograft loss in this subpopulation is faster.[21]

Electron microscopy is inevitable in differentiating MPGN from TG pattern as both have double contouring of the glomerular basement membrane (GBM) on light microscopy. The presence of electron-dense deposits in the GBM points toward MPGN, while electron-lucent material in the subendothelium is characteristic of the TG pattern.[22]

LIVER DISEASE POST-TRANSPLANTATION

Monitoring of liver disease in chronic HCV infection is performed by TE to assess the progression of liver fibrosis.

Patients with cirrhosis or advanced fibrosis require lifelong annual surveillance by liver ultrasound and TE. It is advocated irrespective of the status of sustained virological response (SVR), owing to the risk of developing hepatocellular carcinoma.[5]

Chronic hepatitis is the most common liver disease seen in HCV-infected subpopulation of transplant recipients. A more severe form called fibrosing cholestatic hepatitis causes rapid liver failure.[23] The rate of progression of liver disease to cirrhosis in transplant recipients depends on the severity and duration of HCV infection, comorbidities at the time of transplantation, and differences in the immunosuppressive regimens.[24]

NEW-ONSET DIABETES AFTER TRANSPLANTATION

Screening for new-onset diabetes after transplantation (NODAT) is recommended for all transplant recipients. The chances of occurrence of NODAT in HCV-infected transplant recipients are four times higher than that in the general transplant population (39.4 vs. 9.8%).[25] The derangement in glucose metabolism reported in HCV-infected patients is secondary to insulin resistance. The antiviral treatment before transplant in HCV patients helps to reduce the risk of post-transplant diabetes and also helps to increase insulin sensitivity. Also, tacrolimus-based regimens have an eightfold higher risk of post-transplantation diabetes mellitus (PTDM) than cyclosporine (58 vs. 7.7%).[26]

Post-transplant Lymphoproliferative Disease

The risk of post-transplant lymphoproliferative disease (PTLD) in solid organ transplant recipients in HCV-seropositive patients is three times higher than that of the seronegative recipients. The patients with PTLD in HCV patients also have a higher mortality risk.[27]

Treatment

Hepatitis C virus is known to cause poorer patient and graft outcomes and is associated with an increased risk of NODAT and de novo glomerulopathy. Eradication of HCV pretransplant might mitigate some of these adverse outcomes. DAA have revolutionized the outcomes of HCV-infected patients and are strongly recommended for every prospective transplant recipient by the American Association for the Study of Liver Diseases (AASLD). Interferon-free DAA regimens target the HCV NS5B polymerase, the HCV NS5A protein, and the HCV NS3/4 protease, which are proteins essential for viral replication. Most of these regimens have excellent cure rates of >95% of patients having SVR in 8–24 weeks and are well tolerated.[5] The Hepa-C Spanish Registry documented the data on 103 HCV-positive kidney transplant recipients treated with DAAs after kidney transplant with excellent outcomes. After 12 weeks (SVR12), the SVR rate was 98%, without any worsening of renal functions or proteinuria.[28]

TIMING OF ANTIVIRAL THERAPY

The decision on when to initiate antiviral therapy depends on the following facts:

- The severity of liver fibrosis
- Extrahepatic manifestations of HCV infection
- Type of transplant (living vs. deceased donor)
- Anticipated wait list time on the transplant
- Center-specific policies governing the use of receipt of organs from HCV-infected donors.[5]

Combined liver–kidney transplantation is the definitive management for kidney transplant candidates with decompensated cirrhosis. Before or after transplantation, the decision to institute DAA depends on short-term prognosis, amenability to transplantation, and other comorbidities.

Transplant candidates with rapidly progressive liver fibrosis or advanced disease in the absence of decompensated cirrhosis or severe extrahepatic manifestations should be instituted on immediate antiviral therapy irrespective of transplantation.[29]

For the rest of the candidates with mild to moderate disease, deciding to initiate DAAs depends on living versus deceased donor transplantation.[29] For candidates awaiting deceased donor transplant, delaying antiviral therapy in patients with stable liver functions facilitates the chances of early transplant if HCV-infected donor organ becomes available, followed by antiviral treatment post-transplant.[29]

However, suppose the anticipated waiting list time is long, or the receipt of HCV-infected donor organs is not feasible or is not expected to reduce the wait list by >24 weeks. In that case, DAAs should be instituted at the earliest while awaiting deceased donor transplant to mitigate the risk of HCV-related complications.[5,29]

For candidates awaiting living donor transplants, early antiviral treatment is recommended for all the patients at the earliest. KDIGO guidelines (2018) recommended the initiation of DAAs after transplantation if the time to transplant is <24 weeks or depends on the HCV genotypes.[5] However, the advent of safe pangenotypic regimens after 2018 allows the early institution of DAAs before transplant. HCV-infected potential living kidney donors should be evaluated for the extent of liver fibrosis, and those not having cirrhosis should receive DAAs before donation.[29]

TIMING OF ANTIVIRAL TREATMENT: BEFORE VERSUS AFTER TRANSPLANTATION

In the post-transplant period, antiviral therapy should be started early to prevent the development of post-transplant complications such as NODAT and de novo glomerulopathy, described above. In the early post-transplant period, due to higher calcineurin inhibitor (CNI) dosages, interactions between DAAs and immunosuppression therapy (IST) may occur more frequently. Hence, the optimal time should be once immunosuppressive medications are at stable levels after 6 months **(Flowchart 1)**.[5]

MANAGEMENT OF HEPATITIS C VIRUS INFECTION IN TRANSPLANT RECIPIENTS

Any licensed DAA-based regimens can be used in transplant recipients for 12 weeks, with CNI monitoring during and after treatment. Interferons are contraindicated in transplant recipients infected with HCV as it is associated with an increased risk of allograft rejection.[5] All the following DAA combinations have proven excellent outcomes in studies.

- Sofosbuvir–velpatasvir × 12 weeks for all genotypes[31]
- Sofosbuvir–ledipasvir × 12 weeks for genotypes 1, 4, 5, 6[31]
- Glecaprevir–pibrentasvir for 12 weeks, for all genotypes, but it should not be used in transplant recipients who are on cyclosporine >100 mg dose or those with decompensated cirrhosis (Child–Pugh class B and C). Also, concurrent use of cyclosporine increases the levels of glecaprevir and pibrentasvir.[32]
- Grazoprevir–elbasvir × 12 weeks for genotypes 1, 4.

The coadministration of elbasvir-grazoprevir with cyclosporine is contraindicated because OATP1B1/3 inhibition could lead to elevated grazoprevir concentrations in plasma causing transaminitis.[33,34]

Sofosbuvir-based regimens are preferred with glomerular filtration rate (GFR) >30 mL/min/1.73 m^2. Ribavirin, now rarely preferred, also can be used in transplant recipients with a GFR of 30–50 mL/min/1.73 m^2 at alternating doses of 200 and 400 mg **(Fig. 1)**.[33,34]

TABLE 1: The advantages of initiation of direct antiviral agents before transplantation as compared to delaying the institution after transplantation.[30]

Treatment before transplant	*Treatment after transplant*
• Effective pangenomic regimens • Halt progression of liver disease • Decreases dialysis transmission • Decreases the risk of PTDM • Reduced the risk of de novo GN post-transplant • May improve extrahepatic manifestations	• Increases the chances of HCV-positive organ availability and early transplant • Curtails waiting time for transplant • No enhanced risk of rejection • Reduces overall cost burden

(GN: glomerulonephritis; HCV: hepatitis C virus; PTDM: post-transplantation diabetes mellitus)

DRUG INTERACTIONS BETWEEN IMMUNOSUPPRESSION THERAPY AND DIRECT ANTIVIRAL AGENTS

Direct antiviral therapy can be safely used to treat HCV infection in transplant recipients on standard maintenance immunosuppression. Conversely, all currently

Flowchart 1: Flowchart to proceed with the evaluation of HCV-infected transplant candidates for the type of transplantation and when to start antiviral therapy with respect to transplantation.[5]

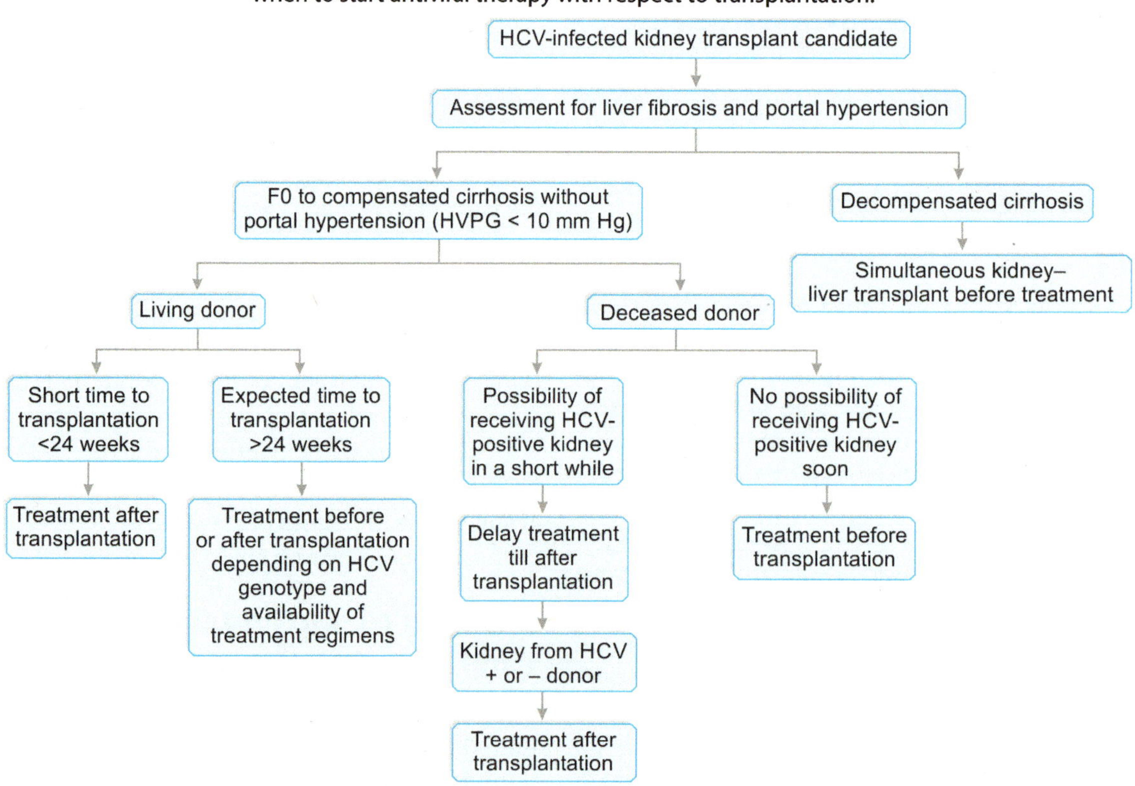

(F0: no fibrosis; HCV: hepatitis C virus; HVPG: hepatic venous pressure gradient)

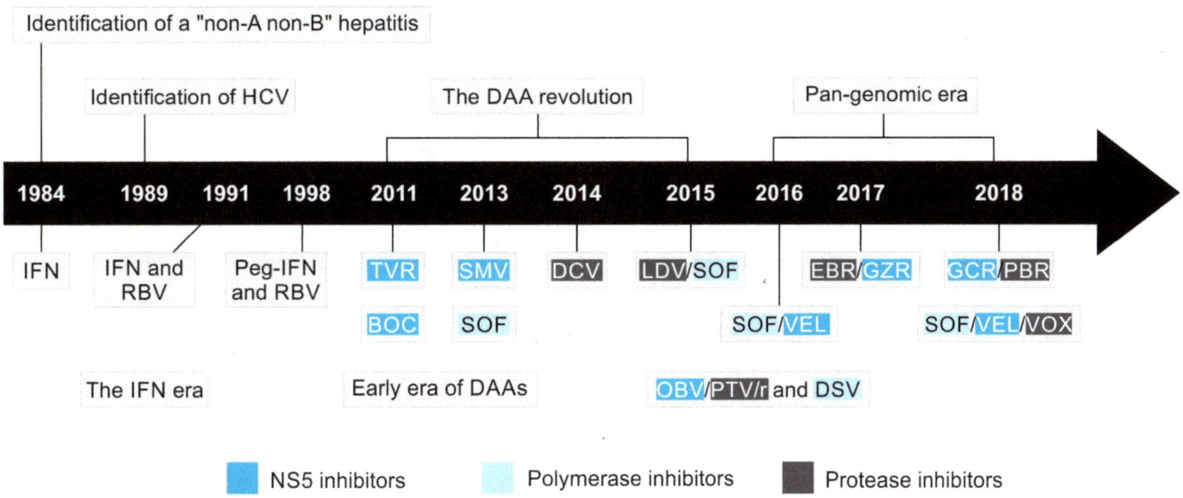

Fig. 1: The timeline and evolution of direct antivirals and HCV treatment over the years. (BOC: boceprevir; DAA: direct antiviral agents; DCV: daclatasvir; DSV: dasabuvir; EBR: elbasvir; GCR: glecaprevir; GZR: grazoprevir; HCV: hepatitis C virus; LDV: ledipasvir; NS5: Non-structural protein; OBV: ombitasvir; Peg-IFN: pegylated Interferon; PBR: pibrentasvir; PTV: paritaprevir; RBV: ritonavir; SMV: simeprevir; SOF: sofosbuvir; TVR: telaprevir; VEL: velpatasvir; VOX: voxilaprevir)

TABLE 2: Drug interactions between immunosuppressive medications and direct antiviral agents in hepatitis C virus-positive transplant patients.

	Tacrolimus	*Cyclosporine*	*MMF*	*Azathioprine*	*Sirolimus*	*Everolimus*
Sofosbuvir	Safe	Safe	Safe	Safe	Safe	Safe
Sofosbuvir–ledipasvir	Safe	Safe	Safe	Safe	Safe	Increases EVR levels
Sofosbuvir–velpatasvir	Safe	Safe	Safe	Safe	Safe	Increases EVR levels
Daclatasvir	Safe	Not recommended if cyclosporine dose >100 mg/day	Safe	Safe	Safe	Increases EVR levels
Glecaprevir–pibrentasvir	Increases levels	*Increases GCR/PBR levels* Not recommended if cyclosporine dose >100 mg/day	Safe	Safe	Increases SRL levels	Increases EVR levels
Elbasvir–grazoprevir	Increases levels	*Increases GZR levels* Not recommended if cyclosporine dose >100 mg/day	Safe	Safe	Increases SRL levels	Increases EVL levels
Sofosbuvir–velpatasvir–voxilaprevir	Safe	Not recommended if cyclosporine dose >100 mg/day	Safe	Safe	Increases SRL levels	Increases EVL levels
Simeprevir	Increases levels	Not recommended if cyclosporine dose >100 mg/day	Safe	Safe	Increases SRL levels	Increases EVL levels
Ombitasvir–paritaprevir–ritonavir	Avoid; if used to decrease tacrolimus dose to 0.5 mg every 7 days and monitor levels	Avoid; if used to reduce cyclosporine to one-fifth dose and monitor levels	Monitor levels	Safe	Not recommended	Not recommended

(EVL: everolimus; EVR: early virological response; GCR: glecaprevir; GZR: grazoprevir; MMF: mycophenolate mofetil; PBR: pibrentasvir; SRL: sirolimus)

practiced conventional induction and maintenance immunosuppressive drugs can be used in HCV-infected kidney transplant recipients. Protease inhibitors, such as paritaprevir and simeprevir, are enzyme inducers and increase the drug levels of CNI and mammalian target of rapamycin (mTOR) inhibitors. Tacrolimus in HCV transplant recipients increases the risk of NODAT compared to cyclosporine.[26]

Table 2 shows drug-drug interactions between certain DAAs and immunosuppressive medications.[35,36]

EXPANDING DONOR POOL

The KDIGO 2018 practice guidelines have not allowed the use of allografts from HCV-infected donors to HCV-infected recipients. However, the possibility of transplanting HCV-infected donor kidneys into HCV-negative transplant candidates have been explored in two small studies. THINKER (Transplanting Hepatitis C Kidneys Into Negative Kidney Recipients) study analyzed the outcomes of the transplant of HCV genotype 1 viremic kidneys transplanted into seronegative recipients, followed by treatment with grazoprevir–elbasvir for 12 weeks.[37] All the recipients achieved sustained virological remission and had comparable graft outcomes with HCV-negative transplant recipients for 12 months post-transplant.[38] EXPANDER (Exploring Renal Transplants Using Hepatitis C Infected Donors for HCV-negative Recipients) trial further included HCV-positive kidneys of any genotype to be transplanted to HCV-negative transplant recipients D+/R–, followed by grazoprevir–elbasvir treatment for 12 weeks. In addition, those who received HCV genotype 2 or 3 donor kidneys were given sofosbuvir (GPZ–EBR + SOF). Outcomes achieved viral loads below the lower limit of quantification in >50% of the recipients.[39]

REFERENCES

1. Choo Ql, Kuo G, Weiner AJ, Overby LR, Bardley DW, Houghton M. Isolation of a cDNA clone derived from a blood borne non-A, non-B viral hepatitis genome. Science. 1989;244(4902):359-62.
2. Hissar SS, Goyal A, Kumar M, Pandey C, Suneetha PV, Sood A, et al. Hepatitis C virus genotype 3 predominates in North and Central India and is associated with significant histopathologic liver disease. J Med Virol. 2006;78(4):452-8.
3. Poynard T, Bedossa P, Opolon P. Natural history of liver fibrosis progression in patients with chronic hepatitis C. The OBSVIRC, METAVIR, CLINIVIR, and DOSVIRC groups. Lancet. 1997;349(9055):825-32.
4. Goel A, Seguy N, Aggarwal R. Burden of hepatitis C virus infection in India: a systematic review and meta-analysis. J Gastroenterol Hepatol. 2019;34(2):321-9.
5. Kidney Disease: Improving Global Outcomes (KDIGO) Hepatitis C Work Group. KDIGO 2018 clinical practice guideline for the prevention, diagnosis, evaluation, and treatment of hepatitis C virus in chronic kidney disease. Kidney Int Suppl. 2018;8(3):91-165.
6. Heo NY, Mannalithara A, Kim D, Udompap P, Tan JC, Kim WR. Long-term patient and graft survival of kidney transplant recipients with hepatitis C virus infection in the United States. Transplantation. 2018;102:454-60.
7. El-Sherif A, Elbahrawy A, Aboelfotoh A, Abdelkarim M, Mohammad AGS, Abdallah AM, et al. High false-negative rate of anti-HCV among Egyptian patients on regular hemodialysis. Hemodial Int. 2012;16:420.
8. Ingsathit A, Kamanamool N, Thakkinstian A, Sumethkul V. Survival advantage of kidney transplantation over dialysis in patients with hepatitis C: a systematic review and meta-analysis. Transplantation. 2013;95:943.
9. Liu CH, Liang CC, Huang KW, Liu CJ, Chen SI, Lin JW, et al. Transient elastography to assess hepatic fibrosis in hemodialysis chronic hepatitis C patients. Clin J Am Soc Nephrol. 2011;6:1057.
10. Taneja S, Borkakoty A, Rathi S, Kumar V, Duseja A, Dhiman RK, et al. Assessment of liver fibrosis by transient elastography should be done after hemodialysis in end stage renal disease patients with liver disease. Dig Dis Sci. 2017;62:3186.
11. Khunpakdee N, Jayanama K, Kaewdoung P, Promson K, Rattanasiri S, Warodomwichit D, et al. Transient elastography in end-stage renal disease patients on hemodialysis: the effect of net fluid withdrawal. Blood Purif. 2015;40:256.
12. Eason JD, Gonwa TA, Davis CL, Sung RS, Gerber D, Bloom D. Proceedings of consensus conference on simultaneous liver kidney transplantation (SLK). Am J Trans. 2008;8(11):2243.
13. Paramesh AS, Davis JY, Mallikarjun C, Zhang R, Cannon R, Shores N, et al. Kidney transplantation alone in ESRD patients with hepatitis C cirrhosis. Transplantation. 2012;94:250.
14. Parsikia A, Campos S, Khanmoradi K, Pang J, Balasubramanian M, Zaki R, et al. Equal 3-year outcomes for kidney transplantation alone in HCV-positive patients with cirrhosis. Int Surg. 2015;100:142.
15. Periera BJ, Wright TL, Schmid CH, Levey AS. The impact of pretransplantation hepatitis C infection on the outcome of renal transplantation. Transplantation. 1995;60(8):799-805.
16. Hanafusa T, Ichikawa Y, Kishikawa H, Kyo M, Fukunishi T, Kokado Y, et al. Retrospective study on the impact of hepatitis C virus infection on kidney transplant patients over 20 years. Transplantation. 1998;66(4):471-6.
17. Kamar N, Ribes D, Izopet J, Rostaing L. Treatment of hepatitis C virus (HCV) after renal transplantation: implications for HCV-positive dialysis patients awaiting a kidney transplant. Transplantation. 2006;82(7):853-6.
18. Cruzado JM, Carrera M, Torras J, Grinyo JM. Hepatitis C virus infection and de novo glomerular lesions in renal allografts. Am J Transplant. 2001;1(2):171-8.
19. Morales JM, Pascual-Capdevilla J, Campistol JM, Fernandez-Zatarain G, Muñoz MA, Andres A, et al. Membranous glomerulonephritis associated with hepatitis C virus infection in renal transplant patients. Transplantation. 1997;63(11):1634.
20. Baid S, Pascual M, Williams Jr WW, Tolkoff-Rubin N, Johnson SM, Collins B, et al. Renal thrombotic microangiopathy associated with anti-cardiolipin antibodies in hepatitis C-positive renal allograft recipients. J Am Soc Nephrol. 1999;10(1):146.
21. Baid-Agrawal S, Farris 3rd AB, Pacual M, Mauiyyedi S, Farrell ML, Tolkoff-Rubin N, et al. Overlapping pathways to transplant glomerulopathy: chronic humoral rejection, hepatitis C infection, and thrombotic microangiopathy. Kidney Int. 2011;80(8):879-85.
22. Gallay BJ, Alpers CE, Davis CL, Schultz MF, Johnson RJ. Glomerulonephritis in renal allografts associated with hepatitis C infection: a possible relationship with transplant glomerulopathy in two cases. Am J Kidney Dis. 1995;26(4):662.
23. De Bustillo EM, Ibarrola C, Colina F, Castellano G, Fuertes A, Andrés A, et al. Fibrosing cholestatic hepatitis in hepatitis C virus infected renal transplant recipients. J Am Soc Nephrol. 1998;9(6):1109-13.

24. Roth D, Gaynor JJ, Reddy KR, Ciancio G, Sageshima J, Kupin W, et al. Effect of kidney transplantation on outcomes among patients with hepatitis C. J Am Soc Nephrol. 2011; 22(6):1152.
25. Fabrizi F, Martin P, Dixit V, Bunnapradist S, Kanwal F, Dulai G. Post-transplant diabetes mellitus and HCV seropositive status after renal transplantation: meta-analysis of clinical studies. Am J Transplant. 2005;5:2433.
26. Bloom RD, Rao V, Weng F, Grossman RA, Cohen D, Mange KC. Association of hepatitis C with posttransplant diabetes in renal transplant patients on tacrolimus. J Am Soc Nephrol. 2002;13:1374-80.
27. Burra P, Buda A, Livi U, Rigotti P, Zanus G, Calabrese F, et al. Occurrence of post-transplant lymphoproliferative disorders among over thousand adult recipients: any role for hepatitis C infection? Eur J Gastroenterol Hepatol. 2006;18:1065.
28. Fernandez I, Munoz-Gomez R, Pascasio JM, Baliellas C, Polanco N, Esforzado N, et al. Efficacy and tolerability of interferon-free antiviral therapy in kidney transplant recipients with chronic hepatitis C. J Hepatol. 2017;66(4):71.
29. Shelton BA, Sawinski D, Linas BP, Reese PP, Mustian M, Hungerpiller M, et al. Population level outcomes and cost-effectiveness of hepatitis C treatment pre- vs post kidney transplantation. Am J Transplant. 2018;18(10):2483.
30. Chute DF, Chung RT, Sise ME. Direct-acting antiviral therapy for hepatitis C virus infection in the kidney transplant recipient. Kidney Int. 2018;93:560-7.
31. Friebus-Kardash J, Gackler A, Kribben A, Witzke O, Wedemeyer H, Treckmann J, et al. Successful early sofosbuvir-based antiviral treatment after transplantation of kidneys from HCV-viremic donors into HCV-negative recipients. Transpl Infect Dis. 2019;21(5):e13146.
32. Reau N, Kwo PY, Rhee S, Brown Jr RS, Agarwal K, Angus P, et al. Glecaprevir/pibrentasvir treatment in liver or kidney transplant patients with hepatitis C virus infection. Hepatology. 2018;68(4):1298.
33. Joint Panel from the American Association of the Study of Liver Diseases and the Infectious Diseases Society of America. HCV guidance: recommendations for testing, managing, and treating hepatitis C. [online] Available from http://www.hcvguidelines.org/. [Last accessed May, 2022].
34. European Association for the Study of the Liver. EASL recommendations on treatment of hepatitis C. J Hepatol. 2018;69(2):461.
35. University of Liverpool. Hepatitis Drug Interactions. Available from http://www.hep-druginteractions.org. [Last accessed May, 2022].
36. UpToDate 2022. Drug interactions between immunosuppressive agents and direct-acting antiviral agents for HCV infection.
37. Goldberg DS, Abt PL, Blumberg EA, Van Deerlin VM, Levine M, Reddy KR, et al. Trial of transplantation of HCV-infected kidneys into uninfected recipients. N Engl J Med. 2017;376:2394-5.
38. Reese PP, Abt PL, Blumberg EA, Van Deerlin VM, Bloom RD, Potluri VS, et al. Twelve-month outcomes after transplant of hepatitis C-infected kidneys into uninfected recipients: a single-group trial. Ann Intern Med. 2018;169:273-81.
39. Durand CM, Bowring MG, Brown DM, Chattergoon MA, Massaccesi G, Bair N, et al. Direct-acting antiviral prophylaxis in kidney transplantation from hepatitis C virus-infected donors to noninfected recipients: an open-label nonrandomized trial. Ann Intern Med. 2018;168: 533-40.

12.2.4 Hepatitis B Virus

Kalpana Shailesh Mehta, Atim Pajai

CASE VIGNETTE

- AK, at the age of 17 years, was diagnosed with chronic glomerulonephritis (CGN) and needed renal replacement therapy (RRT) 5 years later.
- 1 year later, he underwent living-related kidney transplantation (LRKT), with his mother as a donor, with tacrolimus-based immunosuppression. His hepatitis B virus (HBV), hepatitis C virus (HCV), and human immunodeficiency virus (HIV) markers were negative.
- 2 years post-kidney transplantation (KT), he was detected to be hepatitis B surface antigen (HBsAg) positive with viral copies 16,900 IU/mL, alanine aminotransferase (ALT) 53 IU/dL, and serum creatinine 1.9 mg%. His allograft biopsy showed features of interstitial fibrosis and tubular atrophy (IFTA).
- He was initiated on entecavir 0.5 mg on alternate days.
- His viral load 2 years after was 5,500 IU/mL and serum creatinine 3 mg%.
- With continued entecavir, his viral load 3 years after initiation of antiviral was <29 IU/mL. ALT was 25 IU/dL.
- He is presently on maintenance hemodialysis.

INTRODUCTION

India falls into an intermediate endemic zone with the prevalence of HBV 2–4%, with over 40 million HBV carriers. Every year, 115,000 Indians die of HBV-related complications.[1] About two-thirds of the disease burden in India is with low or undetectable viral load, which naturally mitigates the disease severity to some extent. However, this ameliorating effect, along with that of vaccination, may be offset by the rising burden of high-risk groups, including chronic kidney disease (CKD) on dialysis and kidney transplant recipients (KTR) on immunosuppression, who are living longer with their diseases.[2]

The prevalence of HBsAg in hemodialysis populations ranges from 1.3 to 14.6% in Asian Pacific countries. HBV infection, in this patient setting, is usually asymptomatic even in the acute phase. Transaminase levels are lower compared to the general population and seroconversion from hepatitis B e antigen (HBeAg) to anti-hepatitis B e antibody (HBeAb) or from anti-hepatitis B core antibody (HBcAb) immunoglobulin M (IgM) to IgG is delayed or does not occur, even after resolution of the active infection. About 80% of HBV-infected dialysis patients progress silently to a chronic carrier state.[3]

Mortality prior to antiviral therapy was reportedly 50% in those transplanted with positive HBsAg.[4,5] HBV reactivation is one of the main reasons for liver failure in HBV-infected patients. Cytotoxic therapy and immunosuppression in KTR are known risk factors for HBV reactivation, and liver failure is more likely to occur compared to novel infection.[6]

HEPATITIS B VIRUS REACTIVATION POST-KIDNEY TRANSPLANT AND EFFECT ON PATIENT AND GRAFT SURVIVAL

Increased skin breaching, sharing dialysis machines, higher exposure to blood products, immunosuppressive CKD state, and immunosuppression post-transplant make KTR a vulnerable and high-risk group for HBV infection and reactivation, which can affect patient and graft survival.

Reactivation of HBV is well described in association with the use of immunosuppressive agents such as B-cell depleting agents (e.g., rituximab). Reactivation effect is thought to be due to the disruption of the host immune response and possibly with enhanced replication of HBV mediated by some drugs. Cyclosporin has been shown to inhibit HBV replication by binding to mitochondrial cyclophilin and by inhibiting the cellular entry of HBV by blocking sodium taurocholate cotransporting polypeptide. More recent studies have shown that the effect of mycophenolate may vary and that it may enhance HBV replication. Rapamycin [a mammalian target of rapamycin (mTOR) inhibitor] has been shown to enhance HBV production by inducing cellular autophagy. The use of steroids can induce reactivation of HBV secondary to the stimulatory effect on the glucocorticoid-responsive enhancer region of the HBV genome. In another in vitro study using HBV deoxyribonucleic acid (DNA)-transfected hepatoma cells, prednisolone and azathioprine increased intracellular viral DNA and ribonucleic acid (RNA) levels by approximately twofold and fourfold, respectively, but treatment with cyclosporin did not alter the levels of viral RNA or DNA. However, a combination of all three immunosuppressive agents increased the level of intracellular viral DNA eightfold, indicating an additive effect.[7]

Hepatitis B virus infection is associated with more frequent and rapid progression to cirrhosis and hepatocellular carcinoma in solid organ transplant recipients, thus contributing to higher mortality. HBV may also cause de novo membranous glomerulonephritis, potentially impacting renal function after transplantation.[7] Hepatitis B reactivation may rarely manifest as fulminant hepatitis with massive necrosis or as severe fibrosing cholestatic hepatitis.[8]

Mo et al., in their analysis of 77 HBsAg-positive KTR, reported reactivation in 22.4%. The median time to reactivation was 27 months. 52.9% of HBV reactivation was accompanied by hepatitis. Inappropriate antiviral agents and HBV DNA titer ≥1,000 IU/mL before transplant increased the risk of HBV reactivation. 64.7% of reactivated patients were not on antiviral medication at the time of reactivation. With antiviral medication, there was no statistical difference in patient survival between HBsAg-negative patients and HBsAg-positive patients. None of the deaths in HBsAg-negative group was related to liver failure, while HBsAg-positive group had four deaths due to liver failure. There was no difference in death-censored graft survival between HBsAg-negative and HBsAg-positive patients.[9]

Older age: >60 years and anti-T-cell antibodies use were identified as risk factors for HBV reactivation by Chen et al. in 322 occult HBV carriers with significantly lower patient survival in the HBV reactivation group.[10] Rituximab desensitization and the absence of anti-HBs antibodies were risk factors for HBV reactivation in Lee et al.'s cohort of 172 resolved HBV patients,[11] while Kanaan et al. noted no HBV reactivation in patients with HBs antibodies >100 IU/mL.[12]

CHAPTER HIGHLIGHTS

- All those KT candidates with HBsAg inactive carrier and SVR state should undergo liver biopsy prior to transplant. All should receive antiviral therapy with entecavir or tenofovir as the first-line therapy for lifelong. Frequent monitoring with HBV DNA and ALT is essential.
- For those with active carrier states, therapy with one of the available antiviral agents is indicated until HBeAg becomes negative and viral replication is suppressed.

PREVENTION: THE BEST STRATEGY

Vaccination

Vaccination is the mainstay of HBV prevention.[1,3]

- As per the World Health Organization (WHO) recommendation, the first dose of hepatitis B vaccine should be given as soon as possible after birth, preferably within 24 hours. This should be followed by three primary series at 6, 10, and 14 weeks to complete the schedule. This complete series induces protective antibodies in >95% of infants, children, and young adults, which lasts at least 20 years and can be lifelong.
- All children and young adults <18 years and not vaccinated prior should receive vaccine.
- CKD patients should be vaccinated prior to going on dialysis because vaccine immunogenicity is higher in the general population in comparison to dialysis patients (90 vs. 70%).
- Dialysis patients should also be vaccinated against HBV infection and have an annual test regarding their anti-HBs antibody titer. If it is <10 IU/mL, an intensified protocol should be followed vis-à-vis a booster vaccine dose should be administered.

Dialysis Precautions

- Universal precautions in hemodialysis unit
- Mandatory isolation of HBsAg-positive patients from negative ones
- Single use of dialyzers in HBsAg-positive patients
- Aggressive vaccination protocols
- Appropriate use of erythropoietin and hematinics to avoid the use of blood products

KIDNEY TRANSPLANT IN HEPATITIS B SURFACE ANTIGEN-POSITIVE CANDIDATE

Wait-listed transplant candidates must be either inactive carriers or sustained viral responders (SVR) with persistently low or undetectable HBV DNA and should be monitored every 6–12 months with HBV DNA and transaminase levels.[3,13]

- It is advisable to screen all dialysis patients with HBsAg, anti-HBc, and anti-HBs.
- HBV polymerase chain reaction (PCR) should be done in few cases of isolated anti-HBc positivity to detect occult carriers, especially among those on the waiting list.
- *Additional serologic markers:* Anti-HBc (IgM and IgG), HBeAg/anti-HBeAb, anti-hepatitis B surface antibody (HbsAb), quantitative HBV DNA PCR, and liver biochemistry are necessary in case of seropositivity to differentiate between active and inactive liver infection.
- Patients from hepatitis D virus (HDV) endemic areas should be screened with HDV serology if they are positive.
- Accordingly, these wait-listed candidates can be either active carriers, inactive carriers, or with occult infection.
    - *Active carriers:* These are HBsAg positive with HBeAg or HBeAb positive, with HBV viral load above 2,000 IU/mL (approximately 11,200 copies), with or without elevated ALT levels.
    - *Inactive carriers:* These are HBsAg positive and HBeAg negative with persistently low viral load, normal liver enzymes, and low anti-HBc IgM or anti-HBc IgG levels.
    - *Occult HBV carriers:* These are HBsAg negative, most often with detectable anti-HBc but low viral load without liver enzyme elevation.

Hepatitis B Surface Antigen-positive Kidney Transplant Candidate and Active Carrier State

Therapy with one of the available antiviral agents is indicated until HBeAg becomes negative and viral replication is suppressed.

Hepatitis B Surface Antigen-positive Kidney Transplant Candidate and Inactive Carrier State

- These candidates must be referred to a specialist for the complete evaluation of the recipient, including assessment of HBV status, targeted antiviral therapy or prophylaxis, and post-transplant follow-up.[7]

- Kidney Disease Improving Global Outcomes (KDIGO) guidelines recommend performing a liver biopsy in hemodialysis patients that are candidates for a kidney allograft and are positive for HBsAg so that the severity of hepatitis is assessed.[13]
- Noninvasive tools such as aspartate aminotransferase (AST) to platelet ratio index (APRI) score and liver elastography have only 50% accuracy in dialysis patients and are not validated.[3] Liver biopsy should still be considered as the gold standard in this group.
- Screening should be done for hepatocellular carcinoma in candidates with cirrhosis prior to transplantation using techniques (e.g., ultrasound, alpha-fetoprotein) and frequency as per local guidelines.[13]
- HBsAg-positive and/or HBV DNA-positive (SVR) candidates are recommended to undergo isolated KT if they do not have decompensated cirrhosis and are stable on antiviral therapy after specialist evaluation.[13]
- Patients with advanced HBV-related liver disease requiring another organ transplant be considered for combined transplantation after careful consideration of the potential risks and benefits.[7]
- Antiviral prophylaxis must begin before or at worst, immediately after transplantation.[3]
- These candidates ideally should receive antiviral lifelong as immunosuppression continues lifelong.[14]
- Cost, development of resistance with long-term therapy, and nephrotoxicity of certain antivirals (tenofovir and adefovir) may lead to consideration of withdrawal of antivirals in cautiously selected group of patients: Stable renal function, low immunological rejection risk, a minimum of 6–9 months low-dose maintenance immunosuppression, no evidence for HBV activity, and a minimum of 12 months therapy with antiviral agent without developing resistance. Frequent measurement of HBV DNA levels and 3–6 months of testing of liver enzymes are essential, while antiviral treatment ought to be reinstated if immunosuppression grows, i.e., in the case of antirejection therapy.[3]
- Frequent monitoring post-transplant with HBV DNA and transaminases is essential.

HEPATITIS B SURFACE ANTIGEN-POSITIVE/ HEPATITIS B CORE ANTIBODY-POSITIVE PROSPECTIVE KIDNEY DONOR

UK Guidelines Recommendation[7]

The kidneys, heart, and lungs from the HBcAb-positive organ donor can be used for any recipient and the risk of de novo HBV infection is low. (1A)

UK Guidelines Suggestion[7]

- If need demands, the nonliver solid organs of the HBsAg-positive organ donor can be used for any recipient after an individualized assessment of risk and benefit. (2C)
- When an HBcAb-positive donor is used, lamivudine (LAM) prophylaxis may be given for 6 months after transplantation, although the risk of transmission is very low. (2C)

However, it is safer to avoid unnecessary organ discarding, especially in endemic areas, to transplant kidneys from HBsAg-positive donors into HBsAg-positive recipients.

Transplanting kidney from an HBsAg-positive donor to HBV-naïve recipient will result in acquired infection with subsequent implications and is not suggested.[15] It is imperative in such cases to obtain a written informed consent after fully briefing the patient prior to KT and restricting transplant only to those recipients with the recipient's titers of at least 10 IU/mL [with past infection or vaccine]. All such recipients at Laiko General Hospital in Athens receive one booster vaccination dose combined with hepatitis B immunoglobulin (HBIg) just before transplantation and entecavir prophylaxis for 6 months.[3]

The risk of HBV transmission from donors with isolated hepatitis B core antigen (HBcAg) positivity is very low and significantly smaller than that from HBsAg-positive donors.[16] These donors should preferably be checked for the presence of anti-HBc IgM in order to exclude recent infection and recipients should receive antiviral prophylaxis.[7] A recent analysis found seroconversion to HBsAg positivity only in 0.28% and anti-HBc positivity in 2.3%.[17]

POST-KIDNEY TRANSPLANT COURSE

Antivirals

Before the introduction of antiviral therapy, HBV infection was considered to be a contraindication of KT with a mortality of up to 50%.[5]

Although HBsAg-positive patients are associated with substantial HBV reactivation rates, KT can be safely carried out while taking antiviral agents to mitigate reactivation risk, more so with newer generation of antinucleos(t)ide analogs: Entecavir and tenofovir as the risk of resistance is much less than that with LAM and adefovir.[18]

Antivirals are recommended in all prospective KTR with HBsAg positivity, inclusive of even those with HBV DNA negative. It may need to be lifelong in immunocompromised patients as cessation is associated with increased flare-up of liver disease and rarely decompensated liver disease.[18]

Lamivudine

Majority of reports are with LAM; 100 mg/day is highly effective. In one trial, HBV DNA disappeared in all three groups (preemptive, prophylactic, and advanced liver disease) and the recurrence rate was 10% in preemptive and prophylaxis groups versus 42% in non-LAM group.[19] Virological clearance and normalization of ALT were reported in 91 and 81%, respectively, by Fabrizi et al. in their meta-analysis, but resistance was seen in 18%.[20] LAM is no longer preferred as the first line of treatment.[18]

Adefovir Dipivoxil

The standard dose of adefovir is 10 mg/day and needs adjustment as per the glomerular filtration rate (GFR). It is potentially nephrotoxic as it can result in acute tubular injury as seen in HIV patients with high dosages. It is used either as a single-agent therapy or combined with entecavir in HBV-infected patients and LAM-resistant cases. Fontaine et al. treated 11 renal transplant recipients with LAM resistance with adefovir alone. After 12 months, serum HBV DNA declined satisfactorily, with no hepatitis B reactivation observed and no nephrotoxicity.[21] In two other studies, a significant decrease in GFR was noted with adefovir.[22,23]

Entecavir

Entecavir (dosed at 0.5 mg/day) should be considered as the first line of treatment for KT candidates with HBV infection that have no concern for LAM resistance.[18] It is considered much more effective compared to LAM, with high antiviral potency and a high genetic barrier for resistance.

Hu et al. studied 18 naïve renal transplant recipients and nine recipients that had been previously treated with LAM but without resistant mutations. Entecavir was successful in clearing HBV DNA in 70, 74, 96, and 100% of patients after 12, 24, 52, and 104 weeks, respectively.[24]

Complete response to entecavir may take >6 weeks and may not be achieved at all in those with LAM resistance. There are no reported entecavir-resistant cases in KTR, while, in cases with LAM resistance, the chance of entecavir-resistant cases increases annually from year 1 to 5 (6, 15, 36, 46, and 51%, respectively).[3]

Tenofovir Disoproxil Fumarate

Tenofovir (300 mg daily) is less nephrotoxic, allowing higher dosages, and has a strong antiviral effect. It is used in the therapy of naïve patients and those that present LAM resistance. Data of tenofovir use in KTR are scarce. In a recent study, seven transplant patients (three kidneys) with chronic HBV were treated with tenofovir; all showed a decline in HBV DNA, while three achieved clearance. Tenofovir should be considered as the first-line drug in KTR with chronic HBV infection.[3,18]

Dose of tenofovir, LAM, and entecavir may be mentioned.

Interferon

Its use in KTR for treating HBV should be avoided, given the unacceptable high rates of precipitating rejection and availability of other antiviral drugs.[18]

IMMUNOSUPPRESSION POST-TRANSPLANT

All immunosuppressive agents used in renal transplantation could be administered in HBV-positive patients. The total amount of immunosuppression is more important than the effect of a particular agent. Efforts should focus on minimization of the total immunosuppression burden long term. Minimization protocols, especially corticosteroid-avoiding or sparing protocols, are preferable and should be applied to low immunological risk HBV-positive recipients. Close HBV monitoring is mandatory whenever the total immunosuppression status is altered.[3]

POST-TRANSPLANT OUTCOME OF KIDNEY TRANSPLANTATION IN HEPATITIS B VIRUS IN THE ERA OF ANTIVIRAL THERAPY

The natural history and outcome of chronic HBV infection in KTR in the era of antiviral therapy are less well studied. Yap et al., in their cohort of 63 HBsAg-positive KTR, reported an improved 20-year mortality (83 vs. 34%, $p = 0.006$) in patients treated with antiviral therapy.[25]

Immunosuppressive therapy has been shown to have a more deleterious effect in KTR with HBV and HCV coinfection.[26]

INDIAN STUDIES

Agarwal and Tiwari describe their experience of 739 adult KTRs, with 4.7% having HBV infection. LAM was used in all. At 1-year follow-up, ALT was normal in 77% and HBV DNA undetectable in 45.7%.[27]

CONCLUSION

All those KT candidates with HBsAg inactive carrier and SVR state should undergo liver biopsy prior to transplant. All should receive antiviral therapy with entecavir or tenofovir as first-line therapy for lifelong. Frequent monitoring with HBV DNA and ALT is essential.

REFERENCES

1. World Health Organization. (2016). Hepatitis B. [online] Available from https://www.who.int/docs/default-source/searo/india/health-topic-pdf/factsheet-b-hepatitisday2016.pdf?sfvrsn=da61ef0_2. [Last accessed October, 2022].
2. Ray G. Current scenario of hepatitis B and its treatment in India. J Clin Transl Hepatol. 2017;5:277-96.
3. Marinaki S, Kolovou K, Sakellariou S, Boletis JN, Delladetsima IK. Hepatitis B in renal transplant patients. World J Hepatol. 2017;9(25):1054-63.

4. Pirson Y, Alexandre GP, Ypersele C. Long-term effect of hbs antigenemia on patient survival after renal transplantation. N Engl J Med. 1977;296:194-6.
5. Parfrey PS, Forbes RD, Hutchinson TA, Kenick S, Farge D, Dauphinee WD, et al. The impact of renal transplantation on the course of hepatitis B liver disease. Transplantation. 1985;39:610-5.
6. Reddy PN, Sampaio MS, Kuo HT, Martin P, Bunnapradist S. Impact of pre-existing hepatitis B infection on the outcomes of kidney transplant recipients in the United States. Clin J Am Soc Nephrol. 2011;6:1481-7.
7. UK Guidelines for Hepatitis B & Solid Organ Transplantation, 1st edition. British Transplantation Society; 2018. pp. 27-55.
8. Lok AS, Liang RH, Chiu EK, Wong KL, Chan TK, Todd D. Reactivation of hepatitis B virus replication in patients receiving cytotoxic therapy. Report of a prospective study. Gastroenterology. 1991;100:182-8.
9. Mo H, Min S, Han A, Jung IM, Ha J. Outcome after kidney transplantation in hepatitis B surface antigen-positive patients. Sci Rep. 2021;11:11744.
10. Chen GD, Gu JL, Qiu J, Chen LZ. Outcomes and risk factors for hepatitis B virus (HBV) reactivation after kidney transplantation in occult HBV carriers. Transpl Infect Dis. 2013;15:300-5.
11. Lee J, Park JY, Huh KH, Kim BS, Kim MS, Kim SI, et al. Rituximab and hepatitis B reactivation in HBsAg-negative/anti-HBc-positive kidney transplant recipients. Nephrol Dial Transpl. 2017;32:722-9.
12. Kanaan N, Kabamba B, Maréchal C, Pirson Y, Beguin C, Goffin E, et al. Significant rate of hepatitis B reactivation following kidney transplantation in patients with resolved infection. J Clin Virol. 2012;55:233-8.
13. Kidney Disease: Improving Global Outcomes (KDIGO) Transplant Work Group. KDIGO clinical practice guideline for the care of kidney transplant recipients. Am J Transplant. 2009;9(Suppl 3):S1-155.
14. Te H, Doucette K. Viral hepatitis: guidelines by the American Society of Transplantation Infectious Disease Community of Practice. Clin Transplant. 2019;33:e13514.
15. Wolf JL, Perkins HA, Schreeder MT, Vincenti F. The transplanted kidney as a source of hepatitis B infection. Ann Intern Med. 1979;91:412-3.
16. Wachs ME, Amend WJ, Ascher NL, Bretan PN, Emond J, Lake JR, et al. The risk of transmission of hepatitis B from HBsAg(-), HBcAb(+), HBIgM(-) organ donors. Transplantation. 1995;59:230-4.
17. Mahboobi N, Tabatabaei SV, Blum HE, Alavian SM. Renal grafts from anti-hepatitis B core-positive donors: a quantitative review of the literature. Transpl Infect Dis. 2012;14:445-51.
18. Adnan S, Nasia S, Michael RL. Liver disease among liver transplant recipients. In: Knechtle SJ, Marson LP, Morris PJ (Eds). Kidney Transplantation: Principles and Practice, 8th edition. Philadelphia, PA: Elsevier; 2019. pp. 539-65.
19. Han DJ, Kim TH, Park SK, Lee SK, Kim SB, Yang WS, et al. Results on preemptive or prophylactic treatment of lamivudine in HBsAg (+) renal allograft recipients: comparison with salvage treatment after hepatic dysfunction with HBV recurrence. Transplantation. 2001;71(3):387-94.
20. Fabrizi F, Dulai G, Dixit V, Bunnapradist S, Martin P. Lamivudine for the treatment of hepatitis B virus-related liver disease after renal transplantation: meta-analysis of clinical trials. Transplantation. 2004;77(6):85964.
21. Fontaine H, Vallet-Pichard A, Chaix ML, Currie G, Serpaggi J, Verkarre V, et al. Efficacy and safety of adefovir dipivoxil in kidney recipients, hemodialysis patients, and patients with renal insufficiency. Transplantation. 2005;80:1086-92.
22. Lai HW, Chang CC, Chen TH, Tsai MC, Chen TY, Lin CC. Safety and efficacy of adefovir therapy for lamivudine-resistant hepatitis B virus infection in renal transplant recipients. J Formos Med Assoc. 2012;111:439-44.
23. Kamar N, Huart A, Tack I, Alric L, Izopet J, Rostaing L. Renal side effects of adefovir in hepatitis B virus-(HBV) positive kidney allograft recipients. Clin Nephrol. 2009;71:36-42.
24. Hu TH, Tsai MC, Chien YS, Chen YT, Chen TC, Lin MT, et al. A novel experience of antiviral therapy for chronic hepatitis B in renal transplant recipients. Antivir Ther. 2012;17:745-53.
25. Yap DY, Tang CS, Yung S, Choy BY, Yuen MF, Chan TM. Long-term outcome of renal transplant recipients with chronic hepatitis B infection-impact of antiviral treatments. Transplantation. 2010;90(3):325-30.
26. Pouteil-Noble C, Tardy JC, Chossegros P, Mion F, Chevallier M, Gérard F, et al. Co-infection by hepatitis B virus and hepatitis C virus in renal transplantation: morbidity and mortality in 1098 patients. Nephrol Dial Transplant. 1995;10(6):122-4.
27. Agarwal SK, Tiwari SC. Efficacy and tolerability of lamivudine in hepatitis B infected renal transplant recipients: a single center study. Indian J Nephrol. 2009;19(3):91-5.

12.2.5 Human Immunodeficiency Virus

Anwitha Varmudy, Sree Bhushan Raju

CASE VIGNETTE

A 45-year-old male with biopsy proven chronic glomerulonephritis with a baseline serum creatinine of 2.5 mg/dL on conservative treatment, was detected to have HIV positivity during follow-up with CD4 of 210 cells/µL. He was started on ART regimen of Abacavir, Lamivudine, Efavirenz. He progressed to ESRD in next 2 years. He did not develop any opportunistic infection during this period. He underwent ABO compatible renal transplantation with wife as donor in 2018, with 2/6 HLA match. His CD4 count at the time of transplant was 570 cells/µL, with undetectable HIV viral load. He received ATG induction at 3 mg/kg. Post-transplant ART consisted of Dolutegravir, Lamivudine and Abacavir. His immunosuppression included prednisolone, mycophenolate mofetil and tacrolimus. Patient is maintaining a stable graft function with CD4 count of more than 500 cell/µL during 3 years of follow-up.

INTRODUCTION

Acquired immunodeficiency syndrome (AIDS) due to HIV infection was first identified in the United States in 1981. As per the India HIV estimation 2019 report, the prevalence of HIV in adults aged 15–49 years was 0.22%. The total number of people living with HIV (PLHIV) in India was estimated at 23.19 lakh in 2020.[1]

Renal involvement is seen in around 5–30% of HIV-seropositive patients.[2] The first reported renal involvement was in the form of HIV-associated nephropathy (HIVAN) in the United States in 1984.[3] Other podocytopathies such as focal segmental glomerulosclerosis (FSGS) not otherwise specified (NOS), minimal change disease, and diffuse mesangial sclerosis are also seen in this setting. The other manifestations of renal involvement in HIV-seropositive patients include HIV-immune complex kidney disease (HIVICK); vascular dominant lesions such as thrombotic microangiopathy and arteriosclerosis; drug-induced tubular injury due to antiretroviral therapy (ART; e.g., tenofovir, indinavir) and antimicrobials used to treat opportunistic infections (e.g., trimethoprim-sulfamethoxazole, aminoglycosides, acyclovir, amphotericin, and foscarnet);[4] and renal involvement by comorbidities such as diabetic nephropathy, autosomal dominant polycystic kidney disease (ADPKD), and age-related nephrosclerosis. Prerenal AKI may be seen due to diarrheal illnesses. The incidence of HIVAN has declined with the widespread use of combined antiretroviral therapy (cART). However, there has been a concomitant rise in non-HIV-associated chronic kidney disease due to increased lifespan of these individuals. This has led to a progressive rise in need for renal replacement therapy for these patients, including renal transplantation.[2]

Human immunodeficiency virus-infected end-stage renal disease (ESRD) patients have been for a long time excluded from renal transplantation programs. Currently, HIV seropositivity is not considered a contraindication to renal transplantation at some centers, as the overall survival has improved with the use of highly active antiretroviral therapy (HAART), with similar graft survival rates as in HIV-negative patients.[5-8]

Initially, there were few case reports of KT in HIV positive patients, a notable case series of liver and KT in HIV-positive individuals was published in 2003, with a triple immunosuppression regimen of prednisone, cyclosporine, and mycophenolate mofetil (MMF). Of the 10 transplanted patients, 50% developed acute rejection that was treated with antithymocyte globulin (ATG). At 1-year follow-up, an undetectable HIV viral load was maintained in all patients with HAART and stable CD4 count was seen in those not treated for rejection.[9]

HIV/HCV Co-infection

With a 10 times higher transmission of HCV than HIV on percutaneous exposure, HCV/HIV coinfection has become a matter of public health concern. Affecting around 2.3 million individuals worldwide, HIV accelerates HCV-related liver fibrosis. Cirrhosis and hepatocellular carcinoma is seen to occur earlier in this population. HCV coinfection has been shown to reduce or retard $CD4^+$ T-cell recovery after antiretroviral therapy.

Data from the Scientific Registry of Transplant Recipients (SRTR) have shown that transplantation provided a survival benefit in HIV-seropositive individuals after 194 days and for those with hepatitis C virus (HCV) coinfection, the same benefit is observed 392 days post-transplant.[10] However, individuals with HIV face multiple barriers to renal transplantation. A single-center study conducted between 2000 and 2007[11] showed that only 20% of the patients with HIV who were evaluated for transplant were listed. The risk factors associated with failure to reach the wait list included Black race, a history of substance abuse, and uncontrolled HIV infection (CD4 count <200 cells/m^3 or detectable viral load). Data have also shown that gaining entry into the wait list does not ensure transplantation due to multiple barriers.[12,13]

CHAPTER HIGHLIGHTS

- Kidney transplantation (KT) is a safe and viable option of renal replacement therapy in human immunodeficiency virus (HIV)-positive patients who have a well-controlled infection with highly active antiretroviral therapy (HAART).
- Post-transplant immunosuppression and antiretroviral therapy need to be studied in more detail in the future trials so as to adopt regimens that avoid drug interactions that can reduce renal allograft and patient survival.
- Studies have shown good results of KT in HIV-positive recipients from HIV-positive donors.
- The focus should also be on reducing graft rejection rates while avoiding spikes in post-transplant infections and malignancies.

TABLE 1: HIV-positive donor eligibility criteria.

Deceased donors	No evidence of invasive opportunistic complications of HIV infection. Preimplant donor organ biopsy
Living donor	Well-controlled HIV infection defined as: • $CD4^+$ T-cell count ≥500/μL for the 6-month period before donation • HIV-1 RNA <50 copies/mL • No evidence of invasive opportunistic complications of HIV infection Preimplant donor organ biopsy

(HIV: human immunodeficiency virus)

PRETRANSPLANT MANAGEMENT

Kidneys acquired via live donation (related or unrelated donor) are preferred over cadaveric donation. British HIV Association guidelines suggest that extended criteria donors are not used with deceased donors till more experience is garnered in HIV-positive renal transplant recipients. Live donors should be made aware of the HIV-seropositive status of the recipients and that the prognosis for both the graft and the patient may be worse than the average population. All prospective recipients should undergo a psychiatric evaluation. A drug-free period of 2 years is recommended for drug users.[14]

Patients with ESRD and well-controlled HIV meeting the following criteria are considered suitable for transplantation:[14-17]

- Adherent to HAART, with good tolerance to the drugs
- Devoid of any of the AIDS-defining illnesses
- A CD4 count >200 cells/μL
- An HIV viral load <50 HIV-1 RNA copies/mL

Patients with prior or current infections such as incompletely treated mycobacterial, recent influenza, recent respiratory syncytial virus (RSV), recent severe bacterial infection, aspergillosis, other invasive fungal infections, and active cytomegalovirus (CMV) infection, which are all considered to be at risk for post-transplant reactivation, are excluded by British and Italian groups.[14,17]

The Spain and United States groups do not exclude patients with a previous history of esophageal candidiasis, *Mycobacterium tuberculosis*, and pneumocystis pneumonia (PCP) infection.[15,16] It is recommended to screen for HCV and hepatitis B virus (HBV) coinfections due to accelerated progression to end-stage liver disease and mortality post KT in this subset of patients.[18,19] Patients with actively replicating HBV need treatment until they develop undetectable viral load to become candidates for transplantation.[14]

The HIV Organ Policy Equity Act (HOPE Act) was enacted in November 2013, for the development of research criteria concerning the transplantation of HIV-positive organs into HIV-positive individuals. It permitted transplantation from HIV-positive donors to recipients with HIV **(Table 1)**.[20]

POST-TRANSPLANT MANAGEMENT

Monitoring[21]

- Routine post-transplant laboratory testing
- CD4 count and HIV viral load checked at 1-month post-transplant and every 2–3 months thereafter
- Patients with a CD4 count <200 cells/m^3 will require prophylaxis for opportunistic infections
- Patients with detectable viral load will require evaluation for adherence and viral resistance testing in selected cases.

Antiretroviral Therapy

Specific guidelines do not exist for HIV-positive kidney transplant recipients (KTR). Therefore, general guidelines and recommendations for HIV-negative patients should be followed and adjusted to specific patient scenarios.[22,23] One suggested first-line regimen is the combination of abacavir (or tenofovir as an alternative), lamivudine/emtricitabine, and raltegravir.[24] Protease inhibitors (PIs), especially ritonavir and cobicistat, inhibit CYP450, leading to large variations in through levels of calcineurin inhibitors (CNIs), potentially causing rejection. Nonnucleoside reverse transcriptase inhibitors (NNRTIs) are inducers of CYP450 and decrease CNI levels, potentially causing rejection.[25,26] Newer antiretrovirals that do not interact with CYP450 have been developed, such as integrase inhibitors raltegravir, elvitegravir, and dolutegravir. Raltegravir is increasingly being used in HIV-infected KT recipients and is associated with good antiretroviral efficacy.[27] Among integrase inhibitors, it should be noted that dolutegravir inhibits tubular secretion of creatinine, which can falsely elevate serum creatinine levels, and elvitegravir requires cobicistat boosting, which also induces CYP3A4. Therefore, many transplant recipients are on a raltegravir-based regimen.

Treatment of Hepatitis B Virus Coinfection

Patients who are coinfected with HBV require two drugs with anti-HBV activity, usually a tenofovir-based regimen. Tenofovir alafenamide is less nephrotoxic and is the preferred agent for use in this population.[28]

Treatment of Hepatitis C Virus Coinfection

In the general transplant population, treatment of HCV infection has been associated with improved patient and allograft survival.[29] Studies suggest a similar outcome in renal transplant recipients coinfected with HIV/HCV.[30] Post-transplant treatment is also essential. Pretransplant treatment maybe preferred in patients with advanced liver disease at risk of decompensation and in centers that do not use HCV-positive organs, whereas post-transplant treatment can be given in patients with HCV-positive donors, especially if they have less severe fibrosis (METAVIR stage F0–F1).[31]

Post-transplant Immunosuppression—Induction and Maintenance

Human immunodeficiency virus-positive KTR are at increased risk for rejection, with studies showing 1-year cumulative risk of acute rejection being 30% in HIV-positive recipients, compared to 10–15% nationally among the HIV-negative patients.[5]

Current British guidelines recommend induction with an anti-interleukin-2 (anti-IL-2) antibody basiliximab.[32] Maintenance immunosuppressive treatment should constitute CNIs, MMF, and tapering corticosteroids. Patients receiving ATG induction therapy have been found to develop double the number of serious infections and also have an increased risk of death and graft loss compared to patients who did not receive induction therapy.[5,9] Hence, ATG induction therapy is only recommended for patients with a very high immunological risk for rejection.[5,33] Belatacept-based immunosuppressive regimens may benefit HIV-positive kidney transplant patients as they do not expose the patient to metabolic side effects of CNIs while also avoiding drug interactions between CNI and antiretroviral medications.[34,35] Polyclonal antibodies and OKT3 should not be used for induction or rescue therapy due to an increased risk of post-transplant lymphoproliferative disease, CMV, and other infections.[36-38]

Mycophenolate mofetil can increase intracellular levels of abacavir, didanosine, and tenofovir, which may increase their toxicity.[39] It has also been shown to have an inhibitory effect on HIV replication in multiple studies.[40-42] Solid organ transplantation-associated malignancies such as Kaposi sarcoma maybe prevented by the antiproliferative effect of mechanistic target of rapamycin (mTOR) inhibitors.[43]

OUTCOMES

Selhorst et al. followed all PLHIV in South Africa who received KT from HIV-positive donors ($N = 51$). The study reported 5-year overall survival and graft survival of 83.3 and 78.7%, respectively. The outcomes were comparable to the result of transplantation in HIV+ recipients from HIV– donor organs.[44]

An analysis of Organ Procurement and Transplantation Network (OPTN) data including HIV+ and HIV/HCV+ KT showed an excellent patient [adjusted hazard ratio (aHR), 0.90; 95% confidence interval (CI), 0.66–1.24] and allograft survival (aHR, 0.60; 95% CI, 0.40–0.88).[45]

Results of a recently published prospective multicenter pilot study comparing HIV D+/R+ to KT in HIV-negative donor to HIV+ recipient (HIV D–/R+) showed no difference in deaths and 1-year graft survival.[46]

DATA FROM INDIA

From India, Mahesh et al. reported results of eight HIV-positive KTRs with a maximum follow-up of 24 months. In the analysis, one patient succumbed to bronchopneumonia. Other infections were urinary tract infection (UTI), cellulitis, pneumonia, and esophageal candidiasis observed in seven patients; all were treated satisfactorily and no rejection episode was reported.[47]

A case of successful KT involving HIV-positive living donor and recipient has also been reported by Kapuriya et al.[48] Virani et al. reported a case of ABO incompatible living donor KT in an HIV-positive woman. Post-transplantation, the patient received ART-included lamivudine, abacavir, and raltegravir.[49]

INFECTIONS AND POST-TRANSPLANT PROPHYLAXIS

Post-transplant infections are common among recipients who are HIV positive. In the HIV-TR multisite trial,[5] 38% of the recipients had an infection requiring hospitalization. The group induced with rabbit antithymocyte globulin (rATG) and patients coinfected with HCV showed a higher incidence of infections. The majority of the infections were bacterial (69%), with genitourinary (26%), respiratory (20%), and bloodstream (19%) sources being the most common. Opportunistic infections were rare. Consensus guidelines[21] suggest at least 1 year of *Pneumocystis jirovecii* pneumonia (PJP) prophylaxis, some centers administering it lifelong. Trimethoprim–sulfamethoxazole is preferred as it also provides coverage for toxoplasma. Prophylaxis for CMV is given either as a high-dose valganciclovir (900 mg daily, dosed for renal function) for 3–6 months, depending on donor and recipient serostatus, or as is followed in HIV-negative individuals. Recipients require coverage for histoplasma and coccidioidomycosis if they live in endemic areas. Screening for latent tuberculosis should be done pretransplant and those with known exposure require isoniazid treatment if it is not completed pretransplant.

MALIGNANCY

Among transplant recipients, virally mediated cancers such as Kaposi sarcoma, liver, and anogenital cancers are all significantly increased and many "common" cancers such as lung, kidney, colon, skin, and pancreas are also more prevalent.[50]

Current guidelines do not provide specific recommendations for cancer screening in HIV-positive transplant recipients, but as per the current data, regular screening for human papilloma virus-related malignancies (anal and cervical cancers) as well as lung cancer screening among those with significant cigarette exposure can be advised.

REFERENCES

1. National AIDS Control Organisation. HIV facts and figures. [online] Available from http://naco.gov.in/hiv-facts-figures. [Last accessed June, 2022].
2. Prakash J, Ganiger V, Prakash S, Sivasankar M, Sunder S, Singh U. Kidney disease in human immunodeficiency virus-seropositive patients: absence of human immunodeficiency virus-associated nephropathy was a characteristic feature. Indian J Nephrol. 2017;27(4):271-6.
3. Rao TK, Filippone EJ, Nicastri AD, Landesman SH, Frank E, Chen CK, et al. Associated focal and segmental glomerulosclerosis in the acquired immunodeficiency syndrome. N Engl J Med. 1984;310:669-73.
4. Alameddine M, Jue JS, Zheng I, Ciancio G. Challenges of kidney transplantation in HIV positive recipients. Transl Androl Urol. 2019;8(2):148-54.
5. Stock PG, Barin B, Murphy B, Hanto D, Diego JM, Light J, et al. Outcomes of kidney transplantation in HIV-infected recipients. N Engl J Med. 2010;363:2004-14.
6. Pelletier SJ, Norman SP, Christensen LL, Stock PG, Port FK, Merion RM. Review of transplantation in HIV patients during the HAART era. Clin Transpl. 2004:63-82.
7. Kumar MSA, Sierka DR, Damask AM, Fyfe B, McAlack RF, Heifets M, et al. Safety and success of kidney transplantation and concomitant immunosuppression in HIV-positive patients. Kidney Int. 2005;67:1622-9.
8. Touzot M, Pillebout E, Matignon M, Tricot L, Viard JP, Rondeau E, et al. Renal transplantation in HIV-infected patients: the Paris experience. Am J Transplant. 2010;10:2263-9.
9. Stock PG, Roland ME, Carlson L, Freise CE, Roberts JP, Hirose R, et al. Kidney and liver transplantation in human immunodeficiency virus-infected patients: a pilot safety and efficacy study. Transplantation. 2003;76:370-5.
10. Locke JE, Gustafson S, Mehta S, Reed RD, Shelton B, MacLennan PA, et al. Survival benefit of kidney transplantation in HIV infected patients. Ann Surg. 2017;265:604-8.
11. Sawinski D, Wyatt CM, Casagrande L, Myoung P, Bijan I, Akalin E, et al. Factors associated with failure to list HIV-positive kidney transplant candidates. Am J Transplant. 2009;9:1467-71.
12. Tourret J, Guiguet M, Lassalle M, Grabar S, Lièvre L, Isnard-Bagnis C, et al. Access to the waiting list and to kidney transplantation for people living with HIV: a national registry study. Am J Transplant. 2019;19:3345-55.
13. Cohen JB, Locke JE, Shelton B, Reed RD, Mustian M, MacLennan P, et al. Disparity in access to kidney allograft offers among transplant candidates with human immunodeficiency virus. Clin Transplant. 2019;33:e13466.
14. Bhagani S, Sweny P, Brook G. Guidelines for kidney transplantation in patients with HIV disease. HIV Med. 2006;7:133-9.
15. Solid organ transplantation in the HIV-infected patient. Am J Transplant. 2004;4(Suppl. 10):83-8.
16. Miro JM, Torre-Cisnero J, Moreno A, Tuset M, Quereda C, Laaguno M, et al. GESIDA/GESITRA-SEIMC, PNS and ONT consensus document on solid organ transplant (SOT) in HIV-infected patients in Spain (March, 2005). Enferm Infecc Microbiol Clin. 2005;23:353-62.
17. Grossi PA, Tumietto F, Costigliola P, Gabbrielli F, Rizzato L, Venettoni S, et al. Liver transplantation in HIV-infected individuals: results of the Italian national program. Transplantation. 2006;82:446.
18. Pereira BJ. Renal transplantation in patients positive for hepatitis B or C (con). Transplant Proc. 1998;30:2070-2.
19. Parfrey PS, Forbes RD, Hutchinson TA, Beaudoin JG, Dauphinee WD, Hollomby DJ, et al. The clinical and pathological course of hepatitis B liver disease in renal transplant recipients. Transplantation. 1984;37:461-6.
20. Health Resources and Services Administration (HRSA), Department of Health and Human Services (HHS). Organ procurement and transplantation: implementation of the HIV Organ Policy Equity Act. Final rule. Fed Regist. 2015;80(89):26464-7.
21. Blumberg EA, Rogers CC, American Society of Transplantation Infectious Diseases Community of Practice. Solid organ transplantation in the HIV-infected patient: guidelines from the American Society of Transplantation Infectious Diseases Community of Practice. Clin Transplant. 2019;33:e13499.
22. Thompson MA, Aberg JA, Cahn P, Montaner JSG, Rizzardini G, Telenti A, et al. Antiretroviral treatment of adult HIV infection: 2010 recommendations of the International AIDS Society-USA panel. JAMA. 2010;304:321-33.
23. Panel de Expertos de Gesida, Plan Nacional sobre el Sida. AIDS Study Group/Spanish AIDS Plan consensus document on antiretroviral therapy in adults with human immunodeficiency virus infection (updated January 2010). Enferm Infecc Microbiol Clin. 2010;28:362.e1-91.
24. Trullas JC, Cofan F, Tuset M, Ricart MJ, Brunt M, Cervera C, et al. Renal transplantation in HIV-infected patients: 2010 update. Kidney Int. 2011;79:825-42.
25. Brinkman K, Huysmans F, Burger DM. Pharmacokinetic interaction between saquinavir and cyclosporine. Ann Intern Med. 1998;129:914-5.
26. Tseng A, Nguyen ME, Cardella C, Humar A, Conly J. Probable interaction between efavirenz and cyclosporine. AIDS. 2002;16:505-6.
27. Tricot L, Teicher E, Peytavin G, Zucman D, Conti F, Calmus Y, et al. Safety and efficacy of raltegravir in HIV-infected transplant patients cotreated with immunosuppressive drugs. Am J Transplant. 2009;9:1-7.
28. Sawinski D. Kidney transplantation in patients with HIV. Kidney360. 2020;1(7):705-11.
29. Axelrod DA, Schnitzler MA, Alhamad T, Gordon F, Bloom RD, Hess GP, et al. The impact of direct-acting antiviral agents on liver and kidney transplant costs and outcomes. Am J Transplant. 2018;18:2473-82.
30. Camargo JF, Anjan S, Chin-Beckford N, Morris MI, Abbo LM, Simkins J, et al. Clinical outcomes in HIV+/HCV+ coinfected

kidney transplant recipients in the pre- and post-direct-acting antiviral therapy eras: 10-year single center experience. Clin Transplant. 2019;33:e13532.
31. Shelton BA, Berdahl G, Sawinski D, Linas BP, Reese PP, Mustian MN, et al. Optimal timing of hepatitis C treatment among HIV/HCV coinfected ESRD patients: pre- vs post-transplant. Am J Transplant. 2019;19:1806-19.
32. Working Party of the British Transplantation Society. UK Guidelines for kidney and pancreas transplantation in patients with HIV 2015. [online] Available from http://www.bhiva.org/ kidney-transplantation-guidelines.aspx. [Last accessed June, 2022].
33. Suarez JF, Rosa R, Lorio MA, Morris MI, Abbo LM, Simkins J, et al. Pretransplant CD4 count influences immune reconstitution and risk of infectious complications in human immunodeficiency virus-infected kidney allograft recipients. Am J Transplant. 2016;16:2463-72.
34. Ebcioglu Z, Liu C, Shapiro R, Rana M, Salem F, Florman S, et al. Belatacept conversion in an HIV-positive kidney transplant recipient with prolonged delayed graft function. Am J Transplant. 2016;16:3278-81.
35. Cohen EA, Mulligan D, Kulkarni S, Tichy EM. De novo belatacept in a human immunodeficiency virus-positive kidney transplant recipient. Am J Transplant. 2016;16:2753-7.
36. Portela D, Patel R, Larson-Keller JJ, Ilstrup DM, Wiesner RH, Steers JL, et al. OKT3 treatment for allograft rejection is a risk factor for cytomegalovirus disease in liver transplantation. J Infect Dis. 1995;171:1014-8.
37. Boland GJ, Hene RJ, Ververs C, de Haan MA, de Cast GC. Factors influencing the occurrence of active cytomegalovirus (CMV) infections after organ transplantation. Clin Exp Immunol. 1993;94:306-12.
38. Hesse UJ, Wienand P, Baldamus C, Pollok M, Pichlmaier H. The risk of infection following OKT3 and antilymphocyte globulin treatment for renal transplant rejection: results of a single center prospectively randomized trial. Transpl Int. 1992;5(Suppl. 1):S440-3.
39. Izzedine H, Launay-Vacher V, Baumelou A, Deray G. Antiretroviral and immunosuppressive drug-drug interactions: an update. Kidney Int. 2004;66:532-41.
40. Chapuis AG, Paolo Rizzardi G, D'Agostino C, Attinger A, Knabenhans C, Fleury S, et al. Effects of mycophenolic acid on human immunodeficiency virus infection in vitro and in vivo. Nat Med. 2000;6:762-8.
41. Hossain MM, Coull JJ, Drusano GL, Margolis DM. Dose proportional inhibition of HIV-1 replication by mycophenolic acid and synergistic inhibition in combination with abacavir, didanosine, and tenofovir. Antiviral Res. 2002;55:41-52.
42. Sankatsing SU, Hoggard PG, Huitema AD, Sparidans RW, Kewn S, Crommentuyn KML, et al. Effect of mycophenolate mofetil on the pharmacokinetics of antiretroviral drugs and on intracellular nucleoside triphosphate pools. Clin Pharmacokinet. 2004;43:823-32.
43. Stallone G, Schena A, Infante B, Di Paolo S, Loverre A, Maggio G, et al. Sirolimus for Kaposi's sarcoma in renal-transplant recipients. N Engl J Med. 2005;352:1317-23.
44. Selhorst P, Combrinck CE, Manning K, Botha FCJ, Labuschagne JPL, Anthony C, et al. Longer-term outcomes of HIV-positive-to-HIV-positive renal transplantation. N Engl J Med. 2019;381:1387-9.
45. Sawinski D, Forde KA, Eddinger K, Troxel AB, Blumberg E, Tebas P, et al. Superior outcomes in HIV-positive kidney transplant patients compared with HCV-infected or HIV/HCV-coinfected recipients. Kidney Int. 2015;88(2):341–9.
46. Durand CM, Zhang W, Brown DM, Yu S, Desai N, Redd AD, et al. A prospective multicenter pilot study of HIV-positive deceased donor to HIV-positive recipient kidney transplantation: HOPE in action. Am J Transplant. 2021;21(5):1754-64.
47. Mahesh E, John MM, Konana GC, Parampalli RM, Bande SR, Suryadevara S. Renal transplantation in HIV-positive patients—no more a scare! Saudi J Kidney Dis Transpl. 2017; 28:1106-11.
48. Kapuriya M, Vaidya A, Rajkumar V. Successful HIV-positive, live renal donor transplant. A unique method of expanding the donor pool. Transplantation. 2020;104(5):e140-1.
49. Virani ZA, Rajput P, Nandu VP, Shah BV. ABO-Incompatible living donor kidney transplant in a human immunodeficiency virus-positive woman. Indian J Transplant. 2018;12:64-6.
50. Engels EA, Pfeiffer RM, Fraumeni Jr JF, Kasiske BL, Israni AK, Snyder JJ, et al. Spectrum of cancer risk among US solid organ transplant recipients. JAMA. 2011;306:1891-901.

12.2.6 Other Viral Infections

Mayuri Trivedi, Krishna Kumar Agrawaal

INTRODUCTION

Chronic immunosuppression, which is an essential part of kidney transplantation, predisposes the patients to a variety of infections including viral infections which may occur at any stage of the post-transplantation period. Despite significant scientific advances in the field of immunology and kidney transplantation, viral infections continue to be a major cause of mortality and morbidity in these patients. Viral infections not only contribute to potential graft loss due to direct and indirect graft involvement but also impair the overall host defenses and predispose to other infections.[1] In this chapter, we describe some of the common viral infections which affect the recipients of kidney transplantation.

HERPESVIRUS INFECTION

Herpes simplex viruses 1 and 2 (HSV-1 and HSV-2) are double-stranded DNA alpha-herpesvirus found to have more severe infections in the immunocompromised transplant recipients as compared with the immunocompetent hosts.[2]

As the majority of transplant recipients are seropositive for HSV, symptomatic HSV infection in these patients is usually due to reactivation of the previously acquired virus.[3]

Due to the universal antiviral prophylaxis which is commonly prescribed in the early post-transplantation period, the incidence of HSV infection in the first year post-transplantation is not very common. In a study by Jha et al., the incidence was found to be only 11% in the first year post-transplantation.[4] Female gender, prior HSV seropositivity, episodes of rejection, and use of a preemptive approach for cytomegalovirus (CMV) prevention are associated with a higher risk of symptomatic HSV infection.[5] Primary infection from donor-derived allograft can be severe due to loss of immunologic memory. Use of mycophenolate mofetil is associated with an increased risk of HSV reactivation whereas the risk of HSV is reduced with the use of the mammalian target of rapamycin (mTOR) inhibitors.[6,7]

Herpes simplex virus most commonly presents as painful vesicular or ulcerative lesions at orolabial or genital areas. More severe forms of HSV diseases include disseminated mucocutaneous or visceral disease, esophagitis, and hepatitis including fulminant hepatic failure and pneumonitis.[8] In a study by Yousuf et al., which studied the predisposing risk factors for HSV keratitis across Northern India, majority of the patients had solid organ transplants and were on immunosuppression therapy.[9] Viral lesions due to HSV-1 and -2 are the most common skin manifestations in transplant recipients.[10,11] The diagnosis of HSV is essentially clinical. However, in immunocompromised patients, polymerase chain reaction (PCR) is preferred for the diagnosis. Direct fluorescent antibody (DFA) can be done when PCR is not available. Culture is preferred when nucleoside resistance is suspected. The prophylaxis and treatment of HSV are given in **Table 1**. Additionally, local application of acyclovir ointment can be used.[12]

TABLE 1: Treatment of herpes simplex virus in adult transplant recipients.[5]

Indication	*Agents*	*Remarks*
Prevention	• Acyclovir 400–800 mg twice a day • Valacyclovir 500 mg twice a day	• Administer for at least 1 month • Lower doses for recurrent labialis, higher doses for recurrent genital or ocular disease
Mucocutaneous disease	• Acyclovir 400 mg thrice a day • Valacyclovir 1,000 mg twice a day • Famciclovir 500 mg twice a day • Inj. acyclovir 5 mg/kg IV every 8 hours (if unable to take PO or more extensive disease)	Treatment for 5–7 days
Severe disease/ CNS	Inj. acyclovir 10 mg/kg IV infusion every 8 hours	
Acyclovir-resistant HSV	Inj. foscarnet 80–120 mg/kg/day IV in two to three divided doses	

(CNS: central nervous system; HSV: herpes simplex virus)

VARICELLA-ZOSTER VIRUS

Varicella-zoster virus (VZV) is exclusively a human virus that belongs to the alpha herpesvirus family. Primary infection leads to acute varicella or "chickenpox" which is a common contagious disease of the childhood with low risk of mortality.[13] However, in the immunocompromised host, albeit a rare occurrence, it causes a high incidence of mortality and morbidity. After the initial infection, the virus establishes latency in nerve endings and dorsal root ganglia and may cause reactivation of infection known as herpes zoster virus (HZV).[14] In a study from Lucknow by Kaul et al., the incidence of varicella zoster in the postrenal transplantation period was as low as 1.48%. However, the mortality among this group of patients was high at 13.4%, most commonly due to superadded infections.[15]

Primary varicella typically presents with a characteristic disseminated vesicular pruritic rash along with constitutional symptoms such as fever and body ache.[16] Usually, it resolves within 7–10 days but may lead to disseminated multiorgan involvement in immunocompromised patients of renal transplantation. The infection may progress to life-threatening hepatitis, pancreatitis, or encephalitis with high mortality.[17-19]

Herpes zoster (HZ), which occurs due to reactivation of the primary varicella infection may present as a painful dermatomal rash followed by postherpetic neuralgia or as a fulminant disseminated disease.[20] As compared to the general population, the incidence as well as the complications of HZ is much higher in transplantation patients.[21] The complications include disseminated HZ including more than a single dermatomal involvement, multi-organ involvement with dysfunction, or very commonly postherpetic neuralgia.[22]

Age >50 years, use of antithymocyte globulin (ATG) and mycophenolate mofetil, and the duration of CMV prophylaxis showed direct correlation with the severity of the infection.[23] Patients with a previous history of VZV infection are at a higher risk of developing HZ after immunosuppression.[21]

The diagnosis of varicella-zoster (VZ) and HZ is usually a clinical one due to the characteristic dermatological manifestation of the infection. Disseminated pruritic rash (papules, vesicles, and crusted lesions) of varying time lineage along with prodromal symptoms characterize VZ. HZ is characterized by painful vesicular rash that involves ≤2 adjacent dermatomes. However, in the immunocompromised host, the patient may present with disseminated dermatomal involvement or organ involvement like HZ ophthalmicus (trigeminal ganglia) or HZ oticus (geniculate ganglia), also known as Ramsay Hunt syndrome.[21,24] Definitive laboratory testing in the form of PCR or DFA from the skin scrapping or vesicular fluid is usually used only in atypical cases or visceral involvement.[25] The possibility of a false-positive test, especially during the active infection, must be kept in mind while interpreting the serological tests.[21] The treatment options for VZV and HSV are summarized in **Table 2**.

Prophylaxis for VZV is considered in those patients who do not receive CMV prophylaxis with either oral acyclovir or valacyclovir. Vaccination with varicella vaccine is recommended in the pretransplantation period in patients who are seronegative. Caution needs to be exercised in the post-transplant period as the varicella vaccine is a live vaccine.[26] Immunoprophylaxis with VZV immunoglobulin (VZV Ig) or nonspecific intravenous immunoglobulin (IVIG) may be considered in seronegative patients who have been exposed to the virus within the first 96 hours of exposure.[25] Though by itself, secondary immune prophylaxis with IVIG or VZV Ig may not prevent the infection, it helps in reducing its severity and future complications.

TABLE 2: Treatment of varicella-zoster virus/herpes zoster virus in adult transplant recipients.[21]

Indications	*Treatment*	*Comments*
VZV	• Acyclovir 10–15 mg/kg IV every 8 hours (dose modification as per creatinine clearance) • Valacyclovir 2 g orally four times a day (dose modification as per creatinine clearance)	Acyclovir may predispose patients to develop crystal nephropathy and hence the patient has to be hydrated appropriately to prevent tubular accumulation
HZV (dermatomal)	• Acyclovir 800 mg orally five times a day • Valacyclovir 1 g orally three times a day • Famciclovir 500 mg three times a day	• Acyclovir may predispose patients to develop crystal nephropathy and hence the patient has to be hydrated appropriately to prevent tubular accumulation • IV dosing may be used for those who do not tolerate oral route
HZV (disseminated or complicated)	Acyclovir 10–15 mg/kg IV every 8 hourly (dose modification as per creatinine clearance)	

(HZV: herpes zoster virus; VZV: varicella-zoster virus)

CHAPTER HIGHLIGHTS

- Postrenal transplant viral infections are a common cause of mortality and morbidity in this group of immunocompromised hosts.
- Apart from acute graft dysfunction and subsequent graft loss, viral infections can contribute to death due to disseminated sepsis also.
- Specific antivirals may be useful for a few viral infections, but care must be taken regarding their renal dose adjustments to prevent further graft dysfunction.
- A few viral infections may result due to primary infection whereas the rest of the viral diseases are due to reactivation of the latent virus due to an immunocompromised state.
- Systematic screening, clinical examination, and the use of timely diagnostic tests may help early diagnosis and treatment of these infections.
- Primary prophylaxis with antiviral or vaccines whenever available should be widely utilized, which may help in lessening the severity of the infection.

EPSTEIN–BARR VIRUS

Epstein–Barr virus (EBV) is a double-stranded DNA herpes-virus that infects B lymphocyte cells affecting around 90% of the population.[27,28] The EBV infection in renal transplant recipients presents with a spectrum of asymptomatic viremia to infectious mononucleosis to post-transplant lymphoproliferative disorders (PTLD). Case reports from India have found rare hepatic smooth muscle tumor in such recipients.[29] The prevalence of PTLD in India ranges from 1 to 3% in renal transplant recipients with higher rates in pediatric recipients as compared to adults.[30-34]

The risk of PTLD depends on the type of transplanted organ being higher for heart and liver as compared to kidney, exposure to lymphocyte-depleting antibody therapies, EBV infection, and immunity status of donor and recipient, being highest in EBV-seronegative recipients of EBV-seropositive donor organs.[35,36]

Post-transplant lymphoproliferative disorder may be life-threatening in renal allograft recipients. Mostly, it is associated with replication of EBV after either primary infection or reactivation when on immunosuppressive agents.[35]

Immunosuppressive agents used post-transplant can cause disruption of balance between immune systems in latently infected patients and this latent virus leads to reactivation of EBV. For disease monitoring, surveillance, and diagnosis of PTLD, quantification of EBV viral load by PCR is done. An increase in viral load correlates with the development of EBV-related PTLD. Histopathological examination is the gold standard test for the diagnosis of PTLD. High-risk transplant recipients who were EBV-seronegative with an EBV-seropositive donor should be monitored for EBV viral load with PCR for early identification and prompt intervention.[37,38]

The first-line treatment approach in the management of PTLD is the reduction of immunosuppression. Recent evidences suggest that mTOR inhibitors are effective in suppressing EBV-related PTLD. In localized PTLD cases, surgery and radiotherapy can be used as an adjunctive to a reduction in immunosuppression. Rituximab monotherapy has a high response rate in B-cell PTLD. The use of other agents, such as IVIG and interferon-α, has been considered in the treatment of PTLD.[39,40]

JC POLYOMAVIRUS

The JC polyomavirus (JCV) is a member of the polyomaviridae family with double-stranded DNA genomes. The natural hosts for the JCV other than humans also include other primates such as rabbits and rodents.[41] JCV is not seen to infect any other species except humans with particular tropism for the human glial cells, kidney epithelial cells, and B-lymphocytes.[42,43]

The transmission of JCV continues to remain obscure with 70% of the adults showing the presence of JCV-specific antibodies.[44] The primary infection is thought to have occurred during childhood followed by a latency that is attained by the virus in the kidney epithelial cells where it continues to be shed in the urine. In an immunocompromised host, such as a transplantation patient, there is a spread of the virus with selective tropism for the oligodendrocytes which subsequently leads to the demyelinating disease—progressive multifocal leukoencephalopathy (PML).[45,46]

Though a very rare infection, JCV is seen to cause both JCV polyomavirus-associated nephropathy (PyVAN) and PML in patients more commonly following kidney transplantation.[47] The earliest report of virus shedding in the urine is as early as 3 months post kidney transplantation and correlates well with drug-related graft injury, rejection episodes, human leukocyte antigen (HLA) mismatch, and longer cold ischemia times.[48,49]

The classic form of PML involves the white matter and presents as a multifocal progressive disease with motor and gait deficits, visual disturbances, and rarely as unexplained altered sensorium. Atypical presentations include meningitis, encephalitis, progressive cerebellar ataxia, and muscle-wasting syndromes.[50-52] The overall life expectancy and prognosis of this syndrome are very poor, and no effective treatment has been described till date.[47]

JC polyomavirus PyVAN is seen more commonly post renal transplantation and usually may present with asymptomatic urinary virus shedding or unexplained renal dysfunction and graft loss.[53] However, in contrast to the closely related BK virus nephropathy, the immunosuppressive regimen does not seem to correlate with the nephropathy, and therefore a reduction in immunosuppressive drugs post diagnosis remains controversial.[54]

Though not widely available, definitive diagnosis is established with PCR assay of kidney tissue or urine samples. Due to the otherwise slow progressive course and indolent nature of this virus, it is recommended that monitoring for this viral infection be carried out during the first 24 months post-transplantation.[47]

HUMAN PAPILLOMAVIRUS

Human papillomavirus (HPV) is one of the most common sexually transmitted viral diseases and the most common etiology of a variety of genital, anal, and head–face malignancies in post-kidney transplantation patients.[55] It is a small DNA type virus with more than 100 subtypes which are further classified as high risk or low risk depending upon their capacity to cause invasive cervical cancers.[56] In a study from India, which estimated the prevalence of high-risk HPV subtypes in female transplant recipients, it was observed that despite the absence of cervical dysplasia, the prevalence of high-risk subtype of HPV was 1.9 times higher than the control population.[57] The HPV-associated cancers seen in the transplant population are diagnosed at a much younger age as compared to the general population.[55]

The most common manifestations of HPV infection in transplant recipients include anogenital cancers; head, neck, and upper airway benign neoplasms; invasive and intraepithelial cervical neoplasia; anal intraepithelial neoplasia; and cutaneous and anogenital warts.[55] In contrast to the warts, the anogenital and cervical invasive malignancies and intraepithelial neoplasia do not present with clinically obvious lesions. They require the use of high-resolution colposcopy or anoscopy, thus making regular screening for this infection a very important diagnostic tool.[55] In contrast, the warts are easily identifiable bulky outgrowths with symptoms such as irritation, itching, or recurrent bleeding.

Besides the obvious clinical examination, Papanicolaou (Pap) test is the backbone of screening for invasive cervical cancers and has reduced the incidence of cervical cancers up to 70%.[58]

Molecular-based methods such as DNA hybrid capture and PCR on clinical specimens may also aid in the diagnosis.[59]

In general, the treatment options for kidney transplant patients with HPV-related lesions is decided depending upon the size, location, and grade of lesions. The treatment of high-grade premalignant lesions is always a priority.[60] There is scant evidence that supports the reduction of immunosuppression in these patients.[61] However, some institutes have protocolized the changing over of calcineurin inhibitors to mTOR inhibitors in case of a malignant transformation.[61] Prophylactic HPV vaccines, usually targeting subtypes 16 and 18 have been found to be effective and should be offered prophylactically to transplant recipients from 12 to 26 years of age.[62] Most HPV-associated malignancies are easily preventable due to the long preinvasive precursor lesions and therefore routine screening and clinical examination should be a regular protocol in postrenal transplantation patients.

CORONAVIRUS AND COVID-19

Until recently, coronaviruses were mainly responsible for the common cold. In December 2019, the novel coronavirus designated as 2019-nCoV was identified in Hubei province of China which became a global health emergency. The WHO declared this as a pandemic in 2020 and named the disease as COVID-19. Since then, COVID-19 infection has become synonymous for coronavirus infection.[63-66]

Currently, more than 450 million cases of COVID-19 have been diagnosed and kidney transplantation was affected worldwide including India. The first case of COVID was reported in India on January 30, 2020.[67,68] To lower the risk of infection and preservation of hospital resources, there was deferral of nonurgent transplant during the pandemic period. Current guidelines recommend screening of organ donor and recipients for 2019-nCoV.[69]

Acute COVID in organ transplant recipient has higher morbidity and due to other associated comorbidities such as diabetes, hypertension, and cardiovascular diseases, the mortality is also high.[70] Observational studies from India also showed increased graft dysfunction and mortality in COVID-19 patients.[69,71-73] In India, the three waves of the COVID-19 pandemic had a different clinical spectrum in kidney transplant recipients though the mortality was comparable in the first two waves.[74] The current guidelines recommend adjustments to the immunosuppressive regimen based upon time since transplant and the risk of acute allograft rejection.[75] It is recommended to either reduce or hold antimetabolites such as mycophenolate, especially in patients with lymphopenia. As the calcineurin inhibitors such as tacrolimus inhibit interleukin-6 (IL-6) and IL-1, they may be continued.[76] Experimental studies suggest that mTOR inhibitors may have inhibitory activity on SARS-CoV. The decision to reduce immunosuppression is to be taken into consideration based on risk versus benefit and risk of rejection.[77,78]

Post-COVID-19, prospective recipients can undergo kidney transplantation with appropriate pretransplant evaluation and risk–benefit analysis.[79] Pre-exposure prophylaxis with tixagevimab plus cilgavimab is appropriate for solid organ transplant patients (aged ≥12 years) who are receiving immunosuppressive treatment and may not have an adequate immune response to vaccination.[80]

The Food and Drug Administration (FDA) had issued an emergency use authorization (EUA) to use the monoclonal antibody combination casirivimab–imdevimab or bamlanivimab–etesevimab to prevent SARS-CoV-2 infection as a postexposure prophylaxis.[81]

HUMAN T-CELL LEUKEMIA VIRUS

Human T-cell leukemia virus type 1 (HTLV-1) is the first pathogenic retrovirus to be described which causes two devastating disorders: adult T-cell leukemia/lymphoma (ATL) and a neurological disorder, HTLV-1-associated myelopathy (HAM)/tropical spastic paraparesis.[82] HTLV-2 has been linked to HAM but not to ATL. There is usually a 2–3-decade latency after the initial infection before the actual symptoms start. Based on the available literature, 5–10 million people are infected with this virus world over at present.[83] Donor/recipient screening remains almost nonexistent for this virus in the pretransplantation period due to the low positive predictive value of serologic screening tests, and a lack of serologic tests appropriate for use by organ procurement agencies along with the variable prevalence of this infection worldwide.[84] It is recommended that organ procurement organizations and transplant programs should determine local prevalence to guide screening efforts.[85]

CONCLUSION

In conclusion, the postrenal transplantation period continues to remain a high-risk period for the patient to get infected with viral infections due to the immunocompromised status. Most viral infections do not have specific antiviral therapy available for treatment of the infection. Primary prophylaxis and pretransplant screening remain an important step to prevent these infections in the post-transplantation period. Optimizing the immunosuppressive therapy may also help to prevent mortality and morbidity as well as the severity of infection due to viral diseases.

REFERENCES

1. Weikert BC, Blumberg EA. Viral infection after renal transplantation: surveillance and management. Clin J Am Soc Nephrol. 2008;3:S76-86.
2. Naraqi S, Jackson GG, Jonasson O, Yamashiroya HM. Prospective study of prevalence, incidence, and source of herpesvirus infections in patients with renal allografts. J Infect Dis. 1977;136(4):531-40.
3. Looker KJ, Magaret AS, May MT, Turner KME, Vickerman P, Gottlieb SL, et al. Global and regional estimates of prevalent and incident herpes simplex virus type 1 infections in 2012. PLoS One. 2015;10(10):e0140765.
4. Jha V, Chugh S, Chugh KS. Infections in dialysis and transplant patients in tropical countries. Kidney Int. 2000;57:S85-93.
5. Lee DH, Zuckerman RA. Herpes simplex virus infections in solid organ transplantation: guidelines from the American Society of Transplantation Infectious Diseases Community of Practice. Clin Transplant. 2019;33(9):e13526.
6. Vanichanan J, Udomkarnjananun S, Avihingsanon Y, Jutivorakool K. Common viral infections in kidney transplant recipients. Kidney Res Clin Pract. 2018;37(4):323-37.
7. Ethem U, Ahmet T, Muhammed Taha D, Omer Faruk O. Viral infections after kidney transplantation: an updated review. Int J Virol AIDS. 2018;5(1):10-3.
8. Ayyappa A, Sahay M, Ismail K, Vali PS. Fulminant hepatic failure secondary to herpes simplex virus type 2 infection in a renal allograft recipient. Indian J Transplant. 2017;11:163-5.
9. Yousuf M, Akhter M, Sajad. Clinical spectrum of herpes simplex keratitis in patients attending various health institutions in North India. J Med Sci Clin Res. 2018;6(11):134-8.
10. Castello M, Gregorini M, Rampino T, Bosio F, Bedino G, Piotti G, et al. A retrospective analysis of dermatological lesions in kidney transplant patients. Indian J Med Res. 2013;137(6):1188-92.
11. George L, John GT, Jacob CK, Eapen P, Pulimood S, George R. Skin lesions in renal transplant recipients: a single center analysis. Indian J Dermatol Venereol Leprol. 2009;75(3):255-61.
12. Basu G. Infections after kidney transplantation: the bug bear of kidney transplantation in tropics. Open Urol Nephrol J. 2015;8:76-87.
13. Pergam SA, Limaye AP, AST Infectious Diseases Community of Practice. Varicella zoster virus (VZV) in solid organ transplant recipients. Am J Transplant. 2009;9(Suppl. 4):S108-15.
14. Gilden DH, Kleinschmidt-DeMasters BK, LaGuardia JJ, Mahalingam R, Cohrs RJ. Neurologic complications of the reactivation of varicella-zoster virus. N Engl J Med. 2000; 342:635-45.
15. Kaul A, Sharma RK, Bhadhuria D, Gupta A, Prasad N. Chickenpox infection after renal transplantation. Clin Kidney J. 2012;5(3):203-6.
16. Heininger U, Seward JF. Varicella. Lancet. 2006;368:1365-76.
17. Centers for Disease Control and Prevention (CDC). Varicella-related deaths among adults—United States, 1997. MMWR Morb Mortal Wkly Rep. 1997;46:409-12.
18. Rubin RH, Tolkoff-Rubin NE. Viral infection in the renal transplant patient. Proc Eur Dial Transplant Assoc. 1983; 19:513-26.
19. Luby JP, Ramirez-Ronda C, Rinner S, Hull A, Vergne-Marini P. A longitudinal study of varicella-zoster virus infections in renal transplant recipients. J Infect Dis. 1977;135:659-63.
20. Hanna RM, Abd-El-Malak F, Alnaser A, Cader R, Yabu JM. Herpes zoster in kidney transplant recipients: a series of three cases. Case Rep Nephrol Dial. 2020;10:139-46.
21. Pergam SA, Limaye AP, AST Infectious Diseases Community of Practice. Varicella zoster virus in solid organ transplantation. Am J Transplant. 2013;13(Suppl. 4):138-46.
22. Drolet M, Brisson M, Schmader KE, Levin MJ, Johnson R, Oxman MN, et al. The impact of herpes zoster and postherpetic neuralgia on health-related quality of life: a prospective study. CMAJ. 2010;182(16):1731-6.
23. Kho MML, Roest S, Bovée DM, Metselaar HJ, Hoek RAS, van der Eijk AA, et al. Herpes zoster in solid organ transplantation: incidence and risk factors. Front Immunol. 2021;12:645718.
24. Volpi A. Severe complications of herpes zoster. Herpes. 2007;14(Suppl. 2):35-9.
25. American Academy of Pediatrics. Varicella-zoster infections. In: Pickering LK, Baker CJ, Long SS, McMillan JA (Eds). Red Book 2006: Report of the Committee on Infectious Diseases, 27th edition. Elk Grove Village, IL: American Academy of Pediatrics; 2006.
26. Humar A. Reactivation of viruses in solid organ transplant patients receiving cytomegalovirus prophylaxis. Transplantation. 2006;82(2 Suppl.):S9-14.
27. Odumade OA, Hogquist KA, Balfour HH. Progress and problems in understanding and managing primary Epstein-Barr virus infections. Clin Microbiol Rev. 2011;24(1):193-209.
28. Womack J, Jimenez M. Common questions about infectious mononucleosis. Am Fam Physician. 2015;91(6):372-6.
29. Thirunavukkarasu B, Nada R, Ramchandran R, Sakhuja V. Epstein–Barr virus–associated hepatic smooth muscle tumor post–renal transplant. Kidney Int. 2021;99(5):1245.
30. Sakhuja V, Ramachandran R, Kohli HS, Jha V, Gupta KL, Rathi M, et al. Spectrum of lymphoproliferative disorders following renal transplantation in North India. Indian J Nephrol. 2013;23(4):287-91.
31. Chandra A, Kaul A, Aggarwal V, Srivastava D. Native kidney posttransplant lymphoproliferative disorder in a renal transplant recipient. Saudi J Kidney Dis Transpl. 2017;28(4): 942-4.
32. Burns DM, Crawford DH. Epstein-Barr virus-specific cytotoxic T-lymphocytes for adoptive immunotherapy of post-transplant lymphoproliferative disease. Blood Rev. 2004;18:193-209.
33. Green M, Michaels MG. Epstein-Barr virus infection and posttransplant lymphoproliferative disorder. Am J Transplant. 2013;13(Suppl. 3):41-54.
34. Caillard S, Lelong C, Pessione F, Moulin B. Post-transplant lymphoproliferative disorders occurring after renal transplantation in adults: report of 230 cases from the French registry. Am J Transplant. 2006;6:2735-42.

35. Knight JS, Tsodikov A, Cibrik DM, Ross CW, Kaminski MS, Blayney DW. Lymphoma after solid organ transplantation: risk, response to therapy, and survival at a transplantation centre. J Clin Oncol. 2009;27:3354-62.
36. Dharnidharka VR, Lamb KE, Gregg JA, Meier-Kriesche HU. Associations between EBV serostatus and organ transplant type in PTLD risk: an analysis of the SRTR national registry data in the United States. Am J Transplant. 2012;12:976-83.
37. Parker A, Bowles K, Bradley JA, Emery V, Featherstone C, Gupte G, et al. Diagnosis of post-transplant lymphoproliferative disorder in solid organ transplant recipients—BCSH and BTS guidelines. Br J Haematol. 2010;149:675-92.
38. Ghobrial IM, Habermann TM, Maurer MJ, Geyer SM, Ristow KM, Larson TS, et al. Prognostic analysis for survival in adult solid organ transplant recipients with post-transplantation lymphoproliferative disorders. J Clin Oncol. 2005;23:7574-82.
39. Allen UD, Preiksaitis JK, AST Infectious Diseases Community of Practice. Epstein-Barr virus and posttransplant lymphoproliferative disorder in solid organ transplantation. Am J Transplant. 2013;13(Suppl. 4):107-20.
40. Parker A, Bowles K, Bradley JA, Emery V, Featherstone C, Gupte G, et al. Management of post-transplant lymphoproliferative disorder in adult solid organ transplant recipients—BCSH and BTS Guidelines. Br J Haematol. 2010;149:693-705.
41. Imperiale MJ. The human polyomaviruses: an overview. In: Khalili K, Stoner GL (Eds). Human Polyomaviruses: Molecular and Clinical Perspective, Chapter 5. New York, NY: John Wiley & Sons; 2001. pp. 53-71.
42. Khalili K, Del Valle L, Otte J, Weaver M, Gordon J. Human neurotropic polyomavirus, JCV, and its role in carcinogenesis. Oncogene. 2003;22(33):5181-91.
43. Raj GV, Khalili K. Transcriptional regulation: lessons from the human neurotropic polyomavirus, JCV. Virology. 1995; 213(2):283-91.
44. Egli A, Infanti L, Dumoulin A, Buser A, Samaridis J, Stebler C, et al. Prevalence of polyomavirus BK and JC infection and replication in 400 healthy blood donors. J Infect Dis. 2009; 199(6):837-46.
45. Clayson ET, Brando LVJ, Compans RW. Release of simian virus 40 virions from epithelial cells is polarized and occurs without cell lysis. J Virol. 1989;63(5):2278-88.
46. Caldarelli-Stefano R, Vago L, Omodeo-Zorini E, Mediati M, Losciale L, Nebuloni M, et al. Detection and typing of JC virus in autopsy brains and extraneural organs of AIDS patients and non-immunocompromised individuals. J Neurovirol. 1999;5(2):125-33.
47. Delbue S, Ferraresso M, Ghio L, Carloni C, Carluccio S, Belingheri M, et al. A review on JC virus infection in kidney transplant recipients. Clin Dev Immunol. 2013;2013:926391.
48. Nickeleit V, Hirsch HH, Zeiler M, Gudat F, Prince O, Thiel G, et al. BK-virus nephropathy in renal transplants—tubular necrosis, MHC-class II expression and rejection in a puzzling game. Nephrol Dial Transplant. 2000;15(3):324-32.
49. Bohl DL, Storch GA, Ryschkewitsch C, Gaudreault-Keener M, Schnitzler MA, Major EO, et al. Donor origin of BK virus in renal transplantation and role of HLA C7 in susceptibility to sustained BK viremia. Am J Transplant. 2005;5(9):2213-21.
50. Berger JR. Progressive multifocal leukoencephalopathy and newer biological agents. Drug Safety. 2010;33(11):969-83.
51. Behzad-Behbahani A, Klapper PE, Vallely PJ, Cleator GM, Bonington A. BKV-DNA and JCV-DNA in CSF of patients with suspected meningitis or encephalitis. Infection. 2003; 31(6):374-8.
52. Fontoura P, Vale J, Lima C, Scaravilli F, Guimarães J. Progressive myoclonic ataxia and JC virus encephalitis in an AIDS patient. J Neurol Neurosurg Psychiatry. 2002;72(5):653-6.
53. Hirsch HH, Steiger J. Polyomavirus BK. Lancet Infect Dis. 2003;3(10):611-23.
54. Kazory A, Ducloux D. Renal transplantation and polyomavirus infection: recent clinical facts and controversies. Transplant Infect Dis. 2003;5(2):65-71.
55. Grulich AE, van Leeuwen MT, Falster MO, Vajdic CM. Incidence of cancers in people with HIV/AIDS compared with immunosuppressed transplant recipients: a meta-analysis. Lancet. 2007;370(9581):59-67.
56. Chin-Hong PV. Human papillomavirus in kidney transplant recipients. Semin Nephrol. 2016;36(5):397-404.
57. Aggarwal R, Suri V, Awasthi S, Naru J, Nijhawan R, Minz M, et al. Prevalence and genotypes of HPV in female renal transplant recipients in North India. Int J Gynecol Pathol. 2014;33(5):537-42.
58. Vaccarella S, Franceschi S, Engholm G, Lonnberg S, Khan S, Bray F. 50 years of screening in the Nordic countries: quantifying the effects on cervical cancer incidence. Br J Cancer. 2014;111(5):965-9.
59. Carozzi FM, Del Mistro A, Confortini M, Sani C, Puliti D, Trevisan R, et al. Reproducibility of HPV DNA testing by hybrid capture 2 in a screening setting. Am J Clin Pathol. 2005;124(5):716-21.
60. Singh JC, Kuohung V, Palefsky JM. Efficacy of trichloroacetic acid in the treatment of anal intraepithelial neoplasia in HIV-positive and HIV-negative men who have sex with men. J Acquir Immune Defic Syndr. 2009;52(4):474-9.
61. Guba M, Graeb C, Jauch KW, Geissler EK. Pro- and anti-cancer effects of immunosuppressive agents used in organ transplantation. Transplantation. 2004;77(12):1777-82.
62. Kumar D, Unger ER, Panicker G, Medvedev P, Wilson L, Humar A. Immunogenicity of quadrivalent human papillomavirus vaccine in organ transplant recipients. Am J Transplant. 2013;13(9):2411-7.
63. WHO. WHO Director-General's remarks at the media briefing on 2019-nCoV on 11 February 2020. [online] Available from http://www.who.int/dg/speeches/detail/who-director-general-s-remarks-at-the-media-briefing-on-2019-ncov-on-11-february-2020. [Last accessed May, 2022].
64. Zhu N, Zhang D, Wang W, Li X, Yang B, Song J, et al. A novel coronavirus from patients with pneumonia in China, 2019. N Engl J Med. 2020;382:727.
65. Huang C, Wang Y, Li X, Ren L, Zhao J, Hu Y, et al. Clinical features of patients infected with 2019 novel coronavirus in Wuhan, China. Lancet. 2020;395:497-506.
66. Coronaviridae Study Group of the International Committee on Taxonomy of Viruses. The species severe acute respiratory syndrome-related coronavirus: classifying 2019-nCoV and naming it SARS-CoV-2. Nat Microbiol. 2020;5(4):536-44.
67. ArcGIS dashboards. [online] Available from https://www.arcgis.com/apps/dashboards/bda7594740fd40299423467b48e9ecf6. [Last accessed May, 2022].
68. Sahay M, Kute V, Prasad N. Corona, COVID and kidney transplantation. Indian J Transplant. 2020;14(1):1-4.

69. Kumar N, Rana R, Rana DS, Gupta A, Sachdeva MP. SARS-CoV-2 in kidney transplant recipients: a systematic review. Transplantology. 2022;3(1):33-48.
70. Akalin E, Azzi Y, Bartash R, Seethamraju H, Parides M, Hemmige V, et al. Covid-19 and kidney transplantation. N Engl J Med. 2020;382:2475-77.
71. Arumugam V, Sastry B, Solomon D, Gopalakrishnan N, Kannan B, Shankar P, et al. Clinical characteristics and outcome of novel coronavirus disease in kidney transplant recipients: a single-center prospective observational study. Indian J Transplant. 2021;15(3):189-98.
72. Godara S, Saraf K, Sadasukhi TC, Gupta H, Gupta M, Sadasukhi N, et al. COVID-19 infection in kidney transplant recipients: a single centre study from Northern India. Indian J Nephrol. 2021;31(6):531-5.
73. Bhandari G, Tiwari V, Gupta A, Bhargava V, Malik M, Gupta A, et al. COVID-19 infection in renal transplant patients: early report from India. Indian J Nephrol. 2021;31(3):271-5.
74. Kute VB, Meshram HS, Navadiya VV, Chauhan S, Patel DD, Desai SN, et al. Consequences of the first and second COVID-19 wave on kidney transplant recipients at a large Indian transplant centre. Nephrology. 2022;27(2):195-207.
75. Tatapudi RR, Kopparti VR, Poosapati A, Metta S, Gongada AR, Vedulla B. SARS-CoV-2 infection in kidney transplant recipients: a single-centre study of 20 cases from India. Int J Nephrol. 2021;2021:2243095.
76. Kute VB, Bhalla AK, Guleria S, Ray DS, Bahadur MM, Shingare A, et al. Clinical profile and outcome of COVID-19 in 250 kidney transplant recipients: a multicenter cohort study from India. Transplantation. 2021;105(4):851-60.
77. Fishman JA. The immunocompromised transplant recipient and SARS-CoV-2 infection. J Am Soc Nephrol. 2020;31:1147.
78. Guillen E, Pineiro GJ, Revuelta I, Rodriguez D, Bodro M, Moreno A, et al. Case report of COVID-19 in a kidney transplant recipient: does immunosuppression alter the clinical presentation? Am J Transplant. 2020; 20:1875.
79. Kute VB, Ray DS, Yadav DK, Pathak V, Bhalla AK, Godara S, et al. A multicenter cohort study from India of 75 kidney transplants in recipients recovered after COVID-19. Transplantation. 2021;105(7):1423-32.
80. NIH. COVID-19 treatment guidelines. The COVID-19 treatment guidelines panel's statement on tixagevimab plus cilgavimab (Evusheld) for pre-exposure prophylaxis for SARS-CoV-2 infection. [online] Available from https://www.covid19treatmentguidelines.nih.gov/therapies/statement-on-evusheld-for-prep/. [Last accessed January, 2022].
81. Fact sheet for healthcare providers: emergency use authorization for Evusheld™ (tixagevimab co-packaged with cilgavimab). [online] Available from https://www.fda.gov/media/154701/download. [Last accessed May, 2022].
82. Gallo RC, Willems L, Hasegawa H, Global Virus Network's Task Force on HTLV-1. Screening transplant donors for HTLV-1 and -2. Blood. 2016;128(26):3029-31.
83. Gessain A, Cassar O. Epidemiological aspects and world distribution of HTLV-1 infection. Front Microbiol. 2012; 3(3):388.
84. Organ Procurement and Transplantation Network. Guidance for HTLV-1 screening and confirmation in potential donors and reporting potential HTLV-1 infection. [online] Available from https://optn.transplant.hrsa.gov/resources/guidance/guidance-for-htlv-1-screening-and-confirmation-in-potential-donors-and-reporting-potential-htlv-1-infection/. [Last accessed May, 2022].
85. Tedla F, Brar A, John D, Sumrani N. Risk of transmission of human T-lymphotropic virus through transplant. Am J Transplant. 2015;15(4):1123-4.

12.3 Fungal Infections

N Gopalakrishnan, Tanuj M Lamech, Venkatesh Arumugam

CASE VIGNETTE 1

A 40-year-old gentleman received a deceased donor renal transplant 1 month earlier, with antithymocyte globulin as induction agent, followed by triple immunosuppression with steroids, mycophenolate mofetil and tacrolimus. He now presented with fever, headache, and a productive cough. CT imaging showed consolidation of the right lower zone, but sputum and blood cultures were unrevealing. His MMF dose was reduced and he was treated with empirical piperacillin-tazobactam. He developed new-onset generalized tonic-clonic seizures during hospitalization. Neuroimaging revealed a brain abscess. What are the probable differentials in this patient?

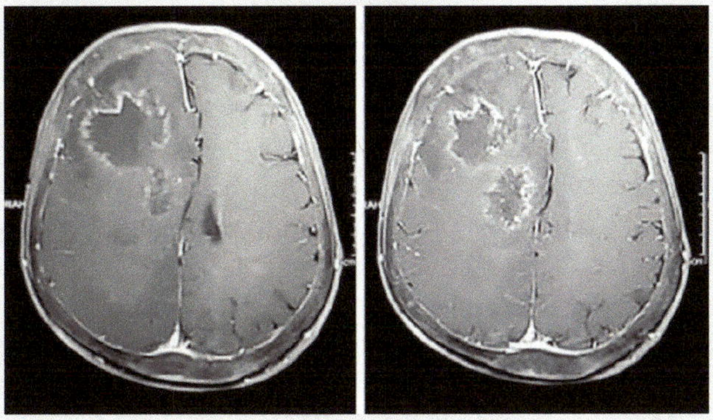

MRI image of brain abscess

INTRODUCTION

Kidney transplant recipients are particularly vulnerable for invasive fungal infections in view of therapeutic immunosuppression. The occurrence of an invasive fungal infection is by itself an indicator of high net immunosuppression. Fungal infections are rarely covered by standard "empirical" antimicrobial prescriptions; diagnosis is difficult due to cost constraints and inadequate availability of specific assays, and therefore targeted therapy is often delayed. Familiarity with the common syndromes of invasive fungal infections, along with a high index of suspicion, is paramount in ensuring patient and graft survival.

For the sake of brevity, only the most commonly encountered systemic mycoses are described in brief—invasive aspergillosis, candidiasis, cryptococcosis, mucormycosis, pheohyphomycosis, and *Pneumocystis* infection. The reader is advised to refer to the many excellent reviews that have been referenced in the text for a more nuanced description of these and other entities.

INVASIVE ASPERGILLOSIS

Aspergillus is a ubiquitous environmental pathogen, and inhalational exposure is unavoidable.[1] Causative agents include *Aspergillus fumigatus* complex, *A. flavus*, *A. niger*, and *A. terreus*. They have characteristically septate hyphae that branch at acute angles. Specific risk factors include neutropenia, critical illness, corticosteroid use, and severe respiratory viral infections, including severe acute respiratory syndrome coronavirus 2 (SARS-CoV-2) and influenza.[2]

Clinical Features

Aspergillus infections can have protean clinical manifestations in both immunocompetent and immunocompromised hosts. However, only the entity of invasive aspergillosis, which is most relevant to the transplant population, is discussed here.

Presentation can be deceivingly indolent, over weeks rather than days, and is often delayed. The initial site of infection is the lung, with subsequent dissemination to other organs either by contiguous or by hematogenous spread. Systemic manifestations include endophthalmitis, cutaneous disease, central nervous system (CNS) disease (presenting as mass lesions or nodules), and even infective endocarditis.

Chest imaging in patients with pulmonary involvement can show consolidation, patchy infiltrates, cavitation, or nodules. Characteristic radiological findings include the "halo sign" (nodules surrounded by ground-glass infiltrates) and the "air crescent sign" (cavitation of the nodule after recovery from neutropenia).

Diagnosis

Aspergillus can be detected by direct microscopy or by the culture of respiratory samples. However, these techniques have limited sensitivity, and even when the organism is isolated, it could represent simple colonization rather than invasive infection. Demonstration of fungal elements on histopathology of tissue sections was the traditional standard for proof of invasion, but obtaining biopsy material is often difficult.

Noninvasive testing includes the detection of galactomannan and 1,3-β-D-glucan, which are fungal wall components. Serum galactomannan at an optical density index ≥0.5 has a sensitivity of 82% and a specificity of 81% for invasive aspergillosis.[1] Bronchoalveolar lavage (BAL) fluid can also be tested for galactomannan to make the diagnosis. 1,3-β-D-glucan appears to be more sensitive than galactomannan but is not specific for *Aspergillus*.[1] It is a component of the cell wall of various pathogenic fungi including molds, yeasts (e.g., *Candida*), and *Pneumocystis*.[3]

CHAPTER HIGHLIGHTS

- Invasive fungal infections are an indicator of high net immunosuppression and associated with significant morbidity and mortality
- The common infections of invasive aspergillosis, candidiasis, cryptococcosis, mucormycosis, pheohyphomycosis, and *Pneumocystis* are discussed in detail
- Accurate diagnosis and targeted antifungal therapy is essential to prevent adverse outcomes

Aspergillus polymerase chain reaction (PCR) has also become available for both serum and BAL samples, but false positivity due to cross-reactivity has been described. Furthermore, PCR of respiratory samples cannot distinguish between invasive infection and incidental colonization.

Management

First-line therapy comprises voriconazole, isavuconazole, or posaconazole **(Table 1)**. Of note, there is randomized controlled trial (RCT) evidence that voriconazole is superior to amphotericin B.[1] Therapeutic drug monitoring is recommended for both voriconazole and posaconazole. The duration of therapy is dictated by the patient's clinical course and is usually continued for at least 12 weeks.

Interactions with calcineurin inhibitors (CNIs) are to be anticipated, and close monitoring of trough levels is prudent. The azoles are strong inhibitors of the CYP3A enzyme system and therefore result in extremely high levels of CNIs, which must be down-titrated. Clinicians must also be aware that long-term use of these azoles is associated with QT prolongation and peripheral neuropathy. Furthermore, prolonged voriconazole administration has been linked with cutaneous squamous cell carcinomas,[3] periostitis, photopsia, CNS disturbances, and photosensitivity.[1]

Immunosuppression is usually reduced, but the risk of precipitating an immune reconstitution syndrome-like entity must be borne in mind.[3]

CANDIDIASIS

Most cases of invasive candidiasis are caused by five species—*Candida* (*C*). *albicans*, *C. glabrata*, *C. tropicalis*, *C. parapsilosis*, and *C. krusei*. However, an alarming increase in the frequency of *C. auris* infections, which are frequently drug-resistant, has been reported around the world over the last decade.[4] Among solid organ transplant recipients, the incidence is highest among small bowel transplants and lowest in kidney transplants.[5]

Clinical Features

The clinical presentation of invasive candidiasis may vary from simple laboratory abnormalities, such as leukocytosis, to frank septic shock and multiorgan dysfunction. Invasive candidiasis should be in the differential diagnosis of an unexplained fever that does not respond to antibacterial therapy. A dilated fundoscopic examination should be performed for all patients, as ocular involvement may occur in 15% of patients with candidemia and may rarely evolve into sight-threatening endophthalmitis.

Among organ transplant recipients, common clinical syndromes include oropharyngeal candidiasis, esophageal candidiasis, asymptomatic candiduria, and symptomatic *Candida* urinary tract infection (UTI).

Diagnosis

Blood cultures have a sensitivity of only around 50% for invasive candidiasis, but this can be enhanced by the use of blood volumes of at least 40–60 mL and the use of special

TABLE 1: Drug dosing recommendations for invasive aspergillosis.[3]

Drug	*Dose (adult)*	*Comments*
Voriconazole	6 mg/kg IV/PO, every 12 hours for 1 day, followed by 4 mg/kg IV/PO every 12 hours	• Target trough level for treatment is >1 mg/L • Clinical experience with the use of IV voriconazole in patients with renal failure has been good. However, due to accumulation of the IV vehicle (cyclodextrin), the manufacturer recommends oral voriconazole in patients with CrCl <50 mL/min
Isavuconazole	Isavuconazonium sulfate 372 mg (isavuconazole 200 mg) IV/PO every 8 hours for six doses, followed by isavuconazonium sulfate 372 mg (isavuconazole 200 mg) IV/PO once daily	• Routine therapeutic drug monitoring is not recommended • Half-life is 130 hours and thus there is a long time to clearance after drug discontinuation • Dose adjustment not required in renal failure, as the IV preparation does not contain cyclodextrin
Posaconazole	• 300 mg PO (delayed-release tablets)/IV twice daily on day 1 followed by 300 mg PO (delayed-release tablets)/IV once daily on day 2 and thereafter • When using suspension 200 mg PO every 8 hours or 400 mg PO every 12 hours	• Target trough level for treatment is >1 mg/L (preferably >1.25 mg/L) • Although the delayed-release tablet can be taken without food, a high-fat meal can increase its serum concentration by 1.5-fold • Dose adjustment not required in renal failure

(CrCl: creatinine clearance; IV: intravenous)

fungal blood culture media that suppress bacteria that may overgrow fungi. Histological examination of tissue specimens stained with Gomori's methenamine silver (GMS) stain or periodic acid–Schiff (PAS) stain may also help make the diagnosis.

β-D-glucan is a fungal cell wall component that is not specific to *Candida* but has high sensitivity and negative predictive value for invasive candidiasis. More recent techniques include detection of mannan antigen and anti-mannan antibody, detection of *C. albicans* germ tube antigen (CAGTA), and PCR-based assays.[4]

Management

First-line therapy for invasive candidiasis is echinocandins, which have been demonstrated to be superior to azoles and amphotericin B. Furthermore, it does not require dose reduction with renal failure and is not dialyzable. However, azoles (fluconazole or voriconazole) maybe preferred in the case of endophthalmitis, meningitis, urinary tract candidiasis, and esophageal candidiasis, as echinocandins have reduced tissue penetration at these sites **(Table 2)**.

Once the patient has stabilized, therapy may be stepped down to an oral azole. Fluconazole is generally preferred if the isolate is susceptible, but voriconazole may be used if fluconazole resistance is documented. Certain species, including *C. glabrata*, *C. krusei*, and *C. auris* are more likely to display fluconazole resistance. Experience with posaconazole and isavuconazole is limited, but excellent in vitro activity has been demonstrated. Therapy is continued for at least 14 days after clearance of candidemia from the bloodstream.

With regard to asymptomatic candiduria, recent guidelines advise against treatment even in kidney transplant recipients with a ureteric stent in place. However, if cystoscopic stent removal is being performed, a 7-day course of therapy is advised to prevent invasive infection. It is recommended that urinary catheters are removed as early as possible in all patients with candiduria.[5]

Among patients with symptomatic *Candida* UTI, fluconazole and voriconazole remain the drugs of choice, with conventional amphotericin B deoxycholate reserved for azole-resistant isolates. Importantly, neither echinocandins nor liposomal amphotericin B formulations achieve sufficient urinary concentrations, and are therefore not recommended for treating *Candida* UTI.

CRYPTOCOCCOSIS

Cryptococcus typically occurs 1–2 years post-transplant. With the advent of molecular techniques, the erstwhile species *C. neoformans* and *C. gattii*, which were the primary causative agents, have now been reclassified into seven distinct species, and other rarer species have also been identified to be pathogenic.[6] *Cryptococcus* is an environmental fungus, and most children have already been exposed by the time they reach 5 years of age.[7] Cryptococcosis post-transplant usually represents the reactivation of a previously quiescent infection.

Clinical Features

Pulmonary manifestations run the gamut from asymptomatic infection to fulminant respiratory failure. Radiologically, the most common pattern is one of solitary or multiple nodules, which may occasionally cavitate.

Neurological involvement manifests subacutely over weeks. Patients present with fever, headache, personality changes, and memory loss, eventually progressing to obtundation. Classic signs of neck stiffness and meningismus are often absent.

Less commonly, other organ systems may also be involved, particularly the skin and eyes. Case reports have even demonstrated cryptococcosis on renal biopsy specimens, with yeast cells invading both the glomerular and the tubulointerstitial compartments.[8]

Diagnosis

The organism can be cultured by routine media such as Sabouraud's agar or visualized directly on tissue specimens with GMS stain or PAS stain. Cryptococcal antigen detection has greatly improved diagnostic accuracy and maybe identified in both serum and cerebrospinal fluid.

TABLE 2: Drug dosing recommendations for candidiasis.[5]

Site of candidiasis	*Initial therapy*	*Alternative therapy*
Candidemia and invasive candidiasis	Echinocandin (caspofungin 70 mg loading dose and then 50 mg IV daily; micafungin 100 mg IV daily; anidulafungin 200 mg loading dose and then 100 mg IV daily)	Fluconazole 12 mg/kg loading dose and then 6 mg/kg IV/PO daily
Esophageal candidiasis	• Fluconazole 200–400 mg PO or IV daily • If fluconazole refractory—itraconazole solution 200 mg daily PO or voriconazole 3 mg/kg q12h PO or IV	Echinocandin (caspofungin 70 mg loading dose then 50 mg IV daily; micafungin 150 mg IV daily; anidulafungin 200 mg IV daily)
Urinary tract infection	Fluconazole 200 mg PO daily (if susceptible)	Amphotericin B deoxycholate 0.3–0.6 mg/kg IV daily

(IV: intravenous)

Management

For disseminated disease, therapy is divided into an induction phase (with lipid formulations of amphotericin B, along with 5-flucytosine, for 2 weeks), a consolidation phase (with oral fluconazole 400–800 mg/day for 8 weeks), and a maintenance phase (with oral fluconazole 200–400 mg/day for 6–12 months) **(Table 3)**. The duration of the induction phase maybe extended, if required, based on clinical circumstances. Particular attention must bepaid to potential drug interactions between fluconazole and CNIs. Therapeutic drug monitoring is recommended for 5-flucytosine, and dose reduction is warranted in the presence of renal failure.

Elevated intracranial pressure is a significant cause of morbidity and even mortality and requires specific therapy. Repeated therapeutic lumbar punctures maybe performed until the opening pressure is normalized, but some cases require surgical procedures such as extraventricular drains or ventriculoperitoneal shunting.

Immunosuppression is reduced and sometimes withdrawn, but this might rarely precipitate an immune reconstitution inflammatory syndrome with apparent clinical worsening. Antifungal therapy should be continued, but a short course of corticosteroids can be considered.

MUCORMYCOSIS

These are invasive fungal infections attributed to species of the order *Mucorales*, subphylum *Mucormycotina*. Common organisms pathogenic to humans include *Rhizopus*, *Mucor*, *Rhizomucor*, *Cunninghamella*, and *Absidia*.[7] They are ubiquitous in nature but cause disease only in patients with specific risk factors—diabetes (particularly diabetic ketoacidosis), iron overload, organ transplant recipients, and other immunocompromised individuals.[9]

Recently, a veritable epidemic of mucormycosis was observed following the second wave of the COVID-19 pandemic in India, particularly between the months of June and August 2021. Most patients presented with rhino-orbital mucormycosis immediately following, or concomitant with, a COVID-19 infection. A clear explanation for this surprising association is still lacking. It has been suggested that upregulation of glucose-regulated protein 78 (GRP78), a heat shock protein, maybe involved in the pathogenesis.[10,11]

TABLE 3: Drug dosing recommendations for cryptococcosis.[6]

Drug	Dose	Duration
Induction phase:		
• Liposomal amphotericin B *And/or*	• 3–4 mg/kg/day • 5 mg/kg/day	Minimum of 2 weeks
• Amphotericin B lipid complex, plus 5-flucytosine*	• 100 mg/kg/day	
Consolidation phase:		
• Fluconazole*	400–800 mg/day	8 weeks
Maintenance phase:		
• Fluconazole*	200–400 mg/day	Minimum of 6–12 months

*Both fluconazole and 5-flucytosine require dose reduction in the presence of renal insufficiency.

Clinical Features

The classical presentation is one of the rhino-orbital-cerebral diseases. Infection of the paranasal sinuses commonly spreads to the orbit and the cavernous sinus, causing focal neurological deficits and pressure effects, including ptosis, chemosis, and ophthalmoplegia. Angioinvasion is a hallmark of the disease.

In the Transplant-Associated Infection Surveillance Network (TRANSNET) study of solid organ transplant recipients, pulmonary mucormycosis accounted for 56% of cases in this population.[12] It may present as consolidations, nodules, mass lesions, and cavities. Diagnosis is often delayed because of frequent misattribution of the clinical presentation to bacterial or tubercular etiologies.

Disseminated mucormycosis carries a grim prognosis, with mortality rates in excess of 90%. Rare instances of graft-transmitted mucormycosis have also been reported.[13]

Diagnosis

Demonstration of the organism from a sterile site, either by culture or by histopathology, confirms the diagnosis. Mucorales are killed by tissue homogenization, which is the standard technique to prepare tissue cultures. Instead, whenever the diagnosis is suspected, tissue must be cut into sections before being placed on culture dishes to improve the diagnostic yield and sensitivity. Histological examination of tissue samples demonstrates characteristic thick-walled, aseptate hyphal elements which branch at right angles.

Management

Amphotericin B remains the standard of care for mucormycosis. The lipid formulations are purported to be less nephrotoxic and more efficacious, though head-to-head comparisons are lacking **(Table 4)**. Add-on therapy with echinocandins has been suggested to improve survival, though this requires confirmation. Posaconazole has been used as salvage therapy or step-down treatment.[7] The duration of therapy is unclear but should continue at least until the resolution of all clinical and imaging evidence of

TABLE 4: Drug dosing recommendations for mucormycosis.[9]

Drug	Dose
Amphotericin B deoxycholate (AmB)	1–1.5 mg/kg/day
Liposomal amphotericin B (L-AmB)	5 mg/kg/day
Amphotericin B lipid complex (ABLC)	5 mg/kg/day

infection, with some suggesting that long-term maintenance therapy be continued with posaconazole or isavuconazole for as long as the patient is on immunosuppression.[14] With the exception of patients with isolated and localized pulmonary involvement, expedient surgical debridement is critical to eradicate the infection.

PHEOHYPHOMYCOSIS

The causative agents of pheohyphomycosis are a group of darkly pigmented fungi that are known as dematiaceous or melanized molds. It is believed that melanin acts as a virulence factor by scavenging free radicals and thus offering protection from the oxidative burst of phagocytes. The most common species that cause clinical disease is *Lomentospora* (formerly *Scedosporium*) *prolificans.*[15]

It commonly presents as superficial infections such as onychomycosis, subcutaneous nodules, and keratitis, often associated with minor trauma. Invasive disease and dissemination are less common but have been known to occur.

Diagnosis is by tissue histopathology or by culture on Sabouraud dextrose agar. Surgical resection is indicated, along with broad-spectrum azoles such as voriconazole and posaconazole. However, members of some species, particularly *Lomentospora prolificans*, are multidrug-resistant. The optimal duration of therapy is unclear.

PNEUMOCYSTIS JIROVECII

Despite universal prophylaxis with trimethoprim-sulfamethoxazole (TMP-SMX), *P. jirovecii* remains an important cause of pneumonia in kidney transplant recipients. Clinical disease may occur de novo through airborne transmission or may represent reactivation of prior infection (initial exposure commonly occurs in childhood).[16] Though classically *Pneumocystis* pneumonia was said to occur between the 2nd and 6th months post-transplant,[17] recent insights have suggested a shift in the epidemiology, with a much lower incidence and delayed onset of disease, with presentation commonly occurring in the second year post-transplant.[18] Risk factors include a high net immunosuppression and recent cytomegalovirus (CMV) infection.

Clinical Features

Symptoms usually develop over a few days, and patients present with marked hypoxemia that is out of proportion to the physical findings. Common clinical features include fever, dyspnea, cough, chest pain, and hypoxemia, which can progress to acute respiratory distress syndrome (ARDS). *Pneumocystis* infection is an independent risk factor for graft failure and mortality.[19]

Diagnosis

The cyst or trophozoite forms can be directly visualized by GMS stain, Giemsa stain, or Wright stain but can also be demonstrated by direct immunofluorescence staining. Respiratory secretions can be obtained by noninvasive or invasive techniques (such as transbronchial or open lung biopsies). Serum 1,3-β-D-glucan and molecular techniques using PCR have been studied, but specificity is limited.

CASE VIGNETTE 2

A 38-year-old deceased donor renal transplant recipient presented 17 months after transplantation with diabetic ketoacidosis, graft dysfunction, and a nonresolving culture-negative lobar pneumonia. Bronchoalveolar lavage was stained with calcofluor white (right) and demonstrated the aseptate hyphae of mucormycosis. The patient underwent a lobectomy and the histopathology specimen (left) showed necrotic lung tissue with fungal hyphae within the alveoli.

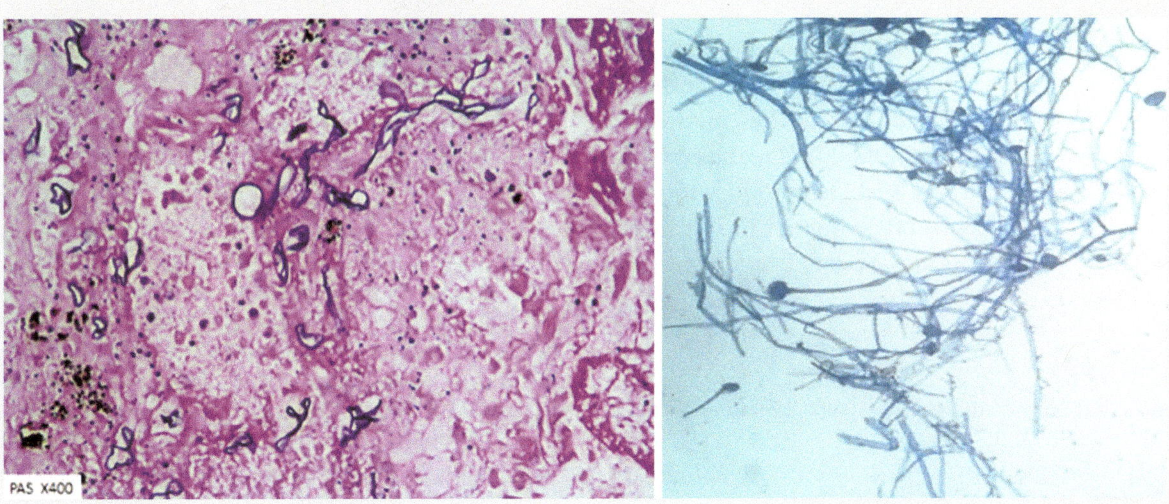

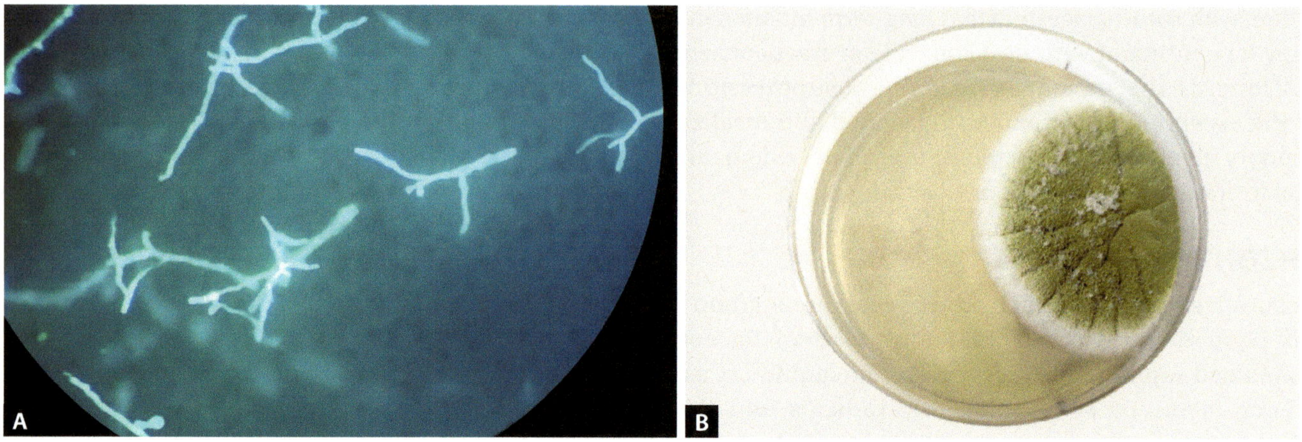

Figs. 1A and B: (A) Calcofluor white stain; (B) Fungal culture.

Treatment

Trimethoprim-sulfamethoxazole is the drug of choice. The trimethoprim component is given at 15–20 mg/kg/day IV in three to four divided doses for 21 days. In milder disease, two double-strength tablets (160 mg TMP/800 mg SMX) can be given orally q8h. Other drugs available as second-line agents include pentamidine, atovaquone, and dapsone. In hypoxemic patients, a short course of steroid therapy can also be given.[16]

Prophylaxis

Primary prophylaxis with TMP-SMX is recommended for all kidney transplant recipients for at least 6–12 months post-transplant.[16]

A burr hole aspiration was performed and the aspirate was sent for microbiological examination. This demonstrated fluorescent hyphae on Calcofluor white stain, and *Aspergillus flavus* on culture. The patient was started on voriconazole and tacrolimus level was closely monitored in view of drug interactions, but he had progressively worsening respiratory failure requiring mechanical ventilation, and he eventually succumbed to his illness **(Figs. 1A and B)**.

CONCLUSION

Awareness of the risk factors and the varied clinical presentations of systemic fungal infections in kidney transplant recipients is an essential skill for the modern-day nephrologist. Comprehension of specific therapies targeted at specific mycoses will enormously impact the choice of antimicrobial therapy in the day-to-day management of transplant patients.

REFERENCES

1. Thompson GR 3rd, Young JH. Aspergillus infections. N Engl J Med. 2021;385(16):1496-509.
2. Kosmidis C, Denning DW. The clinical spectrum of pulmonary aspergillosis. Thorax. 2015;70(3):270-7.
3. Husain S, Camargo JF. Invasive aspergillosis in solid-organ transplant recipients: guidelines from the American Society of Transplantation Infectious Diseases Community of Practice. Clin Transplant. 2019;33(9):e13544.
4. Pappas PG, Lionakis MS, Arendrup MC, Ostrosky-Zeichner L, Kullberg BJ. Invasive candidiasis. Nat Rev Dis Primers. 2018;4:18026.
5. Aslam S, Rotstein C, AST Infectious Disease Community of Practice. Candida infections in solid organ transplantation: guidelines from the American Society of Transplantation Infectious Diseases Community of Practice. Clin Transplant. 2019;33(9):e13623.
6. Baddley JW, Forrest GN, AST Infectious Diseases Community of Practice. Cryptococcosis in solid organ transplantation-guidelines from the American Society of Transplantation Infectious Diseases Community of Practice. Clin Transplant. 2019;33(9):e13543.
7. Cohen J, Powderly W, Opal S. Infectious Diseases, 4th edition. Amsterdam: Elsevier; 2017.
8. Saltarén LE, Pérez RA. Renal cryptococcosis. N Engl J Med. 2020;383(24):2371.
9. Kasper D, Fauci A, Hauser S, Longo D, Jameson J, Loscalzo J. Harrison's Principles of Internal Medicine, 19th edition. New York: McGraw-Hill Education; 2015.
10. Liu M, Spellberg B, Phan QT, Fu Y, Fu Y, Lee AS, et al. The endothelial cell receptor GRP78 is required for mucormycosis pathogenesis in diabetic mice. J Clin Invest. 2010;120(6):1914-24.
11. Fu J, Wei C, He J, Zhang L, Zhou J, Balaji KS, et al. Evaluation and characterization of HSPA5 (GRP78) expression profiles in normal individuals and cancer patients with COVID-19. Int J Biol Sci. 2021;17(3):897-10.
12. Pappas PG, Alexander BD, Andes DR, Hadley S, Kauffman CA, Freifeld A, et al. Invasive fungal infections among organ transplant recipients: results of the Transplant-Associated Infection Surveillance Network (TRANSNET). Clin Infect Dis. 2010;50(8):1101-11.
13. Alexander BD, Schell WA, Siston AM, Rao CY, Bower WA, Balajee SA, et al. Fatal Apophysomyces elegans infection transmitted by deceased donor renal allografts. Am J Transplant. 2010;10(9):2161-7.
14. Sipsas NV, Gamaletsou MN, Anastasopoulou A, Kontoyiannis DP. Therapy of mucormycosis. J Fungi (Basel). 2018;4(3):90.
15. Arcobello JT, Revankar SG. Phaeohyphomycosis. Semin Respir Crit Care Med. 2020;41(1):131-40.

16. Fishman JA, Gans H, AST Infectious Diseases Community of Practice. Pneumocystis jiroveci in solid organ transplantation: guidelines from the American Society of Transplantation Infectious Diseases Community of Practice. Clin Transplant. 2019;33(9):e13587.
17. Martin SI, Fishman JA, AST Infectious Diseases Community of Practice. Pneumocystis pneumonia in solid organ transplantation. Am J Transplant. 2013;13(Suppl. 4):272-9.
18. Park SY, Jung JH, Kwon H, Shin S, Kim YH, Chong YP, et al. Epidemiology and risk factors associated with Pneumocystis jirovecii pneumonia in kidney transplant recipients after 6-month trimethoprim-sulfamethoxazole prophylaxis: a case-control study. Transpl Infect Dis. 2020;22(2):e13245.
19. Kim JE, Han A, Lee H, Ha J, Kim YS, Han SS. Impact of Pneumocystis jirovecii pneumonia on kidney transplant outcome. BMC Nephrol. 2019;20(1):212.

12.4 Parasitic Infections

Dharmendra Bhadauria, B Karthikeyan

CASE VIGNETTE

A 42-year-old female, who is known case of chronic kidney disease (native kidney disease probably chronic glomerulonephritis) underwent live related renal transplant 8 months back presented with a history of diarrhea for one week. During transplant, she received Basiliximab as induction therapy and currently on the triple immunosuppressive regimen (Steroids, Tacrolimus and Mycophenolate mofetil). She had normal graft function over 8 months and it has worsened with the recent history of diarrhea. She had 7–8 bowel movements of watery stools per day with associated dehydration. Her vitals were stable at admission. Her blood investigations revealed mild leukocytosis and elevated serum creatinine 2.1 (baseline serum creatinine-1.2). Tacrolimus levels checked was within therapeutic range. Stool examination and CMV PCR was sent and she was started on Intravenous antibiotics and intravenous fluids. But she had persistent diarrhea and her mycophenolate mofetil dose was reduced. In the meantime, stool examination revealed strongyloides larvae. She had no other features of disseminated disease or hyperinfection syndrome. Patient was treated with combination of Ivermectin and albendazole for 14 days. She had gradual improvement in her bowel movement and repeat stool examination done did not reveal strongyloides. At 2 weeks of follow up, her serum creatinine returned to baseline and had complete resolution of diarrhea.

INTRODUCTION

As organ transplantation awareness increases worldwide, the pool of organ transplant recipients continues to expand with more patients on immunosuppression. These patients on immunosuppression are at a high risk of acquiring infection with unusual and resistant organisms, which may be life-threatening.

Due to migration and travel, parasitic infections are more common in transplant recipients, especially in developing and developed countries. This increase in parasitic infection in transplant recipients challenges donor and recipient screening and infection management clinicians. Even though there are case reports, it is still the most understudied infection in renal transplant patients. The published literature on postrenal transplant parasitic infections from India is also minimal. Newer diagnostic methods and newer treatment options are being developed for these parasitic infestations.

TRANSMISSION

Parasitic diseases can occur in renal transplant patients due to recurrence in a previously infected recipient or by transmission through the transplanted organ from the infected donor or by de novo infection.

Given global travel worldwide, the incidence and prevalence of parasitic infections in transplant recipients are expected to rise.

The various reasons for the increase in parasitic infections are transplant programs in endemic areas, referral of donor/recipients from endemic regions to developed nations, and the increasing popularity of transplant tourism.

The decrease in the use of cyclosporine-based immunosuppression and the increase in the use of immunosuppression that lacks the antiparasitic effect of cyclosporin may result in a higher incidence of parasitic infection in transplant candidates.[1]

Migration and tourism to endemic areas is another risk factor for parasitic infection in transplant patients.

EPIDEMIOLOGY

The United States Renal Data System (USRDS) data indicate that the infection is responsible for 20% of all-cause mortality in transplant recipients.[2] The contribution of parasitic infection to this mortality could not be determined precisely. As parasitic infections are more common in developing and underdeveloped countries and there is less published literature, the exact incidence of post-transplant parasitic infection is unknown. The prevalence is also less reported than bacterial, viral, and fungal infections.

CLINICAL PRESENTATION

Postrenal transplant parasitic diseases can be classified into two clinical profiles:[3]

1. Acute systemic illness like presentation in the form of constitutional symptoms, multiorgan dysfunction with acute allograft dysfunction, e.g., malaria, trypanosomiasis, leishmaniasis, and toxoplasmosis
2. The localized form of presentation like gastrointestinal (GI) manifestation, e.g., *Cryptosporidium*, microspora, and *Strongyloides*.

Dissemination of local infection into systemic disease can be devastating.

MODE OF TRANSMISSION

Transplant recipients can acquire parasitic infection in three different modes.[3]

1. A primary new infection acquired through oral (*Cryptosporidium*) or blood-borne (malaria, babesiosis) transmission.

   Recrudescence of latent infection when patients are started on immunosuppression.

2. The reactivations are commonly observed with leishmaniasis, malaria, strongyloidiasis, and trypanosomiasis.
3. Transmission of disease through the transplanted organ. Examples include leishmaniasis, malaria, *Toxoplasma*, and *Trypanosoma*.

CHAPTER HIGHLIGHTS

- Due to human mobility, parasitic infections are increasing in transplant recipients, especially in developing and developed countries.
- Parasitic infection in transplant recipients poses particular challenges in donor and recipient screening and infection.
- The exact incidence of parasitic infection in transplant recipients is unknown. The prevalence is less reported than bacterial, viral, and fungal infections.

IMMUNOPATHOGENESIS

Innate immunity is responsible for reducing the burden of parasitic infection. This is usually followed by an adaptive response where T helper type 1 (Th1) cells are involved in the acute phase of parasitic infection and T helper type 2 (Th2) cells in the chronic phase.[4] Most of the glomerulopathies due to parasitic infections are associated with immune complex deposition such as immunoglobulin M (IgM) and parasitic antigens; on the contrary, the cell-mediated immune response is related to chronic indolent response leading to granuloma as in schistosomiasis.[5]

Parasitic antigens may trigger autoimmunity, coinfection, or activation of macrophages. Activation of macrophages can lead to a predisposition to amyloidosis and the progression of glomerular diseases.[6]

CLINICAL MANIFESTATION

Due to uncontrolled parasite replication, transplant recipients with reduced immunity can present with local tissue invasion or disseminated disease (DD). Constitutional symptoms such as fever, myalgia, and anemia are commonly encountered at presentation. Some parasites such as malaria, schistosomiasis, trypanosomiasis, toxoplasmosis, and babesiosis may have DD. So other than constitutional symptoms, patient may have cardiac, pulmonary, neurological, and cutaneous involvement.[3] Acute kidney injury due to acute interstitial nephritis or acute tubular necrosis may be misinterpreted as acute allograft rejection.

On the contrary, local tissue invasion is primarily caused by intestinal protozoa such as *Cryptosporidium* and microsporidium.[3] These parasites may cause diarrhea and abdominal pain. Local disease followed by disseminated infection can occur with strongyloidiasis and *Acanthamoeba*.

Tissue and Blood Protozoan Infections

Toxoplasmosis

Toxoplasmosis is a zoonotic disease transmitted by protozoa *Toxoplasma gondii*. It can be sent by contaminated food or water, donor graft, or recrudescence of latent infection. The most encountered means of transmission is by donor's cardiac allograft. Primary disease can be acquired by ingesting cysts in contaminated soil or water, undercooked meat, maternal–fetal transmission, or blood transfusion. In one series, the mortality rate due to toxoplasmosis was 13.6%.[7]

Clinical features: Patients infected with toxoplasmosis may have a variety of clinical features. It can cause fever, myocarditis, hepatosplenomegaly, chorioretinitis, pancytopenia, and disseminated infection. Clinical manifestations usually develop 3 months after renal transplantation.[7]

Diagnosis: Toxoplasma gondii can be isolated from blood, body fluids, or tissue samples. Detection of immunoglobulin G (IgG) via the enzyme-linked immunosorbent assay (ELISA) method is an indirect method of detecting infection.[8] In immunocompromised patients, bronchoalveolar lavage (BAL), lymph node, and brain biopsy are proper diagnostic methods to detect disease. Molecular diagnostic methods using the real-time polymerase chain reaction (PCR) method are the most frequently used test for diagnosis of toxoplasmosis recently.[9] PCR tests can be done in body fluids such as amniotic fluid, cerebrospinal fluid (CSF), BAL, and blood. The acute phase has tachyzoites, while the chronic stage has the parasite in the cyst form.

The presence of multiple ring-enhancing lesions in the brain, especially IgG antibodies to toxoplasma, suggests central nervous system (CNS) toxoplasmosis.[10] CSF analysis may show mononuclear pleocytosis and elevated protein levels. Myocarditis in toxoplasmosis can present with heart failure. Pulmonary involvement can present with fever, dyspnea, cough, and reticulonodular infiltrates. The diagnosis can be confirmed by the demonstration of tachyzoites in BAL.

Treatment: The optimal treatment for toxoplasmosis after renal transplant remains elusive. However, there is enough literature on the treatment of toxoplasmosis in patients with human immunodeficiency virus/acquired immunodeficiency syndrome (HIV/AIDS), which can guide the treatment of transplant recipients.

Treatment of toxoplasmosis includes induction therapy with pyrimethamine and sulfadiazine to suppress tachyzoites, followed by chronic maintenance therapy to prevent recurrence.[11] Induction therapy is usually given for 6 weeks based on response treatment. For regular suppressive therapy, medications with reduced toxicity such as trimethoprim/sulfamethoxazole (TMP/SMX) may be used.[11-13]

Prophylaxis: Transplant centers with low toxoplasma seroprevalence need not do routine screening in transplant recipients and donors. But in areas with high prevalence, regular screening is recommended. The common use of sulfamethoxazole (SMX) for prophylaxis in postrenal transplant recipients has decreased the risk of *Toxoplasma* infection.[14] Many studies showed successful prevention using TMP/SMX three times weekly for varying durations (3 months to lifelong). An alternative drug to TMP–SMX for prophylaxis is dapsone plus pyrimethamine or atovaquone with or without pyrimethamine.[15]

To avoid primary infection, all transplant recipients should avoid contact with undercooked meat, water, soil, or animal feces that might contain toxoplasma cysts.

Chagas Disease

Chagas disease is endemic in most Latin-American countries. It is caused by the protozoan parasite *Trypanosoma cruzi*. Contaminated feces transmit the infection through the triatomine insect vector.[16] It can also be sent by oral ingestion, blood transfusion, organ transplantation, and from mother to fetus.

Clinically human involvement in Chagas disease has two presentations: acute and chronic illness. In immune-competent individuals, spontaneous resolution of infection can occur even if left untreated, but in the absence of specific therapy, the patient may become chronically infested. The latent phase may exist for 10–30 years and lifelong. About one-third of the patients with chronic infection may have irreversible heart involvement, causing cardiomyopathy.[16]

Mode of transmission: Trypanosoma cruzi can be transmitted through skin abrasions, conjunctival lesions, and other amenable surfaces through the infested vector. Infection through blood products has been dramatically reduced due to advanced techniques in the screening of blood products. Vertical transmission from mother to fetus is possible with frequent pregnancies.

Chagasic cardiomyopathy: Chagasic cardiomyopathy is one of the leading causes of heart transplantation in Brazil. The post-transplant outcomes are comparable to nonchagasic cardiomyopathy heart transplant cases. Reactivation of the disease after transplant has been reported in 27–43% of patients.[17] Clinical symptoms may usually range from asymptomatic parasitemia to fever, fatigue, headache, and cutaneous manifestations such as rash and myocarditis, which may be difficult to distinguish from rejection. Skin biopsy from cutaneous lesions will show trypanosomes.

Nonheart transplant: In a patient with a chronic trypanosomal infection, reactivation occurs in the post-transplant's first year. It is most often asymptomatic parasitemia, but fever, fatigue, headache, and cutaneous manifestations such as rash, myocarditis, and encephalitis have been reported in the literature.[18]

Seronegative recipients who receive organs from a seropositive donor may develop acute *T. cruzi* infection post-transplant.[19] Transmission rates are higher in cardiac transplants than in renal and liver transplants.[20]

Diagnosis: Serological testing has limited utility in diagnosing reactivation postorgan transplant. Direct methods for diagnosing Chagas disease include microscopic examination of the fresh buffy coat preparation, Giemsa stained smear, and PCR of the whole blood or biopsy tissue.[21] PCR is the most sensitive method to detect trypanosomal infection. But it may be positive in the absence of disease reactivation in patients with chronic illness, and it may not be helpful.

Polymerase chain reaction is recommended to monitor infection in the seronegative recipient after receiving an organ from a seropositive donor to detect disease reactivation and early treatment before developing the clinically significant disease.

Treatment: Treatment is recommended in patients with acute infection after transplant or reactivation of chronic illness. Nifurtimox and benznidazole are the drugs that are used for the treatment of Chagas disease. Benznidazole is well tolerated and has few drug interactions than nifurtimox in transplant recipients.[22]

Prophylactic treatment is not recommended to prevent transmission or reactivation of potential drug-related toxicity.

Leishmaniasis

Leishmaniasis is a heterogeneous group of protozoan parasites belonging to the *Leishmania* genus and presents with various clinical syndromes. Leishmaniasis is mainly found in tropical and subtropical climatic conditions, and the bite of infected sandflies spreads it. More than 90% of visceral leishmaniasis occurs in south Asian countries such as India, Nepal, Bangladesh, Sudan, and Brazil. Clinically, leishmaniasis can be classified into visceral, cutaneous, and mucocutaneous diseases.[23]

Leishmania infection is primarily asymptomatic and remains latent in the immunocompetent hosts. Severe disease can occur in organ transplant recipients when immunocompromised.[24] The primary mechanisms of acquiring infection in organ transplant candidates are: (1) direct primary infection after transplant, (2) reactivation of any latent infection after transplant, and (3) receiving an infected organ during transplantation.

The *Leishmania donovani* complex causes visceral leishmaniasis, and the clinical features are fever, hepatosplenomegaly, and pancytopenia. Cutaneous and mucocutaneous leishmaniasis is due to *L. mexicana* complex and is less reported in organ transplant recipients. Atypical presentations are not uncommon in renal transplant recipients. A case report from India by Rana et al. showed GI involvement without significant symptoms and signs where amastigotes were identified in duodenal biopsy.[25]

Diagnosis: The gold standard for diagnosing visceral leishmaniasis is a demonstration of amastigotes in histopathology or culture of promastigotes in the bone marrow or splenic aspirates. In organ transplant recipients, bone marrow biopsy has been reported to have greater sensitivity, contrary to the immunocompetent individuals where splenic aspirate has greater sensitivity than bone marrow biopsy. Serological testing for visceral leishmaniasis cannot distinguish between prior exposure and active infection.[26]

A biopsy for culture and histopathological exam should be obtained in suspected cutaneous and mucocutaneous leishmaniasis. Species-specific monoclonal antibodies or isoenzyme analysis help in the identification of species. Quantitative or semiquantitative PCR assays have a high diagnostic yield when applied to histopathological specimens.

Treatment: Drugs that are effective in treating leishmaniasis include pentavalent antimonials, amphotericin, and miltefosine. The pentavalent antimonials (sodium stibogluconate or meglumine antimonate) are the cornerstone of the therapeutic regimens for all forms of leishmaniasis. But due to the increasing development of resistance and significant toxicity associated with the drug, amphotericin B is currently recommended for visceral leishmaniasis.[27] Cure rates in immunocompromised are comparable with immunocompetent hosts using amphotericin B. Relapse can occur at any time in organ transplant recipients. The rate of relapse can approach 24% in organ transplant recipients. Secondary prevention with intermittent weekly amphotericin B doses may help prevent relapse in these patients. The following drug regimens are recommended in the Indian subcontinent:

- Liposomal amphotericin B alone (single dose, the drug of choice for kala-azar eradication)
- Liposomal amphotericin B in a single dose plus 7 days of oral miltefosine or 10 days of paromomycin
- Miltefosine plus paromomycin for 10 days
- Amphotericin B deoxycholate: 0.75–1 mg/kg/day daily or alternate day for 10 days
- Miltefosine orally or intramuscular (IM) paromomycin for 28 days
- Sodium stibogluconate: 20 mg/kg/day intravenous (IV) or IM for 30 days.

The first-line therapy for visceral leishmaniasis is the liposomal amphotericin B. To prevent relapse, secondary prophylaxis with amphotericin is beneficial in selected patients. On the contrary, the pentavalent antimonial is recommended as first-line therapy for severe cases of cutaneous and mucocutaneous leishmaniasis.

Malaria

Malaria is one of the most prevalent diseases worldwide. It causes more than one million deaths every year and causes 300 million acute cases annually. It is transmitted to humans through the bite of a female *Anopheles* mosquito. Rarely, it can transmit through blood transfusion and organ transplantation in endemic areas.[28] Malaria does not offer any protective immunity. Instead, resistance to hyperinflation may be acquired through frequent exposure to the parasite and its prolonged existence in the liver, microvasculature, and circulation. This increases the frequency of asymptomatic cases in endemic areas with parasitemia in the circulation. This poses a high risk of malaria transmission through organ or blood donation, especially in developing countries.[29] On the contrary, malaria is rarely reported in the developed world unless the transplant recipient has visited the endemic area or has received the organ from a donor residing in the endemic zone.

The four different *Plasmodium* species that affect humans are *Plasmodium falciparum*, *P. vivax*, *P. ovale*, and *P. malariae*. In India, most malarial infections are caused by *P. vivax*, followed by *P. falciparum*. Renal involvement is most commonly seen with *P. falciparum* infection.[30] Clinical manifestations that can occur in the early post-transplant period have been described in the kidney, liver, and heart transplant recipients. Even though fever is the most common symptom at presentation, a typical cyclical or paroxysmal pattern may not be present.[31] Malaria can cause acute tubular necrosis, acute interstitial nephritis, and cortical necrosis in the graft kidney. In a study from India by Rajapurkar, associated acute cellular rejection had also been reported in renal transplant patients with malarial infection.[30]

Diagnosis: Diagnosis of malaria involves microscopic observation of thin or thick blood smears. Rapid diagnostic tests using plasmodium antigens are used in diagnosing malarial infection.[32] The alternative techniques that are available for diagnosis are:

- ELISA testing for *P. falciparum* antigen
- Enzyme immunofluorescence assay for species-specific identification
- Deoxyribonucleic acid (DNA) hybridization and messenger ribonucleic acid (mRNA) amplification technique via PCR method.

Post-transplant malaria is usually diagnosed by identifying the malarial parasite in peripheral blood smear during the febrile period.

Treatment: Treatment of malaria relies on specific antimalarial drugs, identifying particular species, their geographical distribution, and their sensitivity to the drugs. In chloroquine-sensitive regions, *P. vivax*, *P. ovale*, *P. malariae*, and uncomplicated *P. falciparum* infections are treated with chloroquine. In chloroquine-resistant areas, malaria can be treated with artesunate-based combination regimens. Complicated *P. falciparum* conditions are treated with IV artesunate therapy.[33] If artesunate is unavailable, IV quinine plus doxycycline, tetracycline, or clindamycin can be given in these cases. Primaquine should be prescribed to prevent relapse in *P. vivax* and *P. ovale* infection after evaluating for glucose-6-phosphate dehydrogenase (G6PD) deficiency.

Malarial infection is potentially fatal in transplant recipients. Early diagnosis and initiation of treatment lead to better outcomes in transplant patients. *P. falciparum* disease, drug toxicity, and other concurrent infection may worsen these patients' outcomes. Treatment with quinine can cause a decrease in cyclosporine levels, so special attention should be given when quinine is used for treatment.[34]

Prevention: Potential screening methods to prevent malarial infection should include thick and thin smears stained with Giemsa, Wright, or Field stains, and rapid diagnostic tests to detect the histidine-rich protein 2 (HRP2) antigen. Transplant recipients traveling to the endemic malarial zone should be given chemoprophylaxis before travel to prevent infection. Chloroquine can increase the cyclosporine levels, and proper dose reduction should be made.

Babesiosis

Babesiosis is a tick-borne protozoal illness caused by *Babesia* sp., which causes lysis of red blood cells. The various species identified are *Babesia microti, B. divergence,* and *B. duncani. B. divergens* is the more virulent among these species. Transmission occurs through ticks or blood transfusion.[35]

The factors associated with increased risk for babesiosis include age, immunocompromised state, and asplenia.[36] Clinical manifestations can range from asymptomatic infections to life-threatening diseases. Early symptoms include fever, malaise, severe hemolytic anemia, adult respiratory distress syndrome, and multiorgan dysfunction. The hemolytic syndrome in transplant recipients can manifest as a post-transplant hemolytic uremic syndrome or hemophagocytic syndrome.[36]

Diagnosis: Laboratory investigations will show hemolytic anemia, thrombocytopenia, and unconjugated hyperbilirubinemia. Babesiosis can be diagnosed by microscopic examination of peripheral smear or blood PCR. Differentiating *Plasmodium* sp. and *Babesia* sp. can be challenging as both have similar morphology on microscopy. Specific epidemiological exposure and PCR testing would help determine the diseases. Histiocytosis and hemophagocytosis can be demonstrated in bone marrow biopsy in babesiosis.[36]

Treatment: Babesiosis is a life-threatening disease in an immunocompromised host; without early appropriate antimicrobial therapy, it is fatal to the transplant recipient. Exchange transfusion is required in patients with >10% parasitemia, severe hemolysis, renal, hepatic, or pulmonary involvement.

Reduction of immunosuppressive medications should be considered in transplant recipients. The optimal therapy in transplant recipients is not precise. Atovaquone plus azithromycin or clindamycin plus quinine are the drug regimens used to treat babesiosis.[37] Azithromycin increases the tacrolimus levels, and quinine causes the slow metabolism of tacrolimus and sirolimus. Henceforth, drug levels need to be monitored in the transplant recipient. Persistent relapsing illness has been documented in the immunocompromised hosts.[38] Continuation of antibiotics for >2 weeks after documenting negative smears can lead to resolution of persistent infection. Monitoring by blood smears helps in identifying response and relapse after completing therapy. Rarely resistance to the atovaquone/azithromycin regimen can occur, mainly in the immunocompromised hosts.[39]

Prevention: Transplant recipients should avoid tick exposure when visiting endemic areas using permethrin repellents and general protective clothing.[40] Frequent tick checks and removal of ticks may help as early reduction decreases the chance of transmission.

Balamuthia

Balamuthia is a free-living amoeba found in soil and causes disease in both immunocompetent and immunocompromised hosts. It causes granulomatous meningoencephalitis[41] and chronic granulomatous skin lesions. Diagnosis is unfortunately often done postmortem after pathological examination of the infected tissue. Brain and skin tissue will have trophozoites and cysts in the granulomatous inflammation. An indirect immunofluorescence assay confirms the diagnosis by staining the tissue. Neither serum nor CSF studies are helpful for diagnosis. As the disease is rare, data are scarce on treating this infection. Experts recommend that treatment include a multidrug regimen for a prolonged period, yet the results are unclear. The different multidrug regimens include amphotericin B, azoles, paromomycin, pentamidine, miltefosine, and albendazole.[42]

Acanthamoeba and Naegleria

Acanthamoeba is a protozoan parasite found in dust, soil, water, contact lens fluid, sewage, and air conditioners. It causes focal disease involving skin, eyes, brain, or lungs that causes keratitis, granulomatous amoebic encephalitis, brain abscess, and pulmonary and cutaneous lesions. Rarely does it cause DD, which is often fatal to transplant recipients?

Naegleria is found in fresh warm water, heated contaminated water, and soil. Infection occurs during swimming in contaminated water. Using organs from donors unknown to be infected with *Naegleria fowleri* at the time of transplantation can cause disease in the recipient.

Diagnosis: The initial manifestation can be a cutaneous lesion and should be biopsied early to increase the chance of survival. CSF examination and culture can be performed for the diagnosis. The culture would take up to 2 weeks for the amoeba to appear on the agar plate. Immunofluorescence methods can do species confirmation. Serology is not helpful for confirmation of diagnosis but can be used for seroprevalence studies.

Treatment: The optimal treatment for acanthamoeba remains elusive—a combination of amphotericin B with rifampicin, sulfonamides, azithromycin, caspofungin, and pentamidine combinations has been tried. After transplantation with amphotericin B and miltefosine, successful treatment of acanthamoeba has been reported.[43,44] Prevention is the best measure in *Naegleria* infections as nearly all these infections are fatal.[45]

Intestinal Protozoan

Intestinal protozoans such as *Cryptosporidium, Cyclospora,* microspore, giardia, and *Blastocystis hominis* can cause gastroenteritis in transplant recipients.[46] Although mycophenolate mofetil (MMF) can cause diarrhea in transplant recipients, *Cryptosporidium* and giardiasis are the common parasites that cause diarrhea worldwide.[47]

Amoebic Dysentery

The causative organism here is *Entamoeba histolytica,* a common cause of diarrhea in endemic regions. The classic presentation includes bloody diarrhea and colicky abdominal pain, typically postprandial. Risk factors include steroid therapy and other immunosuppressive regimens that multiple liver abscesses can complicate.

Giardiasis

Giardia duodenalis is one of the common causes of diarrhea worldwide.[48] Clinically, it causes nonbloody diarrhea, abdominal pain, foul-smelling stools, and malabsorption syndrome. Generally, giardiasis constitutes <1% of the post-transplant parasitic diseases. The excellent response to metronidazole therapy can explain the low incidence.

Cryptosporidiosis

It is a common cause of traveler diarrhea. The source of infection is contaminated water/food with *Cryptosporidium* oocysts and can be transmitted through the orofecal route. Diarrhea is usually self-limiting in immunocompetent hosts, but it may have a long course in transplant recipients. In endemic zones, cryptosporidiosis has been observed in 53% of diarrheal illnesses in transplant recipients.[49] In a study by Bhadauria et al. in India, *Cryptosporidium* was found in 28.5% of all postrenal transplant diarrheal infections. Patients with tacrolimus and MMF combination therapy have a higher risk of cryptosporidial infection than patients on cyclosporine-based treatment.[50]

Microsporidiosis

Microsporidia are intracellular spore-forming protozoa that can live in the intestine of birds, insects, and humans. *Enterocytozoon bieneusi* and *Encephalitozoon intestinalis* are the two well-recognized species that cause human intestinal microsporidiosis. Transmission occurs through ingestion/inhalation of the resistant microsporidia spores from the environment, person–person transmission, or other mammals or insects. Diarrhea is usually mild and self-limiting in immunocompetent hosts, but disseminating infection in immunocompromised individuals can lead to a grave prognosis.[51] Post-transplant diarrhea induced by *E. bieneusi* has been reported in many European countries and the United States.[52,53]

Diagnosis: Stool examination for ova and parasites in intestinal protozoan infections may be helpful in diagnosis but time-consuming. Concentration techniques and special stains may increase the sensitivity to diagnose specific pathogens. Special stains such as trichome and safranin are used to diagnose microspora and *Cyclospora.* ELISA and direct immunofluorescence tests may help in diagnosing cryptosporidia and giardia infections. Electron microscopy of the bowel biopsies may also help diagnose this infection. *E. histolytica* can be analyzed with stool examination for ova and parasites, although this is less sensitive than stool assay using *Entamoeba* antigen testing or PCR. Serology may help identify extraintestinal amoebiasis.

Treatment: Cryptosporidium infections are treated with nitazoxanide. Paromomycin, azithromycin, or a combination of these drugs can be used. *Cyclospora* and isospora infections are treated with TMP/SMX.[54] Ciprofloxacin or nitazoxanide are other alternative drugs if the patient is allergic to sulfa drugs. In an Indian study, it was reported that combination therapy with nitazoxanide and quinolones was associated with better cyst clearance than nitazoxanide alone.[50] *Cystoisospora belli* can also be treated with pyrimethamine along with folinic acid. For microsporidiosis, albendazole and fumagillin are effective.[55] Giardia can be treated with metronidazole. Tinidazole, nitazoxanide, or paromomycin can also be used to treat giardiasis. Refractory giardiasis is treated with metronidazole plus quinacrine.[56] *B. hominis* can be treated with nitazoxanide, metronidazole, iodoquinol, or TMP/SMX.

Intestinal protozoa can be challenging to eradicate, especially in immunocompromised patients. The use of MMF can augment and prolong diarrhea in transplant recipients. Tacrolimus levels may increase during diarrhea and should be carefully monitored.

Prevention: Transplant recipients should avoid drinking untreated well or lake water as most intestinal protozoan infections are transmitted through contaminated water or food. Chlorination does not sterilize *Cryptosporidium*, making it challenging to eradicate.

Intestinal Nematodes

Strongyloides

This parasite is endemic in tropical and subtropical countries and temperate regions. *Strongyloides stercoralis* can complete its life cycle in the human host's environment. Consequently, the parasite has an autoinfective cycle that produces long-term persistent infections. The host's immune response influences the autoinfection rate, and the disease's severity correlates with the worm burden. The major source of the parasite is soil contaminated with human feces. The filariform *Strongyloides* larvae can penetrate the intact skin, enter the blood, and then migrate to the lungs. Then the larvae migrate to the trachea and pharynx, whereby swallowing, the larvae enter duodenal mucosa. In the duodenum, the larvae become an adult parasite. Adult females reproduce asexually or sexually, producing rhabditiform larvae that excrete in stools or filariform larvae, penetrating the intestinal mucosa and perpetuating the infection **(Fig. 1)**.[57] In immunosuppressed hosts, the moulting of rhabditiform larvae to filariform larvae is accelerated, leading to autoinfection of the host.[58] As a result, many adult worms are found in the intestinal lumen. This can lead to lung involvement or a disseminated form of the disease.[59]

The clinical syndromes associated with *Strongyloides* are acute infection, chronic infection with autoinfection, hyperinfection syndrome (HIS), and DD.

Hyperinfection syndrome is characterized by accelerated larvae production, migration, and increased parasite burden leading to clinical manifestations. But the larvae are usually restricted to pulmonary and GI systems. The DD includes the features of HIS components with parasites spreading to other organs. The host's immunosuppressive burden

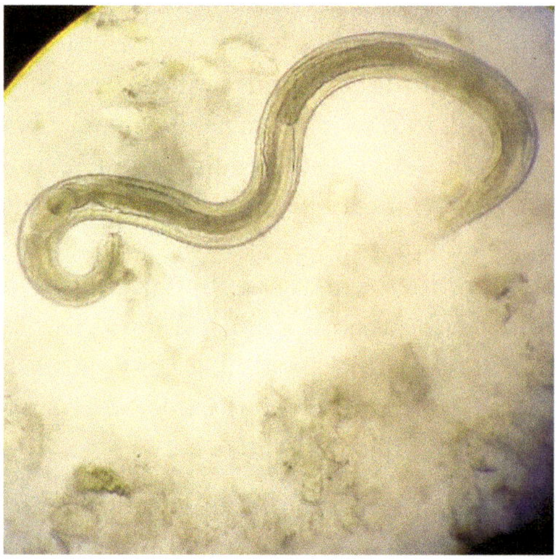

Fig. 1: *Strongyloides* in stool specimen.

is the predominant risk factor for HIS and DD. Human T-lymphotropic virus type 1 (HTLV-1) coinfection can increase the risk of HIS/DD progression.

Strongyloides in transplant recipient has been reported in two forms: (1) Reactivation of latent infection, or (2) donor-transmitted infection. The mortality rates in transplant recipients may exceed up to 50% in HIS and almost 70% in DD.[60]

The clinical manifestation may vary with pulmonary involvement, sepsis, or bacterial meningitis with gram-negative rods from intestinal flora carried on the parasite's surface during tissue migration. GI presentations include acute and severe abdominal pain, bloody diarrhea, adynamic ileus, intestinal obstruction, and GI bleeding. The GI bleeding occurs due to the penetration of larvae through the gut wall. The severity of manifestation is likely high in the early post-transplant stages as the immunosuppression is more intense in this period.

Diagnosis: Even though acute infection shows eosinophilia, patients with chronic infection, HIS, and DD may have normal eosinophil counts. Definite diagnosis is achieved by identifying larvae in clinical specimens, mainly in stool and duodenal aspirates. In patients with DD, larvae can be found in respiratory secretions, urine, peritoneal fluid, CSF, blood specimens, pleural effusion, and other tissue specimens. The duodenal fluid aspirate is more sensitive than the stool specimen but is associated with the intervention procedure.[61] Serological testing with ELISA is more sensitive (80–95%) and specific (90%), but it may not differentiate between active and previous infection.[62] In immunocompromised hosts, the sensitivity and specificity are reduced to 68 and 89%, respectively. Applying combined tests may increase the sensitivity up to 90% in immunocompromised patients. The presence of other helminthic diseases can increase the false positivity rate. A gelatin particle indirect agglutination test reported 98.2% sensitivity and 100% specificity.[63]

Treatment: Ivermectin effectively eradicates adult parasites and larvae from the intestine, and hence the treatment of choice for strongyloidiasis. To treat the less susceptible forms, the dose must be repeated at 2 weeks to prevent the progression to more susceptible forms. The cure rate of albendazole is only 45–75%, and it is used only as second-line therapy for this disease.[64] The treatment experience of hyperinflation syndrome and disseminated infection with ivermectin in transplant recipients is limited, and many case reports mention clinical failure and relapse.[65] Patients with heavy parasitic burdens should be treated with daily doses of ivermectin until clearance of the parasites and also with additional amounts for 7–14 days to reduce the risk of relapse. Anecdotal reports suggest a combination or sequential treatment with ivermectin and albendazole is also very effective. Off-label ivermectin can be effective in patients with concomitant malabsorption due to

Strongyloides. Coinfection with HTLV-1 requires prolonged therapy because no treatment reliably cures strongyloidiasis.

Prevention: In endemic regions, transplant recipients should be advised to wear closed footwear to reduce the risk of infection. To reduce the risk of DD in asymptomatic patients, screening and treatment of disease in recipients before transplant is necessary. To reduce the risk of transmission from infected donors, the donors should be treated before transplant. If untreated, the recipients should receive preemptive therapy before transplant and be monitored for infection post-transplant.

Schistosomiasis

Schistosomiasis is a new waterborne disease prevalent in endemic rural regions and the second most prevalent tropical disease worldwide.[66] *Schistosoma* species are mainly found in warmer climate regions. The species that cause intestinal and hepatic manifestations are *Schistosoma mansoni* and *S. japonicum*, while *S. haematobium* predominantly affects the bladder and kidney.

Schistosoma lays eggs in either portal or perivesical venous plexus, which may exit through urine or stools. After contact with fresh water, the eggs hatch, releasing miracidia that infect snails and mature into cercariae. The cercariae can infect humans by penetrating the human host and will develop into *Schistosoma*. The latter migrate through the lymphatics to the bloodstream and finally settle in hepatic or perivesical venous plexus, thus completing the life cycle. In theory, the transmission of infection through blood transfusion or organ donation can occur but rarely during the short stage of parasite migration. But this type of transmission is not reported. Transplant recipients are either vulnerable to new infection or reinfected.[67]

Schistosoma mansoni infection can lead to pipe stem fibrosis around the hepatic portal veins and portal hypertension. Intestinal schistosomiasis may present with abdominal pain, anorexia, and diarrhea. Urinary schistosomiasis can lead to hematuria, dysuria, and increased frequency of urination. A chronic bladder infection can lead to fibrosis and calcification of the bladder and ureter, resulting in hydroureteronephrosis. This eventually leads to schistosomal nephropathy and, ultimately, end-stage renal disease. Recurrence of schistosomal glomerulopathy in endemic zones has been reported.

Mahmoud et al. reported that treated schistosomiasis has no significant effect on patient/graft survival, with no evidence of reinfection.[68] Increased urinary tract infection and acute/chronic CNI toxicity have been observed. It is unclear whether transplantation and immunosuppression alter the clinical course of schistosomiasis. Recurrence disease after liver transplant has been reported, possibly from reactivation of the previous infection due to immunosuppressive therapy.

The adult schistosomes transmitted through organ transplantation do not replicate in the host, so acute schistosomiasis is often asymptomatic. Chronic schistosomiasis can occur in 60% of the infected individuals, yet only 4–8% of patients have extensive liver involvement. Adult worms usually die after 3–5 years of infection. Hence, both donor and recipient may be unaware of the background schistosomal disease.

Neuroschistosomiasis: Neuroschistosomiasis is the most devastating complication associated with schistosomal disease. Ectopic *Schistosoma* ova may migrate to the CNS through lumbar veins into the internal vertebral venous vasculature. It can either form granuloma by deposition in the adjacent spinal cord or transmit vertically into the brain during coughing or straining, especially *S. japonicum*, due to the small size of their eggs. Hence, *S. japonicum* may get deposited in the cerebral cortex, basal ganglia, internal capsule, and subcortical white matter. On the contrary, *S. mansoni* and *S. haematobium* will cause lumbosacral myelopathy. The clinical presentation of neuroschistosomiasis can be encephalopathy, seizures, headache, motor deficit, and ataxia. Spinal involvement causes lumbar and radicular pain, sensory losses, and bladder dysfunction.[69]

Diagnosis: Schistosomiasis can be diagnosed by tissue biopsy, serological tests, or examining stools or urine for ova and parasites. Many serological tests can show the cross-reaction between species, primarily based on *S. mansoni* antigens.[70] Seroconversion is delayed in transplant recipients and may not occur for several months after infection. Antibody levels should not be used to monitor the response to therapy as it does not correlate with the intensity of infection.

Treatment: Praziquantel is the standard drug of choice for schistosomiasis. Several case reports showed good responses in transplant recipients with praziquantel.[67] Cyclosporine may alter the drug's metabolism, increasing the drug's toxicity. Cyclosporine has been shown to have antischistosomal properties in vitro and some animals. The cure rate with this drug approaches 85%, and even without a complete cure, the egg loading rate will be declined. Oxamniquine is the second-line drug primarily used against *S. mansoni*, and its cure rate can approach 60–90%. In neuroschistosomiasis, praziquantel with steroids is the treatment of choice. Steroids are administered to limit the inflammation and edema formed around the eggs. Anticonvulsant therapy is required in patients with seizures.

Prevention: Schistosomal infection can be prevented by instructing the recipients to avoid contact with fresh water in endemic regions. Screening the donor and recipients from the endemic areas helps prevent the donor-derived and relapsing infection.

Cestodes

Echinococcosis

Echinococcosis is caused by the ingestion of eggs of the cestode *Echinococcus granulosus* or *Echinococcus multilocularis*. *E. granulosus* causes a hydatid cyst, and its primary host is domestic dogs. *E. multilocularis* causes alveolar cyst disease and is a parasite of wild canines. Humans act as intermediate hosts in both species. Hydatid cysts are clinically asymptomatic. Symptoms may occur due to mass effect, cyst infection, rupture, and leakage of cyst contents. The continuous growth of hydatid cysts can result in end-stage liver failure. In end-stage liver failure, liver transplantation has been performed due to hydatid invasion.[71] These patients did not receive antiparasitic medications and did not develop recurrence or death due to hydatid disease.[72]

In *E. multilocularis* infection, larvae may continuously increase, leading to alveolar cyst formation and indefinite cyst growth. They ultimately need surgical removal as they resemble slowly growing metastatic lesions. If not surgically resected, it may be potentially lethal over the years. Liver transplantation should be considered early for patients with hilar involvement, recurrent biliary infections, secondary biliary cirrhosis, ascites, and variceal bleeding caused by portal hypertension.[73] The disease can spread to the lungs and the brain; screening for extrahepatic involvement before transplant is necessary. CNS involvement should be considered as an exclusion criterion for transplant.

Diagnosis: Hydatid cysts are often incidentally discovered during routine radiological imaging studies. History of epidemiological exposure with a lesion in X-ray, ultrasound, computerized tomography (CT), or magnetic resonance imaging (MRI) leads to suspicion of Echinococcosis. Serological studies may help confirm the diagnosis. *E. multilocularis* infection needs to be differentiated from hepatic malignancy. Diagnosis can be achieved by serological tests and by imaging techniques. Liver biopsy is the gold standard for diagnosis but is limited due to the high risk of spreading infection. The use of ELISA to measure anti *E. granulosus* IgG titers may help predict the recurrence of the disease.

Treatment: In potential organ transplant recipients, hydatid cyst should be treated with surgical removal of cysts and albendazole therapy before transplantation. Administration of albendazole 7–10 days before surgery helps reduce cyst contents' seeding if spillage occurs during surgery.[74] Many experts recommend praziquantel in the event of intraoperative cyst spillage. Percutaneous puncture, aspiration, injection, and reaspiration (PAIR) technique can be used to obliterate the cyst before complete surgical removal. Although radical surgical excision is necessary for treating *E. multilocularis* infection, recent reports suggest that long-term treatment with benzimidazole may slow the progression of the disease.[74]

Prevention: Primary prevention involves avoiding contact with the dog fecal material, which may be contaminated with

Flowchart 1: Diagnostic flowchart for the parasitic infestation in organ transplant recipients.

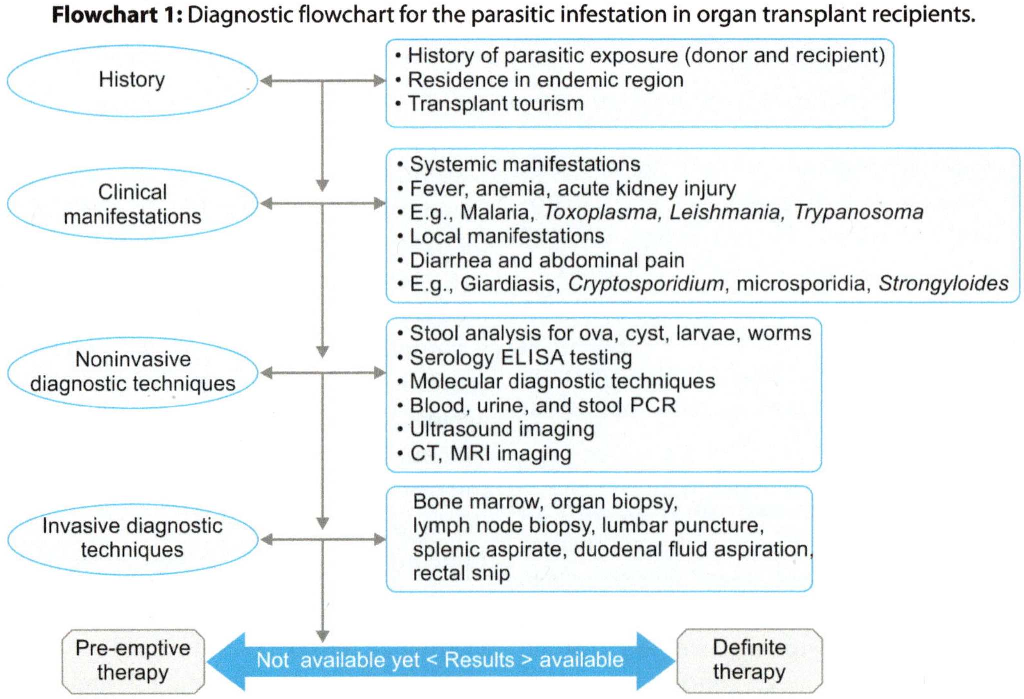

(CT: computerized tomography; ELISA: enzyme-linked immunosorbent assay; MRI: magnetic resonance imaging; PCR: polymerase chain reaction)

TABLE 1: Parasitic infection in organ transplant recipients.

Disease	***Treatment***
Toxoplasmosis	• Pyrimethamine and sulfadiazine is the primary treatment of choice • *Induction therapy:* Pyrimethamine and sulfadiazine for 6 weeks • *Chronic suppression therapy:* TMP/SMX
Chagas disease	Benznidazole (first-line therapy if tolerated) and nifurtimox
Visceral leishmaniasis	• *Antimonials:* Sodium stibogluconate or meglumine • Antimonial-resistant cases can be treated with liposomal amphotericin • First-line therapy for visceral leishmaniasis is liposomal amphotericin
Cutaneous and mucocutaneous leishmaniasis	Antimonial agents, cryotherapy, sodium stibogluconate instillation, topical paromomycin, urea
Malaria	• *P. falciparum* • *Artesunate based:* Artemether-lumefantrine, mefloquine, atovaquone-proguanil • *Quinine-based:* Quinine plus doxycycline or clindamycin or pyrimethamine–sulfadoxine combination • Chloroquine in sensitive areas (Central America and the Middle East) • *P. ovale and P. vivax:* Chloroquine plus primaquine/artemisinin drugs • *P. malariae:* Chloroquine
Babesiosis	• Atovaquone + azithromycin (first line) • Clindamycin + quinine (alternate therapy) • *Exchange transfusion:* If parasitemia >10%, severe hemolysis, MODS
Entamoeba histolytica	• *Active trophozoite:* Metronidazole or tinidazole followed by paromomycin to eradicate cystic forms • *Luminal agent:* Nitazoxanide to prevent transmission and infective complications • *Complete eradication:* Tissue amoebicide (metronidazole) + luminal agent (paromomycin)
Giardiasis	Metronidazole, albendazole, nitazoxanide
Microsporidiosis	• *For Enterocytozoon bieneusi:* Albendazole • *For Cyclospora:* TMP/SMX with reduction of immunosuppression
Diphyllobothriasis	A single dose of praziquantel
Anisakiasis	Albendazole 400–800 mg for 6–21 days
Strongyloidiasis	• Ivermectin (first line) • Albendazole (alternative therapy)
Schistosomiasis	• Praziquantel • Oxamniquine • *For neurological disease:* Praziquantel + glucocorticoids
Echinococcosis	• Surgical resection of cysts + preoperative albendazole • Praziquantel for intraoperative spillage • PAIR technique • *Benzimidazole:* To slow disease progression

(MODS: multiple organ dysfunction syndrome; PAIR: percutaneous puncture, aspiration, injection, and reaspiration; TMP/SMX: trimethoprim/sulfamethoxazole)

echinococcal eggs. Good hand hygiene after dog grooming may reduce the risk of exposure. Direct contact and disease acquisition are rare because wild animals are the definitive hosts for *E. multilocularis*.

The diagnostic flowchart and treatment of parasitic infections in kidney transplant recipients is given in **Flowchart 1 and Table 1** respectively.

CONCLUSION

Post-transplant parasitic infections pose a significant challenge to the treating physician in a transplant recipient. The clinician should have thorough knowledge of the epidemiology of parasitic diseases, and the threshold for suspicion of parasitic diseases should be low, especially if the donor or recipient is from endemic regions for certain parasitic infections. Timely diagnosis through correct laboratory techniques and early treatment would lead to better transplant recipients with these parasitic diseases.

REFERENCES

1. Schwartz BS, Mawhorter SD, AST Infectious Diseases Community of Practice. Parasitic infections in solid organ transplantation. Am J Transplant. 2013;13(Suppl. 4):280-303.
2. USRDS. [online] Available from https://www.usrds.org/. [Last accessed June, 2022].
3. Barsoum RS. Parasitic infections in transplant recipients. Nat Clin Pract Nephrol. 2006;2(9):490-503.

4. Nylén S, Gautam S. Immunological perspectives of leishmaniasis. J Glob Infect Dis. 2010;2(2):135-46.
5. Barsoum R, Nabil M, Saady G, Genin C, Saleh E, Francis M, et al. Immunoglobulin-A and the pathogenesis of schistosomal glomerulopathy. Kidney Int. 1996;50(3):920-8.
6. Barsoum RS, Bassily S, Soliman M, Milad M, Hassaballa AM. Amyloidosis in hepatosplenic schistosomiasis. Trans R Soc Trop Med Hyg. 1978;72(2):215-6.
7. Fernàndez-Sabé N, Cervera C, Fariñas MC, Bodro M, Muñoz P, Gurguí M, et al. Risk factors, clinical features, and outcomes of toxoplasmosis in solid-organ transplant recipients: a matched case-control study. Clin Infect Dis. 2012;54(3):355-61.
8. Montoya JG. Laboratory diagnosis of Toxoplasma gondii infection and toxoplasmosis. J Infect Dis. 2002;185(s1):S73-82.
9. Tlamcani Z, Lemkhenete Z, Lmimouni BE. Toxoplasmosis: the value of molecular methods in diagnosis compared to conventional methods. J Microbiol Infect Dis. 2013;3(2):93-9.
10. Ionita C, Wasay M, Balos L, Bakshi R. MR imaging in toxoplasmosis encephalitis after bone marrow transplantation: paucity of enhancement despite fulminant disease. AJNR Am J Neuroradiol. 2004;25(2):270-3.
11. Kaplan JE, Benson C, Holmes KK, Brooks JT, Pau A, Masur H, et al. Guidelines for prevention and treatment of opportunistic infections in HIV-infected adults and adolescents: recommendations from CDC, the National Institutes of Health, and the HIV Medicine Association of the Infectious Diseases Society of America. MMWR Recomm Rep. 2009;58(RR-4):1-207; quiz CE1-4.
12. Béraud G, Pierre-François S, Foltzer A, Abel S, Liautaud B, Smadja D, et al. Cotrimoxazole for treatment of cerebral toxoplasmosis: an observational cohort study during 1994–2006. Am J Trop Med Hyg. 2009;80(4):583-7.
13. Torre D, Casari S, Speranza F, Donisi A, Gregis G, Poggio A, et al. Randomized trial of trimethoprim-sulfamethoxazole versus pyrimethamine-sulfadiazine for therapy of toxoplasmic encephalitis in patients with AIDS. Italian Collaborative Study Group. Antimicrob Agents Chemother. 1998;42(6):1346-9.
14. Baden LR, Katz JT, Franck L, Tsang S, Hall M, Rubin RH, et al. Successful toxoplasmosis prophylaxis after orthotopic cardiac transplantation with trimethoprim-sulfamethoxazole. Transplantation. 2003;75(3):339-43.
15. Girard PM, Landman R, Gaudebout C, Olivares R, Saimot AG, Jelazko P, et al. Dapsone-pyrimethamine compared with aerosolized pentamidine as primary prophylaxis against Pneumocystis carinii pneumonia and toxoplasmosis in HIV infection. The PRIO Study Group. N Engl J Med. 1993;328(21):1514-20.
16. Rodriques Coura J, de Castro SL. A critical review on Chagas disease chemotherapy. Mem Inst Oswaldo Cruz. 2002;97(1):3-24.
17. Campos SV, Strabelli TMV, Amato Neto V, Silva CP, Bacal F, Bocchi EA, et al. Risk factors for Chagas' disease reactivation after heart transplantation. J Heart Lung Transplant. 2008;27(6):597-602.
18. Gallerano V, Consigli J, Pereyra S, Gómez Zanni S, Danielo C, Gallerano RH, et al. Chagas' disease reactivation with skin symptoms in a patient with kidney transplant. Int J Dermatol. 2007;46(6):607-10.
19. Figueiredo JF, Martinez R, da Costa JC, Moysés Neto M, Suaid HJ, Ferraz AS. Transmission of Chagas disease through renal transplantation: report of a case. Trans R Soc Trop Med Hyg. 1990;84(1):61-2.
20. Kun H, Moore A, Mascola L, Steurer F, Lawrence G, Kubak B, et al. Transmission of Trypanosoma cruzi by heart transplantation. Clin Infect Dis. 2009;48(11):1534-40.
21. Schijman AG, Vigliano C, Burgos J, Favaloro R, Perrone S, Laguens R, et al. Early diagnosis of recurrence of Trypanosoma cruzi infection by polymerase chain reaction after heart transplantation of a chronic Chagas' heart disease patient. J Heart Lung Transplant. 2000;19(11):1114-7.
22. Pinazo M-J, Miranda B, Rodríguez-Villar C, Altclas J, Brunet Serra M, García-Otero EC, et al. Recommendations for management of Chagas disease in organ and hematopoietic tissue transplantation programs in nonendemic areas. Transplant Rev (Orlando). 2011;25(3):91-101.
23. Piscopo TV. Leishmaniasis. Postgrad Med J. 2007; 83(976):649-57.
24. Fernández-Guerrero ML, Aguado JM, Buzón L, Barros C, Montalbán C, Martín T, et al. Visceral leishmaniasis in immunocompromised hosts. Am J Med. 1987;83(6):1098-102.
25. Rana A, Gadde A, Lippi L, Bansal SB. Visceral leishmaniasis after kidney transplant: an unusual presentation and mode of diagnosis. Exp Clin Transplant. 2022;20(3):311-5.
26. Sharma RK, Jha R, Kumar P, Kher V, Gupta A, Kumar A, et al. Visceral leishmaniasis in a renal transplant recipient: diagnostic and therapeutic problems. Am J Nephrol. 1996; 16(4):358-60.
27. Boletis JN, Pefanis A, Stathakis C, Helioti H, Kostakis A, Giamarellou H. Visceral leishmaniasis in renal transplant recipients: successful treatment with liposomal amphotericin B (AmBisome). Clin Infect Dis. 1999;28(6):1308-9.
28. Mungai M, Tegtmeier G, Chamberland M, Parise M. Transfusion-transmitted malaria in the United States from 1963 through 1999. N Engl J Med. 2001;344(26):1973-8.
29. Fischer L, Sterneck M, Claus M, Costard-Jäckle A, Fleischer B, Herbst H, et al. Transmission of malaria tertiana by multi-organ donation. Clin Transplant. 1999;13(6):491-5.
30. Rajapurkar MM. Renal involvement in malaria. J Postgrad Med. 1994;40(3):132.
31. Lee PC, Lee PY, Lei HY, Chen FF, Tseng JY, Ching YT. Malaria infection in kidney transplant recipients. Transplant Proc. 1994;26(4):2099-100.
32. Faye A, Ndiaye P, Diagne-Camara M, Badiane O, Wone I, Diongue M, et al. Economic evaluation of rapid diagnostic tests in malaria treatment. Sante Publique. 2010;22(6):617-23.
33. Visser BJ, Bierhoff M, van Gool T, van Hattem JM, Grobusch MP, van Vugt M. The treatment of malaria. Ned Tijdschr Geneeskd. 2019;163:D3321.
34. Tan HW, Ch'ng SL. Drug interaction between cyclosporine A and quinine in a renal transplant patient with malaria. Singapore Med J. 1991;32(3):189-90.
35. Perdrizet GA, Olson NH, Krause PJ, Banever GT, Spielman A, Cable RG. Babesiosis in a renal transplant recipient acquired through blood transfusion. Transplantation. 2000;70(1): 205-8.
36. Slovut DP, Benedetti E, Matas AJ. Babesiosis and hemophagocytic syndrome in an asplenic renal transplant recipient. Transplantation. 1996;62(4):537-9.
37. Krause PJ, Lepore T, Sikand VK, Gadbaw J, Burke G, Telford SR, et al. Atovaquone and azithromycin for the treatment of babesiosis. N Engl J Med. 2000;343(20):1454-8.
38. Krause PJ, Gewurz BE, Hill D, Marty FM, Vannier E, Foppa IM, et al. Persistent and relapsing babesiosis in immunocompromised patients. Clin Infect Dis. 2008;46(3):370-6.

39. Wormser GP, Prasad A, Neuhaus E, Joshi S, Nowakowski J, Nelson J, et al. Emergence of resistance to azithromycin-atovaquone in immunocompromised patients with Babesia microti infection. Clin Infect Dis. 2010;50(3):381-6.
40. Carroll JF, Benante JP, Kramer M, Lohmeyer KH, Lawrence K. Formulations of deet, picaridin, and IR3535 applied to skin repel nymphs of the lone star tick (Acari: Ixodidae) for 12 hours. J Med Entomol. 2010;47(4):699-704.
41. Schuster FL, Yagi S, Gavali S, Michelson D, Raghavan R, Blomquist I, et al. Under the radar: balamuthia amebic encephalitis. Clin Infect Dis. 2009;48(7):879-87.
42. Martínez DY, Seas C, Bravo F, Legua P, Ramos C, Cabello AM, et al. Successful treatment of Balamuthia mandrillaris amoebic infection with extensive neurological and cutaneous involvement. Clin Infect Dis. 2010;51(2):e7-11.
43. Young AL, Leboeuf NR, Tsiouris SJ, Husain S, Grossman ME. Fatal disseminated Acanthamoeba infection in a liver transplant recipient immunocompromised by combination therapies for graft-versus-host disease. Transpl Infect Dis. 2010;12(6):529-37.
44. Aichelburg AC, Walochnik J, Assadian O, Prosch H, Steuer A, Perneczky G, et al. Successful treatment of disseminated Acanthamoeba sp. infection with miltefosine. Emerg Infect Dis. 2008;14(11):1743-6.
45. Centers for Disease Control and Prevention. (2019). Parasites—Naegleria fowleri—primary amebic meningoencephalitis (PAM)—amebic encephalitis. [online] Available from https://www.cdc.gov/parasites/naegleria/index.html. [Last accessed June, 2022].
46. Azami M, Sharifi M, Hejazi SH, Tazhibi M. Intestinal parasitic infections in renal transplant recipients. Braz J Infect Dis. 2010;14(1):15-8.
47. Udgiri N, Minz M, Kashyap R, Heer M, Gupta CS, Mohandas K, et al. Intestinal cryptosporidiasis in living related renal transplant recipients. Transplant Proc. 2004;36(7):2128-9.
48. Bajer A. Cryptosporidium and Giardia spp. infections in humans, animals and the environment in Poland. Parasitol Res. 2008;104(1):1-17.
49. Raja K, Abbas Z, Hassan SM, Luck NH, Aziz T, Mubarak M. Prevalence of cryptosporidiosis in renal transplant recipients presenting with acute diarrhea at a single center in Pakistan. J Nephropathol. 2014;3(4):127-31.
50. Bhadauria D, Goel A, Kaul A, Sharma RK, Gupta A, Ruhela V, et al. Cryptosporidium infection after renal transplantation in an endemic area. Transpl Infect Dis. 2015;17(1):48-55.
51. Carlson JR, Li L, Helton CL, Munn RJ, Wasson K, Perez RV, et al. Disseminated microsporidiosis in a pancreas/kidney transplant recipient. Arch Pathol Lab Med. 2004;128(3):e41-3.
52. Bednarska M, Bajer A, Welc-Faleciak R, Czubkowski P, Teisseyre M, Graczyk TK, et al. The first case of Enterocytozoon bieneusi infection in Poland. Ann Agric Environ Med. 2013;20(2):287-8.
53. Smith RM, Muehlenbachs A, Schaenmann J, Baxi S, Koo S, Blau D, et al. Three cases of neurologic syndrome caused by donor-derived Microsporidiosis. Emerg Infect Dis. 2017;23(3):387-95.
54. Kappagoda S, Singh U, Blackburn BG. Antiparasitic therapy. Mayo Clin Proc. 2011;86(6):561-83.
55. Lanternier F, Boutboul D, Menotti J, Chandesris MO, Sarfati C, Mamzer Bruneel MF, et al. Microsporidiosis in solid organ transplant recipients: two Enterocytozoon bieneusi cases and review. Transpl Infect Dis. 2009;11(1):83-8.
56. Nash TE, Ohl CA, Thomas E, Subramanian G, Keiser P, Moore TA. Treatment of patients with refractory giardiasis. Clin Infect Dis. 2001;33(1):22-8.
57. Liu LX, Weller PF. Strongyloidiasis and other intestinal nematode infections. Infect Dis Clin North Am. 1993;7(3):655-82.
58. Keiser PB, Nutman TB. Strongyloides stercoralis in the immunocompromised population. Clin Microbiol Rev. 2004;17(1):208-17.
59. Patel G, Arvelakis A, Sauter BV, Gondolesi GE, Caplivski D, Huprikar S. Strongyloides hyperinfection syndrome after intestinal transplantation. Transpl Infect Dis. 2008;10(2):137-41.
60. Ramanathan R, Nutman T. Strongyloides stercoralis infection in the immunocompromised host. Curr Infect Dis Rep. 2008;10(2):105-10.
61. Siddiqui AA, Berk SL. Diagnosis of Strongyloides stercoralis infection. Clin Infect Dis. 2001;33(7):1040-7.
62. Lindo JF, Conway DJ, Atkins NS, Bianco AE, Robinson RD, Bundy DA. Prospective evaluation of enzyme-linked immunosorbent assay and immunoblot methods for the diagnosis of endemic Strongyloides stercoralis infection. Am J Trop Med Hyg. 1994;51(2):175-9.
63. Schaffel R, Nucci M, Carvalho E, Braga M, Almeida L, Portugal R, et al. The value of an immunoenzymatic test (enzyme-linked immunosorbent assay) for the diagnosis of strongyloidiasis in patients immunosuppressed by hematologic malignancies. Am J Trop Med Hyg. 2001;65(4):346-50.
64. Archibald LK, Beeching NJ, Gill GV, Bailey JW, Bell DR. Albendazole is effective treatment for chronic strongyloidiasis. Q J Med. 1993;86(3):191-5.
65. DeVault GA, King JW, Rohr MS, Landreneau MD, Brown ST, McDonald JC. Opportunistic infections with Strongyloides stercoralis in renal transplantation. Rev Infect Dis. 1990;12(4):653-71.
66. Ariza-Heredia E, Razonable RR. Incidental hepatic schistosomiasis in a liver transplant recipient. Transpl Infect Dis. 2012;14(1):75-8.
67. Hoare M, Gelson WTH, Davies SE, Curran M, Alexander GJM. Hepatic and intestinal schistosomiasis after orthotopic liver transplant. Liver Transplant. 2005;11(12):1603-7.
68. Mahmoud KM, Sobh MA, El-Agroudy AE, Mostafa FE, Baz ME, Shokeir AA, et al. Impact of schistosomiasis on patient and graft outcome after renal transplantation: 10 years' follow-up. Nephrol Dial Transplant. 2001;16(11):2214-21.
69. Carod-Artal FJ. Neurological complications of Schistosoma infection. Trans R Soc Trop Med Hyg. 2008;102(2):107-16.
70. Barsoum RS, Esmat G, El-Baz T. Human schistosomiasis: clinical perspective: review. J Adv Res. 2013;4(5):433-44.
71. Moreno-González E, Loinaz Segurola C, García Ureña MA, García García I, Gómez Sanz R, Jiménez Romero C, et al. Liver transplantation for Echinococcus granulosus hydatid disease. Transplantation. 1994;58(7):797-800.
72. Loinaz C, Moreno-González E, Gómez R, García I, González-Pinto I, Jiménez C, et al. Liver transplantation in liver disease: echinococcus granulosus. Transplant Proc. 1998;30(7):3268-9.
73. Bresson-Hadni S, Vuitton DA, Bartholomot B, Heyd B, Godart D, Meyer JP, et al. A twenty-year history of alveolar echinococcosis: analysis of a series of 117 patients from eastern France. Eur J Gastroenterol Hepatol. 2000;12(3):327-36.
74. Guidelines for treatment of cystic and alveolar echinococcosis in humans. WHO Informal Working Group on Echinococcosis. Bull World Health Organ. 1996;74(3):231-42.

12.5 *Pneumocystis jirovecii*

Tukaram Jamale, Nikhil Saxena

CASE VIGNETTE 1

A 25-year-old male patient, 5 months post-transplant on triple immunosuppression [steroids + mycophenolate mofetil (MMF) + Tac] with history of allergy to sulfa group of drugs. He was not on septran prophylaxis. The patient presented with complaints of mild-grade fever for 5 days with progressively worsening dyspnea from grade 1 to grade 3. On examination, the patient had bilateral crepitations all over the lung fields and oxygen saturation was 85% on room air with a respiratory rate of 35 breaths/min.

The patient was put on noninvasive ventilation and computed tomography (CT) scan of the chest was done which showed diffuse bilateral ground-glass opacities and consolidation in the left lower lobe. Sputum examination was inconclusive but β-D-glucan level was 250 pg/mL and lactate dehydrogenase (LDH) was 550 U/L. Bronchoalveolar lavage (BAL) could not be done as the patient was in respiratory distress. In view of the clinical history, radiographic findings, and β-glucan levels, a presumptive diagnosis of Pneumocystis pneumonia (PCP) was made. The patient was started on clindamycin 600 mg 6 hourly IV and primaquine. Corticosteroids were also given at adose of 80 mg/day for 5 days followed by 40 mg/day for 5 days followed by 20 mg OD for 11 days.

The patient improved clinically by the end of 6th day of the therapy and the treatment was continued for 3 weeks.

CASE VIGNETTE 2

A 35-year-old female patient, 3 months post live-related kidney transplant, has a history of acute cellular rejection on postoperative day 10 for which she was treated with methylprednisolone and antithymocyte globulin (ATG). She presented with complaints of low-grade intermittent fever (maximum temp 38°C) and dry cough. Physical examination showed normal vesicular breath sounds on auscultation. Oxygen saturation was 90% on room air.

Investigations:
- *Chest X-ray:* Normal
- *CT chest:* Ground-glass opacities in both lungs
- *Induced sputum for bacterial and fungal culture:* Negative
- Serum β-D-glucan level: 300 pg/mL
- BAL–PCR-detected Pneumocystis.

The patient was started on co-trimoxazole DS 2 tablets 8 hourly. On day 3 of the therapy, she developed leukopenia which was worsening and on day 5 absolute neutrophil count (ANC) was 300/mm^3. Hence, septran was stopped and the patient was started on clindamycin 600 mg 6 hourly along with primaquine 30 mg/day for 3 weeks. By the end of 5th day of the therapy, the patient's hypoxia improved and fever subsided.

INTRODUCTION

Pneumocystis jirovecii is an important cause of opportunistic infection in immunocompromised patients which include those with acquired immunodeficiency syndrome (AIDS), hematologic malignancies, and solid organ transplant recipients.[1]

EPIDEMIOLOGY AND RISK FACTORS

Pneumocystis was discovered in 1909 by Chagas who thought it to be a new stage in the life cycle of *Trypanosoma cruzi*. Research carried out by Delanoes and Carinii in 1912 led to the establishment of a new genus and species, and the organism was named *Pneumocystis carinii*. It emerged as a public health problem during World War II when it caused interstitial pneumonia in malnourished children.[2] In 1988, it was proposed that *Pneumocystis* is a fungus, not a protozoan, based on molecular studies which included gene-sequence homologies, composition of cell walls, and key cellular enzymes.[3] The *Pneumocystis* spp. infects many mammalian species and the human-specific pathogen is *P. jirovecii*.

Pneumocystis pneumonia is an AIDS-defining illness. Its incidence is declining after the introduction of prophylaxis with cotrimoxazole and highly active antiretroviral therapy (HAART).[4] *Pneumocystis* can colonize the airways of immunocompetent individuals without causing the disease. Primary infection occurs in 75% of individuals within 4 years of age.[5]

The incidence of PCP in renal transplant recipients is 0.6–14%,[6] and it increases exponentially with additional immunosuppressive factors such as extra corticosteroids and anti thymocyte globulin. Simultaneous infection with cytomegalovirus (CMV) increases the risk of acquiring PCP as CMV accelerates aging of T cells.[7]

Pneumocystis pneumonia can cause outbreaks of infection in solid organ transplant units.

Patients with human immunodeficiency virus (HIV) and low CD4 counts are at the highest risk of PCP. Among organ transplant recipients, the rates of PCP infection are highest in lung and heart transplant recipients[8] while the lowest rate of infection is in renal transplant recipients[9] **(Box 1)**. Glucocorticoids predispose to PCP by altering the lung surfactant and suppressing cell-mediated immunity.

PATHOPHYSIOLOGY

Three developmental forms of *Pneumocystis* are described: trophic, precyst, and cyst forms. Its life cycle is not fully elucidated as the organism has not been consistently cultured.

BOX 1: Risk factors for Pneumocystis pneumonia in kidney transplant recipients.[10]

- Intensive immunosuppression
- Treatment of acute rejection within last 6 months
- Low lymphocyte counts
- Hypogammaglobulinemia
- Advanced age (>65 years)
- First 6 months post-transplant

CHAPTER HIGHLIGHTS

- *Pneumocystis jirovecii* is an important opportunistic infection in solid organ transplant recipients worldwide.
- Its life cycle consists of three developmental forms: trophic stage, precyst, and cyst.
- Although traditionally, PCP in kidney transplant recipients is known to cause a severe respiratory illness, patients with mild infection can have an indolent disease with mild dyspnea and cough.
- Serum β-D-glucan levels can be used for screening the infection but demonstration of organism in respiratory secretions remains the gold standard.
- The drug of choice for treatment and prophylaxis of PCP is cotrimoxazole.

The trophic form has an asexual phase of cell division (resembling binary fission) and also a sexual phase in which haploid trophic forms conjugate to form a diploid zygote. The zygote forms eight haploid nuclei which undergo compartmentalization to form spores, which emerge and become the trophic forms and enter either phase of division.[11]

The primary mode of transmission is airborne. The most common form of acquiring infection is transmission from an immunocompromised infected host. It can be acquired from environmental exposure and asymptomatic carriers.[12] The trophic form predominates over cysts during an infection.

Microscopy reveals that *Pneumocystis* (trophic stage) attaches to type I pneumocyte which resides within extra-cellular matrix proteins. The binding of *Pneumocystis* to fibronectin and vitronectin triggers altered gene expression that results in increased *Pneumocystis* growth causing diffuse alveolar damage following which they get filled with proteinaceous exudative material. *Pneumocystis* proliferation also provokes a mononuclear cell response which further contributes to lung damage. β-Glucan, a cell wall component of *Pneumocystis*, is responsible for driving inflammation in the lungs.

Stained lung sections show foamy, vacuolated alveolar exudates composed largely of viable and nonviable organisms which are stained by silver and Giemsa stain. In advanced stages, interstitial edema and fibrosis may develop **(Figs. 1A to C)**.

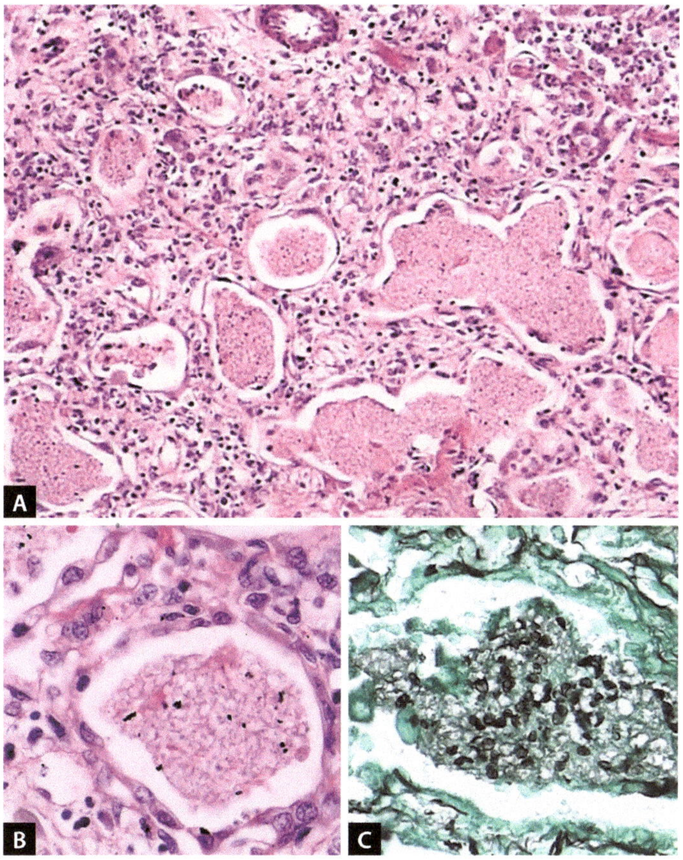

Figs. 1A to C: Histopathology of lung alveoli. (A) Collection of foamy exudates within the alveolar spaces. There is widening of the alveolar septa with few lymphocytes (H&E × 200); (B) Foamy exudates within an alveolar space. There is cuboidal metaplasia of the alveolar lining (H&E × 400); (C) Cyst-like organisms are present within the exudate (Gomori methenamine silver × 400).
Courtesy: Department of Pathology (Cardiovascular and Thoracic Division), Seth GS Medical College, Mumbai.

CLINICAL FEATURES

The most typical time of onset of symptoms of PCP is 6–8 weeks following initiation of immunosuppression. The symptoms may be very subtle with acute or subacute onset. Diarrhea, vomiting, flu-like prodrome, and dry cough are the symptoms that may precede classical presentation which is characterized by dyspnea and fever.[13] Patients may experience pleuritic chest pain and in fulminant cases it may progress to respiratory failure and death. Extrapulmonary manifestations are exceedingly rare and can involve any organ, most notably lymph nodes, spleen, and bone marrow.

Unlike the subacute to chronic respiratory illness in AIDS patients, PCP in kidney transplant recipients can present as an acute or a severe respiratory illness with fever, cough, hypoxia, and poorer outcomes. This is because ofthe more severe inflammatory response despite the lower load of organisms in patients without AIDS.[14,15] However, kidney transplant recipiemts can also have subtle symptoms because of the immunosuppressive medications.[16]

Physical examination findings are nonspecific. Patients may have no adventitious breath sounds in spite of having hypoxemia. Majority of the patients with PCP will have either hypoxemia at rest or with exertion or an increase in alveolar arterial oxygen tension gradient.[17] Without treatment, they may develop diffuse rales and signs of consolidation.

DIAGNOSIS

Serology

β-D-glucan is a component of the cell wall of PCP. Serum β-D-glucan levels are used as a screening tool for PCP infection.[18] Reasons for false-positive tests include the use of intravenous amoxicillin–clavulanic acid, some bacterial infections such as *Pseudomonas*, fungal infections, treatment with immunological preparations such as globulins/albumin, use of cellulose membranes and filters made from cellulose in hemodialysis, and use of cotton gauze swabs.[19] β-D-glucan levels cannot be used to predict the severity of infection and the response to treatment. PCP infection can be ruled out if serum β-D-glucan levels are negative.

Lactate dehydrogenase levels are raised in PCP because of pulmonary damage. Plasma levels of S-adenosylmethionine are low in patients with PCP, but the diagnostic significance of these markers is inferior to that of β-D-glucan.[20] A standard test for serological diagnosis of PCP needs to be established.

Microbiology

Since *Pneumocystis* cannot be readily cultured in the lab, the demonstration of organisms in the respiratory secretions is the gold standard for diagnosis.[21] Before the 1990s, the optimal specimen was obtained via open lung biopsy and later transbronchial lung biopsy was employed. Hematoxylin and eosin staining of lung tissue demonstrates the presence of foamy alveolar infiltrates and mononuclear interstitial infiltrates. The cysts can be identified using methenamine silver stain which has good specificity but low sensitivity. Because trophic forms predominate over cyst forms, Giemsa and Diff-Quik staining of trophic forms has high sensitivity. Direct fluorescent antibody staining using a fluorescein conjugated monoclonal antibody can visualize both trophic forms and cysts.[22]

Organisms can be demonstrated in induced sputum and BAL. The diagnostic yield of microscopy with staining of induced sputum is 50–90% in patients with HIV infection but is lower in patients without AIDS.[23] BAL is difficult to carry out in non-HIV patients with PCP because of the more severe respiratory insufficiency. Also, this subgroup of patients has a lower load of organisms in their respiratory secretions, making the diagnosis more challenging.

Polymerase chain reaction (PCR) can be done on BAL, induced sputum, oropharyngeal, and nasopharyngeal washings. By using quantitative real-time PCR, the copy number variant in PCP patients is significantly higher than in those with PCP colonization, thus differentiating infection from colonization.[24]

TABLE 1: Various tools for the diagnosis of Pneumocystis pneumonia (PCP).

	Sensitivity (%)	*Specificity (%)*
β-D-glucan levels	94.8	86.3
Lactate dehydrogenase[26]	63	43
Polymerase chain reaction	94–100	79–96
Loop-mediated isothermal amplification	95.4	

Note: The cut-off for β-D-glucan used for the diagnosis of PCP in solid organ transplant recipients is not specified and using a higher cut-off than that for human immunodeficiency virus (HIV) patients has been proposed.[27]

Loop-mediated isothermal amplification (LAMP) is a nucleic acid amplification test, which offers rapid, cost effective, and accurate diagnosis of PCP **(Table 1)**[25].

Radiology

In initial stages and in mild infections, the chest radiograph maybe completely normal. The classical chest X-ray shows bilateral symmetric perihilar interstitial infiltrates but it is not specific for PCP. High-resolution computed tomography (HRCT) scan of chest shows diffuse ground-glass opacities in bilateral lungs sparing the lung periphery. A normal HRCT essentially rules out PCP infection.[28] Consolidation, cysts, pneumothorax, and nodules can also be seen in HRCT. Patients receiving aerosolized pentamidine tend to develop upper lobe infiltrates due to reduced deposition of the drug in the upper lobes.

The incidence of lung cysts is reported to be higher in HIV patients. Consolidation is more common in patients without AIDS due to hampered host immunologic response in patients with AIDS.[29] Granulomatous inflammation is seen in 5% of the patients in whom immunodeficiency is not profound and may present as solitary or multiple lung nodules. Features of infective bronchiolitis such as tree in bud pattern are not seen in PCP.

Definitive diagnosis requires identification of the organism by staining, immunofluorescence, or PCR. In cases where the organism load is too less and/or there is inability to obtain an appropriate clinical specimen, a presumptive diagnosis can be made based upon the clinical history, risk factors, β-D-glucan levels, and radiology.

PROGNOSIS AND TREATMENT

Mortality from PCP in patients with HIV infection is 10–20% compared with 35–50% in those without HIV. Mortality is highest in patients with cancer **(Box 2 and Table 2)**.

BOX 2: Poor prognostic indicators.

- PCP in non-HIV patient
- Low serum albumin
- Advanced age
- Need of mechanical ventilation
- Preexisting lung disease
- Development of pneumothorax

(HIV: human immunodeficiency virus; PCP: pneumocystis pneumonia)

TABLE 2: Treatment of *Pneumocystis* pneumonia.

Drug	*Dose*	*Comments*
Cotrimoxazole (drug of choice)	15–20 mg/kg (dosing based upon the TMP component) in three divided doses	Monitoring of drug levels is to be done in patients with low GFR (maintenance of 2 hours post-sulfamethoxazole level between 100 and 150 μg/mL)
Dapsone	100 mg/day	To be avoided in patients with severe reaction to cotrimoxazole (e.g., Stevens–Johnson syndrome) Check G6PD prior
Clindamycin	600 mg IV 8 hourly PO (6 hourly in severe disease)	
Primaquine	30 mg/day	Check G6PD prior
Pentamidine	3–4 mg/kg/day over 1 hour	Monitor blood pressure, blood sugars. Contraindicated in pregnancy
Atovaquone	750 mg 12 hourly	Administered orally. To be given with meals. Absorption decreased in diarrhea and fasting state
Glucocorticoids	High dose required, e.g., 40 mg BD followed by slow taper	Used in moderate-to-severe infection

(GFR: glomerular filtration rate; TMP: trimethoprim)

The drug of choice for treatment of PCP is trimethoprim–sulfamethoxazole (TMP–SMX). It interferes with the folate metabolism. Adverse effects of TMP–SMX include leukopenia, rash, anaphylactoid reactions, hepatitis, and hyperkalemia.[30]

Patients with allergy to TMP–SMX ideally require desensitization, since it is the most effective drug for *P. jirovecii* pneumonia (PJP). However, if the patient has a past history of Steven–Johnson syndrome or toxic epidermal necrolysis with the use of TMP–SMX, then its use should be avoided.[31]

TABLE 3: Patient subgroups based on severity of infection.

	Mild disease	*Moderate disease*	*Severe disease*
A–a O_2 gradient (mm Hg)	<35	≥35 to <45	≥45
Partial pressure of arterial oxygen (mm Hg)	≥70	≥60 to <70	<60

TABLE 4: Choice of regimen in patients with *Pneumocystis* pneumonia who cannot take trimethoprim–sulfamethoxazole.

Mild disease	*Moderate disease*	*Severe disease*
Atovaquone	Clindamycin plus primaquine	Clindamycin plus primaquine
TMP plus dapsone	TMP plus dapsone	Intravenous pentamidine
Clindamycin plus primaquine		

(TMP: trimethoprim)
Note: G6PD to be checked prior to administration of primaquine and dapsone.

Sulfadiazine–pyrimethamine, dapsone–pyrimethamine, clindamycin–primaquine, and dapsone–TMP are also effective against *Pneumocystis.* The suggested duration of treatment is 3 weeks and clinical improvement is expected to happen by the end of first week of therapy.

Side effects of dapsone include gastrointestinal (GI) upset, rash, fever, hemolytic anemia, agranulocytosis, and methemoglobinemia.

Patients who do not tolerate TMP–SMX can be treated with intravenous pentamidine. Care needs to be taken to avoid potentially lethal hypotension, pancreatitis, dysglycemia (life-threatening hypoglycemia that can occur days to weeks after initial infusion followed by hyperglycemia), torsades de pointes, neutropenia, taste disturbances, and renal dysfunction.[32]

Atovaquone can be used as a second-line agent in patients with mild-to-moderate PCP infection. Major side effects include GI distress, rash, hepatitis, and fever.

Patients can be divided into three subgroups based on the severity of infection **(Tables 3 and 4)**.

Patients who do not show improvement after 8 days of therapy are considered to have treatment failures. It may be due to the severity of the disease at the time of diagnosis or due to a simultaneous unidentified infection. In such patients, the following algorithms maybe useful:

- Convert oral TMP–SMX to IV TMP–SMX.
- If patient is on IV TMP–SMX, convert it to clindamycin–TMP.
- If the patient is on alternative regimen for PCP, see if desensitization and therapy with TMP–SMX is an option.[33]

There is no guideline to recommend management of immunosuppression during PCP infection. However, as a general measure, the dose of immunosuppression needs to be reduced. The cyst wall of PCP contains β-D-glucan, the synthesis of which is inhibited by echinocandins. However, the role of echinocandins in treatment is controversial.[34] For patients requiring mechanical ventilation, low tidal volume and plateau pressures should be used as there is potential presence of pneumatoceles which may get converted to pneumothorax.

Corticosteroids should be used with those kidney transplant recipients with moderate-to-severe PCP as defined by PaO_2 <70 mm Hg in room air or an alveolar gradient of >35 mm Hg or hypoxemia on pulse oximetry (sO_2 on room air <92%).[35] A convenient regimen is to give 40 mg 12 hourly for 5 days followed by 40 mg daily for 5 days followed by 20 mg daily for 11 days. Glucocorticoids reduce the pulmonary inflammation that occurs after a specific therapy is started and organisms begin to die.[36]

For the treatment of PCP in pregnancy, the preferred drug is TMP–SMX, but its use in the first trimester is associated with the development of neural tube defects and cardiovascular and urinary tract anomalies in the fetus. Folic acid supplementation is hence advised. TMP–SMX can cause kernicterus if used near term. Pregnant patients not tolerating TMP–SMX should be given TMP–dapsone for treatment.[37]

PROPHYLAXIS

The most effective way for prevention of PCP is to eliminate the cause of immunosuppression by withdrawing immunosuppressive therapy and treatment of underlying cause.

The use of TMP–SMX prophylaxis has resulted in a relative risk (RR) of 0.08 of developing PCP compared to placebo. Kidney Disease Improving Global Outcomes (KDIGO) recommends that all kidney transplant recipients receive PCP prophylaxis with daily TMP–SMX for 3–6 months after transplantation and for at least 6 months during and after the treatment of acute rejection. Other agents which can be used for prophylaxis include dapsone, aerosolized pentamidine, and atovaquone **(Table 5)**.

Aerosolized pentamidine is less effective for prophylaxis as it acts only locally, and untreated areas remain at risk for PCP. Its use has been associated with the transmission of *Mycobacterium tuberculosis* and requires a special equipment.

Patients who have been treated for PCP infection should receive antimicrobial therapy at a reduced dose to prevent recurrent infection (secondary prophylaxis) with the same drugs used to prevent primary infection.[38]

TABLE 5: Prophylaxis of *Pneumocystis* pneumonia.

Drugs used for prophylaxis	*Dose*
Co-trimoxazole	Single-strength pill daily or double-strength pill three times per week
Atovaquone	1.5 g/day
Dapsone	100 mg once daily or in two divided doses
Aerosolized pentamidine	300 mg once a month via Respirgard II nebulizer

REFERENCES

1. Masur H, Morris A. Pneumocystis infections. In Harrison's Principles of Internal Medicine, 19th edition. New York: McGraw Hill; 2016. pp. 1358-62.
2. Walzer PD. The ecology of pneumocystis: perspectives, personal recollections, and future research opportunities. J Eukaryot Microbiol. 2013;60(6):634-45.
3. Edman JC, Kovacs JA, Masur H, Santi DV, Elwood HJ, Sogin ML. Ribosomal RNA sequence shows Pneumocystis carinii to be a member of the fungi. Nature. 1988;334(6182):519-22.
4. Huang L, Cattamanchi A, Davis JL, den Boon S, Kovacs J, Meshnick S, et al. HIV associated Pneumocystis pneumonia. Proc Am Thorac Soc. 2011;8(3):294-300.
5. Chapman JR, Mariott DJ, Chen SCA, MacDonald PS. Post-transplant Pneumocystis jirovecii pneumonia—a re-emerged public health problem? Kidney Int. 2013;84(2):240-3.
6. Rodriguez M, Fishman JA. Prevention of infection due to Pneumocystis spp. in human immunodeficiency virus-negative immunocompromised patients. Clin Microbiol Rev. 2004;17(4):770-82.
7. Meijers RW, Litgens NH, Hesselink DA, Langerak AW, Baan CC, Betjes MGH. Primary Cytomegalus infection significantly impacts circulating T cells in kidney transplant recipients. Am J Transplant. 2015;15(12):3143-56.
8. Dummer JS, Montero CG, Griffith BP, Hardesty RL, Paradis IL, Ho M. Infections in heart-lung transplant recipients. Transplantation. 1986;41(6):725-9.
9. Radisic M, Lattes R, Chapman JF, del Carmen Rial M, Guardia O, Seu F, et al. Risk factors for Pneumocystis carinii pneumonia in kidney transplant recipients: a case control study. Transpl Infect Dis. 2003;5(2):84-93.
10. Fishman JA, Gans H, AST Infectious Diseases Community of Practice. Pneumocystis jiroveci in solid organ transplantation—guidelines from the American Society of Transplantation Infectious Diseases Community of Practice. Clin Transplant. 2019;33(9):e13587.
11. Aliouat-Dennis CM, Martinez A, Aliouat EM, Pottier M, Gantois N, Dei-Cas E. The pneumocystis life cycle. Mem Inst Oswaldo Cruz. 2009;104(3):419-26.
12. Yale SH, Limper AH. Pneumocystis carinii pneumonia in patients without acquired immunodeficiency syndrome: associated illness and prior corticosteroid therapy. Mayo Clin Proc. 1996;71(1):5-13.
13. Sepkowitz KA, Brown AE, Telzak EE, Gottlieb S, Armstrong D. Pneumocystis carinii pneumonia among patients without AIDS at a cancer hospital. JAMA. 1992;267(6):832-7.

14. Tasaka S, Tokuda H. Pneumocystis jirovecii pneumonia in non-HIV-infected patients in the era of novel immunosuppressive therapies. J Infect Chemother. 2012;18(6):793-806.
15. Kovacs JA, Hiemenz JW, Macher AM, Stover D, Murray HW, Shelhamer J, et al. Pneumocystis carinii pneumonia: a comparison between patients with the acquired immunodeficiency syndrome and patients with other immunodeficiencies. Ann Intern Med. 1984;100(5):663-71.
16. Ng VL, Yajko DM, Hadley WK. Extrapulmonary pneumocystosis. Clin Microbiol Rev. 1997;10(3):401-18.
17. Thomas Jr CF, Limper AH. Pneumocystis pneumonia. N Engl J Med. 2004;350(24):2487-98.
18. Carmona AM, Limper AH. Update on the diagnosis and treatment of Pneumocystis pneumonia. Ther Adv Respir Dis. 2011;5(1):41-59.
19. Nakamura H, Tateyama M, Tasato D, Haranaga S, Yara S, Higa F, et al. Clinical utility of serum β-D-glucan and KL-6 levels in Pneumocystis jiroveci pneumonia. Intern Med. 2009;48(4):195-202.
20. de Boer MGJ, Gelinck LBS, van Zelst BD, van de Sande WWJ, Willems LNA, van Dissel JT, et al. β-D-glucan and S-adenosyl methionine serum levels for the diagnosis of Pneumocystis pneumonia in HIV negative patients: a prospective study. J Infect. 2011;62(1):93-100.
21. Bigby TD. Diagnosis of Pneumocystis pneumonia. How invasive? Chest. 1994;105(3): 650-2.
22. Cregan P, Yamamoto A, Lum A, VanDerHeide T, MacDonald M, Pulliam L. Comparison of four methods for rapid detection of Pneumocystis carinii in respiratory specimens. J Clin Microbiol. 1990;28(11):2432-6.
23. Jacobs JA, Dieleman MM, Cornelissen EI, Groen EA, Wagenaar SS, Drent M. Bronchoalveolar lavage fluid lavage cytology in patients with Pneumocystis carinii pneumonia. Acta Cytol. 2001;45(3):317-26.
24. Caliendo AM, Hewitt PL, Allega JM, Keen A, Ruoff KL, Ferraro MJ. Performance of a PCR assay for detection of Pneumocystis carinii from respiratory specimens. J Clin Microbiol. 1998;36(4):979-82.
25. Nakashima K, Aoshima M, Ohkuni Y, Hoshino E, Hashimoto K, Otsuka Y. Loop mediated isothermal amplification method for diagnosing Pneumocystis pneumonia in HIV uninfected immunocompromised patients with pulmonary infiltrates. J Infect Chemother. 2014;20(12): 757- 61.
26. Vogel MN, Weissgerber P, Goeppert B, Hetzel J, Vatlach M, Claussen CD, et al. Accuracy of serum LDH elevation for the diagnosis of Pneumocystis jiroveci pneumonia. Swiss Med Wkly. 2011;141:w13184.
27. Theel ES, Jespersen DJ, Iqbal S, Bestrom JE, Rollins LO, Misner LJ, et al. Detection of (1,3)-β-D-glucan in bronchoalveolar lavage and serum samples collected from immunocompromised host. Mycopathologia. 2013;175(1-2): 33-41.
28. Crans Jr CA, Boiselle PM. Imaging features of Pneumocystis carinii pneumonia. Crit Rev Diagn Imaging. 1999;40(4): 251-84.
29. Hardak E, Brook O, Yigla M. Radiological features of Pneumocystis jirovecii patients with and without AIDS. Lung. 2010;188(2):159-63.
30. Limper AH, Knox KS, Sarosi GA, Ampel NM, Bennett JE, Catanzaro A, et al. An official American Thoracic Society Statement: treatment of fungal infections in adult pulmonary and critical care patients. Am J Respir Crit Care Med. 2011;183(1):96-128.
31. Lau WK, Young LS. Trimethoprim sulfamethoxazole treatment of Pneumocystis carinii pneumonia in adults. N Engl J Med. 1976;295:716-8.
32. Hughes WT, Feldman S, Chaudhary SC, Ossi MJ, Cox F, Sanyal SK, et al. Comparison of pentamidine isethionate and trimethoprim-sulfamethoxazole in the treatment of Pneumocystis carinii pneumonia. J Pediatr. 1978;92(2): 285- 91.
33. Helweg-Larsen J, Benfield T, Atzori C, Miller RF. Clinical efficacy of first and second line treatments for HIV associated Pneumocystis jirovecii pneumonia: a tri-centre cohort study. J Antimicrob Chemother. 2009;64(6):1282-90.
34. Huang YS, Liu CE, Lin SP, Lee CH, Yang CJ, Lin CY, et al. Echinocandins as alternative treatment for HIV-infected patients with Pneumocystis pneumonia. AIDS. 2019;33(8): 1345-51.
35. Ewald H, Raatz H, Boscacci R, Furrer H, Bucher HC, Briel M. Adjunctive corticosteroids for Pneumocystis jiroveci pneumonia in patients with HIV infection. Cochrane Database Syst Rev. 2015;2015(4):CD006150.
36. Gagnon S, Boota AM, Fisch MA, Baier H, Kirksey OW, Voie LL. Corticosteroids as adjunctive therapy for severe Pneumocystis carinii pneumonia in the acquired immunodeficiency syndrome. A double blind placebo controlled trial. N Engl J Med. 1990;323(21):1444-50.
37. Czeizel AE, Rockenbauer M, Sørensen HT, Olsen J. The teratogenic risk of trimethoprim-sulfonamides: a population based case-control study. Reprod Toxicol. 2001;15(6):637-46.
38. Ledergerber B, Mocroft A, Reiss P, Furrer H, Kirk O, Bickel M, et al. Discontinuation of secondary prophylaxis against Pneumocystis carinii pneumonia in patients with HIV infection who have a response to antiretroviral therapy. Eight European Study Groups. N Engl J Med. 2001;344(3):168.

12.6 Urinary Tract Infection

Krishan Lal Gupta, Joyita Bharati

CASE VIGNETTE 1

A 27-year-old male with disseminated tuberculosis had acute kidney injury caused by granulomatous tubulointerstitial nephritis (GTIN). There was no evidence of genitourinary tuberculosis in the form of obstructive uropathy. He progressed to end-stage kidney disease (ESKD) over 4 months despite treatment with antituberculous treatment and steroids. After a hemodialysis vintage of 20 months, he underwent a living donor kidney transplant from an unrelated donor through kidney pair exchange program. Antithymocyte immunoglobulin was followed by tacrolimus, mycophenolate mofetil (MMF), and steroids for immunosuppression. 2 months later, he developed fever with burning micturition. On examination, he was febrile, general condition was good, and vitals were normal. There was no allograft tenderness. Laboratory parameters showed a rise in serum creatinine to 3.8 mg/dL (baseline serum creatinine = 1.4 mg/dL), and urine microscopy was notable for significant pus cells. Urine culture grew >10^5 colony-forming units (CFU) of Escherichia coli having sensitivity to carbapenems only. Ultrasonography (USG) of the kidney and urinary bladder showed echoes in the bladder and bilateral shrunken native kidneys with mild hydronephrosis of the kidney allograft. A diagnosis of complicated urinary tract infection (UTI) was made. On day 3 of intravenous meropenem and hydration, his fever resolved, and serum creatinine subsequently decreased to 2.1 mg/dL. However, 4 weeks after discharge from this admission, he developed another episode of UTI. A contrast-enhanced computed tomography (CT) was done in this episode of UTI, which revealed a dilated and enhanced pelvicalyceal system suggestive of hydroureteronephrosis of the kidney allograft. Voiding cystourethrogram showed grade III vesicoureteric reflux in the kidney allograft. His graft dysfunction persisted with slowly increasing creatinine levels to 4 mg/dL.

CASE VIGNETTE 2

A 28-year-old male with ESKD due to antiglomerular basement membrane disease underwent a living donor kidney transplant with mother as the donor. Induction therapy was omitted, and tacrolimus, MMF, and steroids were used as maintenance immunosuppressive agents. 3 months after transplant, he developed post-transplant diabetes mellitus (PTDM) requiring an insulin basal-bolus regime. 1 year after transplant, the patient developed an uncomplicated UTI caused by E. coli sensitive to most antibiotics. Detailed evaluation of the urinary tract system did not reveal any structural anomaly. The patient had uncontrolled blood sugar levels for the past 1 year. Insulin regimen was modified, and tacrolimus was changed to cyclosporine. After vigilant follow-up and close monitoring, blood sugar levels were adequately controlled and kidney function remained stable at 3 years post-transplant without any recurrence of symptomatic UTI.

INTRODUCTION

Urinary tract infection is typically diagnosed when a patient has lower urinary tract symptoms with or without fever along with a positive urine culture, i.e., >10^5 CFU/mL of an organism. Fever is often the only apparent symptom of UTI in a certain group of patients such as neonates, infants, and bedridden patients on assisted care. In the elderly, altered mentation or behavior could be the only symptom of UTI. Moreover, kidney transplant recipients (KTR) with UTI could present with only fever or nonspecific sepsis syndrome without apparent lower urinary tract symptoms. Patients with UTI typically have pyuria [>5 white blood cells (WBCs)/high power field].

EPIDEMIOLOGY

Infections account for more than 50% of all causes of mortality after kidney transplant, especially in tropical countries. UTI is the most common infection in the first year after kidney transplant, occurring in ~25% of all KTRs,[1,2] and 30% of all hospitalizations for sepsis in KTRs are due to UTI.[3] Among all solid organ transplantation, kidney transplant has the highest risk for UTI.[4] The creation of complex anatomy of the urinary draining system in kidney transplant surgery predisposes KTR to UTI. Additionally, intense immunosuppression and PTDM are responsible for recurrent UTI in a significant proportion of KTRs. The basic diseases of kidney failure such as diabetic kidney disease, renal stone disease, obstructive uropathy, reflux nephropathy, and cystic kidney diseases act as the nidus of repeated UTI after kidney transplant in another significant proportion of KTRs. Most UTIs in KTRs occur in the first 3–6 months after kidney transplant. Recurrent UTI is also commonly seen in KTRs with a wide range of prevalence between 4 and 72%.[5]

RISK FACTORS

Common risk factors for developing UTI in the KTR are female sex, old age, diabetes mellitus, duration of hemodialysis, induction therapy with antithymocyte immunoglobulin, and urological structural anomalies such as ureteric stenosis, indwelling ureteral stents, urethral catheterization of instrumentation, deceased donor transplantation, delayed graft function, previous history of recurrent UTI before transplant, episodes of acute cellular rejection, and vesicoureteral reflux (VUR). It is often a multifactorial risk in KTRs and most such risk factors are present in the KTR with UTI in the early post-transplant period.

CHAPTER HIGHLIGHTS

- Urinary tract infection (UTI) is the most common infection in the first year after kidney transplant.
- Recurrent UTI is evaluated using USG kidney ureter bladder and fasting blood sugar.
- Graft survival is adversely affected by recurrent UTI.
- Treatment is decided based on type of UTI and time point after kidney transplant.

However, after the first 6 months, the epidemiology of UTI shifts toward that of general population such as female sex and diabetes mellitus in addition to specific risk factors such as increased creatinine and high steroid dose.

DEFINITIONS

Types of UTI:[6] Patients with UTI after kidney transplant can present either with *acute simple cystitis*, i.e., lower urinary tract symptoms, hematuria, and suprapubic pain, or with *complicated UTI or acute pyelonephritis*, i.e., fever, allograft site tenderness, pain, chills, constitutional symptoms with or without graft dysfunction. Patients with complicated UTI may have lower urinary tract symptoms as well; however, patients with simple cystitis do not have systemic symptoms of complicated UTI and/or any indwelling device. It is noteworthy that KTRs may not manifest allograft pain or tenderness in the background of a denervated allograft kidney. *UTI in the presence of indwelling devices or structural and/or functional anomalies is classified as complicated UTI. However, an uncomplicated kidney transplant surgery and immunosuppression after the first 3-6 months of kidney transplant are typically not considered structural and functional anomalies associated with complicated UTI, respectively.* Some patients may have *asymptomatic bacteriuria* (*ASB*) when a screening urine culture, done in the absence of symptoms of UTI, shows the presence of $>10^5$ bacterial CFU/mL. ASB is possible with or without pyuria, and could be reflecting contamination or colonization without true infection. Some patients with cystitis and pyelonephritis may have fewer than 10^5 bacterial CFU/mL of a uropathogen in a midstream urine sample. *Recurrent UTI* is defined as three or more episodes of UTI in a 12-month period.

MICROBIOLOGY

Enteric gram-negative bacteria, *E. coli*, are the most common cause of UTI in KTRs. *Staphylococcus saprophyticus*, enterococci, and *Pseudomonas aeruginosa* are other common organisms causing UTI in KTRs. *Staphylococcus aureus* is frequently associated with hematogenous spread to the urinary tract, rather than ascending infection. *Candida* species is a common colonizer of the lower urinary tract; however, *Candida* can cause upper tract involvement too.

TREATMENT

For ASB, treatment with an appropriate antibiotic for 5–7 days is recommended by most experts in the first 3 months' post-transplant. After the first 3 months, ASB screening and treatment are not recommended.[6]

For simple cystitis, oral third-generation cephalosporin, fluoroquinolones (ciprofloxacin or levofloxacin), and amoxicillin–clavulanate are recommended for 5–7 days. Single dose and short courses (<5 days) of antibiotic treatment are not recommended in KTRs with UTI.[6] Nitrofurantoin is also a preferred choice except in patients with creatinine clearance <30 mL/min. Fosfomycin is to be reserved for multidrug resistant cases. In the first 3 months after transplantation *P. aeruginosa* and enterococci are more frequently isolated and empirical treatment must cover these microorganisms, for example, a combination of ciprofloxacin and amoxicillin can be used.

For complicated UTI, piperacillin–tazobactam, carbapenem, or cefepime is recommended intravenously for a period of 14–21 days.[6] In cases of abscesses, antibiotics should be covered or extended until the abscesses are drained or have reduced significantly.

Evaluation of the underlying mechanism of UTI is crucial to successfully manage and prevent further recurrent UTI in a KTR. Structural and functional abnormality should be corrected alongside antibiotic therapy to prevent recurrent episodes, achieve successful cure, and prevent antibiotic resistance from prolonged antibiotic therapy. It is important to check interaction of antimicrobial agents with immunosuppressants, especially with calcineurin inhibitors.

RECURRENT URINARY TRACT INFECTION

The management of recurrent UTI in KTRs is not high-quality evidence-based as few studies are reported in the literature. Risk factors for recurrent UTI in KTR include immunosuppression (especially in the first 3–6 months post-transplant), diabetes mellitus (uncontrolled), anatomical urinary tract abnormality, and bladder atony resulting from prolonged pretransplant anuria.[7] Recurrent UTI is commonly caused by multidrug resistant gram-negative organisms and result in poor graft survival. Patients should be evaluated with the aim to look for common risk factors **(Box 1)**. Post-transplant recurrent UTI may have origin in the native kidneys or the allograft kidney. Recurrent native kidney pyelonephritis commonly develops in the background of polycystic kidney disease, renal stone disease, diabetes mellitus, and reflux/obstructive uropathy. Infection prevention measures such as adequate hydration, timed voiding, and precautionary steps in females of the reproductive age group (as in general population) should be communicated to patients. Topical (vaginal) estrogen cream is a proven therapy to prevent recurrent

BOX 1: Evaluation of recurrent urinary tract infection (UTI) in kidney transplant recipients.

- *USG kidney urinary bladder:* Postvoid residual urine, prostate (in the elderly man), evidence of pyelonephritis, renal stones in native or allograft kidney, hydroureteronephrosis, urinary bladder changes.
- *Fasting blood sugar, HbA1c:*
  - If structural abnormality is present: surgery or corrective measures
  - If no structural abnormality on USG, perform voiding cystourethrography and urodynamic study
  - If vesicoureteral reflux is present: surgery or endoscopic injection
  - If bladder dysfunction is present: medical and/or surgical management
  - *If high blood sugar:* Manage with oral and/or injectable antihyperglycemic agents

(HbA1c: hemoglobin A1C; KTR: kidney transplant recipient; USG: ultrasonography)

UTI in postmenopausal women with atrophic vaginitis. While a small retrospective study in KTR population showed benefit,[8] the role of cranberry products in preventing recurrent UTI in the general population is unclear at present. Apart from voiding cystourethrography and urodynamic studies, cystoscopy should also be considered in the evaluation of recurrent UTI in an individual with suggestive bladder pathology. The treatment of VUR with surgical correction is not routinely advocated in KTRs without recurrent pyelonephritis as mild-to-moderate VUR is common after kidney transplant surgery and is not consistently associated with recurrent UTI. Endoscopic treatment should be attempted in patients with moderate UTI and VUR post-transplant, and open surgical correction is shown to be useful in reducing UTI in KTRs with recurrent pyelonephritis. Treatment of UTI in KTRs with recurrent UTI is the same as general population, i.e., appropriate antibiotic for a week or two (oral or parenteral) based on simple cystitis or pyelonephritis-like presentation. Some experts recommend continuing antibiotics for a longer duration such as 4–6 weeks in case of relapsing UTI with the same pathogen. After treating an episode of UTI successfully, prophylaxis can be started to prevent further episodes, especially in those with recurrent graft pyelonephritis and decreased graft function.

PREVENTION

- Thorough management of structural and functional urinary tract abnormalities in the pretransplant period, for example, nephrectomy of the native kidneys, especially in patients with recurrent UTI in polycystic kidney disease, renal stone disease, and VUR to their native kidneys would reduce recurrence of UTI post-transplant.
- After transplant surgery, removal of the urinary catheter and ureteral stent should be done as soon as appropriate. Indwelling ureteral stents have been shown to increase the risk of UTI, especially if used for longer duration.[9]
- No recommendation can be made about changing immunosuppressive drugs from one class to another to prevent a recurrence of UTI.
- No screening recommendations in the postrenal transplant period for asymptomatic bacteriuria are available. However, in the first 3–6 months post-transplant, most experts treat asymptomatic bacteriuria to avoid complications of UTI in the face of strong immunosuppression.
- In patients with recurrent UTI without previous known cause, further investigations for anatomical abnormalities, stones, anastomotic complications, bladder dysfunction or infection of the native kidneys and blood sugar control should be initiated.
- *Antibiotic prophylaxis in the KTR:* Use of co-trimoxazole prophylaxis for the first 6–12 months after transplant has been shown to reduce bacteriuria, bacteremia, and sepsis in KTRs.[10] Although the dose of co-trimoxazole for preventing *Pneumocystis jiroveci* pneumonia in the early post-transplant period is lower than doses studied for preventing UTI, owing to the side effect profile of co-trimoxazole, the American Society of Transplantation (AST) recommends using lower dose for both *P. jiroveci* pneumonia and UTI.[6] In patients with contraindications for the use of co-trimoxazole, considerations should be made for using alternative agents for preventing UTI for those at high risk of UTI. Alternative agents such as nitrofurantoin should be used in those with glomerular filtration rate (GFR) > 60 mL/min, and cephalosporins (cephalexin) in those not suitable for nitrofurantoin, preferably in the first month after transplant. 6–12 months of nitrofurantoin use was reported to be safe in healthy women;[11] however, longer duration of use is known to be associated with nephropathy and lung toxicity. Use of fluoroquinolones should be avoided due to emergence of resistance to these antibiotics.[12] The choice of antibiotic for long-term prophylaxis in patients with recurrent UTI should be based on patient's culture sensitivity, drug allergies, and creatinine clearance.

IMPACT OF URINARY TRACT INFECTION ON THE PATIENT

Urinary tract infection in a KTR is associated with infectious and noninfectious complications such as bacteremia, sepsis, acute graft dysfunction, acute cellular rejection, allograft loss, and mortality. The cost of kidney transplant also increases substantially in patients with recurrent UTI post-transplant. UTI, if untreated in the early post-transplant period, is associated with acute cellular rejection as bacterial infection is known to activate the immune system.[13] Also, UTI and sepsis are known to result in reduction of immunosuppressive agents leading to graft rejection. Recurrent UTI is associated with poor graft outcomes and increased multidrug-resistant organisms.[14]

CONCLUSION

Urinary tract infection is a common complication after kidney transplant. Besides common risk factors for UTI in the general population, additional factors predispose KTR to frequent UTI. UTI, especially recurrent UTI, is associated with a huge negative impact in the KTR. Preventive measures begin during pretransplant evaluation, such as native kidney nephrectomy in those with high-risk factors for recurrent UTI, antibiotic prophylaxis, minimal use of devices, optimization of immunosuppression, and adequate management of diabetes mellitus. Treatment of UTI in KTRs is essentially the same as in the general population, except ASB, which unlike in general population, is usually treated in the first 3 months after transplant.

REFERENCES

1. Ariza-Heredia EJ, Beam EN, Lesnick TG, Kremers WK, Cosio FG, Razonable RR. Urinary tract infections in kidney transplant recipients: role of gender, urologic abnormalities, and antimicrobial prophylaxis. Ann Transplant. 2013;18: 195-204.
2. Alangaden GJ, Thyagarajan R, Gruber SA, Morawski K, Garnick J, El-Amm JM, et al. Infectious complications after kidney transplantation: current epidemiology and associated risk factors. Clin Transplant. 2006;20(4):401-9.
3. Abbott KC, Oliver 3rd JD, Hypolite I, Lepler LL, Kirk AD, Ko CW, et al. Hospitalizations for bacterial septicemia after renal transplantation in the United States. Am J Nephrol. 2001;21(2):120-7.
4. Vidal E, Torre-Cisneros J, Blanes M, Montejo M, Cervera C, Aguado JM, et al. Bacterial urinary tract infection after solid organ transplantation in the RESITRA cohort. Transpl Infect Dis. 2012;14(6):595-603.
5. Hollyer I, Ison MG. The challenge of urinary tract infections in renal transplant recipients. Transpl Infect Dis. 2018;20(2):e12828.
6. Goldman JD, Julian K. Urinary tract infections in solid organ transplant recipients: guidelines from the American Society of Transplantation Infectious Diseases Community of Practice. Clin Transplant. 2019;33(9):e13507.
7. Bodro M, Linares L, Chiang D, Moreno A, Cervera C. Managing recurrent urinary tract infections in kidney transplant patients. Expert Rev Anti Infect Ther. 2018;16(9): 723-32.
8. Jorgenson MR, Descourouez JL, Siodlak M, Tjugum S, Rice JP, Fernandez LA. Efficacy and safety of probiotics and synbiotics in liver transplantation. Pharmacotherapy. 2018;38(7):758-68.
9. Wilson CH, Rix DA, Manas DM. Routine intraoperative ureteric stenting for kidney transplant recipients. Cochrane Database Syst Rev. 2013:CD004925.
10. Green H, Rahamimov R, Gafter U, Leibovitci L, Paul M. Antibiotic prophylaxis for urinary tract infections in renal transplant recipients: a systematic review and meta-analysis. Transpl Infect Dis. 2011;13(5):441-7.
11. Price JR, Guran LA, Gregory WT, McDonagh MS. Nitrofurantoin vs other prophylactic agents in reducing recurrent urinary tract infections in adult women: a systematic review and meta-analysis. Am J Obstet Gynecol. 2016;215(5):548-60.
12. Khorvash F, Mortazavi M, Hakamifard A, Ataei B. Comparison of the effect of co-trimoxazole and co-trimoxazole plus ciprofloxacin in urinary tract infection prophylaxis in kidney transplant patients. Adv Biomed Res. 2016;5:108.
13. Audard V, Amor M, Desvaux D, Pastural M, Baron C, Philippe R, et al. Acute graft pyelonephritis: a potential cause of acute rejection in renal transplant. Transplantation. 2005;80(8):1128-30.
14. Britt NS, Hagopian JC, Brennan DC, Pottebaum AA, Santos CAQ, Gharabagi A, et al. Effects of recurrent urinary tract infections on graft and patient outcomes after kidney transplantation. Nephrol Dial Transplant. 2017;32(10):1758-66.

12.7 Tuberculosis

Arunkumar S, Sanjay K Agarwal

CASE VIGNETTE

A 36-year-old male renal allograft recipient was admitted for intermittent low-grade fever, malaise, loss of appetite, and loss of weight (3 kg) for the last 1 month. He had received kidney transplantation 2 years earlier with mother as donor. He did not receive any induction therapy, was treated with standard triple drug immunosuppression and had an uneventful postoperative course with a stable serum creatinine of 0.9–1.1 mg/dL. Current immunosuppressive regimen consisted of tacrolimus, mycophenolate mofetil (500 mg twice/day) and low dose prednisolone (5 mg/day). The dose of tacrolimus was titrated to achieve trough whole blood level of 4–6 ng/mL.

Clinically the patient was alert, awake and had stable vitals with normal hydration status. Respiratory examination showed evidence of right sided pleural effusion. Rest of the systemic examination was normal. Leucocyte count was 5600/cmm. Chest X-ray revealed loculated right side pleural effusion. High resolution computed tomography (HRCT) scan revealed mediastinal lymphadenopathy and confirmed pleural effusion. Ultrasound guided pleural fluid aspiration revealed an exudative lymphocyte rich pleural fluid with an ADA level of 50 IU/L. The clinical and imaging features were suggestive of extra-pulmonary tuberculosis (lymph nodal + pleural) and patient was planned for anti-tuberculous therapy. Moxifloxacin based antitubercular therapy (ATT) consisting of isoniazid, pyrazinamide, ethambutol was started for the patient. Patient tolerated the ATT regimen and there was symptomatic improvement by 3rd week of therapy. After 2 months of intensive regimen, he was continued on maintenance regimen of moxifloxacin, isoniazid and ethambutol. Imaging repeated after 2 months revealed resolution of mediastinal lymphadenopathy and mild pleural thickening. A total of 9 months of maintenance therapy is being planned. Patient is on regular follow-up with a serum creatinine of 1.1–1.3 mg/dL and no fresh symptoms.

INTRODUCTION

Infections are the most common cause of mortality following kidney transplantation, especially in developing countries. Tuberculosis (TB) is one such infection commonly seen following renal transplantation (RT). It is an air-borne communicable disease and the leading infectious cause of death worldwide. Renal transplant recipients (RTRs) are more vulnerable to acquire TB, present with diverse and atypical manifestations, and cause significant morbidity and mortality. The management is even more challenging as recommendations for treatment are based mainly on consensus guidelines in the absence of appropriate controlled clinical trials. With RT becoming more common and accessible in TB-endemic countries, the burden of TB is bound to increase in the years to come.

GLOBAL PREVALENCE OF TUBERCULOSIS

Tuberculosis is a global disease reported in every part of the world and remains till today as a public health issue, especially in developing countries. Worldwide, the South-East Asian region reports the maximum (43%) number of new cases followed by the African countries (25%) and then the Western Pacific region (18%).[1] It is estimated that about one-third of the total world's population is infected with TB.[2] The Indian subcontinent contributes to one-fifth of the global TB incidence and is one of the TB-endemic countries.

PREVALENCE OF TUBERCULOSIS IN RENAL TRANSPLANTATION

Renal transplant recipients are at a significantly higher risk of contracting TB compared to general population. Even among solid-organ transplants, RTRs are more likely to be infected with TB, only superseded by lung transplant recipients.[3] Though the prevalence varies according to the geographical region, transplant recipients are 4–30 times more frequently affected by TB.[3] The overall pooled prevalence of postrenal transplant TB is estimated to be 2.5%.[4] Prevalence of post-transplantation TB varies from 0.5–1% in North America to 0.7–5% in Europe, 1.5–3.5% in the Middle East, and 3–15% in Asian countries. Notwithstanding, the underreporting of cases and lack of patient databases, TB disease burden is disproportionately higher in developing countries which are TB endemic, wherein it reaches a high prevalence of approximately 15%.

India being a TB-endemic country with an active transplantation program, numerous centers across the country are expected to be a hotbed of infections. The overall prevalence is reported to be 10–15%.[5-7] Prevalence data from major centers of the country are enlisted in **Table 1**.

End-stage renal disease (ESRD) patients on maintenance dialysis are also at a higher risk for acquiring TB while

TABLE 1: Prevalence of tuberculosis in transplant recipients in various studies across India.

Study	*Center*	*Number of transplant recipients (n)*	*Prevalence of TB (%)*
Sharma et al.[8]	SGPGIMS, Lucknow	350	5.4%
Agarwal et al.[5]	AIIMS, New Delhi	1,664	10.9%
John et al.[6]	CMC, Vellore	1,414	13.3%
Sakhuja et al.[7]	PGIMER, Chandigarh	305	11.8%

CHAPTER HIGHLIGHTS

- Tuberculosis (TB) is common after renal transplantation especially in endemic countries like India accounting for significant morbidity and mortality.
- The prevalence of TB in Indian transplant recipients is around 10-15% and is more common with patients treated with calcineurin based triple drug immunosuppression. Though it is common in first year after transplant, it continues to develop even in late transplant period.
- Post-transplant TB can be due to reactivation of latent infection, can be donor-derived or because of de novo primary infection.
- Transplant recipients with TB present with diverse, atypical manifestations leading to delay in diagnosis and a high index of suspicion is warranted. Though extra-pulmonary TB is frequent, pulmonary TB is still the commonest presentation.
- The most common presenting symptoms are fever, generalized fatigue and weight loss. Depending on the organ system involved, the patient may have organ specific symptoms.
- Combination of clinical, imaging and microbiological findings are often required to confirm tuberculosis and nearly 20% of patients are empirically treated based on clinical suspicion after exclusion of other possible causes of symptoms.
- As rifampicin (RIF) is a potent cytochrome enzyme inducer and affects calcineurin and steroid levels. It is substituted in most transplant recipients with quinolones as part of antituberculous therapy (ATT).
- The inherent limitation of presently available tests to diagnose latent TB precludes recommendations for TB chemoprophylaxis in endemic areas.

on dialysis. The incidence of TB in dialysis population is also approximately 10–12%. A sizeable number of these patients carry TB while being transplanted and complete anti-TB therapy during the RT period, while it was started during the dialysis period.

De novo post-transplant TB (PTTB) is mostly due to reactivation of quiescent foci; hence, it exponentially parallels the prevalence in the general population in that particular region. This increased risk can be explained by the use of immunosuppressive drugs in the RTR, and the intensity of immunosuppression has been shown to be a significant predictive factor. Patients with a history of acute rejection who receives additional potent immunosuppression are at further higher risk. However, immunosuppression is not the only risk factor as seen in one of the largest series from India, wherein the use of more potent tacrolimus-based immunosuppression had significantly decreased the incidence of TB compared to cyclosporine-based immunosuppression.[5] Diabetes mellitus, chronic liver disease, old age, and coexisting infections (cytomegalovirus, *Pneumocystis jirovecii*, *Nocardia*, etc.) are known risk factors for PTTB.[9]

A study while comparing calcineurin inhibitor (CNI)-based immunosuppression versus without CNI had shown that there was a similar incidence of PTTB in both the groups but in patients receiving CNI, PTTB developed earlier in the post-transplant period and miliary TB was more common in the CNI group.[5] Other studies also have shown earlier onset of PTTB in patients receiving CNI-based immunosuppression.

PATHOGENESIS OF TUBERCULOSIS

Tuberculosis, being an airborne disease, is transmitted by inhalation of aerosol droplets containing *Mycobacterium tuberculosis* (MTB). Depending on the immune system and host factors, the bacilli are cleared or lead to primary disease or persist in a latent state. The host immune response by alveolar macrophages causes a nodular granulomatous response called a tubercle. Once bacilli reach the lymph nodes, it results in local lymphadenopathy. An effective cell-mediated immunity controls the infection in the first few weeks. In those with blunted immune responses, there will be progressive destruction of the lung. There can be hematogenous dissemination of bacilli resulting in disseminated TB.

Tuberculosis in transplant recipients occurs via three mechanisms:[10]

1. *Reactivation of latent infection:* The most common cause of PTTB, particularly in endemic regions
2. *Donor-derived:* Transmitted through the donor allograft
3. *De novo primary infection:* Rare; can be a cause in pediatric population.

Reactivation occurs due to the immunosuppressed state, which allows the proliferation of previously dormant bacilli, which were seeded at the time of primary infection and could have been asymptomatic. Nosocomial TB can occur during outbreaks of TB in a renal transplant unit, but is uncommon.

CLINICAL FEATURES

The clinical presentation of infections in RTR is frequently nonspecific, atypical, and involves uncommon sites. TB is no exception, and RTR have a myriad of presenting features. The timing of PTTB is varied. About two-thirds of the PTTB develops in the first year post-transplant with a median time of onset of 9 months (6–11 months).[11,12] This is seen in those with prior history or evidence of TB in the pretransplant period. There are conflicting reports on the role of intensity of immunosuppression on the timing of infection, with some reports suggesting a role of more intensive immunosuppression in causing early onset of TB in the post-transplant period. Late onset of TB occurs in one-third of the transplant recipients.[13] However, PTTB continues to be seen in the late post-transplant period, sometimes without any recent increase in immunosuppression and sometimes following a recent increase in immunosuppression like following antirejection therapy.

Similar to immunocompetent hosts, pulmonary TB is still the most common presentation in RTR. About one-third of RTR with TB have extrapulmonary involvement as compared to 10–15% in the community with TB infection.[3] This is more frequent in the early post-transplant period. The atypical clinical presentation results in delayed or missed diagnosis, which increases patient morbidity and sometimes also mortality.

The most common presenting symptoms are fever, night sweats, weight loss, cough, and generalized fatigue. In one large series, fever was present in only 64% of patients with localized disease but seen in 90% of patients with disseminated disease.[11] RTR may be totally asymptomatic, and TB can be diagnosed incidentally during routine follow-up evaluation in some cases. TB should always be considered as a differential in any RTR with pyrexia of unknown origin (PUO) and any patient with positive lesions on plain X-ray chest. Allograft dysfunction and coinfections [cytomegalovirus, *Pneumocystis jirovecii* pneumonia (PCP), etc.] can be seen in transplant recipients as in RTR, more than a third patients have mixed infection with pulmonary involvement. In addition to the constitutional symptoms, the other combination of symptoms depends on the afflicted organ. The pattern of organ involvement in various major studies across India is enlisted in **Table 2**. Pulmonary TB presents with cough, hemoptysis, shortness of breath, or various radiological evidence of pulmonary infiltrates. Disseminated disease involves more than one organ and most commonly involves the lungs in a majority (85%) of cases. Genitourinary TB usually manifests with urological symptoms, sterile pyuria, and allograft dysfunction. Gastrointestinal tract involvement can present with diarrhea, gastrointestinal bleeding, ulcerative disease, or peritonitis. Renal allograft TB, though rare, has been reported in case reports and is usually diagnosed when granulomas are detected in allograft biopsy. Tenosynovitis, osteoarticular involvement, cutaneous lesions, and pyomyositis are less common manifestations. The organ of involvement in RTR does not seem to be influenced by transplant-related factors. This may depend on host factors and the persistence of dormant tubercular foci in that particular organ.

TABLE 2: Pattern of organ involvement in Indian patients with post-transplant tuberculosis.

Site of TB	*Agarwal et al.*[5]	*John et al.*[6]	*Sakhuja et al.*[7]
Total RTR	1,664	1,414	305
No. of cases of TB	182	166	36
Pleuropulmonary	38.6%	48.2%	41.7%
Pyrexia of unknown origin	13.5%	15.7%	19.4%
Disseminated	5.4%	19.3%	27.8%
Nodal	16.8%	4.8%	–
Allograft	0.8%	–	–

(RTR: renal transplant recipients; TB: tuberculosis)

DIAGNOSIS

Clinicians should have a high index of suspicion for infection in post-transplant patients to prevent delay in diagnosis due to overlapping clinical features. This is particularly difficult in RTR who have subclinical infection. Despite advances in diagnostic techniques, 5–10% of RTR are diagnosed with TB at necropsy and nearly 20% patients are treated on clinical diagnosis without confirming microbiological proof. A careful detailed history about prior history of TB, exposure to individuals with TB, and antitubercular drug use including the dose and duration for adequacy of treatment is paramount in patient evaluation and deciding treatment regimens.

Microbiological diagnosis is essential and is established by the finding of acid-fast bacillus (AFB) in a patient's biological samples such as sputum, urine, pleural or peritoneal fluid, bone marrow specimens, lymph node aspirates and biopsy, bronchoalveolar lavage, lung biopsy, and other tissue biopsies depending on the site of involvement.[14] In RTR, the samples should be subjected to drug-resistance testing. Compared to earlier culture techniques which took a long (6–8 weeks) time, the present culture techniques give results as early as 2 weeks. Polymerase chain reactions (PCR) and nucleic acid amplification testing (NAAT) of patient samples have high specificity. Rapid NAAT techniques such as GeneXpert MTB/rifampicin (RIF) not only diagnose TB but also test for drug resistance to RIF, the most commonly used antitubercular drug. Invasive procedures such as bronchoscopy, tissue biopsy (lymph nodes, etc.) may be needed to establish the diagnosis in difficult situations. Nowadays for mediastinal lymph nodes' enlargement, esophageal ultrasound-guided node biopsies are becoming common for tissue diagnosis. Histopathological examination of tissue samples can reveal the classical necrotizing caseating granuloma with or without positive AFB staining.

Imaging Findings

Post-transplant pulmonary TB can present as consolidations, pleural effusions, lymphadenopathy, tree-in-bud appearance, and military nodules.[15] A chest radiograph is useful for screening patients, but a high-resolution computed tomography (CT) improves the diagnostic yield not only for diagnostic pattern but also for extent of lesion. In a study from India on evaluation of pulmonary infections in KTR, 16.7% patients with a normal chest radiograph were diagnosed based on CT imaging. Overall, transplant patients have lesser preponderance of developing cavitary disease and can also have any lobe involvement. Airway dissemination results in the tree-in-bud appearance. The various radiological features of PTTB are depicted in **Figures 1 and 2**. In patients with PUO and atypical presentation, a positron emission tomography would help in localization and diagnosis.

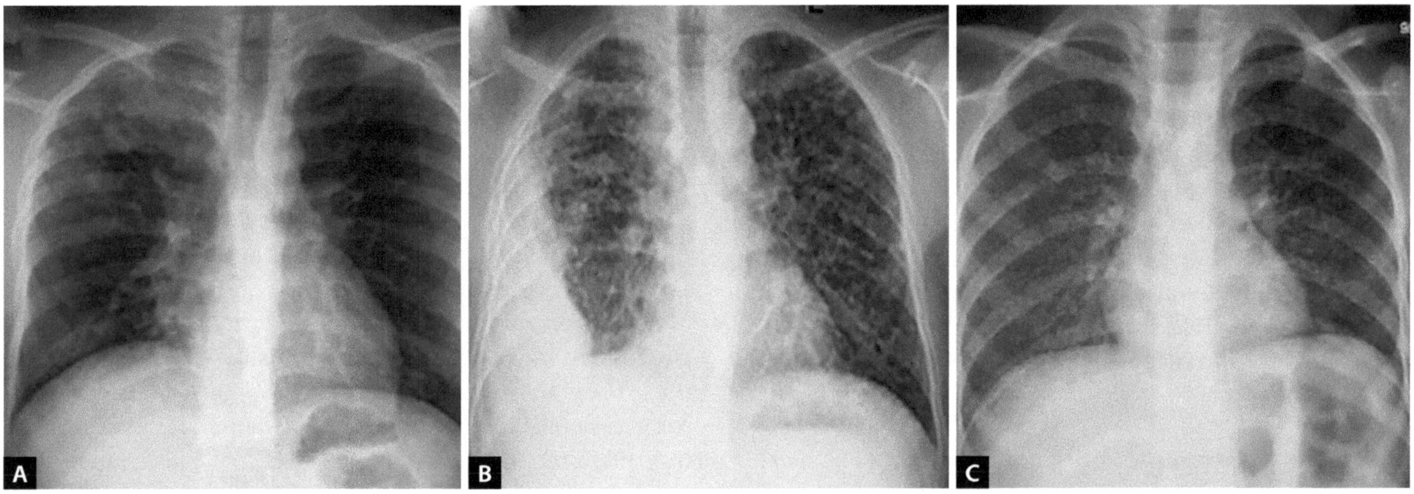

Figs. 1A to C: Chest radiographs showing findings in patients with PTTB. (A) Right upper zone consolidation with prominent hilum; (B) Right-sided loculated pleural effusion with multiple air-space nodules scattered in both lungs; (C) Widespread randomly distributed innumerable tiny nodules in both lungs. (PTTB: post-transplant tuberculosis)

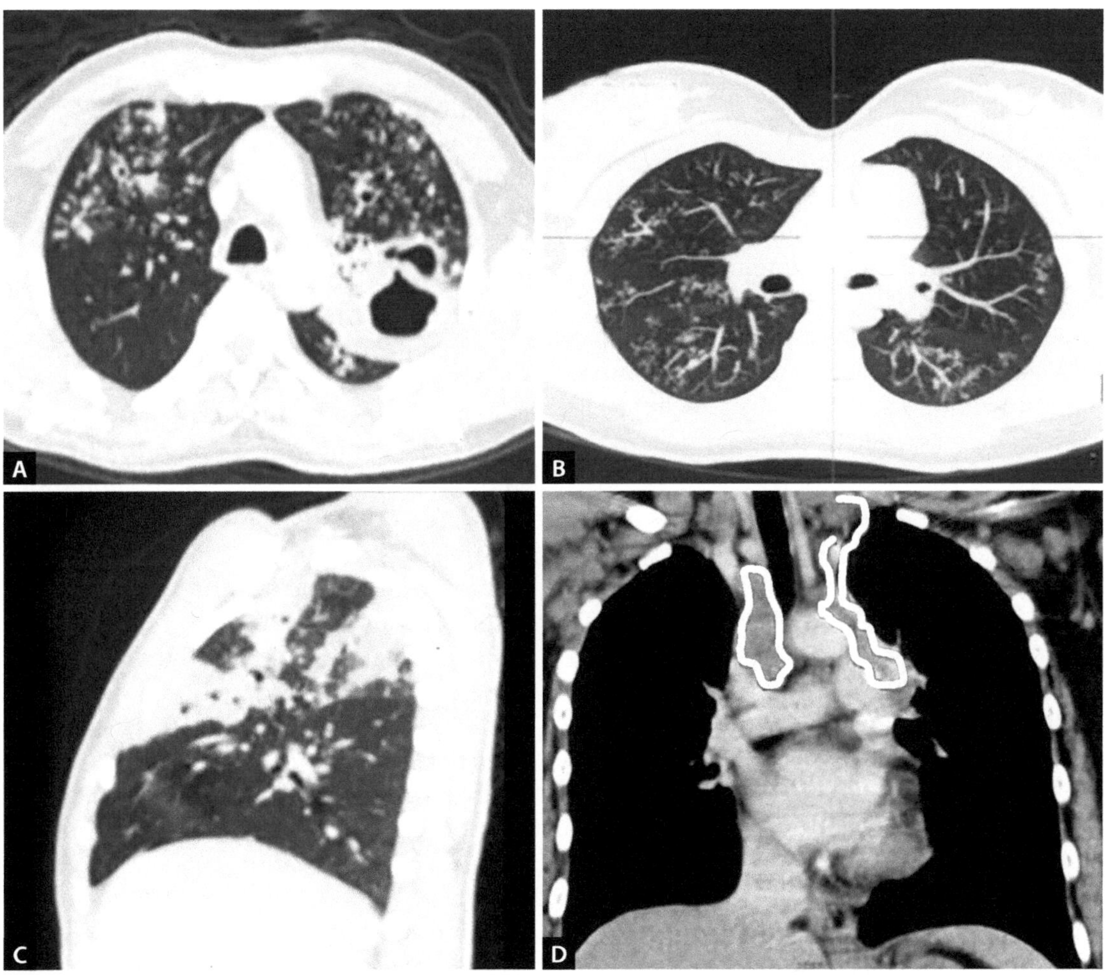

Figs. 2A to D: Computed tomography scan findings in PTTB patients depicting (A) Thick-walled cavitary disease; (B) Tree-in-bud nodules, (C) Consolidation, and (D) Enlarged necrotic mediastinal lymph nodes. (PTTB: post-transplant tuberculosis)

Tuberculin skin testing (TST) using 5 IU of purified protein derivative (tuberculin) has limited utility in diagnosing PTTB on account of the immunological anergy due to use of immunosuppressive medications. The T-SPOT TB and QuantiFERON-TB gold tests are T-cell interferon gamma release assays (IGRAs), which have been evaluated as an alternative to TST. Either of these tests or in combination may be useful for screening of latent TB in pretransplant candidates. However, studies from India have shown that there is poor agreement between these tests in the dialysis population.[16] All these tests cannot differentiate a latent infection from an active infection; they may be false positive in those with prior history of TB or false negative with use of immunosuppressive drugs.[17] A recent change in positivity (earlier documented negative to present positivity) helps in diagnosing TB. Both the IGRA tests have shown some utility in transplant recipients but need further large-scale studies before incorporation into clinical practice. These are more applicable for the diagnosis of latent TB rather than active infection.

MANAGEMENT

The widespread availability of effective antitubercular therapy (ATT) has improved the outcome of patients with TB over the last couple of decades. Though the drug regimens used in normal hosts and immunocompromised hosts are similar, therapy for TB in RTR is fraught with many challenges. The increased risk of drug toxicities and risk of drug–drug interactions require careful individualized planning to improve patient outcomes in RTR.

Conventional ATT therapy is a combination of multiple drugs administered in adequate doses for an appropriate duration. Any deviation from this results in suboptimal outcomes. Therapy is divided into an intensive four-drug phase consisting of isoniazid (INH), RIF, pyrazinamide, and ethambutol for 2 months followed by a continuation phase with INH and RIF for 4 months. Ethambutol has been made a part of the continuation phase (three-drug regimen) in the recent Indian guidelines. In RTR, there are no specific guidelines, and most centers tend to prolong treatment duration to 9–12 months in pulmonary TB and 12–18 months in extrapulmonary TB. This is in line with prior reports wherein treatment duration <9 months increases mortality risk while therapy for >12 months is associated with no recurrence.[18,19] In one large series, treatment duration among transplant recipients ranged from 7.3 months to 18 months revealing the heterogeneity in treatment protocols.[20] Daily dosing is recommended instead of twice or thrice weekly administration in transplant recipients. The European Society of Clinical Microbiology and Infectious Diseases recommends 9 months of therapy if rifamycin is used and 12–18 months of therapy for rifamycin-sparing regimens in solid organ transplant recipients.[21] There is paucity of trials comparing different durations of treatment with anti-TB drugs.

Transplant patients need particular care in the drug regimen as RIF is a potent inducer of cytochrome P450-3A4 enzymes, which is involved in the metabolism of CNI and sirolimus.[22] Being an integral part of the immunosuppressive regimen in RTR, this causes a two- to five-fold decrease in CNI levels which can result in under immunosuppression and allograft rejection. One alternative is to use rifabutin instead of RIF as it is a less potent inducer of microsomal enzymes, which may decrease the degree of induction of enzyme but will not eliminate altogether. Therefore, this would still require modification of CNI dose and constant monitoring of drug levels, which will also increase the overall cost of treatment for RTR. Also, issues with availability and limited experience preclude its use routinely.[23] Quinolones (moxifloxacin/levofloxacin) are the more commonly used alternatives to rifamycin and have proven to be equally effective in managing PTTB, and this is standard of care in most transplant centers in India. Second-line therapy for drug-resistant TB has not been systematically studied in transplant recipients, and hence, individual experiences and case reports are relied upon for managing such patients.[24]

Another issue with rifamycin is that it also affects the level of few antihypertensive agents and can worsen hypertension, which is a common comorbidity in kidney patients and RTR.[25] Therefore, patients requiring multiple antihypertensive drugs may as such become unfit for use of rifamycin.

Multidrug-resistant TB (MDR-TB) refers to *M. tuberculosis* which is resistant to INH and RIF. According to the World Health Organization (WHO), 27 countries account for nearly all of the MDR-TB burden and this includes the Indian subcontinent. Pulmonary TB is the most common form of MDR-TB reported in RTR. Treatment for drug-resistant TB is demanding even in general population with a significant risk of poor compliance due to drug toxicity and prolonged duration of therapy. This is even pronounced in RTR, wherein our experience of treating drug-resistant TB is limited to a couple of case reports and case series. MDR-TB, initially identified by NAAT, should be evaluated by rapid molecular resistance testing to confirm and plan a therapeutic regimen. The WHO recommends starting with at least four anti-TB drugs (based on drug sensitivity) including a parenteral agent during the intensive phase and a total duration of 20 months which is often modified based on response to therapy and treatment compliance.[26] In India, there is a shorter MDR-TB regimen (bedaquiline based) of 9–11 months with 4–6 months of intensive phase followed by continuation phase.[27] The longer MDR-TB regimen is given for 18–20 months and has no separate intensive or continuation phase. Though India has a high burden of MDR-TB, data on treatment and outcome of PTTB are unavailable.

The hepatotoxicity of INH, RIF, and pyrazinamide is a known complication of ATT therapy. Nearly 20% of transplant recipients report varying degrees of hepatotoxicity with these agents and hence require close monitoring.[20] Hepatotoxicity in these patients also requires screening for hepatotropic viral infections, which are common in these patients. The second line agents have more serious toxicities, the most common being nephrotoxicity with aminoglycosides, QT prolongation with quinolones and bedaquiline, and neurotoxicity with cycloserine and ethionamide.

Post-transplant tuberculosis results in significant morbidity and mortality. Graft loss occurs in approximately 25% of transplant recipients with many cases of rejection due to RIF-related CNI drug interactions.[22] The mortality in RTR with TB is reported to be 18–30%, which is appreciably higher than in the general population and also from transplant patients without TB.[11,20] Over the years, there has been a significant decrease in mortality (21–10% in one series) due to TB.[28] There is no data on long-term outcomes in drug-resistant TB in transplant recipients and further studies are required to better understand its impact on patient outcomes.

RECURRENCE OF POST-TRANSPLANT TUBERCULOSIS

Recurrent TB is the diagnosis of TB following treatment completion or cure. It is common in high TB-endemic countries, including India. A recent multicenter study among all sputum-positive PTTB patients revealed a recurrence rate of 10.9% on follow-up.[29] Male patients, diabetics, smokers, and higher degree of sputum AFB positivity have been reported to be risk factors for recurrence.[30] Data on transplant recipients and recurrence of PTTB is lacking. In one of the studies, there was no recurrence of PTTB during 14.6 months of follow-up.[7] Daily regimen of ATT therapy, closer follow-up, and reduced immunological reactivity may be the reasons for reduced recurrence in the transplant setting. The lack of studies in transplant population with longer follow-up limits our data on the true prevalence of recurrent PTTB.

NONTUBERCULOUS MYCOBACTERIA

Being ubiquitous environmental organisms, nontuberculous mycobacteria (NTM) infections are not uncommon in transplant recipients. Over 25 different species have been reported in transplant recipients.[31] Their incidence in RTR ranges between 0.16 and 0.38%.[21] Reports from the Indian subcontinent are limited to a case series and a couple of case reports.[32] The most common presentation is with cutaneous lesions followed by tenosynovitis and arthritis. The clinical suspicion in a patient with AFB who does not respond to ATT points to NTM infection. Longer laborious culture techniques are required to establish the diagnosis. The advent of molecular diagnostics has helped in more rapid diagnosis. Management of NTM disease involves reduction of immunosuppression and surgical drainage/excision with a long course of combination antimicrobial therapy consisting of rifamycins, macrolides, and fluoroquinolones. Drug sensitivity testing is required to tailor the antimicrobial type and duration of therapy.[21]

PREVENTION/CHEMOPROPHYLAXIS IN RENAL TRANSPLANTATION

Considering the high morbidity and mortality associated with PTTB and the diagnostic difficulties, it is prudent to think that treatment of latent TB would be a promising approach. Though there are multiple studies on treatment options for latent TB, data with regard to RTR are limited. The two randomized controlled trials from our subcontinent did show a protective role for INH prophylaxis.[33,34] The study by Agarwal et al. showed a positive trend for protection which was not statistically significant, whereas Naqvi et al.'s study revealed a statistically significant benefit for INH prophylaxis. The only concern in endemic areas is the ability of tests to diagnose latent TB with the tests available today.[16,35] As against low TB-endemic countries, where screening and treatment for latent TB are recommended for all transplant recipients as part of the pretransplant evaluation, only a select subgroup may benefit in high TB-endemic areas.

The choice of therapy is unequivocal with INH being the mainstay of preventive therapy. The various regimens used in transplant recipients are:[3]

- INH for 9 months (6-month/12-month regimen is also tried) with pyridoxine
- RIF for 4 months
- INH + RIF for 3 months (especially in children and adolescents)
- Others: Rifapentine + weekly INH for 3/4 months; rifabutin for 4 months.

CONCLUSION

Tuberculosis in RTR is common and is more challenging to treat than in the general population. Atypical presentations result in diagnostic quandary, and a high index of suspicion is required for timely diagnosis and appropriate management. Microbiological diagnosis is the mainstay of evaluation, and the advent of rapid NAAT has made it easier to diagnose TB. ATT needs to be administered with special attention to drug toxicity and drug–drug interactions. There is a limited role of directly observed therapy (DOT) in these patients. Rifamycin-sparing regimens are the backbone of TB treatment in transplant recipients and are administered for 9–12 months. There are multiple promising new drugs under investigation which may improve the prognosis of transplant patients with TB. The role of chemoprophylaxis is still controversial.

REFERENCES

1. Chakaya J, Khan M, Ntoumi F, Aklillu E, Fatima R, Mwaba P, et al. Global Tuberculosis Report 2020—reflections on the global TB burden, treatment and prevention efforts. Int J Infect Dis. 2021;113:S7-12.

2. Sudre P, ten Dam G, Kochi A. Tuberculosis: a global overview of the situation today. Bull World Health Organ. 1992;70(2):149-59.
3. Subramanian AK, Theodoropoulos NM, Infectious Diseases Community of Practice of the American Society of Transplantation. Mycobacterium tuberculosis infections in solid organ transplantation: guidelines from the infectious diseases community of practice of the American Society of Transplantation. Clin Transplant. 2019;33(9):e13513.
4. Mamishi S, Pourakbari B, Moradzadeh M, van Leeuwen WB, Mahmoudi S. Prevalence of active tuberculosis infection in transplant recipients: a systematic review and meta-analysis. Microb Pathog. 2020;139:103894.
5. Agarwal SK, Bhowmik D, Mahajan S, Bagchi S. Impact of type of calcineurin inhibitor on post-transplant tuberculosis: single-center study from India. Transpl Infect Dis. 2017; 19(1):e12626.
6. John GT, Shankar V, Abraham AM, Mukundan U, Thomas PP, Jacob CK. Risk factors for post-transplant tuberculosis. Kidney Int. 2001;60(3):1148-53.
7. Sakhuja V, Jha V, Varma PP, Joshi K, Chugh KS. The high incidence of tuberculosis among renal transplant recipients in India. Transplantation. 1996;61(2):211-5.
8. Sharma H, Prasad N, Kaul A, Singh DB, Ranjan MP, Ranjan MB, et al. POS-812 factors predicting post renal transplant tuberculosis: a tertiary care centre experience. Kidney Int Rep. 2022;7(2):S348-9.
9. John GT, Shankar V. Mycobacterial infections in organ transplant recipients. Semin Respir Infect. 2002;17(4):274-83.
10. Muñoz P, Rodríguez C, Bouza E. Mycobacterium tuberculosis infection in recipients of solid organ transplants. Clin Infect Dis. 2005;40(4):581-7.
11. Singh N, Paterson DL. Mycobacterium tuberculosis infection in solid-organ transplant recipients: impact and implications for management. Clin Infect Dis. 1998;27(5):1266-77.
12. Lopez de Castilla D, Schluger NW. Tuberculosis following solid organ transplantation. Transpl Infect Dis. 2010;12(2): 106-12.
13. Torre-Cisneros J, Doblas A, Aguado JM, San Juan R, Blanes M, Montejo M, et al. Tuberculosis after solid-organ transplant: incidence, risk factors, and clinical characteristics in the RESITRA (Spanish Network of Infection in Transplantation) cohort. Clin Infect Dis. 2009;48(12):1657-65.
14. Lewinsohn DM, Leonard MK, LoBue PA, Cohn DL, Daley CL, Desmond E, et al. Official American Thoracic Society/ Infectious Diseases Society of America/Centers for Disease Control and Prevention Clinical Practice Guidelines: diagnosis of tuberculosis in adults and children. Clin Infect Dis. 2017;64(2):111-5.
15. Ahmad Z, Bagchi S, Naranje P, Agarwal SK, Das CJ. Imaging spectrum of pulmonary infections in renal transplant patients. Indian J Radiol Imaging. 2020;30(3):273-9.
16. Agarwal SK, Singh UB, Zaidi SH, Gupta S, Pandey RM. Comparison of interferon gamma release assay and tuberculin skin tests for diagnosis of latent tuberculosis in patients on maintenance haemodialysis. Indian J Med Res. 2015;141(4):463-8.
17. Yang Y, Wang H-J, Hu W-L, Bai G-N, Hua C-Z. Diagnostic value of interferon-gamma release assays for tuberculosis in the immunocompromised population. Diagnostics. 2022; 12(2):453.
18. Aguado JM, Herrero JA, Gavaldá J, Torre-Cisneros J, Blanes M, Rufí G, et al. Clinical presentation and outcome of tuberculosis in kidney, liver, and heart transplant recipients in Spain. Spanish Transplantation Infection Study Group, GESITRA. Transplantation. 1997;63(9):1278-86.
19. Park YS, Choi JY, Cho CH, Chang KH, Song YG, Kim YS, et al. Clinical outcomes of tuberculosis in renal transplant recipients. Yonsei Med J. 2004;45(5):865-72.
20. Abad CLR, Razonable RR. Mycobacterium tuberculosis after solid organ transplantation: a review of more than 2000 cases. Clin Transplant. 2018;32(6):e13259.
21. Meije Y, Piersimoni C, Torre-Cisneros J, Dilektasli AG, Aguado JM, ESCMID Study Group of Infection in Compromised Hosts. Mycobacterial infections in solid organ transplant recipients. Clin Microbiol Infect. 2014;20(Suppl. 7): 89-101.
22. Aguado JM, Silva JT, Samanta P, Singh N. Tuberculosis and transplantation. Microbiol Spectr. 2016;4(6).
23. Tabarsi P, Farshidpour M, Marjani M, Baghaei P, Yousefzadeh A, Najafizadeh K, et al. Mycobacterial infection and the impact of rifabutin treatment in organ transplant recipients: a single-center study. Saudi J Kidney Dis Transplant. 2015;26(1):6-11.
24. Abad CL, Razonable RR. Prevention and treatment of tuberculosis in solid organ transplant recipients. Expert Rev Anti Infect Ther. 2020;18(1):63-73.
25. Agrawal A, Agarwal SK, Kaleekal T, Gupta YK. Rifampicin and anti-hypertensive drugs in chronic kidney disease: pharmacokinetic interactions and their clinical impact. Indian J Nephrol. 2016;26(5):322-8.
26. Sharma SK, Dheda K. What is new in the WHO consolidated guidelines on drug-resistant tuberculosis treatment? Indian J Med Res. 2019;149(3):309-12.
27. Saravu K, Pai M. Drug-resistant tuberculosis: progress towards shorter and safer regimens. Lung India. 2019;36(5): 373-5.
28. Sun H-Y, Munoz P, Torre-Cisneros J, Aguado JM, Lattes R, Montejo M, et al. Tuberculosis in solid-organ transplant recipients: disease characteristics and outcomes in the current era. Prog Transplant Aliso Viejo Calif. 2014;24(1):37-43.
29. Velayutham B, Chadha VK, Singla N, Narang P, Gangadhar Rao V, Nair S, et al. Recurrence of tuberculosis among newly diagnosed sputum positive pulmonary tuberculosis patients treated under the Revised National Tuberculosis Control Programme, India: a multi-centric prospective study. PLoS One. 2018;13(7):e0200150.
30. Moosazadeh M, Bahrampour A, Nasehi M, Khanjani N. The incidence of recurrence of tuberculosis and its related factors in smear-positive pulmonary tuberculosis patients in Iran: a retrospective cohort study. Lung India. 2015;32(6):557-60.
31. Piersimoni C. Nontuberculous mycobacteria infection in solid organ transplant recipients. Eur J Clin Microbiol Infect Dis. 2012;31(4):397-403.
32. Alexander S, John GT, Jesudason M, Jacob CK. Infections with atypical mycobacteria in renal transplant recipients. Indian J Pathol Microbiol. 2007;50(3):482-4.
33. Agarwal SK, Gupta S, Dash SC, Bhowmik D, Tiwari SC. Prospective randomised trial of isoniazid prophylaxis in renal transplant recipient. Int Urol Nephrol. 2004;36(3):425-31.
34. Naqvi R, Naqvi A, Akhtar S, Ahmed E, Noor H, Saeed T, et al. Use of isoniazid chemoprophylaxis in renal transplant recipients. Nephrol Dial Transplant. 2010;25(2):634-7.
35. Agarwal SK, Gupta S, Bhowmik D, Mahajan S. Tuberculin skin test for the diagnosis of latent tuberculosis during renal replacement therapy in an endemic area: a single center study. Indian J Nephrol. 2010;20(3):132-6.

12.8 Nocardiosis

Shiv Chadha, Vaibhav Tiwari, Manish Malik, Pallav Gupta

CASE VIGNETTE

A 34-year-old male, who had undergone renal transplantation 2 years back, presented with shortness of breath and high-grade fever of 1-week duration. He was on triple-drug maintenance therapy (prednisolone, tacrolimus, and mycophenolate mofetil).

On evaluation, he was found to be hypotensive [blood pressure (BP) 90/60] and hypoxemic (SpO_2 88%). His laboratory results were significant for leukocytosis (18,000/mm^3) and elevated creatinine level (3.2 mg/dL). His immunosuppression was modified along with intravenous (IV) antibiotics and supportive management was started. His chest computed tomography (CT) scan showed right pleural effusion and consolidation in both parahilar regions with nodular changes in the right upper and middle lobes, left pleural effusion, and consolidation in both parahilar regions with nodular changes in the left upper lobe. Subsequently, his condition deteriorated and was put on mechanical ventilator. Bronchoalveolar lavage (BAL) was done, and BAL fluid showed branched, beaded, filamentous, gram-positive bacilli, weakly acid-fast by modified acid-fast strain suggestive of *Nocardia* species. Later, with the matrix-assisted laser desorption ionization time-of-flight (MALDI-TOF), species identification was done which revealed *Nocardia farcinica.* He was initiated on renal dose-adjusted cotrimoxazole with meropenem. Gradually, his condition improved and he was extubated on sixth day of intensive care unit (ICU) admission. He was discharged after 2 weeks of hospital stay on oral cotrimoxazole for the next 6 months. His last follow-up after 18 months of discharge did not reveal any signs of relapse.

INTRODUCTION

Infectious complications following transplantation can usually be classified according to their time of occurrence. Prolonged and intensive immunosuppression raises the risk of opportunistic infections, and antibiotic prophylaxis is frequently used to lower the risk of the most prevalent illnesses.

During the late post-transplant period (beyond 6 months), transplantation recipients suffer from infections seen in the general community [e.g., community-acquired pneumonia, urinary tract infection (UTI), infection with *Aspergillus*, atypical molds, *Mucor* species, and infection with *Nocardia*].[1]

Nocardiosis is an unprecedented opportunistic infection resulting from *Nocardia* spp., a ubiquitous aerobic actinomycete. *Nocardia* spp. are often aerosolized in dust and inhaled, and a useful immune system is obligatory to clean them.[2,3]

Nocardia can infect immunocompetent patients, but invasive nocardiosis is mostly seen in patients with immune deficiency, such as that caused by corticosteroid therapy, transplantation, human immunodeficiency virus (HIV) infection, cancer, chronic granulomatous disease, or the presence of autoantibodies against granulocyte-macrophage colony-stimulating factor and/or in patients with chronic lung disease.[4]

Solid organ transplantation (SOT) and hematopoietic stem cell transplantation (HSCT) account for 25 and 6% of cases of nocardiosis, respectively.[5]

After organ transplantation, nocardiosis affects 0.04–3.5% (SOT) of patients. The risk of nocardiosis depends on the type of organ transplanted, but the highest infection rate is found in lung transplants (0.8–3.5%) and the lowest infection rate is found in liver and kidney transplants (0.04–1.2%).[4]

After SOT, *Nocardia* infection is a serious infection with a 20% fatality rate.[4] The requirement for long-term treatment (typically 6–12 months) to minimize relapses, as well as the antibiotics' toxicity, especially when paired with immunosuppressive medicines, makes managing these opportunistic infections problematic.[4]

EPIDEMIOLOGY AND RISK FACTORS[6]

The current incidence of nocardiosis after kidney transplantation is lower than previously reported 0.04% (1/2,527) to 0.7% (9/1,255) cases. This tendency is most likely due to factors such as improvement in the patient's general condition as a result of previous transplants and the introduction of trimethoprim-sulfamethoxazole (TMP-SMX) prophylaxis.

Data from India

Incidences of nocardiosis in Indian renal transplants are largely lacking as most of the reports are case reports and case series. A study from Christian Medical College (CMC) Vellore, Tamil Nadu reported an incidence of 1.4% during the 30-year period.[7] All patients had *Nocardia asteroides* in culture. A mortality of 33.3% was recorded in the study.

RISK FACTORS[7]

- Long-term use of corticosteroids (20 mg prednisone per month) or higher doses (>2 pulses of 1 g of methylprednisolone)
- *Cytomegalovirus (CMV) infection in the last 6 months:* Reactivation of CMV occurred in 14–83% of patients with

nocardiosis prior to the onset of the disease. CMV causes further immunosuppression, which increases the risk of opportunistic infections.

- A high median calcineurin inhibitor serum level in the last 30 days (>15 g/mL for tacrolimus or >300 ng/mL for cyclosporine)
- The length of the initial ICU stay following transplantation and the patient's age at the time of diagnosis.

Pediatric nocardiosis appears to be a rare infection, with only 10 pediatric cases in transplanted children.

CLINICAL AND RADIOLOGICAL FEATURES AND PROGNOSIS[5,7-11]

Nocardiosis is the cause of a wide range of clinical and radiological syndromes. Despite the lack of an accepted international classification, in most cases it can be defined as follows:[3]

- Primary cutaneous/subcutaneous
- Invasive nocardiosis

Primary cutaneous nocardiosis accounts for about 10% of all transplant cases and is caused by barefoot walking or, more generally, bacterial inoculation through the contracted skin after gardening. Skin symptoms include limb nodules, pustules, abscesses (single or multiple), and soft-tissue infections (lymphatic cutaneous nocardiosis) that can spread to the lymph nodes.

The most commonly reported species that causes primary cutaneous nocardiosis is *Nippostrongylus brasiliensis, Nocardia nova,* and *Nocardia otitidiscaviarum.* Cutaneous nocardiosis corresponds to either primary cutaneous nocardiosis or disseminated nocardiosis. Clinical and radiological evaluation of possible disseminated signs is essential because there are no specific features that distinguish between primary cutaneous nocardiosis and disseminated nocardiosis with skin lesions.

Invasive nocardiosis accounts for 80–90% of cases and is caused by inhalation of bacteria, most often causing pneumonia. The bacteria can then reach the bloodstream and spread to all organs, including the central nervous system (CNS). Invasive nocardiosis can be defined as lung, CNS, or disseminated nocardiosis. Disseminated infection is defined as the involvement of at least two nonadjacent organs. Lung lesions are found in about 90% of cases of invasive nocardiosis that occur after SOT. Dyspnea may be accompanied by asthenia and low-grade fever. Chest X-ray, or more reliably CT, may show pulmonary infiltrates with pulmonary consolidation, nodules, cups, or less common frosted glassy opacity and thickening of the septum.

Extrapulmonary tuberculosis is described in about one-third of invasive cases, and the most commonly affected site is the CNS. The most typical feature is a brain abscess, which can be single or multiple. Due to its slow development, patients may not show neurological symptoms, emphasizing the crucial importance of systematic radiological assessments such as magnetic resonance imaging (MRI) and CT scans of invasive diseases. Patients may also report frontal lobe signs, seizures, and symptoms associated with intracranial hypertension with or without coma.

PROGNOSIS

After SOT, the mortality rate of nocardiosis is nonuniform and ranges from 0 to 70%, depending on the follow-up period and the patient's general condition. Most frequently, the overall mortality is around 30%.[8,10,12]

DIAGNOSIS[6]

Because clinical or radiological signs are nonspecific, the diagnosis is based on the identification of microorganisms in clinical specimens from pathological sites.[13]

Pus or sputum smears are examined after staining by Gram stain, methenamine silver, and acid-fast techniques for the narrow (<1 μm) branching hyphae, which are only partially acid-fast. Cultures of *N. asteroides* can be obtained on Sabouraud's glucose agar and on other isolation media from which antibacterial antibiotics are withheld. Colonies are compact, folded, and glabrous, ranging from cream to red.

Respiratory specimens are essential for the diagnosis of nocardiosis, as lung lesions occur in about 90% of the cases and should include sputum, bronchial aspirates, and pleural effusion, if any.

Bronchoalveolar lavage should be performed due to the wide differential diagnosis spectrum and the high frequency of coinfection. If negative, especially for nodular pneumonia, a transbronchial or puncture biopsy should be considered.

Nocardia can spread to virtually any organ, so a variety of probes can be used: Blood culture, skin biopsy, or biopsy from the affected area.

Histopathology

The bacteria induce a mixed acute abscess and granulomatous response with fibrosis. Occasionally, the bacteria are clumped together with a surrounding Hoeppli-Splendore (HS) reaction. More often, they are more loosely dispersed and resemble *Actinomyces species.* Hematoxylin and eosin (H&E) stains demonstrate the bacilli poorly. They are 1 μm in diameter, filamentous, branching, beaded, gram-positive, Grocott silver positive, and usually weakly acid fast, but modified Ziehl–Neelsen stain can help in visualization **(Figs. 1A and B)**. This latter feature assists in the distinction of *Nocardia* from *Actinomyces* and related bacilli; specific antisera with immunocytochemistry are also helpful, and culture is definitive. The shape of the organisms distinguishes them from mycobacteria. The Grocott silver method is the most sensitive screening stain for nocardiosis.

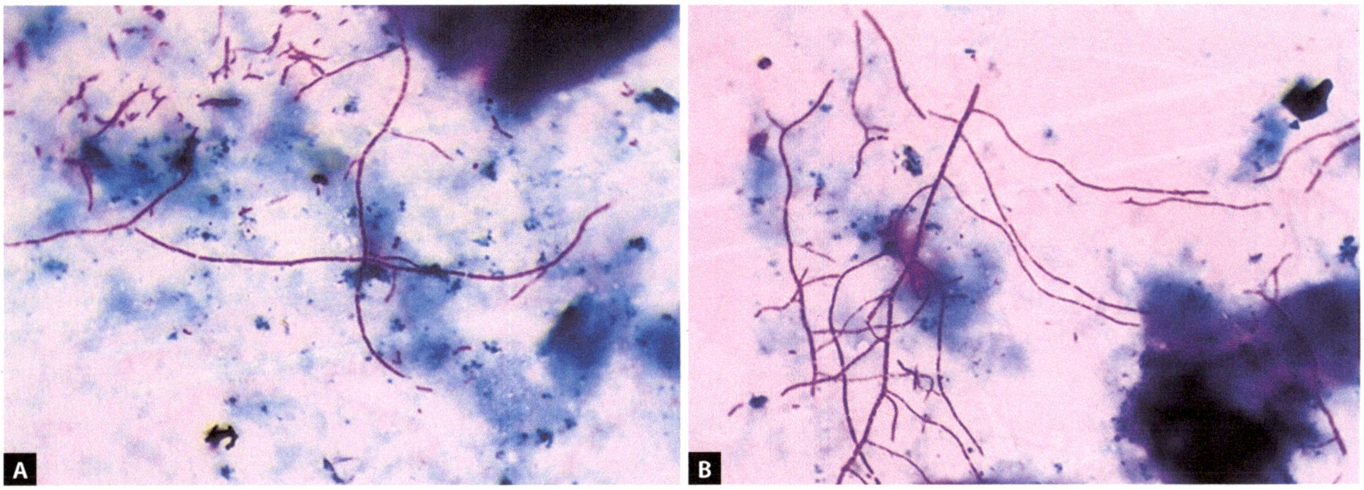

Figs. 1A and B: Modified ZN Stain showing slender acid fast filamentous organism, few of which also show branching.

Polymerase Chain Reaction

Microbiologically, the two conventional diagnostic techniques (i.e., microscopy and culture) have a number of limitations. First, suggestive branching filamentous organisms may not be visible under microscopy despite the presence of culture-proven nocardiosis. Second, cultures may be negative if the incubation time is not long enough (e.g., <2 weeks). *Nocardia* polymerase chain reaction (PCR)-based assay may help transplant physicians to identify *Nocardia* in a rapid and culture-dependent manner. BAL samples can be used for PCR assay, but the result should be interpreted with great caution as it lacks specificity for the diagnosis of invasive pulmonary nocardiosis due to the fact that *Nocardia* airway colonization may lead to positive PCR result.

Antibiotic susceptibility testing (AST) has historically been evaluated using antibiotic disc diffusion on agar plates. Due to the difficulty of interpreting the results, the guidelines of the Clinical and Laboratory Standards Institute (CLSI) consider the determination of the minimum inhibitory concentration (MIC) of microdilution of broth to be the gold standard. Interpretation of the MIC in broth microdilution is difficult and has many technical and interpretation pitfalls.

Due to their severe immunosuppression, transplant patients are exposed to a wide range of opportunistic pathogens. There are no specific signs of nocardiosis, so physicians should keep in mind the diagnosis of nocardiosis until microbiological evidence is available.

Another risk is the high prevalence of coinfection reported in 20–64% of cases of nocardiosis. In fact, 7 of the 35 cases of nocardiosis after SOT (20%) had at least one coinfection, including CMV infection, invasive fungal infection, and bacterial infection. CNS coinfection is an important factor and should be considered if it is clinically exacerbated despite the use of appropriate antibiotics.

WORKUP OF NOCARDIOSIS AFTER TRANSPLANTATION[6]

In suspected nocardiosis patients, the chief work-up includes identifying its degree of involvement with various tissues. Primarily it is classified based on either localized cutaneous/subcutaneous disease or pulmonary involvement with or without dissemination.

If the disease is localized (cutaneous or subcutaneous), a skin biopsy is conducted and later confirmed for either bacterial/mycobacterial or histology examination along with culture examination (Gram staining).

When only pulmonary involvement is seen, specimens from sputum, pleural fluid, and bronchial aspirate/BAL are taken and examined for bacterial examination along with culture. If negative and nodular pneumonia is seen, we need to consider transbronchial or percutaneous lung biopsy.

Treatment[6]

Once *Nocardia* is identified in a clinical specimen, antibacterial treatment is usually initiated before detailed microbiological information such as species identification or AST is available. This initial antibiotic regimen is referred to as "probabilistic treatment."

For Patients of Pulmonary Nocardiosis

- *Stable patient:* Given a single-drug regimen of TMP–SMX or linezolid or multiple-drug regimen of two drugs (imipenem/amikacin) or (TMP–SMX/amikacin) or (TMP–SMX/imipenem) or (TMP–SMX/cefotaxime) or (cefotaxime/amikacin)
- *Critical patients:* Multiple-drug regimen of two drugs as mentioned above is followed.

For Patients with Cutaneous Nocardiosis

For patients of cutaneous nocardiosis, single-drug regimen of TMP–SMX or linezolid is followed.

TABLE 1: Recommended first-line antibiotics against *Nocardia* spp.

Features	*TMP–SMX*	*IMP*	*AMK*	*LZD*	*CTX*	*CRO*
Total daily dose (invasive)	15 (10–20) mg TMP/kg/day	2–3 g/day	15 mg/kg/day	1,200 mg/day	3–12 g/day	2 g/day
Total daily dose (primary cutaneous)	10 mg TMP/kg/day	1.5 g/day	15 mg/kg/day			
Route of administration	PO or IV	IV	IV	PO or IV	IV	IV
Main side effects	Bone marrow suppression, urinary lithiasis	Seizures	Nephrotoxicity	Bone marrow suppression, peripheral neuropathy, lactic acidosis	Nephrotoxicity	

(AMK: amikacin; CRO: ceftriaxone; CTX: cefotaxime; IMP: imipenem; IV: intravenous; LZD: linezolid; TMP–SMX: trimethoprim–sulfamethoxazole)

For Patients with Disseminated Nocardiosis

For patients of disseminated nocardiosis or in which CNS involvement is seen, multiple-drug regimen of two to three drugs including TMP–SMX/amikacin/cefotaxime or TMP–SMX/amikacin/imipenem or imipenem/amikacin or TMP–SMX/amikacin or TMP–SMX/imipenem is followed.

Only five antibiotics can be recommended as first-line medicines against *Nocardia* spp., based on their broad spectrum of action **(Table 1)**.[1,2,4,14-17]

Trimethoprim–Sulfamethoxazole[1-3,6]

- Sulfonamide has been the drug of choice since the 1940s, and TMP-SMX has been prescribed for nocardiosis.
- TMP–SMX reaches high tissue concentrations in the brain, bones, skin, lungs, etc., and is effective against all *Nocardia* species.
- However, common side effects such as allergies, gastrointestinal disorders, nephrotoxicity, and myelosuppression can lead to discontinuation of treatment in 20–50% of cases. It has also been reported to interfere with cyclosporine and increase the risk of nephrotoxicity. Do not use as monotherapy for severe or disseminated disease due to high mortality.
- In case of clinical deterioration, bactericidal antibiotics should also be suggested. Among them, imipenem and amikacin can be considered for their broad-spectrum activity in vitro and their effect on in vivo models of brain or lung nocardiosis.

When CNS is involved, a probabilistic three-drug regimen has been proposed to address the situation of imipenem-resistant strains that can only be treated with amikacin with a two-drug regimen before obtaining the results of AST (imipenem/amikacin, etc.).

Do not use ertapenem as it is less active against *Nocardia* spp. Do not use even if imipenem has been shown to be active in vitro. Meropenem should only be used after a thorough in vitro evaluation of its efficacy, as strains sensitive to imipenem may also be resistant to meropenem.

Linezolid has been advocated more recently because no resistant strain has been found.[18,19] This drug's major properties are high CNS penetration and oral bioavailability. Overall, favorable result rates of >80% have been discovered. Unfortunately, in cases of long-term treatment, neurological or hematological tolerance may limit the usage of this medicine.[16]

Oral Therapy after Intravenous Induction

Oral therapy after IV induction can be either monotherapy or combination therapy. In patients without CNS involvement, oral monotherapy (usually after 3–6 weeks) usually suffices.

In patients with CNS disease and/or multiorgan involvement, particularly if there is also immunocompromise, a combination of oral therapy is preferred after a minimum of 6 weeks of IV therapy and clear evidence of clinical improvement. Patients who are switched to oral therapy should be closely monitored to confirm a continued clinical response.

Oral antibiotic regimens for patients with preserved renal function include the following:

- Sulfonamide (e.g., TMP-SMX 10 mg/kg of the trimethoprim component per day in two or three divided doses) and/or
- Minocycline (100 mg twice daily) and/or
- Amoxicillin–clavulanate (875 mg twice daily).

Dosing must be adjusted in patients with impaired renal function.

Duration of Treatment

A prolonged treatment course is usually required because of the relapsing nature of *Nocardia* infection. In immunocompetent patients with isolated cutaneous infection, treatment duration should be 3–6 months but in immunocompromised patients it should be for 6–12 months. However, in patients with CNS involvement, the treatment duration should be at least 1 year. IV therapy is required to be continued for at least 6 weeks and until clinical improvement has occurred; in contrast, immunocompetent patients may be successfully treated with a shorter duration of IV therapy.

The total duration of the therapy is dependent on the severity of the disease and response to treatment.

Drug Interactions[14]

- Drug-drug interactions between antibiotics and immunosuppressive drugs highlight potential problems. The main problem is coprescribing with cyclosporine, tacrolimus, or mammalian target of rapamycin (m-TOR) inhibitors by interacting with the hepatic cytochrome P450 enzyme.
- Switching from initial treatment to oral treatment is possible after at least 2 weeks of IV treatment, but all of the following criteria must be met:
  - *Reliable strain characterization:* AST and/or species identification
  - Clinical improvement
  - Strains sensitive to at least one drug with good oral bioavailability and penetration into the site of infection
  - No worries about digestion and absorption [e.g., graft vs host disease (GVHD), mucositis]
  - No intolerance to the selected drug

Tetracycline should be avoided in patients under the age of 8 years because of the possible toxicity of teeth and bones in the presence of childhood nocardiosis. For the failure of deep abscess or antibiotic treatment alone, surgical treatment should be considered.

CONCLUSION

Nocardiosis following transplantation is an uncommon and serious disease with numerous challenges and unanswered concerns that must be addressed in order to enhance care.

Whole-genome sequencing will likely become commonplace on the patient side in the near future, and 18F-fluorodeoxyglucose (18F-FDG) positron emission tomography (PET)/CT imaging may be used to customize antibiotic durations, minimizing the risk of antibiotic-related side effects.

Finally, immunomonitoring (such as the validation of a phenotypic test measuring the level of drug-induced immunosuppression) may be used to help transplanted patients determine their risk of opportunistic infections on an individual basis.

REFERENCES

1. Cawcutt K, Zimmer A. Management of infection in patients with kidney transplant. Crit Care Nephrol. 2019:552-60. el.
2. Brown-Elliott BA, Brown JM, Conville PS, Wallace Jr RJ. Clinical and laboratory features of the *Nocardia spp.* based on current molecular taxonomy. Clin Microbiol Rev. 2006;19(2):259-82.
3. Ambrosioni J, Lew D, Garbino J. Nocardiosis: updated clinical review and experience at a tertiary center. Infection. 2010;38(2):89-97.
4. Coussement J, Lebeaux D. Nocardia infection in solid organ transplant recipients: a multicenter European case-control study. Clin Infect Dis. 2016;63(3):338-45.
5. Minero MV, Marín M, Cercenado E, Rabadán PM, Bouza E, Muñoz P. Nocardiosis at the turn of the century. Medicine (Baltimore). 2009;88(4):250-61.
6. Lebeaux D, Morelon E, Suarez F, Lanternier F, Scemla A, Frange P, et al. Nocardiosis in transplant recipients. Eur J Clin Microbiol Infect Dis. 2014;33(5):689-702.
7. Peleg AY, Husain S, Qureshi ZA, Silveira FP, Sarumi M, Shutt KA, et al. Risk factors, clinical characteristics, and outcome of Nocardia infection in organ transplant recipients: a matched case-control study. Clin Infect Dis. 2007;44(10):1307-14.
8. Santos M, Gil-Brusola A, Morales P. Infection by *Nocardia* in solid organ transplantation: thirty years of experience. Transplant Proc. 2011;43(6):2141-4.
9. Farina C, Boiron P, Goglio A, Provost F. Human nocardiosis in northern Italy from 1982 to 1992. Northern Italy Collaborative Group on Nocardiosis. Scand J Infect Dis. 1995;27(1):23-7.
10. Arduino RC, Johnson PC, Miranda AG. Nocardiosis in renal transplant recipients undergoing immunosuppression with cyclosporine. Clin Infect Dis. 1993;16(4):505-12.
11. Welsh O, Vera-Cabrera L, Welsh E, Salinas MC. Actinomycetoma and advances in its treatment. Clin Dermatol. 2012;30(4):372-81.
12. Poonyagariyagorn HK, Gershman A, Avery R, Minai O, Blazey H, Asamoto K, et al. Challenges in the diagnosis and management of Nocardia infections in lung transplant recipients. Transpl Infect Dis. 2008;10(6):403-8.
13. Clark NM, Reid GE, AST Infectious Diseases Community of Practice. Nocardia infections in solid organ transplantation. Am J Transplant. 2013;13(Suppl 4):83-92.
14. Rubin RH, Ikonen T, Gummert JF, Morris RE. The therapeutic prescription for the organ transplant recipient: the linkage of immunosuppression and antimicrobial strategies. Transpl Infect Dis. 1999;1(1):29-39.
15. Wallace Jr RJ, Septimus EJ, Williams Jr TW, Conklin RH, Satterwhite TK, Bushby MB, et al. Use of trimethoprim-sulfamethoxazole for treatment of infections due to Nocardia. Rev Infect Dis. 1982;4(2):315-25.
16. Moylett EH, Pacheco SE, Brown-Elliott BA, Perry TR, Buescher ES, Birmingham MC, et al. Clinical experience with linezolid for the treatment of Nocardia infection. Clin Infect Dis. 2003;36(3):313-8.
17. Shen T, Wu L, Geng L, Wei Z, Zheng S. Successful treatment of pulmonary *Nocardia farcinica* infection with linezolid: case report and literature review. Braz J Infect Dis. 2011;15(5):486-9.
18. Tanioka K, Nagao M, Yamamoto M, Matsumura Y, Tabu H, Matsushima A, et al. Disseminated Nocardia farcinica infection in a patient with myasthenia gravis successfully treated by linezolid: a case report and literature review. J Infect Chemother. 2012;18(3):390-4.
19. Brown-Elliott BA, Ward SC, Crist CJ, Mann LB, Wilson RW, Wallace Jr RJ. In vitro activities of linezolid against multiple *Nocardia* species. Antimicrob Agents Chemother. 2001;45(4):1295-7.

CHAPTER

13

Noninfectious Complications

13.1 Cardiovascular Disease in Kidney Transplant Recipients

Jony Agarwal, Shahzad Alam, Amit Gupta

CASE VIGNETTE 1

1. *A 53-year-old female with no history of coronary artery disease (CAD) underwent live related renal transplant, ABO-compatible, donor-sister, on triple immunosuppression [steroids, tacrolimus, and mycophenolate mofetil (MMF)]. Her nadir creatinine was 0.9 mg/dL, and liver functions were normal. Introduction of which drug after transplant in kidney transplant recipients (KTR) has shown to reduce cardiovascular (CV) risk?*
   a. β-blockers
   b. Aspirin
   c. Statins
   d. Angiotensin-converting enzyme inhibitors/angiotensin-receptor blockers (ACEi/ARBs)
   e. Folic acid and multivitamins

CASE VIGNETTE 2

A 43-year-old male, nondiabetic underwent live-related renal transplant, induction-antithymocyte globulin (ATG), donor-wife, on triple immunosuppression (steroids, tacrolimus, and MMF). On postoperative day 3 of renal transplant, he had uncontrolled glycemic status. How will you manage the condition?

a. Lifestyle modification
b. Modification of immunosuppression
c. Only insulin
d. Insulin and oral hypoglycemic agents (OHAs)
e. All of the above

INTRODUCTION

Cardiovascular diseases (CVD) account for the highest (33%) cause of death in individuals with a working transplant kidney.[1] The risk of CVD is predicted to be 10–20 times higher in patients who get regular hemodialysis than in the general population.[2] While a successful transplant can considerably minimize this risk, kidney transplant recipients (KTR) still have a 3.5–5% annual CV event rate.[3] KTR have around four times higher mortality after the first year when compared with the general population.[4] CVD is usually a continuum of pre-existing cardiac diseases in dialysis patients, which along with conventional risk factors such as diabetes, hypertension and transplant-specific risks such as surgery, immunosuppression, and rejections contribute to increased CV risk. In this chapter, we provide insight, especially into conventional modifiable risk factors, which contribute to increased CV risk, the spectrum of CV diseases, and also some of the possible measures that may be undertaken to reduce the risk.

RISK FACTORS AND PATHOPHYSIOLOGY

Numerous risk factors predispose to CVD, which may be categorized into pre-chronic kidney disease (CKD) risk factors (modifiable and nonmodifiable), hemodialysis-related specific risk, and post-transplant risk **(Table 1)**. The interplay of these risk factors contributes to coronary heart disease, pulmonary hypertension, arrhythmias, valvular heart disease, and heart failure, among other CV disorders. According to studies, control of these parameters is generally poor in KTR.

Structural heart disease is more common after transplant, which is a result of abnormal vascular calcification contributed by abnormal bone mineral disorder in CKD patients.[5] This contributes to accelerated atherosclerosis, decreased vascular compliance, and increased vascular stiffening, which further leads to hypertension, left ventricular hypertrophy (LVH), ischemic vascular disease, and ultimately congestive cardiac failure (CCF).[6]

TABLE 1: Comparison of cardiovascular risk factors among general population, patients on dialysis, and postrenal transplant recipients.

	General population	*On dialysis*	*Post-transplant*
Pre-CKD risk			
• *Conventional modifiable*			
– Hypertension	+	+++	++
– Diabetes	+	+	++
– Dyslipidemia	+	++	+++
– Smoking	+	+	+
– Metabolic syndrome	++	+	+++
• *Nonmodifiable*			
– Age	++	+	++
– Race	+	+	+
– Family history	+	+	+
– Gender (♂ > ♀)	+	+	+
Hemodialysis-related specific risk			
Left ventricular hypertrophy	±	++	+
Proteinuria	±	++	+
Low albumin	±	++	+
Inflammatory markers CRP/IL-2 and IL-6	±	++	+
HD vintage	–	++	+
Obstructive sleep apnea	±	++	+
Deranged coagulation profile	±	++	+
↓ GFR	±	++	+
↓ Physical activity	±	++	+
Coronary calcification	±	++	+
Hyperuricemia	±	++	+
BMD	±	++	+
Post-transplant risk			
Post-transplant new-onset diabetes	–	–	+
Acute rejections	–	–	+
Immunosuppression medications	–	–	+
Delayed graft function	–	–	+
New-onset dyslipidemia	–	–	+
CMV and other infections	±	±	+
Donor age	–	–	+
Donor hypertension	–	–	+
Donor proteinuria	–	–	+
Size mismatch	–	–	+
Donor APOL-1	–	–	+

(APOL-1: apolipoprotein L1; BMD: bone mineral disorder; CKD: chronic kidney disease; CMV: cytomegalovirus; CRP: C-reactive protein; GFR: glomerular filtration rate; HD: hemodialysis; IL: interleukin)

SCREENING FOR CARDIOVASCULAR DISEASE IN RENAL TRANSPLANT CANDIDATES

Patients with end-stage kidney disease (ESKD) have a much higher risk of CAD than the general population.[7] Many people with CAD are asymptomatic and have no clinical symptoms of heart ischemia, making diagnosis difficult. The purpose of a pretransplant assessment is to search for the presence of any active heart disease. As a result, patients undergoing kidney transplantation (KT) must have a proper medical history and physical assessment. Except for those undergoing low-risk surgery, the updated American College of Cardiology/American Heart Association (ACC/AHA) guidelines recommend that a 12-lead electrocardiogram (ECG) be considered in asymptomatic patients without a history of CAD.[8] They also recommend that noninvasive stress testing should be done only for kidney transplant candidates with three or more CAD risk factors, regardless of functional status.[9] However, because of the increased risk of CAD in patients with ESKD, noninvasive stress testing has become a standard in patients being assessed for KT, with the goal of detecting occult CAD and minimizing perioperative cardiac risk. Studies have shown that noninvasive stress testing is sensitive enough for the detection of significant CAD. However, no studies have shown a survival benefit in patients undergoing stress testing for asymptomatic CAD.[10,11] Prior to surgery, coronary revascularization to minimize perioperative cardiac events is not advised in the general population. Over 500 patients with stable CAD who needed elective vascular surgery were randomly assigned to either medical therapy alone or medical therapy with revascularization in the CARP (Coronary Artery Revascularization Prophylaxis) trial, which found no difference in mortality between the two groups.[12] Revascularization should only be performed prior to transplantation in patients for whom it is suggested by current clinical practice recommendations.[9] Also, guidelines recommend delaying elective noncardiac surgery after revascularization until a full course of dual antiplatelet medication has been completed with the aim of reducing perioperative bleeding and the need for transfusion.[8] They advise waiting at least a year following the placement of a drug-eluting stent before doing elective surgery; however, newer data suggest that surgery after 6 months may be possible with no increased risk. The European Society of Cardiology (ESC) and the ACC/AHA suggest that patients who have had coronary artery stenting continue to take 75–100 mg of aspirin daily. A number of studies, including systematic reviews, have looked into the role of perioperative medical therapy. β-blockade maintenance has been demonstrated to be advantageous in several observational studies in the general population,[13-15] and the ACC/AHA and ESC have recommended it.[8,9,16] Similarly, statins should be continued during the perioperative phase, according to these recommendations.

CHAPTER HIGHLIGHTS

- CVDs are associated with significant morbidity and mortality in KTR.
- Conventional risk factors such as diabetes and hypertension along with transplant—specific risk factors such as immunosuppression and rejections contribute to CVD.
- Early identification and treatment of risk factors are key to therapy.
- Lifestyle modification, immunosuppression modification (balancing against risk of rejection), and pharmacotherapy form the pillars of treatment.
- More research is needed in this area along with multidisciplinary approach to yield better results for our KTR.

SPECTRUM OF CARDIOVASCULAR DISEASES

Coronary Artery Disease

Kidney transplant recipients are more likely to develop CAD as compared to the general population. The role of stress test for primary or secondary prevention in the post-transplant period is controversial. However, revascularization therapies such as percutaneous coronary intervention (PCI) or coronary artery bypass grafting (CABG) can be undertaken without the risk of renal graft injury or loss.[17] Biomarkers such as cardiac troponins may help in CV risk stratification. They are higher in conditions such as volume overload, uncontrolled hypertension, and LVH, all of which put a patient at risk of CV problems.[18] Persistent elevation of cardiac troponin T has been linked to an elevated risk of death after transplant and significant adverse CV events, according to Mayo Clinic research.[19] The Framingham risk score is a broad population indicator for predicting coronary heart disease, but its role in kidney transplant patients is unclear as it usually underestimates the risk of adverse CV events.[20,21]

The key to treatment is screening and observation. According to Kidney Disease Improving Global Outcomes (KDIGO) guidelines, KTR should be treated for CVD "at least as rigorously as the general population, including appropriate diagnostic tests and therapies."[3] A few trials have been done regarding the treatment, but an extensive study on KTR is still awaited. Data from the Assessment of Lescol in Renal Transplantation (ALERT) study did not show any benefit in its primary CV end point, but follow-up studies of the ALERT trial have shown a 35% relative reduction in cardiac death, nonfatal myocardial infarct, and stroke with fluvastatin therapy, thus suggesting a beneficial role of statins in KTR.[22] However, there was no significant effect on the incidence of renal graft loss or doubling of serum creatinine or death. Considering the benefits, statins should be initiated and continued in transplant patients with CAD. The role of aspirin for primary prevention lacks randomized controlled trials (RCTs). The FAVORIT (Folic Acid for Vascular Outcome Reduction in Transplantation) trial using folic acid and the post hoc analysis of FAVORIT trial using aspirin did not show any benefit on CVD or mortality outcomes.[23]

Heart Failure

After a kidney transplant, the most common cause of CVD-related hospitalization is congestive heart failure (CHF). In a study by Lentine et al., obesity and anemia emerged as the most prominent risk factors for CCF. The incidence was higher in females.[24] LVH decreases after renal transplant as evident by a decrease in left ventricular mass and volume on echocardiography[25,26] which may be due to better volume control, due to decrease in anemia, and in some cases, also closure of the arteriovenous fistula.[27] However, after a renal transplant, the risk of developing de novo heart failure increases. There is dysfunction of the cardiorenal axis along with global longitudinal strain (an echocardiographic marker of left ventricular function) that continues even after a transplant, leading to acute myocardial infarction (AMI), ventricular dilation, and arrhythmias in heart failure patients.[28,29] De novo heart failure after transplant should be diagnosed in the same way as it is in the general population, which includes a CAD examination. Pretransplant levels of the N-terminal prohormone B-type natriuretic peptide (NT-proBNP) are linked to post-transplant mortality, but post-transplant levels of NT-proBNP are linked to LVH.[30,31] There is currently no evidence that NT-proBNP can be used to aid diagnosis or treatment of de novo heart failure after a transplant. Heart failure treatment guidelines are comparable to those used for the general population.[32] In most studies, anemia is linked to heart failure in KTR.[24] However, the use of parenteral iron or hypoxia-inducible factor prolyl hydroxylase inhibitors in KTR has not been studied.[32]

Arrhythmias and Structural Heart Disease

Kidney transplant recipients have preexisting abnormal cardiac myocytes due to uremia, electrolyte, and volume disturbances in the CKD period, which predispose to an increased risk of arrhythmias and sudden cardiac death. Atrial fibrillation after a transplant is associated with dysfunction and even loss of graft.[33] Anticoagulation after stroke risk assessment should be started, but the risk of drug-drug interaction should be borne in mind. Usage of novel oral anticoagulants needs further study.[34]

In the setting of ESKD, structural heart disease, particularly valvular heart disease, is frequent, with a fivefold higher incidence in dialysis patients than in the general population.[35] It is unclear whether KT slows disease development, but research suggests that valvular disease hospitalizations are less common after KT.[36] Despite this, valvular illness in kidney transplant patients frequently necessitates intervention, which most typically concerns the aortic valve.[37]

Pulmonary Hypertension

Pulmonary hypertension is seen in post-transplant patients and is defined as a mean arterial pressure of >25 mm Hg at rest. The incidence is higher in patients who are on hemodialysis with an arteriovenous fistula as compared to those on dialysis from a catheter or on peritoneal dialysis.[38] After renal transplant, pulmonary hypertension may improve as fluid overload status, LVH, and heart failure tend to improve. Transthoracic echocardiography, which is less expensive as well as noninvasive, is the screening test of choice in symptomatic patients. The 2012 AHA/ ACC guidelines on the evaluation of cardiac disease in KTR recommend right heart catheterization in candidates with pulmonary artery systolic pressure (PASP) >50 mm Hg since echocardiographic estimates of PASP may be erroneous.[39]

Evidence-based treatment is difficult as trials of pulmonary hypertension exclude the transplant population. Treatment guidelines as in the general population can be followed. Also, improvement in symptomatic pulmonary hypertension after arteriovenous fistula ligation might be seen as reported in small case series.[40]

IDENTIFICATION AND TREATMENT OF CONVENTIONAL MODIFIABLE RISK FACTORS

Hypertension

The incidence of hypertension in KTR ranges from 70 to 90%.[41] It is exacerbated by immunosuppressive medicines, such as calcineurin inhibitors (CNI)[42] **(Table 2)**, graft dysfunction, and transplant renal artery stenosis (TRAS). Hypertension, in turn, raises the risk of CVD and death.[41,43] According to Kasiske et al., each 10 mm Hg increase in systolic blood pressure (SBP) is linked to an 18% increase in the chance of death in KTR.[41]

In around 55.5% of recipients, SBP was 140 mm Hg or higher after 1 year in the Collaborative Transplant Study.[44] Despite the rising prevalence of hypertension and its link to negative CV outcomes, the ideal blood pressure (BP) target is uncertain, while experts frequently advocate 130/80 mm Hg.[3,45] Regardless of the severity of albuminuria, the KDIGO guidelines recommend a BP goal of <130/80 mm Hg for KTR.

Management

- Treatment of the underlying cause and underlying associated risk factors such as high body mass index (BMI) and increased immunosuppression.
- Perioperative β-blockers reduce CV events in patients with a history of CAD but lack controlled clinical trials.
- The evidence base currently available is insufficient to recommend one antihypertensive agent over another in KTR. Nondihydropyridine calcium channel blockers (CCBs) are commonly used. However, the optimum antihypertensive medicine is uncertain. Diltiazem and verapamil help in the reduction of intraglomerular pressure and also permit a reduction in CNI doses.
- Diuretics are also used in patients with volume expansion.
- ACEi and ARBs are not used immediately after transplant as these drugs can cause acute renal allograft dysfunction[46,47] and hyperkalemia as well. They are initiated when the graft's function becomes stable or proteinuria of >1 g/day is present.[3,45] Regardless of which antihypertensive drug(s) are used, the goal should be to maintain adequate BP control in order to improve graft and patient survival.
- TRAS should be kept as a possibility when serum creatinine rises to >30% above baseline, and occasionally correcting graft renal artery or iliac artery stenosis is related to improved graft performance and lowering of BP.
- Bilateral native nephrectomy has been found to regulate BP in patients who have failed to respond to medical therapy.[48]

TABLE 2: Effects of immunosuppression medications on cardiovascular risk factors.

	Cardiovascular risk factor			
Immunosuppression medication	***Hypertension***	***Post-transplant diabetes mellitus***	***Dyslipidemia***	***Renal dysfunction***
Steroids	–	✓	✓	–
Tacrolimus	✓	✓	✓	✓
Cyclosporine	✓	✓	✓	✓
Mycophenolate mofetil	–	–	–	–
Azathioprine	–	–	–	–
mTOR inhibitor	–	✓	✓	✓

(–) has no effect on the incidence or severity of the risk factor.
(mTOR: mammalian target of rapamycin)

Diabetes

New-onset diabetes after transplantation (NODAT) is a frequent complication of KT that affects 10–40% of recipients.[49] It is linked to a lower rate of survival after KT, owing to an increase in CV morbidity and mortality.[49,50] As a result, a pretransplant assessment of a candidate's risk of developing NODAT is recommended in order to undertake risk-reduction methods. Fasting blood glucose, glycated hemoglobin (HbA1c), or an oral glucose tolerance test (OGT) can all be used to screen for undiagnosed diabetes mellitus (DM) and impaired glucose tolerance. Although fasting blood glucose is an insensitive test for the diagnosis of NODAT and of diabetes among ESKD patients,[51,52] high fasting blood glucose levels are an indication for OGT during candidate screening. Thus, despite the cost, inconvenience, and potential for day-to-day variability, the use of an OGT may be considered the gold standard for demonstrating pretransplant glycemic status and predicting NODAT.[53]

Calcineurin inhibitors, steroids **(Table 2)**, deceased donor grafts, older recipient age, presence of hypertension, obesity, or significant post-transplant weight increase are all known risk factors. Each clinic visit should include a dipstick urinalysis and blood glucose measurement to check for NODAT. NODAT is diagnosed using conventional American Diabetic Association/World Health Organization (ADA/WHO) guidelines.

Management

Diabetes control in KTR is difficult and frequently necessitates the assistance of a diabetologist.[54] Treatment includes lifestyle changes, modification of immunosuppression, and pharmacotherapy. The KDIGO guidelines suggest an HbA1c target of 7–7.5%, whereas the ADA standards suggest an HbA1c target of <7%.

- Lifestyle modifications include dietary restriction, aerobic exercise, and weight reduction. EXPRED (Exercise and Prediabetes after Transplantation) is an ongoing study that examines the ability of exercise to reverse prediabetes in patients who have been transplanted for at least 12 months.[55]
- *Modification of immunosuppression:* Corticosteroids increase insulin resistance,[56] while CNIs, particularly tacrolimus, cause more diabetes than cyclosporine and affect the pancreatic B cells.[57] In individuals with tacrolimus-induced NODAT, a recent clinical trial assessed the efficacy and safety of switching to cyclosporine.[58] Wissing et al. studied 87 people with NODAT who were given the option of switching to cyclosporine A or continuing tacrolimus.[58] Surprisingly, a change in medication resulted in the reversibility of diabetes in 34% of instances, especially in those treated with lifestyle modification. However, any change in immunosuppression, whether steroid avoidance or changing from tacrolimus to cyclosporine, is not risk-free and may increase the risk of rejection.
- *Pharmacotherapy:* In the early post-transplant period (≤7 days), insulin is the preferred treatment option, followed by OHAs and lifestyle modification after the initial 7 days.
    - Metformin is usually avoided in view of safety concerns (lactic acidosis). However, the TRANSDIAB (transplantation and diabetes) study, which looked at the feasibility and safety of metformin following transplantation in patients with prediabetes, found it to be safe in this population but lacked sufficient power to demonstrate efficacy. More research is needed to determine the impact of metformin, a very inexpensive medicine, in preventing NODAT in those at risk.
    - Dipeptidyl peptidase-4 (DPP-4) inhibitors, namely vildagliptin and sitagliptin, have been demonstrated to be safe in limited studies.[59-61]
    - Glucagon-like peptide 1 (GLP-1) receptor agonists have only been tested in small case series so far.[62,63]
    - An open-label, randomized study (NCT03961256) using exenatide 4–6 months after KT is currently underway.
    - Although large ample studies to answer the long-term efficacy of sodium–glucose cotransporter 2 (SGLT2) inhibitors have yet to be performed, limited studies have begun to address the short-term efficacy and safety of SGLT2 inhibitors in KTR and type 2 diabetes. According to a literature review by Shuster et al.,[64] empagliflozin and canagliflozin were the most commonly used SGLT2 inhibitors, the use of which in kidney transplant patients was found to result in a small or nonsignificant decrease in BP, a slight improvement in glycemic control and insulin resistance, and a moderate-to-significant weight loss. According to one trial, it also resulted in steady graft function and a reduction in proteinuria. Urinary tract infection was the most prevalent side effect. There were no new ischemic lower limb ulcerations or amputations, Fournier's gangrene, nor were there any episodes of diabetic ketoacidosis.

Because immunosuppression is often more intense in the first year after KT, the bulk of studies looking at the use of SGLT2 inhibitors in KT have so far excluded patients during this time.

Prior to commencing SGLT2 inhibitors, KTR should get effective counseling, including avoidance education on sick days to reduce the risk of acute kidney injury (AKI) and ketoacidosis, BP monitoring, genital hygiene, and lower extremities surveillance.[65] SGLT2 inhibitors should also be held in the situation of allograft rejection treatment during which immunosuppression is intensified, similar to waiting 6–12 months post-transplantation.

Dyslipidemia

Dyslipidemia is frequently observed in the post-transplant period, involving over 60% of KTR.[66] Contributing factors include diabetes, metabolic syndrome, obesity, immunosuppression, namely steroids, mammalian target of rapamycin (mTOR) inhibitors, and CNIs (cyclosporine > tacrolimus) **(Table 2)**. In KTR, there is a clear link between dyslipidemia and CVD. With blood cholesterol >200 mg/dL or triglycerides >350 mg/dL, the risk of ischemic heart disease is twice.[21] Furthermore, in KTR, total cholesterol levels at 1 year post-transplant predict death independently.[67] Screening for dyslipidemia should begin soon after transplantation and continue at least once a year.[54,68]

Management

- Lifestyle changes along with lipid-lowering agents
- The KDIGO guidelines propose that all KTR, regardless of their low-density lipoprotein (LDL) levels, take statins. The ALERT trial showed that early initiation of fluvastatin lowered LDL-cholesterol by 32% and had a positive impact on post-transplant CV outcomes.[22]
- Elevated triglyceride levels are treated by dose reduction of mTOR inhibitors and use of pharmacological agents such as fibrates, ezetimibe, and bile acid resins. Refractory cases require switching of mTOR inhibitors to MMF or tacrolimus.
- Statins and CNIs, particularly cyclosporine, have significant drug interactions when used together. This results in increased blood statin levels, which increases the risk for myopathy and rhabdomyolysis. Hence, their concomitant use should be avoided.
- Proprotein convertase subtilisin/kexin type 9 (PCSK9) inhibitors have lately been utilized as an adjunct to statin therapy in patients who do not achieve appropriate cholesterol control.[69] Evolocumab significantly reduced LDL cholesterol levels and the incidence of major CV events in participants previously taking statins in the FOURIER (Further Cardiovascular Outcomes Research with PCSK9 Inhibition in Subjects with Elevated Risk) study.[70] However, the trial excluded transplant patients and those with significant renal impairment. PCSK9 inhibitors have never been used in renal transplant recipients (RTR) because they are a new medication class. As a result, more trials with such individuals are needed before PCSK9 drugs can be considered in KTR.

Obesity

The prevalence of obesity (BMI ≥ 30 kg/m^2) continues to rise among transplant recipients.[71] Obesity itself is an important risk factor for higher CV morbidity and mortality. It also contributes to hypertension, post-transplant diabetes, proteinuria, graft dysfunction, and acute rejection, all of which again predispose to CVD. According to research by Lentine et al., each 5-unit rise in recipient BMI increases the risk of cardiac illness, notably heart failure and atrial fibrillation, by 25%.[72]

Management

- Lifestyle and dietary modifications are the mainstays of therapy.
- Immunosuppression modification, especially corticosteroid reduction, may be done with caution, balancing against the risk of rejection.
- Pharmacotherapy after transplant lacks enough evidence and also carries along the risk of drug–drug interactions.
- Post-transplant bariatric surgery for morbid obesity is an option that has shown to reduce comorbidities and decrease mortality.[73]

Cigarette Smoking

Studies have shown increased CV risk and decreased patient and graft survival with increased smoking.[74,75] Hence, all efforts should be made to stop smoking pre- and postrenal transplant. A post hoc analysis of the FAVORIT trial revealed that persistent smoking increases the chance of all-cause mortality by 70%.[76] **Flowchart 1** summarizes the risk factors, outcome, and treatment of CV.

FUTURE DIRECTIONS

The number of kidney transplants continues to increase as it is the best treatment available for patients with ESKD. There is a considerable risk of CV problems and death after a renal transplant. The effects of immunosuppression typically amplify the increased risk of CVD. Hence, the risk-prediction models designed for the general public frequently underestimate the risk in KTR. The adoption of transplant-specific risk calculators could help to alleviate this issue. The addition of CV biomarkers to these ratings should increase accuracy, although more research is needed in this area. Currently, the management of CVD in KTR is based on expert opinion and experience. Hence, multiple RCTs involving transplant patients are required, which would improve screening, early diagnosis, and treatment. Also, a multidisciplinary team is required with a better understanding of disease to improve outcomes.

CONCLUSION

Cardiovascular disease is frequent following a kidney transplant and is linked to a number of conventional modifiable and nonmodifiable risk factors. The cornerstone of therapy is aggressive conventional modifiable risk

Flowchart 1: Cardiovascular risk factors, outcome, and management postrenal transplant.

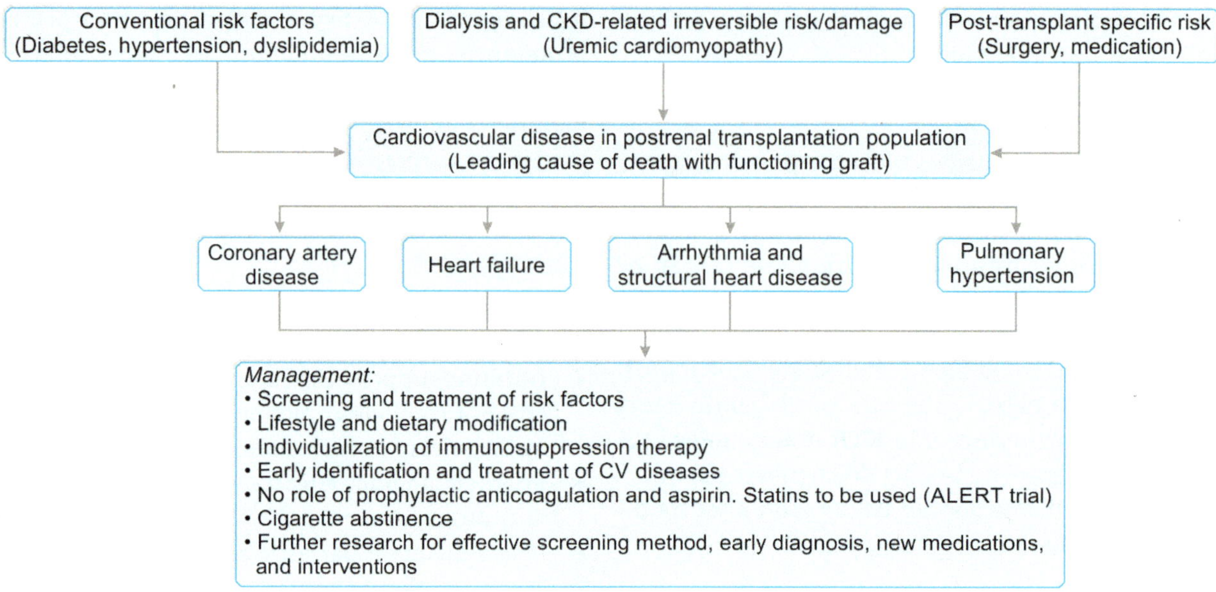

(ALERT: Assessment of Lescol in Renal Transplantation; CKD: chronic kidney disease; CV: cardiovascular)

factor screening and treatment, along with the help of lifestyle and dietary modifications. Individualization of immunosuppression therapy while balancing rejection risk reduces the risk of CVD. Despite advances in CV risk management and outcomes, CVD continues to be a major danger to grafts and patient life after KT. In this population, high-quality evidence is needed to better assess risk and develop ways to enhance outcomes. In addition, practitioners must be able to recognize CV illness quickly when it occurs and collaborate with a multidisciplinary team to offer complete care. More proactiveness and research in this field will hopefully yield the better results we want for all of our KTR.

REFERENCES

1. OPTN/SRTR 2017 Annual Data Report. Scientific Registry of Transplant Recipients. [online] Available from https://srtr.transplant.hrsa.gov/annual_reports/Default.aspx. [Last accessed July, 2022].
2. Baigent C, Burbury K, Wheeler D. Premature cardiovascular disease in chronic renal failure. Lancet. 2000;356(9224):147-52.
3. Kidney Disease: Improving Global Outcomes (KDIGO) Transplant Work Group. KDIGO clinical practice guideline for the care of kidney transplant recipients. Am J Transplant. 2009;9(Suppl. 3):S1-155.
4. Arend SM, Mallat MJ, Westendorp RJ, van der Woude FJ, van Es LA. Patient survival after renal transplantation; more than 25 years follow-up. Nephrol Dial Transplant. 1997;12:1672-9.
5. Goodman WG, Goldin J, Kuizon BD, Yoon C, Gales B, Sider D, et al. Coronary-artery calcification in young adults with end-stage renal disease who are undergoing dialysis. N Engl J Med. 2000;342:1478-83.
6. Berl T, Henrich W. Kidney-heart interactions: epidemiology, pathogenesis, and treatment. Clin J Am Soc Nephrol. 2006;1:8-18.
7. Gill JS, Ma I, Landsberg D, Johnson N, Levin A. Cardiovascular events and investigation in patients who are awaiting cadaveric kidney transplantation. J Am Soc Nephrol. 2005;16:808-16.
8. Fleisher LA, Fleischmann KE, Auerbach AD, Barnason SA, Beckman JA, Bozkurt B, et al. 2014 ACC/AHA guideline on perioperative cardiovascular evaluation and management of patients undergoing noncardiac surgery: a report of the American College of Cardiology/American Heart Association Task Force on practice guidelines. J Am Coll Cardiol. 2014;64:e77-137.
9. Lentine KL, Costa SP, Weir MR, Robb JF, Fleisher LA, Kasiske BL, et al. Cardiac disease evaluation and management among kidney and liver transplantation candidates: a scientific statement from the American Heart Association and the American College of Cardiology Foundation: endorsed by the American Society of Transplant Surgeons, American Society of Transplantation, and National Kidney Foundation. Circulation. 2012;126:617-63.
10. Wang LW, Fahim MA, Hayen A, Mitchell RL, Baines L, Lord S, et al. Cardiac testing for coronary artery disease in potential kidney transplant recipients. Cochrane Database Syst Rev. 2011;2011:CD008691.
11. Wang LW, Masson P, Turner RM, Lord SW, Baines LA, Craig JC, et al. Prognostic value of cardiac tests in potential kidney transplant recipients: a systematic review. Transplantation. 2015;99:731-45.
12. McFalls EO, Ward HB, Moritz TE, Goldman S, Krupski WC, Littooy F, et al. Coronary-artery revascularization before elective major vascular surgery. N Engl J Med. 2004;351:2795-04.
13. Lindenauer PK, Pekow P, Wang K, Mamidi DK, Guiterrez B, Benjamin EM. Perioperative beta-blocker therapy and

mortality after major noncardiac surgery. N Engl J Med. 2005;353:349-61.
14. Wallace AW, Au S, Cason BA. Association of the pattern of use of perioperative beta-blockade and postoperative mortality. Anesthesiology. 2010;113:794-805.
15. Andersson C, Mérie C, Jørgensen M, Gislason GH, Torp-Pederson C, Overgaard C, et al. Association of β-blocker therapy with risks of adverse cardiovascular events and deaths in patients with ischemic heart disease undergoing noncardiac surgery: a Danish nationwide cohort study. JAMA Intern Med. 2014;174:336-44.
16. Kristensen SD, Knuuti J, Saraste A, Anker S, Bøtker HE, De Hert S, et al. 2014 ESC/ESA guidelines on non-cardiac surgery: cardiovascular assessment and management: The Joint Task Force on non-cardiac surgery: cardiovascular assessment and management of the European Society of Cardiology (ESC) and the European Society of Anaesthesiology (ESA). Eur Heart J. 2014;35:2383-431.
17. Ferguson ER, Hudson SL, Diethelm AG, Pacifico AD, Dean LS, Holman WL. Outcome after myocardial revascularization and renal transplantation: a 25-year single-institution experience. Ann Surg. 1999;230:232-41.
18. Jaffe AS, Babuin L, Apple FS. Biomarkers in acute cardiac disease: the present and the future. J Am Coll Cardiol. 2006;48:1.
19. Keddis MT, El-Zoghby ZM, El Ters M, Rodrigo E, Pellika PA, Jaffe AS, et al. Cardiac troponin T before and after kidney transplantation: determinants and implications for posttransplant survival. Am J Transplant. 2013;13:406-14.
20. Ducloux D, Kazory A, Chalopin JM. Predicting coronary heart disease in renal transplant recipients: a prospective study. Kidney Int. 2004;66:441.
21. Kasiske BL, Chakkera HA, Roel J. Explained and unexplained ischemic heart disease risk after renal transplantation. J Am Soc Nephrol. 2000;11:1735.
22. Holdaas H, Fellström B, Jardine AG, Holme I, Nyberg G, Fauchald P, et al. Effect of fluvastatin on cardiac outcomes in renal transplant recipients: a multicentre, randomised, placebo-controlled trial. Lancet. 2003;361:2024-31.
23. Dad T, Tighiouart H, Joseph A, Bostom A, Carpenter M, Hunsicker L, et al. Aspirin use and incident cardiovascular disease, kidney failure, and death in stable kidney transplant recipients: a post hoc analysis of the Folic Acid for Vascular Outcome Reduction in Transplantation (FAVORIT) trial. Am J Kidney Dis. 2016;68:277-86.
24. Lentine KL, Schnitzler MA, Abbott KC, Li L, Burroughs TE, Irish W, et al. De novo congestive heart failure after kidney transplantation: a common condition with poor prognostic implications. Am J Kidney Dis. 2005;46:720-33.
25. Parfrey PS, Harnett JD, Foley RN, Kent GM, Murray DC, Barre PE, et al. Impact of renal transplantation on uremic cardiomyopathy. Transplantation. 1995;60:908-14.
26. Rigatto C, Foley RN, Kent GM, Guttmann R, Parfrey PS. Long-term changes in left ventricular hypertrophy after renal transplantation. Transplantation. 2000;70:570-75.
27. Unger P, Wissing KM, de Pauw L, Neubaeur J, van de Borne P. Reduction of left ventricular diameter and mass after surgical arteriovenous fistula closure in renal transplant recipients. Transplantation. 2002;74:73-9.
28. Laskar SR, Dries DL. The prognostic significance of renal dysfunction in patients with chronic systolic heart failure. Curr Cardiol Rep. 2003;5:205-10.
29. Xu B, Harb S, Hawwa N, Tang W, Nakhaoul G, Fatica R, et al. Impact of end-stage renal disease on left and right ventricular mechanics: does kidney transplantation reverse the abnormalities? JACC Cardiovasc Imaging. 2017;10:1081-83.
30. Yeung SMH, van Londen M, Nakshbandi U, Said MY, Eisenga MF, Hepkema BG, et al. Pretransplant NT-proBNP, dialysis vintage, and posttransplant mortality in kidney transplant recipients. Transplantation. 2020;104:2158-65.
31. Slubowska K, Sadowska A, Kwiatkowski A, Durlik M. N-terminal pro-B-type natriuretic peptide (NT-proBNP) assessment in the first year after renal transplantation and its relationship with graft function and left ventricular hypertrophy. Transplant Proc. 2014;46:2729-32.
32. House AA, Wanner C, Sarnak MJ, Piña IL, McIntyre CW, Komenda P, et al. Heart failure in chronic kidney disease: conclusions from a Kidney Disease: Improving Global Outcomes (KDIGO) Controversies Conference. Kidney Int. 2019;95:1304-17.
33. Lentine KL, Schnitzler MA, Abbott KC, Li L, Xiao H, Burroughs TE, et al. Incidence, predictors, and associated outcomes of atrial fibrillation after kidney transplantation. Clin J Am Soc Nephrol. 2006;1:288-96.
34. Rangaswami J, Mathew RO, Parasuraman R, Tantisattamo E, Lubetzky M, Rao S, et al. Cardiovascular disease in the kidney transplant recipient: epidemiology, diagnosis and management strategies. Nephrol Dial Transplant. 2019;34:760-73.
35. Herzog CA. Kidney disease in cardiology. Nephrol Dial Transplant. 2011;26:46-50.
36. Abbott KC, Hshieh P, Cruess D, Agodoa LYC, Welch PG, Taylor AJ, et al. Hospitalized valvular heart disease in patients on renal transplant waiting list: incidence, clinical correlates and outcomes. Clin Nephrol. 2003;59:79-87.
37. Sharma A, Gilbertson DT, Herzog CA. Survival of kidney transplantation patients in the United States after cardiac valve replacement. Circulation. 2010;121:2733-39.
38. Kosmadakis G, Aguilera D, Carceles O, Da Costa Correia E, Boletris L. Pulmonary hypertension in dialysis patients. Ren Fail. 2013;35:514-20.
39. Lentine KL, Villines TC, Axelrod D, Kaviratne S, Weir MR, Costa SP. Evaluation and management of pulmonary hypertension in kidney transplant candidates and recipients: concepts and controversies. Transplantation. 2017;101:166-81.
40. Clarkson MR, Giblin L, Brown A, Little D, Donohoe J. Reversal of pulmonary hypertension after ligation of a brachiocephalic arteriovenous fistula. Am J Kidney Dis. 2002;40:E8.
41. Kasiske BL, Anjum S, Shah R, Skogen J, Kandaswamy C, Danielson B, et al. Hypertension after kidney transplantation. Am J Kidney Dis. 2004;43:1071-81.
42. Ponticelli C, Cucchiari D, Graziani G. Hypertension in kidney transplant recipients. Transpl Int. 2011;24(6):523-33.
43. Aakhus S, Dahl K, Widerøe TE. Cardiovascular morbidity and risk factors in renal transplant patients. Nephrol Dial Transplant. 1999;14(3):648-54.
44. Opelz G, Wujciak T, Ritz E. Association of chronic kidney graft failure with recipient blood pressure. Collaborative Transplant Study. Kidney Int. 1998;53:217-22.
45. Whelton PK, Carey RM, Aronow WS, Casey Jr D, Collins KJ, Himmelfarb CD, et al. 2017 ACC/AHA/AAPA/ABC/ACPM/AGS/APhA/ASH/ASPC/NMA/PCNA guideline for the

prevention, detection, evaluation, and management of high blood pressure in adults: a report of the American College of Cardiology/American Heart Association Task Force on Clinical Practice Guidelines. Hypertension. 2018;71:e13-115.

46. Ahmad T, Coulthard MG, Eastham EJ. Reversible renal failure due to the use of captopril in a renal allograft recipient treated with cyclosporin. Nephrol Dial Transplant. 1989;4:311-2.
47. Garcia TM, da Costa JA, Costa RS, Ferraz AS. Acute tubular necrosis in kidney transplant patients treated with enalapril. Ren Fail. 1994;16:419-23.
48. Fricke L, Doehn C, Steinhoff J, Sack K, Jocham D, Fornara P. Treatment of posttransplant hypertension by laparoscopic bilateral nephrectomy? Transplantation. 1998;65:1182-7.
49. Yates CJ, Fourlanos S, Hjelmesaeth J, Colman PG, Cohney SJ. New-onset diabetes after kidney transplantation-changes and challenges. Am J Transplant. 2012;12:820-8.
50. Cole EH, Johnston O, Rose CL, Gill JS. Impact of acute rejection and new-onset diabetes on long-term transplant graft and patient survival. Clin J Am Soc Nephrol. 2008;3:814-21.
51. Armstrong KA, Prins JB, Beller EM, Campbell SB, Hawley CM, Johnson DW, et al. Should an oral glucose tolerance test be performed routinely in all renal transplant recipients? Clin J Am Soc Nephrol. 2006;1:100-8.
52. Valderhaug TG, Jenssen T, Hartmann A, Midtvedt K, Holdaas H, Reisaeter AV, et al. Fasting plasma glucose and glycosylated hemoglobin in the screening for diabetes mellitus after renal transplantation. Transplantation. 2009;88:429-34.
53. Caillard S, Eprinchard L, Perrin P, Braun L, Heibel F, Moreau F, et al. Incidence and risk factors of glucose metabolism disorders in kidney transplant recipients: role of systematic screening by oral glucose tolerance test. Transplantation. 2011;91:757-64.
54. Baker RJ, Mark PB, Patel RK, Stevens KK, Palmer N. Renal association clinical practice guideline in postoperative care in the kidney transplant recipient. BMC Nephrol. 2017;18(1):174.
55. Morales Febles R, Negrín Mena N, Rodríguez-Rodríguez AE, Martín LD, Rinne FG, Miranda DM, et al. Exercise and Prediabetes after Renal Transplantation (EXPRED): protocol description. Nephron. 2021;145(1):55-62.
56. Rakel A, Karelis AD. New-onset diabetes after transplantation: risk factors and clinical impact. Diabetes Metab. 2011;37:1-14.
57. Mora PF. New-onset diabetes after renal transplantation. J Investig Med. 2010;58:755-63.
58. Wissing KM, Abramowicz D, Weekers L, Budde K, Rath T, Witzke O, et al. Prospective randomized study of conversion from tacrolimus to cyclosporine A to improve glucose metabolism in patients with posttransplant diabetes mellitus after renal transplantation. Am J Transplant. 2018;18(7):1726-34.
59. Strøm Halden TA, Åsberg A, Vik K, Hartmann A, Jenssen T. Short-term efficacy and safety of sitagliptin treatment in long-term stable renal recipients with new-onset diabetes after transplantation. Nephrol Dial Transplant. 2014;29(4):926-33.
60. Werzowa J, Hecking M, Haidinger M, Lechner F, Döller D, Pacini G, et al. Vildagliptin and pioglitazone in patients with impaired glucose tolerance after kidney transplantation: a randomized, placebo-controlled clinical trial. Transplantation. 2013;95(3):456-62.
61. Haidinger M, Werzowa J, Hecking M, Antlanger M, Stemer G, Pleiner J, et al. Efficacy and safety of vildagliptin in new-onset diabetes after kidney transplantation: a randomized, double-blind, placebo-controlled trial. Am J Transplant. 2014;14(1):115-23.
62. Halden TAS, Egeland EJ, Åsberg A, Hartmann A, Midtvedt K, Khiabani HZ, et al. GLP-1 restores altered insulin and glucagon secretion in posttransplantation diabetes. Diabetes Care. 2016;39(4):617-24.
63. Pinelli NR, Patel A, Salinitri FD. Coadministration of liraglutide with tacrolimus in kidney transplant recipients: a case series. Diabetes Care. 2013:36(10);e171-2.
64. Shuster S, Al-Hadhrami Z, Awad S, Moore S, Shamseddin K. *Efficacy and safety of SGLT2 inhibitors in diabetic kidney transplant patients: review of the current literature. J Endocr Soc.* 2021;5(Suppl. 1):A411-2.
65. Lam D, Shaikh A. Real-life prescribing of SGLT2 inhibitors: how to handle other medications, including glucose-lowering drugs and diuretics. Kidney360. 2021;2:742-6.
66. Kasiske B, Cosio FG, Beto J, Bolton K, Chavers BM, Grimm Jr R, et al. Clinical practice guidelines for managing dyslipidemias in kidney transplant patients: a report from the managing dyslipidemias in Chronic Kidney Disease Work Group of the National Kidney Foundation Kidney Disease Outcomes Quality Initiative. Am J Transplant. 2004;4(Suppl. 7):13-53.
67. Kasiske BL, Guijarro C, Massy ZA, Weiderkehr MR, Ma JZ. Cardiovascular disease after renal transplantation. J Am Soc Nephrol. 1996;7(1):158-65.
68. Kasiske BL, Zeier MG, Chapman JR, Craig JC, Ekberk H, Garvey CA, et al. KDIGO clinical practice guideline for the care of kidney transplant recipients: a summary. Kidney Int. 2010;77(4):299-311.
69. Mayor S. NICE recommends PCSK9 inhibitors for patients not responding to statins. BMJ. 2016;353:i2609.
70. Sabatine MS, Giugliano RP, Keech AC, Honarpour N, Wiviott SD, Murphy SA, et al. Evolocumab and clinical outcomes in patients with cardiovascular disease. N Engl J Med. 2017;376(18):1713-22.
71. Kwan JM, Hajjiri Z, Metwally A, Finn PW, Perkins DL. Effect of the obesity epidemic on kidney transplantation: obesity is independent of diabetes as a risk factor for adverse renal transplant outcomes. PLoS One. 2016;11(11):e0165712.
72. Lentine KL, Rocca-Rey LA, Bacchi G, Wasi N, Schmitz L, Salvalaggio PR, et al. Obesity and cardiac risk after kidney transplantation: experience at one center and comprehensive literature review. Transplantation. 2008;86(2):303-12.
73. Schindel H, Winkler J, Yemini R, Carmeli I, Nesher E, Keidar A. Survival benefit in bariatric surgery kidney recipients may be mediated through effects on kidney graft function and improvement of co-morbidities: a case-control study. Surg Obes Relat Dis. 2019;15:621-7.
74. Nogueira JM, Haririan A, Jacobs SC, Cooper M, Weir MR. Cigarette smoking, kidney function, and mortality after live donor kidney transplant. Am J Kidney Dis. 2010;55:907-15.
75. Kasiske BL, Klinger D. Cigarette smoking in renal transplant recipients. J Am Soc Nephrol. 2000;11:753-9.
76. Weinrauch LA, Claggett B, Liu J, Finn PV, Weir MR, Weiner DE, et al. Smoking and outcomes in kidney transplant recipients: a post hoc survival analysis of the FAVORIT trial. Int J Nephrol Renovasc Dis. 2018;11:155-64.

13.2 Hepatic Dysfunction in Kidney Transplant Recipients

Ashish Kumar

CASE VIGNETTE 1

A 60-year-old, long-standing diabetic male, with end-stage renal disease (ESRD) due to diabetic nephropathy, underwent live-related ABO compatible renal transplant, with son as the donor, 3 years ago. The patient was on maintenance immunosuppression with tacrolimus, mycophenolate mofetil, and prednisolone. He had stable course and suffered no rejection episodes or opportunistic infections. He now presented with mild dull aching pain in the right upper quadrant of the abdomen for the last 3 months. On examination, he had a body mass index (BMI) of 29 kg/m^2 and mild right upper quadrant tenderness. On investigations, he had stable renal functions, but his liver function tests were deranged with serum bilirubin (total) 1.1 mg/dL, alanine aminotransferase (ALT) 85 IU/L, aspartate aminotransferase (AST) 66 IU/L, serum alkaline phosphatase (SAP) 101 IU/L, and gamma-glutamyl transferase (GGT) 59 IU/L. His albumin and international normalized ratio (INR) levels were normal. His hemoglobin A1C (HbA1c) was 7.5% and lipid profile showed a low-density lipoprotein (LDL) cholesterol value of 149 mg/dL, high-density lipoprotein (HDL) cholesterol value of 35 mg/dL, and triglyceride level of 273 mg/dL. He tested negative for hepatitis B and C markers. His ultrasound abdomen revealed grade II fatty liver. His transient elastography revealed liver stiffness measurement (LSM) of 8.1 kPa and controlled attenuated parameter (CAP) of 322 dB/m. A working diagnosis of nonalcoholic steatohepatitis (NASH) was made. He was advised lifestyle modifications (diet and exercise) aimed at weight reduction along with modification in his antidiabetic medications. He was also advised saroglitazar 4 mg tablets at bedtime. In 6 months with strict adherence to lifestyle changes, he was able to lose 8 kg of weight. His pain had vanished, and his transaminases and triglyceride levels had normalized.

CASE VIGNETTE 2

A 56-year-old male with history of ESRD due to immunoglobulin A (IgA) nephropathy underwent deceased donor kidney transplantation 1 year ago. The donor was CMV positive while the recipient was CMV negative. Before transplantation, his laboratory test results were AST 29 U/L, ALT 35 U/L, SAP 127 U/L, and serum total bilirubin 0.9 mg/dL. His immunosuppression included mycophenolate sodium and tacrolimus, target levels 10–12 ng/mL up to 2 months and 8–10 ng/mL 3–6 months post-transplant, with a prednisone taper to 10 mg daily. Valganciclovir was started for CMV prophylaxis with undetectable viral load shortly after transplant. 4 months following transplant, aminotransferases were elevated, and CMV prophylaxis was discontinued assuming valganciclovir was the cause. 8 months post-transplant, he was evaluated for pain in right hypochondrium. His transaminases were elevated with an AST of 201 U/L, ALT of 314 U/L, SAP of 325 U/L, and bilirubin of 1.3 mg/dL. His hepatitis B surface antigen (HBsAg) and antihepatitis C virus (HCV) were negative. The CMV viral load was 457,145 IU/mL. Liver biopsy showed cytoplasmic inclusions. The immunohistochemical stain was positive for CMV. A diagnosis of CMV hepatitis was made. Intravenous ganciclovir was started with which his abdominal pain and aminotransferases improved. Renal function remained stable. CMV viral load became undetectable.

INTRODUCTION

Recipients of kidney transplant have similar risk for all hepatic ailments as the general population; however, certain hepatic disorders may occur with higher frequency in kidney transplant recipients as compared to nontransplant population.[1] Some conditions such as polycystic kidney disease (PKD) have involvement of both kidney and liver as part of the same underlying disease. In other situations, such as chronic infections with hepatotropic viruses, the liver disease may have been acquired separately by kidney transplant recipients. In addition, certain liver conditions are a consequence of the implicit risks of the kidney transplant process, such as hepatic infections due to opportunistic organisms secondary to immunosuppression or hepatic adverse effects of immunosuppressant medications. Finally, the high prevalence of obesity, dyslipidemia, type 2 diabetes mellitus, and metabolic syndrome in the general population as well as the organ transplant patients has resulted in increasing prevalence of NAFLD in the kidney transplant recipients. Although there are numerous causes of hepatic dysfunction in renal transplant recipients **(Table 1)**, the goal of this chapter is to describe common causes along with current approaches to their diagnosis and management.

PREVALENCE OF ABNORMAL LIVER ENZYMES IN RENAL TRANSPLANT RECIPIENTS

The prevalence of liver enzyme elevation after renal transplantation has not been studied adequately. In a retrospective study on 1,589 renal transplants, who had no other apparent liver disease, ALT was the liver enzyme abnormality with the highest prevalence (34%) followed by AST (7%). These were significantly elevated within the first 3 months after transplantation. There was also a significant correlation between liver enzyme values and the cyclosporine blood levels. The investigators recommended the need for vigilant monitoring of liver function tests in all patients after

TABLE 1: Causes of liver disease in renal transplant recipients.

Infections	Hepatotropic viral	• Hepatitis B • Hepatitis C • Hepatitis E
	Nonhepatotropic viral	• Cytomegalovirus • Epstein–Barr virus • Herpes simplex virus • Varicella-zoster virus
	Bacterial	• Hepatic abscess • Mycobacteria
Inherited		• ADPKD • ARPKD • Alpha-1 antitrypsin deficiency • Hemochromatosis • Wilson disease
Drug-induced liver injury	Hepatocellular pattern	• Acetaminophen • Allopurinol • Amiodarone • Fluoxetine • INH • NSAIDs • Rifampin • HMG-CoA reductase inhibitors • Tetracyclines
	Mixed pattern	• Amitriptyline • Azathioprine • Clindamycin • Nitrofurantoin • Phenytoin • TMP/SMX • Verapamil
	Cholestatic pattern	• Amox/Clav • Anabolic steroids • OCPs • Erythromycins • Terbinafine • Tricyclic antidepressants
Metabolic		• NAFLD • Alcoholic liver disease
Autoimmune		• Autoimmune hepatitis • Primary biliary cirrhosis

(ADPKD: autosomal dominant polycystic kidney disease; Amox/Clav: amoxicillin/clavulanic; ARPKD: autosomal recessive polycystic kidney disease; HMG-CoA: β-hydroxy β-methylglutaryl-CoA; INH: isoniazid; NAFLD: nonalcoholic fatty liver disease; NSAIDs: nonsteroidal anti-inflammatory drugs; OCPs: oral contraceptive pills; TMP/SMX: trimethoprim/sulfamethoxazole)

Source: Adapted from Gunderson A, Said A. Liver disease in kidney transplant recipients. Transplant Rev. 2015;29(1):1-7.

renal transplantation.[2] In another observational study on 62 children with renal transplantation, the liver enzyme levels were abnormal in 68% during the first 6 months following, with a peak on day 14. CMV infection and high tacrolimus levels were possible causes.[3] In another study from Turkey on 107 kidney transplant recipients over 7-year period, 38% patients had abnormal liver functions. Drug toxicity due to mycophenolate mofetil and pretransplant positive CMV immunoglobulin M (IgM) tests were found to be a significant independent risk factor for hepatotoxicity.[4] Thus, the prevalence of liver enzyme abnormalities is variable and has multifactorial etiology.

CHAPTER HIGHLIGHTS

- Renal transplant recipients have similar risk for all hepatic ailments to the general population; however, certain hepatic disorders may occur with higher frequency in kidney transplant recipients as compared to nontransplant population.
- Postrenal transplantation, the prevalence of liver enzyme abnormalities is variable and has multifactorial etiology.
- Infections due to hepatitis B and C, and nonhepatotropic viruses such as cytomegalovirus (CMV), herpes simplex virus (HSV), and varicella-zoster virus (VZV) are important causes of post-transplant hepatitis.
- Nonalcoholic fatty liver disease (NAFLD) is an emerging cause of transaminases elevation due to rise in obesity and metabolic syndrome.
- Drug-induced liver injury (DILI) is also frequently encountered in renal transplant recipients because of the use of multiple drugs.

HEPATITIS B VIRUS INFECTION

Hepatitis B virus (HBV) can cause acute as well as chronic liver infections. Acute HBV infection in adults results in self-limiting acute hepatitis characterized by inflammation and in rare cases hepatocellular necrosis. However, most patients are able to clear the virus and produce neutralizing antibodies. In contrast, chronic HBV infection is usually persistent and leads to chronic hepatitis characterized by hepatocellular injury, inflammation, and fibrosis, which can progress to liver cirrhosis.

In the postrenal transplantation settings, prior to effective antiviral therapy, HBV-infected recipients used to have poorer survival compared with non-HBV-infected recipients. A meta-analysis of observational studies, published in 2005, found that HBsAg positive renal transplant recipients had approximately 2.5 times higher mortality as well as reduced graft survival.[5] Studies also documented liver fibrosis progression in HBV-positive renal transplant recipients, with up to 28% developing cirrhosis in 5 years.[6] With the advent of effective antiviral therapy, the prognosis of HBV-infected renal transplant recipients is much better now. A recent study from China on HBV-positive renal transplant recipients revealed an 83% 20-year survival in patients treated with antiviral therapy.[7]

Renal transplant recipients may develop de novo HBV infection after transplantation which is associated with high viral replication and rapid progression of liver disease. The highest risk of post-transplantation de novo hepatitis exists in recipients who are nonimmune for HBV (anti-HBs negative) and receive an organ from HBsAg and hepatitis B e-antigen (HBeAg)-positive donor. The risk of transmission from an HBsAg-negative but anti-HBc-positive-only donor is much less. The risk of de novo HBV infection is significantly reduced if the recipient is vaccinated and has protective titers of anti-HBs, although it is not completely eliminated.[8] Immunosuppressive therapy may also lead to HBV reactivation, especially with the use of rituximab for desensitization of ABO-incompatible or positive crossmatch renal transplantation.[9,10]

All HBsAg-positive renal transplant recipients should receive antiviral therapy, regardless of negative HBV deoxyribonucleic acid (DNA).[11-13] Entecavir (ETV) or tenofovir alafenamide (TAF) are the preferred options, while tenofovir disoproxil fumarate (TDF) should preferably be avoided in view of renal safety issues. Long-term antiviral therapy with these agents has been shown to reduce hepatic complications and improve survival.[14] Interferon and peginterferon are contraindicated because of the risk of organ rejection. Renal function should be serially monitored during antiviral therapy. The optimal duration of therapy is yet to be determined and may need to be given indefinitely. Cessation of antiviral therapy maybe associated with an increased risk of hepatic disease flare and, in rare circumstances, hepatic decompensation.

HEPATITIS C VIRUS INFECTION

The common mode of transmission of HCV infection is transfusion of HCV-infected blood and blood products, hemodialysis machines, and intravenous drug use. Studies have found that the frequency of HCV infection in patients on maintenance hemodialysis is greater than in the general population and may range between 2.6 and 22.9%.[15] Contributing factors for HCV infection among renal transplant candidates include exposure to blood products, length of time on hemodialysis, and the high prevalence of HCV infection in the dialysis facility.[16] With the use of extended criteria donor organs, including those positive for HCV antibody, allograft transmission of HCV has also become a possibility, although this practice is still considered investigational.[17]

Prior to effective antiviral therapy, kidney transplant recipients who are HCV-positive had decreased patient and/or graft survival.[18,19] In a meta-analysis of observational studies published in 2005, the presence of HCV was an independent risk factor for increased mortality and graft failure. The frequent causes of mortality in these patients were decompensated liver cirrhosis and hepatocellular carcinoma (HCC).[20]

The treatment of HCV has advanced over the last decade from interferon-based therapy to the direct-acting antiviral agents (DAAs). The novel DAAs are orally acting drugs, which act directly on the replicative cycle of HCV, and are highly effective in curing HCV infection with cure rates >95% with treatment durations of 2–6 months. The commonly used DAAs have been sofosbuvir, ledipasvir, simeprevir, ombitasvir, and daclatasvir, with or without ribavirin.

Caution needs to be applied as some of the DAAs such as ombitasvir, simeprevir, and ledipasvir can interact with immunosuppressive drugs due to their common mode of metabolism. Hence, serial monitoring of renal functions is of utmost importance.

Patients on dialysis can receive anti-HCV therapy with DAAs with excellent cure rates with almost negligible possibility of relapse post-transplantation. Postrenal transplant anti-HCV therapy with DAAs is also very effective and safe, and considered by many as a superior option than treating HCV on dialysis unless there is a risk of progression of hepatic disease usually in patients with advanced fibrosis due to HCV.

NONHEPATOTROPIC VIRAL INFECTIONS

Cytomegalovirus (CMV) is one of the most common viral infections in transplant recipients. Approximately 50–60% of transplant patients have been shown to excrete CMV in body secretions at some point or develop CMV antigenemia.[21,22] CMV hepatitis is one of the most important clinical manifestations of CMV infection, which is a severe disease, usually with multiple other organ involvement or widespread infection.[22] In view of significant mortality and morbidity of CMV hepatitis in renal transplant patients, prevention of CMV infection and early treatment are of critical importance.

Another nonhepatotropic virus, the HSV, remains latent in ganglia and may reactivate with immunosuppression. The HCV disease in an immunocompromised host is generally more severe and more frequent.[23] In kidney transplant patients, the HSV infection has been reported to have an incidence rate of 30–50% in the absence of prophylaxis.[24] In the first 90 days after the transplant, the risk of HSV reactivation is the highest because of the higher level of immunosuppression required during this phase. The clinical features of HSV infection included stomatitis, fever, and pain in abdomen, usually in association with disseminated infection. HSV hepatitis is frequently encountered in kidney transplant population, which is associated with 67% mortality in this patient population.[25] Liver biopsy is required for the diagnosis of HSV hepatitis which demonstrates viral involvement of liver tissue. In view of high mortality associated with disseminated HSV infection, renal transplant recipients who present with fever, abdominal symptoms, progressive transaminase elevation, with or without evidence of cutaneous HSV infection, should be promptly investigated for HSV hepatitis and early therapy with intravenous acyclovir instituted. For prophylaxis against HSV, oral acyclovir is recommended which has significantly reduced the incidence of HSV infection in renal transplant population.[24]

Varicella-zoster virus is another herpesvirus that causes two distinct diseases: herpes zoster and varicella. Like all herpesviruses, VZV establishes latency and may subsequently reactivate. However, in general, primary VZV infection is a more severe illness than reactivation of VSV. The most common presenting features of VZV infection are fever, cutaneous vesicular lesions, and back or abdominal pain. Varicella hepatitis is rare but has been described in renal transplant recipients. The typical rash may not be initially visible at the time of liver involvement; thus, the diagnosis of varicella hepatitis may be delayed. High-dose acyclovir is an effective treatment for varicella hepatitis. In renal transplant patients, disseminated zoster infection can be a severe and life-threatening. Fifty percent of these patients develop varicella hepatitis and disseminated intravascular coagulation (DIC), and 29% develop viral pneumonia. About one-third of these patients die; however, the mortality rate seems to have decreased over time from >50% to <25% now.[26]

NONALCOHOLIC FATTY LIVER DISEASE

Excessive alcohol consumption and NAFLD are two important causes of fatty liver disease in general population as well as renal transplant recipients. In any patient presenting with ultrasonography (USG) evidence of fatty liver disease, taking detailed history of alcohol consumption is very important. In absence of alcohol abuse, a diagnosis of NAFLD is considered. NAFLD, which is now also known as metabolic associated fatty liver disease (MAFLD), is a condition with excessive fat accumulation in the liver without another clear cause such as alcohol or certain drug use. The syndrome of NAFLD encompasses a histologic spectrum which ranges from bland fat accumulation to the more progressive form, the NASH, which is frequently associated with liver fibrosis and can progress to cirrhosis. Approximately 25–30% of the general adult population and up to 70% of obese and diabetic patients have NAFLD. Obesity, diabetes, hypertension, and hyperlipidemia are significant concerns after kidney transplantation in majority of patients. These same factors are also responsible for development of NAFLD.[27]

Up to 60% of renal transplant recipients may have NAFLD.[28] USG is the diagnostic modality of choice for diagnosing NAFLD after excluding alcohol abuse and other chronic liver conditions. Transient elastography (Fibroscan®) is a new modality that utilizes noninvasive "shear wave technology" and liver attenuation to diagnose the degree of liver stiffness and steatosis. Elevated transaminases are not an accurate way to detect NASH in this population as they do not differ between those with and without NASH in the kidney transplant population.[28]

The mainstay of treatment of NAFLD as well as NASH is weight reduction using lifestyle modifications of diet and exercise. Treatment of the underlying metabolic conditions including obesity, insulin resistance, metabolic syndrome, diabetes mellitus, hypertension, and dyslipidemia is also of paramount importance. Pharmacological therapies for NASH include drugs that can improve insulin resistance, improve glycemic control, improve lipid metabolism, or those with antioxidant effects. Pioglitazone had shown some benefit including histologic improvement and can be used in the treatment of NASH. Vitamin E, which is an antioxidant, has also shown histologic improvement in randomized controlled trials.[29] In India, saroglitazar is an approved treatment of NASH, along with lifestyle modifications,[30] although it has not yet been investigated in renal transplant recipients.

DRUG-INDUCED LIVER INJURY

Drug-induced liver injury is frequently encountered in renal transplant recipients because of the use of multiple drugs. Many of the drugs are metabolized via the same hepatic metabolic pathways, thus increasing the risk of accumulation of hepatotoxic metabolites. Common drug classes used in post-transplant patients that have been attributed in DILI include antibiotics, immunosuppressants, statins, antihypertensives, and antidiabetics. Frequently, more than one drug may be responsible for DILI in a given patient.[31] In addition, many patients also consume complementary and alternative medicines, which can also cause DILI. The mainstay of DILI treatment is identification and withdrawal of the offending drug. Most offending drugs do not have specific antidotes, however, for acetaminophen toxicity *N*-acetylcysteine can be used and for valproic acid toxicity, L-carnitine can be used. There is no proven role of corticosteroids in DILI. Urgent liver transplantation should be considered if the DILI has progressed to acute liver failure.

Among the immunosuppressants, azathioprine hepatotoxicity has been encountered in kidney transplant patients, though it is uncommon. Azathioprine and its metabolite 6-mercaptopurine causes direct hepatotoxicity, endothelial damage, and interlobular bile duct injury. Veno-occlusive disease, now known as sinusoidal obstruction syndrome (SOS), is the most severe manifestation of azathioprine toxicity, which is characterized by fibrosis and obliteration of the central venule and sinusoidal congestion.[32] The clinical features of SOS are ascites, jaundice, elevated liver enzymes, and hepatomegaly. SOS rarely regresses with cessation of azathioprine. Specific therapy for SOS, including defibrotide, ursodeoxycholic acid, heparin, and prostaglandin E_1, have produced mixed results. Liver transplantation maybe required in severe cases.

Tacrolimus and cyclosporine are immunosuppressive drugs that belong to the class of calcineurin inhibitors.

Cyclosporine is metabolized via the cytochrome P-450 system and interactions with drugs that stimulate or inhibit this pathway can result in decreased or increased cyclosporine levels, respectively. Cyclosporine can also cause decrease in bile flow resulting from reduced bile acid secretion and thus can lead to biliary sludge and stone formation in 2–5% of transplant recipients.[33] Transient elevations of aminotransferase and bilirubin levels have also been reported usually in the first 90 days, which respond to dose reduction.[33] Persistent elevations in aminotransferases occur in <5% of kidney transplant recipients. Tacrolimus is usually not associated with cholestasis and biliary stone formation. Also with tacrolimus, there were less incidences of hyperbilirubinemia (0.3%) as compared to cyclosporine (3.3%).[34] Elevations in aminotransferases are generally mild, and completely reversible with dose reduction of tacrolimus.

Another drug that is structurally related to tacrolimus is sirolimus (rapamycin) which is an inhibitor of mammalian target of rapamycin (mTOR). Hepatotoxicity due to sirolimus is uncommon, and elevations of liver enzymes with nonspecific histologic changes have been reported.[35] These resolve with discontinuation of sirolimus.

POLYCYSTIC KIDNEY AND LIVER DISEASE

Autosomal dominant polycystic kidney disease (ADPKD) is a genetic condition that results in the progressive development and enlargement of kidney and liver cysts. Renal cystic disease may progress to chronic kidney disease (CKD) that requires renal transplantation. Polycystic liver disease (PLD) is usually an extrarenal manifestation of ADPKD, occurring in 20–94% of cases, and is characterized by numerous cysts which occupy at least 50% of the hepatic parenchymal volume.[36,37] The cysts first appear during puberty and progressively increase in size and number with age. The cysts are usually lined by secretory biliary epithelium.

Polycystic liver disease is diagnosed using USG, which is considered the diagnostic modality of choice. Genetic testing for PKD is not usually required, unless patients have kidney failure in absence of renomegaly, or there is markedly asymmetric PKD.

In patients with ADPKD, the hepatic cysts do not require any specific treatment if they are asymptomatic. However, massively enlarging hepatic cysts produce compartmental syndrome in the abdomen which is unable to accommodate the enlarging cystic mass. These patients then experience early satiety, abdominal pain, or dyspnea. In addition, complications such as infection, rupture of cyst, hemorrhage into cyst, or cyst torsion can occur. Liver function and portal flow and pressure are usually normal. Rare hepatic manifestations of ADPKD are biliary obstruction, ascites, portal hypertension, variceal bleeding, and hepatic encephalopathy.

In moderate-to-severe PLD, somatostatin analogs—octreotide and lanreotide—have been shown to lead to reduction in total hepatic volume.[38-40] Large cysts causing symptoms can also be treated with aspiration sclerotherapy, fenestration, or resection. For patients with debilitating symptoms, liver transplantation is the only option.

REFERENCES

1. Gunderson A, Said A. Liver disease in kidney transplant recipients. Transplant Rev. 2015;29(1):1-7.
2. Einollahi B, Ghadian A, Ghamar-Chehreh E, Alavian SM. Non-viral related liver enzymes elevation after kidney transplantation. Hepat Mon. 2014;14(2):e9036.
3. Alfandary H, Davidovits M, Dagan A. Transient abnormal liver enzyme level in the early stage after renal transplantation in children. Indian J Transplant. 2018;12(2):90.
4. Dizdar OS, Ersoy A, Aksoy S, Ozel Coskun BD, Yildiz A. Analysis of liver function test abnormalities in kidney transplant recipients: 7 year experience. Pak J Med Sci. 2016;32(6):1330-5.
5. Fabrizi F, Martin P, Dixit V, Kanwal F, Dulai G. HBsAg seropositive status and survival after renal transplantation: meta-analysis of observational studies. Am J Transplant. 2005;5(12):2913-21.
6. Fornairon S, Pol S, Legendre C, Carnot F, Mamzer-Bruneel MF, Brechot C, et al. The long-term virologic and pathologic impact of renal transplantation on chronic hepatitis B virus infection. Transplantation. 1996;62(2):297-9.
7. Yap DYH, Tang CSO, Yung S, Choy BY, Yuen MF, Chan TM. Long-term outcome of renal transplant recipients with chronic hepatitis B infection-impact of antiviral treatments. Transplantation. 2010;90(3):325-30.
8. De Feo TM, Grossi P, Poli F, Mozzi F, Messa P, Minetti E, et al. Kidney transplantation from anti-HBc+ donors: results from a retrospective Italian study. Transplantation. 2006;81(1): 76-80.
9. Arora A, Anand AC, Kumar A, Singh SP, Aggarwal R, Dhiman RK, et al. INASL guidelines on management of hepatitis B virus infection in patients receiving chemotherapy, biologicals, immunosupressants, or corticosteroids. J Clin Exp Hepatol. 2018;8(4):403-31.
10. Lee J, Park JY, Huh KH, Kim BS, Kim MS, Kim SI, et al. Rituximab and hepatitis B reactivation in HBsAg-negative/ anti-HBc-positive kidney transplant recipients. Nephrol Dial Transplant. 2017;32(4):722-9.
11. Cholongitas E, Tziomalos K, Pipili C. Management of patients with hepatitis B in special populations. World J Gastroenterol. 2015;21(6):1738-48.
12. Fabrizi F, Martin P, Messa P. Novel perspectives on the hepatitis B virus vaccine in the chronic kidney disease population. Int J Artif Organs. 2015;38(12):625-31.
13. Gajurel K, Stapleton JT. Hepatitis viruses in kidney transplantation. Semin Nephrol. 2016;36(5):386-96.
14. European Association for the Study of the Liver. EASL 2017 clinical practice guidelines on the management of hepatitis B virus infection. J Hepatol. 2017;67(2):370-98.
15. Fissell RB, Bragg-Gresham JL, Woods JD, Jadoul M, Gillespie B, Hedderwick SA, et al. Patterns of hepatitis C prevalence and seroconversion in hemodialysis units

from three continents: the DOPPS. Kidney Int. 2004;65(6): 2335-42.
16. Liver Disease Among Renal Transplant Recipients. (2022). [online] Available from https://coek.info/pdf-liver-disease-among-renal-transplant-recipients-.html. [Last accessed May, 2022].
17. Stevens PE, Levin A, Kidney Disease: Improving Global Outcomes Chronic Kidney Disease Guideline Development Work Group Members. Evaluation and management of chronic kidney disease: synopsis of the kidney disease: improving global outcomes 2012 clinical practice guideline. Ann Intern Med. 2013;158(11):825-30.
18. Legendre C, Garrigue V, Le Bihan C, Mamzer-Bruneel MF, Chaix ML, Landais P, et al. Harmful long-term impact of hepatitis C virus infection in kidney transplant recipients. Transplantation. 1998;65(5):667-70.
19. Mathurin P, Mouquet C, Poynard T, Sylla C, Benalia H, Fretz C, et al. Impact of hepatitis B and C virus on kidney transplantation outcome. Hepatology. 1999;29(1):257-63.
20. Fabrizi F, Martin P, Dixit V, Bunnapradist S, Dulai G. Hepatitis C virus antibody status and survival after renal transplantation: meta-analysis of observational studies. Am J Transplant. 2005;5(6):1452-61.
21. Kotton CN, Fishman JA. Viral infection in the renal transplant recipient. J Am Soc Nephrol. 2005;16(6):1758-74.
22. Sagedal S, Hartmann A, Nordal KP, Osnes K, Leivestad T, Foss A, et al. Impact of early cytomegalovirus infection and disease on long-term recipient and kidney graft survival. Kidney Int. 2004;66(1):329-37.
23. Walker DP, Longson M, Mallick NP, Johnson RW. A prospective study of cytomegalovirus and herpes simplex virus disease in renal transplant recipients. J Clin Pathol. 1982; 35(11):1190-3.
24. Jirasiritham S, Sumethkul V, Chiewsilp P, Gojaseni P. Prevention of recurrent herpes infection after renal transplantation by low-dose oral acyclovir. Transplant Proc. 1994;26(4):2125-6.
25. Kusne S, Schwartz M, Breinig MK, Dummer JS, Lee RE, Selby R, et al. Herpes simplex virus hepatitis after solid organ transplantation in adults. J Infect Dis. 1991;163(5):1001-7.
26. Fehr T, Bossart W, Wahl C, Binswanger U. Disseminated varicella infection in adult renal allograft recipients: four cases and a review of the literature. Transplantation. 2002; 73(4):608-11.
27. Byrne CD, Targher G. NAFLD: a multisystem disease. J Hepatol. 2015;62(1 Suppl):S47-64.
28. Mikolasevic I, Racki S, Lukenda V, Milic S, Pavletic-Persic M, Orlic L. Nonalcoholic fatty liver disease in renal transplant recipients proven by transient elastography. Transplant Proc. 2014;46(5):1347-52.
29. Said A, Akhter A. Meta-analysis of randomized controlled trials of pharmacologic agents in non-alcoholic steatohepatitis. Ann Hepatol. 2017;16(4):538-47.
30. Gawrieh S, Noureddin M, Loo N, Mohseni R, Awasty V, Cusi K, et al. Saroglitazar, a PPAR-α/γ agonist, for treatment of NAFLD: a randomized controlled double-blind phase 2 trial. Hepatology. 2021;74(4):1809-24.
31. Chalasani N, Fontana RJ, Bonkovsky HL, Watkins PB, Davern T, Serrano J, et al. Causes, clinical features, and outcomes from a prospective study of drug-induced liver injury in the United States. Gastroenterology. 2008;135(6): 1924-34, 1934.e1-4.
32. Marubbio AT, Danielson B. Hepatic veno-occlusive disease in a renal transplant patient receiving azathioprine. Gastroenterology. 1975;69(3):739-43.
33. Lorber MI, Van Buren CT, Flechner SM, Williams C, Kahan BD. Hepatobiliary complications of cyclosporine therapy following renal transplantation. Transplant Proc. 1987;19(1 Pt. 2):1808-10.
34. Margreiter R, European Tacrolimus vs Ciclosporin Microemulsion Renal Transplantation Study Group. Efficacy and safety of tacrolimus compared with ciclosporin microemulsion in renal transplantation: a randomised multicentre study. Lancet. 2002;359(9308):741-6.
35. Niemczyk M, Wyzgał J, Perkowska A, Porowski D, Paczek L. Sirolimus-associated hepatotoxicity in the kidney graft recipient. Transpl Int. 2005;18(11):1302-3.
36. Wong MY, McCaughan GW, Strasser SI. An update on the pathophysiology and management of polycystic liver disease. Expert Rev Gastroenterol Hepatol. 2017;11(6):569-81.
37. Drenth JPH, Chrispijn M, Nagorney DM, Kamath PS, Torres VE. Medical and surgical treatment options for polycystic liver disease. Hepatology. 2010;52(6):2223-30.
38. Hogan MC, Masyuk TV, Page LJ, Kubly VJ, Bergstralh EJ, Li X, et al. Randomized clinical trial of long-acting somatostatin for autosomal dominant polycystic kidney and liver disease. J Am Soc Nephrol. 2010;21(6):1052-61.
39. Caroli A, Antiga L, Cafaro M, Fasolini G, Remuzzi A, Remuzzi G, et al. Reducing polycystic liver volume in ADPKD: effects of somatostatin analogue octreotide. Clin J Am Soc Nephrol. 2010;5(5):783-9.
40. van Keimpema L, Nevens F, Vanslembrouck R, van Oijen MGH, Hoffmann AL, Dekker HM, et al. Lanreotide reduces the volume of polycystic liver: a randomized, double-blind, placebo-controlled trial. Gastroenterology. 2009;137(5): 1661-8.e1-2.

13.3 Neurological Disorders in Kidney Transplant Recipients

Priti Meena, Arvind Canchi

CASE VIGNETTE 1

A 45-year-old male on triple-drug immunosuppression 5 years post-live-related renal transplant presents with fever, altered sensorium, and leukopenia for 10 days.

a. What is differential diagnosis?
b. How would you evaluate?

Ans. Refer to text

CASE VIGNETTE 2

*A 30-year-old female on triple-drug immunosuppression developed lethargy, unexplained fever, and altered mental status 1-year postrenal transplantation. Axial T2-weighted magnetic resonance images of the brain show regions of hyperintensity lesions **(Fig. 1)**.*

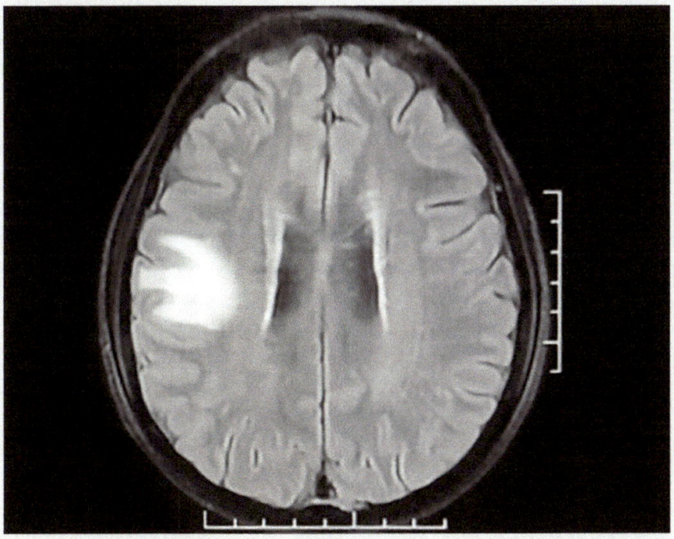

Fig. 1

a. What is differential diagnosis?

Ans. Refer to text

INTRODUCTION

Neurological diseases are commonly seen in kidney transplant recipients (KTRs) and can result in increased morbidity and mortality. However, they are often underdiagnosed. A meta-analysis by Mohammadi et al. reported a prevalence of neurological disorders in KTRs as 7.9%.[1] This chapter describes neurological conditions in KTRs as disorders existing prior to the transplantation and those occuring post-transplantation, in the early, subacute, and late periods following transplantation.

PRE-EXISTING NEUROLOGICAL DISEASE

Sometimes, neurological complications of kidney failure may manifest after kidney transplantation. Comorbidities related to kidney failure such as malnutrition, chronic inflammation, cerebrovascular accidents (CVAs), vascular calcification, diabetes mellitus, hypertension, or other underlying diseases such as systemic lupus erythematosus (SLE) predispose patients to neurological manifestations post-transplantation. In diabetes mellitus, peripheral nerves are affected that can lead to painful sensory neuropathy. SLE patients can have multiple neurological manifestations, such as seizure, myelopathy, meningitis, or mononeuropathies.[2] Human immunodeficiency virus (HIV) patients can experience features of dementia, neuropathies, and myelopathies.[3]

Long-standing uremia can itself cause polyneuropathy and autonomic dysfunction that may not completely recover even after the restoration of normal kidney function.[4] Multiple factors such as older age, inflammation, CVA, diabetes mellitus, and oxidative stress result in reduced cerebral perfusion and eventually cerebral ischemia in end-stage renal disease (ESRD) patients rendering them susceptible to cognitive impairment and dementia.[5]

IMMEDIATE NEUROLOGICAL COMPLICATIONS

Neurological complications occurring immediately after transplantation surgery can be due to impairment in central nervous system (CNS) or peripheral nervous system (PNS).

Central Nervous System Dysfunction

Perioperative sedation in KTRs may result in mild symptoms such as behavioral changes or confusion, but sometimes there may be severe symptoms such as encephalopathy or coma as a consequence of hypoxic-ischemic insult. High doses of corticosteroids could be a reason for acute psychosis after transplantation.[6]

Electrolyte Imbalance

Electrolyte disturbances such as dysnatremia, hyperkalemia, hypophosphatemia, and hypomagnesemia are frequently observed following transplant surgery. Severe hyponatremia could be symptomatic and manifests as confusion, obtundation, or seizures. Severe hypomagnesemia can lead to confusion, muscle weakness, tetany, and seizures.[7] Usually, symptoms resolve after the correction of existing electrolyte imbalance. Correction of sodium disorders needs to be done meticulously to avoid central pontine myelinolysis.

Hypertensive Encephalopathy

Factors such as medications [steroids/calcineurin inhibitor (CNI)], allograft rejection, and renal artery stenosis can cause uncontrolled hypertension in the immediate post-transplant period which sometimes could lead to hypertensive encephalopathy.[8]

Kidney transplant recipients can also experience posterior reversible encephalopathy syndrome (PRES). Patients usually present with severe headache, visual defects, seizure, or altered mental sensorium. Characteristic magnetic resonance imaging (MRI) findings are vasogenic edema in bilateral deep cortical and subcortical regions of the parietal and occipital lobes.[9] High doses of steroids, CNI, and younger age group also predispose for PRES. Management is conservative and involves blood pressure control.[10]

Peripheral Nervous System Dysfunction

During kidney transplantation surgery, peripheral nerve injuries can occur in up to 5% of the recipients.[11] Commonly affected nerves are femoral nerve, lumbosacral plexus, and lateral femoral cutaneous nerve.[12] Compression by a local site hematoma formation or prolonged retraction causing stretching of the nerve can result in nerve damage. Within 24–48 hours following surgery, rarely acute femoral neuropathy may develop.[13] Nerve damage can happen due to ischemia, owing to "steal phenomenon" in cases in which renal graft artery is anastomosed to the internal iliac artery, as the proximal end-to-end anastomosis diverts blood away from the vasa nervorum.[14] Damage to the lateral femoral cutaneous nerve can result in numbness over the lateral aspect of the thigh.[15] Some patients might complain of pain in the gluteal region due to lumbosacral plexopathy in cases where the internal iliac artery is used for graft revascularization. Most neuropathies resolve spontaneously; however, sometimes they can take months to recover.[12,13]

Seizure

Studies have shown the incidence of seizure to be approximately 17% in KTRs.[16] It may be due to numerous possible etiologies, e.g., electrolyte disorders, withdrawal of antiepileptic agents, PRES, CNI toxicity, liver dysfunction, CVA, meningitis, or brain malignancies. Computed tomography (CT) or MRI of the head can help in the identification of possible etiology. Cerebrospinal fluid (CSF) analysis plays an essential role to rule out an infectious cause. Management includes identifying and treating the underlying etiology along with the use of antiepileptic drug(s) (AEDs). Of note, AED selection in a KTR is challenging due to factors such as drug interactions, tolerability, metabolism, and excretion. AEDs such as barbiturates, phenytoin, and carbamazepine, in particular, are the inducers of hepatic cytochrome P450 enzymes. Therefore, they can have drug interactions with immunosuppressive agents and result in increased metabolism of CNIs and steroids.[17] Newer AEDs such as levetiracetam, pregabalin, lacosamide, and gabapentin are preferred due to their favorable adverse effect profiles and less drug interactions. **Table 1** shows pharmacokinetics of some important AEDs.

TABLE 1: Summary of pharmacokinetics of antiepileptic drugs.

Drugs	*Route of elimination*	*Metabolism*
Phenobarbital	Hepatic	Inducer of CYP3A
Levetiracetam	Renal	None
Carbamazepine	Hepatic	Inducer of CYP3A
Lacosamide	Renal	Hepatic (CYP450) metabolism
Lamotrigine	Hepatic	Induces CYP34A
Phenytoin	Hepatic (95–99%), Renal (1–5%)	Inducer of CYP3A, metabolized by CYP2C9
Topiramate	Renal	Variable
Valproate	Hepatic	Hepatic (CYP450) metabolism, inhibit CYP2C9

CHAPTER HIGHLIGHTS

- Neurological diseases are commonly encountered in kidney transplant recipients (KTRs) and are the cause of substantial morbidity and mortality.
- Neurological complications could be due to infections, immunosuppressive agents, cancers, and other comorbid conditions.
- Neurological adverse effects of calcineurin inhibitor may be present in 10–28% of KTRs.

SUBACUTE NEUROLOGICAL COMPLICATIONS

Infections

Central nervous system-related infections can be present in up to 5–10% of KTRs and can occur at any time following transplantation.[18] In KTRs, development of an infection depends on two important factors: (1) Epidemiologic exposure of the organism and (2) net immunosuppressive status of the patient.[19] Extensive use of immunosuppressive therapy for the management of allograft rejection, malnutrition, diabetes mellitus, and poor graft functions are some important predisposing factors.[20] Clinical manifestations of infections vary from fever, headache, confusion, convulsion, meningismus to altered sensorium. In **Case Vignette 1**, the possibility of any CNS infection should be ruled out with the help of CNS imaging and CSF analysis. Leukopenia in the patient points toward OR hints at the possibility of

TABLE 2: Common central nervous system (CNS) infections postrenal transplantation.

Diseases	Organism		Diagnosis	Treatment
Meningitis	Bacterial	*Listeria monocytogenes*, *Haemophilus influenzae*, *Neisseria meningitidis*, and *Streptococcus pneumoniae*	• CSF—pleocytosis, increased protein, and reduced glucose • Gram-stain positive • Rapid antigen latex agglutination test • PCR for *Neisseria meningitidis* and *Streptococcus pneumoniae*	Antibiotics based on culture and sensitivity
		Mycobacterium tuberculosis	• CSF—acid-fast bacilli + • Raised adenosine deaminase • Raises total leukocyte with lymphocyte predominance, low glucose, increased protein	Antitubercular therapy
	Fungal	CSF—lymphocytic or monocytic pleocytosis, elevated protein, and low glucose		
		Cryptococcus neoformans	CSF cryptococcal antigen, India ink	IV amphotericin B and fluconazole
		Aspergillus spp.	• Galactomannan assay • (1,3)-β-D-glucan assay • DNA PCR assay in serum or BAL samples • Branching, septated hyphae	Voriconazole, amphotericin B
		Candida spp.	Pseudohyphae and budding yeast	Fluconazole, echinocandin, or amphotericin B
Encephalitis		Cytomegalovirus	• CSF PCR positive • MRI—enhancing ventriculoencephalitis	Ganciclovir
		Varicella-zoster virus	• MRI—mixed lesion (ischemic or hemorrhagic infarcts) • Demyelinating lesions at gray–white matter junction • CSF PCR positive	Acyclovir, ganciclovir
		Human herpes virus-6	• CSF PCR positive • Focal or diffuse encephalitis	Ganciclovir or foscarnet
Focal brain infections	Parasite	*Toxoplasma gondii*	MRI—multiple ring-enhancing lesions, predilection to basal ganglia, thalami, and corticomedullary junction	Pyrimethamine and folinic acid
	Bacterial	*Nocardia asteroides*	• Gram-positive, weakly acid-fast, branching rod-shaped bacteria • MRI—single or multiple lesions with contrast enhancement and little mass effect	Trimethoprim/ sulfamethoxazole and neurosurgical intervention
	Fungal	Mucormycosis, *Aspergillus*, *Candida*, *Cryptococcus*	Begin with paranasal sinuses, producing periorbital edema and may invade the intracavernous carotid artery, cerebral artery emboli, mycotic aneurysm, and stroke	Antifungals

(BAL: bronchoalveolar lavage; CSF: cerebrospinal fluid; DNA: deoxyribonucleic acid; IV: intravenous; MRI: magnetic resonance imaging; PCR: polymerase chain reaction)

viral infections such as cytomegalovirus. However, due to an immunosuppressive state, there may only be minimal signs and symptoms. CNS infections can be meningitis, encephalitis, or focal brain abscess. Frequently experienced CNS infections in transplant recipients are summarized in **Table 2.**[19-22] Sometimes, intracranial lesions as shown in **Case Vignette 2** can be the manifestations of infections such as tuberculosis, nocardiosis, and fungal infections, clinically presenting as focal neurological weakness, ataxia, confusion, and altered sensorium. CNS malignancies, mostly Epstein–Barr virus (EBV)-related post-transplant lymphoproliferative disorder (PTLD), are also differential diagnosis for such lesions. This patient had raised CSF-adenosine deaminase (ADA) levels; hence, he was started on antitubercular agents. The patient responded well to the therapy.

Progressive Multifocal Leukoencephalopathy

Progressive multifocal leukoencephalopathy is a potentially fatal and dreadful CNS condition. It is caused by the John Cunningham (JC) virus, a virus of human polyoma family. The incidence in KTR is 0.027%, and the median time of infection following transplant is around 17 months.[23] It causes cerebral white matter demyelination and oligodendrocyte lysis. Common manifestations are motor weakness, seizure, visual deficits, and mental deficits (cognitive changes, emotional liability, and memory loss). The condition is devastating and highly progressive leading to mortality within a short span of time. MRI findings are characterized by multifocal and asymmetric lesions in cortical and subcortical areas with a minute or no mass effect or enhancement. Typically parieto-occipital regions are involved.[24] Although brain biopsy is the gold standard method for diagnosis, CSF examination for JC virus using deoxyribonucleic acid (DNA) by the polymerase chain reaction (PCR) technique can aid in diagnosis.[25] Currently, other than cessation or reduction of immunosuppressive therapy, there is no approved efficacious therapy for PML. Treatment attempts with cytarabine and interferons have been made but with less clear efficacy rates.[26]

Drug Toxicity

Calcineurin Inhibitors

Tacrolimus (TAC) and cyclosporine (CsA) are the key components of immunosuppressive therapy in a transplant recipient. They can be responsible for neurological adverse effects in 10–28% of KTRs.[27,28] As compared to CsA, neurotoxicity is more frequently experienced with TAC.[27] CNS side effects of CNIs usually appear during the first month of initiation. Side effects are more frequent at higher doses but can also occur at therapeutic drug levels. Both nerve and muscle can get affected. Symptoms of neurological side effects of CNI are shown in **Table 3**. Visual hallucinations and cortical blindness could occur, in the rare instance.[28] Few cases of axonal, demyelinating and multifocal demyelinating neuropathy have also been reported with TAC **(Table 4)**.[29] Factors such as advanced liver failure, low cholesterol levels, and hypomagnesemia can predispose for the development of CNI-induced neurological damage.

TABLE 3: Neurological side effects of calcineurin inhibitors.

Central toxicity	***Peripheral toxicity***
Insomnia, visual disturbances, headache, and mood changes	Paresthesias, peripheral neuropathy, and myopathy
PRES, akinetic mutism, toxic encephalopathy, and convulsions	Axonal and demyelinating neuropathy, Guillain–Barré syndrome

(PRES: posterior reversible encephalopathy syndrome)

TABLE 4: Severity of neurological side effects of calcineurin inhibitors.

	Side effects
Mild	Tremor, headache, insomnia, vivid dream imagery, photophobia
Moderate	Visual and cortical disturbances
Severe	Encephalopathy, convulsion, coma, and flaccid quadriparesis

Mechanisms of Neurotoxicity

- Being highly lipophilic drugs, CsA and TAC can readily cross the blood–brain barrier and damage the white matter. Calcineurin is also expressed in several areas of the brain such as cerebral cortex, striatum, substantia nigra, cerebellum, and hippocampus.[30] CsA and TAC can induce vasoconstriction and vasospasm by gaining access to astrocytes and cerebral vascular smooth muscle followed by disruption of endothelin integrity. Additionally, CNIs can result in increased expression of endothelin and decreased nitric oxide production.[31]
- Other mechanisms for neurotoxicity of CsA and TAC are alteration of mitochondrial function and apoptotic or necrotic cell death via activation of anaerobic glycolysis, proteases, phospholipases, and generation of free radicals.[32]

The use of delayed-release TAC formulations, strict monitoring of blood levels, and vigilance to pharmacological interactions may help in reducing drug-induced neurotoxicity.

Calcineurin-induced Pain Syndrome

It is a condition characterized by incapacitating pain in bilateral legs mostly affecting the knee and feet but sparing the hip areas. It usually presents within the first year of transplantation. There is worsening of symptoms with physical activity and stress, whereas improvement may occur with rest. Bone marrow edema of affected areas may be seen in imaging studies.[33] The exact pathophysiology is unclear. The postulated hypothesis is that CNIs affect sensory neural function via two-pore potassium channels leading to altered neuronal resting membrane potential. The condition mostly is self-resolving. However, calcium channel blockers may be helpful.

Corticosteroids

Many neuropsychiatric symptoms ranging from insomnia, concentration impairment, mood disorders, and irritability to severe psychosis can be associated with the use of steroids. Symptoms usually occur at the time of treatment initiation. With long-term use, proximal myopathy may develop.[34]

Bortezomib

Bortezomib use can be associated with the development of painful sensory neuropathy by causing dysregulation of neurotrophins and blocking nerve growth factor-mediated neuronal survival induced through nuclear factor kappa B (NF-κB) inhibition.[35]

CENTRAL NERVOUS SYSTEM MALIGNANCY

The most common CNS malignancies in KTRs are lymphomas and metastatic tumors, which are usually de novo malignancies. The common PTLD subtype in a post-transplant setting is diffuse large B-cell lymphoma, followed by Burkitt lymphoma and plasmablastic lymphoma.

Of all cases of PTLD, CNS is involved in approximately 30% of the patients.[36] The overall immunosuppressive state and EBV seropositivity are the two critical factors for the development of malignancies in a KTR. In an analysis by Snanoudj et al., the median duration of occurrence of lymphoma postrenal transplantation was 18 months.[37] Clinical presentation varies according to the site of brain involvement. Lowering the doses or cessation of immunosuppressive agents is the primary step of management. Other treatment options are rituximab-based chemotherapy, intrathecal chemotherapy, radiation, or surgery, according to the stage and extension of the malignancy (*See* Chapter 13.7 for details).

CHRONIC NEUROLOGICAL COMPLICATIONS

Cerebrovascular Disease

Cerebrovascular accidents, including ischemic, hemorrhagic stroke, or transient ischemic attacks, are frequent complications in a KTR and the incidence of CVA is approximately 5 and 9.4% during the first and second year post-transplant, respectively.[38] After infections, strokes are one of the common causes of mortality in a transplant recipient.[39] Increased risk of stroke is attributed to prolonged steroid use, hypertension, diabetes mellitus, obesity, smoking, poor graft function, and dyslipidemia.[40] It is important to rule out fungal infections such as aspergillosis and mucormycosis particularly in cases of ischemic strokes as the hyphae can result in distal embolization and invade cerebral arteries. Correction of reversible predisposing factors is crucial in improving clinical outcomes.

Cognitive and Psychiatric Disorders

Prevalence of cognitive decline in kidney transplant patients (KTPs) ranges from 22 to 58%.[41] Unlike in the general population, cognitive impatient can affect younger patients. Chu et al. reported a greater cognitive decline in KTPs with higher baseline frailty over 4 years in KTPs.[42] Etiopathogenesis of cognitive decline is usually multifactorial due to the effects of immunosuppressive agents, less physical activity, malnutrition, altered gut microbiome along with traditional risk factors such as hypertension, hypercholesterolemia, metabolic syndrome, diabetes, and hyperuricemia.[43] Cognitive impairment can result in poor quality of life, adherence breach to immunosuppressive medications, higher healthcare costs, and poor graft survival. Treatment of cognitive impairment is mostly comprehensive and supportive care including management of associated factors such as depression and optimal effective immunosuppression strategies. Polypharmacy and the use of psychotropic drugs should be avoided.

REFERENCES

1. Mohammadi M, Salarzaei M, Parooie F. Neurological complications after renal transplantation: a systematic review and meta-analysis. Ther Apher Dial. 2019;23:518-28.
2. Tsokos GC. Systemic lupus erythematosus. N Engl J Med. 2011;365(22):2110-21.
3. McArthur JC, Brew BJ, Nath A. Neurological complications of HIV infection. Lancet Neurol. 2005;4:543-55.
4. Savica V, Musolino R, Di Leo R, Santoro D, Vita G, Bellinghieri G. Autonomic dysfunction in uremia. Am J Kidney Dis. 2001;38(Suppl. 1): S118-21.
5. Kalirao P, Pederson S, Foley RN, Kolste A, Tupper D, Zaun D, et al. Cognitive impairment in peritoneal dialysis patients. Am J Kidney Dis. 2011;57(4):612-20.
6. Abbott KC, Agodoa LY, O'Malley PG. Hospitalized psychoses after renal transplantation in the United States: incidence, risk factors, and prognosis. J Am Soc Nephrol. 2003;14: 1628-35.
7. De Waele L, Van Gaal PJ, Abramowicz D. Electrolytes disturbances after kidney transplantation. Acta Clin Belg. 2019; 74(1):48-52.
8. Stott VL, Hurrell MA, Anderson TJ. Reversible posterior leukoencephalopathy syndrome: a misnomer reviewed. Intern Med J. 2005;35:83-90.
9. Haughey D, Narsipur SS. Posterior reversible encephalopathy syndrome after renal transplant: a simple solution for a complicated patient. Case Rep Nephrol Dial. 2014;5(1): 20-5.
10. Cengiz N, Adibelli Z, Yakupoğlu YK, Türker H. Neurological complications after renal transplantation: a retrospective clinical study. Noro Psikiyatr Ars. 2015;52(4):331-5.
11. Van Veer H, Coosemans W, Pirenne J, Monbaliu D. Acute femoral neuropathy: a rare complication after renal transplantation. Transplant Proc. 2010;42:4384-8.
12. Li QS, Huo WQ, Nie ZL, Wang HF, Liang PH, Jin FS. Acute femoral neuropathy following renal transplantation: a retrospective, multicenter study in China. Transplant Proc. 2010;42:1699-703.
13. van der Voort van Zyp NCM, Davin JC, Idu M, Aronson DC. Kidney transplant survival rates and surgical complications in kidney transplants in children; experiences in the Emma Children's hospital AMC. Ned Tijdschr Geneeskd. 2005;149:584-8.
14. Dhillon SS, Sarac E. Lumbosacral plexopathy after dual kidney transplantation. Am J Kidney Dis. 2000;36(5):1045-8.
15. Sharma KR, Cross J, Santiago F, Ayyar DR, Burke 3rd G. Incidence of acute femoral neuropathy following renal transplantation. Arch Neurol. 2002;59:541-5.
16. Lin P, Tian X, Wang X. Seizures after transplantation. Seizure. 2018;61:177-85.
17. Títoff V, Moury HN, Títoff IB, Kelly KM. Seizures, antiepileptic drugs, and CKD. Am J Kidney Dis. 2019;73:90-101.
18. Fishman JA. Infection in solid-organ transplant recipients. N Engl J Med. 2007;357:2601-14.

19. Karuthu S, Blumberg EA. Common infections in kidney transplant recipients. Clin J Am Soc Nephrol. 2012;7:2058-70.
20. Tunkel AR, Glaser CA, Bloch KC, Sejvar JJ, Marra CM, Roos KL, et al. The management of encephalitis: clinical practice guidelines by the Infectious Diseases Society of America. Clin Infect Dis. 2008;47:303-27.
21. Khoury JA, Brennan DC. Infectious complications in kidney transplant recipients: review of the literature. Saudi J Kidney Dis Transpl. 2005;16:453-97.
22. Hu JH, Zhao H, Huang YP, Zhang X, Gao HN, Yang MF, et al. Opportunistic post-transplantation virus infections in renal transplant recipients. Transplant Proc. 2011;43(10):3715-9.
23. Sarbu N, Shih RY, Jones RV, Horkayne-Szakaly I, Oleaga L, Smirniotopoulos JG. White matter diseases with radiologic-pathologic correlation. Radiographics. 2016; 36(5):1426-47.
24. Wang Y, Kirby JE, Qian Q. Effective use of JC virus PCR for diagnosis of progressive multifocal leukoencephalopathy. J Med Microbiol. 2009;58:253-5.
25. Aksamit AJ. Treatment of non-AIDS progressive multifocal leukoencephalopathy with cytosine arabinoside. J Neurovirol. 2001;7:386.
26. Sospedra M, Schippling S, Yousef S, Jelcic I, Bofill-Mas S, Planas R, et al. Treating progressive multifocal leuko-encephalopathy with interleukin 7 and vaccination with JC virus capsid protein VP1. Clin Infect Dis. 2014;59: 1588.
27. Pirsch JD, Miller J, Deierhoi MH, Vincenti F, Filo RS. A comparison of tacrolimus (fk506) and cyclosporine for immunosuppression after cadaveric renal transplantation. FK506 Kidney Transplant Study Group. Transplantation. 1997;63:977-83.
28. Wijdicks EF. Neurotoxicity of immunosuppressive drugs. Liver Transpl. 2001;7:937-42.
29. Meena P, Bhargava V, Rana DS, Bhalla AK, Gupta A, Malik M, et al. Tacrolimus-associated Guillain-Barré syndrome. Am J Ther. 2020;28(2):e268-70.
30. Serkova NJ, Christians U, Benet LZ. Biochemical mechanisms of cyclosporine neurotoxicity. Mol Interv. 2004;4:97-107.
31. Illsinger S, Janzen N, Lücke T, Bednarczyk J, Schmidt KH, Hoy L, et al. Cyclosporine A: impact on mitochondrial function in endothelial cells. Clin Transplant. 2011;25: 584-93.
32. Asai A, Qiu J, Narita Y, Chi S, Saito N, Shinoura N, et al. High level calcineurin activity predisposes neuronal cells to apoptosis. J Biol Chem. 1999;274:34450-8.
33. Collini A, De Bartolomeis C, Barni R, Ruggieri G, Bernini M, Carmellini M. Calcineurin-inhibitor induced pain syndrome after organ transplantation. Kidney Int. 2006;70(7):1367-70.
34. Faravelli I, Velardo D, Podestà MA, Ponticelli C. Immuno-suppression-related neurological disorders in kidney transplantation. J Nephrol. 2021;34(2):539-55.
35. Schmidt N, Alloway RR, Walsh RC, Sadaka B, Shields AR, Girnita AL, et al. Prospective evaluation of the toxicity profile of proteasome inhibitor-based therapy in renal transplant candidates and recipients. Transplantation. 2012;94:352-61.
36. Morscio J, Tousseyn T. Recent insights in the pathogenesis of post-transplantation lymphoproliferative disorders. World J Transplant. 2016;6:505-16.
37. Snanoudj R, Durrbach A, Leblond V, Caillard S, De Ligny BH, Noel C, et al. Primary brain lymphomas after kidney transplantation: presentation and outcome. Transplantation. 2003;76:930-7.
38. Meena P, Bhargava V, Rana D, Bhalla A, Gupta A. An approach to neurological disorders in a kidney transplant recipient. Kidney360. 2020;1(8):837-44.
39. U.S. Renal Data System. USRDS 2014 Annual Data Report: Volume One: Chronic Kidney Disease in the United States and Volume Two: End-stage Renal Disease in the United States. Bethesda, MD: National Institutes of Health, National Institute of Diabetes and Digestive and Kidney Diseases; 2014.
40. Willicombe M, Kumar N, Goodall D, Clarke C, McLean AG, Power A, et al. Incidence, risk factors, and outcomes of stroke post-transplantation in patients receiving a steroid sparing immunosuppression protocol. Clin Transplant. 2015;29:18-25.
41. Gupta A, Mahnken JD, Johnson DK, Thomas TS, Subramaniam D, Polshak T, et al. Prevalence and correlates of cognitive impairment in kidney transplant recipients. BMC Nephrol. 2017;18:158.
42. Chu NM, Gross AL, Shaffer AA, Haugen CE, Norman SP, Xue Q-L, et al. Frailty and changes in cognitive function after kidney transplantation. J Am Soc Nephrol. 2019;30:336-45.
43. Jurgensen A, Qannus AA, Gupta A. Cognitive function in kidney transplantation. Curr Transplant Rep. 2020;7:145-53.

13.4 Hypertension in Kidney Transplant Recipients

Santosh Varughese, Jeethu Joseph Eapen

CASE VIGNETTE

Mr C is a 34-year-old gentleman who underwent kidney transplantation with his 58-year-old mother being his voluntary kidney donor. He developed an acute cellular rejection in his first month which responded well to steroids. His serum creatinine is 1.6 mg/dL. He is on prednisolone 10 mg once daily, tacrolimus 2 mg twice daily, and mycophenolate mofetil (MMF) 1,000 mg twice daily. His current problem is that blood pressure (BP) is 150/90 mm Hg despite being on amlodipine 10 mg once daily, bisoprolol 5 mg twice daily, and prazosin XL 10 mg twice daily.

His problem of post-transplant hypertension is quite common in kidney transplant recipients.

INTRODUCTION

Hypertension is arguably the most common post-transplant medical problem encountered in kidney transplant recipients. The presence of pretransplant hypertension often lulls both the patient and the physician into complacency arising out of familiarity. Using ambulatory blood pressure monitoring (ABPM), it is estimated that almost 95% of all kidney transplant recipients maybe hypertensive[1] with 85% requiring antihypertensive drugs.[2] Since elevated BP adversely affects both recipient survival[3] and graft survival,[4,5] it is incumbent upon transplant physicians to pay meticulous attention to control of BP in kidney transplant recipients.

ETIOPATHOGENESIS

The etiology of post-transplant hypertension is multifactorial and results from a complex interplay of varying pathophysiological factors including donor and recipient characteristics, graft kidney function, effect of immunosuppressive medications, and complications of kidney transplantation.

Donor Factors

Donor factors that increase the risk of hypertension are older age, presence of hypertension in the kidney donor,[6,7] lower donor organ quality as in extended criteria donor transplants,[8] genetic polymorphisms,[9-14] and donor–recipient size mismatches.[15,16] A donor of relatively smaller physical size, female gender, or different ethnicity from the recipient or older age—all these have the potential to lead to "underdosing" of the nephron mass and consequent maladaptive glomerular hypertrophy, hyperfiltration, and intraglomerular hypertension.[15] The decrease in filtration size leads to sodium retention and subsequent rise in system BP.[17]

Recipient Factors

The majority of kidney transplant recipients are hypertensive prior to transplantation as a consequence of the chronic kidney disease itself. Most of these recipients continue to be hypertensive after transplant surgery, possibly as a consequence to stiffness of vessels and decreased compliance.[18] Recipient factors associated with post-transplant hypertension are recipient age, genetic factors, increased body mass index, and presence of additional conditions such as obstructive sleep apnea or more rarely endocrine tumors such as pheochromocytomas or adrenal adenoma.

Renal Allograft-related Factors

Transplant physicians have long observed that any injury to the renal allograft can either cause or worsen hypertension. The most common causes are rejection episodes—both cellular and antibody mediated, thrombotic microangiopathy (recurrence, de-novo, or drug induced), recurrence of glomerular disease [e.g., immunoglobulin A (IgA) nephropathy], and chronic allograft injury (chronic antibody-mediated rejection and interstitial fibrosis/tubular atrophy). Acute rejection assorted stimulation of the renin–angiotensin–aldosterone system (RAAS) is the likely etiology of hypertension in these patients. Therefore, new-onset hypertension must be evaluated and monitored for the acute rejection episode. Hypertension associated with an acute rejection episode is easily corrected with treatment of the rejection. Antibodies to the angiotensin II type I receptor (AT1 receptors) may cause an antibody-mediated rejection without donor-specific antibodies and hypertension. Hypertension in this group may be prevented by AT1 receptor blockers.[19-21] The hypertension that results from chronic allograft injury is similar to chronic kidney disease of the native kidney. Of the recurrent glomerular diseases, focal segmental glomerulosclerosis is associated with worsening of BP control.[22]

Rarer conditions that cause treatable hypertension include renal artery kinking (*parvus et tardus* waveform on Doppler) and Page kidney (external compression of the kidney by a hematoma, including that caused by an allograft biopsy), urinoma, or lymphocele. Early recognition of these conditions is crucial as they are amenable to surgical treatment and control of hypertension.

Immunosuppression-related Factors

Glucocorticoids are the most common drug implicated in post-transplant hypertension, accounting for about 15%

of post-transplant hypertension,[23,24] with maximal effect on those who had pretransplant hypertension. The hypertensive effect is dose dependent with a dose of 20 mg or more of prednisolone being more likely to cause hypertension than a dose of 5 mg daily.[25] Glucocorticoids cause hypertension by increased sensitivity to the action of vasoconstrictor agents (the predominant cause) and mineralocorticoid receptor activation leading to salt and water restrictions.[26] Lowering or avoidance of glucocorticoids may decrease risk of hypertension[27] but the results are not uniform,[28,29] and the increased rejection risk from steroid avoidance or reduction may offset the advantage thereof of increased BP.[30,31]

The near-uniform use of calcineurin inhibitors (CNI) both causes and worsens post-transplant hypertension, (4 from 12) cyclosporine more than tacrolimus.[32] The etiology of CNI-induced hypertension is the direct vascular effect. The afferent arteriolar vasoconstriction causes renal sodium retention.[33,34] Tacrolimus also causes a sodium-sensitive hypertension due to activation of sodium chloride cotransporter activation.[35] Among the CNI agents, cyclosporine has been implicated more often than tacrolimus in registry data and clinical trials.[36-38] Change of CNI agent from cyclosporine to tacrolimus seems to improve BP control.[38] MMF, another nearly ubiquitous immunosuppressive drug used in kidney transplantation, may prevent development of salt-sensitive hypertension.[39,40] Decrease in tubulointerstitial fibrosis and T-cell infiltration has been seen in animal studies.[40] The lowering of BP was observed in a nontransplant clinical study,[41] but this is as yet unproven in the transplantation setting.[42] In fact, the 30–80% hypertension incidence in transplant recipients receiving MMF is likely related to the presence of concomitant glucocorticoids, CNI, and other comorbidities.[42]

The purported mechanisms of post-transplant hypertension and relevant management strategies are described in **Flowchart 1**.[42]

Secondary Hypertension

In the myriad causes of post-transplant hypertension, the clinician must not forget the relatively rarer causes of secondary hypertension, of which the most common is

Flowchart 1: Mechanism of post-transplant hypertension and management strategies.[42]

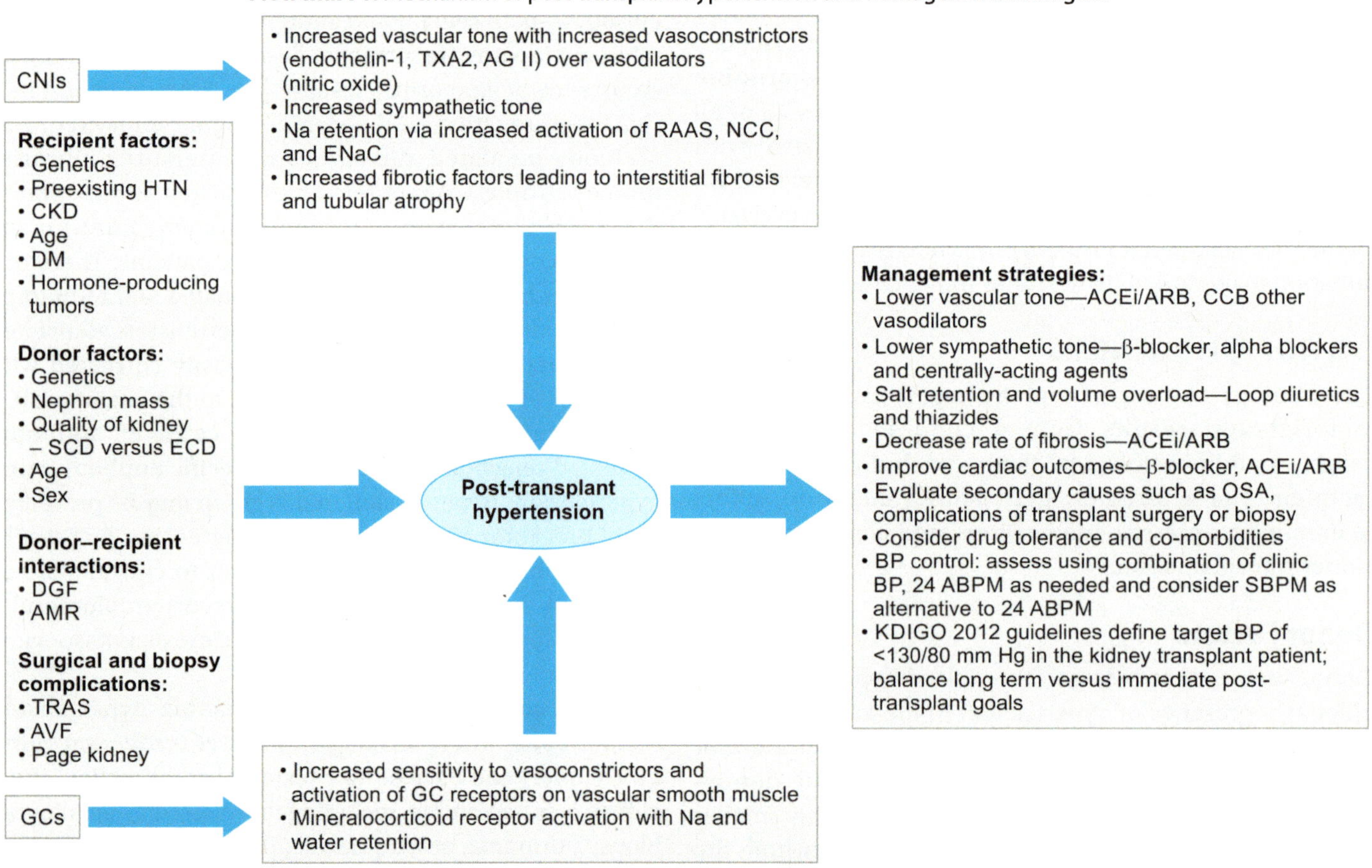

(ABPM: ambulatory blood pressure monitoring; ACEi: ACE inhibitor; AMR: antibody-mediated rejection; ARB: angiotensin receptor blocker; AVF: arteriovenous fistula; BP: blood pressure; CCB: calcium channel blocker; CKD: chronic kidney disease; CNIs: calcineurin inhibitors; DGF: delayed graft function; DM: diabetes mellitus; ECD: expanded criteria donor; ENaC: epithelial sodium channel; GCs: glucocorticoids; HTN: hypertension; KDIGO: Kidney Disease: Improving Global Outcomes; Na: sodium; NCC: sodium–chloride cotransporter; OSA: obstructive sleep apnea; RAAS: renin-angiotensin-aldosterone system; SBPM: self blood pressure monitoring; SCD: standard criteria donor; TRAS: transplant renal artery stenosis; TXA2: thromboxane A2)

BOX 1: Cause of secondary hypertension in kidney transplant recipients (modified).[18]

Kidney-related causes:
- Acute rejection
- Transplant renal artery stenosis
- Ischemic nephropathy
- Hydronephrosis

Nonkidney-related causes:
- Primary hyperaldosteronism
- Obstructive sleep apnea

transplant renal artery stenosis (TRAS) which conforms to Goldblatt's single clip model of renovascular hypertension. **Box 1** lists the common causes of secondary hypertension after kidney transplantation. Clues to presence of secondary hypertension are resistant hypertension, hypokalemia (rather than hyperkalemia), accelerated target organ damage, and/or declining graft function.

Transplant Renal Artery Stenosis

Transplant renal artery stenosis may occur in a wide range of kidney transplant recipients with values ranging from 1 to 23% reported in literature,[43] and the most common site is at the anastomosis. TRAS maybe also present at more proximal locations like the external iliac artery.[44] The typical clinical presentation is worsening of graft function with use of angiotensin-converting-enzyme inhibitor (ACEi) or angiotensin receptor blocker (ARB) therapy. Edema may also be a common clinical finding. Presence of bruit may not always be pathognomonic and may occur due to a small arteriovenous fistula following graft kidney biopsy.[18] Diagnosis is by renal artery Doppler, computerized tomography of the renal artery with contrast, or magnetic resonance angiography. Carbon dioxide angiography is another investigational technique that reduces the risk of contrast-induced allograft injury. Treatment of TRAS is controversial and challenging. Worsening hypertension with graft dysfunction is an indication for intravascular intervention with percutaneous angioplasty, with or without stenting, being the treatment of choice when medical therapy appears inadequate.[43] Surgical revision is reserved for the very early occurrence of TRAS or when the stenotic lesions are not amenable for percutaneous angioplasty or when the stenosis recurs despite angioplasty.

DEFINITION, DIAGNOSIS, AND GOALS OF THERAPY

The diagnosis of hypertension and the goals of therapy are based on presence, or lack thereof, of proteinuria and other comorbid conditions such as diabetes mellitus and atherosclerotic vascular disease.[45,46]

The recent KDIGO (Kidney Disease: Improving Global Outcomes) guideline on control of BP[47] has not made any change to the previous target of systolic BP <130 mm Hg and diastolic BP <80 mm Hg.[48] A reasonable target for BP control in all transplant recipients is at least <140/90 mm Hg with <130/80 mm Hg in those with spot urine protein to creatinine ratio 500–1,000 mg/g creatinine (as per the Canadian Society of Nephrology)[49] and <125/75 mm Hg (as per the European Best Practices Guidelines Expert Group on Renal Transplantation).[50] The Systolic Blood Pressure Intervention Trial (SPRINT) trial in nondiabetic patients with high cardiovascular risk found lower rates of cardiovascular events (both fatal and nonfatal) in patients whose target systolic BP <120 mm Hg compared to a target <140 mm Hg.[51,52] The applicability of this finding to kidney transplant recipients remains unclear as this study population did not have any kidney transplant recipients. In the absence of autoregulation, the transplanted kidneys maybe more susceptible to ischemic injury if the pressure head is too low. Therefore, a target BP <130/80 mm Hg is reasonable as stated in the KDIGO guidelines.

Blood pressure variability is common and clinic BPs may considerably differ from home BP reading. There are possibilities of both white coat hypertension and masked hypertension.[53] Hence, BP recordings in the transplant clinic alone may be insufficient to guide therapy. Masked hypertension may cause progression of native kidney disease,[53] but this is yet unproven in kidney transplant recipients. Home BP monitoring and ABPM have been proposed as alternatives to clinic BP alone and there is good correlation between home BP and ABPM recordings.[54] A study by David et al. from Christian Medical College Vellore, South India, using ABPM in kidney transplant recipients concluded that ABPM was the best tool for diagnosis and monitoring hypertension in kidney transplant recipients as was home BP monitoring, both being better than office BP recordings alone.[55] When in doubt, it may be prudent to rely more on ABPM or home BP monitoring than office BP recording alone.[18]

TREATMENT

Treatment of hypertension in the kidney transplant recipient is aimed at preventing cardiovascular disease and hypertensive injury to the graft. Long-term graft survival is likely to be adversely affected by post-transplant hypertension.[4,5] In an experimental animal model of chronic rejection, control of hypertension improved graft function, increased survival, reduced degree of proteinuria, and decreased hypertensive injury to the glomeruli in the graft.[56]

All kidney transplant recipients with hypertension should be advised nonpharmacological management including dietary salt restriction, regular exercise, weight control, and avoidance of smoking. In one study, restriction of salt to 80–100 mmol/day of sodium caused a significant drop in both systolic and diastolic BP in comparison to the BP in the control group not on a salt-restricted diet.[57] The benefit of salt restriction may be more obvious in patients receiving CNI compared to those who were only on azathioprine.[58]

In the initial weeks to months of the post-transplant period, development of hypertension maybe influenced by volume overload, high glucocorticoid dose, higher target CNI levels, and decreased allograft function. Lowering of glucocorticoids and CNI dose and achievement of ideal volume status may help in lowering BP.[18]

The choice of antihypertensive drug therapy in kidney transplant recipients is determined on basis of efficacy, absent or negligible drug interactions with immunosuppressive drugs, tolerability, and presence of associated comorbidities. The commonly used drugs are calcium channel blockers (CCBs), β-blockers, α-1 blockers, diuretics, ACEi, and ARBs. Nearly universally, CCBs are considered *the* therapeutic agent of choice in the post-transplant period since they could potentially counteract the CNI-induced vasoconstriction.[59] This pharmacological efficacy of CCBs is irrespective of the patients' age or gender nor is it appreciably affected by salt intake, unlike ACEi and ARB.

There has been no incontrovertible evidence of superiority of using ACEi or ARBs in kidney transplant recipients. There is an ongoing prospective randomized controlled trial involving 528 kidney transplant recipients from 11 Canadian transplant centers. Patients with estimated glomerular filtration rate (GFR) between 20 and 55 mL/min/1.73 m^2 are being randomized to receive either ramipril 5 mg twice daily or placebo. This study aims to look for changes in GFR, proteinuria, BP as well as incidence of hyperkalemia, anemia, and other adverse events, cardiovascular events and health-related quality of life.[60]

Important Drug Interactions

Grapefruit juice inhibits enterocyte CYP3A4 activity and increases the bioavailability of both CNIs and CCBs.[18] The CCB most susceptible to this interaction is felodipine in which there is doubling of its bioavailability.[18] Common dihydropyridine CCBs such as nifedipine and amlodipine as well as nondihydropiridine CCBs (e.g., diltiazem and verapamil) have inherently high bioavailability, and there is only 20–30% increase in blood levels but symptomatic hypotension may occasionally occur.[18]

It is very important to remember that the nondihydropiridine CCBs diltiazem and verapamil cause significant suppression of CYP3A4 activity. This can be used clinically to increase the therapeutic drug level of CNIs making it an economically prudent therapeutic option. Diltiazem given at a dose of 120 mg/day allows up to 60% reduction in dose of CNI, but interpatient variability could still occur, necessitating close therapeutic monitoring.[18] **Table 1** lists the interactions of antihypertensive medications with the cytochrome P450 enzyme system.

TABLE 1: Antihypertensive medications and the cytochrome P450 system.[18]

Drug class	*Cytochrome P_{450} interaction potential*	*Interactions*
ACE inhibitors	No significant interactions; most ACE inhibitors are prodrugs that undergo hepatic and/or enterocyte metabolism	Prodrug conversion to active diacid ACE inhibitors is minimally effected by hepatic disease as occurs in heart failure
Diuretics	Hydrochlorothiazide and chemically related diuretics are not metabolized. Furosemide and spironolactone are metabolized to glucuronide and sulfated metabolites, respectively. Eplerenone is metabolized by CYP3A4	Neither has a significant effect on the cytochrome P_{450} system. Coadministration of verapamil with eplerenone results in an approximately two-fold increase in the area-under-the-curve for eplerenone
Angiotensin receptor blockers	Losartan and irbesartan are primarily metabolized by CYP2C9. Losartan undergoes metabolism to an active metabolize E-3174 via CYP2C9, which creates the potential for interaction with inhibitors or simulators of this P_{450} isozyme	Coadministration of losartan with enzyme inducers, such as rifampin and phenobarbital decrease losartan and E-3174 levels, whereas enzyme inhibitors, such as fluconazole, decrease the levels of E-3174. These changes are inconsequential and seem not be affect the BP lowering effect of losartan
β-adrenergic blocking agents	Pharmacokinetics of a number of β-adrenergic blocking agents are strongly affected by cytochrome P_{450} inducers and inhibitors as relates to CYP2D6	Rifampin increases propranolol clearance by 2-3-fold; quinidine and diphenhydramine increase blood levels of β-blockers, such as timolol or metoprolol
CCBs	These drugs serve as substrates for and inhibitors of CYP3A4. Verapamil and diltiazem are known inhibitors of CYP3A4. Symptomatic hypotension can occur when CYP3A4 and inhibitors are given with dihydropyridine CCBs	Concomitant use of azole antifungals with dihydropyridine CCBs should be done with caution; most CCBs inhibit the metabolism of cyclosporine; diltiazem inhibits the metabolism of triazolam and methylprednisolone

(ACE: angiotensin-converting enzyme; BP: blood pressure; CCBs: calcium channel blockers)

HYPERTENSION IN PEDIATRIC KIDNEY TRANSPLANT RECIPIENT

Since over three decades, similar to adults, hypertension has been known to be a complication in pediatric kidney transplantation.[61] Also, like adults, hypertension is the most common modifiable risk factor for occurrence of cardiovascular disease in pediatric kidney transplant recipient.[18] The number of pediatric kidney transplant recipients requiring pharmacological antihypertensive therapy in the immediate post-transplant period may exceed 80% and by 5 years, the numbers reduce approximately to 70% in deceased donor kidney transplant recipients and 60% in living donor kidney transplant recipients, who continue to require drugs for optimal BP control after 5 years.[62] Nearly half the normotensive pediatric kidney transplant recipient become hypertensive in the initial 2 years after transplantation.[63] This number may reach as high as 70–80% when ABPM is used to diagnose hypertension.[18] There appears to be a 50% higher prevalence of masked hypertension, i.e., normal clinic BP with elevated BP on ABPM.[64-67] Many pediatric kidney transplant recipients may also be nondippers.[67,68]

Similar to adults, in pediatric kidney transplant recipients too, hypertension is associated with lower graft function, with higher systolic BP at 3 months post-transplant being associated with lower GFR at the end of the first year.[69] Requirement of more antihypertensive agents appears to be also associated with higher graft failure rates,[70] although it is difficult to exclude that hypertension maybe a consequence of poor allograft function rather than the other way around. For each 10% increase in systolic BP at the end of the first year, there was a doubling of risk of future graft failure.[71]

As per the KDIGO guidelines, BP in pediatric kidney transplant recipients should be maintained <90th percentile for age, gender, and height.[72] ACEi and ARB are advised as first-line therapy. Annual ABPM measurement of BP is also likely to result in improved BP control.[73] Steroid avoidance protocol may also allow for better BP control though this has not been studied.[18]

RESISTANT HYPERTENSION

Resistant hypertension is defined as office BP that remains above the target with concurrent use of three antihypertension drugs at maximal doses, one of which is a diuretic.[74,75]

Though clinical trials peg the incidence of resistant hypertension around 20–30% of transplant recipients,[76] true incidence (based on office BP readings) is likely to be around 6.4%[77] and by ABPM as high as 20%.[78] It is also likely more common in older recipients, in diabetics, in those with lower GFR, and in those requiring higher doses of steroids.[76] Resistant hypertension is more common among populations with higher obesity rates, increased life expectancy, and a sedentary lifestyle.[76] Resistant hypertension in kidney transplant recipients is associated with decreased 5-year patient survival and graft survival compared to recipients with BP controlled to <130/80 mm Hg—patient survival 60 versus 79% and graft survival 80 versus 93%, respectively.[79] The astute clinician must distinguish true resistant hypertension from pseudo-resistance which occurs from inaccurate measurement of BP, nonadherence to prescribed therapy, inappropriate drug choices or doses, white coat hypertension, and secondary causes of resistant hypertension due to obstructive sleep apnea, hyperaldosteronism, coarctation of aorta, thyroid diseases, intake of exogenous substances, pheochromocytoma, and of these perhaps the most common, renal artery stenosis.

CONCLUSION

Hypertension is common in the post-transplant period in both adults and children. Control of BP is likely to result in improved cardiovascular morbidity and mortality. BP must be optimized using nonpharmacological and pharmacological methods (where needed) with CCBs being the drug of first choice and ACEi or ARB being more advantageous in those with proteinuria. ABPM maybe helpful to diagnose masked hypertension as well as for adequate BP control in adult and pediatric kidney transplant recipients.

Secondary causes such as TRAS, hyperaldosteronism, obstructive sleep apnea, and rarer causes need to be considered in evaluating patients with resistant hypertension.

REFERENCES

1. Fontán MP, Rodríguez-Carmona A, Falcón TG, Rivera CF, Valdés F. Early immunologic and nonimmunologic predictors of arterial hypertension after renal transplantation. Am J Kidney Dis. 1999;33(1):21-8.
2. Wadei HM, Textor SC. Hypertension in the kidney transplant recipient. Transplant Rev. 2010;24(3):105-20.
3. Mange KC. Blood pressure and the survival of renal allografts from living donors. J Am Soc Nephrol. 2004;15(1):187-93.
4. Sanders CE, Curtis JJ. Role of hypertension in chronic renal allograft dysfunction. Kidney Int Suppl. 1995;52:S43-7.
5. Cheigh JS, Haschemeyer RH, Wang JC, Riggio RR, Tapia L, Stenzel KH, et al. Hypertension in kidney transplant recipients. Effect on long-term renal allograft survival. Am J Hypertens. 1989;2(5 Pt. 1):341-8.
6. Włodarczyk Z, Glyda M, Kościanska L, Kołodziejczyk J, Sulikowska B, Manitius J. Prevalence of arterial hypertension following kidney transplantation: a multifactorial analysis. Ann Transplant. 2003;8(2):43-6.
7. Guidi E, Menghetti D, Milani S, Montagnino G, Palazzi P, Bianchi G. Hypertension may be transplanted with the kidney in humans: a long-term historical prospective follow-up of recipients grafted with kidneys coming from donors with or without hypertension in their families. J Am Soc Nephrol. 1996;7(8):1131-8.

8. Blanca L, Jiménez T, Cabello M, Sola E, Gutierrez C, Burgos D, et al. Cardiovascular risk in recipients with kidney transplants from expanded criteria donors. Transplant Proc. 2012; 44(9):2579-81.
9. Freedman BI, Murea M. Target organ damage in African American hypertension: role of APOL1. Curr Hypertens Rep. 2012;14(1):21-8.
10. Grisk O, Steinbach AC, Ciecholewski S, Schlüter T, Klöting I, Schmidt H, et al. Multidrug resistance-related protein 2 genotype of the donor affects kidney graft function. Pharmacogenet Genomics. 2009;19(4):276-88.
11. Hauser IA, Schaeffeler E, Gauer S, Scheuermann EH, Wegner B, Gossmann J, et al. ABCB1 genotype of the donor but not of the recipient is a major risk factor for cyclosporine-related nephrotoxicity after renal transplantation. J Am Soc Nephrol. 2005;16(5):1501-11.
12. Joy MS, Hogan SL, Thompson BD, Finn WF, Nickeleit V. Cytochrome P450 3A5 expression in the kidneys of patients with calcineurin inhibitor nephrotoxicity. Nephrol Dial Transplant. 2007;22(7):1963-8.
13. Lee BT, Kumar V, Williams TA, Abdi R, Bernhardy A, Dyer C, et al. The APOL1 genotype of African American kidney transplant recipients does not impact 5-year allograft survival. Am J Transplant. 2012;12(7):1924-8.
14. Reeves-Daniel AM, DePalma JA, Bleyer AJ, Rocco MV, Murea M, Adams PL, et al. The APOL1 gene and allograft survival after kidney transplantation. Am J Transplant. 2011;11(5):1025-30.
15. Brenner BM, Milford EL. Nephron underdosing: a programmed cause of chronic renal allograft failure. Am J Kidney Dis. 1993;21(5 Suppl. 2):66-72.
16. Johnson RJ, Herrera-Acosta J, Schreiner GF, Rodriguez-Iturbe B. Subtle acquired renal injury as a mechanism of salt-sensitive hypertension. N Engl J Med. 2002;346(12): 913-23.
17. Mizuno M, Siddique K, Baum M, Smith SA. Prenatal programming of hypertension induces sympathetic overactivity in response to physical stress. Hypertension. 2013; 61(1):180-6.
18. Weir MR, Burgess ED, Cooper JE, Fenves AZ, Goldsmith D, McKay D, et al. Assessment and management of hypertension in transplant patients. J Am Soc Nephrol. 2015;26(6): 1248-60.
19. Dragun D, Müller DN, Bräsen JH, Fritsche L, Nieminen-Kelhä M, Dechend R, et al. Angiotensin II type 1-receptor activating antibodies in renal-allograft rejection. N Engl J Med. 2005;352(6):558-69.
20. Wei F, Jia XJ, Yu SQ, Gu Y, Wang L, Guo XM, et al. Candesartan versus imidapril in hypertension: a randomised study to assess effects of anti-AT1 receptor autoantibodies. Heart Br Card Soc. 2011;97(6):479-84.
21. Xia Y, Kellems RE. Receptor-activating autoantibodies and disease: preeclampsia and beyond. Expert Rev Clin Immunol. 2011;7(5):659-74.
22. Curtis JJ. Distinguishing the causes of post-transplantation hypertension. Pediatr Nephrol Berl Ger. 1991;5(1):108-11.
23. Hricik DE, Lautman J, Bartucci MR, Moir EJ, Mayes JT, Schulak JA. Variable effects of steroid withdrawal on blood pressure reduction in cyclosporine-treated renal transplant recipients. Transplantation. 1992;53(6):1232-5.
24. Veenstra DL, Best JH, Hornberger J, Sullivan SD, Hricik DE. Incidence and long-term cost of steroid-related side effects after renal transplantation. Am J Kidney Dis. 1999;33(5): 829-39.
25. Ratcliffe PJ, Dudley CR, Higgins RM, Firth JD, Smith B, Morris PJ. Randomised controlled trial of steroid withdrawal in renal transplant recipients receiving triple immunosuppression. Lancet. 1996;348(9028):643-8.
26. Taler SJ, Textor SC, Canzanello VJ, Schwartz L, Porayko M, Wiesner RH, et al. Role of steroid dose in hypertension early after liver transplantation with tacrolimus (FK506) and cyclosporine. Transplantation. 1996;62(11):1588-92.
27. Giessing M, Fuller TF, Tuellmann M, Slowinski T, Budde K, Liefeldt L. Steroid- and calcineurin inhibitor free immunosuppression in kidney transplantation: state of the art and future developments. World J Urol. 2007;25(3): 325-32.
28. Curtis JJ, Galla JH, Kotchen TA, Lucas B, McRoberts JW, Luke RG. Prevalence of hypertension in a renal transplant population on alternate-day steroid therapy. Clin Nephrol. 1976;5(3):123-7.
29. McDonald FD, Horensten ML, Mayor GB, Turcotte JG, Selezinka W, Schork MA. Effect of alternate-day steroids on renal transplant function. A controlled study. Nephron. 1976;17(6):415-29.
30. Knight SR, Morris PJ. Steroid avoidance or withdrawal after renal transplantation increases the risk of acute rejection but decreases cardiovascular risk. A meta-analysis. Transplantation. 2010;89(1):1-14.
31. Hricik DE. Antihypertensive and renal effects of enalapril in post-transplant hypertension. Clin Nephrol. 1987;27(5): 250-9.
32. Verghese PS, Dunn TB, Chinnakotla S, Gillingham KJ, Matas AJ, Mauer MS. Calcineurin inhibitors in HLA-identical living related donor kidney transplantation. Nephrol Dial Transplant. 2014;29(1):209-18.
33. Gardiner SM, March JE, Kemp PA, Fallgren B, Bennett T. Regional haemodynamic effects of cyclosporine A, tacrolimus and sirolimus in conscious rats. Br J Pharmacol. 2004;141(4):634-43.
34. Roullet JB, Xue H, McCarron DA, Holcomb S, Bennett WM. Vascular mechanisms of cyclosporin-induced hypertension in the rat. J Clin Invest. 1994;93(5):2244-50.
35. Hoorn EJ, Walsh SB, McCormick JA, Fürstenberg A, Yang CL, Roeschel T, et al. The calcineurin inhibitor tacrolimus activates the renal sodium chloride cotransporter to cause hypertension. Nat Med. 2011;17(10):1304-9.
36. Campistol JM, Romero R, Paul J, Gutiérrez-Dalmau A. Epidemiology of arterial hypertension in renal transplant patients: changes over the last decade. Nephrol Dial Transplant. 2004;19(Suppl. 3):iii62-6.
37. Krämer BK, Del Castillo D, Margreiter R, Sperschneider H, Olbricht CJ, Ortuño J, et al. Efficacy and safety of tacrolimus compared with ciclosporin A in renal transplantation: three-year observational results. Nephrol Dial Transplant. 2008;23(7):2386-92.
38. Morales JM, Domínguez-Gil B. Impact of tacrolimus and mycophenolate mofetil combination on cardiovascular risk profile after kidney transplantation. J Am Soc Nephrol. 2006;17(12 Suppl. 3):S296-303.

39. Cross NB, Webster AC, Masson P, O'Connell PJ, Craig JC. Antihypertensive treatment for kidney transplant recipients. Cochrane Database Syst Rev. 2009;(3):CD003598.
40. Heinze G, Mitterbauer C, Regele H, Kramar R, Winkelmayer WC, Curhan GC, et al. Angiotensin-converting enzyme inhibitor or angiotensin II type 1 receptor antagonist therapy is associated with prolonged patient and graft survival after renal transplantation. J Am Soc Nephrol. 2006;17(3):889-99.
41. Herrera J, Ferrebuz A, MacGregor EG, Rodriguez-Iturbe B. Mycophenolate mofetil treatment improves hypertension in patients with psoriasis and rheumatoid arthritis. J Am Soc Nephrol. 2006;17(12 Suppl. 3):S218-25.
42. Thomas B, Taber DJ, Srinivas TR. Hypertension after kidney transplantation: a pathophysiologic approach. Curr Hypertens Rep. 2013;15(5):458-69.
43. Beecroft JR, Rajan DK, Clark TWI, Robinette M, Stavropoulos SW. Transplant renal artery stenosis: outcome after percutaneous intervention. J Vasc Interv Radiol. 2004;15(12):1407-13.
44. Voiculescu A, Hollenbeck M, Plum J, Rüdiger Hetzel G, Mödder U, Pfeiffer T, et al. Iliac artery stenosis proximal to a kidney transplant: clinical findings, duplex-sonographic criteria, treatment, and outcome. Transplantation. 2003; 76(2):332-9.
45. Mangray M, Vella JP. Hypertension after kidney transplant. Am J Kidney Dis. 2011;57(2):331-41.
46. Gill JS. Cardiovascular disease in transplant recipients: current and future treatment strategies. Clin J Am Soc Nephrol. 2008;3(Suppl. 2):S29-37.
47. Kidney Disease: Improving Global Outcomes (KDIGO) Blood Pressure Work Group. KDIGO 2021 clinical practice guideline for the management of blood pressure in chronic kidney disease. Kidney Int. 2021;99(3S):S1-87.
48. Kidney Disease: Improving Global Outcomes (KDIGO) Blood Pressure Work Group. KDIGO clinical practice guideline for the management of blood pressure in chronic kidney disease. Kidney Int Suppl. 2012;2(5):337.
49. Ruzicka M, Quinn RR, McFarlane P, Hemmelgarn B, Ramesh Prasad GV, Feber J, et al. Canadian Society of Nephrology commentary on the 2012 KDIGO clinical practice guideline for the management of blood pressure in CKD. Am J Kidney Dis. 2014;63(6):869-87.
50. EBPG Expert Group on Renal Transplantation. European best practice guidelines for renal transplantation. Section IV: long-term management of the transplant recipient. IV.5.2. Cardiovascular risks. Arterial hypertension. Nephrol Dial Transplant. 2002;17(Suppl. 4):25-6.
51. SPRINT Research Group, Wright JT, Williamson JD, Whelton PK, Snyder JK, Sink KM, et al. A randomized trial of intensive versus standard blood-pressure control. N Engl J Med. 2015;373(22):2103-16.
52. SPRINT Research Group, Lewis CE, Fine LJ, Beddhu S, Cheung AK, Cushman WC, et al. Final report of a trial of intensive versus standard blood-pressure control. N Engl J Med. 2021;384(20):1921-30.
53. Minutolo R, Gabbai FB, Agarwal R, Chiodini P, Borrelli S, Bellizzi V, et al. Assessment of achieved clinic and ambulatory blood pressure recordings and outcomes during treatment in hypertensive patients with CKD: a multicenter prospective cohort study. Am J Kidney Dis. 2014;64(5):744-52.
54. Agena F, dos Santos Prado E, Souza PS, da Silva GV, Carvalhinho Lemos FB, Mion Jr D, et al. Home blood pressure (BP) monitoring in kidney transplant recipients is more adequate to monitor BP than office BP. Nephrol Dial Transplant. 2011;26(11):3745-9.
55. David V, Jeyaseelan L, Deborah M, Jacob S, Alexander S, Varughese S, et al. Prospective blood pressure measurement in renal transplant recipients. Indian J Nephrol. 2014;24(3): 154.
56. Paul LC, Benediktsson H. Post-transplant hypertension and chronic renal allograft failure. Kidney Int Suppl. 1995;52: S34-7.
57. Keven K, Yalçin S, Canbakan B, Kutlay S, Sengül S, Erturk S, et al. The impact of daily sodium intake on posttransplant hypertension in kidney allograft recipients. Transplant Proc. 2006;38(5):1323-6.
58. Curtis JJ, Luke RG, Jones P, Diethelm AG. Hypertension in cyclosporine-treated renal transplant recipients is sodium dependent. Am J Med. 1988;85(2):134-8.
59. Grześk G, Wiciński M, Malinowski B, Grześk E, Manysiak S, Odrowąż-Sypniewska G, et al. Calcium blockers inhibit cyclosporine A-induced hyperreactivity of vascular smooth muscle cells. Mol Med Rep. 2012;5(6):1469-74.
60. Knoll GA, Cantarovitch M, Cole E, Gill J, Gourishankar S, Holland D, et al. The Canadian ACE-inhibitor trial to improve renal outcomes and patient survival in kidney transplantation—study design. Nephrol Dial Transplant. 2008;23(1):354-8.
61. Ingelfinger JR, Grupe WE, Levey RH. Post-transplant hypertension in the absence of rejection or recurrent disease. Clin Nephrol. 1981;15(5):236-9.
62. Weaver DJ, Somers MJG, Martz K, Mitsnefes MM. Clinical outcomes and survival in pediatric patients initiating chronic dialysis: a report of the NAPRTCS registry. Pediatr Nephrol Berl Ger. 2017;32(12):2319-30.
63. Sinha MD, Gilg JA, Kerecuk L, Reid CJD, British Association for Paediatric Nephrology. Progression to hypertension in non-hypertensive children following renal transplantation. Nephrol Dial Transplant. 2012;27(7):2990-6.
64. Calzolari A, Giordano U, Matteucci MC, Pastore E, Turchetta A, Rizzoni G, et al. Hypertension in young patients after renal transplantation: ambulatory blood pressure monitoring versus casual blood pressure. Am J Hypertens. 1998;11(4 Pt. 1): 497-501.
65. Giordano U, Matteucci MC, Calzolari A, Turchetta A, Rizzoni G, Alpert BS. Ambulatory blood pressure monitoring in children with aortic coarctation and kidney transplantation. J Pediatr. 2000;136(4):520-3.
66. Matteucci MC, Giordano U, Calzolari A, Turchetta A, Santilli A, Rizzoni G. Left ventricular hypertrophy, treadmill tests, and 24-hour blood pressure in pediatric transplant patients. Kidney Int. 1999;56(4):1566-70.
67. Seeman T, Dusek J, Vondrák K, Simková E, Kreisinger J, Feber J, et al. Ambulatory blood pressure monitoring in children after renal transplantation. Transplant Proc. 2004; 36(5):1355-6.
68. McGlothan KR, Wyatt RJ, Ault BH, Hastings MC, Rogers T, DiSessa T, et al. Predominance of nocturnal hypertension in pediatric renal allograft recipients. Pediatr Transplant. 2006;10(5):558-64.

69. Mitsnefes MM, Omoloja A, McEnery PT. Short-term pediatric renal transplant survival: blood pressure and allograft function. Pediatr Transplant. 2001;5(3):160-5.
70. Sorof JM, Sullivan EK, Tejani A, Portman RJ. Antihypertensive medication and renal allograft failure: a North American Pediatric Renal Transplant Cooperative Study report. J Am Soc Nephrol. 1999;10(6):1324-30.
71. Mitsnefes MM, Khoury PR, McEnery PT. Early post-transplantation hypertension and poor long-term renal allograft survival in pediatric patients. J Pediatr. 2003;143(1):98-103.
72. Kasiske BL, Zeier MG, Chapman JR, Craig JC, Ekberg H, Garvey CA, et al. KDIGO clinical practice guideline for the care of kidney transplant recipients: a summary. Kidney Int. 2010;77(4):299-311.
73. Balzano R, Lindblad YT, Vavilis G, Jogestrand T, Berg UB, Krmar RT. Use of annual ABPM, and repeated carotid scan and echocardiography to monitor cardiovascular health over nine yr in pediatric and young adult renal transplant recipients. Pediatr Transplant. 2011;15(6):635-41.
74. Calhoun DA, Jones D, Textor S, Goff DC, Murphy TP, Toto RD, et al. Resistant hypertension: diagnosis, evaluation, and treatment. A scientific statement from the American Heart Association Professional Education Committee of the Council for High Blood Pressure Research. Hypertension. 2008;51(6):1403-19.
75. Mancia G, De Backer G, Dominiczak A, Cifkova R, Fagard R, Germano G, et al. 2007 Guidelines for the management of arterial hypertension: the task force for the management of arterial hypertension of the European Society of Hypertension (ESH) and of the European Society of Cardiology (ESC). J Hypertens. 2007;25(6):1105-87.
76. Arias M, Fernandez-Fresnedo G, Gago M, Rodrigo E, Gómez-Alamillo C, Toyos C, et al. Clinical characteristics of resistant hypertension in renal transplant patients. Nephrol Dial Transplant. 2012;27(Suppl. 4):iv36-8.
77. Gago Fraile M, Fernandez Fresnedo G, Gómez-Alamillo C, de Castro SS, Arias M. Clinical and epidemiological characteristics of refractory hypertension in renal transplant patients. Transplant Proc. 2009;41(6):2132-3.
78. Franco-Esteve A, Gómez Huertas E, Cabello V. Prevalencia y significado clínico de la hipertensión arterial en trasplante renal. Estudio Retenal. Nefrologia. 2011;31:141.
79. Fernández-Fresnedo G, Gago-Fraile M, Gómez-Alamillo C, Sanz de Castro S, Arias-Rodriguez M. Risk of cardiovascular disease associated with refractory hypertension in renal transplant recipients. Transplant Proc. 2010;42(8):2908-9.

13.5 Diabetes Mellitus After Kidney Transplantation

Niwrutti Hase, Aniket Hase

CASE VIGNETTE 1

A 56-year-old male was a kidney transplant recipient (KTR) for his end-stage kidney disease due to chronic glomerulonephritis. His sister, 52-years old, human leukocyte antigens (HLA) identical, and ABO compatible, was the donor. The dialysis duration was 1 year. He was nondiabetic but hypertensive requiring three drugs to control, hepatitis C virus (HCV), human immunodeficiency virus (HIV): nonreactive. Cytomegalovirus (CMV) status: R+, D+, pre, transplant body mass index (BMI): 30 kg/m^2, and had impaired glucose tolerance test (IGTT). Complement-dependent cytotoxicity (CDC) and flow cytometry-crossmatch were negative. Immediate post-transplant period during the first week, venous plasma glucose ranged between 250 and 350 mg/dL. He received methylprednisolone 500 mg intravenously (IV) for 3 days and then he was on tacrolimus (TAC), mycophenolate, and prednisolone 20 mg. His TAC trough level was 15 ng/mL. He required regular insulin infusion for initial control. He was on regular insulin premeal and glargine at bedtime. At discharge, as his requirement was <20 units, he was initiated on oral repaglinide 1 mg before each meal. At the end of 5 weeks, because of recurrent hypoglycemia, his antidiabetic drugs were stopped. His blood glucose was well controlled.

a. Can this patient be labeled as post-transplantation diabetes mellitus (PTDM)?
b. What are the risk factors for PTDM in this case?
c. How will you follow up and monitor this patient?

Ans.

a. He should not be labeled as PTDM. This is post-transplant transient hyperglycemia.
b. Recipient age, obesity, impaired glucose tolerance (IGT), high-dose steroid, and transient post-transplant hyperglycemia.
c. This patient is at high risk for PTDM. Blood glucose should be monitored weekly for the first month. This patient should undergo oral glucose tolerance test (OGTT) at 3 months. After 6 months, he can do HbA1c every 3 months.

CASE VIGNETTE 2

A 27-year-old male KTR, post-transplant 1 year and 4 months, was referred for round pneumonia and low-grade fever of 1-week duration. The donor was his 52-year-old mother, ABO compatible, one haploid match CDC, and flow cytometry cross-match negative. He was not on induction therapy but on TAC, mycophenolate mofetil (MMF), and prednisolone. He had developed PTDM. Initially, he was treated with insulin, and currently, he is on gliclazide and metformin. His diabetes was well controlled (HbA1c: 5.6%). He had a COVID-19 illness 2 months back. MMF was stopped, TAC reduced by 50%, and he received methylprednisolone and remdesivir. He made an uneventful recovery. Now he presented with low-grade fever, loss of weight, and uncontrolled diabetes. X-ray and computed tomography (CT) scan of the chest showed round pneumonia. Sputum for acid-fast bacillus (AFB) was negative and Legionella, Mycoplasma, *and* Nocardia *were negative. As shadow was peripheral, CT-guided biopsy was done. The wet mount showed fungal hyphae of suggestive mucormycosis. He was treated with IV liposomal amphotericin. As pneumonia increased, the patient underwent lung resection of the mass. Histopathology confirmed fungal hyphae of mucor. The species identified was* Rhizopus Arrhizus. *The patient made an uneventful recovery.*

Currently, urine shows proteinuria, blood glucose fasting 140 mg/dL, postprandial 230 mg/dL, and serum creatinine 1.6 mg/dL.

a. How will you manage the diabetes of this patient?
b. What are the complications of PTDM?
c. What are the risk factors for mucormycosis in PTDM?
d. What is the role of sodium–glucose cotransporter-2 (SGLT-2) inhibitor and glucagon-like peptide-1 agonists (GLP-1A) in treating this patient?

Ans.

a. During acute illness, metformin should be stopped. This patient should be managed on insulin.
b. PTDM is a risk factor for infections, cardiovascular events, and long-term micro- and macrovascular complications. Long-term graft and patient survival are also decreased.
c. *Risk factors for mucormycosis:* Diabetes mellitus with ketoacidosis, patient on glucocorticoids, solid organ transplant on immunosuppressive, iron overload, and hematologic malignancies.
d. SGLT-2 inhibitors in kidney transplants with PTDM currently have limited safety and efficacy data. SGLT-2 inhibitors should be avoided in patient with recurrent urinary tract infections (UTI). Some may consider their use on a case-by-case basis.

INTRODUCTION

Post-transplantation diabetes mellitus is a common metabolic complication reported in solid organ transplantation. PTDM was first recognized by Starzl et al. in liver transplantation in 1964.[1] By the 1970s, it was described as a metabolic complication of kidney transplantation.[2] The aim of this chapter is to review epidemiology, definition, diagnostic criteria, etiopathogenesis, risk factors, complications, prevention, and management of PTDM.

NOMENCLATURES

Various nomenclatures have been used to describe diabetes detected in post-transplant periods such as steroid diabetes, post-transplantation diabetes, new onset of diabetes,

CHAPTER HIGHLIGHTS

- Post-transplant diabetes mellitus (PTDM) is a common complication in kidney transplant recipients.
- This chapter highlights the epidemiology, diagnostic criteria, risk factors, pathogenesis management, and short-term and long-term outcome of post-transplant diabetes mellitus.

transplant-associated hyperglycemia, new onset of diabetes after transplant (NODAT), and PTDM.[3]

- *NODAT:* This term was established by the international consensus guidelines in 2003 to describe heterogeneous conditions of abnormal glucose tolerance with variable onset duration and severity. NODAT does not include the patients who may have diabetes prior to transplant that was unrecognized or undiagnosed.[4]
- *PTDM:* In 2014, the international panel recommended changing the terminology NODAT back to PTDM to address shortcomings of the definition of NODAT. PTDM describes diabetes after transplantation irrespective of the timing of diagnosis or whether it was present but undetected prior to transplantation or not. The term PTDM should be utilized for clinically stable patients who develop persistent post-transplant hyperglycemias. The PTDM term excludes patients with transient post-transplant hyperglycemia.[5] PTDM is currently the preferred terminology to describe post-transplant diabetes.
- *Transient post-transplant hyperglycemias:* Hyperglycemias due to stress, high-dose steroid, and acute infections and during acute rejection therapy are very common and detected in approximately 90% of KTRs in an early period. This hyperglycemia is transient and resolves in most patients within a few weeks. Transient hyperglycemias should not be labeled as PTDM.[5,6]

INCIDENCE AND PREVALENCE OF POST-TRANSPLANTATION DIABETES MELLITUS

Historically reported incidence and prevalence of PTDM varied according to diagnostic criteria used, population studied, immunosuppressive regimen used, and time from the transplant.[7] After the introduction of calcineurin inhibitors (CNIs) and before the 2003 consensus guidelines for uniform practice, the reported rate of PTDM varied from 2 to 53%.[8] In Norwegian single-center analysis of patients undergoing OGTT at 10 weeks, post-transplantation, the odd of developing PTDM halved between 1997 and 2007.[9] The data from the Organ Procurement and Transplant Network/Scientific Registry of Transplant Recipient (OPTN/SRTR) showed that the prevalence of PTDM at 1-year post-transplantation decreased from 10% in 2004 to under 4% in 2016, while the 5-year incidence rates decreased from approximately 16% in 2007 to 10% in 2012.[10] Long-term studies have reported 2–5 years' incidence rate ranging from 18 to 33%.[11]

Indian literature reports wide variation in prevalence ranging from 16.7 to 54.5%.[12-14] A recent study by Jayam J in the South Indian population reported an incidence of 22.6%.[15]

SCREENING AND DIAGNOSIS OF POST-TRANSPLANTATION DIABETES MELLITUS

- All potential KTRs should be screened for abnormal glucose metabolism by fasting blood glucose and OGTT before transplant to predict their risk of PTDM (Grade 2C).[16]
- Afternoon capillary blood glucose monitoring is recommended to identify patients with postoperative hyperglycemias. Afternoon blood glucose levels ≥200 mg/dL (11.1 mmol/L) are more sensitive than fasting plasma glucose (FPG) to diagnose postoperative hyperglycemia. During the first 4–6 weeks after transplantation, especially in centers using high corticosteroid doses usually administered in the morning, typically experience postprandial hyperglycemic peaks in the afternoon. The fasting blood glucose may be normal.[16]
- A formal diagnosis of PTDM can be made from 6 weeks post-transplantation using OGTT. OGTT is the gold standard for diagnosing PTDM (Grade 1B).[16]
- The HbA1c should not be used to screen for PTDM prior to 3-month post-transplantation because anemia and graft dysfunction in the early 3 months give falsely low values.
- It is recommended that the definition and diagnosis of PTDM should be based on the currently accepted definition and criteria by American Diabetes Association (ADA), World Health Organization (WHO), International Diabetes Federation (IDF), and American College of Endocrinology (ACE) for diagnosing diabetes and IGT in the general population **(Table 1)**.[4]
- Post-transplantation 6 weeks in a stable patient combining the result of fasting venous plasma glucose >126 mg/dL (≥7 mmol/L and/or HbA1c >6.5% (48 mmol/mol) will detect the majority of patients with PTDM (Grade 2C).[16]

PATHOGENESIS OF POST-TRANSPLANTATION DIABETES MELLITUS

The pathogenesis of PTDM is complex and multifactorial. It is the interaction between traditional "pretransplant" risk factors such as increasing age, obesity, metabolic syndrome, genetic susceptibility, and family history of DM and "post-transplantation" trigger factors including immunosuppressive drugs, surgical stress, HCV, CMV infections, and hypomagnesemia. This interaction results in IGT, hyperglycemia, and PTDM due to deficient insulin action. The deficient insulin action is due to insulin resistance and pancreatic β-cell damage resulting in dysfunctional insulin release **(Flowchart 1)**.

TABLE 1: Screening and diagnosis of post-transplantation diabetes mellitus (PTDM).

Time post-transplant (days)	*Screening test/result/criteria*	*Diagnosis*
0–45	Fasting blood glucose ≥126 mg/dL Afternoon capillary blood glucose ≥200 mg/dL	Transient postoperative hyperglycemia. Do not diagnose as PTDM
46–365	Oral glucose tolerance test (OGTT) (The test should be performed as described by WHO, using a glucose load containing the equivalent of 75 g anhydrous glucose dissolved in water) • Fasting venous plasma glucose ≥126 mg/dL (Fasting is defined as no caloric intake for at least 8 hours) • 2 hours venous plasma glucose ≥200 mg/dL after glucose load) *or* • Classical symptoms of diabetes plus random venous plasma glucose ≥200 mg/dL (The classic symptoms of diabetes include polyuria, polydipsia, and unexplained weight loss. Random is defined as any time of day without regard to time since last meal)	PTDM
>365	• Fasting venous blood glucose ≤100 mg/dL • Fasting venous plasma glucose ≥100 mg/dL and ≤126 mg/dL • 2-hour postload glucose on the 75 g OGTT 140–199 mg/dL • HbA1c ≥ 6.5% (The test should be performed in a laboratory using a method that is NGSP certified and standardized to the DCCT assay) • HbA1c 5.7–6.4%	• Normal plasma glucose • Impaired fasting glucose (IFG) • Impaired glucose tolerance (IGT) • PTDM – Do not use this test <365 days will underdiagnose PTDM • Prediabetes

(DCCT: Diabetes Control and Complications Trial; NGSP: National Glycohemoglobin Standardization Program; PTDM: post-transplantation diabetes mellitus; WHO: World Health Organization)

Flowchart 1: Pathophysiology: post-transplantation diabetes mellitus (PTDM).

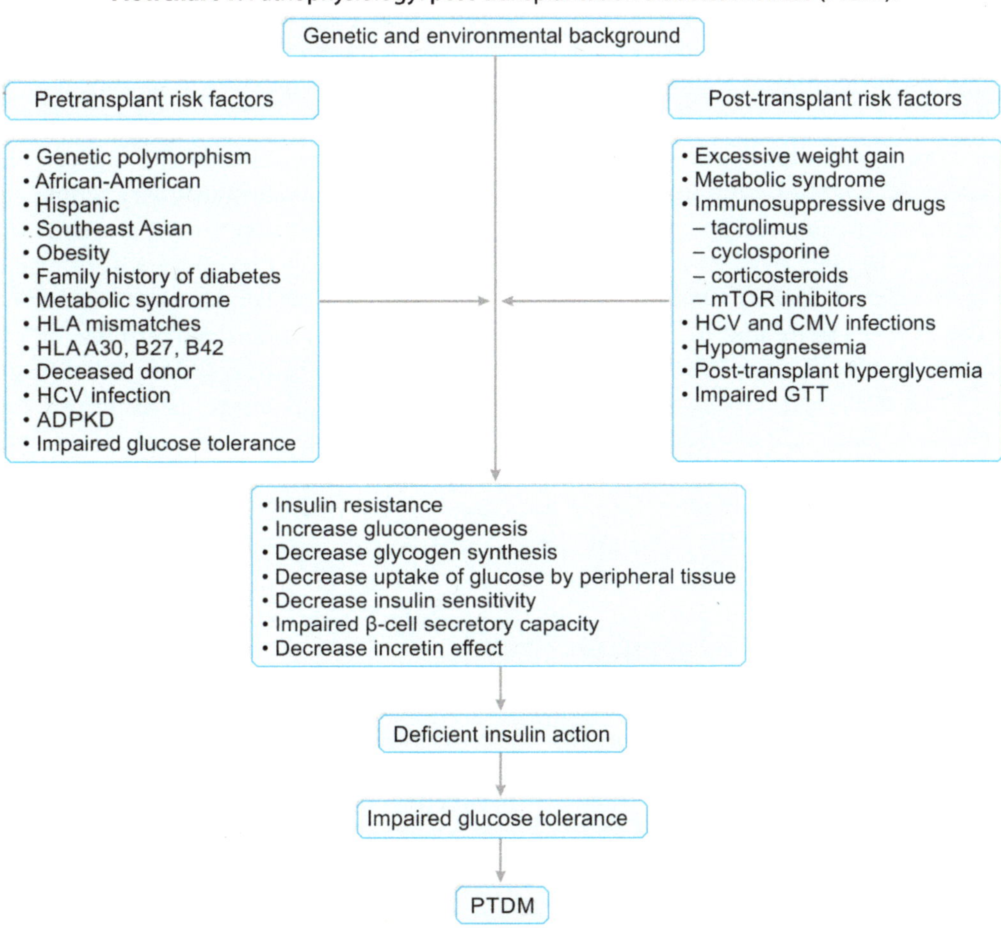

(ADPKD: autosomal dominant polycystic kidney disease; CMV: cytomegalovirus; GTT: glucose tolerance test; HCV: hepatitis C virus; HLA: human leukocyte antigens; mTOR: mammalian target of rapamycin)

RISK FACTORS

Nonmodifiable Risk Factors

Age

The risk of PTDM significantly increases with advancing age at the time of transplantation.[17] Analysis of US Renal System Data (USRDS) by Kasiske et al. showed a strong association between age and PTDM. The risk was highest for those who were ≥60 years.[18]

Race/Ethnicity

African-Americans, Hispanic, and Southeast Asians are at an increased risk for developing PTDM as compared to White.[19,20] The difference may be related to genetic diversity and altered pharmacokinetics and immunosuppressant effect on glucose metabolism.

Family History of Diabetes

There is strong evidence suggesting that individuals with a family history of diabetes among first-degree relatives have an increased risk of PTDM with one study showing a seven-fold increase.[21,22]

Genetic Susceptibility

Several studies have reported a risk associated between PTDM in KTRs and some common single nucleotide polymorphisms (SNP) in genes encoding proteins involved in β-cell apoptosis, adenosine triphosphate (ATP) sensitive potassium channel, adiponectin, leptin, elements of innate immune system and protein involed in inflammatory pathway.[23,24] Genetic risk factor studies have demonstrated an association between single-nucleotide polymorphism in the *HNF-4A* gene and insulin receptor substrate gene with the development of PTDM in KTRs of Hispanic ethnicity.[22] Khan et al. reported two SNPs in genes coding potassium channel (rs2283228 and S210 of *KCNJ11*) associated with PTDM in the Asian Indian population.[25] Meta-analysis of genetic association studies found the relationship between interleukin-7 (IL7) (rs1494558), potassium voltage-gated channel subfamily Q member 1 (*KCNQ1*) (rs2237892), and transcription factor 7 like 2 (*TCF7L2*) (rs7903146) and PTDM development.[25,26] Large genome-wide analysis studies are lacking and their importance for development is not yet known; routine genetic testing is not recommended.

Other Nonmodifiable Risk Factors

Some studies have reported male gender, presence of HLA such as HLA A30, B27, and B12, deceased donor, and polycystic kidney disease as a cause of renal failure as a risk factor to PTDM with no clear evidence.[26,27]

POST-TRANSPLANTATION

Modifiable Risk Factors

One of the major risk factors for PTDM in the post-transplant period is immunosuppressive drugs used for induction and maintenance.

Diabetogenic immunosuppressive drugs include:

- Corticosteroids
- CNIs
    - TAC
    - Cyclosporine A (CsA)
- Mammalian target of rapamycin (mTOR) inhibitors
    - Sirolimus
    - Everolimus.

Corticosteroids

Corticosteroids are well known to cause hyperglycemia and predispose to the development of diabetes. This was first described by Starzl in KTRs as steroid diabetes in 1964.[1] The hyperglycemic effect of glucocorticoid is dose-dependent. High-dose pulse used for induction and treatment of acute rejection has greater diabetogenic potential than long-term low-dose maintenance therapy. Single-center studies have demonstrated that oral prednisolone reduction to 5 mg daily significantly improves glucose tolerance during the first year after transplantation.[28] While a 0.01 mg/kg/day increase in prednisolone dose is associated with a 5% risk of developing PTDM.[29] Studies have shown that complete withdrawal of 5 mg/day of prednisolone did not influence insulin sensitivity significantly.[30] Split dosing of corticosteroids may reduce glycemic variability and peak hyperglycemia.[31] Complete withdrawal of corticosteroid has not been clearly shown to reduce the incidence of PTDM. A significant percentage of patients suffer an episode of acute rejection following the withdrawal of steroids requiring reinstitution of the steroid.[32] Thus, adjustment of immunosuppressive therapy aimed at improving glucose tolerance must be selected after careful assessment of risk, benefit, and long-term outcome. The mechanism of glucocorticoid-induced hyperglycemia is mainly due to insulin resistance and decreased insulin secretion **(Table 2)**.

Calcineurin Inhibitors

Calcineurin inhibitors are the backbone of maintenance immunosuppressive therapy. Both TAC and CsA are associated with the increased risk of PTDM. The DIRECT study confirms the increased diabetogenicity of TAC compared to CsA in post kidney transplantation in randomized controlled trial.[32] Maes et al. have shown that high TAC trough levels, particularly >15 ng/mL, the first month after the transplant, were a significant risk factor for PTDM beyond

TABLE 2: Immunosuppressive drug: pathogenic mechanisms for hyperglycemia.

Immunosuppressive drugs	*Pathogenic mechanism*	*Additional remark*
• Glucocorticoids	• Decreased insulin receptor number and affinity • Decreased and impaired insulin production and secretion from β-cell • Increased hepatic gluconeogenesis and decreased glycogen synthesis • Lipolysis and protein catabolism	• Effect is dose-dependent • No benefit in decreasing dose below 5 mg/day • Split dose may decrease peak and variability of glucose
• *CNIs* – Calcineurin inhibitors – Tacrolimus – CyA	• Impaired insulin secretion • Increase islet cell apoptosis, decreased β-cell mass • Activation of a transcription factor nuclear factor of activated T cell (NFAT) and cAMP response binding proteins • Decrease in insulin synthesis • Hypomagnesemia	• Dose-dependent • TAC more diabetogenic than CyA • Steroid + CNIs have an additive effect
• *mTOR inhibitors* – Sirolimus – Everolimus	• Impaired insulin secretion • Decreased insulin secretion • Insulin signal transduction • Induce apoptosis of islet cells • Impaired pancreatic ductal cell proliferation • Impaired glucose-stimulated insulin secretion • Action insulin receptor pathways	• Dose-dependent • Steroid + CNIs + mTOR inhibitor is additive effect

Notes: Impaired glucose metabolism: TAC +++, CsA ++, sirolimus +, everolimus +, basiliximab +, belatacept ±, MMF –, azathioprine –.
(-) = no effect on glucose metabolism

(cAMP: cyclic adenosine monophosphate; CNIs: calcineurin inhibitors; CsA: cyclosporine A; CyA: cyclosporine; MMF: mycophenolate mofetil; mTOR: mammalian target of rapamycin; TAC: tacrolimus)

the first year.[33,34] The diabetogenic effect of TAC is dose-dependent and is aggravated with hypertriglyceridemia and insulin resistance.[35] A potential interaction between HCV status and the use of TAC as a risk factor for PTDM has been suggested. Bloom et al. have reported that among HCV positive cohorts, PTDM occurs more often in the TAC compared to CsA-treated group (57.8 vs. 7.7%; $p < 0.0001$). In contrast among HCV-negative cohort, the rate of PTDM was similar between TAC and CsA groups (10 vs. 9.4%; $p = 0.521$).[36] There is limited evidence supporting conversion from TAC to CsA in established PTDM. CNI induce PTDM by multiple mechanisms **(Table 2)**.

Mammalian Target of Rapamycin Inhibitors

Mammalian target of rapamycin inhibitors such as sirolimus everolimus are antiproliferative immunosuppressive drugs used in combination with or without CNIs. Extensive clinical evidence suggests that sirolimus is an independent risk factor for the development of PTDM. USRDS data showed that the incidence of PTDM was higher with sirolimus combined with CNIs than MMF.[37] Hyperglycemia and hyperinsulinemia induced by sirolimus are dose-dependent. TOR inhibitors are less diabetogenic than CNIs.

Effect of Antimetabolites and Other Agents of Post-transplantation Diabetes Mellitus

The antimetabolites azathioprine and mycophenolic acid analogs have not been shown to be diabetogenic. Belatacept costimulatory blockade-based regimens do not seem to have an adverse effect on glucose metabolism.[38] A single-center retrospective study of 264 KTRs showed that induction with basiliximab was associated with a significantly greater risk of developing PTDM compared to no induction.[39]

Perioperative impaired glucose tolerance: Abnormal oral glucose tolerance [insulin-like growth factor (IGF) and IGTT] pretransplant predicts the PTDM. Cosio et al. demonstrated in their study consisting of 490 KTRs that higher pretransplant blood glucose is a risk factor for PTDM at 1 year, using patients with pretransplant FPG levels between 90 and 100 mg/dL as the reference group. Patients with blood glucose <90 mg/dL had a lower risk of PTDM [odds ratio (OR) = 0.46, $p = 0.01$]. In contrast, the risk of PTDM increased as pretransplant FPG level increased (FPG = 100–125, OR = 7.6, $p < 0.0001$). Among patients with impaired fasting glucose (IFG) pretransplant, 70% had hyperglycemia at 1 year (IGF 43% and PTDM 27.1%).[40] Hyperglycemia in the immediate post-transplant period is also a risk factor for PTDM. In a retrospective study of 377 patients conducted by Chakkera et al., among 249 patients who developed postoperative hyperglycemia, 102 (29%) developed PTDM within the first year of transplant. In contrast, only one of 28 (4%) developed PTDM who did not have postoperative hyperglycemia.[41] The risk of PTDM was highest among patients who required insulin.

Central obesity: Central obesity (BMI > 30 kg/m^2) is strongly associated with PTDM.[42] Central obesity and metabolic syndrome are associated with hypertriglyceridemia, IGT, and hyperuricemia. Adipocyte-derived cytokine release and low-grade inflammation associated with obesity and metabolic syndrome induce insulin resistance and PTDM independent of sex, age, and immunosuppressive therapy.[43]

Hepatitis C virus infection: Hepatitis C virus infection is a potentially modifiable risk factor as effective treatment with directly acting antiviral therapy prior to transplant may decrease the incidence of PTDM. A meta-analysis of 10 studies including 2,502 KTRs found that HCV-positive patients were nearly four times more likely to have PTDM as compared with HCV-negative patients.[44,45] The possible mechanism includes islet cell dysfunction and insulin resistance.

Cytomegalovirus infection: Association of CMV infection and PTDM was reported by Lehr et al. in 1985.[46] Hjelmesaeth et al. in their study of 160 consecutive nondiabetic KTRs found that asymptomatic CMV infection was associated with a four-fold increased risk of PTDM.[47] The possible pathogenic mechanisms suggested include (1) Impaired pancreatic β-cell insulin release and (2) CMV-induced release of proinflammatory cytokines may lead to apoptosis and functional disturbances of β cells.[48]

Hypomagnesemia: Van Laecke et al. demonstrated that hypomagnesemia during the first month post-transplantation was associated with the development of PTDM, independent of the immunosuppressive regimen used. While the association between the use of CNIs was strongly related to hypomagnesemia, NODAT disappeared after adjustment for Mg levels suggesting that the diabetogenic effect of CNIs is at least in part related to hypomagnesemia.[49] However, oral magnesium supplementation has been ineffective in correcting the defect.

MANAGEMENT OF POST-TRANSPLANTATION DIABETES MELLITUS

Prevention

Prevention is ideal. The Association of British Clinical Diabetologist and Renal Association (ABCD/RA) guidelines on detection and management of diabetes post solid organ transplantation and the 2004 updated international guidelines on PTDM recommend that the risk for development of PTDM should be evaluated as part of the pretransplant workup for all potential KTRs (Grade 1B).[4,16] All potential transplant recipients should be screened for abnormal glucose regulation by fasting blood glucose and OGTT. IGTT and IFG are the most important predictor of post-transplant hyperglycemia.[50] Low calories, low saturated fat, high fiber, and complex carbohydrate diet are recommended. Mediterranean style diet may be associated with lower PTDM risk.[51] Physical activity, the exercise of at least 150 minutes a week, is recommended as a prevention strategy for PTDM.[21] Patients with BMI > 30 kg/m^2 should be recommended to lose weight prior to surgery. Sharif et al. demonstrated the potential benefit from lifestyle modification in KTRs with IGT; 13/25 patients reverted to normal glucose tolerance after 9 months with only one progressing to PTDM.[52]

MANAGEMENT OF HYPERGLYCEMIA IN PERITRANSPLANT (FIRST 6 WEEKS AFTER TRANSPLANTATION) PERIOD AND CONFIRMED POST-TRANSPLANTATION DIABETES MELLITUS CASES

See **Box 1** for stepwise approach to management of PTDM.

Glycemic targets

- Glycemic targets should be HbA1c of 7% but can be individualized (Grade 1B).[16]
- For patients whose goal is prevention of complications, are young, and without comorbidity a lower goal of HbA1c of <6.5% is preferred while for those with multiple comorbidities, limited life expectancy, increased burden of hypoglycemia a higher target of HbA1c 7.5–8.5% might be preferred.[54]

Lifestyle Modification

Diet and Exercise

Diet-medical nutritional therapy is considered a cornerstone in the management of diabetes and obesity. Kidney Disease: Improving Global Outcomes (KDIGO) 2020 guidelines on the management of diabetes in chronic kidney disease (CKD) suggest a diet high in vegetables, fruits, grains, fibers, legumes, plant-based proteins, unsaturated fats, and nuts and lower in processed meat, refined carbohydrates, saturated fats, and sweetened beverages.[55] Physical exercise at moderate intensity for a cumulative duration of at least 150 minutes per week or level compatible with physical and cardiovascular tolerance will help to maintain body weight and improve glucose tolerance.

Pharmacologic Therapy

- When lifestyle changes fail to achieve glycemic control, pharmacologic therapy is recommended.
- According to the prepared but not yet accepted guidelines on detection and management of diabetes in post solid organ transplant by ABCD/RA: Metformin should be considered first-line oral therapy for patients with confirmed PTDM and stable estimated glomerular filtration rate (eGFR) ≥30 mL/min/1.73 m^2 and BMI ≥25 kg/m^2 (Grade 1C). In a large US survey of 14,144 renal transplant recipients with pretransplant diabetes, only 4.7% of them received metformin in the first 12 months post-transplant period; subjects on metformin had significantly lower all-cause, infection, and malignancy-related mortality.[56]

BOX 1: Stepwise approach to management of post-transplantation diabetes mellitus (PTDM).

Step 1

Pretransplant baseline evaluation:

- Complete history and family history
- Determine the baseline blood glucose status by fasting venous plasma glucose and oral glucose tolerance
- *Assess risk factors for diabetes:* Family history of DM in a first-degree relative, IFG, impaired OGT, obesity, metabolic syndrome, and HCV infection

High-risk potential kidney transplant recipient:

- Counsel for risk of PTDM
- *Risk reduction: Lifestyle modification:* Diet advice, weight control, stop smoking, regular exercise, treatment of cardiometabolic risk factors, and HCV infection treatment

Potential kidney transplant recipient no risk: Monitor all potential recipients annually while on the waiting list

Step 2

Intraoperative management:

- *Monitor blood glucose:* Maintain blood glucose between 140 and 180 mg/dL
- If blood glucose is >180 mg/dL—continuous intravenous infusion of regular insulin to maintain blood glucose between 140 and 180 mg/dL

Step 3

Management of hyperglycemia in the first 6 weeks post-transplant period:

- Immediate post-transplant monitor blood glucose every 2 hours
- *Normal blood glucose:* Monitor blood glucose weekly for a month, then 3 monthly for a year, and then annually
- Blood glucose >180 mg/dL
- Consider continuous intravenous regular insulin infusion to maintain blood glucose between 140 and 180 mg till the patient is critical or nil by mouth
- Consider subcutaneous insulin once the patient start taking it orally
  Injecting NPH in morning and evening or basal glargine at bedtime and premeal insulin analogs lispro or aspart
  - Preferred regimen will be the administration of intermediate-acting neutral protamine Hagedorn (NPH) insulin as a single daily dose (initially 5–10 units and adjusted upon afternoon blood glucose level) at the time as steroid dose in the morning. The peak action of NPH matches the typical afternoon peak glucose that is observed with steroid-induced hyperglycemia[53]
- At the time of discharge insulin requirement <20 units consider lifestyle modification diet and oral antidiabetic drugs. If insulin requirement is >20 units, continue insulin therapy.
- Oral antidiabetic drugs preferred are those that have a lower risk of hypoglycemia renal excretion and no interaction with immunosuppressive drugs. Preferred drugs are meglitinide–repaglinide or dipeptidyl peptidase-4 inhibitors (DPP-4i)–linagliptin, vildagliptin, sitagliptin
- Alternatives are sulfonylureas such as glipizide or gliclazide, which has the least risk of hypoglycemia and does not require dose adjustment with renal impairment. There is no drug interaction with immunosuppressive drugs

Step 4—after 45 days

- *Hyperglycemia resolves:* Screen for diabetes using OGTT or HbA1c
- If hyperglycemia persists or OGTT/HbA1c values are diagnostic of diabetes as per ADA/WHO criteria treat as PTDM
- *Reinforce lifestyle modification:* Diet therapy, exercise, weight control, optimizing steroid dose, steroid reduction, steroid minimization without affecting risk of rejection
- Consider oral antidiabetic drugs initially as monotherapy–individualized—metformin, or sulfonylurea, or repaglinide, or DPP-4 inhibitors—or novel agents protecting heart and kidney–GLP-1RA–with care and monitoring
- If no control with oral drugs, consider insulin
- Treatment of dyslipidemias
- Control of BP, target <130/90 mm Hg, cardiac protection

Step 5—long-term monitoring

- HbA1c every 3 months, diabetic education, self-monitoring of blood glucose
- Annual evaluation for diabetic complications—retinopathy, neuropathy, albuminuria lipid levels, and cardiac evaluation
- Goal of the treatment should be to improve glycemic control to reduce microvascular complications, reduce cardiovascular risk, improve quality of life, graft, and patient survival

(ADA: American Diabetes Association; BP: blood pressure; DM: diabetes mellitus; GLP-1RA: glucagon-like peptide-1 receptor agonists; HCV: hepatitis C virus; IFG: impaired fasting glucose; OGTT: oral glucose tolerance test; WHO: World Health Organization)

- Sulfonylureas, meglitinide, dipeptidyl peptidase-4 (DPP-4) inhibitors, pioglitazone, and glucagon-like peptide 1 receptor (GLP-1R) analog can be safely used in patients with PTDM (Grade 2C).
- SGLT-2 inhibitors should be used with caution in patients with stable eGFR ≥ 30 mL/min/1.73 m^2 and poor glycemic control in patients at low risk of UTI after careful coordination and discussions with nephrologist and diabetologist (Grade 1C).
- Insulin therapy should be considered in all patients who have inadequate control or those who have symptoms of hyperglycemia (Grade 1C).
- Pharmacology, advantages, disadvantages, and mechanisms of action drug-drug interaction of antidiabetic drugs are summarized in **Tables 3 and 4**.
- Hypertension is common along with diabetes. The KDIGO guidelines suggest a target blood pressure of 130/80 mm Hg for patients with renal allografts. The preferred drug in the early period of transplant is calcium channel blockers.[57] ACE inhibitors/angiotensin receptor blockers (ARBs) are preferred in patients with proteinuria and stable renal function.[16]
- All patients irrespective of lipid level should receive statins (Grade 1C). Target low-density lipoprotein (LDL) cholesterol < 100 mg/dL and non-high-density lipoprotein (HDL) cholesterol < 130 mg/dL.[58-60]

Modification of Immunosuppression to Prevent or to Treat Post-transplantation Diabetes Mellitus

- Immunosuppressive therapy should be individualized according to immunologic risk rather than glycemic risk (Grade 1C).[16]

TABLE 3: Antidiabetic drugs.

Drug	*Evidence in PTDM*	*Potential interactions with IS*
• Metformin	• First-line drug for patients with eGFR >30 mL/min/1.73 m^2 with BMI ≥30 kg/m^2, patients with cardiovascular disease • KTR high risk for hypoglycemia[16]	• Not reported
• Sulfonylureas • Glipizide • Gliclazide • Glibenclamide • Glimepiride	• No data in PTDM • Avoid in KTR with overweight, cardiovascular disease, and who are high risk for hypoglycemia	• Cyclosporine increases level of glibenclamide and risk of hypoglycemia • No interaction with glipizide • Increased CsA level with glibenclamide and glimepiride
• Meglitinide • Repaglinide • Nateglinide	• Small observation studies • Risk of hypoglycemia	• CsA increased repaglinide level and risk of hypoglycemia
• Thiazolidinediones • Pioglitazone • Rosiglitazone	• Avoid in overweight KTR • Patient with fluid retention and heart failure • No evidence to use in PTDM	• No reported interactions
• Alpha-glucosidase inhibitors (acarbose)	• No data in PTDM	• Not reported • May produce hypoglycemias with insulin
• Insulin	• Insulin is indicated in early post-transplant hyperglycemia and PTDM which is not controlled by lifestyle modification and oral antidiabetics • Early basal insulin reduces the risk of PTDM by β-cell protection	• No interactions

(BMI: body mass index; CsA: cyclosporine A; eGFR: estimated glomerular filtration rate; IS: immunosuppressive drug; KTR: kidney transplant recipient; PTDM: post-transplantation diabetes mellitus)

TABLE 4: Novel antidiabetic drugs.

Drug	*Mechanism of action*	*Advantages*	*Disadvantages*	*Evidence in PTDM*	*Drug interaction with immunosuppressive*
• DPP-4i • Sitagliptin • Saxagliptin • Linagliptin • Vildagliptin	• Decrease inactivation of incretin (GLP-1) • Increase glucose-dependent insulin secretion • Decrease glucose-dependent glucagon secretion	• No weight gains • Promote weight loss • Decrease albuminuria	• Risk of pancreatitis • Risk of cancer • All except linagliptin require adjustment in renal failure	• Linagliptin, sitagliptin, and vildagliptin used in PTDM with good tolerability[70] • Improve β-cell function in KTR	• Sitagliptin increases the level of CsA • Vildagliptin decreases TAC level • No interaction with linagliptin

Contd...

Contd...

Drug	Mechanism of action	Advantages	Disadvantages	Evidence in PTDM	Drug interaction with immunosuppressive
• GLP-1RA • Liraglutide • Exenatide • Dulaglutide • Semaglutide • Lixisenatide	• Increase glucose-dependent insulin secretion • Decrease glucose-dependent glucagon secretion • Delay gastric emptying • Increase satiety and decrease appetite	• No weight gains • Promote weight loss • Decrease BP • No hypoglycemia • Reduction in cardiovascular mortality • No dose adjustment in severe renal failure for liraglutide and semaglutide	• High drug cost • GI side effects, dyspepsia, diarrhea • Exenatide, lixisenatide, and dulaglutide require dose adjustment in renal failure	• Well tolerated in KTR • Preferred with obese and patients with cardiovascular disease • Evidence only as case series[71]	• Not reported
• SGLT-2i • Empagliflozin • Canagliflozin • Dapagliflozin • Ertugliflozin	• Prevent glucose reabsorption in PCT • Increase natriuresis • Activate tubule-glomerular feedback	• Weight loss • Decrease BP • No hypoglycemias • Cardiorenal protection	• Polyuria • Increased risk for UTI • Ketosis, increase bone mass loss with canagliflozin • Increase creatinine at initiation	• Safety and efficacy data are limited but studies have shown their potential benefit in case series. Large trials are awaited in KTR[71]	• CsA increases the level of canagliflozin

(BP: blood pressure; CsA: cyclosporine A; DPP-4i: dipeptidyl peptidase-4 inhibitors; GI: gastrointestinal; GLP-1RA: glucagon-like peptide-1 receptor agonists; KTR: kidney transplant recipient; PCT: proximal convoluted tubule; PTDM: post-transplantation diabetes mellitus; SGLT-2i: sodium–glucose cotransporter-2 inhibitors; TAC: tacrolimus; UTI: urinary tract infection)[70,71]

- At present, there is no evidence to suggest changing immunosuppressive therapy from TAC to CsA or conversion to mTOR inhibitor when PTDM is detected (Grade 2B).[61]
- A Cochrane systematic review including 7,800 KTRs published in 2017 confirmed no difference in the occurrence of PTDM between steroid withdrawal and steroid maintenance up to 5 years post-transplant. However, it did show a significant increased risk of acute rejection with steroid withdrawal either earlier than 14 days (58%) or later (77%) versus steroid maintenance.[62]

IMPACT OF POST-TRANSPLANTATION DIABETES MELLITUS

- Clinical studies evaluating the impact of PTDM on patient and allograft survival have reported variable results. Many studies have shown that PTDM in KTR increases the risk of fatal and nonfatal cardiac events by two to three-fold as compared with nondiabetic KTRs.[63]
- The studies in the era of high-dose glucocorticoid and CsA reported 1 year and 5 years of patient survival 83 and 87%, respectively, in patients with PTDM as compared to 98 and 93% in nondiabetic kidney transplants.[64,65] However, in the era of intensive glucose control and steroid minimization, the study of 628 patients with kidney transplants found no association between PTDM and death with a functioning graft.[66] Most but not all studies have shown decreased allograft survival.[66] Mile et al. in their retrospective study showed that 12-year graft survival was 47% in PTDM as compared with 70% in nondiabetic KTRs ($p = 0.04$) and cox regression analysis revealed that diabetes was a significant predictor of graft loss [$p = 0.04$, risk ratio (RR) = 3.72]. Patient survival was similar in diabetic and nondiabetic—71 versus 74%.[67] In a recent multicentric study by Malik et al., 632 nondiabetic KTRs transplanted between 2010 and 2013 showed that PTDM occurred in 29% of older recipients, and higher BMI was associated with PTDM. PTDM was not associated with graft failure or mortality during the 6 years follow-up.[68]
- KTRs with PTDM can develop metabolic, microvascular, and macrovascular complications of diabetes. The USRDS data from primary renal transplant recipients transplanted during 1995–2000 who developed PTDM showed diabetic complications: Ketoacidosis 8.1%, hyperosmolar coma 3.2%, renal involvement 31.3%, ophthalmic complications 8.3%, neurologic complications 16.3%, peripheral circulatory disorder 4.2%, and hypoglycemia and shock 4.1%. Complications developed in the mean of 500–600 days from diagnosis of PTDM.[69]

REFERENCES

1. Starzl TE, Marchioro TL, Rifkind D, Holmes JH, Rowlands Jr DT, Waddell WR. Factors in successful renal transplantation. Surgery. 1964;56:296-318.
2. Pham PT, Sidhu HS, Pham PM, Pham PC, Feingold KR, Anawalt B, et al. Diabetes mellitus after solid organ transplantation. [Updated 2019 Apr 15]. In: Feingold KR, Anawalt B, Boyce A, et al. (Eds). Endotext [Internet]. South Dartmouth (MA): MDText.com, Inc.; 2000.

3. Stoumpos S, Jardine AG, Mark PB. Cardiovascular morbidity and mortality after kidney transplantation. Transpl Int. 2015;28(1):10-21.
4. Davidson J, Wilkinson A, Dantal J, Dotta F, Haller H, Hernández D, et al. New-onset diabetes after transplantation: 2003 international consensus guidelines. Proceedings of an international expert panel meeting. Barcelona, Spain, 19 February 2003. Transplantation. 2003;75:SS3.
5. Sharif A, Hecking M, de Vries APJ, Porrini E, Hornum M, Rasoul-Rockenschaub S, et al. Proceedings from an international consensus meeting on posttransplantation diabetes mellitus: recommendations and future directions. Am J Transplant. 2014;14(9):1992-2000.
6. Hecking M, Haidinger M, Döller D, Werzowa J, Tura A, Zhang J, et al. Early basal insulin therapy decreases new-onset diabetes after renal transplantation. J Am Soc Nephrol. 2012;23:739-49.
7. Arner P, Gunnarsson R, Blomdahl S, Groth CG. Some characteristics of steroid diabetes: a study in renal-transplant recipients receiving high-dose corticosteroid therapy. Diabetes Care. 1983;6(1):23-5.
8. Hjelmesaeth J, Asberg A, Müller F, Hartmann A, Jenssen T. New-onset post transplantation diabetes mellitus: insulin resistance or insulinopenia? Impact of immunosuppressive drugs, cytomegalovirus and hepatitis C virus infection. Curr Diabetes Rev. 2005;1(1):1-10.
9. Valderhaug TG, Hjelmesaeth J, Rollag H, Leivestad T, Røislien J, Jenssen T, et al. Reduced incidence of new-onset post transplantation diabetes mellitus during the last decade. Transplantation. 2007;84(9):1125-30.
10. Hart A, Smith JM, Skeans MA, Gustafson SK, Wilk AR, Castro S, et al. OPTN/SRTR 2017 annual data report: kidney. Am J Transplant. 2019;19(Suppl. 2):19.
11. Porrini EL, Díaz JM, Moreso F, Delgado Mallén PI, Torres IS, Ibernon M, et al. Clinical evolution of post-transplant diabetes mellitus. Nephrol Dial Transplant. 2016;31:495-505.
12. Prakash J, Rathore SS, Singh TB, Choudhury TA. New-onset diabetes after transplantation (NODAT): analysis of pre-transplant risk factors in renal allograft recipients. Indian J Transplant. 2012;6:77-82.
13. Sharma A, Minz M, Singh S. Incidence of glucose metabolic abnormalities in Indian living renal allograft recipients on tacrolimus-based triple-drug immunosuppression. Transplant Proc. 2008;40:2414-5.
14. Bora GS, Guleria S, Reddy VS, Tandon N, Gupta N, Gupta S, et al. Risk factors for the development of new-onset diabetes mellitus in a living related renal transplant program. Transplant Proc. 2010;42:4072-3.
15. Jayam J, Balakrishnan MA, Srinivasa Prasad ND, Sujit S, Fernando ME. Prevalence and risk factors for posttransplant diabetes mellitus: data from government tertiary care center. Indian J Transplant. 2018;12:119-24.
16. Chowdhury TA, Wahba M, Mallik R, Peracha J, Patel D, De P, et al. Association of British Clinical Diabetologists and Renal Association guidelines on the detection and management of diabetes post solid organ transplantation. Diabet Med. 2021;38(6):e14523.
17. Jenssen T, Hartmann A. Post-transplant diabetes mellitus in patients with solid organ transplants. Nat Rev Endocrinol. 2019;15:172-88.
18. Kasiske BL, Snyder JJ, Gilbertson D, Maras AJ. Diabetes mellitus after kidney transplantation in the United States. Am J Transplant. 2003;3(2)178-85.
19. Montori VM, Basu A, Erwin PJ, Velosa JA, Gabriel SE, Kudva YC. Post transplantation diabetes: a systematic review of the literature. Diabetes Care. 2002;25(3):583-92.
20. Peracha J, Nath J, Ready A, Tahir S, Parekh K, Hodson J, et al. Risk of post-transplantation diabetes mellitus is greater in South Asian versus Caucasian kidney allograft recipients. Transpl Int. 2016;29:727-39.
21. Pham PTT, Pham PMT, Pham SV, Pham PAT, Pham PCT. New-onset diabetes after transplantation (NODAT): an overview. Diabetes Metab Syndr Obes. 2011;4:175-86.
22. Martinez-Castelao A, Hernandez MD, Pascual J, Morales JM, Marcen R, Errasti P, et al. Detection and treatment of post kidney transplant hyperglycemia: a Spanish multicenter cross-sectional study. Transplant Proc. 2005;37(9):3813-6.
23. Chen Y, Sampaio MS, Yang JW, Min D, Hutchinson IV. Genetic polymorphisms of the transcription factor NFATc4 and development of new-onset diabetes after transplantation in Hispanic kidney transplant recipients. Transplantation. 2012;93(3):325-30.
24. Cosio FG, Pesavento TE, Osei K, Henry ML, Ferguson RM. Posttransplant diabetes mellitus: increasing incidence in renal allograft recipients transplanted in recent years. Kidney Int. 2001;59(2):732-7.
25. Khan IA, Poornima S, Jahan P, Rao P, Hasan Q. Type 2 diabetes mellitus and the Association of Candidate Genes in Asian Indian population from Hyderabad, India. J Clin Diagn Res. 2015;9(11):GC01-5.
26. Zielińska K, Kukulski L, Wróbel M, Przybyłowski P, Zielińska M, Strojek K. New onset diabetes after transplantation (NODAT)—scientific data review. Clin Diabetol. 2020;9(5):356-66.
27. Culliford A, Phagura N, Sharif A. Autosomal dominant polycystic kidney disease is a risk factor for posttransplantation diabetes mellitus: an updated systematic review and meta-analysis. Transplant Direct. 2020;6:e553.
28. Hjelmesaeth J, Hartmann A, Kofstad J, Egeland T, Stenstrøm J, Fauchald P. Tapering off prenisolone and cyclosporine the first year after renal transplantation: the effect on glucose tolerance. Nephrol Dial Transplant. 2001; 16:829-35.
29. Midtvedt K, Hjelmesaeth J, Hartmann A, Lund K, Paulsen D, Egeland T, et al. Insulin resistance after renal transplantation: the effect of steroid dose reduction and withdrawal. J Am Soc Nephrol. 2004;15(12):3233-9.
30. Luan FL, Steffick DE, Ojo AO. New-onset diabetes mellitus in kidney transplant recipients discharged on steroid-free immunosuppression. Transplantation. 2011;91(3):334-41.
31. Yates CJ, Fourlanos S, Colman PG, Cohney SJ. Divided dosing reduces prednisolone-induced hyperglycaemia and glycaemic variability: a randomized trial after kidney transplantation. Nephrol Dial Transplant. 2014;29:698-705.
32. Vincenti F, Friman S, Scheuermann E, Rostaing L, Jenssen T, Campistol JM, et al. Results of an international, randomized trial comparing glucose metabolism disorders and outcome with cyclosporine versus tacrolimus. Am J Transplant. 2007; 7:1506-14.

33. Maes BD, Kuypers D, Messiaen T, Evenepoel P, Mathieu C, Coosemans W, et al. Posttransplant diabetes mellitus in FK-506-treated renal transplant recipients: analysis of incidence and risk factors. Transplantation. 2001;72(10): 1655-61.
34. Sharif A, Shabir S, Chand S, Cockwell P, Ball S, Borrows R. Meta-analysis of calcineurin inhibitors in kidney transplantation. J Am Soc Nephrol. 2011;22:2107-18.
35. Porrini E, Delgado P, Alvarez A, Cobo M, Pérez L, González-Posada JM, et al. The combined effect of pre-transplant triglyceride levels and the type of calcineurin inhibitor in predicting the risk of new onset diabetes after renal transplantation. Nephrol Dial Transplant. 2008;23:1436-41.
36. Bloom RD, Rao V, Weng F, Grossman RA, Cohen D, Mange KC. Association of hepatitis C with posttransplant diabetes in renal transplant patients on tacrolimus. J Am Soc Nephrol. 2002;13(5):1374-80.
37. Johnston O, Rose CL, Webster AC, Gill JS. Sirolimus is associated with new-onset diabetes in kidney transplant recipients. J Am Soc Nephrol. 2008;19(7):1411-8.
38. Vanrenterghem Y, Bresnahan B, Campistol J, Durrbach A, Grinyó J, Neumayer HH, et al. Belatacept-based regimens are associated with improved cardiovascular and metabolic risk factors compared with cyclosporine in kidney transplant recipients (BENEFIT and BENEFITEXT studies). Transplantation. 2011;91:976-83.
39. Aasebo W, Midtvedt K, Valderhaug TG, Leivestad T, Hartmann A, Reisaeter AV, et al. Impaired glucose homeostasis in renal transplant recipients receiving basiliximab. Nephrol Dial Transplant. 2010;25:1289-93.
40. Cosio FG, Kudva Y, van der Velde M, Larson TS, Textor SC, Griffin MD, et al. New onset hyperglycemia and diabetes mellitus are associated with increased cardiovascular risk after kidney transplantation. Kidney Int. 2005;67(6):2415-21.
41. Chakkera HA, Knowler WC, Devarapalli Y, Weil EJ, Heilman RL, Dueck A, et al. Relationship between inpatient hyperglycemia and insulin treatment after kidney transplantation and future new onset diabetes mellitus. Clin J Am Soc Nephrol. 2010;5:1669-75.
42. Rodríguez-Rodríguez AE, Porrini E, Hornum M, Donate-Correa J, Morales-Febles R, Khemlani Ramchand S, et al. Post-transplant diabetes mellitus and prediabetes in renal transplant recipients: an update. Nephron. 2021;145:317-29.
43. Hjelmesaeth J, Flyvbjerg A, Jenssen T, Frystyk J, Ueland T, Hagen M, et al. Hypoadiponectinemia is associated with insulin resistance and glucose intolerance after renal transplantation: impact of immunosuppressive and antihypertensive drug therapy. Clin J Am Soc Nephrol. 2006;1:575-82.
44. Fabrizi F, Martin P, Dixit V, Bunnapradist S, Kanwal F, Dulai G. Post-transplant diabetes mellitus and HCV seropositive status after renal transplantation: a meta-analysis of clinical studies. Am J Transplant. 2005;5:2433.
45. Bloom RD, Lake JR. Emerging issues in hepatitis C virus-positive liver and kidney transplant recipients. Am J Transplant. 2006;6:2232.
46. Lehr H, Jao S, Waltzer WC, Anaise D, Rapaport FT. Cytomegalovirus induced diabetes mellitus in a renal transplant recipient. Transplant Proc. 1985;17(5):2152-4.
47. Hjelmesaeth J, Sagedal S, Hartmann A, Rollag H, Egeland T, Hagen M, et al. Asymptomatic cytomegalovirus infection is associated with increased risk for new-onset diabetes and impaired insulin release after renal transplantation. Diabetologia. 2004;47(9);1550-6.
48. Hjelmesaeth J, Muller F, Jenssen T, Rollag H, Sagedal S, Hartmann A. Is there a link between cytomegalovirus infection and new-onset post-transplant diabetes mellitus? Potential mechanisms of virus-induced β-cell damage. Nephrol Dial Transplant. 2005;20(11):2311-5.
49. Van Laecke S, Van Biesen W, Verbeke F, De Bacquer D, Peeters P, Vanholder R. Post transplantation hypomagnesemia and its relation with immunosuppression as predictors of new-onset diabetes after transplantation. Am J Transplant. 2009;9(9):2140-9.
50. Juan Khong M, Ping Chong Ch. Prevention and management of new-onset diabetes mellitus in kidney transplantation. Neth J Med. 2014;72:127-32.
51. Osté MC, Corpeleijn E, Navis GJ, Keyzer CA, Soedamah-Muthu SS, van den Berg E, et al. Mediterranean style diet is associated with low risk of new-onset diabetes after renal transplantation. BMJ Open Diabetes Res Care. 2017; 5(1):e000283.
52. Sharif A, Moore R, Baboolal K. Influence of lifestyle modification in renal transplant recipients with postprandial hyperglycemia. Transplantation. 2008;85:353-8.
53. Burt MG, Roberts GW, Aguilar-Loza NR, Frith P, Stranks SN. Continuous monitoring of circadian glycemic patterns in patients receiving prednisolone for COPD. J Clin Endocrinol Metab. 2011;96:1789.
54. American Diabetes Association. Glycaemic targets: standards of medical care in diabetes. Diabetes Care. 2018; 41(Suppl. 1):S55-64.
55. Kidney Disease: Improving Global Outcomes (KDIGO) Diabetes Work Group. KDIGO 2020 clinical practice guidelines for diabetes management in chronic kidney disease. Kidney Int. 2020;98:s47-57.
56. Vest LS, Koraishy FM, Zhang Z, Lam NN, Schnitzler MA, Dharnidharka VR, et al. Metformin use in the first year after kidney transplant, correlates, and associated outcomes in diabetic transplant recipients: a retrospective analysis of integrated registry and pharmacy claims data. Clin Transplant. 2018;32(8):e13302.
57. Cross NB, Webster AC. Angiotensin-converting enzyme inhibitors-beneficial effects seen in many patient groups may not extend to kidney transplant recipients. Transplantation. 2016;100(3):472-3.
58. Kidney Disease: Improving Global Outcomes Transplant Work Group. KDIGO clinical practice guideline for the care of kidney transplant recipients. Am J Transplant. 2009; 9(Suppl. 3):S1-155.
59. Holdaas H, Fellstrom B, Cole E, Nyberg G, Olsson AG, Pedersen TR, et al. Long-term cardiac outcomes in renal transplant recipients receiving fluvastatin: the ALERT extension study. Am J Transplant. 2005;5(12):2929-36.
60. Palmer SC, Navaneethan SD, Craig JC, Perkovic V, Johnson DW, Nigwekar SU, et al. HMG CoA reductase inhibitors (statins) for kidney transplant recipients. Cochrane Database Syst Rev. 2009;(2):CD005019.
61. Subramaniam S, Zell JA, Kunz PL. Everolimus causing severe hypertriglyceridemia and acute pancreatitis. J Natl Compr Canc Netw. 2013;11(1):5-9.

62. Haller MC, Royuela A, Nagler EV, Pascual J, Webster AC. Steroid avoidance or withdrawal for kidney transplant recipients. Cochrane Database Syst Rev. 2016;2016(8): CD005632.
63. Ducloux D, Kazory A, Chalopin JM. Posttransplant diabetes mellitus and atherosclerotic events in renal transplant recipients: a prospective study. Transplantation. 2005;79:438.
64. Boudreaux JP, McHugh L, Canafax DM, Ascher N, Sutherland DE, Payne W, et al. The impact of cyclosporine and combination immunosuppression on the incidence of posttransplant diabetes in renal allograft recipients. Transplantation. 1987;44:376.
65. Sumrani N, Delaney V, Ding Z, Davis R, Daskalakis P, Friedman EA, et al. Posttransplant diabetes mellitus in cyclosporine-treated renal transplant recipients. Transplant Proc. 1991;23:1249.
66. Gaynor JJ, Ciancio G, Guerra G, Sageshima J, Hanson L, Roth D, et al. Single-centre study of 628 adults, primary kidney transplant recipients showing no unfavorable effect of new-onset diabetes after transplant. Diabetologia. 2015;58:334.
67. Miles AM, Sumrani N, Horowitz R, Homel P, Maursky V, Markell MS, et al. Diabetes mellitus after renal transplantation: as deleterious as non-transplant-associated diabetes? Transplantation. 1998;65:380.
68. Malik RF, Jia Y, Mansour SG, Reese PP, Hall IE, Alasfar S, et al. Post-transplant diabetes mellitus in kidney transplant recipients: a multicenter study. Kidney360. 2021;2:1296-307.
69. Buuuough TE, Swindle J, Takemoto S, Lentine KL, Machnicki G, Irish WD, et al. Diabetic complications associated with new-onset diabetes mellitus in renal transplant recipients. Transplantation. 2007;83:1027.
70. Bae J, Lee MJ, Choe EY, Jung CH, Wang HJ, Kim MY, et al. Effects of dipeptidyl peptidase-4 inhibitors on hyperglycemia and blood cyclosporine levels in renal transplant patients with diabetes: a pilot study. Endocrinol Metab. 2016;31(1):161-7.
71. Montero N, Oliveras L, Soler MJ, Cruzado JM. Management of post-transplant diabetes mellitus: an opportunity for novel therapeutics. Clin Kidney J. 2021;15(1):1-9.

13.6 Mineral Bone Disease in Kidney Transplant Recipients

Vinant Bhargava, Anurag Gupta, Shyam Bansal

IMPORTANT QUESTIONS

a. What are common biochemical abnormalities of serum calcium, phosphorus, and parathyroid hormone (PTH) levels during the early (1–3 months) postrenal transplantation period?
b. How do you diagnose and manage low-turnover bone diseases in kidney transplant recipient (KTR)?
c. What is the best approach to manage hyperparathyroidism (HPT) in a KTR?

INTRODUCTION

Musculoskeletal manifestations in kidney transplant recipient (KTR) are associated with significant fracture risk, poor quality of life, morbidity, and mortality.[1,2] Bone disease is usually a continuum of preexisting bone disease in the end-stage kidney disease (ESKD). However, it can also be due to transplant-related factors, such as immunosuppressive agents. The pathogenesis of bone disease in transplant patients is complex and heterogeneous.

Postrenal transplant alterations in bone density and mineral metabolism lead to a range of bone mineral diseases—renal osteodystrophy, osteoporosis, bone fracture, osteonecrosis, and bone pain syndrome **(Fig. 1)**.[3-7] In a KTR, calcium and phosphate disorders, vitamin D deficiency, and hyperparathyroidism (HPT) (secondary and tertiary) produce a series of mineral and bone-related disorders.[3,5-7] Management of bone disease after transplant is related to correcting biochemical abnormalities.[8]

EPIDEMIOLOGY

The prevalence of bone mineral disease in KTR is widely underrecognized. The pooled prevalence of low bone mineral density (BMD) (osteoporosis and osteopenia) in the spine ranges from 14.5 to 88.0% and 3.2% in the pelvis. The fracture risk ranges from 2- to 14-fold in KTRs compared to the general population.[2] The prevalence of osteopenia and osteoporosis ranges from 5 to 35% at different sites, with osteomalacia reported in up to 52.7% of cases. India lacks a national end-stage renal disease (ESRD) registry, and most estimates are extrapolated from small cross-sectional or hospital-based registries.[9] A few small cohort studies in KTR have documented BMD decline from as early as 3–8 months after transplantation.[10-12] The prevalence of osteopenia and osteoporosis significantly increases from the pretransplant stage to 6 months post-transplant **(Fig. 2)**.[12]

PATHOPHYSIOLOGY AND RISK FACTORS

Bone remodeling is primarily controlled by osteoclasts and osteoblasts. PTH, vitamin D, acidosis, interleukins (IL), such as IL-1, IL-6, tumor necrosis factor, and macrophage migration inhibitory factor (MIF)-1 alpha promote osteoclasts while osteoprotegerin reduces bone absorption.[5] Before renal transplantation, the serum phosphate, PTH, and fibroblast growth factor 23 (FGF-23) levels are elevated with a progressive decline in kidney function.[13,14] These parameters remain elevated even after a few months of renal transplant, despite an improvement in the renal functions. Within a year, these parameters return to normalcy.[15,16]

In KTRs, four components could contribute to bone mineral disease:[3,17-20]

1. Ongoing bone mineral disease due to ESKD that persists in the post-transplant period
2. Immunosuppression therapy
3. Changes in the serum phosphate, calcium, PTH, and FGF-23 levels following transplantation
4. De novo bone mineral disease due to persistent HPT and decline in kidney function.

SPECTRUM

Bone mineral disease in KTRs can include both high-turnover bone disease such as osteitis fibrosa cystica (due to secondary HPT) and low-turnover bone disease such as adynamic bone disease.[17,19,20] Osteoporosis, osteomalacia, and osteonecrosis are not uncommonly reported.

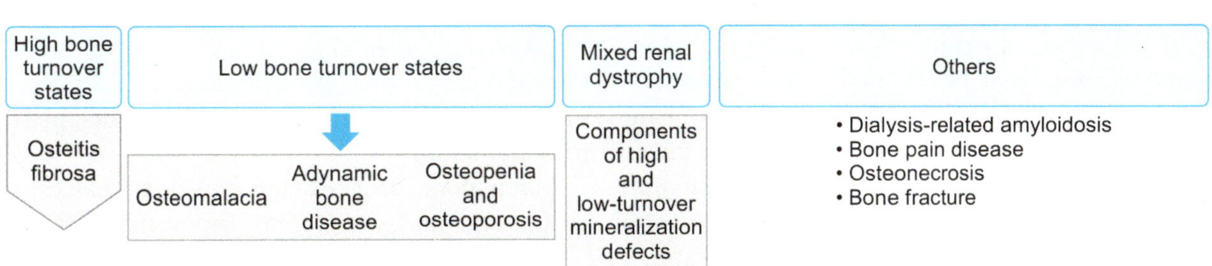

Fig. 1: Spectrum of bone disorders after kidney transplant.

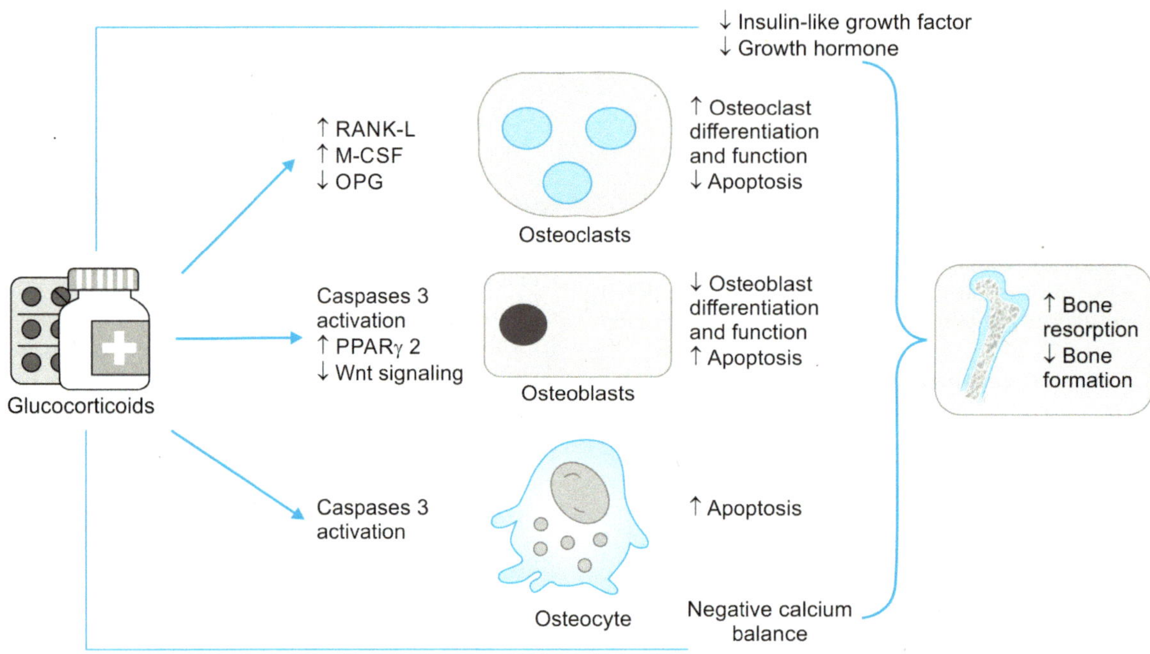

Fig. 2: Direct and indirect effects of glucocorticoids on bone health.[19,22,23] (M-CSF: macrophage colony-stimulating factor; OPG: osteoprotegerin; PPARγ: peroxisome proliferator-activated receptor gamma; RANKL: receptor activator of nuclear factor kappa-B ligand)

Disorders of calcium and phosphate metabolism, and vitamin D deficiency are frequently seen causing several alterations in bone metabolism **(Fig. 1)**.

CHAPTER HIGHLIGHTS

- Mineral bone diseases in kidney transplant recipient (KTR) are associated with significant fracture risk and poor quality of life with substantial morbidity and mortality.
- Disorders of calcium, phosphate, parathyroid hormone (PTH), and vitamin D are commonly encountered in KTR.
- A spectrum of abnormalities in bone, such as osteomalacia, osteopenia, osteonecrosis, and osteoporosis, are common in the post-transplant period.
- Cardiovascular calcifications may be observed with low bone turnover in KTR.
- Therapies directed at mineral bone diseases in KTR are challenging due to heterogeneity of bone disorders and transplant-related factors.

BIOCHEMICAL ABNORMALITIES

In the natural history of renal transplantation, elevated levels of circulating phosphate, PTH, and serum FGF-23 correspond to a decline in renal function post-transplantation. However, despite the restoration of renal function, in the recovery period of post-transplantation, FGF-23 and PTH continue to be elevated for several months leading to hypophosphatemia[16,17] (due to insignificant urinary phosphorus losses). Eventually, FGF-23 levels declined dramatically after 3 months post-transplantation with comparable estimated glomerular filtration rate (eGFR). Serum phosphorus levels start to normalize after a few months following transplantation, which correlates with decline in FGF-23 levels with improved glomerular filtration rate (GFR). Nevertheless, >50% of the KTRs may develop hypophosphatemia.

Hyperparathyroidism activates osteoclast through its direct and indirect actions by inhibiting the sclerostin and activating the receptor activator of nuclear factor kappa-B ligand (RANKL) signaling pathway. The effects of HPT and raised FGF-23 culminate in hypophosphatemia and negate the PTH-mediated osteoblastogenesis.[17,20] Prekidney transplantation PTH ≥ 300 pg/mL increases the risk of persistent HPT and tertiary HPT by one-and-a-half times and by more than twofold, respectively. With restoration of kidney functions, most of the stimuli of parathyroid hyperplasia abate, which results in a gradual decline in PTH concentrations (unlike FGF-23 levels that decline precipitously). Up to >80% of patients can still have inappropriately high PTH even after 1 year post-transplant. Raised PTH levels after transplant factors may be attributable to factors such as pretransplant use of cinacalcet, presence of nodular hyperplasia, and longer dialysis vintage. A significant proportion of patients (up to 66%) develop hypercalcemia after renal transplant. The primary drivers of hypercalcemia could be persistent HPT, high vitamin D levels, decrease in skeletal resistance to PTH following resolution of uremia, use of calcium and vitamin D supplements or rarely, abrupt discontinuation of cinacalcet post-transplantation.

A functional decline of the graft kidney can cause de novo HPT, consequently setting off bone mineral disease.[17,19,21]

Several risk factors have been associated with post-transplantation bone loss and fractures **(Fig. 3)**.

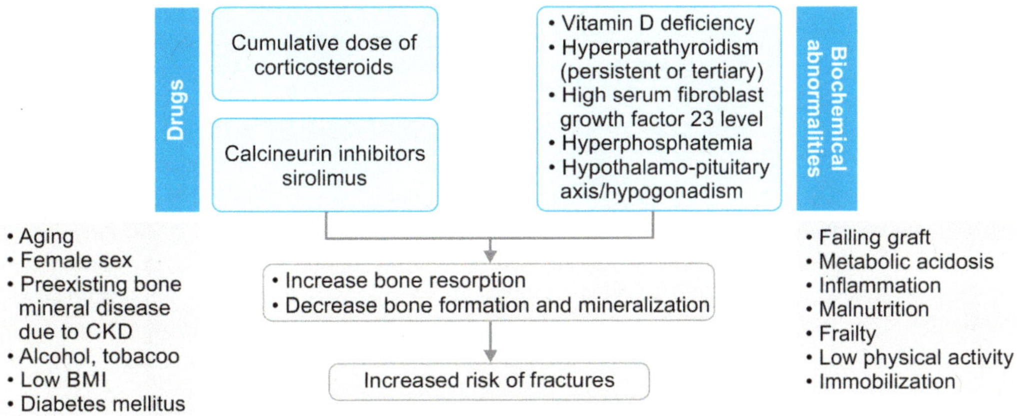

Fig. 3: Risk factors with post-transplantation bone loss and fractures. (BMI: body mass index; CKD: chronic kidney disease)

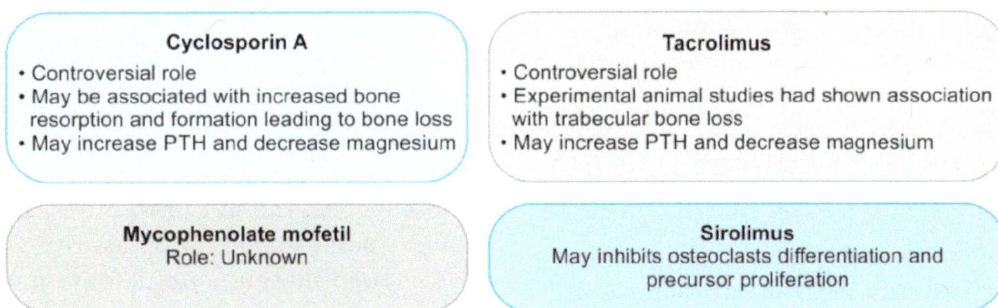

Fig. 4: Effect of other immunosuppressants on bone metabolism.[18,21] (PTH: parathyroid hormone)

ROLE OF IMMUNOSUPPRESSIVE MEDICATIONS

Glucocorticoids are a fundamental component of the immunosuppressive regimen in renal transplantation, directly and indirectly affecting bone mineral disease **(Fig. 3)**.[19,22-24] The effects of immunosuppressants on bone metabolism are summarized in **Figures 2 and 4**.[18,21,25-29]

SCREENING AND MONITORING PATIENTS FOR OSTEOPOROSIS AND FRACTURE RISK

All KTRs should be subjected to screening for osteoporosis and fracture risk **(Table 1)**.[30]

The Fracture Risk Assessment Tool (FRAX) has been used in the general population to accurately estimate the 10-year probability of major osteoporotic fractures and could be used in renal transplant patients at high risk of fracture **(Fig. 5)**.[3,33]

WHO classification	***T-score***
Osteoporosis	–2.5 or below
Osteopenia (low bone mass)	–1.0 and –2.5
Normal	–1.0 or above

(WHO: World Health Organization)

TABLE 1: Methods of assessment of fracture risk in kidney transplant recipient (KTR).

Assessment of biochemical abnormalities	Serum parathyroid hormone, calcium, phosphate, and 25-hydroxyvitamin D levels
Assessment of clinical risk factors for fracture[31,32]	Age/gender, pretransplant fracture history, low body weight, diabetes, obesity, and years of pretransplant kidney failure
Assessment of bone mineral density Dual-energy X-ray absorptiometry (DEXA scan)	• Noninvasive, cost-effective screening method • May not distinguish between cortical and trabecular bone, differentially affected in secondary hyperparathyroidism

BONE BIOPSY

Although unpopular, bone biopsy with double-tetracycline labeling, the gold standard can accurately diagnose post-transplantation bone disease subtype.[34] As per the Kidney Disease Improving Global Outcomes (KDIGO 2017) guidelines, it is reasonable to consider a bone biopsy to guide treatment. Histologic descriptions of bone turnover (T), mineralization (M), and volume (V) can be assessed by bone histomorphometry. However, being an invasive

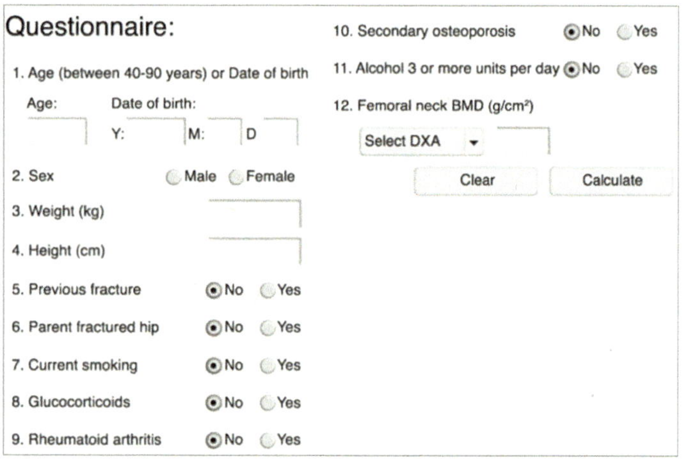
Questionnaire:
1. Age (between 40-90 years) or Date of birth
Age: Date of birth: Y: M: D
2. Sex Male Female
3. Weight (kg)
4. Height (cm)
5. Previous fracture No Yes
6. Parent fractured hip No Yes
7. Current smoking No Yes
8. Glucocorticoids No Yes
9. Rheumatoid arthritis No Yes
10. Secondary osteoporosis No Yes
11. Alcohol 3 or more units per day No Yes
12. Femoral neck BMD (g/cm²)
Select DXA
Clear Calculate

Fig. 5: The World Health Organization fracture risk assessment tool.[33]

TABLE 2: Frequency of monitoring for kidney bone-mineral disorders.[34]

Kidney function stage	Parameters	Frequency
CKD G1T–G3bT	Serum calcium and phosphate	Every 6–12 months
	PTH	Once, with subsequent intervals depending on baseline level and CKD progression
CKD G4T	Serum calcium and phosphate	Every 3–6 months
	PTH	Every 6–12 months
CKD G5T	Serum calcium and phosphate	Every 1–3 months
	PTH	Every 3–6 months
CKD G3aT–G5T	Alkaline phosphatases	Annually, or more frequently in the presence of elevated PTH

(CKD: chronic kidney disease; PTH: parathyroid hormone)

procedure, difficult to interpret and limited data on follow-up makes bone biopsy a less preferred approach in clinical practice.

KDIGO GUIDELINES ON MONITORING POST-TRANSPLANT PATIENTS FOR BONE DISEASE

The KDIGO 2017 guidelines recommend the assessment of fracture risk by measuring BMD measurements using dual-energy X-ray absorptiometry (DEXA) in patients with chronic kidney disease (CKD) G1T–G5T with risk factors for osteoporosis, if results will alter therapy.

Kidney Disease Improving Global Outcomes also recommends measuring serum, PTH, calcium phosphate, and calcidiol in patients in the immediate postkidney transplant period. The suggested frequency of monitoring is presented in **Table 2.**[34]

OTHER BIOMARKERS

Efforts are being made to identify several biomarkers for bone-mineral disorder in KTR. Sclerostin, Dickkopf-related protein 1 (Dkk-1), and serum RANKL were elevated while osteoprotegerin receptor was significantly reduced in KTR.[35] However, researchers are skeptical in using biomarkers because circulating biomarkers after renal transplantation cannot be easily extrapolated to concomitant changes occurring in the bone.[36] Bone biomarkers were not associated with bone metabolism changes detected in bone biopsy specimens.[37]

PREVENTION OF OSTEOPOROSIS

Preventive measures against osteoporosis include lifestyle changes such as regular weight-bearing exercise, smoking cessation, and reducing alcohol consumption.[38] In addition, correction of aberrant biochemical parameters—calcium, PTH, and vitamin D levels—is crucial in preventing osteoporosis. Optimizing glycemic control is essential in patients with diabetes. Another preventive measure is the use of steroid-sparing immunosuppressive regimens.[39]

Although there are no definite pharmacotherapeutic strategies for preventing osteoporosis, bisphosphonates, calcitonin, and vitamin D analogs are considered in several clinical trials to prevent and treat osteoporosis or bone loss after renal transplantation.[40,41] Higher order evidence from systemic and meta-analysis confirms the beneficial role of bisphosphonates in preventing osteoporosis by improving the lumbar spine and femoral neck BMD after 1 year post-transplantation.[40] Bisphosphonates reduced the loss of vertebral and femoral BMD by 6% from baseline at 1 year after renal transplantation.[42]

Calcium and vitamin D supplements must be initiated, specifically in those with a baseline BMD signifying osteopenia or osteoporosis. Bisphosphonates are initiated when patients show a declining BMD despite being on calcium and vitamin D supplements.[41]

A single subcutaneous dose of denosumab every 6 months was associated with significant improvement in BMD both at lumbar and femoral sites.[43] Furthermore, the increase in BMD was greater with denosumab compared with bisphosphonates.[44] Besides improving BMD, denosumab improved trabecular bone texture in de novo postrenal transplant patients.[45] Discontinuation of denosumab after two doses decreased the BMD in the lumbar spine and hip.[46] Among those at risk of osteoporosis, denosumab improved bone quality and BMD.[47]

Glucocorticoids are associated with bone loss and fracture risk. Early post-transplant withdrawal of glucocorticosteroids has shown to preserve the bone mass. Data from the largest kidney transplantation registry, the United States

Renal Data System, showed a 31% reduction in fracture risk by withdrawing corticosteroids. Further, a significantly lower incidence of fractures leading to hospitalizations (1.6% absolute reduction) was observed over 7 years among those discharged without a corticosteroid prescription.[48] Alternatively, steroid-free protocols are warranted for patients with pretransplant osteopenia or osteoporosis.[41]

MANAGEMENT OF KIDNEY BONE MINERAL DISEASE

The KDIGO guidelines on post-transplantation bone disease recommend treatment based on the extent of bone loss and levels of bone turnover markers [PTH and bone-specific alkaline phosphatase (BSAP)] **(Flowchart 1)**.[2,3,49] Before initiating treatment, abnormal calcium, phosphorus, and vitamin D levels should be considered.[49] Therapeutic interventions for overcoming the biochemical abnormalities range from medications to surgical intervention.[2] Patients having osteoporosis with no evidence of low-turnover bone disease can be given antiresorptive therapy, such as bisphosphonates. Denosumab is another alternative. Teriparatide could be a potential option in patients with low BMD and low-turnover bone disease.

Total parathyroidectomy with or without autotransplantation for HPT can correct hypercalcemia but it increases the risk of hypocalcemia.[20,50-52] There are always concerns that parathyroidectomy may adversely affect the graft function. In clinical practice, PTH surgery is limited to KTRs with profoundly high PTH and calcium levels, symptomatic cases [fractures, electrocardiogram (ECG) changes, neurologic sequelae, etc.], or failure of medical management. The optimal timing, choice of surgery, and PTH levels at which PTH surgery is to be done are still unclear. Therefore, this should be decided on a case-by-case basis. A recent retrospective analysis suggested that the extent of parathyroidectomy is important and excessive elevation of intact parathyroid hormone (iPTH) should be avoided by timely parathyroidectomy, before reaching extremely high values.[53] Parathyroidectomy is advisable over cinacalcet in KTRs who require long-term management of post-transplantation bone mineral diseases.

OSTEONECROSIS

Osteonecrosis is another disabling bone complication affecting up to one-third of KTRs. Corticosteroids play a key role in the genesis of osteonecrosis. The underlying pathophysiological mechanism leading to osteonecrosis is probably diminished blood flow to the bone, leading to necrosis and eventually bone destruction. Other attributable factors are fat emboli due to alterations in circulating lipids, enhanced apoptosis of osteoblasts, osteocytes and endothelial cells in addition to procoagulant state and modulation of vasoactive mediators. Usually, weight-bearing long bones are affected and femoral head is the most commonly affected region. The prime strategy of management is early diagnosis as there is no proven therapy. Surgical options include core decompression and osteotomy. Bone grafting is an option for symptomatic patients with progressive early stage osteonecrosis. In case of bone collapse, hemiarthroplasty or total-hip arthroplasty may be offered.

Flowchart 1: Managing mineral and bone disease after kidney transplantation.[2]

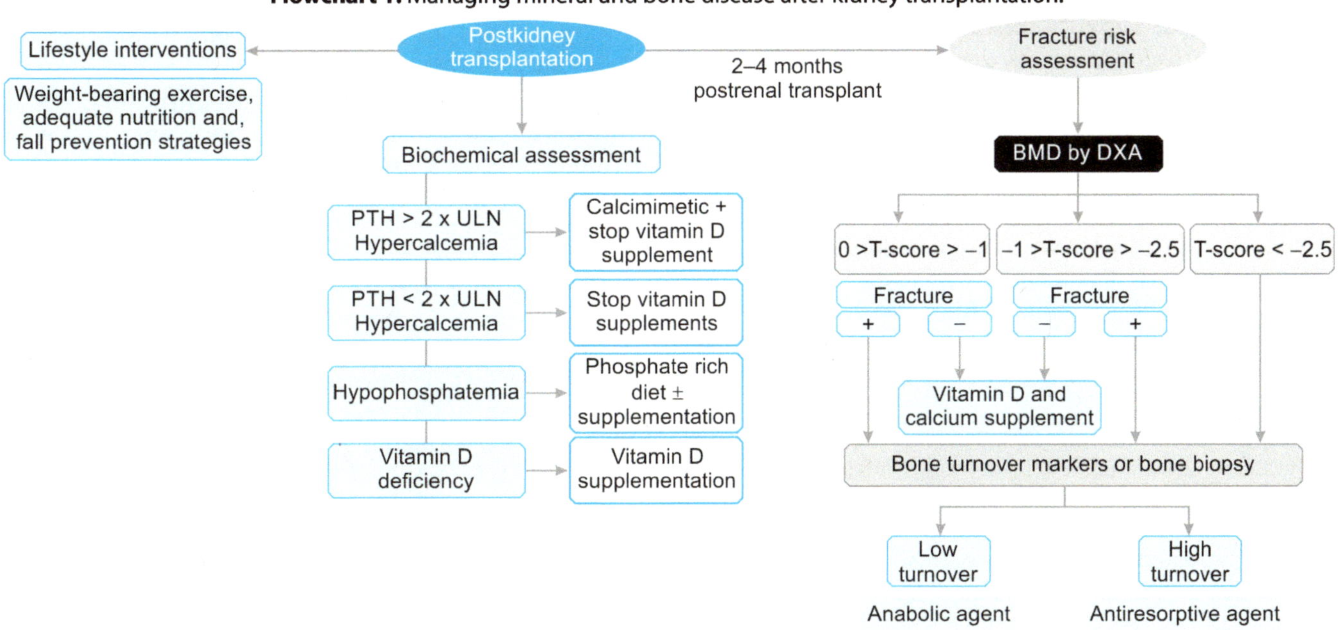

(BMD: bone mineral density; DXA: dual-energy X-ray absorptiometry; LLN: lower limit of normal; PTH: parathyroid hormone; ULN: upper limit of normal; VDRA: vitamin D receptor activator)

CALCINEURIN INHIBITOR-INDUCED PAIN SYNDROME

Calcineurin inhibitor-induced pain syndrome (CIPS) is characterized by deep aching pain mostly occurring in the lower extremities symmetrically. The symptoms generally correlates with the drug levels. The prevalence among KTR is reported to be 0.8–5.8%. The proposed theory for the underlying mechanism is the intraosseous vasoconstrictive effect of calcineurin inhibitors (CNIs) leading to increased marrow pressure and edema. Calcineurin is also involved in nociceptive processes by activating the nitric oxide pathway. Diagnosis is challenging. Plain X-ray could be normal. Bone scintigraphy shows increased tracer uptake in the affected bones and joints. Magnetic resonance imaging (MRI) is suggestive of patchy edema of the bone marrow. The condition is self-limiting. However, treatment with pregabalin and calcium channel blocker, such as nifedipine, can be tried.

INDIAN LITERATURE

Recently, Ramakrishna et al. prospectively analyzed biochemical tests and dual-energy absorptiometry at baseline and 8 months after renal transplantation.[11] The study showed that higher iPTH and low 25-hydroxyvitamin D [25(OH) Vit-D] were associated with lower femoral BMD and reduced forearm BMD, respectively. The spinal BMD worsened but there was an improvement in the forearm BMD at 8 months after transplantation. Cumulative steroid dose had a significant negative impact on BMD at spine. Two patients had avascular necrosis of the femur.

REFERENCES

1. Hassan AB, Ghalib KW, Jahrami HA, El-Agroudy AE. Prevalence of musculoskeletal manifestations in adult kidney transplant's recipients: a systematic review. Medicina. 2021;57(6):525.
2. Khairallah P, Nickolas TL. Bone and mineral disease in kidney transplant recipients. Clin J Am Soc Nephrol. 2022; 17(1):121-30.
3. Bouquegneau A, Salam S, Delanaye P, Eastell R, Khwaja A. Bone disease after kidney transplantation. Clin J Am Soc Nephrol. 2016;11(7):1282.
4. Kalantar-Zadeh K, Molnar MZ, Kovesdy CP, Mucsi I, Bunnapradist S. Management of minerals and bone disorders after kidney transplantation. Curr Opin Nephrol Hypertens. 2012;21(4):389.
5. Shah A, Aeddula NR. Renal osteodystrophy. In: StatPearls. StatPearls Publishing; 2021. [online] Available from http://www.ncbi.nlm.nih.gov/books/NBK560742/. [Last accessed December, 2021].
6. Vangala C, Pan J, Cotton RT, Ramanathan V. Mineral and bone disorders after kidney transplantation. Front Med. 2018;5: 211.
7. Zhang R, Chouhan KK. Metabolic bone diseases in kidney transplant recipients. World J Nephrol. 2012;1(5):127.
8. Altman AM, Sprague SM. Mineral and bone disease in kidney transplant recipients. Curr Osteoporos Rep. 2018; 16(6):703-11.
9. Thurlow JS, Joshi M, Yan G, Norris KC, Agodoa LY, Yuan CM, et al. Global epidemiology of end-stage kidney disease and disparities in kidney replacement therapy. Am J Nephrol. 2021;52(2):98-107.
10. Rathi M, Kumar D, Bhadada SK, Khandelwal N, Kohli HS, Jha V, et al. Sequential changes in bone biochemical parameters and bone mineral density after renal transplant. Saudi J Kidney Diseases Transpl. 2015;26(4):671.
11. Ramakrishna MP, Arun CS, Sreedharan S, Pavithran PV, Bhavani N, Bhaskaran R, et al. Changes in bone mineral density in patients undergoing kidney transplantation. Indian J Transpl. 2021;15(3):199-204.
12. Govindarajan S, Khandelwal N, Sakhuja V, Jha V. Bone mineral density in patients with end-stage renal disease and its evolution after kidney transplantation. Indian J Nephrol. 2011;21(2):85.
13. Jørgensen HS, Behets G, Bammens B, Claes K, Meijers B, Naesens M, et al. Natural history of bone disease following kidney transplantation. J Am Soc Nephrol. 2022;33(3):638-52.
14. Segaud N, Legroux I, Hazzan M, Noel C, Cortet B. Changes in bone mineral density after kidney transplantation: 2-year assessment of a French cohort. Osteoporos Int. 2018; 29(5):1165-75.
15. Baia LC, Heilberg IP, Navis G, de Borst MH. Phosphate and FGF-23 homeostasis after kidney transplantation. Nat Rev Nephrol. 2015;11(11):656-66.
16. Haffner D, Leifheit-Nestler M. CKD-MBD post kidney transplantation. Pediatr Nephrol. 2021;36(1):41-50.
17. Evenepoel P. Recovery versus persistence of disordered mineral metabolism in kidney transplant recipients. Semin Nephrol. 2013;33(2):191-203.
18. Kulak CAM, Borba VZC, Kulak Júnior J, Custódio MR. Bone disease after transplantation: osteoporosis and fractures risk. Arq Bras Endocrinol Metab. 2014;58:484-92.
19. Malluche HH, Monier-Faugere MC, Herberth J. Bone disease after renal transplantation. Nat Rev Nephrol. 2010;6(1): 32-40.
20. Torregrosa JV, Ferreira AC, Cucchiari D, Ferreira A. Bone mineral disease after kidney transplantation. Calcif Tissue Int. 2021;108(4):551-60.
21. Hirukawa T, Kakuta T, Nakamura M, Fukagawa M. Mineral and bone disorders in kidney transplant recipients: reversible, irreversible, and de novo abnormalities. Clin Exp Nephrol. 2015;19(4):543-55.
22. Compston J. Glucocorticoid-induced osteoporosis: an update. Endocrine. 2018;61(1):7.
23. Mazziotti G, Formenti AM, Adler RA, Bilezikian JP, Grossman A, Sbardella E, et al. Glucocorticoid-induced osteoporosis: pathophysiological role of GH/IGF-I and PTH/VITAMIN D axes, treatment options and guidelines. Endocrine. 2016;54(3):603-11.
24. Kovvuru K, Kanduri SR, Vaitla P, Marathi R, Gosi S, Anton DFG, et al. Risk factors and management of osteoporosis post-transplant. Medicina. 2020;56(6):302.
25. Weisinger JR, Carlini RG, Rojas E, Bellorin-Font E. Bone disease after renal transplantation. Clin J Am Soc Nephrol. 2006;1(6):1300-13.

26. Battaglia Y, Bellasi A, Bortoluzzi A, Tondolo F, Esposito P, Provenzano M, et al. Bone mineral density changes in long-term kidney transplant recipients: a real-life cohort study of native vitamin D supplementation. Nutrients. 2022;14(2):323.
27. Sutton W, Chen X, Patel P, Karzai S, Prescott JD, Segev DL, et al. Prevalence and risk factors for tertiary hyperparathyroidism in kidney transplant recipients. Surgery. 2022;171(1):69-76.
28. Messa P, Cafforio C, Alfieri C. Calcium and phosphate changes after renal transplantation. J Nephrol. 2010;23(Suppl. 16): S175-81.
29. Ralston MR, Stevenson KS, Mark PB, Geddes CC. Clinical factors associated with severe hypophosphataemia after kidney transplant. BMC Nephrol. 2021;22(1):407.
30. Marcén R, Caballero C, Uriol O, Fernández A, Villafruela JJ, Pascual J, et al. Prevalence of osteoporosis, osteopenia, and vertebral fractures in long-term renal transplant recipients. Transplant Proc. 2007;39(7):2256-8.
31. O'Shaughnessy EA, Dahl DC, Smith CL, Kasiske BL. Risk factors for fractures in kidney transplantation. Transplantation. 2002;74(3):362-6.
32. Khosravi M, Soltanian N, Monfared A, Ghanbari A, Ramezanzade E, Kazemnezhad Leyli E. Bone mineral density and related factors in renal transplant recipients, in the North of Iran. Iran J Kidney Dis. 2020;14(5):405-11.
33. Watts NB. The Fracture Risk Assessment Tool (FRAX®): applications in clinical practice. J Womens Health (Larchmt). 2011;20(4):525-31.
34. Kidney Disease: Improving Global Outcomes (KDIGO) CKD-MBD Update Work Group. KDIGO 2017 clinical practice guideline update for the diagnosis, evaluation, prevention, and treatment of chronic kidney disease-mineral and bone disorder (CKD-MBD). Kidney Int Suppl. 2017;7(1):1.
35. Magalhães J, Quelhas-Santos J, Pereira L, Neto R, Castro-Ferreira I, Martins S, et al. Could bone biomarkers predict bone turnover after kidney transplantation? A proof-of-concept study. J Clin Med. 2022;11(2):457.
36. Araújo MJCLN, Bacelar Marques ID, Graciolli FG, Fukuhara L, Dos Reis LM, Custódio M, et al. Comparison of serum levels with bone content and gene expression indicate a contradictory effect of kidney transplantation on sclerostin. Kidney Int. 2019;96(5):1100-4.
37. Keronen S, Martola L, Finne P, Burton IS, Kröger H, Honkanen E. Changes in bone histomorphometry after kidney transplantation. Clin J Am Soc Nephrol. 2019;14(6): 894-903.
38. Damasiewicz MJ, Ebeling PR. Management of mineral and bone disorders in renal transplant recipients. Nephrology (Carlton). 2017;22(Suppl. 2):65-9.
39. Gosmanova EO, Gosmanov AR. Osteoporosis in patients with diabetes after kidney transplantation. Rev Endocr Metab Disord. 2017;18(1):97-106.
40. Wang J, Yao M, Xu J-h, Shu B, Wang Y-j, Cui X-j. Bisphosphonates for prevention of osteopenia in kidney-transplant recipients: a systematic review of randomized controlled trials. Osteoporos Int. 2016;27(5):1683-90.
41. Zhang R, Alper B, Simon E, Florman S, Slakey D. Management of metabolic bone disease in kidney transplant recipients. Am J Med Sci. 2008;335(2):120-5.
42. Versele EB, Van Laecke S, Dhondt AW, Verbeke F, Vanholder R, Van Biesen W, et al. Bisphosphonates for preventing bone disease in kidney transplant recipients: a meta-analysis of randomized controlled trials. Transpl Int. 2016;29(2):153-64.
43. Cianciolo G, Tondolo F, Barbuto S, Iacovella F, Zavatta G, Altieri P, et al. Denosumab-induced hypocalcemia and hyperparathyroidism in de novo kidney transplant recipients. Am J Nephrol. 2021;52(8):611-9.
44. McKee H, Ioannidis G, Lau A, Treleaven D, Gangji A, Ribic C, et al. Comparison of the clinical effectiveness and safety between the use of denosumab vs bisphosphonates in renal transplant patients. Osteoporos Int. 2020;31(5): 973-80.
45. Bonani M, Frey D, Graf N, Wüthrich RP. Effect of denosumab on trabecular bone score in de novo kidney transplant recipients. Nephrol Dial Transplant. 2019;34(10):1773-80.
46. Kobel C, Frey D, Graf N, Wüthrich RP, Bonani M. Follow-up of bone mineral density changes in de novo kidney transplant recipients treated with two doses of the receptor activator of nuclear factor κB ligand inhibitor denosumab. Kidney Blood Press Res. 2019;44(5):1285-93.
47. Bonani M, Meyer U, Frey D, Graf N, Bischoff-Ferrari HA, Wüthrich RP. Effect of denosumab on peripheral compartmental bone density, microarchitecture and estimated bone strength in de novo kidney transplant recipients. Kidney Blood Press Res. 2016;41(5):614-22.
48. Nikkel LE, Mohan S, Zhang A, McMahon DJ, Boutroy S, Dube G, et al. Reduced fracture risk with early corticosteroid withdrawal after kidney transplant. Am J Transpl. 2012; 12(3):649.
49. Kidney Disease: Improving Global Outcomes (KDIGO) CKD-MBD Work Group. KDIGO clinical practice guideline for the diagnosis, evaluation, prevention, and treatment of chronic kidney disease-mineral and bone disorder (CKD-MBD). Kidney Int Suppl. 2009;113:S1-130.
50. Chen J, Jia X, Kong X, Wang Z, Cui M, Xu D. Total parathyroidectomy with autotransplantation versus subtotal parathyroidectomy for renal hyperparathyroidism: a systematic review and meta-analysis. Nephrology (Carlton). 2017;22(5):388-96.
51. Liu ME, Qiu NC, Zha SL, Du ZP, Wang YF, Wang Q, et al. To assess the effects of parathyroidectomy (TPTX versus TPTX+AT) for secondary hyperparathyroidism in chronic renal failure: a systematic review and meta-analysis. Int J Surg. 2017;44:353-62.
52. Qiu Z, Lin C, Zhang Y, Lin C, Deng J, Wu M. Analysis of the efficacy and safety of teriparatide and alendronate in the treatment of osteoporosis after renal transplantation. Iran J Kidney Dis. 2021;15(6):451-6.
53. Patecki M, Scheffner I, Haller H, Gwinner W. Long-term renal graft outcome after parathyroidectomy—a retrospective single centre study. BMC Nephrol. 2020;21:53.

13.7 Malignancy in Kidney Transplant Recipients

Arunkumar S, Sandeep Mahajan

CASE VIGNETTE

A 51-year-old female renal allograft recipient was admitted for loss of appetite, on and off diarrhea and loss of weight (6 kg) for 3 months duration. She had received kidney transplantation 8 years earlier for diabetes mellitus related end-stage renal disease. The donor was her husband and she received antithymocyte globulin (ATG) induction. Patient was on standard triple drug immunosuppression and had an uneventful postoperative course with stable serum creatinine of 1.1–1.3 mg/dL. Current immunosuppressive regimen consisted of tacrolimus, mycophenolate mofetil (500 mg thrice/day) and low dose prednisolone (5 mg/day). The dose of tacrolimus was titrated to achieve trough whole blood level of 5 ng/mL.

Clinically the patient had stable vitals with normal hydration status. Stool examination was inconclusive and she was planned for endoscopy. Patient developed acute abdominal pain during hospital stay and was taken up for emergency laparotomy with suspicion of intestinal perforation. During the procedure, a small bowel resection of the perforated segment with primary anastomosis of the small intestine was done. Pathological analysis of this sample revealed diffuse large B-cell lymphoma (DLBCL). Epstein-Barr virus (EBV) RNA on tissue sample was negative. A diagnosis of EBV negative post-transplant lymphoproliferative disorder (DLBCL type) was made. Mycophenolate mofetil was stopped and dose of tacrolimus was halved and 5 mg wysolone was continued. Patient did not have any hematological involvement and PET CT was suggestive of diffuse uptake in the small intestine with regional lymphadenopathy. After medical oncology consultation, patient was planned for rituximab therapy at a dose of 375 mg/m^2. Patient received 4 doses of rituximab and repeat PET CT showed partial resolution. Patient thereafter received 4 cycles of cyclophosphamide, doxorubicin, vincristine and prednisolone following which she attained remission. Patient is on regular follow-up with a serum creatinine of 2–2.2 mg/dL and no fresh symptoms.

INTRODUCTION

The use of better and more advanced immunosuppressive agents has improved the graft survival rates and overall life expectancy of kidney transplant recipients (KTR). This has, however, concurrently increased the risk for malignancy in this population. Cardiovascular diseases, infections, and malignancies are the most common cause of morbidity and mortality in KTR. With aggressive management of cardiovascular diseases and infections, older age of recipients, and longer graft survival, post-transplant malignancy (PTM) is expected to be a major factor affecting patient outcomes in the years to come. Early diagnosis improves the outcome of KTR with malignancy, but the absence of an optimal screening program often results in cancer diagnosis in later stages and results in adverse outcomes. The management of these patients is often challenging and requires a marked change in the immunosuppressive regimen which in turn affects graft and patient outcomes.

PREVALENCE

Cancer occurrence after transplantation is two to three times more common than in the general population. This incidence increases steadily with time after transplantation and is particularly high for virus-related cancers. The absence of dedicated transplant registries limits our full understanding of the problem. Data from the Israel Penn Transplant Tumor Registry (IPTTR) [earlier known as the Cincinnati Transplant Tumor Registry (CTTR)] and some of the national registries have helped us in discerning the extent of PTM to some extent. A cohort study with registry linkage data from over 175,000 solid organ recipients reported a standardized incidence ratio of 2.10 [95% confidence interval (CI), 2.06–2.14] with an excess absolute risk of 719 cases per 100,000 person-years in transplant recipients. Nearly 32 different cancers were more common in transplant recipients with non-Hodgkin's lymphoma, cancers of the lung, liver, and kidney being the most common.[1] Breast and prostate cancer were, however, less common in transplanted patients. Post-transplant lymphoproliferative disorder (PTLD) and squamous cell carcinomas (SCC) were the most frequent tumors in the IPTTR/CTTR patient database. Also, 44% of the patients had multiple tumors which have a poorer prognosis.[2] The classical evidence of time-related risk of PTM is seen in Australian KTR whose risk of skin cancers increased from 7% after 1 year to 45% after 11 years and 70% after 20 years of transplantation.[3] In the Australia and New Zealand Dialysis and Transplant (ANZDATA) registry, 33% of KTR had nonskin cancer at 30 years of follow-up. The risk of mortality is also high in KTR with a standardized mortality ratio of 2.7 and some cancers such as non-Hodgkin's lymphoma (NHL), melanomas, and urogenital cancers have 5–10 times increased risk of death.[4]

The absence of a national transplant registry limits our data on the overall prevalence of malignancies in India. Most of the reports are case reports of rare malignancies or management of immunosuppression in PTM. In one study from South India, the incidence of PTM was 1.9% among 626 KTR and the most common malignancy reported was PTLD.[5] There are a couple of studies on the spectrum of PTLD in KTR wherein the incidence reported is 1.7%[6] and 1.45%,[7] similar to the reported incidence (1–3%) in all other studies. Pediatric data is limited to one report from AIIMS, New Delhi, in which 4.2% of the patients had PTLD in line with the existing literature describing an increased incidence of PTLD in children compared to adults.[8]

CHAPTER HIGHLIGHTS

- Malignancies are serious complications due to chronic exposure to immunosuppression in transplant recipients.
- In addition to conventional risk factors and immunosuppression, prior history of malignancy and viral infection predisposes to post-transplant malignancies.
- Post-transplant malignancies can be de novo, donor-derived, or recurrent.
- Skin cancer and lymphoproliferative disorders are the most common post-transplant malignancies.
- Presentation is varied, and a high degree of clinical suspicion with comprehensive evaluation is paramount for early diagnosis.
- Careful down-titration of immunosuppression, use of mTORi, and coordinated cancer care with surgery/chemotherapy ± radiotherapy improve outcomes of these patients.

PATHOGENESIS

Three different mechanisms can explain the occurrence of PTM:

1. *De novo malignancies:* New cancers in transplant recipients, especially in organs other than the transplanted organs
2. *Donor-related cancers:* Direct transmission of malignancy which preexisted in the donor in the transplanted organ or arising in the transplanted organ sometime after transplantation
3. *Recurrent malignancy:* Recurrence of preexisting malignancy of recipient.

The classification of PTM on the basis of origin and the common malignancies in each class is given in **Table 1**.[9]

The risk factors for PTM are:

- *Recipient related:* Conventional risk factors (age, sun exposure), previous cancer, viral infections, genetic risk factors
- *Donor related:* History of malignancy, micrometastasis
- *Immunosuppression related:* Depends on the class of drug, extent, and duration of immunosuppression.

Immunosuppression: By far the most important risk factor for PTM is the immunosuppressive therapy used. As illustrated in **Flowchart 1**, immunosuppressive drugs play an important role in all stages of oncogenesis. Immune surveillance offers protection against cancer and this is reduced by these drugs. The intensity of antilymphocyte activity parallels the risk of oncogenicity with the highest risk conferred by T-cell depleting induction therapy with antithymocyte globulin (ATG) and maintenance therapy with calcineurin inhibitors (CNI) and azathioprine. When compared to ATG, interleukin (IL)-2 receptor antibodies (basiliximab) are associated with a reduced risk for PTM.[10] CNI therapy results in disordered cytokine release [IL-6, transforming growth factor (TGF)-β] which promotes tumor cell growth and tumor angiogenesis. However, follow-up studies of patients on CNI and CNI withdrawal regimens do not show a difference in the risk of malignancy. Azathioprine affects deoxyribonucleic acid (DNA) repair and increases the risk of melanomas, cancer of the bladder, brain, and breast. Triple immunosuppressive regimen with corticosteroids, cyclosporine, and azathioprine is reported to have an increased risk of PTM.[11]

Mycophenolate mofetil (MMF) and mammalian target of rapamycin inhibitors (mTORi) have tumor antiproliferative effects. MMF acts by inhibition of inosine monophosphate

TABLE 1: Classification of post-transplant malignancy (PTM) on the basis of origin and the common malignancies.

De novo malignancy	*Donor-related cancers*	*Recurrent malignancy*
• PTLD • Kaposi sarcoma • Nonmelanoma skin cancer • Anogenital cancer	• Renal cell carcinoma • Malignant melanoma • Choriocarcinoma	• Hepatocellular carcinoma • Neuroendocrine metastases • Cardiac angiosarcoma

(PTLD: post-transplant lymphoproliferative disorder)

Flowchart 1: Etiopathogenesis of post-transplant malignancy and role of immunosuppression.

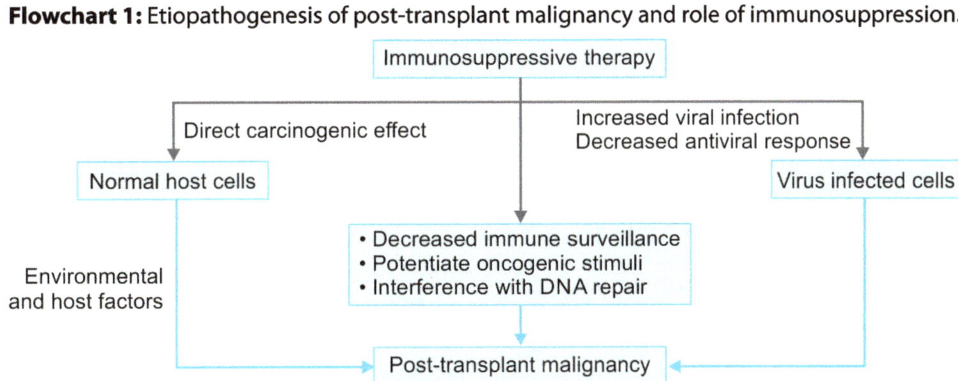

(DNA: deoxyribonucleic acid)

dehydrogenase which is also present in solid tumors and may be protective but does not have a preventive benefit in clinical trials. mTORi (sirolimus and everolimus) inhibits vascular endothelial growth factor (VEGF) and thereby has anticancer properties. Studies have shown a reduced incidence of malignancies and nonmelanoma skin cancer with mTORi-based regimens.[12] Corticosteroids are an integral part of the immunosuppressive regimen for long and have a complex effect on the immune system. Though there are reports of their role in the development of Kaposi's sarcoma, steroids are generally not considered to be oncogenic and continued in patients with malignancy too. Belatacept, a T-cell co-stimulation pathway blocker, is a promising alternative to CNI maintenance therapy but was found to increase the risk of PTLD particularly in Epstein–Barr virus (EBV) seronegative recipients and is contraindicated in this subset of patients.[13]

Oncogenic viruses: Chronic viral infections are implicated in several malignancies similar to what is seen in the general population, but transplant recipients are at a higher risk (nearly 100-fold) of developing cancer, especially with continued immunosuppression.[14] The various infection-associated malignancies are shown in **Figure 1**. These viruses cause persistent infection which in the presence of impaired immune surveillance disrupts the normal cell cycle and promotes tumorigenesis.

Preexisting malignancy: Prior history of malignancy is a known risk factor and an adequate interval of 2–5 years based on the type of cancer was recommended in most guidelines.[15] With the advent of more advanced treatments, there are reports that this waiting period may be reduced. Also, studies did show that patients with low-risk malignancies (thyroid, kidney, bladder, prostate, and oropharynx) did not have a worse outcome when transplanted within 5 years.[16] The latest Kidney Disease Improving Global Outcomes (KDIGO) guidelines do recommend a waiting period of 2 years for most early cancers and 5 years for invasive cancers after curative therapy. Renal transplantation is contraindicated in patients with invasive melanoma and stage 4/anaplastic thyroid cancer. A notable change is the absence of waiting time for treated nonmetastatic basal cell and SCC of the skin, melanoma (in situ), carcinomas in situ, superficial bladder cancer, prostate cancer (Gleason score ≤6), and low-grade thyroid cancer <2 cm.[17]

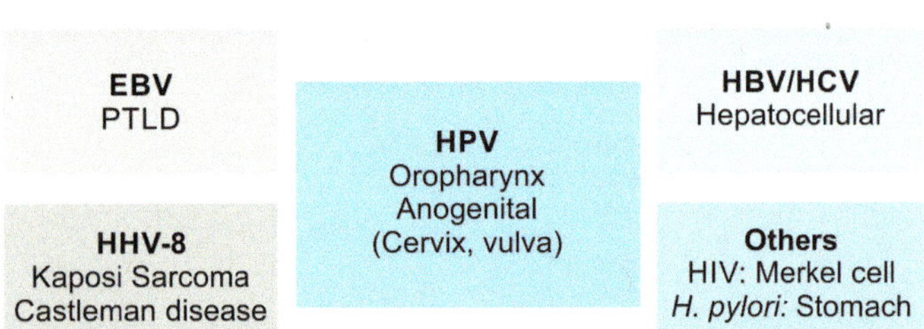

Fig. 1: Infection-related post-transplant malignancies. (EBV: Epstein–Barr virus; *H. pylori*: *Helicobacter pylori*; HBV: hepatitis B virus; HCV: hepatitis C virus; HHV-8: human herpesvirus 8; HIV: human immunodeficiency virus; HPV: human papilloma virus; PTLD: post-transplant lymphoproliferative disorder)

Donor-related cancer: Inadvertent transmission of malignancy through transplanted organ, though rare, is a serious event adversely affecting patient outcomes. An autopsy-based study revealed that 7% of deceased donors had unsuspected malignancy with a risk of transmission to recipient.[18] The IPTTR registry reports 45% donor cancer transmission to cardiothoracic transplant recipients among which choriocarcinoma and melanoma have the worst prognosis.[19] The risk of transmission is least with nonmelanoma skin cancer, carcinoma in situ, and low-grade central nervous system (CNS) tumors. Irrespective of this risk, a routine autopsy is not possible in all cases for logistical reasons and organ procurement even from prospective donors with a high risk of cancer offers substantial survival benefit of up to 7.1 (6.4–7.8) years per recipient.[20] Hence, this risk should not be a deterrent to renal transplantation.

COMMON CANCERS AFTER RENAL TRANSPLANTATION

The risk of all types of malignancies are increased in the transplant recipient. Of all cancers, skin cancers and PTLD are the most common cancer types in all registry studies. The timing of cancer in transplanted patients is also much earlier in KTR. The mean time of diagnosis from transplantation ranges from 6 years for Kaposi's sarcoma, PTLD, and endocrine cancers to 10 years for gastrointestinal cancers.[21]

Skin Cancer

Nonmelanoma skin cancer is the most common malignancy in solid organ transplant recipients (including KTR) and is 60–250-fold more common than in the general population.[22] SCC and basal cell carcinoma (BCC) account for over 90% of the cases. While BCC is more common in the general population, SCC is more common in transplant recipients. In addition to the transplant-related risk factors discussed above, the other risk factors for skin cancers include exposure to ultraviolet rays, fair skin, older age, and the presence of premalignant skin lesions. Among the immunosuppressive drugs, azathioprine is associated with higher rates of skin cancer and mTORi are protective. The timing after transplantation varies with elderly fair-skinned recipients affected as early as 2–3 years after transplant while younger recipients present at a later time period.

Management of skin cancers requires a reduction in cumulative immunosuppression. Superficial, localized lesions can be managed with topical fluorouracil and imiquimod, cryotherapy, electrodesiccation and curettage, or photodynamic therapy. Surgical excision with clear margins is the most definitive therapy and can be accomplished with Mohs micrographic surgery. For patients with multiple and recurrent lesions, systemic retinoids are advised.[23] Radiation therapy is reserved for inoperable lesions. Patients with premalignant lesions such as Bowen's disease, actinic keratosis, and keratoacanthomas need to be treated and followed up.

Though less common, melanoma is more common in KTR than in the general population. It is one of the malignancies which can be donor-derived. Being a more aggressive malignancy, wide local excision with sentinel lymphadenectomy (especially if >1 cm lesion) is advised. The advent of immunotherapy has changed the outlook for advanced melanoma. Newer therapeutic options such as ipilimumab (immune checkpoint inhibitor) and BRAF inhibitors such as dabrafenib and vemurafenib have resulted in better outcomes. Data regarding their use is limited in transplant recipients, and there are reports of rejection with the use of these newer drugs.[24]

Kaposi sarcoma (KS) presents as angiomatous lesions most commonly in the lower limbs and often presents in the first couple of years after transplantation. Mucocutaneous involvement is the predominant presentation in over 90% of transplant recipients. Human herpesvirus 8 (HHV-8) infection is a critical component in the pathogenesis of KS. The most important therapeutic strategy is reducing/discontinuing immunosuppression and switching to mTORi.[25] In nonresponsive cases, chemotherapy is attempted.

Post-transplant Lymphoproliferative Disorder

Post-transplant lymphoproliferative disorder is the second most common malignancy in transplant recipients following skin cancers. Though it is seen only in 0.8–2.5% of KTR, among all malignancies, PTLD constitutes nearly 20% of the total burden.[26] They are 50-fold more common in transplant recipients than in the general population. The timing of presentation is bimodal with an early peak in 1–2 years and a later peak at 5–7 years after transplantation. Monomorphic B-cell and large cell NHL are the predominant types in transplant recipients.[27] EBV infection is the most important risk factor seen in 60–80% of all PTLD cases. EBV-negative PTLD presents later after transplantation and carries a worse prognosis. Persisting EBV infection in B lymphocytes due to impaired immunological surveillance causes uncontrolled activation and proliferation of B cells. Greater intensity of immunosuppression, induction with depleting agents, and use of belatacept increase the risk for PTLD. Alemtuzumab induction has some protective effects compared to depleting agents used for induction.

Histological categorization of PTLD according to the World Health Organization (WHO) 2017 classification recognizes six subclasses—polymorphic PTLD, monomorphic PTLD (B-cell, T-cell, or natural killer cell type), classic Hodgkin's lymphoma, and three types of non-destructive PTLD (infectious mononucleosis-like, plasmacytic hyperplasia, and florid follicular hyperplasia).[28] Clinical presentation is heterogeneous ranging from mildly symptomatic cases with constitutional symptoms to a fulminant presentation. Early PTLD (in the first post-transplant year) more commonly presents in younger transplant recipients, involves the graft, and responds to immunosuppression reduction while late cases present as extranodal disease and require specific therapy.[29] Accurate staging is important for planning therapy and can be done using a combination of computed tomography (CT) imaging with 18F-fluorodeoxyglucose positron emission tomography scan.

The cornerstone of management is reduction of immunosuppression and is sufficient in 20–80% of EBV-positive cases.[29] Complete cessation of the antiproliferative agent with 50% dose reduction of calcineurin inhibitor is done. The role of mTORi in PTLD is debated and is not part of the standard immunosuppressive regimen of these patients. Patients with no response or in partial remission following immunosuppression reduction/withdrawal are treated with four doses of rituximab. Rituximab monotherapy is the first-line treatment for polymorphic PTLD and nondestructive PTLD. Other chemotherapy regimens include combinations of cyclophosphamide, doxorubicin, vincristine, and prednisolone (CHOP) or R-CHOP (rituximab + CHOP). Monomorphic PTLD and other rituximab non-responsive PTLDs are managed with a combination of chemotherapy regimens. Risk stratified sequential therapy with use of immunosuppression reduction and rituximab initially, followed by chemotherapy (R-CHOP) in poorly responsive cases, has become the standard of care following the PTLD-1 study. Response to rituximab therapy is an important prognostic factor for overall survival.[30] CNS PTLD requires local radiotherapy and methotrexate therapy. Adoptive immunotherapy with EBV-specific cytotoxic lymphocytes is a promising therapeutic option.

Other Cancers

Renal cell carcinomas (RCCs) are common de novo malignancies, particularly in KTR. They are more common in the native kidneys, and the risk is more in elderly male patients with a longer dialysis duration and acquired cystic kidney disease.[31] Localized RCC is managed with nephron-sparing surgery or nephrectomy. Immunotherapy is useful for metastatic disease but data is limited in the transplant population and has an inherent risk of precipitating graft rejection.[32]

A general approach in the management of PTM is to discontinue the antimetabolite. mTORi are useful, especially in KTR with skin cancers. Checkpoint inhibitors are a valuable addition to the therapeutic armamentarium of cancer therapy. However, they have to be used with caution in transplant recipients due to the fear of graft rejection. The other management guidelines are similar to the nontransplant population.

CANCER SCREENING AND SURVEILLANCE

Malignancies are increasingly common among patients with end-stage renal disease (ESRD). Active malignancies are an absolute contraindication to renal transplantation, and hence pretransplant screening for malignancies is essential. Prospective recipient screening should be performed as per age and gender-specific guidelines followed in the general population. Chest radiograph is recommended for all patients while a CT scan should be done for those with a history of heavy tobacco use (≥30 years). In patients with history of acquired cystic disease of the kidneys, chronic smokers, analgesic nephropathy or history of cyclophosphamide use, urine cytology, and ultra-sonographic screening of the native kidneys are done to screen for malignancy. Bowel cancer screening for patients with inflammatory bowel disease and screening for hepatocellular carcinoma with ultrasound and α-fetoprotein for patients with cirrhosis has to be done.[17] The use of mammography, fecal occult blood test, prostate-specific antigen measurement, and gynecologic examination are according to age-specific guidelines as in the general population.

Considering the severity of PTM, more frequent screening of KTR for common malignancies may be beneficial. However, there are no specific recommendations for the same. In order to reduce the heightened risk of malignancy in these patients, optimal use of immunosuppression needs to be ensured. EBV-directed antiviral prophylaxis has not been shown to be of proven benefit. Immunizations against oncogenic viruses (HPV and Hepatitis B) should be administered at recommended intervals. Exposure to sun rays is preferably avoided in fair-skinned patients and regular use of sunscreens has to be advised. Annual skin screening by the primary care physician or a dermatologist is advisable. A Papanicolaou (Pap) cytology with pelvic exam should be done every 3–5 years. Patients with liver disease or high-risk conditions (hepatitis C/hepatitis C infected recipients) should be subjected to ultrasound screening and/or α-fetoprotein every 6–12 months.[33] Screening for other malignancies should follow the guidelines for the general population.

CONCLUSION

Post-transplant malignancies are common in KTR and a leading cause of morbidity and mortality. A combination of potent immunosuppression with additional factors such as chronic viral infection, age, and history of preexisting cancer predisposes KTR to malignancies. Skin cancer is most common followed by PTLD in transplant recipients. An important limitation is the absence of controlled trials on cancer screening and management of PTM. A personalized approach to titration of immunosuppressive therapy and planning tumor-directed definitive therapy is paramount to improve patient outcomes. The availability of newer drugs, genomic profiling, and focused screening for malignancies is bound to improve the management of transplant recipients with malignancy.

REFERENCES

1. Engels EA, Pfeiffer RM, Fraumeni JF, Kasiske BL, Israni AK, Snyder JJ, et al. Spectrum of cancer risk among U.S. solid organ transplant recipients: the transplant cancer match study. JAMA. 2011;306(17):1891-901.
2. Penn I. Cancers in renal transplant recipients. Adv Ren Replace Ther. 2000;7(2):147-56.
3. Bouwes Bavinck JN, Hardie DR, Green A, Cutmore S, MacNaught A, O'Sullivan B, et al. The risk of skin cancer in renal transplant recipients in Queensland, Australia. A follow-up study. Transplantation. 1996;61(5):715-21.
4. Au EH, Chapman JR, Craig JC, Lim WH, Teixeira-Pinto A, Ullah S, et al. Overall and site-specific cancer mortality in patients on dialysis and after kidney transplant. J Am Soc Nephrol. 2019;30(3):471-80.
5. Jagadesh GS, Kurian G, R RN, Mathew A, P ZP, Sreedharan S. SAT-346 post-transplant malignancy - our centre. Kidney Int Rep. 2020;5(3):S145.
6. Gupta D, Mendonca S, Tewari R, Ahuja A, Singh L, Joshi A, et al. Posttransplant lymphoproliferative disorder in renal transplant recipients: experience from a Tertiary Care Center. Saudi J Kidney Dis Transplant. 2021;32(2):418.
7. Sakhuja V, Ramachandran R, Kohli HS, Jha V, Gupta KL, Rathi M, et al. Spectrum of lymphoproliferative disorders following renal transplantation in North India. Indian J Nephrol. 2013;23(4):287-91.
8. Thergaonkar RW, Bhardwaj S, Sinha A, Dinda AK, Kumar R, Bagga A, et al. Posttransplant lymphoproliferative disorder: experience from a pediatric nephrology unit in North India. Indian J Nephrol. 2018;28(5):374.
9. Katabathina VS, Menias CO, Tammisetti VS, Lubner MG, Kielar A, Shaaban A, et al. Malignancy after solid organ transplantation: comprehensive imaging review. Radiographics. 2016;36(5):1390-407.
10. Wimmer CD, Rentsch M, Crispin A, Illner WD, Arbogast H, Graeb C, et al. The janus face of immunosuppression - de novo malignancy after renal transplantation: the experience of the Transplantation Center Munich. Kidney Int. 2007; 71(12):1271-8.
11. Penn I, First MR. Development and incidence of cancer following cyclosporine therapy. Transplant Proc. 1986; 18(2 Suppl. 1):210-5.
12. Knoll GA, Kokolo MB, Mallick R, Beck A, Buenaventura CD, Ducharme R, et al. Effect of sirolimus on malignancy and survival after kidney transplantation: systematic review and meta-analysis of individual patient data. BMJ. 2014;349: g6679.

13. Vincenti F, Rostaing L, Grinyo J, Rice K, Steinberg S, Gaite L, et al. Belatacept and long-term outcomes in kidney transplantation. N Engl J Med. 2016;374(4):333-43.
14. Piselli P, Busnach G, Fratino L, Citterio F, Ettorre GM, De Paoli P, et al. De novo malignancies after organ transplantation: focus on viral infections. Curr Mol Med. 2013;13(7):1217-27.
15. Batabyal P, Chapman JR, Wong G, Craig JC, Tong A. Clinical practice guidelines on wait-listing for kidney transplantation: consistent and equitable? Transplantation. 2012; 94(7):703-13.
16. Knoll GA, Chadban SJ. Preexisting cancer in transplant candidates: time for a change in practice? Transplantation. 2018;102(7):1037-8.
17. Chadban SJ, Ahn C, Axelrod DA, Foster BJ, Kasiske BL, Kher V, et al. KDIGO clinical practice guideline on the evaluation and management of candidates for kidney transplantation. Transplantation. 2020;104(4S1 Suppl. 1): S11-103.
18. Sens MA, Zhou X, Weiland T, Cooley AM. Unexpected neoplasia in autopsies: potential implications for tissue and organ safety. Arch Pathol Lab Med. 2009;133(12):1923-31.
19. Buell JF, Trofe J, Hanaway MJ, Lo A, Rosengard B, Rilo H, et al. Transmission of donor cancer into cardiothoracic transplant recipients. Surgery. 2001;130(4):660-6.
20. Desai R, Collett D, Watson CJE, Johnson P, Evans T, Neuberger J. Estimated risk of cancer transmission from organ donor to graft recipient in a national transplantation registry. Br J Surg. 2014;101(7):768-74.
21. Knechtle S, Marson L, Morris P. Kidney Transplantation—Principles and Practice, 8th edition. Elsevier; 2019. p. 752
22. Mittal A, Colegio OR. Skin cancers in organ transplant recipients. Am J Transplant. 2017;17(10):2509-30.
23. Chen K, Craig JC, Shumack S. Oral retinoids for the prevention of skin cancers in solid organ transplant recipients: a systematic review of randomized controlled trials. Br J Dermatol. 2005;152(3):518-23.
24. Rossi E, Schinzari G, Maiorano BA, Esposito I, Acampora A, Romagnoli J, et al. Immune-checkpoint inhibitors in renal transplanted patients affected by melanoma: a systematic review. Immunotherapy. 2022;14(1):65-75.
25. Hosseini-Moghaddam SM, Soleimanirahbar A, Mazzulli T, Rotstein C, Husain S. Post renal transplantation Kaposi's sarcoma: a review of its epidemiology, pathogenesis, diagnosis, clinical aspects, and therapy. Transpl Infect Dis. 2012;14(4):338-45.
26. Opelz G, Döhler B. Lymphomas after solid organ transplantation: a collaborative transplant study report. Am J Transplant. 2004;4(2):222-30.
27. Zamani Z, Haider MZ, Taqi M, Mirza HM, Kumar D, Shahid H, et al. A systematic review of post-transplant lymphoproliferative disorder after renal transplantation. J Clin Oncol. 2021;39(15_suppl):e19577-e19577.
28. Swerdlow SH, Campo E, Pileri SA, Harris NL, Stein H, Siebert R, et al. The 2016 revision of the World Health Organization classification of lymphoid neoplasms. Blood. 2016;127(20):2375-90.
29. Dierickx D, Habermann TM. Post-transplantation lymphoproliferative disorders in adults. N Engl J Med. 2018; 378(6):549-62.
30. Trappe RU, Dierickx D, Zimmermann H, Morschhauser F, Mollee P, Zaucha JM, et al. Response to rituximab induction is a predictive marker in B-cell post-transplant lymphoproliferative disorder and allows successful stratification into rituximab or R-CHOP consolidation in an international, prospective, multicenter phase II trial. J Clin Oncol. 2017; 35(5):536-43.
31. Al-Adra D, Al-Qaoud T, Fowler K, Wong G. De novo malignancies after kidney transplantation. Clin J Am Soc Nephrol. 2022;17(3):434-43.
32. Dahle DO, Skauby M, Langberg CW, Brabrand K, Wessel N, Midtvedt K. Renal cell carcinoma and kidney transplantation: a narrative review. Transplantation. 2022;106(1):e52.
33. Acuna SA, Huang JW, Scott AL, Micic S, Daly C, Brezden-Masley C, et al. Cancer screening recommendations for solid organ transplant recipients: a systematic review of clinical practice guidelines. Am J Transplant. 2017;17(1): 103-14.

13.8 Hematological Disorders in Kidney Transplant Recipients

Rajendra Prasad Mathur, Chandani Bhagat

CASE VIGNETTE

A 32-year-old male had undergone kidney transplant (KTP) 3 months back. The patient was found to have severe anemia on a routine follow-up visit with hemoglobin (Hb) 4.7 g/dL. Diagnostic workup revealed positive immunoglobulin M (IgM) titers for parvovirus B19 antigen. Bone marrow examination showed normal cellular marrow. The patient was given intravenous immunoglobulin (IVIg) therapy at a dose of 2 g/kg body weight. The patient required changes in the maintenance immunosuppression with a reduction in the dose of tacrolimus and withholding of mycophenolate mofetil. However, the patient was not responding and a hematologist's opinion was taken, following which the dose of prednisolone was increased to 1 mg/kg/day body weight. He was also started on injection bortezomib 2 mg/kg body weight on days 1, 4, 8, and 11. The patient responded after 2 weeks with an increase in Hb to 7.3 g/dL. He has been kept on regular follow-up.

INTRODUCTION

For patients with end-stage kidney disease (ESKD), KTP is the best option as treatment. A successful KTP offers improved quality and duration of life. The rate of serious complications following kidney transplantation has declined significantly with better immunosuppressive drugs and matching protocols. However, like any other type of surgery, recipients after kidney transplantation are also at a risk of developing complications as a result of immunosuppressive treatment, progression of graft dysfunction, and rejection process.

Kidney transplant recipients (KTR) are susceptible to hematological disorders due to chronic immunosuppressive therapy. Post-transplant anemia (PTA), post-transplant erythrocytosis (PTE), post-transplant lymphoproliferative disorders (PTLD), and post-transplant cytopenias (PTC, including leukopenia, thrombocytopenia, and pancytopenia) are the most common hematological disorders after kidney transplantation.[1]

Uncommon but serious blood disorders after KTP include hemophagocytic syndrome (HPS), thrombotic microangiopathy (TMA), therapy-related myelodysplastic syndromes (t-MDS), and therapy-related acute myeloid leukemia (t-AML).[2,3]

In order to develop therapeutic strategies for the management of these life-threatening hematological complications, a detailed study of the pathogenesis of these disorders is necessary.

POST-TRANSPLANT ANEMIA

Anemia is common after kidney transplantation. It is classified as acute (within 6 months post-KTP) and chronic (>6 months post-KTP). The World Health Organization's (WHO) definition of PTA as Hb level <12 g/dL in women and <13 g/dL in men[1,4] is also accepted by Kidney Disease: Improving Global Outcomes (KDIGO) and American Society of Transplantation.

Prevalence and Causes of Post-transplant Anemia

Twenty to fifty-one percent of transplanted patients usually present with PTA in the early post-transplant period. Iron deficiency, pretransplant status, donor factors, old age, ischemia time, delayed graft function, and allograft from extended criteria donor are contributing causes.[5,6] Impaired graft function, iron deficiency, female gender, use of angiotensin-converting enzyme inhibitors (ACEIs), antibiotics, antivirals, and immunosuppressive treatment lead to late PTA in 23–35% of patients.[5,7]

Risk Factors Associated with Post-transplant Anemia

Perioperatively, all patients are anemic due to chronic kidney disease (CKD)-associated reduced endogenous erythropoietin synthesis and iron deficiency. Restrictive use of erythropoietin-stimulating agents (ESA) in patients on maintenance hemodialysis to maintain Hb above 9 g/dL has accentuated the problem.[8] Blood loss by frequent blood draws may cumulate to approximately 500 mL in a 3-month period.[9-12] Anemia usually resolves within the first few months after transplantation with normalization of erythropoietin levels.[13]

Hepcidin is an acute-phase reactant protein, which mediates the changes in iron metabolism during inflammation. It is induced by the proinflammatory cytokine interleukin 6 (IL-6).[14] In situations with oxidative stress, increased hepatic synthesis of hepcidin results in decreased bioavailability of iron molecules.[15] Elevated hepcidin levels among KTRs may be due to low-grade inflammation and impaired renal function; however, it may not be a significant pathogenetic factor for anemia in this population.[16-21]

According to Kalantzi et al.,[22] the concentration of erythropoietin produced by a newly implanted kidney allograft peaks after 4 days and then after 16 weeks of transplant.

TABLE 1: Important causes of anemia in renal transplant recipients.

Infections associated with PTA		• Though any infection may aggravate anemia but the following have been most commonly associated with PTA – *Bacterial:* Tuberculosis – *Viral:* CMV, EBV, varicella, HHV-6, HHV-8, BK virus, parvovirus B19
Drugs associated with PTA	Inhibition of the red blood cell synthesis pathway at the level of bone marrow is the main cause for PTA	• ***Antiproliferative agents:*** Azathioprine (AZA), mycophenolic acid (MPA) – *Mechanism of action:* Direct antiproliferative effect on bone marrow[26,27,35-37] – ***MPA:*** Inhibition of enzyme inosine monophosphate dehydrogenase, which is the rate-limiting enzyme for the de novo purine synthesis – **AZA**-associated with macrocytic anemia[38] - *Genetic polymorphisms in MPA metabolism also play a role as studies have shown that reducing exposure of MPA did not result in improvement of PTA*[39]
		• ***mTOR inhibitors:*** Sirolimus and to a similar extent everolimus are associated with dose-dependent anemia up to 57% in some studies, much more than calcineurin inhibitors (CNI) – *Mechanism of action:* SRL causes microcytosis with anemia. Erythropoietin resistance, IL-10-dependent inflammatory autoregulation, and interference of SRL with hepcidin lead to functional iron deficiency[40-46] – *Treatment:* Complete reversibility has been seen with stoppage of medication • ***CNI:*** Do not cause PTA but may be associated with thrombotic microangiopathy[47] • ***Belatacept:*** Not associated with PTA
		• ***Induction therapy:*** OKT3 and rabbit antithymocyte globulin (rATG) – *Mechanism of action:* Toxic effects on the bone marrow[38] • ***Alemtuzumab:*** High incidence of severely acquired red cell aplasia and autoimmune hemolytic anemia • ***Basiliximab:*** Decreased incidence of anemia versus rATG induction • ***Other drugs:*** ACEIs and ARBs • ***Dapsone, trimethoprim:*** Inhibition of G6PD and folic acid synthesis[48] • ***Proton-pump inhibitors:*** Decreased absorption of iron[49]

(ACEIs: angiotensin-converting enzyme inhibitors; ARBs: angiotensin receptor blockers; CMV: cytomegalovirus; EBV: Epstein–Barr virus; G6PD: glucose-6-phosphate dehydrogenase; HHV: human herpesvirus; IL-10: interleukin-10; mTOR: mammalian target of rapamycin; OKT3: muromonab CD3; PTA: post-transplant anemia; SRL: sirolimus)

Anemia late after transplantation is predominantly caused by a decline in renal allograft function.[23,24] Kamar and Rostaing showed that transplant status had the strongest association with anemia, and the observed incidence of anemia in transplant patients was almost 10-fold higher than in the glomerular filtration rate (GFR)-matched general population.[25]

A decreased rate of erythropoietin production from grafts received from donors of >60 years is a contributing cause of PTA.[26-28] The other factors associated with PTA include acute rejection episodes, recent infections, hypoalbuminemia, C-reactive protein (CRP) elevation, metabolic acidosis, and African-American race.[29-31] While iron deficiency is a common risk factor for PTA, it is difficult to assess iron status in transplant patients as shown by Mix et al.[32] Transferrin and ferritin may be raised in conditions of inflammation and are not suitable markers for PTA; however, assessment of hypochromic red blood cells (RBCs) (≥2.5%) has been shown to be a significant marker for PTA by Lorenz et al.[31] Long-term studies have shown that even after Hb correction, iron deficiency may persist in up to 62% of patients and more so in females because of persistent menstruation and lack of androgens.[33,34] Important causes of anemia in renal transplant recipients are given in **Table 1**.

Flowchart 1: Post-transplant anemia and associated outcomes.

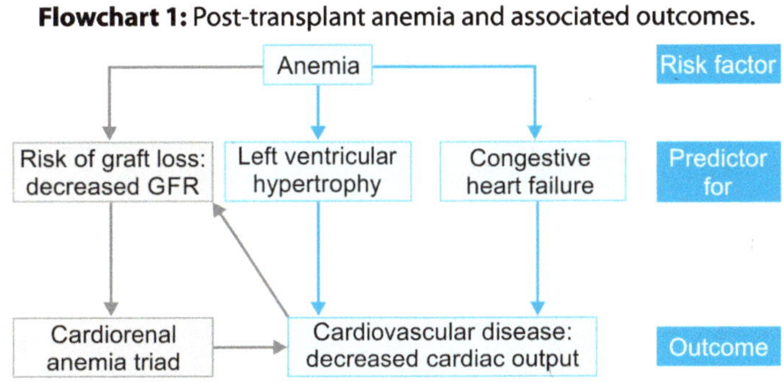

(GFR: glomerular filtration rate)

Post-transplant Anemia and Associated Outcomes

Post-transplant anemia and associated outcomes[50-54] are shown in **Flowchart 1**.

Treatment of Post-transplant Anemia

CAPRIT (Correction of Anemia and Progression of Renal Insufficiency in Transplant Patients) study:[55]

- Complete (13–15 g/dL) correction of Hb versus partial (10.5 g/dL).
- Complete correction patients had a slower decline in GFR and improved quality of life.

- No increase in the risk for cardiovascular events.
- *Limitation of the study:* Patients had a low cardiovascular risk profile.

KDIGO guidelines:[56]

- Assess iron stores during follow-up of transplant patients.
- Replete iron stores even in patients with no iron deficiency.
- ESA to be started to maintain Hb >10 g/dL.

CHAPTER HIGHLIGHTS

- Hematological disorders are common in KTR.
- PTA is the most common hematological disorder.
- PTE, PTLD, and PTC (including leukopenia, thrombocytopenia, and pancytopenia) are the other hematological disorders seen in KTR.
- Graft loss is a serious issue associated with some disorders, and hence a close observation of KTR is necessary to detect such disorders at the earliest.
- Urgent identification and multidisciplinary management are necessary.

POST-TRANSPLANT ERYTHROCYTOSIS

Definition

Post-transplant erythrocytosis is defined as Hb value >17 g/dL (or hematocrit >51%) after kidney transplantation.

Incidence

- Seen in patients with good graft function and still having native kidneys with a history of erythrocytosis prior to transplant [autosomal dominant polycystic kidney disease (ADPKD) patients].[57]
- Incidence falling from 19% (1993–1996) to 8% (1997 and 2005).[58]
- The use of ACEIs/angiotensin receptor blockers (ARBs) and antiproliferative immunosuppression are the important causes of the decline.

Risk Factors[59]

- Male gender
- No history of acute rejection
- Renal artery stenosis
- Smoking
- Cyclosporine treatment
- Simultaneous kidney and pancreas transplantation
- Chronic obstructive pulmonary disease (COPD)
- Malignancies such as hepatocellular carcinoma, renal cell carcinoma (RCC), breast cancer, and pheochromocytoma.

Pathophysiological Mechanism[60,61]

- Unregulated excess production of erythropoietin by native kidneys
- Increased sensitivity to erythropoietin in patients with suppressed erythropoietin levels
- Increased production of insulin-like growth factor-1 (IGF-1), IGF-1-binding proteins, serum-soluble stem cell factor (sSCF), hypoxia-inducible factor (HIF) mutations, and activation of angiotensin-II receptor.

Treatment[62,63]

- Hb levels <17.5 g/dL should be targeted in normotensive patients
- ACEI or ARB—preferred initial treatment if Hb <18.5 g/dL
- Inhibition of renin–angiotensin–aldosterone system (RAAS) leads to decreased erythropoietin production
- Phlebotomy if no response with ACEI/ARB or Hb >18.5 g/dL
- Theophylline can reduce Hb levels by 10–15%; however, it has a narrow therapeutic window.

POST-TRANSPLANT LEUKOPENIA AND PANCYTOPENIA

- Multifactorial etiology **(Fig. 1)**.[64]
- Identification of cause necessary to direct treatment
- Frequently observed following KTP.
- Data regarding incidence and treatment are scarce.
- Myelosuppression secondary to immunosuppressive drugs [mycophenolic acid (MPA) and valganciclovir (VGCV)] and infections [cytomegalovirus (CMV)].
- Usually occur during the first few months of transplant when high-dose immunosuppression is being administered.
- Differential analysis of low total leukocyte count (TLC) helps in differentiating lymphopenia from neutropenia.
- Lymphopenia is a common side effect of rabbit antithymocyte globulin (rATG), while neutropenia predisposes patients to severe infections, which is the second-most common cause of mortality.[65]

Drug-induced Leukopenia and Pancytopenia

Immunosuppressive Drugs

- *MPA:* Dose-dependent leukopenia. Exacerbation with ganciclovir, VGCV, SRL, and lymphocyte depleting agents.[66]
- Tacrolimus enhances the myelosuppressive effect by increasing the bioavailability of MPA.[67,68]
- Azathioprine (AZA) causes bone marrow suppression and cytopenia.
- Allopurinol causes severe cytopenia by decreasing AZA metabolism.

	Anemia	Leukopenia	Pancytopenia
Drugs	Azathioprine, Mycophenolate mofetil, Thymoglobulin, Alemtuzumab, Trimethoprim-sulfamethoxazole, Ganciclovir, Valganciclovir, mTor inhibitor, ACE inhibitors	Azathioprine, Mycophenolate mofetil, Thymoglobulin, Alemtuzumab, Trimethoprim-sulfamethoxazole, Ganciclovir, Valganciclovir	Azathioprine, Mycophenolate mofetil, Thymoglobulin, Trimethoprim-sulfamethoxazole, Ganciclovir, Valganciclovir
Viral infections	Parvovirus, Cytomegalovirus, HIV, Human herpes virus-6, EBV	Parvovirus, Cytomegalovirus, HIV, Human herpes virus-6	Parvovirus, Cytomegalovirus, HIV, Human herpes virus-6, EBV
Nutritional deficiencies	Iron, Vitamin B-12, Folate, Copper, Zinc, deficiency	Deficiencies in vitamin B12, Folate, Copper	Vitamin B12 and Folate deficiency
Other Hematological causes	TMA, Hemolysis		Post-transplant lymphoproliferative disorder, Multiple myeloma, Immunological diseases: SLE, Hemophagocytic syndrome

Fig. 1: Etiology of cytopenia after kidney transplant. (ACE: angiotensin-converting enzyme; EBV: Epstein–Barr virus; HIV: human immunodeficiency virus; mTOR: mammalian target of rapamycin; SLE: systemic lupus erythematosus; TMA: thrombotic microangiopathy)

Opportunistic Infections Causing Pancytopenia

Opportunistic infections may suppress bone marrow activity:

- CMV is commonly associated with bone marrow toxicity in the first 6 months of transplant, characterized by fever, anemia (64%), leukopenia (21%), thrombocytopenia (47%), and atypical lymphocytes.[69]
- CMV may cause specific organ damage leading to pneumonitis, enteritis, hepatitis, and retinitis.
- Allograft dysfunction may occur leading to an increase in creatinine.

Other Infections

Other infections include human herpesvirus-6 (HHV-6), HHV-8, EBV, Parvovirus which are less common causes of cytopenia.

Clinical Implications and Treatment Strategies

- TLC <3,000–4,000 cells/mm^3 and absolute neutrophil count <500/mm^3 are criteria for starting treatment.[70]
- Definite cause is mostly difficult to find.
- Early discontinuation of MPA is necessary. The amount of dose reduction of MPA is not clearly defined.
- In cases of severe agranulocytosis to prevent graft rejection, replacement of MPA with AZA may be done.[71]
- Granulocyte colony-stimulating factor (G-CSF) is safe to use in severe neutropenia with no increase in the risk of graft loss; however, the indication to start G-CSF is not well defined and long-term data is not available.
- Thorough surveillance for early CMV disease or reactivation.
- Discontinuation of prophylactic VGCV; it should be started only as treatment for CMV in low dose (450 mg/day).

POST-TRANSPLANT THROMBOCYTOPENIA

- Frequently seen as part of pancytopenia or TMA
- Isolated post-transplant thrombocytopenia (PTT) is rare
- Data on the prevalence and significance of low platelet count in relation to increased risk of bleeding is lacking.
- *Risk factors:* Infections causing PTA and post-transplant thrombocytopenia (PTL) (CMV, parvovirus); drugs such as SRL (benign), MPA, AZA, rATG, OKT3, and VGCV.
- *Treatment:* Discontinuation of the drug. Transfusion of platelets in severe cases.[72] Second-line drugs for PTT[73] include corticosteroids and thrombopoietin receptor agonists (eltrombopag and romiplostim).

THROMBOTIC MICROANGIOPATHY[74,75]

- *TMA:* Triad of thrombosis, thrombocytopenia, and hemolysis.
- The histopathological lesion, initiated by platelet aggregation.
- Hemolysis may occur in the kidney, brain, and other organs.
- *Laboratory findings:* Anemia, thrombocytopenia, reticulocytosis, increased lactate dehydrogenase (LDH) levels, and fragmentocytes in blood smear.

Post-transplant TMA (TA-TMA) is of two types: Recurrent and de novo. The pretransplant hemolytic uremic syndrome (HUS) may recur in the graft kidney, which is known as recurrent TA-TMA. Such recurrences are usually of atypical HUS or may be associated with antiphospholipid syndrome (APS). Recurrent TA-TMA may occur usually within days or few weeks of transplant. The recurrence rate is high (50–100%) with a high risk of graft loss (90%). In view of the high risk of recurrence and graft loss, prospective KTRs suffering from atypical HUS are offered grafts from deceased donors versus living donors.[76]

Management

Plasmapheresis may be tried for APS cases. Eculizumab is a monoclonal antibody against C5 complement protein and prevents recurrence in patients with CFH and CFI mutations.[77] It has been approved by the Food and Drug Administration (FDA) and is useful for both recurrent atypical HUS and APS nephropathy. Eculizumab resolved TMA lesions and improved graft function; however, the graft continued to have chronic vascular changes.

However, if the TMA presents for the first time in the graft kidney, it is classified as de novo TA-TMA. This may be secondary to ischemia–reperfusion injury, immunosuppressive drugs such as calcineurin inhibitors (CNI)/SRL, antibody-mediated rejection, and viral infections [CMV, parvovirus, BK virus, hepatitis C virus (HCV)].[78,79] Cyclosporin has been associated with an increased incidence of TMA (3–14%) as compared to tacrolimus (1%) due to higher chances of endothelial damage.

Treatment of de novo TA-TMA: Stop CNI and SRL.[80] In progressive cases, plasma exchange or eculizumab to refractory cases may be given.[81]

POST-TRANSPLANT LYMPHOPROLIFERATIVE DISORDERS

Post-transplant lymphoproliferative disorders occur due to lymphoid or plasmacytic proliferations. According to the WHO 2016 classification, diagnosis of PTLD is by biopsy and histopathological categorization, which recognizes six subclasses of PTLD:

1. Plasmocytic hyperplasia PTLD
2. Infectious mononucleosis PTLD
3. Florid follicular hyperplasia PTLD
4. Polymorphic PTLD
5. Monomorphic PTLD [B or T/natural killer (NK) cell types]
6. Classical Hodgkin lymphoma PTLD (cHL-PTLD).

The first three entities are considered early lesions and are usually nondestructive.[82] Lymphoma is more common among immunocompromised (21%) as compared to immunocompetent individuals (4%).[83] KTRs have the lowest incidence (10-year incidence being 1–2% in adults and 3% in childhood recipients).[84]

Risk Factors

- Epstein–Barr virus (EBV) seronegativity of the recipient. Early lesions are usually associated with EBV infection.
- Early onset PTLD is dependent on induction immunosuppression, while late-onset PTLD depends on a cumulative dose of immunosuppression.[64]

Clinical Presentation

Post-transplant lymphoproliferative disorders range from asymptomatic to fulminant organ failure, spontaneous tumor lysis syndrome, and extranodal involvement most commonly in the gastrointestinal tract (20–30%), solid allografts (10–15%), and the central nervous system (5–20%).[85] Biopsy should always incorporate in situ hybridization (ISH) assay for EBV-encoded ribonucleic acid (RNA) (EBER) and/or immune-histochemistry for viral antigens, e.g., LMP1, EBNA1.

Treatment

The aim of the treatment is to prevent graft function and resolve PTLD. Immunosuppressive reduction is the first-line therapy. The dose of CNI should be reduced to half, while antimetabolites such as AZA and mycophenolate should be stopped. In severe cases, all immunosuppression is stopped except steroids.

- EBV-negative disease is less responsive to decrease in immunosuppression.[86] Belatacept-based immunosuppression in EBV-negative patients increases the incidence of PTLD by nine times.
- Other treatment strategies include rituximab, chemotherapy, and EBV-specific cytotoxic lymphocytes. Local therapies such as surgery and radiotherapy may be given for extranodal involvement.

OTHER HEMATOLOGICAL COMPLICATIONS AFTER KIDNEY TRANSPLANTATION

Passenger Lymphocyte Syndrome

Graft versus host disease due to minor ABO/Rhesus system incompatibility leads to early hemolysis. Transfer of lymphocytes, especially from blood group O donors to blood group A, B, and AB recipients, produces antibodies against recipient cell surface (ABO) antigens.[87] IgG antibodies against recipient RBCs appear within 7–10 days. KTR have fewer incidences of passenger lymphocyte syndrome (PLS) (14%) due to lesser number of lymphocytes being transfused and lesser antibody formation (16%), and symptoms usually resolve over a short time.[88]

Hemophagocytic Syndrome[89-91]

Hemophagocytic syndrome (HPS) is a rare disorder (incidence 0.4%) but life-threatening with mortality rate

BOX 1: Diagnostic criteria for hemophagocytic syndrome (five out of eight criteria should be fulfilled).

1. Fever
2. Cytopenia affecting at least two blood cell lines
3. Elevated ferritin (>500 mg/dL)
4. Elevated triglycerides (>3 mmol/L) and/or low fibrinogen (<1.5 g/L)
5. Splenomegaly
6. Elevated sIL-2RA (>2,400 U/mL)
7. NK cell activity is reduced or undetectable
8. Hemophagocytosis in the bone marrow, lymph nodes, or cerebrospinal fluid

(NK: natural killer; sIL-2RA: soluble interleukin 2 receptor alpha)

up to 47%. It can be primary or secondary to opportunistic infections. Uncontrolled activation of macrophages and cytotoxic T cells leads to phagocytosis of erythrocytes, leukocytes, platelets, and precursors. It usually develops in the initial months after kidney transplantation. In cases secondary to parasitic infections or malignancy, HPS may develop after years.

Clinical Presentation

Symptoms include fever, hepatosplenomegaly, pancytopenia, hemophagocytosis, hyperferritinemia, and coagulopathy. Renal manifestations are acute kidney infection (AKI) and nephrotic syndrome (collapsing focal and segmental glomerulosclerosis and minimal change disease).

Diagnostic Criteria

For diagnostic criteria, see **Box 1**.

Treatment

- Decreasing/stopping immunosuppression.
- Treating underlying infection or malignancy.
- KTR may be given IVIg in a high dose.
- In severe cases, graft nephrectomy may be needed.

Myeloid Neoplasms Following Kidney Transplant

Common examples are AML, t-MDS, and t-AML. Clonal disorders are secondary to genotoxic agents and radiation.[92] Incidence of MDS and AML, are 3.8% and 1.8% respectively.[93]

Presentation: Cytopenias and multilineage dysplasia, with the potential progression of MDS to AML.

Etiology: Immunosuppressive drugs, infections, drugs with oncogenicity, antigenic stimulation by graft.[94]

Treatment: Difficult, tapering of immunosuppression, and medical oncologist review for chemotherapy.

TABLE 2: Management plan for hematological disorders after kidney transplant.

PTA	Oral or IV iron ± ESA to keep Hb 12–13 g/dL
PTE	• ACEI or ARB • *Nonresponders:* Phlebotomy • *Other treatments:* Theophylline, ketanserin—antagonist of peripheral serotonin-5-HT2 receptor, rapamycin (mTOR) inhibitors • To keep Hb < 17 or PCV < 51%
TA-TMA	• Reduction/cessation of immunosuppression • Treatment of underlying infection or antibody-mediated rejection (plasma exchange ± IVIg) • *Non-responders:* Eculizumab, rituximab, or belatacept
HPS	• Reduction or cessation of immunosuppression and treatment of underlying disease • *Other treatments:* High-dose IVIg, IV methylprednisolone • Nephrectomy for life-threatening HPS

(ACEI: angiotensin-converting enzyme inhibitor; ARB: angiotensin receptor blocker; ESA: erythropoietin-stimulating agents; Hb: hemoglobin; HPS: hemophagocytic syndrome; mTOR: mammalian target of rapamycin; IV: intravenous; IVIg: intravenous immunoglobulin; PCV: packed cell volume; PTA: post-transplant anemia; PTE: post-transplant erythrocytosis; TA-TMA: post-transplant thrombotic microangiopathy)

CONCLUSION

Post-KTP hematological disorders are a common cause of morbidity and mortality. Since most of the disorders are managed by decreasing the dose of immunosuppressive drugs, a close watch is needed to detect early signs of graft dysfunction, and specialized care under a nephrologist is necessary. **Table 2** provides an overview of the management of important hematological disorders following a KTP. Besides the above common hematological disorders, one should also be vigilant about the relatively rare, but potentially fatal complications such as HPS, transplant-associated TMA, and myeloid neoplasms. The nephrologist often has to face the challenging task to keep the delicate balance between the reduction of immunosuppression for control of infections, cytopenia, malignancy, and the possible risk of rejection of allograft due to reduced immunosuppression. In a life-threatening situation, it is always better to save the life than the graft!

REFERENCES

1. Kasiske BL, Vazquez MA, Harmon WE, Brown RS, Danovitch GM, Gaston RS, et al. Recommendations for the outpatient surveillance of renal transplant recipients. American Society of Transplantation. J Am Soc Nephrol. 2000;11(Suppl. 15):S1-86.
2. Ardalan MR, Shoja MM, Tubbs RS, Esmaili H, Keyvani H. Postrenal transplant hemophagocytic lymphohistiocytosis and thrombotic microangiopathy associated with parvovirus B19 infection. Am J Transplant. 2008;8:1340-4.

3. Reindl-Schwaighofer R, Oberbauer R. Blood disorders after kidney transplantation. Transplant Rev (Orlando). 2014;28:63-75.
4. World Health Organization. Report of WHO Scientific Group. WHO Technical Report Series, No. 405. Geneva: WHO; 1968. pp. 1-40.
5. Schechter A, Gafter-Gvili U, Shepshelovich D, Rahamimov R, Gafter U, Mor E, et al. Postrenal transplant anemia: severity, causes and their association with graft and patient survival. BMC Nephrol. 2019;20:51.
6. Gafter-Gvili A, Cohen E, Avni T, Grossman A, Vidal L, Garty M, et al. Predicting the emergence of anemia—a large cohort study. Eur J Intern Med. 2015;26:338-43.
7. Turkowski-Duhem A, Kamar N, Cointault O, Lavayssiere L, Ribes D, Esposito L, et al. Predictive factors of anemia within the first year post renal transplant. Transplantation. 2005;80:903-9.
8. Besarab A, Caro J, Jarrell BE, Francos G, Erslev AJ. Dynamics of erythropoiesis following renal transplantation. Kidney Int. 1987;32:526-36.
9. Poesen R, Bammens B, Claes K, Kuypers D, Vanrenterghem Y, Monbaliu D, et al. Prevalence and determinants of anemia in the immediate postkidney transplant period. Transpl Int. 2011;24:1208-15.
10. Zheng S, Coyne DW, Joist H, Schuessler R, Godboldo-Brooks A, Ercole P, et al. Iron deficiency anemia and iron losses after renal transplantation. Transpl Int. 2009;22:434-40.
11. Sun CH, Ward HJ, Paul WL, Koyle MA, Yanagawa N, Lee DB. Serum erythropoietin levels after renal transplantation. N Engl J Med. 1989;321:151-7.
12. Karthikeyan V, Karpinski J, Nair RC, Knoll G. The burden of chronic kidney disease in renal transplant recipients. Am J Transplant. 2004;4:262-9.
13. Vanrenterghem Y. Anaemia after renal transplantation. Nephrol Dial Transplant. 2004;19(Suppl. 5):V54-8.
14. Nemeth E, Valore EV, Territo M, Schiller G, Lichtenstein A, Ganz T. Hepcidin, a putative mediator of anemia of inflammation, is a type II acute-phase protein. Blood. 2003;101: 2461-3.
15. Han O. Molecular mechanism of intestinal iron absorption. Metallomics. 2011;3:103-9.
16. Eisenga MF, Dullaart RP, Berger SP, Sloan JH, de Vries APJ, Bakker SJL, et al. Association of hepcidin-25 with survival after kidney transplantation. Eur J Clin Invest. 2016;46: 994-1001.
17. Malyszko J, Koc-Zorawska E, Malyszko JS, Glowinska I, Mysliwiec M, Macdougall IC. GDF15 is related to anemia and hepcidin in kidney allograft recipients. Nephron Clin Pract. 2013;123:112-7.
18. Chan W, Ward DG, McClean A, Bosch JA, Jones D, Kaur O, et al. The role of hepcidin-25 in kidney transplantation. Transplantation. 2013;95:1390-5.
19. Malyszko J, Malyszko JS, Mysliwiec M. A possible role of hepcidin in the pathogenesis of anemia among kidney allograft recipients. Transplant Proc. 2009;41:3056-9.
20. Malyszko J, Malyszko JS, Pawlak K, Mysliwiec M. Hepcidin, iron status, and renal function in chronic renal failure, kidney transplantation, and hemodialysis. Am J Hematol. 2006;81:832-7.
21. Malyszko J, Malyszko JS, Pawlak K, Mysliwiec M. Hepcidin, an acute-phase protein and a marker of inflammation in kidney transplant recipients with and without coronary artery disease. Transplant Proc. 2006;38:2895-8.
22. Kalantzi M, Kalliakmani P, Papachristou E, Papasotiriou M, Savvidaki E, Zavvos V, et al. Parameters influencing blood erythropoietin levels of renal transplant recipients during the early post-transplantation period. Transplant Proc. 2014;46:3179-82.
23. Chadban SJ, Baines L, Polkinghorne K, Jefferys A, Dogra S, Kanganas C, et al. Anemia after kidney transplantation is not completely explained by reduced kidney function. Am J Kidney Dis. 2007;49:301-9.
24. Imoagene-Oyedeji AE, Rosas SE, Doyle AM, Goral S, Bloom RD. Post-transplantation anemia at 12 months in kidney recipients treated with mycophenolate mofetil: risk factors and implications for mortality. J Am Soc Nephrol. 2006;17:3240-7.
25. Kamar N, Rostaing L. Negative impact of one-year anemia on long-term patient and graft survival in kidney transplant patients receiving calcineurin inhibitors and mycophenolate mofetil. Transplantation. 2008;85:1120-4.
26. Jones H, Talwar M, Nogueira JM, Ugarte R, Cangro C, Rasheed H, et al. Anemia after kidney transplantation; its prevalence, risk factors, and independent association with graft and patient survival: a time-varying analysis. Transplantation. 2012;93:923-8.
27. Winkelmayer WC, Chandraker A, Alan Brookhart M, Kramar R, Sunder-Plassmann G. A prospective study of anaemia and long-term outcomes in kidney transplant recipients. Nephrol Dial Transplant. 2006;21:3559-66.
28. Molnar MZ, Czira M, Ambrus C, Szeifert L, Szentkiralyi A, Beko G, et al. Anemia is associated with mortality in kidney-transplanted patients—a prospective cohort study. Am J Transplant. 2007;7:818-24.
29. Ourahma S, Mercadal L, Tezenas du Montcel S, Assogba D, Bitker M-O, Mallet A, et al. Anemia in the period immediately following renal transplantation. Transplant Proc. 2007;39: 1446-50.
30. Shibagaki Y, Shetty A. Anaemia is common after kidney transplantation, especially among African Americans. Nephrol Dial Transplant. 2004;19:2368-73.
31. Lorenz M, Kletzmayr J, Perschl A, Furrer A, Horl WH, Sunder-Plassmann G. Anemia and iron deficiencies among long-term renal transplant recipients. J Am Soc Nephrol. 2002;13:794-7.
32. Mix TC, Kazmi W, Khan S, Ruthazer R, Rohrer R, Pereira BJG, et al. Anemia: a continuing problem following kidney transplantation. Am J Transplant. 2003;3:1426-33.
33. Jimeno L, Rodado R, Campos M, Lanuza M. Iron deficiency—an underrecognized problem in nonanemic and erythrocytic kidney transplant recipients: risks and effects of ACEI and of iron treatment. Transplant Proc. 2005;37:1007-8.
34. Unal A, Sipahioglu MH, Akcakaya M, Tokgoz B, Sav T, Oymak O, et al. An underappreciated problem in renal transplant recipients: anemia. Transplant Proc. 2008;40:1399-403.
35. Shah N, Al-Khoury S, Afzali B, Covic A, Roche A, Marsh J, et al. Post-transplantation anemia in adult renal allograft recipients: prevalence and predictors. Transplantation. 2006;81:1112-8.

36. Winkelmayer WC, Kewalramani R, Rutstein M, Gabardi S, Vonvisger T, Chandraker A. Pharmacoepidemiology of anemia in kidney transplant recipients. J Am Soc Nephrol. 2004;15:1347-52.
37. Khosroshahi HT, Asghari A, Estakhr R, Baiaz B, Ardalan MR, Shoja MM. Effects of azathioprine and mycophenolate mofetil-immunosuppressive regimens on the erythropoietic system of renal transplant recipients. Transplant Proc. 2006; 38:2077-9.
38. Zazgornik J. Azathioprine induced macrocytosis and red cell aplasia in renal transplant patients. Nephrol Dial Transplant. 1997;12:628.
39. Kuypers DR, de Jonge H, Naesens M, de Loor H, Halewijck E, Dekens M, et al. Current target ranges of mycophenolic acid exposure and drug-related adverse events: a 5-year, open-label, prospective, clinical follow-up study in renal allograft recipients. Clin Ther. 2008;30:673-83.
40. Jacobson PA, Schladt D, Oetting WS, Leduc R, Guan W, Matas AJ, et al. Genetic determinants of mycophenolate-related anemia and leukopenia after transplantation. Transplantation. 2011;91:309-16.
41. Augustine JJ, Knauss TC, Schulak JA, Bodziak KA, Siegel C, Hricik DE. Comparative effects of sirolimus and mycophenolate mofetil on erythropoiesis in kidney transplant patients. Am J Transplant. 2004;4:2001-6.
42. Friend P, Russ G, Oberbauer R, Murgia MG, Tufveson G, Chapman J, et al. Incidence of anemia in sirolimus-treated renal transplant recipients: the importance of preserving renal function. Transpl Int. 2007;20:754-60.
43. Fishbane S, Cohen DJ, Coyne DW, Djamali A, Singh AK, Wish JB. Post-transplant anemia: the role of sirolimus. Kidney Int. 2009;76:376-82.
44. Kim MJ, Mayr M, Pechula M, Steiger J, Dickenmann M. Marked erythrocyte microcytosis under primary immunosuppression with sirolimus. Transpl Int. 2006;19:12-8.
45. Augustine JJ, Rodriguez V, Padiyar A, Bodziak KA, Schulak JA, Hricik DE. Reduction in erythropoietin resistance after conversion from sirolimus to enteric coated mycophenolate sodium. Transplantation. 2008;86:548-53.
46. Sofroniadou S, Kassimatis T, Goldsmith D. Anaemia, microcytosis and sirolimus—is iron the missing link? Nephrol Dial Transplant. 2010;25:1667-75.
47. Carson JM, Newman ED, Farber JL, Filippone EJ. Tacrolimus-induced thrombotic microangiopathy: natural history of a severe, acute vasculopathy. Clin Nephrol. 2012;77:79-84.
48. Marathias KP, Agroyannis B, Mavromoustakos T, Matsoukas J, Vlahakos DV. Hematocrit-lowering effect following inactivation of renin-angiotensin system with angiotensin converting enzyme inhibitors and angiotensin receptor blockers. Curr Top Med Chem. 2004;4:483-6.
49. Douwes RM, Gomes-Neto AW, Eisenga MF, Vinke JSJ, de Borst MH, van den Berg E, et al. Chronic use of proton-pump inhibitors and iron status in renal transplant recipients. J Clin Med. 2019;8:1382.
50. Djamali A, Becker YT, Simmons WD, Johnson CA, Premasathian N, Becker BN. Increasing hematocrit reduces early post-transplant cardiovascular risk in diabetic transplant recipients. Transplantation. 2003;76:816-20.
51. Kovesdy CP, Trivedi BK, Kalantar-Zadeh K, Anderson JE. Association of anemia with outcomes in men with moderate and severe chronic kidney disease. Kidney Int. 2006;69:560-4.
52. Akbari A, Hussain N, Karpinski J, Knoll GA. Chronic kidney disease management: comparison between renal transplant recipients and nontransplant patients with chronic kidney disease. Nephron Clin Pract. 2007;107:c7-13.
53. Kamar N, Rostaing L, Ignace S, Villar E. Impact of post-transplant anemia on patient and graft survival rates after kidney transplantation: a meta-analysis. Clin Transplant. 2012;26:461-9.
54. Efstratiadis G, Konstantinou D, Chytas I, Vergoulas G. Cardiorenal anemia syndrome. Hippokratia. 2008;12:11-6.
55. Choukroun G, Kamar N, Dussol B, Etienne I, Cassuto-Viguier E, Toupance O, et al. Correction of postkidney transplant anemia reduces progression of allograft nephropathy. J Am Soc Nephrol. 2012;23:360-8.
56. Streja E, Kovesdy CP, Greenland S, Kopple JD, McAllister CJ, Nissenson AR, et al. Erythropoietin, iron depletion, and relative thrombocytosis: a possible explanation for hemoglobin-survival paradox in hemodialysis. Am J Kidney Dis. 2008;52:727-36.
57. Kolonko A, Pinocy-Mandok J, Kocierz M, Kujawa-Szewieczek A, Chudek J, Malyszko J, et al. Anemia and erythrocytosis after kidney transplantation: a 5-year graft function and survival analysis. Transplant Proc. 2009;41:3046-51.
58. Kiberd BA. Post-transplant erythrocytosis: a disappearing phenomenon? Clin Transplant. 2009;23:800-6.
59. Malyszko J, Oberbauer R, Watschinger B. Anemia and erythrocytosis in patients after kidney transplantation. Transpl Int. 2012;25:1013-23.
60. Brox AG, Mangel J, Hanley JA, St Louis G, Mongrain S, Gagnon RF. Erythrocytosis after renal transplantation represents an abnormality of insulin-like growth factor-I and its binding proteins. Transplantation. 1998;66:1053-8.
61. Vlahakos DV, Marathias KP, Agroyannis B, Madias NE. Post-transplant erythrocytosis. Kidney Int. 2003;63:1187-94.
62. Hiremath S, Fergusson D, Doucette S, Mulay AV, Knoll GA. Renin angiotensin system blockade in kidney transplantation: a systematic review of the evidence. Am J Transplant. 2007;7:2350-60.
63. Barenbrock M, Spieker C, Rahn KH, Zidek W. Therapeutic efficiency of phlebotomy in post-transplant hypertension associated with erythrocytosis. Clin Nephrol. 1993;40:241-3.
64. Malyszko J, Basak G, Batko K, Capasso G, Capasso A, Drozd-Sokolowska J, et al. Haematological disorders following kidney transplantation. Nephrol Dial Transplant. 2022;37:409-20.
65. Ojo AO, Hanson JA, Wolfe RA, Leichtman AB, Agodoa LY, Port FK. Long-term survival in renal transplant recipients with graft function. Kidney Int. 2000;57:307-13.
66. The Tricontinental Mycophenolate Mofetil Renal Transplantation Study Group. A blinded, randomized clinical trial of mycophenolate mofetil for the prevention of acute rejection in cadaveric renal transplantation. Transplantation. 1996;61:1029-37.
67. Zucker K, Tsaroucha A, Olson L, Esquenazi V, Tzakis A, Miller J. Evidence that tacrolimus augments the bioavailability of mycophenolate mofetil through the inhibition of mycophenolic acid glucuronidation. Ther Drug Monit. 1999;21:35-43.
68. Knoll GA, MacDonald I, Khan A, Van Walraven C. Mycophenolate mofetil dose reduction and the risk of acute

rejection after renal transplantation. J Am Soc Nephrol. 2003;14:2381-6.
69. Razeghi E, Hadadi A, Mansor-Kiaei M, Molavi M, Khashayar P, Pourmand G. Clinical manifestation, laboratory findings, and the response of treatment in kidney transplant recipients with CMV infection. Transplant Proc. 2007;39:993-6.
70. Hurst FP, Belur P, Nee R, Agodoa LY, Patel P, Abbott KC, et al. Poor outcomes associated with neutropenia after kidney transplantation: analysis of United States Renal Data System. Transplantation. 2011;92:36-40.
71. Mourad G, Morelon E, Noel C, Glotz D, Lebranchu Y. The role of thymoglobulin induction in kidney transplantation: an update. Clin Transplant. 2012;26:E450-64.
72. Zuber J, Le Quintrec M, Sberro-Soussan R, Loirat C, Fremeaux-Bacchi V, Legendre C. New insights into postrenal transplant hemolytic uremic syndrome. Nat Rev Nephrol. 2011;7:23-35.
73. Schiffer CA, Anderson KC, Bennett CL, Bernstein S, Elting LS, Goldsmith M, et al. Platelet transfusion for patients with cancer: clinical practice guidelines of the American Society of Clinical Oncology. J Clin Oncol. 2001;19:1519-38.
74. Khalil MAM, Khalil MAU, Khan TFT, Tan J. Drug-induced hematological cytopenia in kidney transplantation and the challenges it poses for kidney transplant physicians. J Transplant. 2018;2018:1-22.
75. Yang Y, Yu B, Chen Y. Blood disorders typically associated with renal transplantation. Front Cell Dev Biol. 2015;3:18.
76. Zimmerhackl LB, Hofer J, Cortina G, Mark W, Würzner R, Jungraithmayr TC, et al. Prophylactic eculizumab after renal transplantation in atypical hemolytic-uremic syndrome. N Engl J Med. 2010;362:1746-8.
77. Canaud G, Kamar N, Anglicheau D, Esposito L, Rabant M, Noël L-H, et al. Eculizumab improves post-transplant thrombotic microangiopathy due to antiphospholipid syndrome recurrence but fails to prevent chronic vascular changes. Am J Transplant. 2013;13:2179-85.
78. Ponticelli C, Banfi G. Thrombotic microangiopathy after kidney transplantation. Transpl Int. 2006;19:789-94.
79. Caires RA, Marques IDB, Repizo LP, Sato VAH, Carmo LPF, Machado DJB, et al. De novo thrombotic microangiopathy after kidney transplantation: clinical features, treatment, and long-term patient and graft survival. Transplant Proc. 2012;44:2388-90.
80. Weclawiak H, Kamar N, Ould-Mohamed A, Cardeau-Desangles I, Rostaing L. Biological agents in kidney transplantation: belatacept is entering the field. Expert Opin Biol Ther. 2010;10:1501-8.
81. Ashman N, Chapagain A, Dobbie H, Raftery MJ, Sheaff MT, Yaqoob MM. Belatacept as maintenance immunosuppression for postrenal transplant de novo drug-induced thrombotic microangiopathy. Am J Transplant. 2009;9:424-7.
82. Swerdlow SH, Campo E, Pileri SA, Harris NL, Stein H, Siebert R, et al. The 2016 revision of the World Health Organization classification of lymphoid neoplasms. Blood. 2016;127:2375-90.
83. Siegel RL, Miller KD, Jemal A. Cancer statistics, 2016. CA Cancer J Clin. 2016;66:7-30.
84. Dierickx D, Habermann TM. Post-transplantation lymphoproliferative disorders in adults. N Engl J Med. 2018;378:549-62.
85. Luskin MR, Heil DS, Tan KS, Choi S, Stadtmauer EA, Schuster SJ, et al. The impact of EBV status on characteristics and outcomes of post-transplantation lymphoproliferative disorder. Am J Transplant. 2015;15:2665-73.
86. Reshef R, Vardhanabhuti S, Luskin MR, Heitjan DF, Hadjiliadis D, Goral S, et al. Reduction of immunosuppression as initial therapy for post-transplantation lymphoproliferative disorder. Am J Transplant. 2011;11:336-47.
87. Achkar R, Chiba AK, Zampieri-Filho JP, Pestana JOM, Bordin JO. Hemolytic anemia after kidney transplantation: a prospective analysis. Transfusion. 2011;51:2495-9.
88. Yorgin PD, Scandling JD, Belson A, Sanchez J, Alexander SR, Andreoni KA. Late post-transplant anemia in adult renal transplant recipients. An under-recognized problem? Am J Transplant. 2002;2(5):429-35.
89. Ramos-Casals M, Brito-Zeron P, Lopez-Guillermo A, Khamashta MA, Bosch X. Adult haemophagocytic syndrome. Lancet. 2014;383:1503-16.
90. Karras A, Thervet E, Legendre C. Hemophagocytic syndrome in renal transplant recipients: report of 17 cases and review of literature. Transplantation. 2004;77(2):238-43.
91. Asci G, Toz H, Ozkahya M, Cagirgan S, Duman S, Sezis M, et al. High-dose immunoglobulin therapy in renal transplant recipients with hemophagocytic histiocytic syndrome. J Nephrol. 2006;19:322-6.
92. McNerney ME, Godley LA, Le Beau MM. Therapy-related myeloid neoplasms: when genetics and environment collide. Nat Rev Cancer. 2017;17:513-27.
93. Morton LM, Gibson TM, Clarke CA, Lynch CF, Anderson LA, Pfeiffer R, et al. Risk of myeloid neoplasms after solid organ transplantation. Leukemia. 2014;28:2317-23.
94. Rashidi A, Fisher SI. Acute myeloid leukemia following solid organ transplantation: entity or novelty? Eur J Haematol. 2014;92:459-66.

CHAPTER 14

Recurrent and de novo Glomerulonephritis After Kidney Transplantation

Sabina Yusuf, Suceena Alexander

CASE VIGNETTE

A 25-year-old male patient was diagnosed with chronic kidney disease (CKD) in September 2018. Both his kidneys were contracted and echogenic at the time of diagnosis and his native kidney disease (NKD) was unknown. He progressed to end-stage kidney disease (ESKD) in 2019 and was started on hemodialysis in December 2019. He was found to have hepatitis C virus (HCV) infection in January 2021 with HCV ribonucleic acid (RNA) polymerase chain reaction (PCR) 42,000,000 IU/mL. He was treated with direct-acting antivirals (DAAs) and attained sustained virologic response (SVR). He underwent live-related, ABO-compatible kidney transplantation in August 2021. He received induction therapy with basiliximab followed by triple-drug immunosuppression with prednisolone, tacrolimus, and mycophenolate mofetil (MMF). His peri- and postoperative course was uneventful; he achieved nadir creatinine on postoperative day (POD) 5 and was subsequently discharged on POD 7. Therapeutic drug monitoring was done and doses of tacrolimus and MMF were adjusted. 1-month post-transplant, while his serum creatinine was stable, his urinalysis showed 3+ protein and no active sediments. 24-hour urine protein was 2.8 g with serum albumin of 3.5 g/dL. His HCV RNA PCR at 1-month post-transplant was 26,000 IU/mL. He was again started on DAAs and graft biopsy was done. Graft biopsy was reported as membranous nephropathy (MN) and was positive for phospholipase A2 receptor (PLA2R) immunohistochemistry. Serum anti-PLA2R was negative. He was started on angiotensin receptor blockers (ARBs). He completed his DAA treatment and attained SVR in 12 weeks. The dose of his ARBs was also titrated and he attained complete remission of proteinuria while his renal functions remained stable. This case highlights the development of de novo MN in a renal allograft recipient following reactivation of HCV infection in the post-transplant period. Although PLA2R positivity helps in differentiating primary from secondary and recurrent from de novo MN, PLA2R positivity has been noted in cases of MN associated with viral infections also[1] and though rare but can be present in de novo MN as well. Larsen and Walker reported 8% PLA2R positivity in de novo MN biopsies.[2] Immunoglobulin G (IgG) subclass was not done in this patient due to unavailability of the test at the time.

INTRODUCTION

Glomerulonephritis (GN) accounts for 10–25% cases of ESKD worldwide as reported through various registries.[3] Glomerular diseases can occur in the graft kidney also and affect long-term graft outcomes. Overall, 18–22% of kidney allografts are lost due to GN, either recurrent or de novo.[4] The occurrence in the first allograft risks the recurrence in subsequent allografts further jeopardizing the chance of a successful long-term renal replacement therapy. Our understanding of the pathogenesis of these diseases are limited, which has clinical implications in kidney transplantation owing to the recurrent nature of some glomerular diseases. This chapter focuses on the most common forms of primary glomerular diseases that are seen after kidney transplantation, their impact on graft survival, and optimal management strategies as per our current knowledge and understanding.

CLASSIFICATION OF GLOMERULONEPHRITIS AFTER KIDNEY TRANSPLANTATION

In clinical practice transplant, GN can be classified into three categories:

1. *Recurrent GN:* Allograft GN is the same as NKD as confirmed by kidney biopsy.
2. *GN with unknown NKD:* Allograft GN is confirmed by kidney biopsy in a patient with unknown NKD.
3. *De novo GN:* Allograft GN, which is biopsy proven, is different from the NKD.

The diagnosis of NKD remains unknown for a large number of patients who reach ESKD and undergo kidney transplantation. Lack of NKD is a far greater problem in our part of the world where patients lack adequate access to medical care. In the study conducted in south India, patients with unknown NKD formed 60% of the cohort of patients with post-transplant GN (Yusuf et al., unpublished data, 2021) **(Table 1)**.

CHAPTER HIGHLIGHTS

- Glomerular diseases can occur in the graft kidney also and affect long-term graft outcomes.
- Approximately, 18–22% of kidney allografts are lost due to recurrent or de novo glomerulonephritis.
- The risk for recurrence depends on the type of glomerulonephritis (GN).
- Recurrence can occur for both primary and secondary GN.

EPIDEMIOLOGY

The epidemiology of GN after kidney transplant mirrors that of the native kidney glomerular disease distribution in the CKD population. Immunoglobulin A nephropathy (IgAN) has been found to be the most common glomerular disease causing ESKD in various populations around the world including ours and is also the most common glomerular disease to occur in the graft kidney **(Table 2)**. Analysis of data from various registries has revealed that prevalence rates of GN in native kidneys and in allografts are higher in children and in the white population.[3] Higher prevalence in children is related to the lower prevalence of diabetes as a cause of ESKD. Predominance of white patients has been explained by the lack of information on kidney biopsy in black patients and higher prevalence of hypertensive nephrosclerosis and diabetic nephropathy in these patients. Studies conducted to identify the factors associated with an increased risk of GN after transplant have found that the type and severity of the original disease, the age at onset, the interval from onset to ESKD, the clinical course of the previous transplantation, the donor source, and the immunosuppressive regimen may influence the likelihood of recurrence.

Immunoglobulin A Nephropathy

Immunoglobulin A nephropathy is one of the most common types of GN seen in the graft kidney. The incidence of recurrent IgAN has been variably reported between 9 and 53%.[9,10] One of the major reasons for this large discrepancy is the variable biopsy practices followed in different centers around the world and the durations of follow-up, which vary from study to study. The recurrence of IgAN post-transplant can be histological only or clinical. Histological recurrence is diagnosed in a protocol biopsy in an asymptomatic patient while clinical recurrence is associated with urinary abnormalities and/or graft dysfunction. Histological recurrence is more common and occurs earlier post-transplant while clinical recurrence is rare before 5 years of transplant.[4]

Few pathogenetic mechanisms for recurrent IgAN that have been elucidated include higher levels of circulating galactose-deficient IgA1 and IgA-IgG immune complexes and lower levels of circulating complexes of IgA-soluble CD89, the myeloid cell receptor for IgA.[11] Younger age and a rapidly progressive disease before transplantation have been associated with an increased risk of recurrence. Studies on association of recurrence with living-related donation[12-16]

TABLE 1: Native kidney glomerular disease frequencies in end-stage kidney disease (ESKD) among various populations worldwide.

Authors	*Year*	*IgAN (%)*	*FSGS (%)*	*MN (%)*	*MPGN (%)*	*Unknown or presumed GN (in patients with PTGN) (%)*
An et al.[5] (Korea)	1995–2010	66.1	8.2	2.1	4.1	33.2
Lim et al.[6] (ANZDATA)	1990–2012	55.9	2.7	7.5	7.3	10
Chailimpamontree et al.[7] (Canada)	1990–2005	12.1	9.7	0.9	2.1	7.8
Allen et al.[8] (ANZDATA)	1985–2014	37.9	21.3	5.4	5.7	–
Yusuf et al. (CMC, Vellore) (unpublished data)	1971–2018	26.5	21.8	1.8	11.9	56.5

(ANZDATA: Australia New Zealand Dialysis Transplant Data System; CMC: Christian Medical College; FSGS: focal segmental glomerulosclerosis; GN: glomerulonephritis; IgAN: immunoglobulin A nephropathy; MN: membranous nephropathy; MPGN: membranoproliferative glomerulonephritis; PTGN: post-transplant glomerulonephritis)

TABLE 2: Frequencies of various types of glomerulonephritis after kidney transplant.

Authors	*Year*	*Incidence of PTGN (%)*	*IgAN (%)*	*FSGS (%)*	*MN (%)*	*MPGN (%)*
An et al.[5] (Korea)	1995–2010	9.2	77.1	11.4	2.8	4.2
Chailimpamontree et al.[7] (Canada)	1990–2005	7.1	42.3	36.8	4.9	5.5
Allen et al.[8] (ANZDATA)	1985–2014	2.7	40.7	26.1	8.9	11
Yusuf et al. (CMC, Vellore) (unpublished data)	1971–2018	4.8	52.5	20.9	2.3	4

(ANZDATA: Australia New Zealand Dialysis Transplant Data System; CMC: Christian Medical College; FSGS: focal segmental glomerulosclerosis; IgAN: immunoglobulin A nephropathy; MN: membranous nephropathy; MPGN: membranoproliferative glomerulonephritis; PTGN: post-transplant glomerulonephritis) and use of induction therapy[17-19] have shown inconsistent results. Propensity of thymoglobulin to influence the Tregs has been proposed as a possible mechanism of protection. The risk has also been found to be higher in patients receiving steroid-free immunosuppression post-transplantation.[20,21]

Recurrence of IgAN is associated with a high risk of graft failure[14,22] and rates varying from 45 to 70% have been reported. The optimal treatment for recurrent IgAN remains unknown. The nature of immunosuppressive medication has not been shown to impact the risk of graft failure from recurrent IgAN.[23] Angiotensin-converting enzyme inhibitors (ACEIs) have been found to reduce proteinuria and blood pressure in transplant recipients with IgAN and may be prescribed.[24] There are case reports of patients treated with tonsillectomy for disease recurrence; however, because of the limited evidence available, it cannot be recommended as a treatment option.[25,26] Crescentic IgAN in the graft has been treated with more aggressive immunosuppression in the form of cyclophosphamide and rituximab, but again these treatment options are largely unproven and have not been found to be effective in reversing the disease process.[27-30]

De novo IgAN has been reported to be less common than recurrent IgAN. Some authors argue that de novo IgAN might be considered as "transmitted disease," which means that the recipient received an allograft that already had a "latent" form of IgAN.[31] This argument is supported by the finding that mesangial IgA deposition was found in nearly 16% 0-hour protocol biopsies in a Japanese study.[32] De novo IgAN is frequently asymptomatic. Course and prognosis are usually quiescent except in the presence of crescents in the allograft, in which the prognosis is poor.

Primary Focal Segmental Glomerulosclerosis

The occurrence of focal segmental glomerulosclerosis (FSGS) after renal transplantation has been described as early as 1972.[33] The true incidence of recurrent FSGS, however, is difficult to ascertain given the diversity of etiologic mechanisms and the possibility of misclassification of primary versus secondary FSGS. Studies have reported recurrence rates of FSGS varying from 30% in adults to 50% in pediatric patients[34] with an exponential increment of risk (up to 80%) at subsequent renal grafts **(Table 3)**.[35-38]

Increased concentrations of circulating permeability factors such as soluble urokinase-type plasminogen activator receptor (suPAR)[39] and cardiotrophin-like cytokine factor 1 (CLCF-1)[40] have been implicated in the pathogenesis of primary FSGS and its recurrence. Research studies on serum factors predicting the risk of FSGS recurrence have identified autoantibodies against a panel of nearly 800 unique antigens significantly increased in the sera of patients with recurrent FSGS. In this panel, the anti-CD40 antibody has been found to have the strongest correlation with FSGS recurrence prediction.[41] Clinical risk factors for recurrence include young age, mesangial proliferation in the native kidneys, a rapid progression to ESKD, a pretransplant bilateral nephrectomy, White ethnicity, and specific aspects of genetic background.[42] Recurrence usually presents with significant proteinuria (urinary protein creatinine ratio >0.5)[43,44] occurring as early as the

TABLE 3: Summary of the frequency of recurrence, time to recurrence, risk factors for recurrence, and graft outcomes in different types of recurrent glomerulonephritis (GN) after transplantation.

Type of GN	*Recurrence rates*	*Median time of recurrence*	*Risk factors for recurrence*	*Risk of graft loss*
IgAN	10–60%	2–5 years post-tx	Younger age, living-related donor, steroid-free immunosuppression post-transplantation, genetic variants in CFHR5, HLA alleles HLA-B35, HLA-DR4, HLA-B8, HLA-DR3 in recipient	45–70%
FSGS	• 20–30% • 80% in repeat tx after first graft loss from recurrent FSGS	• Early days to weeks post-tx • Late months to years post-tx	Younger age, rapid progression to ESKD, pretransplant native kidney nephrectomy, history of recurrence in prior graft	20–50%
IC-MPGN	• Polyclonal 20–30% • Monoclonal 60–65%	• 1–5 years post-tx • Early post-tx	Low-serum complement levels, presence of monoclonal protein, poor response to treatment and rapid progression to ESKD	• 10% • 50%
C3-MPGN	• DDD 50–100% • C3GN 70%	4 months to 2 years post-tx	HLA antigens B8, DR3, DR4; higher proteinuria; presence of crescents in native kidney biopsy	• 25% • 50%
MN	• Anti-PLA2R Ab positive 70% • Anti-PLA2R Ab negative 30%	1–4 years post-tx	High pretransplant circulating levels of anti-PLA2R antibody	10–30%

(anti-PLA2R Ab: antiphospholipase A2 receptor antibody; C3GN: C3 glomerulonephritis; C3-MPGN: complement-mediated membranoproliferative glomerulonephritis; DDD: dense deposit disease; ESKD: end-stage kidney disease; FSGS: focal segmental glomerulosclerosis; HLA: human leukocyte antigen; IC-MPGN: immune complex-mediated membranoproliferative glomerulonephritis; IgAN: immunoglobulin A nephropathy; MN: membranous nephropathy; tx: transplant) first 48–72 hours post-transplant. However, glomerular and tubular proteinuria not related to FSGS (proteinuria from the native kidneys or secondary to ischemia-reperfusion injury to the graft) may also occur post renal transplantation. Non-FSGS proteinuria decreases in the first 3 weeks but can persist up to 9 weeks post-transplant.[43,45,46] A renal biopsy is often needed for definitive diagnosis. A subacute course of FSGS recurrence has also been described, where proteinuria and graft dysfunction develop slowly and progress over months and years. In the later post-transplantation period, classification between recurrent and de novo FSGS can be blurred especially when significant chronic changes are found on biopsies. The general perception is that the degree of podocyte effacement is more pronounced in the primary versus secondary forms.

The spectrum of outcomes in recurrent FSGS varies from immediate graft loss to slowly progressive proteinuria with chronic allograft dysfunction to complete remission with no long-term consequences on the graft and is dependent on multiple factors including the severity of proteinuria and graft dysfunction at presentation, response to the treatment employed, and the presence of other risk factors. The incidence of graft loss varies from 20 to 50% in the first 5 years post-transplant.[47] The management of recurrent FSGS following kidney transplantation remains extremely challenging. Due to lack of randomized trials, treatment recommendations are based on small study cohorts, case series, and case reports **(Table 4)**. In general, plasmapheresis-based approaches are used for the early aggressive recurrence. At least 8–12 plasmapheresis treatments have been required for induction of remission, although dependence on long-term plasmapheresis dependence has also been reported. Based on its off-target binding SMPDL-3b (sphingomyelin phosphodiesterase acid like 3B) on podocytes and effect on acid sphingomyelinase activity, use of rituximab has gained popularity in recent reports.[48,49] Two to six doses of 375 mg/m^2/dose of rituximab every 1–2 weeks have been used in published reports. Use of intravenous galactose, anti-tumor necrosis factor (TNF) alpha agents, cyclophosphamide, abatacept, and belatacept has also been reported; however, they are not found to be beneficial.

Unlike recurrent FSGS, de novo FSGS usually presents more than 12 months after renal transplantation. Variable amounts of proteinuria, hypertension, and progressive decline in allograft function are the usual presenting features.[31] Donor–recipient size discrepancy, presence of diabetes, hypertension, BK polyomavirus, parvovirus B19 infection, and calcineurin inhibitor (CNI) toxicity have been implicated causative. CNI withdrawal and introduction of MMF or mammalian target of rapamycin (mTOR) inhibitors early in the course of disease have been reported to induce stabilization or even improvement of allograft function albeit at an increased risk of rejection.

Membranoproliferative Glomerulonephritis

The overall reported rate of recurrence of membranoproliferative glomerulonephritis (MPGN) in the literature is quite variable (27–65%).[50-53] MPGN can be idiopathic or secondary to a variety of diseases. The introduction of a new classification of MPGN, which considers the differences in the pathogenesis and histological findings of MPGN subtypes (i.e., immune complex-mediated MPGN and complement-mediated MPGN), has enabled a more accurate assessment of the nature and course of the disease, including the risk of disease recurrence after kidney transplantation.

For immune complex-mediated MPGN, the patterns and types of Ig deposits have diagnostic and prognostic significance. While MPGN with polyclonal Ig deposits has a relatively low risk of recurrence, usually presenting late during the first 5 years and progressing relatively slowly,[54] MPGN with monoclonal glomerular deposits (typically IgG3κ and IgG3λ) with or without the presence of serum monoclonal proteins recurs often (66%) very early post-transplantation and often follows an aggressive course with a high risk of graft failure.[55-58] The most important aspect of recurrent MPGN is the identification of the processes responsible for the original native disease. A thorough pre-transplant screening for monoclonal gammopathy and close monitoring post-transplant for signs of disease recurrence is essential. A diagnosis of monoclonal gammopathy in association with MPGN justifies intensive chemotherapy and/or autologous stem cell transplantation before kidney transplantation. Appropriate counseling of patients such that they are cognizant of the risk of disease recurrence post-transplant, weighing between this risk of premature allograft failure (if disease recurs) and that associated with remaining on dialysis is also required. The approach to the treatment of recurrent disease is not well established. Cyclophosphamide and high-dose MMF have been used in case reports.[59] In MPGN with monoclonal deposits, plasmapheresis and anti-CD 20 antibodies have been proven to be effective in uncontrolled trials.

In complement-mediated MPGN [C3 glomerulonephritis (C3GN) and dense deposit disease (DDD)], DDD has the higher rate of recurrence approaching nearly 100%.[60] Clinical presentation of recurrent C3GN includes proteinuria, hematuria, and higher serum creatinine. DDD usually recurs later than C3GN and presents clinically only with allograft dysfunction.[61] Presence of monoclonal paraprotein,[61] lower serum complement level,[54] human leukocyte antigens B8, DR3, B49, and DR4,[62] higher proteinuria, and the presence of crescents in the native kidney biopsy[63] have been associated with increased risk of recurrence of C3GN after transplant. A precise assessment of the underlying mechanism responsible for the MPGN is essential for prevention,

TABLE 4: Treatment strategies for recurrent focal segmental glomerulosclerosis (FSGS) after transplantation.

Strategy	*Study*	*Study participants*	*Treatment received*	*Outcomes*
Plasma exchange	Kashgary et al.[65]	423 patients with recurrent FSGS	Systematic review of 43 case series and 34 case reports	Complete remission in 47% and partial remission in 28%
	Hickson et al.[66]	13/30 patients with recurrent FSGS	Daily for 3–7 days followed by thrice weekly for 4–12 weeks followed by as needed	Remission in 9/13 (69%)
	Ponticelli et al.[42]	147 patients (70 patients <18 years, 77 patients ≥18 years)	Analysis of PE response in 22 studies	Partial/complete remission of proteinuria in 49/70 (70%) children and 49/77 (63%) adults
	Gohh et al.[67]	10 patients (1 patient <18 years, 9 patients ≥ 18 years)	Prophylactic course of eight PE sessions in the perioperative period in patients at high risk of recurrence	7/10 free of recurrence
Intravenous cyclosporine	Canaud et al.[68]	10 patients (≥18 years)	Intravenous CyA (C0 levels between 200 and 400 ng/mL), followed by oral CyA (C2 levels 1,200–1,400 ng/mL), high dose oral and a course of PE sessions for 9 months	Complete remission of proteinuria in 10/10; proteinuria relapse in 1/10 successfully treated with rituximab (two doses)
	Salomon et al.[69]	16 patients (<18 years; one regrafted with a subsequent recurrence)	Intravenous CyA (trough levels: 250–350 ng/mL)	Complete remission in 14/17 (82%); partial remission in 2/17 (12%)
Galactose	Sgambat et al.[70]	Seven patients (<18 years) with steroid-resistant nephrotic syndrome (2/7 with recurrent FSGS)	High galactose diet (0.2 g/kg per dose twice daily orally)	Reduction in permeability factor without effect on proteinuria values
Rituximab	Fornoni et al.[49]	41 patients (14 controls vs. 27 treated)	Rituximab within 24 hours after surgery (one dose, 375 mg/m^2) in patients at high risk of recurrence	Nephrotic proteinuria within 1 month in 7/27 patients in rituximab group versus 9/14 patients in control group ($p < 0.005$)
	Audard et al.[71]	Four patients (≥18 years)	Rituximab induction in patients at high risk of recurrence (first graft lost due to recurrence)	No evidence of significant proteinuria at the end of follow-up
CTLA4-Ig abatacept	Yu et al.[72]	Four patients (2/4 <18 years, 2/4 ≥ 18 years) with FSGS recurrence; One patient (≥18 years) with FSGS on native kidneys	1–2 doses of abatacept	Complete remission in 2/5; partial remission in 3/5
Ofatumumab	Wang et al.[73]	1/5 patients with post-transplant recurrent FSGS	Ofatumumab at 300 mg/1.73 m^2 for the first dose, followed by 5 weekly doses of 2,000 mg/1.73 m^2 after failed therapy with rituximab and PE	Complete remission
	Bernard et al.[74]	One patient with recurrent FSGS in second transplant	Two infusions of ofatumumab 8 months apart	Partial remission

(CTLA4: cytotoxic T lymphocyte-associated antigen 4; CyA: cyclosporine; PE: plasma exchange)

anticipatory management, and treatment of recurrent C3GN/DDD. Patients with complement dysregulation (e.g., factor H deficiency) should receive replacement infusions (fresh frozen plasma) before and after transplantation,[64] although no controlled trials of the efficacy of this approach have yet been conducted. Plasmapheresis (with fresh frozen plasma replacement) and/or rituximab have been found to be helpful in patients with a neutralizing autoantibody to factor H. Eculizumab (monoclonal antibody to C5a) may also be beneficial, but this has not yet been shown in a randomized trial.[64] Patients with genetic causes for factor H or I deficiency may require combined liver and kidney transplantation to avoid recurrences,[75] but this is mainly derived from experience with hereditary forms of complement-mediated thrombotic microangiopathy (TMA) also associated with factor H deficiency.[76]

Occurrence of a de novo MPGN pattern of injury in the graft is often related to the development of a systemic disease. Various causative factors implicated are HCV infection, cryoglobulinemia, and CNI toxicity or rejection (usually associated with a clinical pattern of de novo TMA). Patients present with variable degrees of proteinuria and graft dysfunction. Patients with nonnephrotic proteinuria and normal graft function may have a slow and largely silent course, but in other cases, the development of MPGN accelerates loss of the graft.[77] Steroids and reinforcement of immunosuppression have been used with inconsistent and usually poor results. De novo C3GN is very rare and the existing literature is restricted to case reports. An acquired complement abnormality after renal transplantation has been postulated to be the cause.

Membranous Nephropathy

Idiopathic MN recurs at a rate of 30–50% following kidney transplantation.[78] A direct relationship between the anti-PLA2R titer level and risk of disease recurrence post-transplant has been observed with a positive predictive value for disease recurrence of 83%.[79,80] Patients with anti-PLA2R antibodies pretransplantation have a 60–76% risk of histologic recurrence, whereas antibody-negative patients have a significantly lower risk (28–30%). Histologic recurrence of primary MN occurs most often during the first-year post-transplantation, but a second period of high risk occurs around 5 years.[81,82]

Serum anti-PLA2R antibody titers should be monitored in patients who have high levels of circulating anti-PLA2R antibodies prior to transplantation and in those who develop an early recurrence of disease post-transplant. Anti-PLA2R antibody also helps in differentiating recurrent from de novo MN or other causes of proteinuria and in monitoring the response to treatment.[83]

The treatment of disease recurrence is largely extrapolated from treatment in the general population. Continuation of CNI or changing from mTOR inhibitor-based regimen to CNI, use of renin-ARBs, and considering the addition of anti-CD20 antibodies are advocated. Rituximab is an effective treatment for disease recurrence with complete or partial remission seen in up to 80% of patients with the use of rituximab for early disease recurrence post-transplant.[84-87] Use is recommended irrespective of the anti-PLA2R antibody status. Many patients, however, may have only histological recurrence and current literature has no recommendations in place to guide the decision and initiation of treatment in them. However, early intervention (proteinuria approaching 1 g) in contrary to native MN is recommended.[86] Serial follow-up of anti-PLA2R antibody titer should be used to anticipate the magnitude of response to therapy as well as the possibility of relapse. In cases where rituximab has been found to be ineffective, use of alkylating agents and bortezomib has been proposed.[88] Use of rituximab to decrease anti-PLA2R antibody levels prior to renal transplantation is controversial since treatment of early recurrent MN with rituximab is quite successful. However, such therapy may be considered in patients with previous allograft loss due to recurrent MN.

De novo MN usually occurs several years after renal transplantation. Presence of a dominant glomerular staining for IgG1 (in place of IgG4) and absence of staining for PLA2R help to differentiate this entity from recurrent disease on kidney biopsy specimens. Viral, ischemic, immunological (by donor-specific antibodies), and mechanical injury can induce podocyte damage and expose various cryptogenic antigens leading to development of de novo disease. Decline in the levels of a novel regulatory podocyte protein (named Pdlim2) has been described to have a pathogenetic role.[89] However, a thorough search for underlying malignancy and a hidden viral infection is recommended in all patients in view of the clear general association between MN and both cancer and infection. Prognosis of de novo MN is variable depending on the etiology with a poorer prognosis attributable to associated antibody-mediated rejection if present. Therapy of de novo MN is unclear. There is lack of enough data to support the use of rituximab in de novo MN therapy and there is no clear base supporting the introduction of cytotoxic therapy or the intensified immunosuppressive agents.

Thrombotic Microangiopathy

Post-transplant TMA (PT-TMA) has been found to occur at a rate of 0.8–14%.[90,91] TMA in the graft may be a de novo disease or recurrence of a previous complement-mediated TMA (c-TMA) which may or may not have been diagnosed before kidney transplantation. In both de novo and recurrent TMA, various factors operating post-transplant, especially in the early post-transplant period, may trigger complement activation and produce TMA.[92] The most important of these factors include ischemia reperfusion injury, drugs (CNIs and mTOR inhibitors), and infections. Patients with an underlying genetic dysregulation of complement components (recurrent c-TMA) have 36 times higher risk of developing TMA compared to those with de novo disease (29% vs. 0.8%).[91] Features like the presence of systemic (rather than localized) TMA and a positive family history of TMA point toward a recurrent rather than de novo disease.

Although rare, the manifestations of PT-TMA can be devastating and lead to poor patient and graft outcomes. PT-TMA may vary from a limited form confined to the kidney to a full-blown systemic variant.[93-95] The systemic form comprises 20–60% cases and occurs early post-transplant, usually in the first 3 months. It presents acutely with acute kidney injury (AKI) and laboratory features of thrombocytopenia and microangiopathic hemolytic anemia [raised lactate dehydrogenase (LDH), low haptoglobin, and formation of schistocytes]. The localized form, on the other hand, can appear any time post-transplant and can be either acute manifesting as AKI or chronic causing a slowly worsening graft function. Difficult-to-control hypertension and proteinuria are other presentations of a chronic TMA that may be diagnosed only when a kidney biopsy is performed.[96,97]

The overall prognosis for PT-TMA is quite poor resulting in a graft loss rate of nearly 40% in the first 2 years.[90,91] In the pre-eculizumab era, recurrence of c-TMA appeared in 60% of transplant patients and resulted in 90% graft loss in the first year.[98] Eculizumab has been used as the first-line therapy to prevent recurrence; use of a first dose 1 hour before reperfusion and a second dose 24 hours after transplantation has been advocated to reduce secondary complement activation due to ischemia-reperfusion. Prophylactic plasmapheresis has not been found to be effective in preventing recurrence in patients with high- or moderate-risk mutations. In the treatment of established recurrent disease, little success has been achieved after plasmapheresis; nevertheless, good results have been observed with an early introduction of eculizumab after recurrence.[99] The duration of eculizumab treatment in cases of c-TMA recurrence can be lifelong (depending on the genetic mutation).

De novo TMA is much more frequent than recurrent c-TMA (90 vs. 10% of all cases) and is caused by various pathogenic mechanisms as outlined above. Complement genetic mutations have been reported in 30% in a series of patients with de novo TMA,[100] indicating an overlap between recurrent and de novo TMA. The risk of development of de novo TMA may be minimized by preventing complement overactivation by maintaining adequate renal perfusion during organ procurement and avoiding a prolonged cold ischemia time. Once developed, the treatment of de novo TMA is based on identifying the potential cause and correcting it. In TMA secondary to use of immunosuppressive drugs, treatment consists of reducing or stopping the culprit drug, switching from tacrolimus to cyclosporine or to mTORi or vice versa. Use of belatacept (cytotoxic T lymphocyte antigen 4-immunoglobulin fusion protein) has also been advocated since it may allow discontinuation of CNIs and mTORi albeit with an increased risk of rejection. TMA unresponsive to these measures should be treated with plasmapheresis. Eculizumab has been used in case reports in these patients if they fail to recover after a course of plasmapheresis.

Secondary Glomerulonephritis

Secondary GN due to various systemic diseases may also recur postrenal transplant. Recurrence is less common compared to primary glomerular diseases, occurs late post-transplant, and is an infrequent cause of allograft failure. Rates of recurrence of antineutrophil cytoplasmic antibody (ANCA)-associated vasculitis in the allograft have been reported to be 17%. The titers of ANCA, ANCA subtype, or disease severity prior to renal transplant do not predict the risk of disease recurrence post-transplant. Allograft loss from disease recurrence varies from 7 to 10%;[101] overall long-term outcomes of patients with ANCA vasculitis who undergo a kidney transplant are comparable to those transplanted for other causes of ESKD. Lupus nephritis has been seen to recur in 2–10% patients[102-104] post-transplant. Most of the data on recurrent lupus nephritis is based on single center and registry studies; the exact incidence and outcomes of disease are largely unclear. Factors that have been associated with an increased risk of recurrence include young age, female gender, black non-Hispanic ancestry, living-related donation, and presence of antiphospholipid (aPL) autoantibodies.[105] Graft and patient outcomes have been reported to be inferior in patients who experience recurrence compared to those who do not; however, the association is inconsistent given the unavailability of large-scale data. In patients with antiglomerular basement membrane (GBM) disease, disease recurrence after kidney transplant is <5% in the era of modern immunosuppression. However, if transplantation is done in the presence of circulating antibodies, recurrence rate is as high as 50%. De novo anti-GBM disease after transplantation can occur in those with Alport syndrome as a result of development of anti-GBM antibody in patients with genetic deficiency of type IV collagen proteins in their native kidneys.[106]

CHALLENGES IN DIAGNOSIS

Proteinuria and hematuria are the hallmark features of GN occurring after transplant. However, urinalysis is not included as part of routine post-transplant surveillance in many centers and in majority of the patients who undergo a graft biopsy, tissue specimens are not processed for immunofluorescence (IF) and electron microscopy (EM). Finally, the interpretation of the glomerular disease on a graft biopsy is also problematic. The histology of early GN after transplant may be different from advanced GN seen in native biopsies. For example, early cases of FSGS may not have glomerulosclerosis or subepithelial electron dense deposits may not be seen in early MN. Furthermore, the coexistence of CNI toxicity and acute or chronic alloimmune injury makes it difficult to distinguish the manifestations of these from lesions caused by GN. Hence, while interpreting graft biopsies it is essential to keep early histological changes in mind and conduct a careful histologic evaluation, including IF and EM examinations to avoid erroneous diagnosis.

CONCLUSION

In the past, recurrent or de novo glomerular diseases were considered infrequent causes of graft loss. However, with the current immunosuppressive therapy, reducing the incidence of acute and chronic rejection and prolonging long-term renal survival, glomerular diseases after renal transplantation have become significant contributors to late graft loss. A careful research into the pathogenesis and underlying biomolecular mechanisms of native and allograft glomerular diseases is warranted for appropriate treatment and optimization of renal transplant outcomes.

REFERENCES

1. Nikolopoulou A, Teixeira C, Cook HT, Roufosse C, Cairns THD, Levy JB, et al. Membranous nephropathy associated with viral infection. Clin Kidney J. 2021;14(3):876-83.
2. Larsen CP, Walker PD. Phospholipase A2 receptor (PLA2R) staining is useful in the determination of de novo versus recurrent membranous glomerulopathy. Transplantation. 2013;95(10):1259-62.
3. Golgert WA, Appel GB, Hariharan S. Recurrent glomerulonephritis after renal transplantation: an unsolved problem. Clin J Am Soc Nephrol. 2008;3(3):800-7.
4. Cosio FG, Cattran DC. Recent advances in our understanding of recurrent primary glomerulonephritis after kidney transplantation. Kidney Int. 2017;91(2):304-14.
5. An JN, Lee JP, Oh YJ, Oh YK, Ha J, Chae D-W, et al. Incidence of post-transplant glomerulonephritis and its impact on graft outcome. Kidney Res Clin Pract. 2012;31(4):219-26.
6. Lim WH, Wong G, McDonald SP, Chakera A, Luxton G, Isbel NM, et al. Long-term outcomes of kidney transplant recipients with end-stage kidney disease attributed to presumed/advanced glomerulonephritis or unknown cause. Sci Rep. 2108;8(1):9021.
7. Chailimpamontree W, Dmitrienko S, Li G, Balshaw R, Magil A, Shapiro RJ, et al. Probability, predictors, and prognosis of post-transplantation glomerulonephritis. J Am Soc Nephrol. 2009;20(4):843-51.
8. Allen PJ, Chadban SJ, Craig JC, Lim WH, Allen RDM, Clayton PA, et al. Recurrent glomerulonephritis after kidney transplantation: risk factors and allograft outcomes. Kidney Int. 2017;92(2):461-9.
9. Jiang SH, Kennard AL, Walters GD. Recurrent glomerulonephritis following renal transplantation and impact on graft survival. BMC Nephrol. 2018;19(1):344.
10. Odum J, Peh CA, Clarkson AR, Bannister KM, Seymour AE, Gillis D, et al. Recurrent mesangial IgA nephritis following renal transplantation. Nephrol Dial Transplant. 1994;9(3):309-12.
11. Berthelot L, Robert T, Vuiblet V, Tabary T, Braconnier A, Dramé M, et al. Recurrent IgA nephropathy is predicted by altered glycosylated IgA, autoantibodies and soluble CD89 complexes. Kidney Int. 2015;88(4):815-22.
12. Maixnerova D, Hruba P, Neprasova M, Bednarova K, Slatinska J, Suchanek M, et al. Outcome of 313 Czech patients with IgA nephropathy after renal transplantation. Front Immunol. 2021;12:726215.
13. Cazorla-López JM, Wu J, Villanego-Fernández F, Naranjo-Muñoz J, Vigara-Sánchez LA, García-García-Doncel A, et al. IgA nephropathy after renal transplant: recurrences and de novo cases. Transplant Proc. 2020;52(2):515-8.
14. Moroni G, Longhi S, Quaglini S, Gallelli B, Banfi G, Montagnino G, et al. The long-term outcome of renal transplantation of IgA nephropathy and the impact of recurrence on graft survival. Nephrol Dial Transplant. 2013;28(5): 1305-14.
15. Ponticelli C, Traversi L, Feliciani A, Cesana BM, Banfi G, Tarantino A. Kidney transplantation in patients with IgA mesangial glomerulonephritis. Kidney Int. 2001;60(5): 1948-54.
16. Nijim S, Vujjini V, Alasfar S, Luo X, Orandi B, Delp C, et al. Recurrent IgA nephropathy after kidney transplantation. Transplant Proc. 2016;48(8):2689-94.
17. Rodas LM, Ruiz-Ortiz E, Garcia-Herrera A, Pereira A, Blasco M, Ventura-Aguiar P, et al. IgA nephropathy recurrence after kidney transplantation: role of recipient age and human leukocyte antigen-B mismatch. Am J Nephrol. 2020;51(5):357-65.
18. Berthoux F, El Deeb S, Mariat C, Diconne E, Laurent B, Thibaudin L. Antithymocyte globulin (ATG) induction therapy and disease recurrence in renal transplant recipients with primary IgA nephropathy. Transplantation. 2008;85(10):1505-7.
19. Pascual J, Mezrich JD, Djamali A, Leverson G, Chin LT, Torrealba J, et al. Alemtuzumab induction and recurrence of glomerular disease after kidney transplantation. Transplantation. 2007;83(11):1429-34.
20. Sutherland S, Li L, Concepcion W, Salvatierra O, Sarwal MM. Steroid-free immunosuppression in pediatric renal transplantation: rationale for and [corrected] outcomes following conversion to steroid based therapy. Transplantation. 2009;87(11):1744-8.
21. Von Visger JR, Gunay Y, Andreoni KA, Bhatt UY, Nori US, Pesavento TE, et al. The risk of recurrent IgA nephropathy in a steroid-free protocol and other modifying immunosuppression. Clin Transplant. 2014;28(8):845-54.
22. Clayton P, McDonald S, Chadban S. Steroids and recurrent IgA nephropathy after kidney transplantation. Am J Transplant. 2011;11(8):1645-9.
23. Mulay AV, van Walraven C, Knoll GA. Impact of immunosuppressive medication on the risk of renal allograft failure due to recurrent glomerulonephritis. Am J Transplant. 2009;9(4):804-11.
24. Oka K, Imai E, Moriyama T, Akagi Y, Ando A, Hori M, et al. A clinicopathological study of IgA nephropathy in renal transplant recipients: beneficial effect of angiotensin-converting enzyme inhibitor. Nephrol Dial Transplant. 2000;15(5):689-95.
25. Hotta K, Fukasawa Y, Akimoto M, Tanabe T, Sasaki H, Fukuzawa N, et al. Tonsillectomy ameliorates histological damage of recurrent immunoglobulin A nephropathy after kidney transplantation. Nephrology (Carlton). 2013;18(12): 808-12.
26. Kennoki T, Ishida H, Yamaguchi Y, Tanabe K. Proteinuria-reducing effects of tonsillectomy alone in IgA nephropathy recurring after kidney transplantation. Transplantation. 2009;88(7):935-41.
27. Zagkotsis G, Vourlakou C, Paraskevopoulos A, Apostolou T. Recurrence of crescentic IgA nephropathy after renal transplantation. CEN Case Rep. 2018;7(2):268-73.
28. Tang Z, Ji S-M, Chen D-R, Wen J-Q, Chen J-S, Liu Z-H, et al. Recurrent or de novo IgA nephropathy with crescent formation after renal transplantation. Ren Fail. 2008;30(6):611-6.
29. Lafayette RA, Canetta PA, Rovin BH, Appel GB, Novak J, Nath KA, et al. A randomized, controlled trial of rituximab in IgA nephropathy with proteinuria and renal dysfunction. J Am Soc Nephrol. 2017;28(4):1306-13.

30. Courtney AE, McNamee PT, Nelson WE, Maxwell AP. Does angiotensin blockade influence graft outcome in renal transplant recipients with IgA nephropathy? Nephrol Dial Transplant. 2006;21(12):3550-4.
31. Ponticelli C, Moroni G, Glassock RJ. De novo glomerular diseases after renal transplantation. Clin J Am Soc Nephrol. 2014;9(8):1479-87.
32. Suzuki K, Honda K, Tanabe K, Toma H, Nihei H, Yamaguchi Y. Incidence of latent mesangial IgA deposition in renal allograft donors in Japan. Kidney Int. 2003;63(6):2286-94.
33. Hoyer JR, Vernier RL, Najarian JS, Raij L, Simmons RL, Michael AF. Recurrence of idiopathic nephrotic syndrome after renal transplantation. Lancet Lond Engl. 1972;2(7773): 343-8.
34. Vinai M, Waber P, Seikaly MG. Recurrence of focal segmental glomerulosclerosis in renal allograft: an in-depth review. Pediatr Transplant. 2010;14(3):314-25.
35. Bertelli R, Ginevri F, Caridi G, Dagnino M, Sandrini S, Di Duca M, et al. Recurrence of focal segmental glomerulosclerosis after renal transplantation in patients with mutations of podocin. Am J Kidney Dis. 2003;41(6):1314-21.
36. Newstead CG. Recurrent disease in renal transplants. Nephrol Dial Transplant. 2003;18(Suppl. 6):vi68-74.
37. Couser W. Recurrent glomerulonephritis in the renal allograft: an update of selected areas. Exp Clin Transplant. 2005;3(1):283-8.
38. Fuentes GMC, Meseguer CG, Carrion AP, Hijosa MM, Garcia-Pose A, Melgar AA, et al. Long-term outcome of focal segmental glomerulosclerosis after pediatric renal transplantation. Pediatr Nephrol. 2010;25(3):529-34.
39. Wei C, El Hindi S, Li J, Fornoni A, Goes N, Sageshima J, et al. Circulating urokinase receptor as a cause of focal segmental glomerulosclerosis. Nat Med. 2011;17(8):952-60.
40. McCarthy ET, Sharma M, Savin VJ. Circulating permeability factors in idiopathic nephrotic syndrome and focal segmental glomerulosclerosis. Clin J Am Soc Nephrol. 2010; 5(11):2115-21.
41. Delville M, Sigdel TK, Wei C, Li J, Hsieh S-C, Fornoni A, et al. A circulating antibody panel for pretransplant prediction of FSGS recurrence after kidney transplantation. Sci Transl Med. 2014;6(256):256ra136.
42. Ponticelli C. Recurrence of focal segmental glomerular sclerosis (FSGS) after renal transplantation. Nephrol Dial Transplant. 2010;25(1):25-31.
43. Chua AN, Alexander SR, Sarwal MM, Millan M, Salvatierra O, Yorgin PD. Proteinuria in pediatric renal transplant recipients during the first 60 post-transplant days. Pediatr Transplant. 2006;10(8):957-61.
44. Mizuiri S, Kawamura T, Miyagi M, Arai K, Sakai K, Aikawa A, et al. Post-transplant early recurrent proteinuria in patients with focal glomerulosclerosis—angiotensin II immunostaining and treatment outcome. Clin Transplant. 2005;19: 12-9.
45. D'Cunha PT, Parasuraman R, Venkat KK. Rapid resolution of proteinuria of native kidney origin following live donor renal transplantation. Am J Transplant. 2005;5(2):351-5.
46. Myslak M, Amer H, Morales P, Fidler ME, Gloor JM, Larson TS, et al. Interpreting post-transplant proteinuria in patients with proteinuria pre-transplant. Am J Transplant. 2006;6(7):1660-5.
47. Abbott KC, Sawyers ES, Oliver JD, Ko CW, Kirk AD, Welch PG, et al. Graft loss due to recurrent focal segmental glomerulosclerosis in renal transplant recipients in the United States. Am J Kidney Dis. 2001;37(2):366-73.
48. Cravedi P, Kopp JB, Remuzzi G. Recent progress in the pathophysiology and treatment of FSGS recurrence. Am J Transplant. 2013;13(2):266-74.
49. Fornoni A, Sageshima J, Wei C, Merscher-Gomez S, Aguillon-Prada R, Jauregui AN, et al. Rituximab targets podocytes in recurrent focal segmental glomerulosclerosis. Sci Transl Med. 2011;3(85):85ra46.
50. Andresdottir MB, Assmann KJ, Hoitsma AJ, Koene RA, Wetzels JF. Recurrence of type I membranoproliferative glomerulonephritis after renal transplantation: analysis of the incidence, risk factors, and impact on graft survival. Transplantation. 1997;63(11):1628-33.
51. Karakayali FY, Ozdemir H, Kivrakdal S, Colak T, Emiroğlu R, Haberal M. Recurrent glomerular diseases after renal transplantation. Transplant Proc. 2006;38(2):470-2.
52. O'Meara Y, Green A, Carmody M, Donohoe J, Campbell E, Browne O, et al. Recurrent glomerulonephritis in renal transplants: fourteen years' experience. Nephrol Dial Transplant. 1989;4(8):730-4.
53. Vangelista A, Frascà GM, Martella D, Bonomini V. Glomerulonephritis in renal transplantation. Nephrol Dial Transplant. 1990;5(Suppl. 1):42-6.
54. Lorenz EC, Sethi S, Leung N, Dispenzieri A, Fervenza FC, Cosio FG. Recurrent membranoproliferative glomerulonephritis after kidney transplantation. Kidney Int. 2010; 77(8):721-8.
55. Nasr SH, Sethi S, Cornell LD, Fidler ME, Boelkins M, Fervenza FC, et al. Proliferative glomerulonephritis with monoclonal IgG deposits recurs in the allograft. Clin J Am Soc Nephrol. 2011;6(1):122-32.
56. Nasr SH, Markowitz GS, Stokes MB, Seshan SV, Valderrama E, Appel GB, et al. Proliferative glomerulonephritis with monoclonal IgG deposits: a distinct entity mimicking immune-complex glomerulonephritis. Kidney Int. 2004;65(1):85-96.
57. Sumida K, Ubara Y, Marui Y, Nakamura M, Takaichi K, Tomikawa S, et al. Recurrent proliferative glomerulonephritis with monoclonal IgG deposits of IgG2λ subtype in a transplanted kidney: a case report. Am J Kidney Dis. 2013;62(3): 587-90.
58. Czarnecki PG, Lager DJ, Leung N, Dispenzieri A, Cosio FG, Fervenza FC. Long-term outcome of kidney transplantation in patients with fibrillary glomerulonephritis or monoclonal gammopathy with fibrillary deposits. Kidney Int. 2009;75(4): 420-7.
59. Lien YH, Scott K. Long-term cyclophosphamide treatment for recurrent type I membranoproliferative glomerulonephritis after transplantation. Am J Kidney Dis. 2000;35(3): 539-43.
60. Braun MC, Stablein DM, Hamiwka LA, Bell L, Bartosh SM, Strife CF. Recurrence of membranoproliferative glomerulonephritis type II in renal allografts: the North American Pediatric Renal Transplant Cooperative Study experience. J Am Soc Nephrol. 2005;16(7):2225-33.
61. Zand L, Lorenz EC, Cosio FG, Fervenza FC, Nasr SH, Gandhi MJ, et al. Clinical findings, pathology, and outcomes

of C3GN after kidney transplantation. J Am Soc Nephrol. 2014;25(5):1110-7.
62. Sethi S, Fervenza FC. Membranoproliferative glomerulonephritis—a new look at an old entity. N Engl J Med. 2012; 366(12):1119-31.
63. Moroni G, Casati C, Quaglini S, Gallelli B, Banfi G, Montagnino G, et al. Membranoproliferative glomerulonephritis type I in renal transplantation patients: a single-center study of a cohort of 68 renal transplants followed up for 11 years. Transplantation. 2011;91(11):1233-9.
64. Smith RJH, Alexander J, Barlow PN, Botto M, Cassavant TL, Cook HT, et al. New approaches to the treatment of dense deposit disease. J Am Soc Nephrol. 2007;18(9):2447-56.
65. Kashgary A, Sontrop JM, Li L, Al-Jaishi AA, Habibullah ZN, Alsolaimani R, et al. The role of plasma exchange in treating post-transplant focal segmental glomerulosclerosis: a systematic review and meta-analysis of 77 case-reports and case-series. BMC Nephrol. 2016;17(1):104.
66. Hickson LJ, Gera M, Amer H, Iqbal CW, Moore TB, Milliner DS, et al. Kidney transplantation for primary focal segmental glomerulosclerosis: outcomes and response to therapy for recurrence. Transplantation. 2009;87(8):1232-9.
67. Gohh RY, Yango AF, Morrissey PE, Monaco AP, Gautam A, Sharma M, et al. Preemptive plasmapheresis and recurrence of FSGS in high-risk renal transplant recipients. Am J Transplant. 2005;5(12):2907-12.
68. Canaud G, Dion D, Zuber J, Gubler M-C, Sberro R, Thervet E, et al. Recurrence of nephrotic syndrome after transplantation in a mixed population of children and adults: course of glomerular lesions and value of the Columbia classification of histological variants of focal and segmental glomerulosclerosis (FSGS). Nephrol Dial Transplant. 2010;25(4): 1321-8.
69. Salomon R, Gagnadoux M-F, Niaudet P. Intravenous cyclosporine therapy in recurrent nephrotic syndrome after renal transplantation in children. Transplantation. 2003;75(6): 810-4.
70. Sgambat K, Banks M, Moudgil A. Effect of galactose on glomerular permeability and proteinuria in steroid-resistant nephrotic syndrome. Pediatr Nephrol Berl Ger. 2013;28(11): 2131-5.
71. Audard V, Kamar N, Sahali D, Cardeau-Desangles I, Homs S, Remy P, et al. Rituximab therapy prevents focal and segmental glomerulosclerosis recurrence after a second renal transplantation. Transpl Int. 2012;25(5):e62-66.
72. Yu C-C, Fornoni A, Weins A, Hakroush S, Maiguel D, Sageshima J, et al. Abatacept in B7-1-positive proteinuric kidney disease. N Engl J Med. 2013;369(25):2416-23.
73. Wang C, Liverman RS, Garro R, George RP, Glumova A, Karp A, et al. Ofatumumab for the treatment of childhood nephrotic syndrome. Pediatr Nephrol Berl Ger. 2017;32(5):835-41.
74. Bernard J, Bruel A, Allain-Launay E, Dantal J, Roussey G. Ofatumumab in post-transplantation recurrence of a pediatric steroid-resistant idiopathic nephrotic syndrome. Pediatr Transplant. 2018;22(4):e13175.
75. Licht C, Weyersberg A, Heinen S, Stapenhorst L, Devenge J, Beck B, et al. Successful plasma therapy for atypical hemolytic uremic syndrome caused by factor H deficiency owing to a novel mutation in the complement cofactor protein domain 15. Am J Kidney Dis. 2005;45(2):415-21.
76. Saland JM, Ruggenenti P, Remuzzi G. Liver-kidney transplantation to cure atypical hemolytic uremic syndrome. J Am Soc Nephrol. 2009;20(5):940-9.
77. Cruzado JM, Carrera M, Torras J, Grinyó JM. Hepatitis C virus infection and de novo glomerular lesions in renal allografts. Am J Transplant. 2001;1(2):171-8.
78. Passerini P, Malvica S, Tripodi F, Cerutti R, Messa P. Membranous nephropathy (MN) recurrence after renal transplantation. Front Immunol. 2019;10:1326.
79. Tomas NM, Beck LH, Meyer-Schwesinger C, Seitz-Polski B, Ma H, Zahner G, et al. Thrombospondin type-1 domain-containing 7A in idiopathic membranous nephropathy. N Engl J Med. 2014;371(24):2277-87.
80. Debiec H, Lefeu F, Kemper MJ, Niaudet P, Deschênes G, Remuzzi G, et al. Early-childhood membranous nephropathy due to cationic bovine serum albumin. N Engl J Med. 2011;364(22):2101-10.
81. Dabade TS, Grande JP, Norby SM, Fervenza FC, Cosio FG. Recurrent idiopathic membranous nephropathy after kidney transplantation: a surveillance biopsy study. Am J Transplant. 2008;8(6):1318-22.
82. Grupper A, Cornell LD, Fervenza FC, Beck LH, Lorenz E, Cosio FG. Recurrent membranous nephropathy after kidney transplantation: treatment and long-term implications. Transplantation. 2016;100(12):2710-6.
83. Debiec H, Martin L, Jouanneau C, Dautin G, Mesnard L, Rondeau E, et al. Autoantibodies specific for the phospholipase A2 receptor in recurrent and de novo membranous nephropathy. Am J Transplant. 2011;11(10):2144-52.
84. El-Zoghby ZM, Grande JP, Fraile MG, Norby SM, Fervenza FC, Cosio FG. Recurrent idiopathic membranous nephropathy: early diagnosis by protocol biopsies and treatment with anti-CD20 monoclonal antibodies. Am J Transplant. 2009; 9(12):2800-7.
85. Ruggenenti P, Chiurchiu C, Brusegan V, Abbate M, Perna A, Filippi C, et al. Rituximab in idiopathic membranous nephropathy: a one-year prospective study. J Am Soc Nephrol. 2003;14(7):1851-7.
86. Fervenza FC, Abraham RS, Erickson SB, Irazabal MV, Eirin A, Specks U, et al. Rituximab therapy in idiopathic membranous nephropathy: a 2-year study. Clin J Am Soc Nephrol. 2010; 5(12):2188-98.
87. Dahan K, Debiec H, Plaisier E, Cachanado M, Rousseau A, Wakselman L, et al. Rituximab for severe membranous nephropathy: a 6-month trial with extended follow-up. J Am Soc Nephrol. 2017;28(1):348-58.
88. Barbari A, Chehadi R, Kfoury Assouf H, Kamel G, Jaafar M, Abdallah A, et al. Bortezomib as a novel approach to early recurrent membranous glomerulonephritis after kidney transplant refractory to combined conventional rituximab therapy. Exp Clin Transplant. 2017;15(3):350-4.
89. Sistani L, Dunér F, Udumala S, Hultenby K, Uhlen M, Betsholtz C, et al. Pdlim2 is a novel actin-regulating protein of podocyte foot processes. Kidney Int. 2011;80(10):1045-54.
90. Zarifian A, Meleg-Smith S, O'donovan R, Tesi RJ, Batuman V. Cyclosporine-associated thrombotic microangiopathy in renal allografts. Kidney Int. 1999;55(6):2457-66.
91. Reynolds JC, Agodoa LY, Yuan CM, Abbott KC. Thrombotic microangiopathy after renal transplantation in the United States. Am J Kidney Dis. 2003;42(5):1058-68.

92. Noris M, Remuzzi G. Glomerular diseases dependent on complement activation, including atypical hemolytic uremic syndrome, membranoproliferative glomerulonephritis, and C3 glomerulopathy: core curriculum 2015. Am J Kidney Dis. 2015;66(2):359-75.
93. Schwimmer J, Nadasdy TA, Spitalnik PF, Kaplan KL, Zand MS. De novo thrombotic microangiopathy in renal transplant recipients: a comparison of hemolytic uremic syndrome with localized renal thrombotic microangiopathy. Am J Kidney Dis. 2003;41(2):471-9.
94. Satoskar AA, Pelletier R, Adams P, Nadasdy GM, Brodsky S, Pesavento T, et al. De novo thrombotic microangiopathy in renal allograft biopsies-role of antibody-mediated rejection. Am J Transplant. 2010;10(8):1804-11.
95. Nadasdy T. Thrombotic microangiopathy in renal allografts: the diagnostic challenge. Curr Opin Organ Transplant. 2014; 19(3):283-92.
96. George JN, Nester CM. Syndromes of thrombotic microangiopathy. N Engl J Med. 2014;371(7):654-66.
97. Eremina V, Jefferson JA, Kowalewska J, Hochster H, Haas M, Weisstuch J, et al. VEGF inhibition and renal thrombotic microangiopathy. N Engl J Med. 2008;358(11):1129-36.
98. Bresin E, Daina E, Noris M, Castelletti F, Stefanov R, Hill P, et al. Outcome of renal transplantation in patients with non-Shiga toxin-associated hemolytic uremic syndrome: prognostic significance of genetic background. Clin J Am Soc Nephrol. 2006;1(1):88-99.
99. Zuber J, Le Quintrec M, Morris H, Frémeaux-Bacchi V, Loirat C, Legendre C. Targeted strategies in the prevention and management of atypical HUS recurrence after kidney transplantation. Transplant Rev. 2013;27(4):117-25.
100. Le Quintrec M, Lionet A, Kamar N, Karras A, Barbier S, Buchler M, et al. Complement mutation-associated de novo thrombotic microangiopathy following kidney transplantation. Am J Transplant. 2008;8(8):1694-701.
101. Nachman PH, Segelmark M, Westman K, Hogan SL, Satterly KK, Jennette JC, et al. Recurrent ANCA-associated small vessel vasculitis after transplantation: a pooled analysis. Kidney Int. 1999;56(4):1544-50.
102. Mojcik CF, Klippel JH. End-stage renal disease and systemic lupus erythematosus. Am J Med. 1996;101(1):100-7.
103. Stone JH, Amend WJ, Criswell LA. Outcome of renal transplantation in systemic lupus erythematosus. Semin Arthritis Rheum. 1997;27(1):17-26.
104. Goral S, Ynares C, Shappell SB, Snyder S, Feurer ID, Kazancioglu R, et al. Recurrent lupus nephritis in renal transplant recipients revisited: it is not rare. Transplantation. 2003;75(5):651-6.
105. Lionaki S, Skalioti C, Boletis JN. Kidney transplantation in patients with systemic lupus erythematosus. World J Transplant. 2014;4(3):176-82.
106. Hudson BG, Tryggvason K, Sundaramoorthy M, Neilson EG. Alport's syndrome, Goodpasture's syndrome, and type IV collagen. N Engl J Med. 2003;348(25):2543-56.

CHAPTER 15

Kidney Transplantation in Primary Hyperoxaluria

Susan Uthup

INTRODUCTION

Primary hyperoxalurias (PHs) are a rare group of autosomal recessive disorders characterized by abnormal hepatic glyoxylate metabolism leading to excessive hepatic production and accumulation of poorly soluble oxalate and glycolate. These get deposited as calcium oxalate in various organs and tissues. As oxalate is typically excreted in the urine, kidney becomes the prime target of injury. The insoluble glycolate and oxalate cause recurrent nephrolithiasis, nephrocalcinosis, progressive kidney damage, and end-stage kidney disease (ESKD). There are three types of PH. Primary hyperoxaluria type 1 (PH1) is the most common and severe form followed by PH2 and then PH3. The morbidity and mortality due to these disorders are quite high.

EPIDEMIOLOGY

Primary hyperoxaluria affects approximately 1 in 58,000 individuals worldwide. The prevalence is approximately 3 in 1,000,000.[1] Type 1, the most common form, accounts for 80% cases. Types 2 and 3 account for about 10% of cases each.

OXALATE METABOLISM

Oxalate is synthesized in the liver from its main precursor glyoxylate. Three primary steps are involved in oxalate production. In the mitochondria, hydroxyproline from collagen is converted to 4-hydroxy-2-oxoglutarate (HOG). It is then converted into glyoxylate and pyruvate by 4-hydroxy-2-oxoglutarate aldolase (HOGA1). In peroxisomes, pyruvate and glycine are formed by transamination of glyoxylate and L-alanine by alanine-glyoxylate aminotransferase (AGT). Pyridoxine acts as the cofactor in the AGT pathway. Peroxisomal cytosolic enzyme glyoxylate reductase/hydroxypyruvate reductase/deglycerate dehydrogenase (GRHPR) converts glyoxylate to glycolate. In the cytosol, glyoxylate can be converted into insoluble oxalate by lactate dehydrogenase (LDH). Hepatic peroxisomal AGT diverts glyoxylate from oxalate production pathway. Deficiency in AGT or GRHPR leads to the accumulation of glyoxylate in the cytosol and its increased conversion into oxalate by LDH. Oxalate is an end product of metabolism and is not degradable by any known biologic system in humans. Elimination of oxalate depends almost entirely on renal excretion. Oxalate is freely filtered and then undergoes bidirectional transport along the renal tubule, the major role being played by the proximal tubule. The upper limit of normal for urinary oxalate secretion is approximately 0.5 mmol/24 hours. Elevated urinary oxalate levels can also result from excessive intake of oxalate-rich food such as chocolate, cocoa, leafy green vegetables, black teas, nuts and peanut butter (dietary oxaluria), gastrointestinal disorders that can lead to malabsorption such as small bowel disease, or cystic fibrosis or absence of intestinal oxalate degrading bacteria (*Oxalobacter formigenes*) (enteric oxaluria).

PATHOGENESIS

In deficiency in AGT or GRHPR, there will be an increase in the glyoxylate pool. LDH converts glyoxylate to oxalate and glycolate. The relatively insoluble calcium oxalate salt crystallizes in body fluids and tissues whenever and wherever the solubility product is exceeded. The urinary excretion of oxalate is increased, and calcium oxalate supersaturation in the hypertonic interstitium of the renal medulla leads to crystal aggregation. Crystals that get attached to proximal tubular epithelial cells will be transported to the renal interstitium via transcytosis. This leads to crystal deposition, inflammation, necrosis, and nephrocalcinosis. Crystals not absorbed initially continue traveling through the nephron and lead to crystal aggregation and nephrolithiasis.

In the most severe form of PH1, urinary oxalate excretion exceeds 1 mmol/1.73 m^2/day (normal <0.5 mmol/1.73 m^2/day). Progressive renal parenchymal inflammation and fibrosis lead to ESKD. Infection and obstruction from kidney stones also contribute to renal damage. There is rapid progression to ESKD by young adulthood in 50%

of affected persons.[1,2] Plasma oxalate levels increase as the glomerular filtration rate (GFR) falls below 30–40 mL/min/1.73 m^2. The supersaturation threshold for calcium oxalate in plasma is 30 µmol/L. When oxalate levels exceed this threshold, systemic oxalosis results. Calcium oxalate gets deposited in tissues such as retina, myocardium, vessel walls, skin, bone, and brain.

CLASSIFICATION

Three types of PH have been well described.

1. *Primary hyperoxaluria type 1* (*PH1*) is the most common and severe form that accounts for 70–80% cases. It is due to deficiency or mistargeting of the liver-specific peroxisomal enzyme AGT, a pyridoxal 5'-phosphate (PLP)-dependent enzyme required for the transamination of glyoxylate to glycine. PH1 manifests as infantile oxalosis with severe renal insufficiency and calcified kidney **(Figs. 1A and B)** in early infancy or more commonly as recurrent urolithiasis, nephrocalcinosis, and ESRD by the second or third decade of life.[3] PH1 is due to mutations in *AGXT*. *AGXT* gene that encodes the hepatic peroxisomal enzyme AGT is located at the tip of the long arm of chromosome 2 (2q36-37). The defects in the gene maybe single nucleotide substitutions (75%) including missense, nonsense, and splice-site mutations or deletions or insertions. This causes a major deficiency of the enzyme or complete loss of its activity. In 15%, immunoreactive AGT protein is present but the catalytic activity is lacking. In the mistargeting phenotype where AGT is localized in the mitochondria instead of in the peroxisomes, the protein and catalytic activity both will be 50% below normal values.
2. *Primary hyperoxaluria type 2* (*PH2*) (10%) is less severe than PH1 and accounts for about 10% of cases. It is caused by deficiency of peroxisomal cytosolic enzyme glyoxylate reductase/hydroxypyruvate reductase/deglycerate dehydrogenase (*GRHPR*), which normally converts glyoxylate to glycolate. The accumulated glyoxylate and hydroxypyruvate are converted by LDH to oxalate and L-glycerate. These metabolites are excreted in excessive amounts in the urine resulting in hyperoxaluria and recurrent urolithiasis. PH2 is due to variants of *GRHPR* gene on chromosome 9p11 and the most common one is deletion of a single base pair in exon 2 that encodes *GRHPR*.[4]
3. *Primary hyperoxaluria type 3* (*PH3*) (5%) is the least severe form due to a deficiency of liver-specific mitochondrial enzyme 4-hydroxy-2-oxoglutarate aldolase (HOGA). It is due to mutation involving *HOGA1* gene located on chromosome 10. It encodes the liver-specific mitochondrial hydroxy-oxoglutarate aldolase enzyme that catalyzes the cleavage of HOG to pyruvate and glyoxylate hypercalciuria and recurrent nephrolithiasis is the typical presentation. PH3 is due to mutations in *HOGA1* (PH3) gene.[4,5]

ACQUIRED (SECONDARY) HYPEROXALURIA

Hyperoxaluria may also be an acquired (secondary) phenomenon due to increased oxalate absorption from the intestine known as enteric hyperoxaluria (EH) or ingestion of oxalate or its precursors. Intake of drugs such as methoxyflurane or toxins such as ethylene glycol (antifreeze) that are metabolized to oxalate can cause marked hyperoxaluria and can result in acute renal failure. Pyridoxine deficiency may also result in secondary hyperoxaluria.

Enteric hyperoxaluria is due to intestinal malabsorption with a resultant increased absorption of oxalate in the colon. This can occur in various circumstances such as small bowel resection, small bowel bypass for obesity, primary small bowel disease with malabsorption, chronic pancreatitis, and

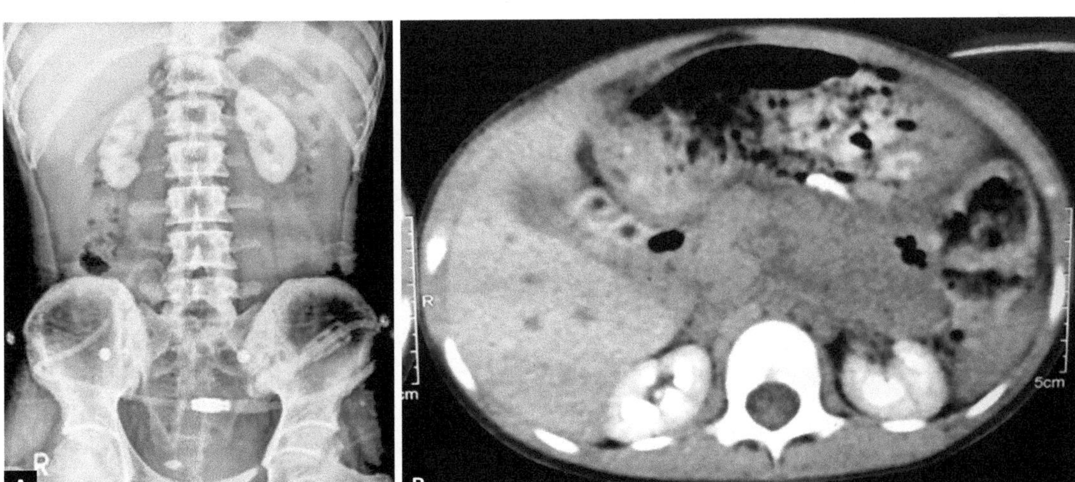

Figs. 1A and B: (A) Plain X-ray kidney, ureter, and bladder (KUB) in an infant showing bilateral nephrocalcinosis and vertebral osteosclerosis; (B) Noncontrast computed tomography (CT) abdomen showing calcified kidneys in a 4-year-old child with primary hyperoxaluria type 1 (PH1).

liver diseases such as cirrhosis. EH is the most common cause of moderate hyperoxaluria in adults.[6,7]

CLINICAL FEATURES

Primary Hyperoxaluria Type 1

Primary hyperoxaluria type 1 is the most severe and common form of hyperoxaluria. There is early progression to ESKD in affected individuals, though there may be marked heterogeneity in disease expression. Based on the age of manifestation, there are five different presentations of PH1. Infantile oxalosis (26%) presents before 6 months of age with severe renal failure and nephrocalcinosis **(Figs. 1A and B)**. 30% present in childhood with recurrent stones, obstruction, infection, and acute kidney injury (AKI). With the relief of obstruction, there maybe a partial recovery but the progression to ESKD will be rapid. 30% present in young adults with recurrent kidney stones. 10% present in ESKD and will be diagnosed with post-transplant disease recurrence. In 10–15%, the diagnosis was made after family screening.[8]

Systemic Oxalosis

When GFR falls below 30 mL/min/1.73 m^2, oxalate accumulates in the blood and gets deposited in various organs and tissues. The clinical features are due to involvement of various organ systems. In patients on dialysis especially for more than a year, bone pain and spontaneous fractures are common. Digital gangrene may occur due to oxalate deposition in vessels. Difficulties may occur with establishing and maintaining vascular access for hemodialysis (HD). Hypothyroidism, peripheral neuropathy, livedo reticularis, peripheral gangrene, calcinosis cutis and dental involvement with tooth pain, root resorption, and pulp exposure are other systemic manifestations of hyperoxaluria.

Primary Hyperoxaluria Type 2

It is usually a milder disease with slower progression. Patients with PH2 typically present in the first two decades of life with urolithiasis. Urine oxalate excretion tends to be lower compared to patients with PH1. The disease manifests in childhood or young adulthood with kidney stones and its complications such as infection or obstruction. 25% may progress to ESKD by the third or fourth decade of life.

Primary Hyperoxaluria Type 3

Primary hyperoxaluria type 3 is typically present in early childhood with recurrent nephrolithiasis, hematuria, obstruction, and infection.

DIAGNOSIS

The diagnosis of PH is made by systemic evaluation based on clinical suspicion or family screening. Patients with recurrent kidney stones, nephrocalcinosis with or without reduction in GFR, or dumbbell-shaped calcium oxalate monohydrate crystals (whewellite) in the urine should be evaluated for PH. Sometimes, the clinical presentation will be unexplained severe renal failure, and a renal biopsy done will show deposition of colorless oxalate crystals in the renal tubules suggestive of hyperoxaluria **(Figs. 2A and B)**. These crystals will be birefringent on polarized light **(Fig. 3)**.

If the GFR is normal, the diagnosis is strongly suggested by a 24-hour urine oxalate value of >1 mmol (90 mg)/1.73 m^2/day and an elevated urine glycolate. Normal urinary oxalate excretion is <0.5 mmol/1.73 m^2/day (45 mg/1.73 m^2/day). In PH types 1 and 2, urinary excretion of oxalate will be as high as 1.5–3 mmol/1.73 m^2/day (135–270 mg/1.73 m^2/day).

In dietary hyperoxaluria and EH, urinary oxalate excretion is elevated, but these levels are usually typically below 1 mmol/day (90 mg/day).

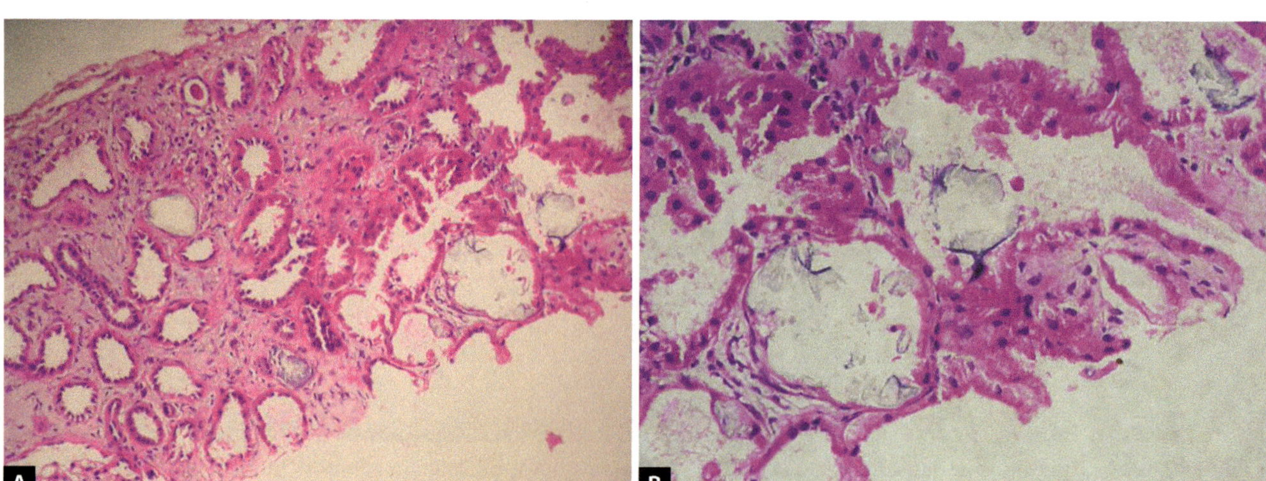

Figs. 2A and B: Renal histology H and E stain—tubular oxalate crystal deposition suggestive of hyperoxaluria.

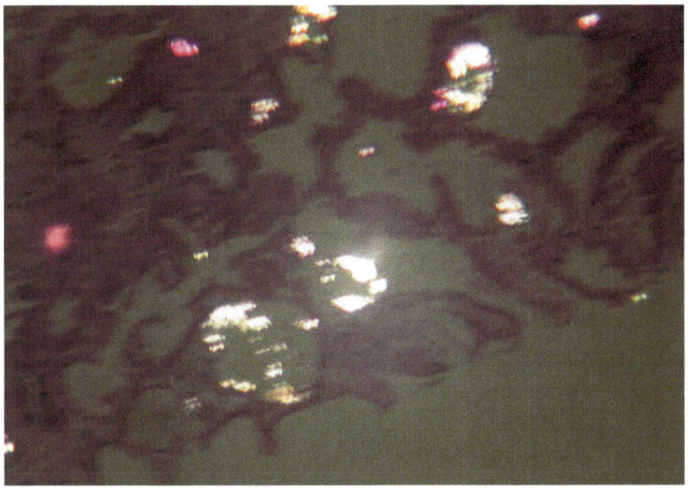

Fig. 3: Birefringent fan-shaped calcium oxalate crystal deposition in renal tubules in hyperoxaluria.

TABLE 1: Normative values for oxalate:creatinine (mmol/mmol) in different age groups.

Age	*Oxalate:creatinine (mmol/mmol)*
Infants <6 months	<0.32–0.36
6 months to 2 years	<0.13–0.17
2–5 years	<0.098–0.1
6–12 years	<0.07–0.08
>16 years	<0.04

In infants and small children, 24-hour urine collection is difficult and hence, an oxalate:creatinine ratio in spot urine samples is used to screen for hyperoxaluria. The normative values for oxalate:creatinine (mmol/mmol) in different age groups are given in **Table 1**.

Urinary oxalate measurements may be falsely low in patients with kidney failure. Plasma oxalate levels may be useful as is an inverse relation between plasma oxalate and kidney function in the early stages of chronic kidney disease (CKD). Plasma oxalate concentration remains normal as long as the GFR is >40 mL/min/1.73 m^2. When GFR is low, increased plasma oxalate and glycolate concentrations support the diagnosis of PH. There will be dense nephrocalcinosis visible on plain X-ray of the kidneys in children who present in severe kidney failure due to PH **(Figs. 1A and B)**.

Metabolic evaluation is helpful in the differentiation between three types of PH. In PH type 1, urinary excretion of glycolate is increased. In PH type 2, L-glyceric acid and in PH type 3, the HOG level is elevated. In recent years, molecular studies have replaced other evaluations. In the past when genetic studies were not universal, the diagnosis of PH types 1 and 2 was confirmed by a liver biopsy demonstrating absent or significantly reduced AGT or GRHPR activity. Quantification of enzymatic activity, an immunoblot to analyze the protein, and an immunoelectronic examination of these enzymes can be done. Now genetic studies have replaced such invasive investigations and confirmation is by genetic testing for any of three known causative genes (*AGXT*, *GRHPR*, and *HOGA1*). Prenatal diagnosis is also possible by the analysis of deoxyribonucleic acid (DNA) from chorionic villi or amniotic cells.

Once the diagnosis is confirmed, further evaluation is mandatory to assess the impact of oxalate on various systems. The evaluation should include a complete hemogram, thyroid function tests, X-ray of long bones, slit-lamp examination, cardiac assessment including electrocardiogram (ECG) and echocardiography, and assessment of GFR.

MANAGEMENT

The aim of medical management is to reduce calcium oxalate excretion in urine as soon as possible so as to preserve renal function and minimize nonrenal sequels. Traditionally available treatment in this regard is limited and includes supplementation of high-dose pyridoxine, potassium citrate, and neutral phosphates. In ESKD, initiation of dialysis followed by combined liver and kidney transplantation is the treatment option and is associated with many potential complications, including operative risks, graft rejection, and post-transplant organ failure, as well as the need for lifelong immunosuppression.[9]

Recent research on the molecular basis of oxalate production has led to the development of newer strategies for the management of this disease. New therapeutics specifically target the oxalate synthetic pathways and reduce the production and accumulation of oxalate in the plasma and tissues. These include substrate reduction therapy (SRT), chaperone therapy, enzyme restoration therapy, intestinal oxalate degradation, and targeting of the inflammasome. Currently, available treatment modalities and the recent advances in the therapeutic paradigms for PHs will be discussed below.

Aggressive Fluid Therapy

An aggressive increase in fluid intake (>2–3 L/day/1.73 m^2) is ensured to decrease tubular fluid oxalate concentration and diminish intratubular oxalate deposition. The goal is to maintain urinary oxalate concentration below 0.4 µmol/L throughout the entire 24-hour day. As infants and small children cannot achieve this high-fluid intake, nasogastric tube or placement of gastrostomy maybe needed.

Restriction of Dietary Oxalate

Diet rich in oxalate such as tea, chocolate, spinach, and rhubarb is avoided in PH though dietary oxalate contributes to <5% of oxalate in urine. Most of the oxalate is from an endogenous source, and these dietary measures are of little help.

High-dose Pyridoxine

Pyridoxal 5'-phosphate, the natural cofactor of AGT, is an excellent chaperone that acts on protein stability, catalytic activity, and peroxisomal import of AGT. Approximately 10–30% of patients with PH type 1 will respond to pyridoxine therapy with a significant reduction of urinary oxalate excretion. There is a strong genotype–phenotype correlation in responsiveness, which mainly occurs in patients with the *Gly170Arg* and *Phe152Ile* mutations.[8]

The most common mutation in the *AGXT* gene, *p.Gly170Arg*, leads to the mistargeting of misfolded AGT (AGT-LRM) to the mitochondria. Treatment with high-dose vitamin B6 increases cytosolic PLP and can partially restore the peroxisomal targeting of AGT. Pyridoxine increases the expression, catalytic activity and peroxisomal import of AGT, restoring the function of the enzyme lost in PH1.[10] It is started at a dose of 5–7 mg/kg/day and then slowly increased to a maximum daily dose of 20 mg/kg. Pyridoxine is not effective in patients with PH2.

INCREASED URINARY PHOSPHATE, CITRATE, AND MAGNESIUM CONCENTRATION

Pyrophosphate, citrate, potassium, and magnesium are inhibitors of calcium oxalate precipitation in urine. Neutral phosphate (orthophosphate), 30–40 mg/kg with a maximum dose of 60 mg/kg/day, potassium citrate–citric acid (0.15 g/kg), and/or magnesium oxide (500 mg/day/m^2) are commonly prescribed to treat kidney stone disease. They inhibit crystallization by maintaining urine pH above 7. In patients with lower GFR who are at risk for hyperkalemia, sodium citrate can be used. Orthophosphates (neutral phosphates) reduce calcium oxalate crystallization and delay stone formation in patients with PH. Orthophosphate should be avoided if GFR is <30 mL/min/1.73 m^2 to prevent phosphate accumulation and exacerbation of secondary hyperparathyroidism.[11]

Oxalobacter formigenes enhance oxalate elimination by the gastrointestinal tract which is another potential method in reducing tissue and body oxalate levels. One proposed mechanism is the administration of *O. formigenes*, an obligate anaerobic colonic bacterium that promotes endogenous oxalate intestinal excretion. No serious adverse effects were reported. However, *O. formigenes* therapy is not routinely administered until there is compelling evidence that it can effectively and safely prevent or slow the progression of ESKD in patients with PH.[12]

RECENT ADVANCES IN MEDICAL MANAGEMENT

New therapeutic options have been developed in recent years that target oxalate synthesis and metabolism, thus decreasing the production, accumulation, and deposition of plasma oxalate in the body **(Table 2)**. The trials are underway and some molecules have completed the phase 3 trial and will possibly revolutionize the management of PH.[3] The drugs that have been clinically tested maybe classified as follows:

- Substrate reduction therapy that targets the key enzymes in oxalate production
- Intestinal oxalate degradation using oral enzymes or probiotics
- Chaperone therapy for misfolded proteins.

TABLE 2: Targeted treatment in primary hyperoxaluria.

Treatment	*Drug*	*Mechanism*
Substrate reduction therapy	• Lumasiran • Nedosiran • Stiripentol • CHK-336	• Glycolate oxidase inhibition • Lactate dehydrogenase (LDH) inhibition • LDH inhibition • LDH inhibition
Restoration of functional enzyme conformation	• Pyridoxine • Betaine	Protein-folding chaperones
Intestinal oxalate degradation	• Oxabact • Nephure • Oxazyme • Reloxaliase	• Probiotics • Oral enzyme therapy

Substrate Reduction Therapy

Substrate reduction therapy is a definitive therapeutic approach in the treatment of metabolic disorders by targeting key enzymes involved in the metabolic pathway. The ideal SRT should target a key step in the pathway, and the inhibition of the target should be associated with minimal off-target adverse effects. Glycolate oxidase and LDH are two such target enzymes in the oxalate-synthetic pathway that can be targeted in the treatment of PH.[3]

Ribonucleic Acid Interference Agents

Ribonucleic acid interference (RNAi) agents are a group of drugs that silences liver-specific glycolate oxidase enzyme and deplete glyoxylate—the substrate for oxalate synthesis in the hepatocyte peroxisomal compartment. RNAi therapeutic strategies for PH1 are particularly attractive because these compounds can be delivered easily to the liver. As the metabolic defect in PH is localized to the liver, the current treatment strategies necessitate liver transplantation (LT) for a cure. The direct hepatic delivery and action of RNAi agents will revolutionize the treatment of PH negating the need for transplantation in the future.[13]

Lumasiran is an RNAi therapeutic agent that silences glycolate oxidase enzyme. In 2020, the US Food and Drug Administration approved lumasiran as the initial therapy for PH1 based on phase 3 trials on PH1 patients including children below 6 years. Lumasiran downregulates glycolate oxidase and reduces glyoxylate production and, ultimately, oxalate synthesis. It causes a >50% reduction in urinary oxalate excretion.

ILLUMINATE-A trial is a multinational double-blind, placebo-controlled study done on genetically confirmed PH1 patients who had a variable degree of kidney impairment [estimated GFR (eGFR) ≥30 mL/min/1.73 m^2]. The drug is administered subcutaneously over a 6-month period. ILLUMINATE-A phase 3 trial of lumasiran showed an impressive reduction in urinary oxalate excretion in PH1.[14]

There are no significant short-term adverse effects. However, long-term follow-up is needed to assess the impact on progression to ESKD as well as to assess long-term side effects. If future trials also demonstrate that lumasiran can prevent and potentially reverse systemic oxalosis in patients with kidney failure, it could represent the beginning of a new era in the treatment of PH1, thereby ending the need for LT sacrificing a fully functional liver with only one metabolic defect.[15,16] The major drawback of lumasiran is the very high cost.[14,17,18]

Nedosiran is a second-generation RNAi agent targeting the messenger RNA (mRNA) encoding hepatic LDH. It may be a safe therapeutic option for the treatment of all types of PH. Phase 3 trial is currently underway.[19]

Dequalinium chloride (DECA) may be beneficial as it may restore normal peroxisomal trafficking of AGT, thereby inhibiting the misdirected AGT transport into the mitochondria. Stiripentol (Diacomit) is an antiepileptic drug initially used for Dravet syndrome. It is a potent inhibitor of LDH and may be useful in PH to reduce the oxalate levels.[20-22]

Intestinal Oxalate Degradation Using Oral Enzymes or Probiotics

Intestinal degradation of oxalate may help to decrease oxalate absorption, thus reducing plasma and urine oxalate levels. Probiotic administration and oral enzyme administration have been tried in this regard. Natural intestinal bacterial flora like *O. formigenes* consumes oxalate as an energy source. *O. formigenes*-derived bioactive factors have been tried as a novel therapeutic for the prevention and/or treatment of hyperoxaluria.[23-25]

Oxalate-degrading enzymes have also been tried as an alternative strategy for intestinal oxalate removal. These enzymes are purified from nonhuman sources and oral administration causes degradation of intestinal oxalate in a safe and tolerable manner. Oxalate decarboxylase (OxDC) is an enzyme that converts oxalate into formate and carbon dioxide. It is purified from fungi and bacteria and is available in multiple formulations (Nephure, Oxazyme).[3]

Urological Interventions

Intervention is required when stones obstruct the urinary tract. Nephrostomy, ureteroscopy, and ureteral JJ stent are preferred interventions for stone removal. Open surgical removal may precipitate acute renal failure. Extracorporeal shock wave lithotripsy (ESWL) is not preferred in PH as calcium oxalate stones are resistant to fragmentation by ESWL. The concomitant nephrocalcinosis makes imaging interpretation challenging and may lead to unnecessary delivery of shock waves. Also, ESWL may harm the kidney because of nephrocalcinosis and microlithiasis. Thus, endoscopic techniques are considered better than ESWL. Repeated surgical interventions may also contribute to renal injury and ESKD.[26]

KIDNEY REPLACEMENT THERAPY IN PRIMARY HYPEROXALURIA

Dialysis

More than 50% of babies with infantile oxalosis present with ESKD. More than 80% of children will need renal replacement by the age of 3 years. Older children may preserve kidney function till adulthood if aggressively managed. Aggressive and intensive dialysis therapy should be started as there is a high risk of systemic oxalosis once ESKD is reached. The daily oxalate production is 3,500–7,500 μmol. Maximal oxalate elimination by conventional HD and peritoneal dialysis (PD) is approximately 950–1,440 μmol, respectively. Predialysis plasma oxalate (POx) level ranges between 100 and 200 μmol/L. Conventional HD reduces oxalate levels by 60–80%. But plasma oxalate returns to 80% of the predialysis value within 24 hours and 95% at 48 hours after dialysis. Thus, the oxalate levels always exceed the supersaturation threshold of 30 μmol/L in the interdialytic period. Intensive 5-hour daily HD sessions using high-flux dialyzers, nocturnal HD, or a combination of HD and PD in small children maybe more efficient compared to longer, thrice-weekly regimens.[27-30]

Transplantation Strategies

The transplantation strategies include combined LKT, sequential liver-kidney transplant, and isolated liver transplant followed by isolated kidney transplant (IKT). Management of children with PH should be individualized with respect to the timing of the transplantation and the type of graft. The most important parameters to be considered when deciding on transplantation are age and weight at presentation, duration on dialysis, and availability of size-matched graft. Preemptive transplantation should be considered as a viable option for a better long-term outcome.[30,31]

The optimum transplantation strategy is a combined LKT when the GFR falls below 40 mL/min/1.73 m^2 before marked tissue oxalate deposition occurs.[31-33] Sequential LKT (first liver followed by the kidney) is the optimum strategy in small children with CKD stage 5 as the combined procedure may not be feasible due to medical and anatomical reasons.

Initial LT coupled with intensive dialysis will allow the removal of tissue oxalate. After sequential transplantation too, the medical management should be continued till the urinary oxalate excretion returns to normal. However, the outcome is not superior and the optimum strategy remains controversial. Bilateral native nephrectomy at the time of transplantation also reduces the oxalate load. The recurrence of oxalate nephropathy in the kidney allograft remains a concern even after the correction of the metabolic defect.[33-38]

Preemptive LT when GFR is between 40 and 60 mL/min/1.73 m^2 is curative as it corrects the underlying enzymatic defect. The correction of metabolic defects demands complete removal of the native liver and orthotopic transplantation. Though the native liver is otherwise normal, any remaining defective hepatic cells with reduced or absent AGT enzyme activity will continue to produce large amounts of oxalate.[31,32]

Isolated kidney transplant results are suboptimal as the enzyme defect is not corrected. There will be oxalate deposition and failure of the allograft. It maybe considered as an option in patients who respond to pyridoxine therapy, but the graft survival is poor. Patients with PH who are homozygous for the G170R mutation of AGXT can maintain near-normal urine oxalate excretion rates for many years post-transplant while on pyridoxine treatment. Unlike AGT, which is found exclusively in hepatocytes, the deficient GRHPR enzyme in type 2 hyperoxaluria is found in multiple body tissues. So, IKT is the recommended approach in PH2.[30,36]

Timing of Transplant

In the infantile form of PH1, the presentation will be in the first few months of life with kidney failure. The tissue oxalate load will be high and often dialysis is started immediately after birth. A combined LKT though indicated is often not feasible due to the difficulty in obtaining size-matched liver and kidney in time, technical difficulties associated with limited abdominal space for the transplanted organs, and the high risk of infectious complications. Often, the time on dialysis is prolonged. The morbidity and mortality are high due to rising oxalate load. Delaying the transplant until these babies achieve at least 7 kg is a rational approach. Performing a segmental LT from a living donor and then subsequently a kidney from a deceased or a living donor several months later is an optimal strategy in some children. While waiting for a KT after LT, the PD is resumed early. Surgical techniques are streamlined so that intestinal manipulation will be minimum and antiadhesive materials will be used. The patency of the PD catheter is also ensured by using a heparin lock solution. The LT-related complications such as biliary leak or stricture, bleeding, and vessel thrombosis may also complicate the graft function.[37,38]

Pretransplant Evaluation

Recognition of PH before transplantation is important in view of the intensive treatment strategies that may be instituted for preserving native kidney function, minimizing systemic oxalosis, and identifying the need for combined or sequential LKT. Also, decisions regarding allograft protective strategies post-op including continuation of dialysis, high-volume diuresis, and use of inhibitors of calcium oxalate crystallization maybe taken. PH should be considered as the native kidney disease in all transplant candidates with recurrent calcium oxalate stones, nephrocalcinosis, or interstitial renal disease of undetermined etiology. Molecular genotyping helps to confirm the disease and plan strategies for individual patients.

When living donor liver transplantation (LDLT) is considered, the heterozygous carriers of PH are not considered as donors due to the decreased enzyme function. In CLKT, if both organs are from the same donor, the acute rejection rate will be low. The kidney graft function and survival will be better when compared with isolated KT or LT. This immune-protective effect is due to human leukocyte antigens (HLA) produced by the transplanted liver allograft which could neutralize circulating alloantibodies. Soluble HLA delivered by the liver allograft could inhibit natural killer and cytotoxic T cells. Kupffer cells and biliary epithelial cells from the liver allograft also demonstrate an ability to clear circulating antigens.[37]

Oxalate Reduction Strategies Before and After Transplant

Prior to transplantation, strategies should be instituted to reduce tissue oxalate stores and protect the allograft from oxalate-mediated injury. These strategies include aggressive medical management (high fluid intake and the administration of neutral phosphate, potassium citrate–citric acid, and/or magnesium oxide), administration of pyridoxine in responsive patients, and intensified dialysis to achieve reduction in oxalate stores.

In PH1 patients on dialysis and RNAi, POx levels are maintained at <20 mmol/L before considering KT. Intensive 5-hour daily HD sessions using high-flux dialyzers, nocturnal HD, hemodiafiltration, or a combination of HD and PD are instituted to maintain the interdialytic plasma oxalate level below 30–45 mmol/L, the threshold of calcium oxalate supersaturation. In the post-transplant period, dialysis is continued. After correcting the metabolic defect, conventional HD could be sufficient to maintain POx values <20 mmol/L.

After the transplant, urinary oxalate excretion is monitored and the medical management is discontinued when it returns to normal.[30-32] After transplantation whether combined, sequential LKT, or an isolated transplant, systemic oxalate from tissue stores is mobilized and there is a risk of oxalate deposition in the renal parenchyma. So the recipient should be closely monitored. The hydration status should be optimized as to maintain a high urine volume. Medications inhibiting oxalate crystal formation should be continued. Daily HD is continued until the renal clearance maintains POx well below 30 μmol/L. It takes years for the oxalate levels in urine to return to normal, and the kidney allograft may still be at risk for oxalosis. Thus after kidney transplantation also, it is essential to closely monitor oxalate levels in both plasma and urine. Hyperhydration and treatment with crystallization inhibitors also should be continued to protect the new kidney allograft from oxalate deposition until normalization of oxalate levels. Pyridoxine supplementation can be discontinued at the time of LT, since normal AGT activity will have been restored.[38,39]

POST-TRANSPLANT OUTCOME IN PRIMARY HYPEROXALURIA

Early diagnosis, genetic testing, supportive therapy, intensified dialysis followed by LKT, and perioperative management targeted to protect the allograft from oxalate-mediated injury have improved the outcome of PH over the years.[40] The United States Renal Data System shows 3- and 5-year death-censored graft survival of 95 and 78% after combined LKT, respectively.[40] European experience demonstrated 1-, 3- and 5-year kidney graft survivals after combined LKT in PH1 children of 82, 79, and 76%, respectively.[41] French experience shows a 10-year kidney graft survival of 87%.[42]

CONCLUSION

Though the overall outcome in patients with PH has improved substantially over the past decade, significant challenges still remain. A high index of suspicion and appropriate diagnostic evaluation is required for timely recognition of PH prior to transplantation in patients presenting with ESKD at any age. Nephrocalcinosis and/or a history of calcium stone disease are usually clues for targeted testing and treatment. Detection of the genotype in PH is important in making decisions regarding kidney alone versus combined liver and kidney transplantation. Since hyperoxaluria often persists for years following correction of the metabolic defect, timely diagnosis pretransplant coupled with preventive strategies is required to protect the kidney allograft from oxalate-mediated injury. Protection of the kidney allograft from oxalate injury remains crucial in deciding the long-term outcome. Small interfering RNA (siRNA) strategies to prevent oxalate-related damage in PH1 have shown positive results in recent trials. Initiation of these molecules pretransplant will reduce the risk of recurrence in the future. Genetic counseling and prenatal diagnosis in familial cases definitely will help in the primary prevention of this disorder associated with high morbidity and mortality.

REFERENCES

1. Hopp K, Cogal AG, Bergstralh EJ, Seide BM, Olson JB, Meek AM, et al. Phenotype-genotype correlations and estimated carrier frequencies of primary hyperoxaluria. J Am Soc Nephrol. 2015;26:2559-70.
2. Hoppe B, Beck BB, Milliner DS. The primary hyperoxalurias. Kidney Int. 2009;75:1264.
3. Shee K, Stoller ML. Perspectives in primary hyperoxaluria—historical, current and future clinical interventions. Nat Rev Urol. 2022;19(3):137-46.
4. Edvardsson VO, Goldfarb DS, Lieske JC, Beara-Lasic L, Anglani F, Milliner DS, et al. Hereditary causes of kidney stones and chronic kidney disease. Pediatr Nephrol. 2013; 28(10):1923-42.
5. Danpure CJ. Advances in the enzymology and molecular genetics of primary hyperoxaluria type 1. Prospects for gene therapy. Nephrol Dial Transplant. 1995;10(Suppl. 8):24.
6. Hoppe B, Langman CB. A United States survey on diagnosis, treatment, and outcome of primary hyperoxaluria. Pediatr Nephrol. 2003;18:986.
7. Sas DJ, Enders FT, Mehta RA, Tang X, Zhao F, Seide BM, et al. Clinical features of genetically confirmed patients with primary hyperoxaluria identified by clinical indication versus familial screening. Kidney Int. 2020;97:786.
8. Harambat J, Fargue S, Acquaviva C, Gagnadoux MF, Janssen F, Liutkus A, et al. Genotype-phenotype correlation in primary hyperoxaluria type 1: the p.Gly170Arg AGXT mutation is associated with a better outcome. Kidney Int. 2010;77:443.
9. Hulton SA. The primary hyperoxalurias: a practical approach to diagnosis and treatment. Int J Surg. 2016;36:649.
10. Fargue S, Rumsby G, Danpure CJ. Multiple mechanisms of action of pyridoxine in primary hyperoxaluria type 1. Biochem Biophys Acta. 2013;1832:1776.
11. Cochat P, Koch Nogueira PC, Mahmoud MA, Jamieson NV, Scheinman JI, Rolland MO. Primary hyperoxaluria in infants: medical, ethical, and economic issues. J Pediatr. 1999;135(6):746-50.
12. Hoppe B, Pellikka PA, Dehmel B, Banos A, Lindner E, Herberg U. Effects of Oxalobacter formigenes in subjects with primary hyperoxaluria type 1 and end-stage renal disease: a phase II study. Nephrol Dial Transplant. 2021;36(8):1464-73.
13. Milliner DS. siRNA therapeutics for primary hyperoxaluria: a beginning. Mol Ther. 2016;24:666.
14. Garrelfs SF, Frishberg Y, Hulton SA, Koren MJ, O'Riordan WD, Cochat P, et al. Lumasiran, an RNAi therapeutic for primary hyperoxaluria type 1. N Engl J Med. 2021;384:1216-26.
15. Liebow A, Li X, Racie T, Hettinger J, Bettencourt BR, Najafian N, et al. An investigational RNAi therapeutic targeting glycolate oxidase reduces oxalate production in models of primary hyperoxaluria. J Am Soc Nephrol. 2017;28:494.
16. Jaklevic MC. First drug approved for rare genetic disorder affecting kidneys. JAMA. 2021;325:214.
17. Frishberg Y, Van't Hoff W, Hulton S, Haslett P, Erbe DV, McGregor T, et al. A phase 1/2 trial of lumasiran (ALN-GO1), an investigational RNAi therapeutic for primary hyperoxaluria type 1. Pediatr Nephrol. 2018;33:1807.
18. Luzzatto L, Hyry HI, Schieppati A, Costa E, Simoens S, Schaefer F, et al. Outrageous prices of orphan drugs: a call for collaboration. Lancet. 2018;392:791-4.

19. Wood KD, Holmes RP, Knight J. RNA interference in the treatment of renal stone disease: current status and future potentials. Int J Surg. 2016;36:713.
20. Le Dudal M, Huguet L, Perez J, Vandermeersch S, Bouderlique E, Tang E, et al. Stiripentol protects against calcium oxalate nephrolithiasis and ethylene glycol poisoning. J Clin Invest. 2019;129:2571.
21. Martin-Higueras C, Feldkötter M, Hoppe B. Is stiripentol truly effective for treating primary hyperoxaluria? Clin Kidney J. 2021;14:442.
22. Wyatt CM, Drüeke TB. Stiripentol for the treatment of primary hyperoxaluria and calcium oxalate nephropathy. Kidney Int. 2020;97:17.
23. Miyata N, Steffen J, Johnson ME, Fargue S, Danpure CJ, Koehler CM. Pharmacologic rescue of an enzyme trafficking defect in primary hyperoxaluria 1. Proc Natl Acad Sci U S A. 2014;111:14406-11.
24. Belostotsky R, Lyakhovetsky R, Sherman MY, Shkedy F, Tzvi-Behr S, Bar R, et al. Translation inhibition corrects aberrant localization of mutant alanine-glyoxylate aminotransferase: possible therapeutic approach for hyperoxaluria. J Mol Med. 2018;96:621-30.
25. Mesa-Torres N, Yunta C, Fabelo-Rosa I, Gonzalez-Rubio JM, Sánchez-Ruiz JM, Salido E, et al. The consensus-based approach for gene/enzyme replacement therapies and crystallization strategies: the case of human alanine-glyoxylate aminotransferase. Biochem J. 2014;462:453-63.
26. Carrasco Jr A, Granberg CF, Gettman MT, Milliner DS, Krambeck AE. Surgical management of stone disease in patients with primary hyperoxaluria. Urology. 2015;85:522.
27. Illies F, Bonzel KE, Wingen AM, Latta K, Hoyer PF. Clearance and removal of oxalate in children on intensified dialysis for primary hyperoxaluria type 1. Kidney Int. 2006;70:1642-8.
28. Hoppe B, Graf D, Offner G, Latta K, Byrd DJ, Michalk D, et al. Oxalate elimination via hemodialysis or peritoneal dialysis in children with chronic renal failure. Pediatr Nephrol. 1996; 10:488.
29. Marangella M, Petrarulo M, Cosseddu D, Vitale C, Linari F. Oxalate balance studies in patients on hemodialysis for type I primary hyperoxaluria. Am J Kidney Dis. 1992;19:546.
30. Chadban SJ, Ahn C, Axelrod DA, Foster BJ, Kasiske BL, Kher V, et al. KDIGO clinical practice guideline on the evaluation and management of candidates for kidney transplantation. Transplantation. 2020;104(4S1):S11-103.
31. Danpure CJ. Primary hyperoxaluria. In: Scriver CR, Beaudet AL, Sly WS, Valle D, (Eds). The Metabolic and Molecular Bases of Inherited Disease, 8th edition. McGraw-Hill; New York: 2001. pp. 3323-67.
32. Devresse A, Cochat P, Godefroid N, Kanaan N. Transplantation for primary hyperoxaluria type 1: designing new strategies in the era of promising therapeutic perspectives. Kidney Int Rep. 2020;5:2136-45.
33. Filler G, Hoppe B. Combined liver-kidney transplantation for hyperoxaluria type II? Pediatr Transplant. 2014;18:237.
34. Del Bello A, Cointault O, Delas A, Kamar N. Primary hyperoxaluria type 2 successfully treated with combined liver-kidney transplantation after failure of isolated kidney transplantation. Am J Transplant. 2020;20:1752.
35. Eytan Mor MD, Weismann I. Current treatment for primary hyperoxaluria type 1: when should liver/kidney transplantation be considered? Pediatr Transplant. 2009;13:805-7.
36. Sasaki K, Sakamoto S, Uchida H, Shigeta T, Matsunami M, Kanazawa H, et al. Two-step transplantation for primary hyperoxaluria: a winning strategy to prevent progression of systemic oxalosis in early onset renal insufficiency cases. Pediatr Transplant. 2015;19(1):E1-6.
37. Scheinman JI. Liver transplantation in oxalosis prior to advanced chronic kidney disease. Pediatr Nephrol. 2010; 25:2217.
38. Brinkert F, Ganschow R, Helmke K, Harps E, Fischer L, Nashan B, et al. Transplantation procedures in children with primary hyperoxaluria type 1: outcome and longitudinal growth. Transplantation. 2009;87:1415.
39. Milliner DS, Harris PC, Sas DJ, Cogal AG, Lieske JC. Primary hyperoxaluria type 1. In: Adam MP, Mirzaa GM, Pagon RA, Wallace SE, Bean LJH, Gripp KW, Amemiya A (Eds). GeneReviews®. Seattle (WA): University of Washington, Seattle; 1993-2022.
40. Metry EL, van Dijk LMM, Peters-Sengers H, Oosterveld MJS, Groothoff JW, Ploeg RJ, et al. Transplantation outcomes in patients with primary hyperoxaluria: a systematic review. Pediatr Nephrol. 2021;36:2217-26.
41. Bergstralh EJ, Monico CG, Lieske JC, Herges RM, Langman CB, Hoppe B, et al. Transplantation outcomes in primary hyperoxaluria. Am J Transplant. 2010;10:2493-501.
42. Compagnon P, Metzler P, Samuel D, Camus C, Niaudet P, Durrbach A, et al. Long-term results of combined liver-kidney transplantation for primary hyperoxaluria type 1: the French experience. Liver Transpl. 2014;20:1475.

CHAPTER

16

Chronic Allograft Injury

Arpita Ray Chaudhury, Saugat Dasgupta

CASE VIGNETTE

A 25-year male, diagnosed chronic kidney disease (CKD) at the age of 17 years with urinary frothing and hypertension, diagnosed as IgA nephropathy in pretransplant biopsy; treated with hemodialysis for the next 2 years via AVF with 2 units blood transfusion during dialysis period; underwent live related kidney transplant at the age of 19 years with mother donor, put on standard triple drug immunosuppression following basiliximab induction, nadir creatinine being 0.89 mg/dL. Pretransplant immunological work up was suggestive of low risk. He did well for the next 6 years with creatinine of 1.1–1.3 mg/dL. At the age of 25 years he again noticed urinary frothing with uPCR 1.8 and on biochemical evaluation creatinine value increased to 1.5 mg/dL and over next 3 months it gradually increased to 2.2 mg/dL, when he agreed for graft biopsy evaluation.

He was compliant during entire post-transplant period, except for few months when following a mild covid infection, he was home isolated, discontinued mycophenolate (MMF) and tacrolimus dose was lowered in view of a tacrolimus level reported 8 ng/mL, and missed the frequency of regular visit to hospital. His tacrolimus dose revised and MMF was reinitiated after 3 months in 2021 May. His blood pressure was controlled on single antihypertensive (cilnidipine 10 mg); blood sugar, lipid profile, electrolytes and routine blood parameters were within normal limits. Post-transplant period was unremarkable for infections requiring hospital admission. Tacrolimus trough level was 5–6 ng/mL in the last 1 year.

Biopsy suggestive of mesangio-proliferative glomerulonephritis with IgA predominance in IF, MEST Score being (M1E0S1T1C0), along with features of chronic antibody-mediated rejection (ABMR) and borderline T cell-mediated rejection (TCMR) (g1, ptc1, i1, t1, v0, c4d 2, cv1, ci1, ct1, cg2) with moderate IFTA.

A diagnosis of chronic ABMR and TCMR with basic disease recurrence has been given ***(Figs. 1A to D)****. After detailed infection screening and optimizing maximally tolerated RAASi therapy and background immunosuppression, patient was put on monthly Tocilizumab trial for C AMR management.*

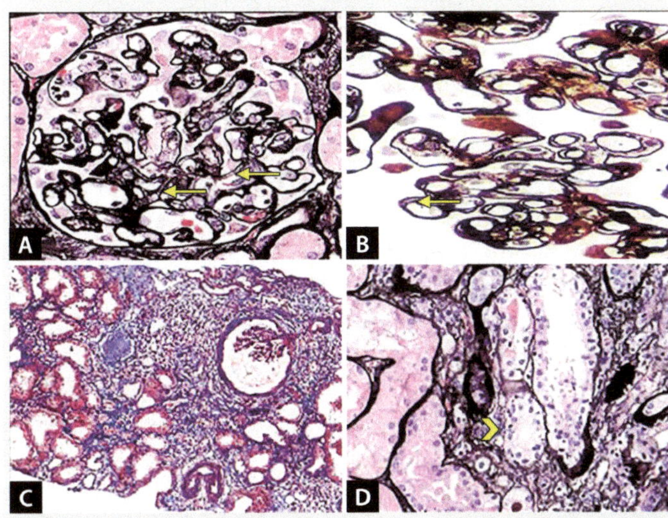

Figs. 1A to D: Kidney biopsy: (A) Double contours (arrows) present in and gt; 50% [cg3] of this affected glomerulus [Jones silver methenamine stain, original magnification 400x]; (B) High power view shows new basement membrane formation. [Jones silver methenamine stain, original magnification 1000x]; (C). Moderate interstitial fibrosis and tubular atrophy with interstitial inflammation in scarred area [Masson trichrome stain, original magnification 400x; (D) The most affected tubules show moderate tubulitis (arrow head). [Jones silver methenamine stain, original magnification 1000x].

INTRODUCTION

Kidney allograft failure is one of the common causes of end-stage kidney disease (ESKD). In the United States, almost 20% of the transplanted kidney recipients are second or third renal allograft recipients, which adds to ever-increasing transplant demand and leads to substantial morbidity and mortality along with adding financial burden of reinitiation of dialysis. Though there is considerable improvement in short-term graft survival with less frequent acute rejections, long-term graft survival did not increase beyond 50% in deceased and 70% in live donors, including both deaths with a functioning allograft and death-censored graft loss.

Flowchart 1: Early intervention for chronic allograft injury (CAI).

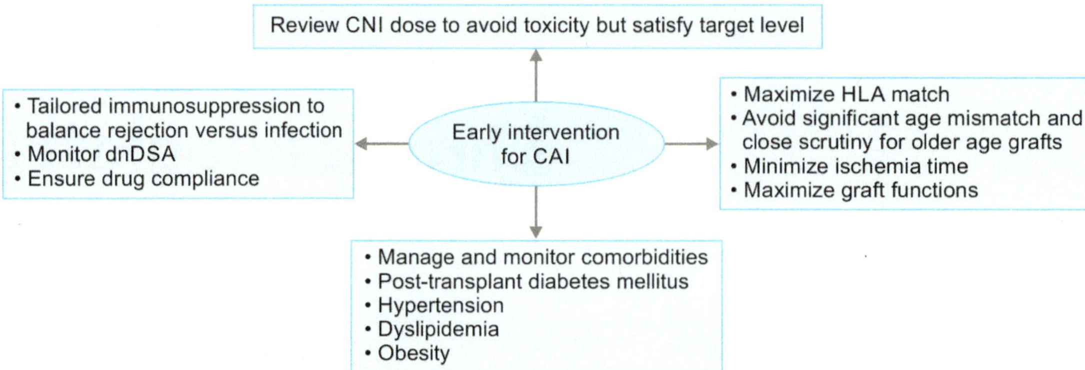

(CNI: calcineurin inhibitor; dnDSA: de novo donor-specific antibodies; HLA: human leukocyte antigen)

The natural corollary brings us to the question of why grafts fail?

Earlier, in registry data, renal allograft damage and then subsequent failure of allograft were plainly attributed to "chronic rejection," and all other causes of graft injury were not recognized. The first Banff Conference on Allograft Pathology (1991) referred to chronic allograft nephropathy (CAN) as a histologic description of significant interstitial fibrosis and tubular atrophy (IF/TA) in a kidney transplant recipient (KTR) without providing any description of specific etiologies. The previous terminology CAN was thereby removed at the 8th Banff Conference (2005). To emphasize nonspecific scarring of all causes of chronic allograft dysfunction (CAD) with fibrosis, CAN was replaced by "IF/TA without evidence of specific etiology," a diagnosis that would initiate the search for the underlying process amalgamating the biopsy findings in different compartments with specific morphological features related to various contributory causes[1] such as polyomavirus nephropathy (PVN), calcineurin inhibitor (CNI) toxicity, and recurrent or de novo glomerular disease.

For describing CAD, in the chapter, we will use the accepted terminology chronic allograft injury (CAI) **(Flowchart 1)**.

CHAPTER HIGHLIGHTS

- Chronic allograft injury (CAI) includes both immune-mediated and nonimmune-mediated injuries to the renal allograft.
- Both immunological and nonimmunological factors of the donor and the recipient culminate to cause CAI.
- The targets of injury are the kidney tubular epithelium, the endothelium, and the glomerulus.
- The process of tissue remodeling and repair results in a maladaptive response resulting in matrix deposition and/or fibrosis leading to graft dysfunction and failure.
- There is an utmost need for new biomarkers to detect the onset and etiology of CAI.

NATURAL HISTORY OF CHRONIC ALLOGRAFT INJURY

The natural history of CAI was first looked at by the Nankivell's group[2] in a prospective study evaluating 961 kidney biopsies from 120 KTRs with type 1 diabetes with a follow-up for 10 years. The natural history of CAI could be divided into two distinct phases. The first year was characterized by new-onset tubulointerstitial damage and rapidly increasing Banff scores for IF/TA. Early subclinical rejections were common (45.7%) during the first 3 months. Ischemic injury, prior severe rejection, and subclinical rejection were found to be the important reasons during the initial phase of early tubulointerstitial damage. In the later phase of CAI, in their observation beyond 1 year, reported chronic rejection (defined as persistent subclinical rejection for 2 years or longer) was uncommon (5.8%). The reporting era was predominantly cyclosporin-based and included patients who were both dual transplants and renal transplants alone. Later, tacrolimus (TAC) and mycophenolate (MMF)-based immunosuppressive regimens, stringent screening for preexisting donor-specific antibodies (DSA), and meticulous tailoring of immunosuppression significantly improved the incidence of early rejections. The authors implicated CNI-induced nephrotoxicity as the main cause of late ongoing injury, which was almost universal at 10 years.

The concept changed over time and in the early part of the second decade of 21st century evidence grew where chronic antibody-mediated rejection (ABMR) accounted for >50% of causes of late graft failure.[3] Of note, CNI nephrotoxicity, posttransplant diabetes mellitus (PTDM), and hypertension three together may explain glomerulosclerosis and arteriolar hyalinosis. The same group published their observations in 200 nondiabetic study recipients with pristine donor kidneys at transplantation, and after comparison of the TAC versus cyclosporine-dominant era, they concluded that the incidence of acute mild arteriolopathy, striped interstitial fibrosis, glomerular congestion, and tubular microcalcification were all ameliorated in TAC biopsies; however, the inexorable progression of chronic arteriolar hyalinosis was unchanged from the cyclosporine A (CsA) era.[4] It also seems difficult to attribute arteriolar hyalinosis and hyaline nodules to CNI toxicity in the usual context of kidney transplantation, as most KTRs also have hypertension and PTDM.

PATHOPHYSIOLOGY OF CHRONIC ALLOGRAFT DAMAGE

With the growing body of literature, it is irrefutable that chronic allograft failure is the consequence of several immune and nonimmune mechanisms which are responsible for progressive injury to the individual nephrons. Finally, the whole organ gets compromised. The hypertrophy remaining nephrons can only compensate partially for losses via hyperfiltration; moreover, the cells of various anatomic compartments of the kidney (glomerular, tubular, interstitial, and microvascular) have a limited repertoire of responses to injury.

Early damage is usually driven by injuries during procurement, preservation, and implantation, followed by cellular and antibody-mediated alloimmunity and additional nonimmune processes. Subsequent tubular injury is often less intense and is the result of residual alloimmunity and inflammation, accompanied by glomerular and microvascular changes. Later disease drivers include late acute rejection from nonadherence, CNI nephrotoxicity, chronic ABMR or chronic active T cell-mediated rejection (CA-TCMR), recurrent glomerulonephritis (GN), acute kidney injury (AKI) from intercurrent illness, and pathologic effects of hypertension, dyslipidemia, and diabetes mellitus.

MECHANISM OF CHRONIC ALLOGRAFT INJURY

- *Inflammatory cytokines:* Acute as well as repeated episodes of tissue injury induce the production of excessive inflammatory cytokines leading to interstitial and vascular fibrosis [mediated by transforming growth factor beta 1 (TGF-β1)]. Upregulated or altered expression of vascular endothelial growth factor (VEGF), endothelin-1, plasminogen-activating factor-1, monocyte chemoattractant protein 1 (MCP-1), platelet-derived growth factor (PDGF)-A and B, RANTES (regulated upon activation, normal T cell expressed and secreted), bone morphogenetic protein-7 (BMP-7), hepatocyte growth factor, connective tissue growth factor (CTGF), and advanced glycation end products have all been described in experimental and human "chronic rejection."
- *Reactive oxygen species (ROS):* ROS released from tubular cell mitochondria can cause cellular injury, apoptosis, and senescence.
- *Glomerular hyperfiltration:* The hyperfiltration theory postulates that an increased share of the kidney's metabolic and protein reabsorption load falls to a diminishing number of remaining nephrons, causing glomerular hypertension and secondary glomerulosclerosis. It has been projected in some research that incompatibility of donor and recipient weight (kidney weight and recipient weight ratio <2.3 g/kg) can be associated with lower graft survival.[5] However, there is a lack of robust evidence to support this theory in human transplantation as many registry studies do not show any effect of donor–recipient size mismatch on the graft survival.
- *Failed resolution of chronic inflammation:* Partial or incomplete resolution of acute injury to the renal allograft can cause enhanced allorecognition and immune-mediated injury. The total inflammatory burden, including inflammation in both scarred and unscarred tissue, is an independent risk factor for graft failure.
- *Epithelial–mesenchymal transition (EMT) induced fibrosis:* EMT is a sequence of phenotypical changes transforming the tubular epithelial cells into spindle-shaped mesenchymal or myofibroblast-like cells. Whenever there is a sublethal tubular hypoxic tissue injury, for example, due to subclinical rejections, CNI induced, or any oxidative stress, the genetically programmed steps of EMT may begin resulting in impaired cell-to-cell adhesion, loss of tight and adherent junctions, desmosomes, and E-cadherin (an epithelial marker). However, this theory is still debated and requires more supporting evidence.
- *Donor age and replicative senescence:* The senescent phenotype of CAI resembles aging and reflects intrinsic alterations of cell-cycling pathways.
- *Cortical ischemia and angioregression:* The tubular epithelial cells are highly metabolically active, and they are susceptible to ischemia from upstream vascular and glomerular disease. These are supplied by a network of peritubular capillaries (PTC) downstream from glomerular efferent arterioles. Vasoconstriction-induced CNIs, arteriolar hyalinosis, and small arterial vascular disease can result in reduced postglomerular capillary blood flow. As an adaptive survival response, hypoxic tubular cells can switch to anaerobic glycolysis and activate antiapoptotic molecular programs.
- *Donor quality and procurement injury:* Inherited donor abnormalities can potentially alter the function of allograft, its histology, and response to injury and also have been projected to influence long-term graft survival. Important donor pathologic features are as follows:
    - The extent of glomerulosclerosis (>20% is severe)
    - Glomerulomegaly (with implied nephron loss and hyperfiltration)
    - Microvascular disease (abnormality mostly associated with donor age, diabetes, hypertension, and death from cerebrovascular disease).

Donation after brain death also has an impact on graft outcomes, mostly due to the potentiation of graft immunogenicity and other nonspecific pathophysiologic changes. Pro-inflammatory mediators released during brain death can alter the immunogenicity of the transplanted organ and can cause higher rejection rates. Injury to the tissue leads to the expression of innate danger receptors or toll receptor system ligands, subsequently resulting in promoting maturation, activation, and rejection of immune cells.

Furthermore, some genetic risk factors of donors can also alter graft outcomes. For instance, some studies show that the presence of two APOL1 high-risk alleles negatively affects graft survival.[6] The plausible mechanism is that high-risk APOL1 may induce podocyte injury and lead to glomerular injury.[7]

- *Delayed graft function (DGF) and ischemic injury:* The incidence of DGF is gradually increasing as the number of kidneys from older deceased donors with vascular comorbidity (expanded criteria donors) or after circulatory death are increasingly being utilized for transplantation.

HISTOPATHOLOGY OF A CHRONICALLY FAILING ALLOGRAFT

It typically shows chronic IF/TA, glomerulosclerosis, and vascular abnormalities. These features are the end result of tissue injury and the fibrotic healing response induced by it. CAI may be best characterized as an "obliterative lumenopathy," manifesting in a progressive concentric narrowing and fibrosis of endothelial- and/or epithelial-lined structures (e.g., blood vessels and tubular lumens) that are critical to maintaining allograft function.

Chronic alloimmune activity can be characterized by:

- Persistent cellular interstitial inflammation in scarred and nonscarred areas
- Fibrointimal arterial hyperplasia
- Transplant glomerulopathy (associated with circulating DSA and microvascular tissue C4d).

Atubular glomeruli may develop due to their disconnection with downstream collapsed tubules. Inflammatory necrosis with obliterative fibrosis can destroy tubular integrity.

HIGHLIGHTS OF THE MAIN ETIOLOGIC CONTRIBUTORS OF CHRONIC ALLOGRAFT INJURY

- Post-transplant hypertension occurs in 70–90% of recipients and is associated with graft failure and death.
- Some studies showed that posttransplant hypertriglyceridemia, but not hypercholesterolemia, may be associated with CAI. The underlying mechanism is yet to be elucidated; possibly hyperlipidemia may trigger rejection possibly by promoting antidonor T helper (Th)17-cell response through costimulatory molecule blockade.[8,9]
- Immune-mediated injury associated with clinical and subclinical rejection has been shown to be associated progression of IF/TA. Overall, the rate of de novo DSA development is 15–20% at 5 years posttransplant, and it is associated with worse graft survival, affecting especially younger patients, noncompliant, and/or with greater DR mismatches. In the DeKAF (Deterioration of Kidney Allograft Function) study, the authors reported that 57% of cases with allograft dysfunction were due to antibody-mediated injury and the severity of injury correlated with the intensity of the antibody response.[10]
- In the Australia/New Zealand registry,[11] recurrent GN was the third leading cause of ESKD in KTRs, with a 10-year incidence of 8.4%. The type of immunosuppression does not seem to be a risk factor for recurrence.[12,13] A recent study suggested that genetic analyses may be a reasonable approach to help stratify the risk of recurrence as evident by the lack of recurrence in all patients with genetic-identified primary focal segmental glomerulosclerosis (FSGS).[14] The type of underlying GN and duration of the exposure of graft to the nephritogenic factors are strong determinants of the recurrence of GN post-transplantation. Higher rates of recurrence are observed in pediatric transplant recipients, and KTRs who lost their first allograft from recurrent.[15-18]
- *CNI toxicity:* CNI use has been linked with nephrotoxicity in both acute and long-term exposure. The mechanism of CNI nephrotoxicity is complex. (Detailed explanation available in Chapter 9.3). CNIs are implicated in the activation of the renin–angiotensin system, with effects on kidney vasculature as well as on juxtaglomerular cells. There can be an increase in profibrotic cytokines [TGF-β1 and tissue inhibitor of metalloproteinase 1 (TIMP-1)].[19]
- *BK nephropathy:* With the increased use of more potent immunosuppressive drugs in the past years, BK nephropathy has become a major cause of both acute and chronic allograft dysfunction. BK virus, with a tropism for uroepithelium, undergoes replication under the immunosuppressive milieu resulting in a marked inflammatory response, leading to tubular epithelial cell injury and, ultimately, IF/TA. (Detailed explanation available in Chapters 11 and 12.2.2)

MANAGEMENT STRATEGY

The management of patients with CAI depends primarily on the underlying cause of injury.

Key points in the management are as follows:

- Obtaining a careful history in regards to the primary renal disease, the early posttransplant course (e.g., severe DGF might indicate significant irreversible early allograft damage), and episodes of acute rejection (if any).
- Meticulous follow-up of CNI levels at regular intervals and checking for noncompliance.
- Appropriate treatment and ensuring complete resolution of rejection episodes are imperative since insufficient

graft function recovery results in poor long-term graft outcomes.

- CAI is largely characterized by biopsy findings; thus, repeated biopsies at 1, 3, and 12 months may be helpful for early diagnosis, as is done in protocol biopsies for research studies.[20] However, this approach is limited by cost and reimbursement issues and the invasive nature of the test.
- *Management of nonimmune causes of injury:* Diagnosis and management of recurrent or de novo glomerular disease, viral infections [especially BK virus and cytomegalovirus (CMV)] and control of hypertension, smoking cessation, dyslipidemia, and blood sugar levels. Angiotensin-converting-enzyme inhibitors or angiotensin receptor blockers are advised to manage hypertension and proteinuria.
- Limiting procurement and perioperative ischemic injury may improve organ quality and ameliorate graft immunogenicity. Better organ preservation techniques and solutions, optimal intensive care unit management, pulsatile ex vivo machine perfusion, rapid transfer of organs, and prompt implantation to reduce organ stresses are some important measures.

CHALLENGES

Considering rising creatinine as a surrogate marker has its limitations as serum creatinine values usually underestimate deterioration in glomerular filtration rate (GFR) and are a poor predictor of CAI and graft loss.[21] Kidney function deterioration of >10% at 3 months post-transplant is associated with a 2.5-times relative risk of 10-year graft loss and predicts a 15% reduction in long-term graft survival.[22]

EARLY DETECTION OF CHRONIC ALLOGRAFT INJURY

- Gene expression profiles may be useful in terms of predicting graft failure and progression as already noted, and further clinical validation is awaited.[23]
- *Documentation of DSA:* Ongoing researches are now suggesting the role of donor-derived cell-free deoxyribonucleic acid (DNA) to detect allograft injury or gene transcripts in peripheral blood mononuclear cells (PBMCs) associated with subclinical inflammation.[24,25] Such assays can have a potential role in guiding patient management, follow-up, and early detection of injury.
- A multicomposite measure model called the integrated risk prediction score (iBOX) from data derived from both surveillance and medically indicated biopsies in a large cohort of kidney transplants, and the use of machine learning algorithms have identified independent risk factors for graft loss **(Table 1)**. It has been suggested to predict the risk of graft failure. These include allograft function, proteinuria, the level of donor-specific human leukocyte antigen (HLA) antibody, and the histopathologic variables of the severity of IF/TA, microvascular injury, inflammation, and tubulitis. The iBOX may assist in the risk assessment of a patient's clinical course and is under consideration in clinical trial design as a surrogate endpoint of late graft failure.[26]

TABLE 1: Risk factors of allograft loss.

Donor risks (nonimmune factors)	*Recipient risks (nonimmune factors)*	*Alloimmune factors*
Deceased donor kidney (vs. living donor)	Female sex, obesity	Young recipient age
Autonomic storm, inotropic use, donor kidney injury	Organ size mismatch (especially pediatric recipients)	Race and ethnicity with altered disposition of immunosuppressive agents
Donation after circulatory death (vs. donation after brain death)	Ascending urinary tract infection and graft pyelonephritis	Variable medication trough levels (noncompliance or possibly malabsorption)
Donor quality: Extended criteria donor (ECD) or with poor KDPI	Transplant ureteric obstruction	Recipient's genetic alloimmune and inflammatory response
Ischemia–reperfusion injury	BK virus nephropathy	Histoincompatibility (HLA or eplet mismatches)
Prolonged organ ischemia	CNI nephrotoxicity	Recipient presensitization (High cPRA) or donor specific antibodies
Acute tubular necrosis (implantation biopsy) and delayed graft function	Recurrent renal disease or de novo glomerulonephritis	Acute rejection that is severe, steroid-resistant, vascular, antibody-mediated, or late occurring rejection
	Recipient hypertension, hyperlipidemia, smoking, and proteinuria	Subclinical rejection, chronic T-cell mediated rejection, late de novo anti-HLA antibody formation (donor-specific antibodies), and chronic antibody-mediated rejection with transplant glomerulopathy
	Preexisting or post-transplantation diabetes mellitus	Therapy nonadherence

(CNI: calcineurin inhibitor; cPRA: calculated panel-reactive antibody; HLA: human leukocyte antigen; KDPI: kidney donor profile index)

MANAGING IMMUNOSUPPRESSION TO REDUCE CHRONIC ALLOGRAFT INJURY

Treatment of chronic ABMR, to prevent late graft failure, has been discussed in Chapter 10.2.

Calcineurin inhibitor nephrotoxicity remains a contributory cause, and various molecules have been tried for minimizing or withdrawing CNIs. Proliferation signal inhibitors (PSI) therapy is commonly practiced for CNI sparing. Following on from early studies utilizing everolimus (EVL) and full-dose CNI, EVL in combination with low-dose CNI has been shown to provide a low incidence of acute rejection in de novo renal transplant recipients maintaining renal function.[27,28] However, the early withdrawal of CNIs from sirolimus-based regimens has been associated with an increased incidence of acute rejection in a meta-analysis of six trials and is not advised in the first 3 months.[29] Two independent multicenter studies and one meta-analysis strengthen the evidence for PSI addition with CNI minimization. In the open-label multicenter ASCERTAIN study, the estimated glomerular filtration rate (eGFR) at 24 months after conversion was not significantly different between three groups—EVL with CNI elimination, CNI minimization, and continued CNI unchanged—at a mean of 5.4 years after transplantation. However, recipients with baseline creatinine clearance >50 mL/min had a greater increase in measured GFR after CNI elimination.[30] In the open-label multicenter APOLLO study, adjusted eGFR within the on-treatment population was significantly higher in the EVL continuation group than in the CNI continuation group at 12 months after conversion at a mean of 7 years post transplantation.[31] The review by Su et al. showed that CNI minimization was not associated with increased biopsy-proven acute rejection (BPAR) ($p = 0.25$; RR 0.85), while CNI elimination was associated with more BPAR grade 1 ($p < 0.00001$; RR 4.20). Use of EVL reduced the risk of CMV infection ($p = 0.0002$; RR 0.47). There was a higher risk of discontinuation of EVL ($p < 0.00001$; RR 1.69) and nonfatal adverse events.[32] In spite of significant advances in transplantation and better mechanistic insights, there are no specific therapies that ameliorate calcineurin inhibitor nephrotoxicity.[33]

Belatacept is an alternative to CNI that has shown promise in recent clinical trials. It is a CTLA4Ig fusion protein that blocks the CD80/CD86 interaction with CD28, preventing T-cell activation. Its use is contraindicated in patients with negative Epstein-Barr virus (EBV) status for concerns of a higher risk of posttransplant lymphoproliferative disorder. Early withdrawal of CNIs mandates careful monitoring of patients to avoid acute rejection episodes.[34,35]

Recently the growing body of literature has shown successful use of sodium-glucose cotransporter 2 (SGLT2) inhibitors in KTRs with PTDM without any significant differences in adverse events, immunosuppressive drug levels, or eGFR.[36]

CONCLUSION

It has been recognized that IF/TA is perpetuated by immune injury as well as nonimmune injuries. Some proposed measures to decrease CAI are an appropriate selection of donors, better organ preservation methods, preemptive approaches such as detection and management of rejections prior to clinical detection, maximizing HLA molecular match instead of traditional HLA antigen match, addressing nonadherence to the transplant medication, and weaning immunosuppressive drugs based on immunological risk profiles. At the same time hypertension, diabetes, and dyslipidemia management remains of paramount importance to protect the graft, along with screening for BK virus nephropathy (BKVN) and identifying the recurrence or de novo GN early.

REFERENCES

1. Solez K, Colvin RB, Racusen LC, Sis B, Halloran PF, Birk PE, et al. Banff'05 Meeting Report: differential diagnosis of chronic allograft injury and elimination of chronic allograft nephropathy ('CAN'). Am J Transplant. 2007;7:518-26.
2. Nankivell BJ, Borrows RJ, Fung CLS, O'Connell PJ, Allen RD, Chapman JR. The natural history of chronic allograft nephropathy. N Engl J Med. 2003;349:2326-33.
3. El-Zoghby ZM, Stegall MD, Lager DJ, Kremers WK, Amer H, Gloor JM, et al. Identifying specific causes of kidney allograft loss. Am J Transplant. 2009;9(3):527-35.
4. Nankivell BJ, P'Ng CH, O'Connell PJ, Chapman JR. Calcineurin inhibitor nephrotoxicity through the lens of longitudinal histology: comparison of cyclosporine and tacrolimus eras. Transplantation. 2016;100:1723-31.
5. Giral M, Foucher Y, Karam G, Labrune Y, Kessler M, Hurault de Ligny B, et al. Kidney and recipient weight incompatibility reduces long-term graft survival. J Am Soc Nephrol. 2010;21:1022-9.
6. Freedman BI, Pastan SO, Israni AK, Schladt D, Julian BA, Gautreaux MD, et al. APOL1 genotype and kidney transplantation outcomes from deceased African American donors. Transplantation. 2016;100:194-202.
7. Beckerman P, Bi-Karchin J, Park AS, Qiu C, Dummer PD, Soomro I, et al. Transgenic expression of human APOL1 risk variants in podocytes induces kidney disease in mice. Nat Med. 2017;23:429-38.
8. Guijarro C, Massy ZA, Kasiske BL. Clinical correlation between renal allograft failure and hyperlipidemia. Kidney Int Suppl. 1995;52:S56-9.
9. Bagley J, Yuan J, Chandrakar A, Iacomini J. Hyperlipidemia alters regulatory T cell function and promotes resistance to tolerance induction through costimulatory molecule blockade. Am J Transplant. 2015;15:2324-35.
10. Gaston RS, Cecka JM, Kasiske BL, Fieberg AM, Leduc R, Cosio FC, et al. Evidence for antibody-mediated injury as a major determinant of late kidney allograft failure. Transplantation. 2010;90:68-74.

11. Briganti EM, Russ GR, McNeil JJ, Atkins RC, Chadban SJ. Risk of renal allograft loss from recurrent glomerulonephritis. N Engl J Med. 2002;347:103-9.
12. Mulay AV, van Walraven C, Knoll GA. Impact of immunosuppressive medication on the risk of renal allograft failure due to recurrent glomerulonephritis. Am J Transplant. 2009;9:804-11.
13. Gallon L, Leventhal J, Skaro A, Kanwar Y, Alvarado A. Resolution of recurrent focal segmental glomerulosclerosis after retransplantation. N Engl J Med. 2012;366:1648-9.
14. Bierzynska A, McCarthy HJ, Soderquest K, Sen ES, Colby E, Ding WY, et al. Genomic and clinical profiling of a national nephrotic syndrome cohort advocates a precision medicine approach to disease management. Kidney Int. 2017;91:937-47.
15. Le Quintrec M, Lionet A, Kamar N, Karras A, Barbier S, Buchler M, et al. Complement mutation-associated de novo thrombotic microangiopathy following kidney transplantation. Am J Transplant. 2008;8:1694-701.
16. Moroni G, Longhi S, Quaglini S, Gallelli B, Banfi G, Montagnino G, et al. The long-term outcome of renal transplantation of IgA nephropathy and the impact of recurrence on graft survival. Nephrol Dial Transplant. 2013;28:1305-14.
17. Dabade TS, Grande JP, Norby SM, Fervenza FC, Cosio FG. Recurrent idiopathic membranous nephropathy after kidney transplantation: a surveillance biopsy study. Am J Transplant. 2008;8:1318-22.
18. Zand L, Lorenz EC, Cosio FG, Fervenza FC, Nasr SH, Gandhi MJ, et al. Clinical findings, pathology, and outcomes of C3GN after kidney transplantation. J Am Soc Nephrol. 2014;25:1110-7.
19. Vincenti F, Rostaing L, Grinyo J, Rice K, Steinberg S, Gaite L, et al. Belatacept and long-term outcomes in kidney transplantation. N Engl J Med. 2016;374:333-43.
20. Chapman JR, O'Connell PJ, Nankivell BJ. Chronic renal allograft dysfunction. J Am Soc Nephrol. 2005;16:3015-26.
21. Dominguez J, Kompatzki A, Norambuena R, Arenas J, Dell'Oro A, Bustamante A, et al. Benefits of early biopsy on the outcome of kidney transplantation. Transplant Proc. 2005;37:3361-3.
22. Marqués GG, Goenaga PE, Royo FJL, Escolá JM, García Fernández N, Unanua AP. Evolution of the renal function is a better predictor of long-term survival than serum creatinine. Transplant Proc. 2005;37:3701-4.
23. Park WD, Griffin MD, Cornell LD, Cosio FG, Stegall MD. Fibrosis with inflammation at one year predicts transplant functional decline. J Am Soc Nephrol. 2010;21:1987-97.
24. Bloom RD, Bromberg JS, Poggio ED, Bunnapradist S, Langone AJ, Sood P, et al. Cell-free DNA and active rejection in kidney allografts. J Am Soc Nephrol. 2017;28:2221-32.
25. Friedewald JJ, Kurian SM, Heilman RL, Whisenant TC, Poggio ED, Marsh C, et al. Development and clinical validity of a novel blood-based molecular biomarker for subclinical acute rejection following kidney transplant. Am J Transplant. 2019;19:98-109.
26. Loupy A, Aubert O, Orandi BJ, Naesens M, Bouatou Y, Raynaud M, et al. Prediction system for risk of allograft loss in patients receiving kidney transplants: international derivation and validation study. BMJ. 2019;366:l4923.
27. Vitko S, Tedesco H, Eris J, Pascual J, Whelchel J, Magee JC, et al. Everolimus with optimized cyclosporine dosing in renal transplant recipients: 6-month safety and efficacy results of two randomized studies. Am J Transplant. 2004;4:626-35.
28. Tedesco-Silva Jr H, Vitko S, Pascual J, Eris J, Magee JC, Whelchel J, et al. 12-month safety and efficacy of everolimus with reduced exposure cyclosporine in de novo renal transplant recipients. Transpl Int. 2007;20:27-36.
29. Mulay AV, Hussain N, Fergusson D, Knoll GA. Calcineurin inhibitor withdrawal from sirolimus-based therapy in kidney transplantation: a systematic review of randomized trials. Am J Transplant. 2005;5:1748-56.
30. Holdaas H, Rostaing L, Serón D, Cole E, Chapman J, Fellstrøm B, et al. Conversion of long-term kidney transplant recipients from calcineurin inhibitor therapy to everolimus: a randomized, multicenter, 24-month study. Transplantation. 2011;92:410-8.
31. Budde K, Rath T, Sommerer C, Haller H, Reinke P, Witzke O, et al. Renal, efficacy and safety outcomes following late conversion of kidney transplant patients from calcineurin inhibitor therapy to everolimus: the randomized APOLLO study. Clin Nephrol. 2015;83:11-21.
32. Su L, Tam N, Deng R, Chen P, Li H, Wu L. Everolimus-based calcineurin-inhibitor sparing regimens for kidney transplant recipients: a systematic review and meta-analysis. Int Urol Nephrol. 2014;46:2035-44.
33. Pascual J, Boletis IN, Campistol JM. Everolimus (Certican) in renal transplantation: a review of clinical trial data, current usage, and future directions. Transplant Rev. 2006;20:1-18.
34. Wiebe C, Nickerson PW. More precise donor-recipient matching: the role of eplet matching. Curr Opin Nephrol Hypertens. 2020;29:630-5.
35. Halden TAS, Kvitne KE, Midtvedt K, Rajakumar L, Robertsen I, Brox J, et al. Efficacy and safety of empagliflozin in renal transplant recipients with posttransplant diabetes mellitus. Diabetes Care. 2019;42:1067-74.
36. Hesp AC, Schaub JA, Prasad PV, Vallon V, Laverman GD, Bjornstad P, et al. The role of renal hypoxia in the pathogenesis of diabetic kidney disease: a promising target for newer renoprotective agents including SGLT2 inhibitors? Kidney Int. 2020;98:579-89.

CHAPTER 17

Management of Patients with Failed Renal Allograft

Jasmine Sethi, Vinay Sakhuja

CASE VIGNETTE

A 55-year-old male known with type 2 (T2) diabetes mellitus with a history of live-related renal transplant 3 years back with his wife as a donor [complement-dependent cytotoxicity (CDC), flow X match negative] was on tacrolimus 2 mg twice daily, mycophenolate mofetil (MMF) 720 mg twice daily, and prednisolone 5 mg once daily. His basic disease was presumed diabetic kidney disease. His baseline creatinine was between 1.2 and 1.4 mg/dL. His post-transplant period was uneventful till 4 months back when he had moderate–severe COVID-19 pneumonia requiring ventilatory support, dexamethasone, and remdesivir. During this illness, his creatinine had risen to 2.3 mg/dL. His MMF and calcineurin inhibitor (CNI) were stopped, and prednisolone was continued at 15 mg daily. CNI was restarted 1 month later with prednisolone tapered to 10 mg OD. But his serum creatinine had a rising trend with a peak of 5.6 mg/dL. His C0 Tac level was 4.2 ng/mL. The patient was initiated on dialysis and biopsied. MMF and therapeutic dose CNI were reinitiated. The allograft biopsy showed features of T cell-mediated rejection (TCMR) IIb. The patient was explained the option of antithymocyte globulin (ATG); however, in view of financial constraints, it could not be given. A steroid pulse was administered; however, the patient had steroid refractory TCMR and ultimately was declared graft loss after 2 weeks. His residual renal function (RRF) was around 600–700 mL/day.

How should we proceed with immunosuppression?

Ans. In view of no immediate transplant prospects and live donors, the patient was counseled and registered on the deceased donor list. His MMF was stopped immediately. CNI continued to preserve his RRF with a plan to taper it over 3–6 months. Prednisolone was tapered as per **Flowchart 1**. An arteriovenous (AV) fistula was created, and a right tunneled jugular catheter was inserted for the time being. Chronic kidney disease (CKD) was managed with erythropoietin and phosphorus binders.

Flowchart 1: Flowchart for managing patients with failed renal allograft.

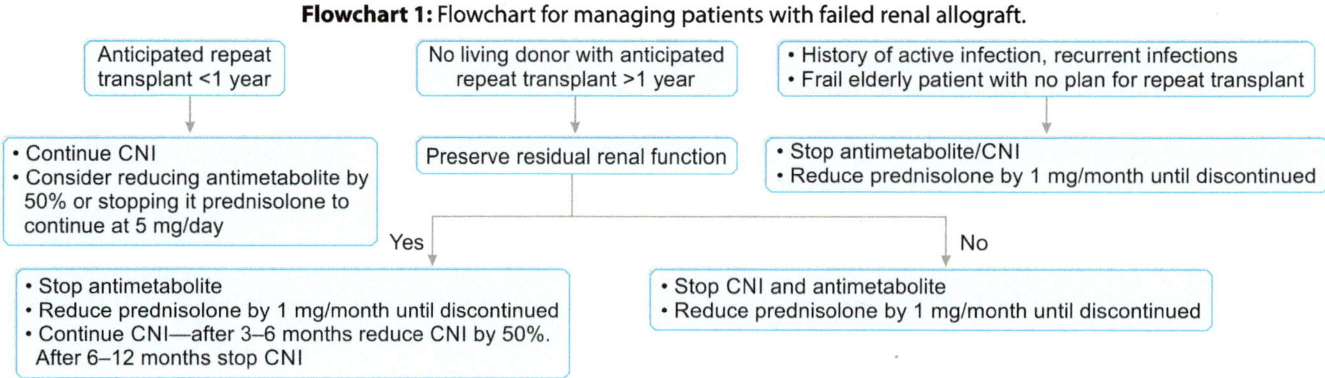

(CNI: calcineurin inhibitor)

INTRODUCTION

Patients with a failed or a failing renal transplant are increasing in number with a substantial number of them initiating dialysis after graft failure. Physician practices vary regarding the timing and extent of immunosuppression (IS) withdrawal. This patient cohort of failed allograft is a unique group with a high degree of morbidity and mortality and specific medical issues. In addition to increased mortality, these patients also experience a higher degree of hospitalizations, infectious complications, severe anemia, lower quality of life scores, and depression. In this chapter, we discuss the challenges and management of patients with renal allograft failure including relisting for repeat transplantation, withdrawal of IS, transplant nephrectomy, and timing of dialysis initiation.

CAUSES OF LATE ALLOGRAFT FAILURE AND PATIENT OUTCOMES AFTER GRAFT FAILURE

Important causes of late allograft failure include chronic rejection, recurrence of the original disease, BK virus nephropathy, and CNI toxicity. A recent study has shown chronic antibody-mediated rejection (ABMR) to be the most common histological cause of allograft dysfunction.[1] Published literature shows a higher prevalence of patients returning to dialysis after graft loss (DAGL) and higher mortality rates in patients who return to DAGL compared to both patients awaiting their first transplant and those who remain dialysis independent, with poor graft function.[2] Patients returning to DAGL are found to have a 3-year mortality rate of 33%.[3] The plausible reasons for such increased mortality could be suboptimal control of the comorbid disease burden, high rates of dialysis catheter use as initial vascular access rather than AV fistula, and last a lack of close follow-up in a significant proportion of these patients. Another reason for high morbidity and mortality in these patients is the persistence of a chronic inflammatory state.[4] In a recent analysis from the United States Renal Data System (USRDS) registry of patients returning to DAGL, a higher mortality was found in patients who did not have an AV fistula at dialysis initiation and had hypoalbuminemia (serum albumin <3.5 g/dL).[5]

CHAPTER HIGHLIGHTS

- Optimal IS strategy in patients with failed allografts should be balanced considering the potential risks (infections) and benefits (avoiding sensitization).
- Patients with failing allograft should be evaluated with a timely placement of vascular access.
- Routine allograft nephrectomy should not be performed in asymptomatic patients who are eligible for repeat transplant due to the significantly increased risk of HLA antibody sensitization.

MANAGEMENT OF IMMUNOSUPPRESSION

One of the most important aspects of managing a patient with failed/failing renal allograft is to decide when and how to safely stop maintenance IS without precipitating rejection or adverse effects related to drug withdrawal. Cessation of IS after graft failure may be immediate, rapid, or can be slowly tapered; moreover, it should be based on the patient's characteristics, the presence of RRF, and the probability of a retransplant. Furthermore, the timing of graft loss is an important determinant. When the failure of transplant occurs during the early period following transplantation due to reasons such as primary non-function (PNF), arterial or venous thrombosis, hyperacute or early refractory acute rejection, in these cases stopping of immunosuppressive agents (and nephrectomy) is usually preferred to avoid the risk of graft rupture and hemorrhage. Conversely, when the occurrence of graft failure is after 12–24 months of transplantation, it is suggested to continue the immunosuppressive therapy, with the maintenance of low-dose IS after weighing both benefits and risks, as discussed below. **Table 1** shows the arguments of continuing IS in the setting of allograft failure.

TABLE 1: Pros and cons for continuing immunosuppression in the setting of transplant failure.

Cons	*Pros*
Increased risk of infection	Reduce sensitization
Increased risk of malignancies	Preservation of residual renal function
Immunosuppression drug-related adverse effects	Reduced risk of graft intolerance syndrome requiring transplant nephrectomy
Altered drug dosing of immunosuppressive agents in severe renal impairment	Reduced risk of secondary adrenal insufficiency
Increased risk of cardiovascular disease	

REASONS FOR WITHDRAWAL OF IMMUNOSUPPRESSION

The reasons for discontinuation of IS in patients returning to dialysis after a failed kidney transplant include a higher risk of infections (bacterial, viral, and opportunistic infections), malignancies, and metabolic complications of the immunosuppressive medication. In an analysis of 197 patients returning to dialysis, the risk of infection was significantly higher in patients remaining on low-dose IS, compared with those in whom IS was withdrawn (1.7 vs. 0.5 infections/patient-year, respectively).[6] Mortality and cardiovascular disease (odds ratios of 3.4 and 4.9) were also increased in the group on IS. Similarly, an increased risk of malignancy is seen in patients who are exposed to IS. Some studies showed that patients who returned to dialysis and maintained a low dose of IS had a lesser chance of occurrence of malignancies such as melanoma, non-Hodgkin's lymphoma, and lip cancer.[7] Last, the inherent metabolic adverse effects of agents used in maintenance IS should also be considered. For instance, the use of CNIs is associated with an increased risk of hypertension, new-onset diabetes after transplantation (NODAT), and dyslipidemia. Continuous use of corticosteroids could be responsible for adverse effects such as an increased risk of hyperglycemias, hypertension, osteoporosis, muscle wasting, and cataracts.

COMPLICATIONS ASSOCIATED WITH IMMUNOSUPPRESSION WITHDRAWAL

Sensitization

Kidney transplant recipients with a failing renal allograft have an increased risk of developing de novo human leukocyte antigen (HLA) sensitization, which occurs most commonly in the setting of restarting dialysis after a failing renal transplant when IS is withdrawn or modified. IS withdrawal with or without transplant nephrectomy has been shown to be an independent predictor of allosensitization. This was well illustrated in a retrospective study of 119 patients with renal allograft failure who had available panel reactive antibody (PRA) testing, the percentage of those who were highly sensitized increased from 21% at the time of graft failure to 68% after withdrawal of IS. In contrast, only 8% of patients who maintained immunosuppression became highly sensitized.[8]

Rejection/Graft Intolerance Syndrome

A major side effect associated with the abrupt stopping of IS is the precipitation of symptomatic rejection termed graft intolerance syndrome. Graft intolerance syndrome characteristically develops within the first year of dialysis initiation after allograft failure. Treatment usually consists of an initial 5–7-days course of steroids or graft nephrectomy if there is no response to steroids. However, some nephrologists prefer immediate graft nephrectomy even with mild symptoms of rejection after drug withdrawal.

Loss of Residual Renal Function

Loss of RRF in general is associated with better survival in both peritoneal dialysis (PD) and hemodialysis. It is speculated that a continuation of maintenance IS in patients with a failed kidney allograft may preserve RRF and thereby improve survival. Liberty of more liberal fluid intake and improved quality of life are other beneficial effects of preservation of RRF. Davies showed a significant rapid decline in RRF in patients initiated on PD after graft failure compared with end-stage kidney disease (ESKD) patients who had not received renal transplantation, indicating the importance of maintaining low-dose IS to preserve residual allograft function.[9] However, there is a lack of robust evidence that the continuation of immunosuppressive agents actually preserves RRF and improves patient survival after graft loss.

STRATEGIES FOR TAPERING IMMUNOSUPPRESSIVE AGENTS

There is no single weaning protocol for immunosuppressive medication.

- According to the British Transplantation Society guideline, antiproliferative agents (azathioprine and MMF) can be stopped immediately, followed by a slow tapering of CNIs or mammalian target of rapamycin inhibitors (generally over several weeks).[10]
- In patients who have early allograft failure (<1 year following transplantation), most centers prefer to perform allograft nephrectomy and immediate withdrawal of IS.
- In the event of late graft failure (>1 year after transplant) and if the retransplantation is planned within 1 year, most centers withdraw antimetabolite, reduce the dose of CNI to target a 24-hour trough level of 2–5 ng/mL for tacrolimus and 50–75 ng/mL for cyclosporine, and prednisolone is continued at a dose of 5 mg/day till the time of retransplantation. Our suggestions for managing patients with a failed allograft are shown in **Flowchart 1**.

GRAFT NEPHRECTOMY

Possible indications for transplant nephrectomy may be related to:[11]

- Graft issues
- Issues related to IS (e.g., sepsis, recurrent urinary tract infection, malignancy, medication-related side effects)
- The presence of signs of chronic inflammation.

The principal indications for allograft nephrectomy are summarized in **Table 2**, and the pros and cons are summarized in **Table 3**.

TABLE 2: Indications of allograft nephrectomy.

Early graft loss	If graft loss occurs <12 months after transplant
Risk of graft rupture	• Vascular thrombosis • Severe acute rejection resistant to immunosuppression
Retransplantation	To create space for new graft
Infectious complications	• Severe graft pyelonephritis • Resistant BK virus nephropathy • Post-transplant lymphoproliferative disease in the graft
Graft intolerance syndrome	• Localizing symptoms—pain, swelling of graft • Chronic inflammation—refractory anemia, increased inflammatory markers

TABLE 3: Advantages and disadvantages of allograft nephrectomy.

Possible benefits of graft nephrectomy	***Risks associated with graft nephrectomy***
Removes possible focus of chronic inflammation	Chances of residual renal function loss
Possible survival benefit	Allosensitization
	Surgery-related morbidity and mortality associated with surgery

Allograft nephrectomy has been demonstrated to be associated with allosensitization: De novo donor-specific antibodies (DSAs) were detected as soon as 5 days after transplantectomy, suggesting that the antibodies were performed, but the increase in PRAs and DSAs could be explained by proinflammatory cytokine production and upregulation of HLA alloantibodies caused by allograft nephrectomy.[12,13]

Thus, it is suggested to not routinely perform a transplant nephrectomy after graft failure.

EFFECTS OF TRANSPLANT NEPHRECTOMY ON RETRANSPLANTATION

Results of allograft nephrectomy are variable with few studies indicating its nonfavorable impact on various clinical outcomes of a second transplant. A meta-analysis involving 1,923 patients showed lower 3- and 5-year graft survival with higher chances of acute rejection, and higher PRA and delayed graft function (DGF).[14] However, it is difficult to draw definite conclusions as many of the included studies were affected by methodologic challenges.

Common hypotheses to explain sensitization after allograft nephrectomy are as follows:[15]

- *"Sponge theory":* The graft continuously adsorbs antibodies; thus, transplant nephrectomy could result in increased levels of preformed HLA antibodies in the serum. Rapid IS tapering post allograft nephrectomy may promote the formation of DSAs.
- Second, allograft nephrectomy by itself causes damage and triggers the immune system leading to the synthesis of HLA antibodies.

Conversely, in some retrospective studies, there were no significant differences in the rate of acute graft rejection, graft survival, and PRA levels between those receiving nephrectomy prior to retransplantation or not.[16]

DIALYSIS AFTER GRAFT FAILURE

The optimal timing of dialysis initiation in patients who have failed renal allograft has been evaluated by several observational studies, but conclusions are limited due to inherent biases. Data from the USRDS registry involving 4741 patients showed that each 1 mL/min/1.73 m^2 increase in estimated glomerular filtration rate at reinitiation of dialysis was associated with a 4% increased risk of mortality on dialysis in failed kidney transplant patients. The explanation for this paradoxical finding might be that in such settings, dialysis is initiated early in sicker patients, at higher levels of RRF.[3] Ideally, the dialysis initiation should be well planned with the creation of an AV fistula as these patients may experience a more rapid decline in renal function with an earlier onset of uremic symptoms.[17] Dialysis modality should be individualized to each patient because there are no compelling data to support one form of replacement therapy over another.

CONCLUSION

In summary, kidney allograft failure is a period of higher risk of mortality compared with other transition periods for patients with ESKD. Risk mitigation is a complex challenge for patients and their care teams. A multidisciplinary approach with early action and frequent intervention leading to comprehensive care is key to mitigating the high mortality experienced by patients with failed allografts who return to dialysis.

REFERENCES

1. Einecke G, Sis B, Reeve J, Mengel M, Campbell PM, Hidalgo LG, et al. Antibody-mediated microcirculation injury is the major cause of late kidney transplant failure. Am J Transplant. 2009;9(11):2520-31.
2. Rao PS, Schaubel DE, Jia X, Li S, Port FK, Saran R. Survival on dialysis post-kidney transplant failure: results from the scientific registry of transplant recipients. Am J Kidney Dis. 2007;49(2):294-300.
3. Gill JS, Abichandani R, Kausz AT, Pereira BJG. Mortality after kidney transplant failure: the impact of non-immunologic factors. Kidney Int. 2002;62(5):1875-83.
4. López-Gómez JM, Pérez-Flores I, Jofré R, Carretero D, Rodríguez-Benitez P, Villaverde M, et al. Presence of a failed kidney transplant in patients who are on hemodialysis is associated with chronic inflammatory state and erythropoietin resistance. J Am Soc Nephrol. 2004;15(9):2494-501.
5. Brar A, Markell M, Stefanov DG, Timpo E, Jindal RM, Nee R, et al. Mortality after renal allograft failure and return to dialysis. Am J Nephrol. 2017;45:180-6.
6. Smak Gregoor PJ, Zietse R, van Saase JL, op de Hoek CT, Ijzermans JN, Lavrijssen AT, et al. Immunosuppression should be stopped in patients with renal allograft failure. Clin Transplant. 2001;15(6):397-401.
7. van Leeuwen MT, Webster AC, McCredie MRE, Stewart JH, McDonald SP, Amin J, et al. Effect of reduced immunosuppression after kidney transplant failure on risk of cancer: population based retrospective cohort study. BMJ. 2010;340:c570.
8. Augustine JJ, Woodside KJ, Padiyar A, Sanchez EQ, Hricik DE, Schulak JA. Independent of nephrectomy, weaning immunosuppression leads to late sensitization after kidney transplant failure. Transplantation. 2012;94(7):738-43.
9. Davies SJ. Peritoneal dialysis in the patient with a failing renal allograft. Perit Dial Int. 2001;21:S280-4.
10. Andrews PA, Standards Committee of the British Transplantation Society. Summary of the British Transplantation Society guidelines for management of the failing kidney transplant. Transplantation. 2014;98:1130-3.
11. Fiorentino M, Gallo P, Giliberti M, Colucci V, Schena A, Stallone G, et al. Management of patients with a failed

kidney transplant: what should we do? Clin Kidney J. 2020;14(1):98-106.
12. Del Bello A, Congy N, Sallusto F, Cardeau-Desangles I, Fort M, Esposito L, et al. Anti-human leukocyte antigen immunization after early allograft nephrectomy. Transplantation. 2012;93(9):936-41.
13. Khakhar AK, Shahinian VB, House AA, Muirhead N, Hollomby DJ, Leckie SH, et al. The impact of allograft nephrectomy on percent panel reactive antibody and clinical outcome. Transplant Proc. 2003;35(2):862-3.
14. Lin J, Wang R, Xu Y, Chen J. Impact of renal allograft nephrectomy on graft and patient survival following retransplantation: a systematic review and meta-analysis. Nephrol Dial Transplant. 2018;33:700-8.
15. Bunthof KLW, Hazzan M, Hilbrands LB. Review: management of patients with kidney allograft failure. Transplant Rev (Orlando). 2018;32(3):178-86.
16. Surga N, Viart L, Wetzstein M, Mazouz H, Collon S, Tillou X. Impact of renal graft nephrectomy on second kidney transplant survival. Int Urol Nephrol. 2013;45:87-92.
17. Beltran S, Gavela E, Kanter J, Sancho A, Avila A, Górriz JL, et al. Beginning hemodialysis: Do patients with a failed renal transplant start in worse condition? Transplant Proc. 2009;41:2129-31.

CHAPTER 18

Radiological Imaging and Biopsy Technique in Kidney Allograft

Ujjwal Gorsi, Prabhjyot Singh Chowhan

INTRODUCTION

Worldwide, the most commonly transplanted solid organ is the kidney. Advancements in surgical techniques, immunosuppressive drugs, follow-up imaging, and histopathologic assessment of graft biopsies have all led to improved survival of graft kidneys. With the ever-rising need for kidney transplantation, the radiologist's role continues to grow as part of a multidisciplinary team. Surveillance imaging and protocol biopsies are commonly done in the initial couple of years post transplantation for picking up graft rejection and chronic graft nephropathy, entities that could be clinically occult in the early stages.[1] In the immediate postoperative period, Doppler ultrasonography (US) is the imaging technique of choice for assessing the graft kidney. It helps to establish a baseline evaluation that can be used for future comparisons. In cases with graft dysfunction, radiological modalities such as contrast-enhanced ultrasonography (CEUS) or magnetic resonance imaging (MRI) can help reach a definitive diagnosis and exclude nonrejection causes of graft dysfunction. Nuclear medicine can also come in use in the assessment of allograft function and perfusion, particularly in the immediate postoperative period. Renal scintigraphy provides both quantitative and qualitative information not only on cortical perfusion but also on parenchymal extraction and excretion. When imaging is equivocal and a histopathologic evaluation is required to guide management, US-guided biopsy is a safe and usually low-risk procedure. The complications related to kidney transplant surgery can be classified according to their time of occurrence since transplant and/or based on the disease categories, such as iatrogenic, immunologic, infectious, urinary, and neoplastic complications. As radiological features are often nonspecific, it is vital to know the patient's detailed history and time since transplant to form a reasonable differential diagnosis and guide a more specific diagnostic evaluation.

SURGICAL TECHNIQUE—THE BASICS

The renal transplant surgery has traditionally been conducted as an open procedure. Over the years, however, robot-assisted techniques have now evolved as safe alternatives.[2] In a subset of cases, laparoscopic approaches can also be used to avoid open surgery. The most common site for positioning the transplant kidney is the right iliac fossa (RIF). The left iliac fossa (LIF) is usually reserved for a second renal transplant in cases of a previous RIF graft or utilized in combined kidney-pancreas transplantation.[3,4] In cases of deceased-donor transplantation, the donor renal artery (RA) is harvested along with a portion of aorta (known as Carrel patch), and then an end-to-side anastomosis is performed with the recipient external iliac artery (EIA). Also, an end-to-side anastomosis of the donor RA and recipient EIA is performed in cases of a living kidney donor. End-to-end anastomosis with the recipient's internal iliac artery is performed in patients in whom the EIA has already been utilized for another transplant or in cases where there is extensive atherosclerotic involvement of the EIA. The donor renal vein is usually anastomosed in an end-to-side manner to the recipient external iliac vein (EIV). As far as ureteric anastomosis is concerned, a myotomy of the bladder wall is done, and the donor ureter is sutured to the mucosa of the bladder over the lateral or anterior wall.

IMAGING MODALITIES

Ultrasonography

Ultrasonography, with its many benefits, including a lack of ionizing radiation and the capability to evaluate graft vasculature without administration of contrast, is now the initial modality to be used for evaluating the graft kidney. Also, a good acoustic window is often available as most of the graft kidneys are placed in the RIF in an extraperitoneal plane. On grayscale evaluation, one must document the longest dimension of the graft kidney, assess the pelvicalyceal system for any hydronephrosis, and look for any perinephric collection(s). **Figure 1** shows the grayscale US appearance of a normal graft kidney. A detailed Doppler assessment of the vasculature should also be done along with spectral analysis. Peak systolic velocity (PSV) must be evaluated at the main RA anastomosis, distal to it, as well as in the EIA proximal to the anastomotic site in order to enable computation of the RA to EIA PSV ratio. Resistive index (RI) in the interlobar arteries must be obtained; normal values range between 0.7 and 0.8. The graft renal vein must be examined from the hilum up to the anastomosis. Patency of the EIV should also be assessed. **Figures 2A and B** demonstrate the normal Doppler features of a transplant kidney.

CHAPTER HIGHLIGHTS

- Complications that develop following renal transplantation usually have a predictable time course and typical clinical and imaging findings.
- The key role of radiological imaging in renal transplant recipients is to evaluate the graft integrity, anatomy, and function and to rule out nonrejection related causes of graft dysfunction.
- When imaging is equivocal and a histopathologic evaluation is required to guide management, ultrasound guided biopsy by the cortical tangential technique is a safe and usually low-risk procedure.

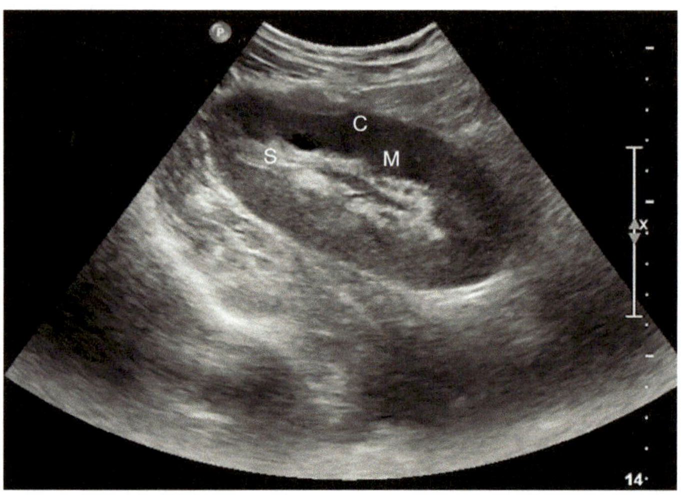

Fig. 1: Ultrasound appearance of normal renal allograft showing the renal sinus (S), cortex (C), and medulla (M).

Contrast-enhanced ultrasonography can also be used to assess graft kidneys. It involves administration of ultrasound contrast agents (UCAs), which are basically gas-containing microbubbles. CEUS can help assess parenchymal perfusion, look for infarcted areas, and can also help assess the flow dynamics of renal masses and thus enable better characterization. A major benefit of using CEUS over contrast-enhanced computed tomography (CECT) is that UCAs are not excreted by the kidneys (but rather by the lungs) and therefore do not cause contrast-induced nephropathy.

Ultrasonography elastography is another rather new modality that evaluates tissue stiffness. Its role in the assessment of graft kidneys is still not established as early studies have shown dismal interobserver agreement and no definite correlation between the measured tissue stiffness and the clinical, laboratory, and/or histologic findings.[5,6]

Computed Tomography

Computed tomography (CT) acts as a complementary modality in the assessment of kidney transplant complications. For example, if a patient's PSVs are elevated on US evaluation, CT angiography (CTA) may be done (if his/her kidney function allows) to establish a diagnosis of renal artery stenosis (RAS) noninvasively. CT with contrast administration can help in characterizing focal lesions that are picked up on US. In addition, CT urography can be conducted to confirm a urinoma. However, in cases with

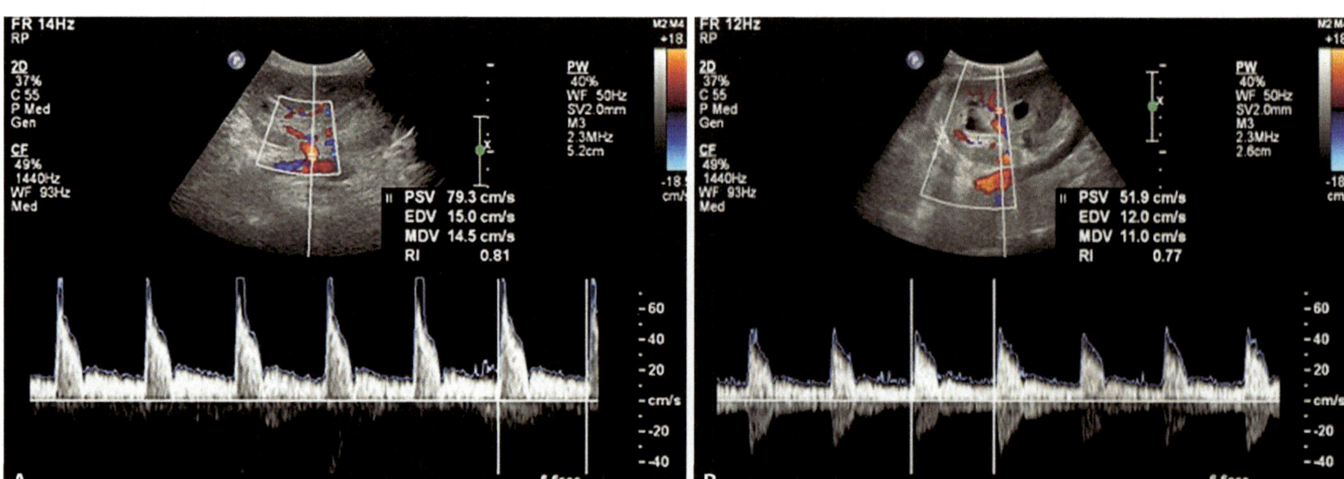

Figs. 2A and B: Doppler features of a normal transplant kidney. (A) The image above shows the tracing at the level of the renal hilum and demonstrates a low resistance arterial vascular bed with streamlined systolic flow and continuous forward diastolic flow; (B) Normal intrarenal artery waveform on spectral Doppler ultrasound shows a brisk systolic upstroke with a subsequent slow decay in diastole, forward flow being maintained until the next cardiac cycle.

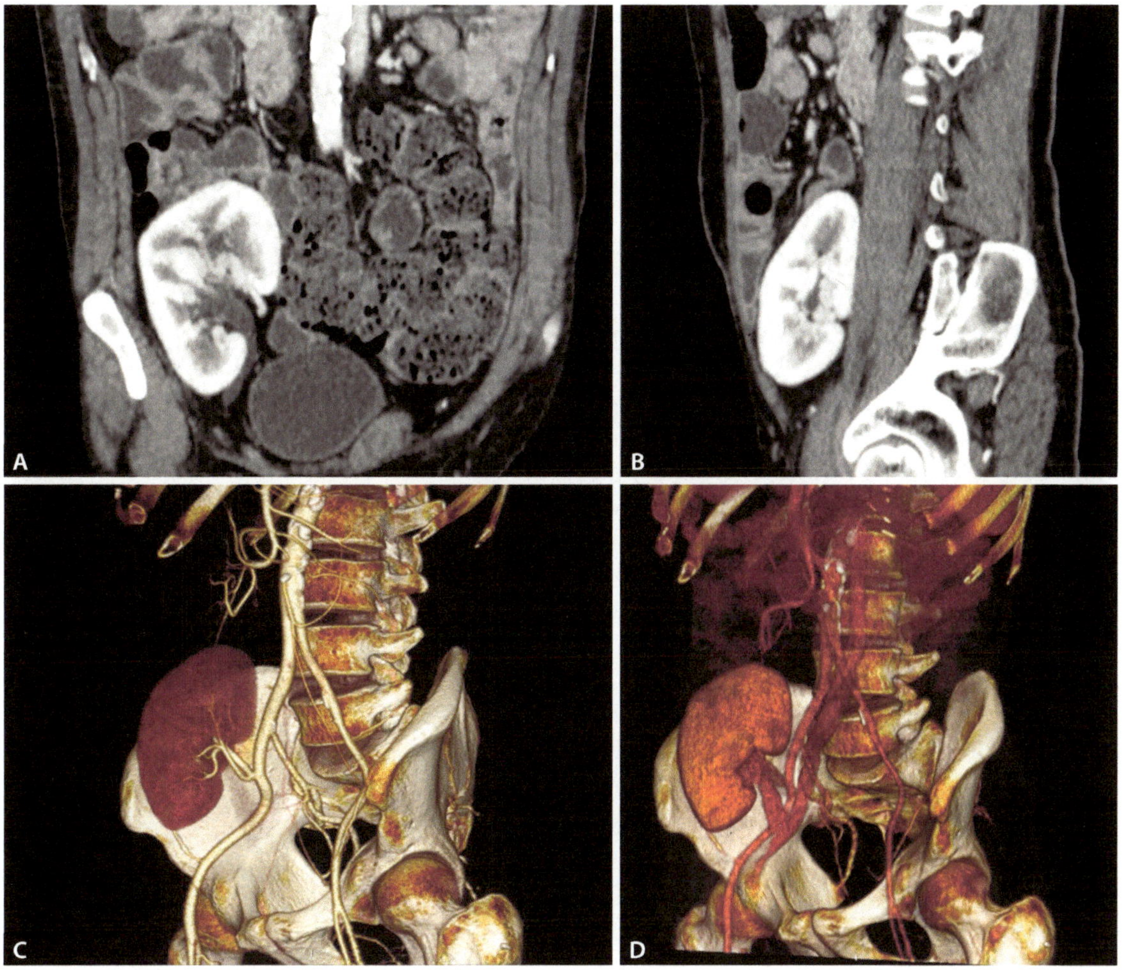

Figs. 3A to D: Normal transplant kidney on CT. (A and B) Postcontrast venous phase (A) coronal and (B) sagittal reformatted images showing the uniformly enhancing parenchyma of the graft kidney; (C and D) Volume-rendered images showing (C) end-to-side anastomosis of the transplant renal artery with the recipient external iliac artery (EIA) and (D) end-to-side anastomosis of the transplant renal vein with the recipient external iliac vein (EIV).

deranged kidney function, contrast administration must be avoided in order to minimize the chances of developing contrast-induced nephropathy. Noncontrast CT (NCCT) can help assess the entire extent of a perinephric collection if it is partly obscured by bowel gas at US. Also, NCCT has a higher accuracy than US for picking up calculi, especially the smaller ones. **Figures 3A to D** show the normal appearance of a transplanted kidney on CECT.

Magnetic Resonance Imaging

Magnetic resonance imaging has emerged as an important problem-solving tool in kidney transplant patients in whom US findings are indeterminate. The modality provides multiple advantages over CT. First, it does not subject the patient to any ionizing radiation. Second, among all the imaging modalities, it has the greatest contrast resolution. Third, angiographic images can be generated with MRI without using contrast. In addition, MR urography is a technique that can be used to study the collecting system without any injection of contrast and thus can be utilized in patients with deranged renal function.

Nuclear Medicine

Nuclear medicine studies have proven to be useful in the evaluation of graft perfusion and for collecting system injury following kidney transplant. Technetium 99m (^{99m}Tc) mercaptoacetyltriglycine (MAG_3) or ^{99m}Tc diethylenetriaminepentaacetic acid (DTPA) is typically used. The radiopharmaceutical is administered by the intravenous route and successive acquisitions are made to assess the vascular (flow) phase, parenchymal (functional) phase, and washout (excretory) phase. These studies are good alternatives for patients who cannot undergo contrast CT and/or MRI.

Fluorodeoxyglucose (FDG) positron emission tomography (PET)/CT is another useful imaging modality in post-transplant patients. It has been shown to be an accurate tool for the workup of patients with diagnostically unresolved symptoms of malignancy and/or infection because of its high sensitivity and negative predictive value.[7] It is also sensitive and specific in the detection of post-transplant lymphoproliferative disorder (PTLD) and can upstage or detect occult PTLD compared with conventional CT imaging.[8] Since it is a type of functional imaging, it also plays a role in monitoring treatment response in cases with PTLD. Recent studies have also shown that FDG PET/CT could noninvasively detect subclinical allograft rejection, with an excellent negative predictive value that may help avoid the need for invasive systematic biopsies.[9]

Digital Subtraction Angiography

Some important indications of graft kidney angiography are acute anuria and graft dysfunction with hypertension not responding to medication, in which definitive diagnosis of rejection or RAS is required in order to plan subsequent management. In acute rejection, a pruned-tree appearance can be appreciated secondary to the loss of second- and third-order branches. The arteriogram is essentially normal in acute tubular necrosis (ATN). In chronic rejection, arteriography demonstrates small graft size with irregularity, attenuation, and occlusion of interlobar arteries and a patchy nephrogram due to areas of cortical infarction.

As discussed earlier, angiography is also indicated in patients with hypertension who do not respond to medical management. In such situations, it may demonstrate the degree of RAS. Hemodynamically significant (>50%) stenosis can be treated in the same sitting with percutaneous transluminal angioplasty (PTA) with covered metal stents or drug-eluting stents.

Patients undergoing biopsy of the graft kidney can develop arteriovenous fistulas (AVFs) and pseudoaneurysms due to vascular injury. Endovascular techniques such as transcatheter embolization are the treatment of choice for both symptomatic AVFs and pseudoaneurysms. Superselective embolization done using metallic coils or placement of stent grafts diminishes the loss of functioning graft parenchyma and ensures long-term graft survival.

Dual-energy X-ray Absorptiometry

Bone and mineral disorders are commonly seen in renal transplant patients and are associated with a high risk of fracture, morbidity, and mortality. There is a wide spectrum of overlapping bone abnormalities seen after transplant surgery, including osteoporosis and persisting high- or low-turnover bone disease. Reduction of fracture risk and other bone-associated complications needs proper identification of these aberrations along with the risk incurred by the immunosuppressive therapy. A dual-energy X-ray absorptiometry (DEXA) scan is a relatively accurate, noninvasive, and cost-effective screening method for estimating bone mass and can help predict fracture risk in renal transplant recipients. A study of 238 renal transplant patients showed that 19% of cases developed a fracture over a 12-year follow-up period, and patients with osteopenia and osteoporosis had a markedly higher risk as compared to those with normal bone mineral density.[10] DEXA, however, has a few limitations, including: (1) An inability to differentiate cortical from trabecular bone, (2) confounding signals from concomitant vascular calcification, and (3) observations that glucocorticoid-induced fractures occur at greater bone mineral density values as compared to patients with nonglucocorticoid-induced osteoporosis.[11]

RENAL TRANSPLANT COMPLICATIONS

The Timeline

Based on the time after which they develop postsurgery, these complications may be categorized into early (including hyperacute and acute), intermediate, and late complications. The major complication categories include perioperative/iatrogenic complications, allograft rejection, perinephric collections, urinary complications, vascular complications, infections, and neoplastic complications. All of these broad categories further comprise a multitude of complications, many of which have a predictable time course and typical clinical and imaging findings. It is important to know that not all complications occur singularly and that multiple complications could occur at the same time in the same patient. However, categorizing complications based on time since transplant permits better discrimination between the differential diagnoses during workup.

Perioperative Complications

The standard practice of performing postoperative US allows quick detection of perioperative complications. This category of complications includes those related to surgical methods, anatomic implications of extraperitoneal positioning of renal grafts such as renal allograft compartment syndrome (RACS), and complications such as hemorrhage, pseudoaneurysm formation and AVFs. Surgical technique-associated complications are usually related to the vascular anastomoses, and these may subsequently result in thrombosis of the graft artery or vein.[12] Vascular thrombosis and RACS characteristically develop in the immediate postoperative period.

Renal Allograft Compartment Syndrome

An infrequent and under-recognized cause of early graft dysfunction, RACS develops due to increased intracompartment pressure and subsequent ischemia of the graft kidney because of its extraperitoneal positioning.[13] This may occur because of extrinsic compression as a result of size discrepancy between the extraperitoneal space and the renal allograft or because of extrinsic vascular compression.[14] Extrinsic pressure from a perinephric collection may also occur.

In the immediate postoperative period, markedly reduced or absent flow in the cortex of the graft kidney on Doppler US is suggestive of RACS, which commonly occurs within 2 hours of surgery.[14] Immediate identification is critical, as the allograft may be saved if reoperated upon immediately. However, intraperitoneal positioning of the graft kidney comes with its own set of complications as such positioning is associated with greater mobility, making the graft prone to torsion.[15]

Vascular Complications

While these can develop any time after surgery, vascular complications are especially important in the early postoperative phase, as timely rectification of these complications may permit rescue of the transplanted kidney. Transplant RA or vein thrombosis may develop immediately post-transplant or up to day 5. RAS is routinely encountered ~3 months or later after transplant, as its causes tend to be multifactorial.

Renal Artery Thrombosis

With a prevalence of around 0.4%, renal artery thrombosis (RAT) is a rare albeit serious complication and can lead to graft loss.[16,17] It mostly occurs within minutes to hours of transplant surgery and can develop due to anastomotic occlusion, hyperacute rejection, RA kinking, or the presence of an intimal flap.[18] Few case reports also suggest extrinsic RA compression and vasculitis as uncommon causes of RAT.[18,19]

Clinical signs of this entity include an abrupt fall in urine output with worsening hypertension. Even though the transplant kidney is denervated, patients may experience pain at the graft site due to irritation of the peritoneum as a result of graft infarction and the associated inflammation along the peritoneal margins.[18]

Infarction of the graft kidney may be global or segmental. On grayscale evaluation, a segmental infarct will be seen as a hypoechoic mass-like area, which may either be poorly defined or have a well-defined echogenic wall with a corresponding wedge-shaped area of avascularity on Doppler evaluation. However, it is important to correlate with the symptoms and urinalysis, as these features may also be noted in cases of pyelonephritis and graft rupture.[18]

In cases of global infarct, Doppler US will show absent blood flow throughout the graft. **Figure 4** shows the appearance of global renal allograft infarction on CECT. Early and precise diagnosis is of paramount importance, as urgent intervention is needed for graft salvage. In cases where the US results are nondiagnostic and there is no clinical indication for immediate reexploration, MR angiography (MRA), digital subtraction angiography (DSA), or renal scintigraphy can be considered. MRA and DSA will demonstrate reduced or absent flow to the graft kidney and an abrupt cutoff in the transplant RA. At scintigraphy, decreased or absent graft perfusion can be appreciated. However, this finding is not specific for RAT and may also be noted with rejection.[20]

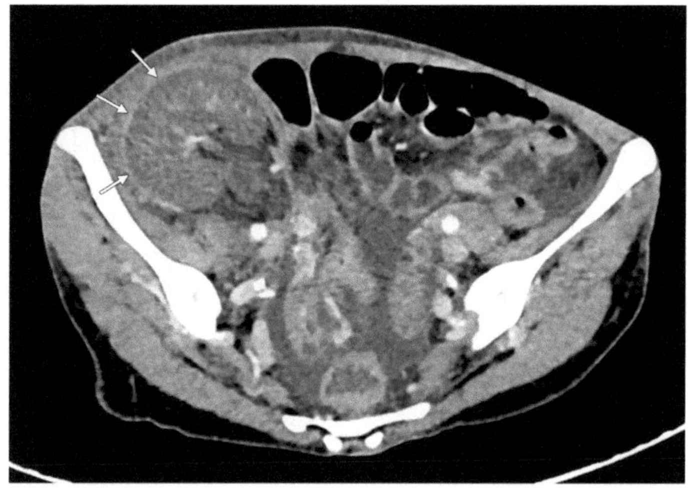

Fig. 4: Global infarction of renal allograft. Axial CECT image showing a globular nonenhancing transplant kidney with the characteristic "cortical-rim" sign (arrows).

Renal Vein Thrombosis

This complication mostly develops within the initial five postoperative days, with peak occurrence within the first 48 hours. However, a few cases of delayed renal vein thrombosis (RVT) have also been reported in the literature.[18,21] While the clinical findings include acute onset pain and reduced urine output, early US will show edematous enlargement of the transplant kidney with loss of corticomedullary differentiation, and perinephric fluid. Spectral Doppler evaluation will show reversal of diastolic flow in the transplant RA; however, flow reversal may also be appreciated in cases with graft rejection, those with graft torsion, and/or in cases with ATN.[22] For RAT, early and precise diagnosis is crucial for graft salvage. To reestablish the venous flow, open surgical thrombectomy is often performed. However, in those with late thrombosis, endovascular thrombolysis may be considered.[23]

Transplant Renal Artery Stenosis

The most common vascular complication of kidney transplant surgery, RAS affects ~3% of all kidney transplant surgeries and usually develops 3 months to 2 years after the transplant surgery. The most common presentation is hypertension not responding to treatment—often occurring in isolation (53%) or in combination with a fall in kidney function (44%).[24]

Direct signs on US can be observed at the narrowing site and include elevated PSV, abnormal RA to EIA PSV ratio, and color aliasing due to the turbulent flow.[25] Historically, a PSV >250 cm/s in the transplant RA or an RA to EIA ratio of >1.8 had been used as indicators of significant transplant RAS.

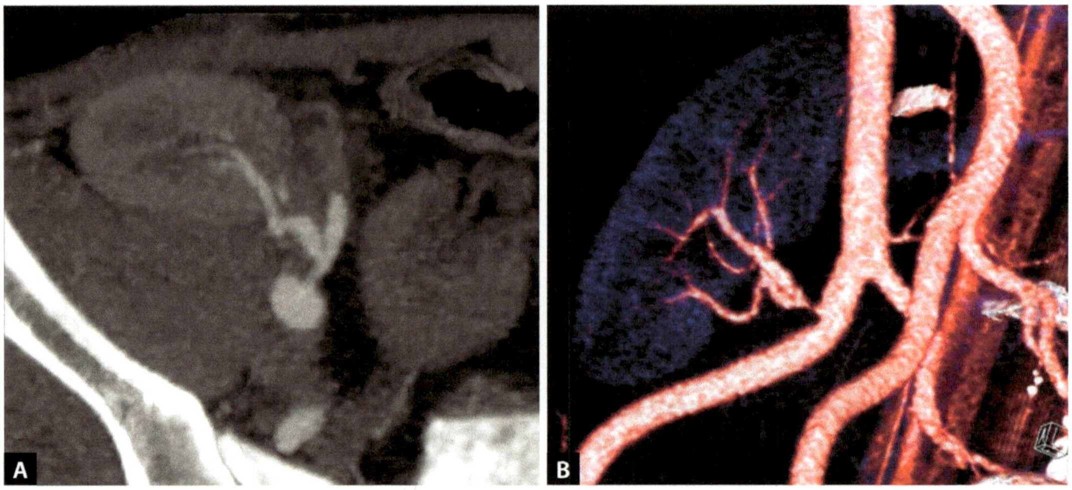

Figs. 5A and B: Transplant renal artery stenosis. (A) Axial maximum intensity projection image; and (B) Volume-rendered image showing focal stenosis at the anastomotic site between the graft renal artery and the recipient right external iliac artery (EIA).

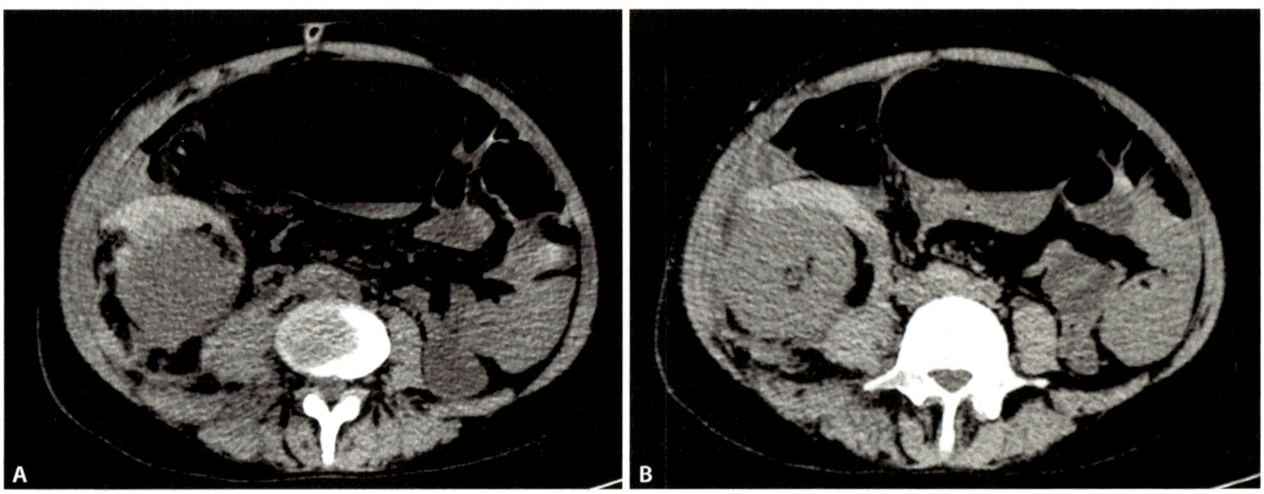

Figs. 6A and B: Perinephric hematoma. Noncontrast CT images at two different axial sections showing a hyperdense collection in a renal transplant recipient on day 4 of surgery.

However, recent data suggest that these values may lead to false-positive diagnoses. A study conducted in 2017[26] found that 26% of renal transplant cases without RAS had PSVs >250 cm/s within the first 9 months post-transplant surgery.

In the absence of other signs or waveform alterations, an anastomotic site PSV of 340–400 cm/s has been advocated as a more reliable cutoff for transplant RAS.[26] Indirect signs may be seen downstream to the stenosis and include a tardus–parvus waveform at spectral analysis. Relatively decreased RI values may also be noted. **Figures 5A and B** demonstrate the characteristic radiological appearance of transplant RAS on CT.

Perinephric Collections

Four major types of collections may be seen around the graft kidney: hematoma, urinoma, abscess, and lymphocele (roughly occurring in that order with respect to time since transplant). Imaging features at grayscale evaluation may often overlap, but Doppler evaluation along with ancillary clinical information can help make the differentiation. When still in doubt with regard to the differentiation between these collections, diagnostic aspiration, and fluid analysis can be considered.

Perinephric Hematoma

These are frequently encountered in the immediate postoperative period and should be documented on the baseline postoperative US. Although most resolve spontaneously, a small subset (such as those causing significant mass effect and/or those associated with continuous bleeding warranting transfusion) may require surgical evacuation.[27] Depending on the evolution of the blood products, hematomas could appear hyperechoic, hypoechoic, or anechoic. Hyperacute hematomas can appear anechoic but will usually contain mobile echogenic debris within. Acute hematomas appear heterogeneously hyperechoic, and over time, develop central hypoechoic or cyst-like areas, indicating clot lysis. At NCCT evaluation **(Figs. 6A and B)**, acute hematomas appear

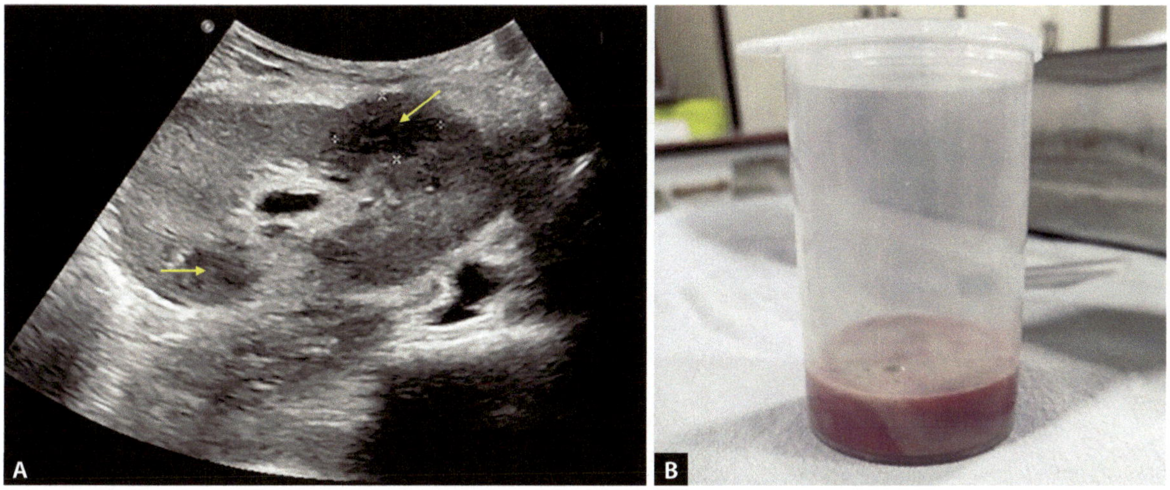

Figs. 7A and B: (A) Grayscale USG showing two heterogeneously hypoechoic lesions (yellow arrows) in a transplanted kidney. The patient had a fever of 102°F with leukocytosis; (B) A diagnostic aspiration was done from the lesion at the lower pole that yielded pus. Culture showed growth of *Staphylococcus* and gram-negative bacteria.

hyperdense (>30 HU), and at MRI, they appear hyperintense on T1-weighted images. It is also important to differentiate a perirenal collection from a subcapsular one as the latter is more likely to exert mass effect on the graft parenchyma.

Urinoma

A leak from the renal collecting system, ureter, or ureteroneocystostomy site can lead to urinoma formation and is usually detected in the first 10 days after transplant surgery. Urinomas frequently develop as a result of sparse blood supply to the ureter or elevated pressures due to obstruction.[18]

On US, urinomas are seen as hypoechoic collections and often mimic seromas and/or lymphoceles. The collecting system may further be evaluated with CT or MR urography to detect any leakage of contrast. Renal scintigraphy or retrograde urography may also be done. Scintigraphy performed with ^{99m}Tc MAG$_3$ shows incremental extraurinary radiopharmaceutical pooling in a region that first appears photopenic and may exhibit mass effect by the urinoma on the renal allograft.

Fluid aspirated from a urinoma usually shows higher potassium and creatinine levels than in the blood serum, whereas a lymphocele aspirate will show these concentrations to be comparable to those in the serum. It is important to identify urinomas as these may lead to electrolyte imbalances or become superinfected.[28]

Perinephric Abscess

Formation of a perinephric abscess usually occurs within the first weeks to months after transplant surgery.[29] A perinephric abscess may form secondary to an infection of the graft kidney or of any adjacent organ or via local dissemination of an infection in the abdominal wall. Fever and elevated total leukocyte count in association with a collection in the perinephric space should point toward this complication. On grayscale, these usually appear heterogeneously hypoechoic with septations and debris within **(Figs. 7A and B)**, with Doppler showing flow within the septations and thickened walls. CT **(Figs. 8A and B)** and MRI may help in evaluating the extent of the collection and in detecting adjacent structures' involvement. Early intervention with systemic antibiotics with or without percutaneous drainage (PCD) is critical, given the immunocompromised status.

Lymphocele

The most common of the perinephric collections after renal transplant, lymphoceles typically occur 2 weeks to 6 months post-transplantation, and frequently lead to graft hydronephrosis.[18] These collections develop along the lymphatic pathways and are usually asymptomatic.[30] On US, they appear anechoic with well-defined margins and may occasionally show thin internal septations. On cross-sectional imaging, these collections typically display a thin, almost imperceptible wall and internal simple fluid attenuation on CT and high signal on T2-weighted MR images. In cases where lymphoceles cause mass effects, PCD or peritoneal fenestration may need to be performed. PCD is usually associated with high rates (~90%) of reaccumulation; thus, sclerosing agents have been tried as alternatives with differing degrees of success.[31]

Obstructive Urologic Complications

In recent years, the incidence of ureteral complications has reduced multifold owing to improvements in surgical techniques, utilization of shorter ureters, and reduction

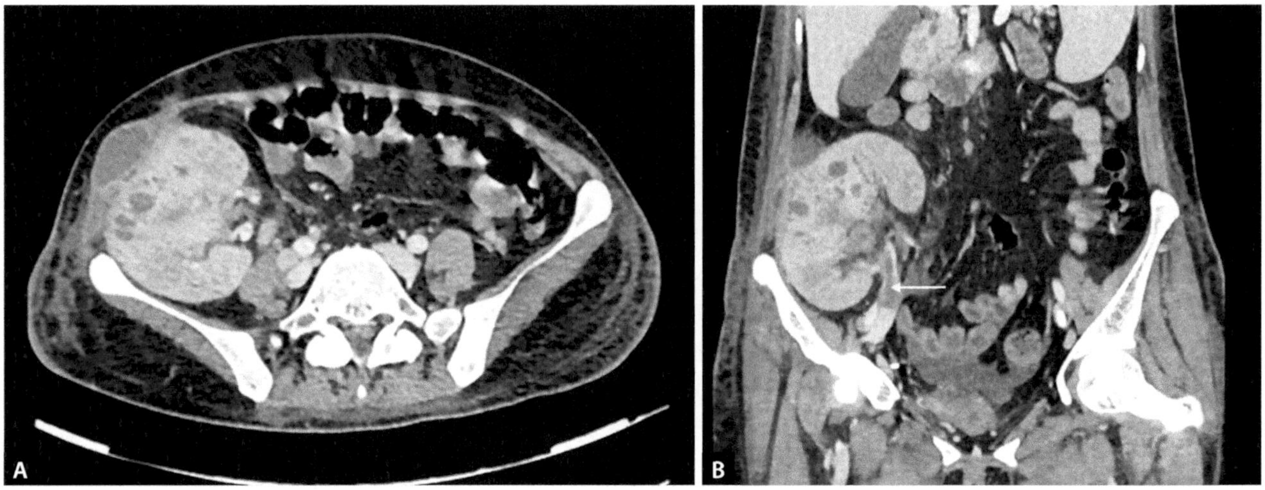

Figs. 8A and B: Renal abscesses with perinephric extension. (A) Axial; and (B) Coronal reformatted CECT images of a renal transplant recipient who presented with fever and right iliac fossa (RIF) pain ~2 weeks after transplantation. The images show reduced nephrographic density of the graft kidney with multiple ill-defined variable-sized hypodense lesions within and an associated peripherally enhancing collection in the perinephric space. Note should be made of transplant renal vein thrombosis (arrow in B)

in steroid usage.[32] Ureteric obstruction may uncommonly develop in the first couple of days post-transplant, but it most frequently develops after the first postoperative month and usually occurs due to ureteric stenosis.[32] The obstruction can develop due to ischemia leading to stricture formation, due to compression from a perinephric collection, or due to intraluminal causes such as calculi.[32]

Ultrasonography assessment for ureteric obstruction must include evaluation of the collecting system and transplant ureter from the urinary bladder to the hilum of the transplanted kidney, and one must also always look for periureteral collections and for the presence of stones or debris within the graft pelvicalyceal system. **Figure 9** demonstrates hydroureteronephrosis in a transplanted kidney secondary to a bladder site anastomotic stricture. Whenever new hydronephrosis is identified, one must always correlate with the urinalysis and exclude superimposed pyonephrosis which would require urgent intervention. In patients with pyonephrosis, US will show urothelial thickening and layered debris within the dilated collecting system **(Fig. 10)**.

Because of the dependent positioning of the graft in the RIF/LIF, the shorter length of transplant ureter, and loss of the normal obliquity, there is an increased tendency for vesicoureteral reflex (VUR) that may lead to mild pelvicaliectasis. However, there is no indication for any intervention in the absence of graft dysfunction and secondary features of obstruction.[33] Stenosis of the graft ureter is usually managed with retrograde balloon dilatation and stent deployment.[34] **Figures 11A to D** show a stricture of the proximal transplant ureter that was managed with antegrade ureteric stenting. For distal lesions, excision of the stricture with ureteric reimplantation can be done. In cases where the scarring is extensive or obstructs the pelviureteric junction, one may have to resort to donor-to-native ureteroureterostomy or pyelovesicostomy.[35]

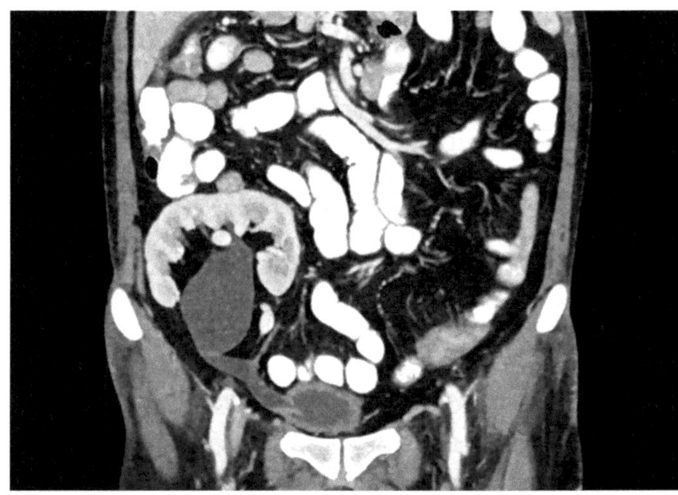

Fig. 9: Hydroureteronephrosis of graft kidney secondary to bladder site anastomotic stricture. Coronal reformatted CECT image showing significant dilatation of the graft pelvicalyceal system and ureter with focal narrowing of the distal ureter at the site of anastomosis with the urinary bladder.

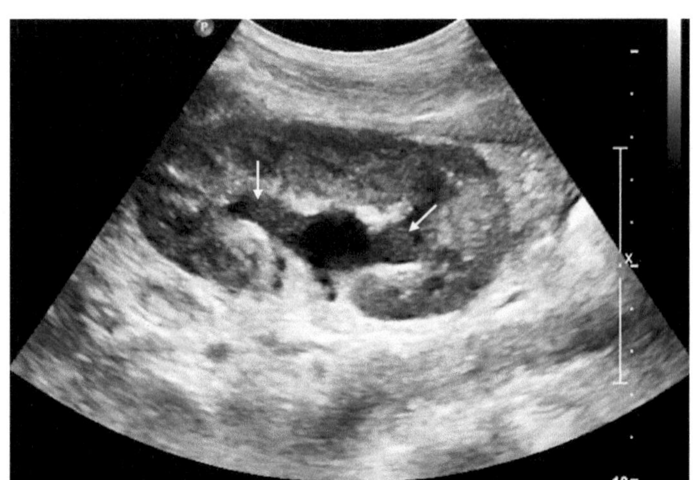

Fig. 10: Pyonephrosis of graft kidney. The image shows dilated renal pelvicalyceal system with echogenic debris within (arrows).

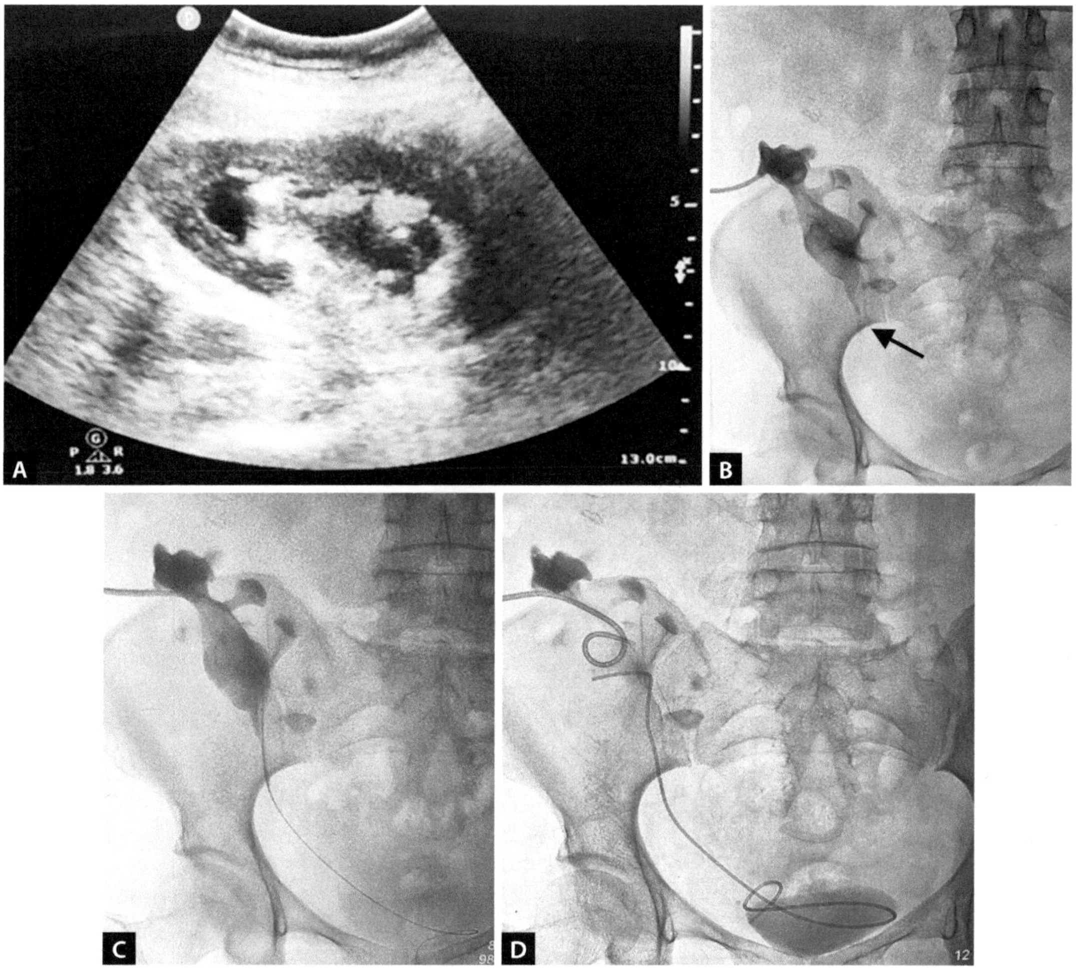

Figs. 11A to D: Transplant ureteric stricture. (A) grayscale US image showing hydronephrosis of the graft kidney with echogenic contents within. A retrograde double J (DJ) stenting was attempted for this patient. However, it was unsuccessful; (B) A percutaneous nephrostomy was then done for this patient and the nephrostogram revealed a stricture in the proximal transplant ureter (arrow); (C) The stricture was negotiated using guidewires and catheters and access into the bladder was attained; (D) A DJ catheter was then inserted in an antegrade fashion over a guidewire.

Allograft Parenchymal Complications

These include delayed graft function, ATN, allograft rejection, and drug-related nephrotoxic effects. In these cases, the most important role of radiology is to exclude other causes that can cause graft dysfunction.

Delayed Graft Function

This complication is said to occur if the patient develops a need for dialysis within the first week of transplant surgery.[36] The most important risk factor here is the cold ischemia time. Other predisposing conditions include graft infarction, rejection, ATN, and perigraft collections. While the grayscale evaluation of the graft parenchyma may show no significant parenchymal changes, Doppler could reveal diminished or absent diastolic flow with increased RIs. These findings are, however, nonspecific and could be seen in cases of rejection as well.

Rejection of Renal Allograft

The Banff classification of allograft pathology classifies graft rejection into six categories based on the histopathology plus the clinical, serological, and molecular parameters.[37] However, before the proposal of this system of classification in 1991, rejection was mainly classified based on the time since transplant surgery into hyperacute, acute, accelerated acute, and chronic types.[38] While the new classification system retains some temporal correlation, it is now established that there is significant overlap between the acute and chronic phases of rejection.

In view of the evolving nomenclature, terms linked to time since surgery continue to be used in day-to-day practice. Hyperacute rejection occurs within minutes to hours and is frequently picked up intraoperatively. This rare condition occurs due to small vessel thrombosis that develops immediately after vascular anastomosis, leading to abrupt global graft ischemia.

Acute rejection develops around 5–7 days post-transplant surgery and occurs due to activation of T cells.[38] Accelerated acute rejection (occurring within the first 5 days) is usually more severe and is mediated by antibodies and is usually seen in cases with prior transfusions or other causes of pre-sensitization.[38] In patients with chronic rejection, there is a gradual progressive decline in graft function, which usually begins months to years after the transplant surgery.

In allograft rejection, the radiological findings are often nonspecific, emphasizing the importance of protocol biopsy, which is required for reaching a conclusive diagnosis. However, US is still an important component of the diagnostic workup as it is needed to rule out other potential causes of kidney dysfunction. In cases of rejection, gray-scale evaluation may show edematous thickening of the cortex with loss of corticomedullary differentiation. Doppler studies may show reduced cortical flow and elevated intraparenchymal RIs. When assessed in the early postoperative phase (1 week to 3 months), increased RI (>0.74) has been seen to be associated with reduced long-term survival of the graft kidney at 1 year.[39] However, RI alone is not sufficient to differentiate rejection from other causes of dysfunction.[40] Increased RI may also be seen in cases of ATN, drug nephrotoxicity, and ureteric obstruction.[41,42] Therefore, it is key to have a sound knowledge of the patient's history before conducting a US evaluation of the graft kidney.

Contrast-enhanced ultrasonography can help in the assessment of the graft perfusion at a microvascular level and may help predict impending graft dysfunction.[43] In acute rejection, delayed cortical perfusion can be noted on CEUS.[44] This modality can also help identify the most viable portions of graft cortex during biopsy.[45]

Computed tomography is not routinely indicated in patients with suspected allograft rejection, as both ATN and rejection show edematous graft enlargement along with patchy enhancement on CT. MRI scores over CT not only provide a detailed evaluation of the anatomy of the graft kidney but also allow functional assessment. Diffusion-weighted imaging (DWI) is a promising noninvasive tool for the assessment of transplant kidneys. Blood oxygenation level dependent (BOLD) and arterial spin labeling MRI sequences can give information on the perfusion and oxygenation of the graft, which play a vital role in the assessment of graft kidney function.[46-48]

Acute Tubular Necrosis

Acute tubular necrosis is another important cause of early transplant kidney dysfunction, and clinical and radiological evaluation usually do not allow distinction between ATN and rejection. Scintigraphy may help but there is significant overlap in the findings of the two entities. Researchers have also investigated the use of fluorine 18 (^{18}F) FDG PET/CT for this differentiation. However, percutaneous biopsy continues to be the gold standard investigation.[49]

Drug-related Nephrotoxicity

Kidney transplant immunosuppression regimens can be divided into three phases: induction therapy, maintenance, and treatment of rejection.[50,51] Maintenance drugs comprise antimetabolite agents, calcineurin inhibitors, and/or corticosteroids. Calcineurin inhibitors are particularly associated with nephrotoxic effects with irreversible damage.[52] It is, however, still a challenge to distinguish between drug toxicity and other causes of graft dysfunction.

Infectious Complications

Transplant patients are more prone to developing infections due to the immunosuppressive drugs. In the early phase (first month postoperative), most infections are nosocomial or surgery related and include microbes such as methicillin-resistant *Staphylococcus aureus* (MRSA) and vancomycin-resistant enterococci (VRE).[53] In the second to sixth month, recipients are more susceptible to opportunistic infections, cytomegalovirus (CMV) being the most common agent, followed by polyomavirus (mainly BK virus) and Epstein–Barr virus (EBV).[53] After 6 months, routine infections are more commonly seen, e.g., urinary tract infection and community-acquired pneumonia. However, in view of continued immunosuppression, these cases continue to be at risk of developing infections with pathogens such as *Nocardia* and fungal infections with *Aspergillus* and *Mucor* species.

Imaging of the graft kidney with a suspected infection is done with the aim to exclude complications. On US, abscesses appear as perinephric or intrarenal collections with heteroechoic contents within along with a peripheral hypervascular rim. However, in most cases of suspected graft infection, the US evaluation is often normal. It is important to look for the presence of echogenic debris or mobile masses within the renal collecting system, which could suggest pyonephrosis or a fungus ball, respectively. In a febrile patient, a striated nephrogram is suggestive of pyelonephritis on CECT, but this finding may also be noted in RVT and in cases with obstructive uropathy. On rare occasions, necrotizing infections may become life threatening by rapidly progressing to emphysematous pyelonephritis. Such patients often require surgical removal of the transplanted kidney.

Neoplastic Complications

After cardiovascular and infective causes, malignancy is the third most frequent cause of mortality in renal transplant recipients. Compared with the general population, these patients have a greater risk of malignancy (approximately three to five times) with some cancers

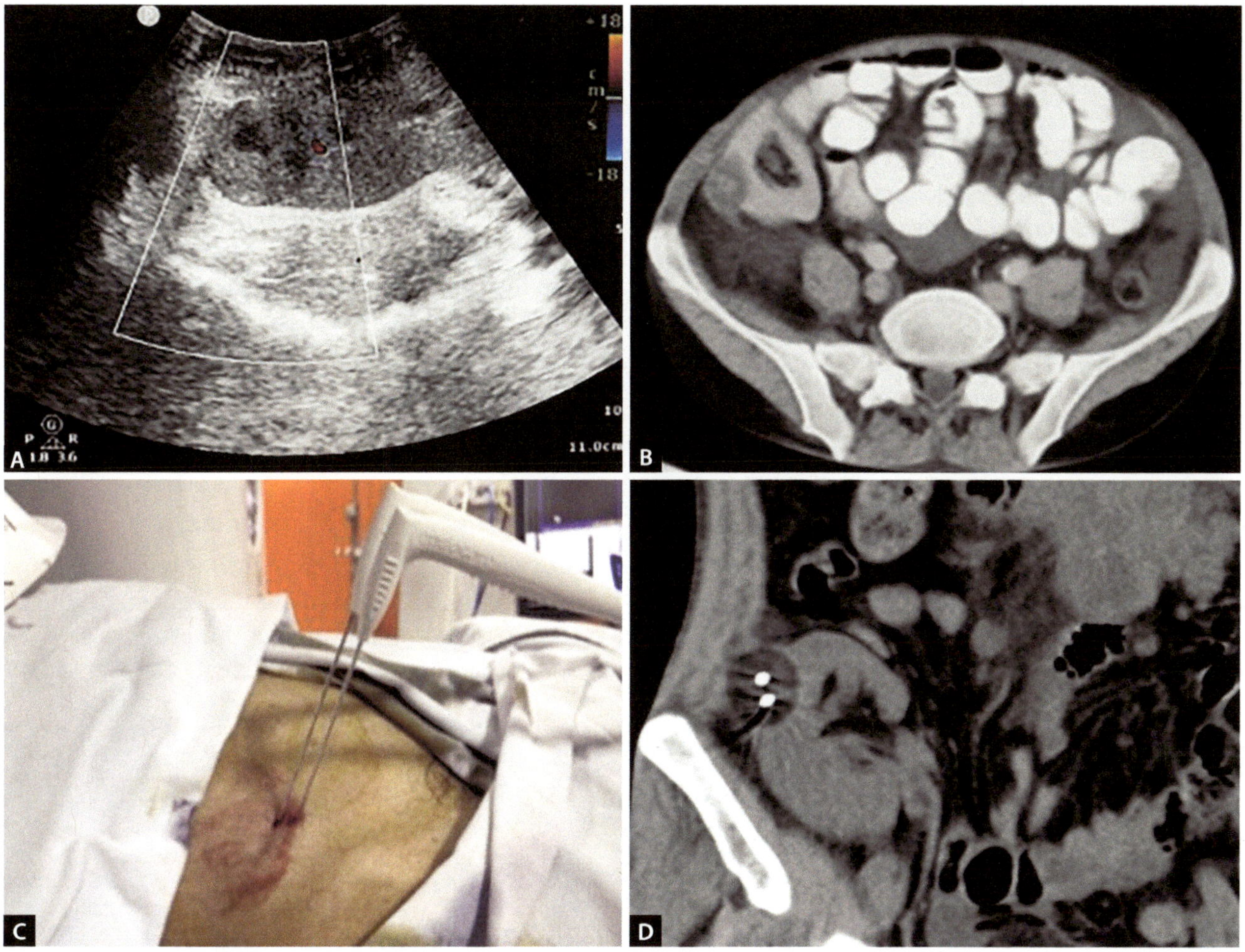

Figs. 12A to D: Incidentally detected renal cell carcinoma (RCC) in graft kidney on surveillance imaging. (A) US showing a well-defined exophytic heteroechoic mass lesion arising from the upper polar cortex of the graft kidney and showing no significant internal vascularity on Doppler; (B) The lesion appears hypoenhancing on CECT. Tissue sampling confirmed the lesion to be an RCC. The patient was then taken up for cryoablation of the lesion; (C) Intraprocedural image showing two cryoprobes in situ; (D) Coronal reformatted noncontrast CT (NCCT) image showing the cryoprobes in situ with the surrounding iceball formation. An A0 ablation was achieved in this case.

(e.g., nonmelanomatous skin cancer, colon cancer, and lymphoma) having a significantly greater risk (~20–500 times).[54-56] However, with some cancers, such as those of the breast, prostate, and brain, no increased incidence is noted.[57] The incidence of primary renal malignant neoplasm **(Figs. 12A to D)** in the transplant kidney is around six times that in the native kidney for all types, but the risk for papillary subtypes is substantially higher (~13 times).[58] A greater risk of urothelial cancers also exists in transplant recipients who develop infections with the BK virus.[59]

Post-transplant lymphoproliferative disorder is a common condition that affects transplant patients. Since the entity may not show any clinical signs or symptoms in the early stages, it is critical to keep a high degree of suspicion for it especially when evaluating the graft kidney at surveillance imaging, as the early stage is the time when it is most amenable to treatment. However, when compared with the incidence of PTLD in recipients of lung, heart, and pancreas transplants (up to 20%), the incidence is lower in kidney transplant recipients (~1–3% of recipients).[60] But when it does occur in these cases, the graft kidney is the most common organ to get involved.[61] PTLD develops most commonly in the setting of active EBV infection in the immunocompromised host and can present as a spectrum ranging from mild polyclonal B-cell proliferation to diffuse multiorgan monoclonal lymphoma.[62]

In the advanced stages, isolated or multiple low-density mass lesions may be appreciated on CT in the graft and/or other solid organs. In the graft kidney, PTLD usually presents as a mass encasing the hilum and often leads to obstruction of the outflow tract. US and cross-sectional imaging may highlight graft hydronephrosis in these cases with or without vessel encasement. On MRI, the lesions often appear hypointense on both T1- and T2-weighted images and display no significant enhancement. Elevated FDG uptake is often seen on PET/CT.[60]

In some situations, cancers may develop in the recipient due to an undetected donor-related malignancy present in the renal allograft at the time of transplant surgery. Since the prognosis changes based on the type of cancer in the graft kidney, there is a need for continued investigation into the benefits and risks of accepting kidneys from donors with a history of cancer.

BIOPSY OF THE GRAFT KIDNEY

Percutaneous biopsy of the graft kidney is a commonly done procedure that yields critical information (both diagnostic and prognostic) and guides management of kidney transplant patients. Biopsies may be conducted as part of routine follow-up (known as protocol biopsies) or to evaluate graft dysfunction (known as cause biopsies). The objective of renal graft biopsy is to yield material from the cortex for pathologic evaluation (the medulla has no significant contribution to the evaluation). The highest yields for sufficient material have been reported with the cortical tangential technique that was first illustrated by Patel et al.[63] In this approach, the needle is advanced within the cortex parallel to the capsule of the graft. This ensures that the tip does not hit the kidney's pelvicalyceal system and/or the hilar vessels.

For biopsies from the RIF grafts, the patients are made to lie in a right anterior oblique position. This displaces the overlying tissues away from the graft and shifts the incision scar medially. This provides a greater amount of skin lateral to the incision site and thus provides a greater amount of space for placing the probe and targeting the underlying kidney. The opposite approach may be utilized for LIF grafts. The basic concept is that your puncture site should be lateral to the incision scar. This is because of a couple of reasons. First, a medial approach is associated with the risk of injuring the inferior epigastric vessels. Second, performing the biopsy via a lateral approach avoids the need to traverse through the scar tissue, which can often be hard to pierce and can cause failure of the biopsy device.

Graft Kidney Biopsy Complications

Minor complications included intrarenal AVFs and small perinephric hematomas. The incidence of biopsy-related intrarenal AVFs is reported to be around 11%;[64] but the actual incidence remains unclear, as many institutions

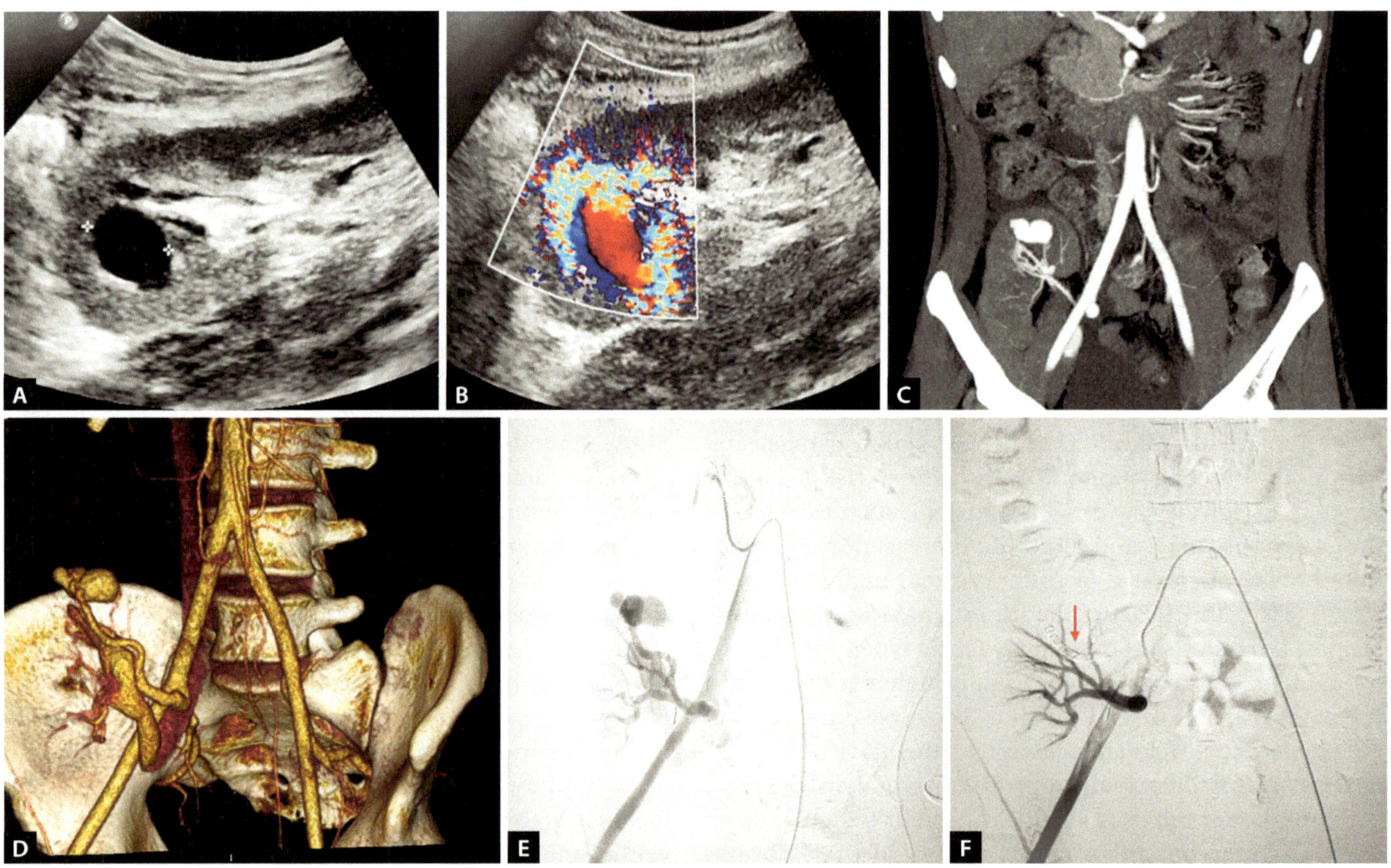

Figs. 13A to F: Transplant Kidney arteriovenous fistula (AVF). (A) Grayscale US image showing a lobulated anechoic structure in the upper pole of the transplant kidney; (B) Color Doppler image showing blood flow within the lesion with a draining vein that shows aliasing on Doppler due to the turbulent high velocity flow; (C) Arterial phase coronal reformatted maximum intensity projection image; and (D) Volume rendered image showing the presence of a lobulated contrast-filled outpouching arising from one of the branches of the transplant renal artery. Note the opacification of a dilated draining vein, the right external iliac vein, and the inferior vena cava in the arterial phase, confirming the lesion to be an AVF; (E and F) The patient was taken up for digital subtraction angiography. The right common iliac run (E) shows the filling of the AV fistula and the early draining vein. The feeder artery was embolized using metallic coils (red arrow) and the postembolization run (F) showed complete obliteration of the AVF.

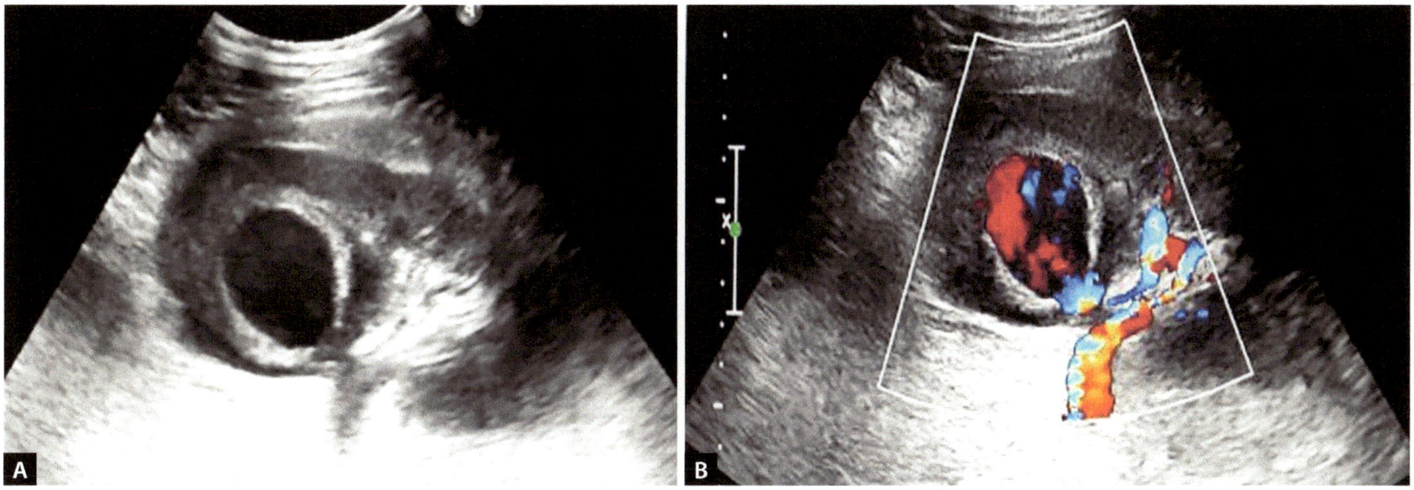

Figs. 14A and B: Transplant kidney pseudoaneurysm. (A) Grayscale US image showing a cystic anechoic structure at the upper polar region of the renal allograft; (B) Doppler evaluation showing the characteristic yin-yang pattern of blood flow within the lesion.

do not conduct immediate postbiopsy imaging routinely. Hematuria is another minor complication that is usually self-limiting. In studies that did not perform graft biopsies using the cortical tangential approach, hematuria has been reported to occur in 3–8% of cases; however, its incidence with the cortical tangential approach is significantly lesser, occurring in <1% of patients.[63,65] Clinically significant hemorrhagic complications can result in marked postbiopsy pain and allograft dysfunction (as with large subcapsular collections) and/or lead to hemodynamic instability.

It is important to differentiate a pseudoaneurysm from a small and hemodynamically insignificant postbiopsy AVF. On Doppler, both entities can be seen as focal lesions with disordered flow that extend beyond the boundaries of normal vessels. A feeder artery is routinely seen in AVFs and they show a high-velocity, low-resistance waveform. The disordered flow is due to high-velocity turbulent flow associated with a segmental or interlobar artery, accompanied by a vein that shows aliasing on Doppler along with an arterialized waveform. **Figures 13A to F** demonstrate a typical AVF of the transplant kidney and its endovascular management.

In comparison, pseudoaneurysms are contained bleeds from parenchymal arteries that develop because of vessel wall injury. These could need intervention, especially if large (>2 cm) or if expanding in size.

On grayscale US, an intrarenal pseudoaneurysm may mimic a simple cyst or may look like a mildly complex cyst **(Figs. 14A and B)**. Therefore, Doppler evaluation should always be done for all anechoic cystic lesions that are picked up on grayscale US. On color Doppler, postbiopsy pseudoaneurysms will show a to-and-fro pattern of flow at the site of the neck and a typical "yin-yang" sign of swirling blood within the sac.

If intervention is planned, a CTA may be done as it helps to better delineate the anatomy of such vascular lesions. MRA with steady-state free precession (SSFP) sequences could also be utilized for mapping the vascular anatomy in patients with deranged renal function in whom contrast cannot be given.

Overall, biopsy of the graft kidney is a relatively safe procedure wherein the benefits frequently outweigh the risks. Sound knowledge of the procedure-related complications and their radiological features is key in their prompt identification and management.

CONCLUSION

The purpose of imaging the graft kidney is to evaluate its integrity, anatomy, and function and to rule out nonrejection-related causes of graft dysfunction. US is the primary modality for the surveillance and initial diagnostic imaging in such cases. Good clinical history-taking and temporal correlation of the occurrence of complications with the time since surgery supplemented with the findings of advanced imaging tools such as CT, MRI, and CEUS can help form a reasonable differential diagnosis and guide a more specific diagnostic evaluation. However, when the diagnosis is still uncertain, US-guided biopsy may need to be performed, which, with the cortical tangential approach, is now a safe and usually low-risk procedure.

REFERENCES

1. Wilkinson A. Protocol transplant biopsies: are they really needed? Clin J Am Soc Nephrol. 2006;1(1):130-7.
2. Breda A, Territo A, Gausa L, Tuğcu V, Alcaraz A, Musquera M, et al. Robot-assisted kidney transplantation: the European experience. Eur Urol. 2018;73(2):273-81.

3. Becker BN, Odorico JS, Becker YT, Groshek M, Werwinski C, Pirsch JD, et al. Simultaneous pancreas-kidney and pancreas transplantation. J Am Soc Nephrol. 2001;12(11):2517-27.
4. Ooms LSS, Roodnat JI, Dor FJMF, Tran TCK, Kimenai HJAN, Ijzermans JNM, et al. Kidney retransplantation in the ipsilateral iliac fossa: a surgical challenge. Am J Transplant. 2015;15(11):2947-54.
5. Grenier N, Poulain S, Lepreux S, Gennisson J-L, Dallaudière B, Lebras Y, et al. Quantitative elastography of renal transplants using supersonic shear imaging: a pilot study. Eur Radiol. 2012;22(10):2138-46.
6. Ozkan F, Yavuz YC, Inci MF, Altunoluk B, Ozcan N, Yuksel M, et al. Interobserver variability of ultrasound elastography in transplant kidneys: correlations with clinical-Doppler parameters. Ultrasound Med Biol. 2013;39(1):4-9.
7. Wareham NE, Lundgren JD, Da Cunha-Bang C, Gustafsson F, Iversen M, Johannesen HH, et al. The clinical utility of FDG PET/CT among solid organ transplant recipients suspected of malignancy or infection. Eur J Nucl Med Mol Imaging. 2017;44(3):421-31.
8. Metser U, Lo G. FDG-PET/CT in abdominal post-transplant lymphoproliferative disease. Br J Radiol. 2016; 89(1057):20150844.
9. Lovinfosse P, Hanssen O, Weekers L, Jadoul A, Huynen A, Bonvoisin C, et al. Exclusion of subclinical kidney allograft rejection by FDG PET/CT imaging systematically performed at 3 months post kidney transplantation. J Nucl Med. 2019; 60(Suppl. 1):1226.
10. Akaberi S, Simonsen O, Lindergård B, Nyberg G. Can DXA predict fractures in renal transplant patients? Am J Transplant. 2008;8(12):2647-51.
11. Van Staa TP, Laan RF, Barton IP, Cohen S, Reid DM, Cooper C. Bone density threshold and other predictors of vertebral fracture in patients receiving oral glucocorticoid therapy. Arthritis Rheum. 2003;48(11):3224-9.
12. Reyna-Sepúlveda F, Ponce-Escobedo A, Guevara-Charles A, Escobedo-Villarreal M, Pérez-Rodríguez E, Muñoz-Maldonado G, et al. Outcomes and surgical complications in kidney transplantation. Int J Organ Transplant Med. 2017;8(2):78-84.
13. Ortiz J, Parsikia A, Horrow MM, Khanmoradi K, Campos S, Zaki R. Risk factors for renal allograft compartment syndrome. Int Surg. 2014;99(6):851-6.
14. Ball CG, Kirkpatrick AW, Yilmaz S, Monroy M, Nicolaou S, Salazar A. Renal allograft compartment syndrome: an under-appreciated postoperative complication. Am J Surg. 2006; 191(5):619-24.
15. Lubner MG, Simard ML, Peterson CM, Bhalla S, Pickhardt PJ, Menias CO. Emergent and nonemergent nonbowel torsion: spectrum of imaging and clinical findings. RadioGraphics. 2013;33(1):155-73.
16. Ayvazoglu Soy EH, Akdur A, Kirnap M, Boyvat F, Moray G, Haberal M. Vascular complications after renal transplant: a single-center experience. Exp Clin Transplant. 2017; 15(Suppl. 1):79-83.
17. Srivastava A, Kumar J, Sharma S, Abhishek, Ansari MS, Kapoor R. Vascular complication in live related renal transplant: an experience of 1945 cases. Indian J Urol. 2013; 29(1):42-7.
18. Akbar SA, Jafri SZH, Amendola MA, Madrazo BL, Salem R, Bis KG. Complications of renal transplantation. RadioGraphics. 2005;25(5):1335-56.
19. Kiykim AA, Ozer C, Yildiz A, Tiftik N, Senli M, Kelebek E, et al. Development of transplant renal artery thrombosis and signs of haemolytic-uraemic syndrome following the change from cyclosporin to tacrolimus in a renal transplant patient. Nephrol Dial Transplant. 2004;19(10):2653-6.
20. Sharfuddin A. Renal relevant radiology: imaging in kidney transplantation. Clin J Am Soc Nephrol. 2014;9(2):416-29.
21. Ponticelli C, Moia M, Montagnino G. Renal allograft thrombosis. Nephrol Dial Transplant. 2009;24(5):1388-93.
22. Lockhart ME, Wells CG, Morgan DE, Fineberg NS, Robbin ML. Reversed diastolic flow in the renal transplant: perioperative implications versus transplants older than 1 month. Am J Roentgenol. 2008;190(3):650-5.
23. Keller AK, Jorgensen TM, Jespersen B. Identification of risk factors for vascular thrombosis may reduce early renal graft loss: a review of recent literature. J Transplant. 2012; 2012:793461.
24. de Morais RH, Muglia VF, Mamere AE, Garcia Pisi T, Saber LT, Muglia VA, et al. Duplex Doppler sonography of transplant renal artery stenosis. J Clin Ultrasound. 2003;31(3):135-41.
25. Al-Katib S, Shetty M, Jafri SMA, Jafri SZH. Radiologic assessment of native renal vasculature: a multimodality review. RadioGraphics. 2017;37(1):136-56.
26. Robinson KA, Kriegshauser JS, Dahiya N, Young SW, Czaplicki CD, Patel MD. Detection of transplant renal artery stenosis: determining normal velocities at the renal artery anastomosis. Abdom Radiol NY. 2017;42(1):254-9.
27. Kolofousi C, Stefanidis K, Cokkinos DD, Karakitsos D, Antypa E, Piperopoulos P. Ultrasonographic features of kidney transplants and their complications: an imaging review. ISRN Radiol. 2013;2013:480862.
28. Titton RL, Gervais DA, Hahn PF, Harisinghani MG, Arellano RS, Mueller PR. Urine leaks and urinomas: diagnosis and imaging-guided intervention. RadioGraphics. 2003;23(5):1133-47.
29. Sugi MD, Joshi G, Maddu KK, Dahiya N, Menias CO. Imaging of renal transplant complications throughout the life of the allograft: comprehensive multimodality review. RadioGraphics. 2019;39(5):1327-55.
30. Ranghino A, Segoloni GP, Lasaponara F, Biancone L. Lymphatic disorders after renal transplantation: new insights for an old complication. Clin Kidney J. 2015;8(5):615-22.
31. Richard HM. Perirenal transplant fluid collections. Semin Interv Radiol. 2004;21(4):235-7.
32. Karam G, Hétet J-F, Maillet F, Rigaud J, Hourmant M, Soulillou J-P, et al. Late ureteral stenosis following renal transplantation: risk factors and impact on patient and graft survival. Am J Transplant. 2006;6(2):352-6.
33. Kumar S, Ameli-Renani S, Hakim A, Jeon JH, Shrivastava S, Patel U. Ureteral obstruction following renal transplantation: causes, diagnosis and management. Br J Radiol. 2014; 87(1044):20140169.
34. Kriegshauser JS, Naidu SG, Heilman RL, Huettl EA, Ferlic EA, Castle EP, et al. Primary percutaneous treatment of transplant ureteral strictures using tandem stents. J Vasc Interv Radiol. 2013;24(6):874-80.

35. Abdul-Muhsin HM, McAdams SB, Nuñez RN, Katariya NN, Castle EP. Robot-assisted transplanted ureteral stricture management. Urology. 2017;105:197-201.
36. Humar A, Ramcharan T, Kandaswamy R, Gillingham K, Payne WD, Matas AJ. Risk factors for slow graft function after kidney transplants: a multivariate analysis. Clin Transplant. 2002;16(6):425-9.
37. Haas M, Loupy A, Lefaucheur C, Roufosse C, Glotz D, Seron D, et al. The Banff 2017 Kidney Meeting Report: revised diagnostic criteria for chronic active T cell-mediated rejection, antibody-mediated rejection, and prospects for integrative endpoints for next-generation clinical trials. Am J Transplant. 2018;18(2):293-307.
38. Bhowmik DM, Dinda AK, Mahanta P, Agarwal SK. The evolution of the Banff classification schema for diagnosing renal allograft rejection and its implications for clinicians. Indian J Nephrol. 2010;20(1):2-8.
39. McArthur C, Geddes CC, Baxter GM. Early measurement of pulsatility and resistive indexes: correlation with long-term renal transplant function. Radiology. 2011;259(1):278-85.
40. Allen KS, Jorkasky DK, Arger PH, Velchik MG, Grumbach K, Coleman BG, et al. Renal allografts: prospective analysis of Doppler sonography. Radiology. 1988;169(2):371-6.
41. Venz S, Kahl A, Hierholzer J, Gutberlet M, Windrich B, Bechstein WO, et al. Contribution of color and power Doppler sonography to the differential diagnosis of acute and chronic rejection, and tacrolimus nephrotoxicity in renal allografts. Transpl Int. 1999;12(2):127-34.
42. Friedewald SM, Molmenti EP, Friedewald JJ, Dejong MR, Hamper UM. Vascular and nonvascular complications of renal transplants: sonographic evaluation and correlation with other imaging modalities, surgery, and pathology. J Clin Ultrasound. 2005;33(3):127-39.
43. Benozzi L, Cappelli G, Granito M, Davoli D, Favali D, Montecchi MG, et al. Contrast-enhanced sonography in early kidney graft dysfunction. Transplant Proc. 2009;41(4):1214-5.
44. Zeisbrich M, Kihm LP, Drüschler F, Zeier M, Schwenger V. When is contrast-enhanced sonography preferable over conventional ultrasound combined with Doppler imaging in renal transplantation? Clin Kidney J. 2015;8(5):606-14.
45. Kazmierski B, Deurdulian C, Tchelepi H, Grant EG. Applications of contrast-enhanced ultrasound in the kidney. Abdom Radiol NY. 2018;43(4):880-98.
46. Thoeny HC, Zumstein D, Simon-Zoula S, Eisenberger U, De Keyzer F, Hofmann L, et al. Functional evaluation of transplanted kidneys with diffusion-weighted and BOLD MR imaging: initial experience. Radiology. 2006;241(3):812-21.
47. Artz NS, Sadowski EA, Wentland AL, Grist TM, Seo S, Djamali A, et al. Arterial spin labeling MRI for assessment of perfusion in native and transplanted kidneys. Magn Reson Imaging. 2011;29(1):74-82.
48. Sadowski EA, Fain SB, Alford SK, Korosec FR, Fine J, Muehrer R, et al. Assessment of acute renal transplant rejection with blood oxygen level-dependent MR imaging: initial experience. Radiology. 2005;236(3):911-9.
49. Lovinfosse P, Weekers L, Bonvoisin C, Bovy C, Grosch S, Krzesinski J-M, et al. Fluorodeoxyglucose F(18) positron emission tomography coupled with computed tomography in suspected acute renal allograft rejection. Am J Transplant. 2016;16(1):310-6.
50. Kalluri HV, Hardinger KL. Current state of renal transplant immunosuppression: present and future. World J Transplant. 2012;2(4):51-68.
51. Halloran PF. Immunosuppressive drugs for kidney transplantation. N Engl J Med. 2004;351(26):2715-29.
52. Naesens M, Kuypers DRJ, Sarwal M. Calcineurin inhibitor nephrotoxicity. Clin J Am Soc Nephrol. 2009;4(2):481-508.
53. Fishman JA. Infection in organ transplantation. Am J Transplant. 2017;17(4):856-79.
54. Einollahi B, Rostami Z, Nourbala MH, Lessan-Pezeshki M, Simforoosh N, Nemati E, et al. Incidence of malignancy after living kidney transplantation: a multicenter study from Iran. J Cancer. 2012;3:246-56.
55. Zeier M, Hartschuh W, Wiesel M, Lehnert T, Ritz E. Malignancy after renal transplantation. Am J Kidney Dis. 2002;39(1):E5.
56. Briggs JD. Causes of death after renal transplantation. Nephrol Dial Transplant. 2001;16(8):1545-9.
57. Sprangers B, Nair V, Launay-Vacher V, Riella LV, Jhaveri KD. Risk factors associated with post-kidney transplant malignancies: an article from the Cancer-Kidney International Network. Clin Kidney J. 2018;11(3):315-29.
58. Karami S, Colt JS, Stewart PA, Schwartz K, Davis FG, Ruterbusch JJ, et al. A case-control study of occupational sunlight exposure and renal cancer risk. Int J Cancer. 2016; 138(7):1626-33.
59. Hickman LA, Sawinski D, Guzzo T, Locke JE. Urologic malignancies in kidney transplantation. Am J Transplant. 2018;18(1):13-22.
60. Camacho JC, Moreno CC, Harri PA, Aguirre DA, Torres WE, Mittal PK. Posttransplantation lymphoproliferative disease: proposed imaging classification. RadioGraphics. 2014;34(7): 2025-38.
61. Rajiah P, Lim YY, Taylor P. Renal transplant imaging and complications. Abdom Imaging. 2006;31(6):735-46.
62. Vrachliotis TG, Vaswani KK, Davies EA, Elkahammas EA, Bennett WF, Bova JG. CT findings in post-transplantation lymphoproliferative disorder of renal transplants. Am J Roentgenol. 2000;175(1):183-8.
63. Patel MD, Phillips CJ, Young SW, Kriegshauser JS, Chen F, Eversman WG, et al. US-guided renal transplant biopsy: efficacy of a cortical tangential approach. Radiology. 2010;256(1):290-6.
64. Furness PN, Philpott CM, Chorbadjian MT, Nicholson ML, Bosmans J-L, Corthouts BL, et al. Protocol biopsy of the stable renal transplant: a multicenter study of methods and complication rates. Transplantation. 2003;76(6):969-73.
65. Redfield RR, McCune KR, Rao A, Sadowski E, Hanson M, Kolterman AJ, et al. Nature, timing, and severity of complications from ultrasound-guided percutaneous renal transplant biopsy. Transpl Int. 2016;29(2):167-72.

CHAPTER 19

HLA Incompatible Kidney Transplantation

Alan Almeida, Ayan Dey

CASE VIGNETTE

Mr B is a 52-year-old gentleman who has been on hemodialysis for the past 1 year. His native kidney disease was diabetic nephropathy. He is a working professional and is desirous of kidney transplantation (KT). He has been explained the advantages of KT over maintenance dialysis.

His daughter is pregnant and despite being desirous to donate her kidney, she cannot be considered as a potential donor currently. He has no siblings and his parents have multiple comorbidities, besides being age-barred. His wife has come forward to donate her kidney, but the preliminary workup revealed complement-dependent cytotoxicity (CDC) crossmatch positivity. He has registered for deceased-donor transplantation in his city. His blood group is O positive and he has been told that the waiting period could stretch beyond 3–5 years based on current data. There are no potential swap/domino transplants feasible.

No donor is available for Mr. B, even from his extended family. He and his wife wish to explore the option of going ahead with KT, even though the crossmatch turned up positive.

INTRODUCTION

Since the first successful KT in 1954,[1] there has been a sustained refinement in the understanding of immunological and physiological barriers that need to be overcome. The rising prevalence of chronic kidney disease (CKD) and end-stage renal disease (ESRD) worldwide translates into an ever-increasing gap between demand and supply, which can be reduced by expanding the donor pool. With the advent of potent immunosuppressants, transplant physicians have ventured into ABO-incompatible kidney transplantation (ABOiKT) with gratifying results. Transplanting across human leukocyte antigen (HLA)-incompatible recipients and donors, which traditionally had been a strict "no-go" venture, is now becoming an increasingly viable option.

NEED FOR HUMAN LEUKOCYTE ANTIGEN-INCOMPATIBLE KIDNEY TRANSPLANTATION

As of 2021, more than 90,000 patients await KT in the United States.[2] While living-donor renal transplantation coexists with deceased-donor kidney transplantation (DDKT) worldwide. In developing countries like India,[3] living-donor kidney transplants (LDKT) predominate. The 7,500 kidney transplants performed annually at 250 kidney transplant centers, 90% being LDKT, are woefully low for the estimated approximately 220,000 people requiring KT in India.[4]

Renal transplantation has better rehabilitation and survival than maintenance dialysis,[5] but the average waiting time for a DDKT is greater than 5 years.[6] It, therefore, becomes advisable to explore all possible options for KT. Besides promoting DDKT and living-related/altruistic donations, swap/domino transplants and ABOiKT have been increasingly performed, albeit inadequately. Transplantation across HLA-incompatible recipients and donors has traditionally been avoided due to higher chances of rejection in the allograft kidney.

The approach has changed in recent years. With an increasing armamentarium of immunosuppressants and buoyed by long-term success rates of ABOiKT, nephrologists have now ventured into HLA-incompatible kidney transplantation (HLAiKT). There is increasing evidence suggesting not only a lower rate of complications, including rejections, but also an increasing survival advantage of even HLAiKT over dialysis.[7] This has further expanded the donor pool for ESRD patients **(Fig. 1)**.

UNDERSTANDING HUMAN LEUKOCYTE ANTIGEN AND ITS CLINICAL SIGNIFICANCE IN KIDNEY TRANSPLANTATION

Human leukocyte antigens representing the most complex immunogenetic system in humans play a key role in host defense mechanisms.[8] These cell surface proteins are encoded by genes in the major histocompatibility complex (MHC),

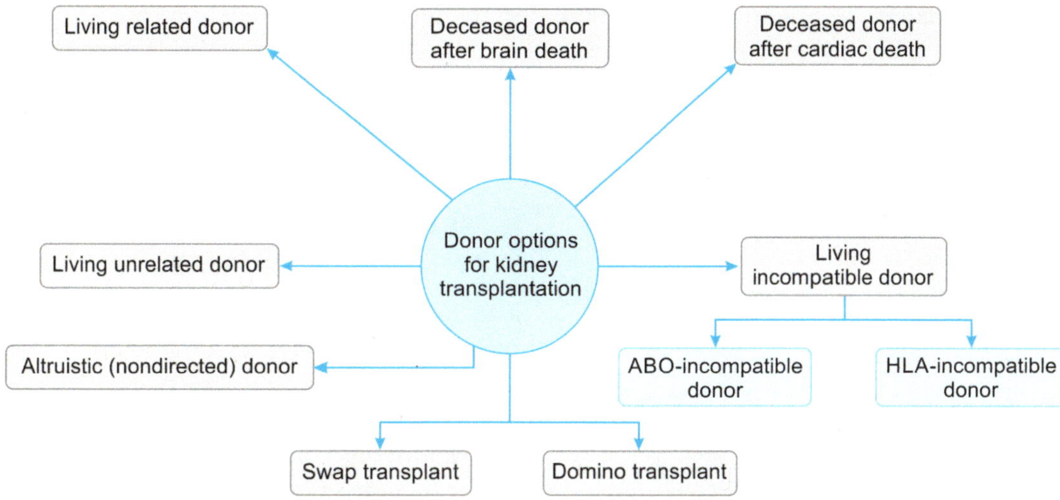

Fig. 1: Options of donor source for kidney transplantation. (HLA: human leukocyte antigen)

CHAPTER HIGHLIGHTS

- Improving short and long-term outcomes of ABO incompatible kidney transplants have encouraged venturing into HLA incompatible kidney transplantation.
- In an ABO compatible recipient and donor pair, the presence of a positive crossmatch between the recipient's serum and donor lymphocytes, suggests sensitization to donor HLA antigens.
- Significant heterogeneity in protocols for desensitization exists across centers worldwide. The basic principles, however, remain the same. Targeted antibody removal from the recipient's circulation followed by minimization of ongoing antibody production along with suppression of the cell and antibody mediated responses is undertaken.
- The commonest protocols include plasmapheresis (circulating antibody removal) with administration of IVIg (to avoid rebound antibody production) along with anti-CD20 antibodies like Rituximab (to downregulate B cell synthesis). Pretransplant induction is done with pulse steroids, antithymocyte globulin (ATG), calcineurin inhibitors (CNI) and antimetabolites like mycophenolate mofetil (MMF).
- Depending on the preliminary crossmatch technique positivity, predetermined thresholds are used to objectively assess the level of desensitization achieved. General rule of thumb is to achieve an acceptable crossmatch titre, defined by a negative CDC crossmatch (>1:2 dilution of patient sera), a negative flow cytometry crossmatch, or a positive flow cytometry crossmatch with mean channel shift <250.
- Long-term studies are emerging which show a definite survival benefit for patients with HLA sensitization, as compared to waiting for a compatible organ and remaining on dialysis.
- There remain challenges with HLAiKt with heterogeneity in standardizing crossmatch positivity (titres and methods), higher early hospital readmission rate, higher infection rates and added financial burden on patients.

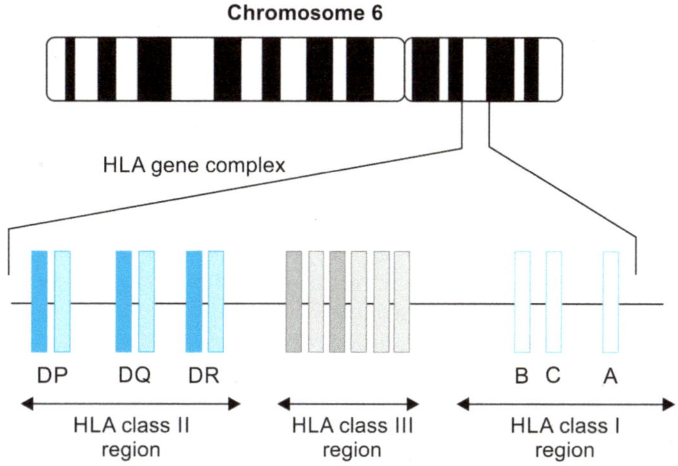

Fig. 2: Gene map of the human leukocyte antigen (HLA) region. The HLA region is located on the short arm of chromosome 6, at 6p21.31.

located at 6p21 position on the short arm of chromosome 6 **(Figs. 2 and 3)**.

There are two classes of HLA, class I and class II, based on the structure and antigen they produce. Whereas class I antigens (HLA-A, B, and C) are expressed on all nucleated cells, class II antigens (HLA-DP, DQ, and DR) are expressed on antigen-presenting cells such as B cells, macrophages, dendritic cells, Langerhans cells, and capillary endothelium. HLA class I molecules present nonself-antigens to cytotoxic CD8 T cells. HLA class II molecules, on the other hand, present the antigens to CD4 T helper cells. These molecules bind to peptide foreign antigens within their peptide grooves and present fragments of antigens to T lymphocytes, which trigger cell-mediated immune responses as well as have downstream effects of stimulating B cells that trigger antibody-mediated responses. The uniqueness of the HLA system is used by the human body to distinguish "self" from "nonself."

The law of transplantation dictates that grafts between genetically identical individuals have better outcomes, while grafts between genetically different individuals have higher chances of rejection. Transplant rejection of the kidney occurs when the immune system of the recipient recognizes the allogeneic kidney as "nonself." This remains a major immunological barrier to organ transplantation. Identifying preexisting circulating anti-HLA antibodies against donor antigens [donor-specific antibody (DSA)] in the recipients is crucial, so as to avoid hyperacute graft rejections, thus ensuring better graft and patient survival. The probability of the recipient harboring DSA increases with sensitizing events such as prior organ transplant, pregnancies, or blood transfusions.

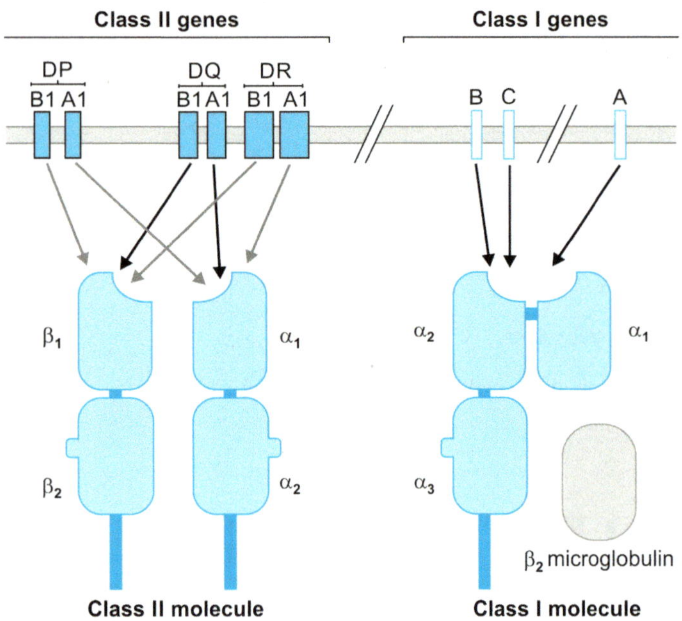

Fig. 3: Structure of the human leukocyte antigen (HLA) molecule. Class I molecules consist of a transmembrane heavy α-chain (45 kDa), which is divided into three extracellular domains α_1, α_2, and α_3. A small β_2-microglobulin (12 kDa) is noncovalently bound to the α-chain. Class II molecules are composed of a transmembrane α-chain, which is divided into two domains α_1 and α_2 and a transmembrane β-chain consisting of two domains β_1 and β_2.

METHODS TO DETECT HUMAN LEUKOCYTE ANTIGEN COMPATIBILITY

The initial assessment of a potential renal transplant recipient involves HLA typing of the donor and recipient, screening for alloantibodies against HLA, and obtaining a history of sensitizing events. The most widely used methods for identifying compatibility between the recipient and donor include (1) screening of recipients to identify anti-HLA antibodies and (2) crossmatch techniques which can identify DSA **(Table 1)**.

Screening for HLA antibodies is done by CDC, flow cytometry, or solid-phase assays. The most commonly used method is the solid-phase assay,[9] which uses beads coated with class I and class II antigens. These beads are incubated with the recipient's serum followed by addition of secondary antibodies [immunoglobulin G (IgG)] tagged with unique immunofluorescence. If screening is positive, then a single antigen bead (SAB) assay[10] is performed wherein each bead is coated with a specific antigen and has a specific signature to identify specific HLA antibodies to class I and class II antigens.

TABLE 1: Crossmatching techniques.

Name	*Method of the test*	*Pros and cons*
Complement-dependent cytotoxicity (CDC)	• Cytotoxic crossmatch technique where recipient serum is incubated with donor lymphocytes along with complement. Presence of antibodies in the serum causes lysis of cells • If the recipient has DSA, there will be cell lysis and a positive crossmatch is interpreted if the percentage of lysed cells is >20%	• Still the gold standard test for crossmatching • Needs a high level of circulating complement fixing DSA • Less sensitive, but positivity means there is a high titer of circulating DSA
Luminex crossmatch	• Beads coated with class I and class II HLA antibodies are incubated with lysate (lysed donor lymphocytes) followed by incubation with recipient serum. Addition of secondary IgG antibodies which are tagged with unique immunofluorescence is done to detect specific antibodies • Very low titers of anti-HLA antibodies in the serum can also be detected by the Luminex assay	• More sensitive test as compared to CDC • Faster turnaround time for the test • Donor lysate can be stored for many years • Can give nonspecific positivity with higher chances of picking clinically insignificant titers of circulating antibodies
Flow cytometric crossmatch (FXM)	• Recipient serum is incubated with viable donor lymphocytes and secondary fluorescein-labeled antibodies against human IgG • Positivity depends on mean channel shift (MCS) as compared to controls in the laboratory	• Identifies complement and noncomplement binding antibodies • Rapid and easily reproducible • Very sensitive test which can detect low titer of nonspecific antibodies
Virtual crossmatch	• Crossmatching based on complete HLA typing of the donor and current HLA antibody status in the recipient • Compatibility can be assessed without the need of viable donor cells	• Quicker method and allows timelier organ allocation decisions, even across provinces and states • Allows transplantation access to highly sensitized patients • Not universally available

(DSA: donor-specific antibody; HLA: human leukocyte antigen; IgG: immunoglobulin G)

HUMAN LEUKOCYTE ANTIGEN-INCOMPATIBLE KIDNEY TRANSPLANTATION

Human leukocyte antigen-incompatible kidney transplantation[11] involves a recipient and potential donor who is ABO compatible but with a positive crossmatch between the recipient's serum and donor lymphocytes. This suggests that the donor possesses HLA capable of provoking an immune response from the recipient on transplantation, predisposing to immediate, early, or late rejection. The transplanted kidney is highly susceptible to graft dysfunction, negatively impacting graft and patient survival.

Protocols for Desensitization for Human Leukocyte Antigen-incompatible Kidney Transplantation

Overcoming the immunological barrier for HLAiKT and ensuring successful engraftment of the "foreign" transplanted kidney depends on a robust desensitization protocol. The aims of desensitization are to increase the success rate of HLAiKT and to prevent antibody-mediated rejections (ABMR) post renal transplant. While the actual protocols differ among institutions and regions, the basic principles remain the same **(Flowchart 1)**.[12]

Targeted removal of antibody from the recipient's circulation to levels precluding a clinically significant immunological attack is mandatory. As the next step, it is necessary to ensure a minimization of the ongoing production of such antibodies with interventions that avoid rebound immunological responses in the recipient. Finally, suppression of the cell and antibody-mediated responses on a continued basis is needed to ensure long-term graft survival and minimization of clinical or subclinical rejections.

The most common protocols include plasmapheresis (circulating antibody removal) followed by anti-CD20 antibody (rituximab) administration to downregulate B-cell synthesis, which is directly related to antibody production. Pretransplant induction from an earlier point in time (weeks before transplant) with pulse steroids, antithymocyte globulin (ATG), calcineurin inhibitors (CNI), and antimetabolites such as mycophenolate mofetil (MMF) ensures that the immune system is downregulated at the time of transplantation and beyond.

Intravenous immunoglobulin (IVIg), which modulates and suppresses both cell and antibody responses, is used post plasmapheresis to avoid rebound antibody production. Frequent antibody titer monitoring [e.g., mean fluorescence intensity (MFI) with flow cytometry crossmatch (FXM)-and Luminex-based assays and dilution titers with CDC technique] remains necessary to ensure that predetermined safe levels are achieved to avoid catastrophic hyperacute rejection episodes.

Newer agents, such as bortezomib and carfilzomib (proteasome inhibitors), which directly cause plasma cell suppression and decrease antibody production, are also being increasingly used. Anti-CD25 monoclonal antibodies (such as daclizumab and alemtuzumab) are being explored further as they are more specific in targeting immune cells and their responses. Specific targeted therapy agents, such as eculizumab (C5 inhibitor), tocilizumab (anti-interleukin 6 receptor monoclonal antibody), imlifidase[13] (IgG-degrading enzyme derived from *Streptococcus pyogenes*), and obinutuzumab (third-generation anti-CD20 monoclonal antibody), are also being tried as desensitizing agents in ongoing clinical trials.

There remains significant heterogeneity across centers worldwide in the timing and dosing of these medications pretransplant **(Table 2)**.

Targets of Desensitization and Monitoring Post-transplant

Depending on the preliminary crossmatch technique positivity, predetermined thresholds objectively assess the level of desensitization achieved. Patients with CDC crossmatch positivity need robust desensitization with

Flowchart 1: Principles of desensitization protocols.

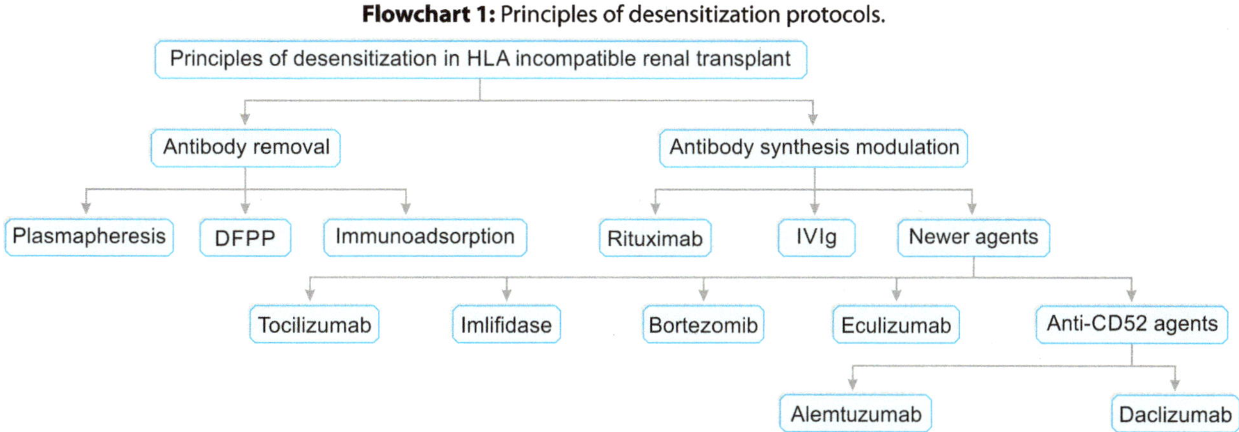

(DFPP: double filtration plasmapheresis; HLA: human leukocyte antigen; IVIg: intravenous immunoglobulin)

TABLE 2: Protocols for desensitization for human leukocyte antigen-incompatible kidney transplantation (HLAiKT).*

Center	***Antibody removal technique***	***New antibody formation blockage***	***Induction regime***	***Maintenance regime***	***Outcomes***
Cedars-Sinai[14]	High-dose IVIg	Rituximab	Alemtuzumab, ATG or anti-CD25	CNI, MMF, and steroids	2-year follow-up, 95% patient survival
Mayo Clinic[15]	Plasmapheresis and low-dose IVIg	Not used since 2005	ATG	CNI, MMF, and steroids	2-year follow-up, 89% patient survival
John Hopkins[16]	Plasmapheresis and low-dose IVIg	Rituximab (splenectomy in the past)	ATG	CNI, MMF, and steroids	8-year follow-up, 80% patient survival
University of Illinois[17]	Plasmapheresis and low-dose IVIg	None (rituximab in the past)	ATG	CNI, MMF, and steroids	2-year follow-up, 93% patient survival
University of Maryland[18]	Plasmapheresis and low-dose IVIg	None	ATG	CNI, MMF, and steroids	5-year follow-up, 85% patient survival
University Hospital Coventry and Warwickshire[19]	Double filtration plasmapheresis	None	Anti-CD 25 (ATG in the past)	CNI, MMF, and steroids	5-year follow-up, 94% patient survival
Seoul National University Hospital[20]	Plasmapheresis and bortezomib	Rituximab	ATG	CNI, MMF, and steroids	7-year follow-up, 96% patient survival
University of Wisconsin Hospital[21]	MFI-based protocol: plasmapheresis and low-dose IVIg	None	Basiliximab	CNI, MMF, and steroids	1-year follow-up, 100% patient survival
Medanta Kidney and Urology Institute[22]	Double filtration plasmapheresis and low-dose IVIg	None	ATG	CNI, MMF, and steroids	3-year follow-up, 100% patient survival

*Protocols may have been modified since publication of these data.
(ATG: antithymocyte globulin; CNI: calcineurin inhibitors; IVIg: intravenous immunoglobulin; MMF: mycophenolate mofetil)

Flowchart 2: Sample desensitization and immune monitoring protocols used in some centers.

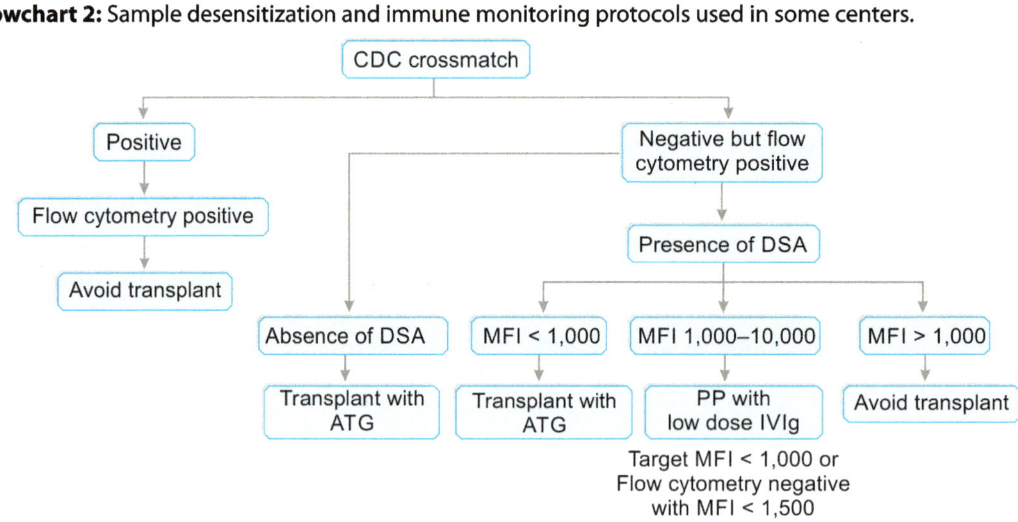

(ATG: antithymocyte globulin; CDC: complement-dependent cytotoxicity; DSA: donor-specific antibody; IVIg: intravenous immunoglobulin; MFI: mean fluorescence intensity; PP: plasmapheresis)

closer monitoring of de novo DSA formation postrenal transplant as compared to CDC-negative, flow cytometry or Luminex-based crossmatch positivity. While the thresholds for desensitization are not standardized, the general rule of thumb is to achieve an acceptable crossmatch titer, defined by a negative CDC crossmatch (≥1:2 dilution of patient sera), a negative flow cytometry crossmatch, or a positive flow cytometry crossmatch with mean channel shift ≤250. Few centers have now developed immunosuppression protocols and monitoring strategies based on their own laboratory data and successful anecdotal experiences **(Flowchart 2).**[23]

Post renal transplantation, patients can be monitored in a manner similar to HLA-compatible renal transplants. However, a high index of suspicion must exist for ABMR with certain centers conducting serial protocol biopsies. Routine monitoring of monthly DSA levels for the initial 3 months post-transplant followed by retests at months 6, 9, and 12, and annually thereafter, are recommended. Persistent or de novo DSAs are evaluated with a renal allograft biopsy to exclude the possibility of ABMR and treated accordingly.

Outcome of Human Leukocyte Antigen-incompatible Kidney Transplantation

Patient survival after HLAiKT has been documented from various centers worldwide with varying success rates over a median follow-up of 4 years post transplant (*see* **Table 2**). The lower than expected patient survival rates of HLAiKT (as compared to LDKT and ABOiKT) could be attributed to the cumulative medical and surgical burden that patients may have to bear, with regard to longer dialysis vintage and/or previous transplantation. There is also a dichotomy of graft outcomes dependent upon the strength of baseline immunological barrier, with worse medium-term outcomes for patients who are CDC positive at baseline versus those who are CDC negative.[19] It is postulated that a better sense of patient survival could be gauged if the outcomes are compared to patients who remain on waiting list for renal transplant and continue on renal replacement therapy.

Seminal work done by Montgomery et al.[16] showed that desensitization with plasmapheresis and IVIg confers a significant survival benefit for patients with HLA sensitization, as compared to waiting for a compatible organ and remaining on dialysis. By 8 years, this survival advantage more than doubled in more than 200 patients over a follow-up of more than 10 years [80.6% compared to 30.5% and 49.1% for matched-control patients remaining on dialysis or eventually receiving compatible kidney transplants, respectively ($p < 0.001$ for both comparisons)]. Similarly, Orandi et al.[7] conducted a multicenter study of 1,025 HLAiKT recipients and found higher short- and long-term patient survival (up to 8 years) compared with waitlisted matched controls. These findings were consistent among recipients who had a positive Luminex assay with negative flow cytometric crossmatch, positive flow cytometric crossmatch, or positive cytotoxic crossmatch.

Efforts to minimize desensitization have been done, so as to avoid the drawbacks of potent immunosuppression in the long term. Patient and graft survival remained comparable in the few studies between highly sensitized recipients desensitized before transplant and less-sensitized recipients not receiving pretransplant desensitization. Toyoda et al.[24] analyzed 910 deceased-donor and living-donor transplant recipients, 372 of whom received pretransplant desensitization because of HLA sensitization or ABO-incompatible transplantation. There was no statistical difference in graft or patient survival up to 5 years between HLA-sensitized recipients of pretransplant desensitization and lower immunologic risk recipients.

Higher degrees of incompatibility are associated with higher risks of graft loss and death. In a study by Orandi et al.,[25] patients with DSA but a negative crossmatch were observed to have a similar risk of death or graft loss compared with compatible recipients. By contrast, crossmatch positivity, detected either by flow cytometry or by CDC method, was associated with a 1.65- or 1.80-fold higher risk of graft loss along with a 1.32- or 1.51-fold higher risk of death compared with compatible recipients, respectively. Five-year unadjusted graft loss (%) was 17, 20, 29, and 40 for compatible recipients, recipients with DSA but negative flow crossmatch, recipients with positive flow crossmatch but negative cytotoxic crossmatch, and recipients of a positive cytotoxic crossmatch kidney transplant, respectively. Similarly, the 5-year unadjusted mortality (%) was 9, 10, 13, and 19 for compatible recipients, recipients with DSA but a negative flow crossmatch, recipients with a positive flow crossmatch but negative cytotoxic crossmatch, and recipients of a positive cytotoxic crossmatch kidney transplant, respectively.

Studies from the United Kingdom have failed to show any long-term survival benefit in patients undergoing HLAiKT in comparison to those who remained on dialysis.[26] However, reasonable success in short- and medium-term outcomes in graft survival has been observed in these studies. In contrast, data from the United States showed better outcomes for HLAi LDKT in comparison to HLAi DDKT or dialysis. These disparities suggest that survival benefit of HLAi LDKT could vary according to the individual situation, including health severity of the dialysis population, quality of dialysis care, median waiting time to HLAi DDKT, quality of HLAi LDKT techniques, and activity of donor exchange programs.

Challenges with Human Leukocyte Antigen-incompatible Kidney Transplantation

Advances in antibody detection and screening, HLA typing, and desensitization of patients have aided in curtailing the risks associated with HLAi renal transplants.[27] Despite this, graft failure due to rejection remains a major obstacle in achieving more successful long-term outcomes in HLAi renal transplantation. A few studies suggested a higher early hospital readmission rate for HLAiKT as compared to compatible transplants and also ABOiKT.[28] Further challenges in terms of heterogeneity in standardizing crossmatch positivity (titers and methods) among centers, lack of uniform guidelines to guide objective evidence of desensitization successes, and variable posttransplant monitoring protocols remain (**Fig. 4**). As aggressive immunosuppression is inevitable in sensitized patients, infectious complications occur more frequently in HLAi LDKT.[29,30] Several studies reported that highly sensitized

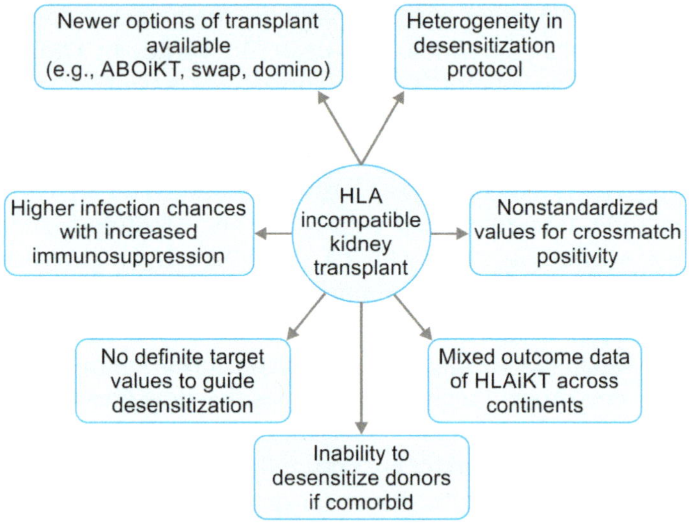

Fig. 4: Challenges with human leukocyte antigen-incompatible kidney transplantation (HLAiKT).
(ABOiKT: ABO-incompatible kidney transplantation)

patients who received rituximab tend to be at a higher risk for bacterial/viral infections and posttransplant lymphoproliferative disorder (PTLD). Viral infections are particularly common in positive crossmatch KT patients. Finally, desensitization protocols add to the financial burden to ESRD patients, especially in developing countries that do not provide universal health coverage.

CONCLUSION

There is considerable heterogeneity in desensitization protocols utilized globally for ensuring successful HLAiKT. However, it is heartening to note that HLAiKT has resulted in comparable success rates to deceased-donor KT and ABOiKT across the various centers around the world. Better immune monitoring techniques, increasing efforts to standardize the immunological responses by laboratories, potent immunosuppressants, and growing awareness of HLAiKT have translated to wider options for ESRD patients. Coupled with the fact that there is clear evidence of better long-term outcomes with HLAiKT as compared to continuing renal replacement therapy, it is imperative that ESRD patients are offered HLAiKT when feasible.

Unlike a few decades ago, when CDC crossmatch positivity precluded further workup and transplantation, HLAiKT offers a beacon of hope to sensitized patients worldwide. The success of HLAiKT rests on the nephrology community embracing the growing armamentarium of interventions and medications, thereby allowing more and more patients to have a better quality of life post renal transplantation.

REFERENCES

1. Nagy J. A note on the early history of renal transplantation: Emerich (Imre) Ullmann. Am J Nephrol. 1999;19(2):346-9.
2. National data—OPTN. (2022). [online] Available from https://optn.transplant.hrsa.gov/data/view-data-reports/national-data. [Last accessed January, 2022].
3. Transplantindia.com. (2022). [online] Available from http://www.transplantindia.com [Last accessed January, 2022].
4. Shroff S. Current trends in kidney transplantation in India. Indian J Urol. 2016;32(3):173.
5. Keith D, Ma J. A longitudinal analysis of disparities in access to the kidney transplant waiting list in the United States. Transplantation. 2014;98:831.
6. Wolfe R, Ashby V, Milford E, Ojo A, Ettenger R, Agodoa L, et al. Comparison of mortality in all patients on dialysis, patients on dialysis awaiting transplantation, and recipients of a first cadaveric transplant. N Engl J Med. 1999;341(23):1725-30.
7. Orandi B, Luo X, Massie A, Garonzik-Wang J, Lonze B, Ahmed R, et al. Survival benefit with kidney transplants from HLA-incompatible live donors. N Engl J Med. 2016;374(10):940-50.
8. Alelign T, Ahmed M, Bobosha K, Tadesse Y, Howe R, Petros B. Kidney transplantation: the challenge of human leukocyte antigen and its therapeutic strategies. J Immunol Res. 2018;2018:1-18.
9. Lachmann N, Todorova K, Schulze H, Schönemann C. Luminex® and its applications for solid organ transplantation, hematopoietic stem cell transplantation, and transfusion. Transfusion Med Hemother. 2013;40(3):182-9.
10. Tait B. Detection of HLA antibodies in organ transplant recipients—triumphs and challenges of the solid phase bead assay. Front Immunol. 2016;7:570.
11. Krishnan N, Zehnder D, Briggs D, Higgins R. Human leukocyte antigen antibody incompatible renal transplantation. Indian J Nephrol. 2012;22(6):409.
12. Sharif A, Alachkar N, Kraus E. Incompatible kidney transplantation: a brief overview of the past, present and future. QJM. 2012;105(12):1141-50.
13. Jordan S, Legendre C, Desai N, Lorant T, Bengtsson M, Lonze B, et al. Imlifidase desensitization in crossmatch-positive, highly sensitized kidney transplant recipients: results of an international phase 2 trial (Highdes). Transplantation. 2021;105(8):1808-17.
14. Vo A, Peng A, Toyoda M, Kahwaji J, Cao K, Lai C, et al. Use of intravenous immune globulin and rituximab for desensitization of highly HLA-sensitized patients awaiting kidney transplantation. Transplantation. 2010;89(9):1095-102.
15. Gloor J, Winters J, Cornell L, Fix L, DeGoey S, Knauer R, et al. Baseline donor-specific antibody levels and outcomes in positive crossmatch kidney transplantation. Am J Transplant. 2010;10(3):582-9.
16. Montgomery R, Lonze B, King K, Kraus E, Kucirka L, Locke J, et al. Desensitization in HLA-incompatible kidney recipients and survival. N Engl J Med. 2011;365(4):318-26.
17. Thielke J, West-Thielke P, Herren H, Bareato U, Ommert T, Vidanovic V, et al. Living donor kidney transplantation across positive crossmatch: the University of Illinois at Chicago experience. Transplantation. 2009;87(2):268-73.
18. Haririan A, Nogueira J, Kukuruga D, Schweitzer E, Hess J, Gurk-Turner C, et al. Positive cross-match living donor kidney transplantation: longer-term outcomes. Am J Transplant. 2009;9(3):536-42.

19. Higgins R, Lowe D, Hathaway M, Williams C, Lam FT, Kashi H, et al. Human leukocyte antigen antibody-incompatible renal transplantation: excellent medium-term outcomes with negative cytotoxic crossmatch. Transplantation. 2011; 92(8):900-6.
20. Koo T, Lee J, Min S, Lee Y, Kim M, Ha J, et al. Presence of a survival benefit of HLA-incompatible living donor kidney transplantation compared to waiting or HLA-compatible deceased donor kidney transplantation with a long waiting time. Kidney Int. 2021;100(1):206-14.
21. Niederhaus S, Muth B, Lorentzen D, Wai P, Pirsch J, Samaniego-Picota M, et al. Luminex-based desensitization protocols: the University of Wisconsin initial experience. Transplantation. 2011;92(1):12-7.
22. Tiwari A, Aggarwal G, Dorwal P, Chauhan R, Arora D, Dara R, et al. Successful renal transplantation across HLA barrier: report from India. Indian J Nephrol. 2017;27(3):210.
23. Bansal S, Gade A, Sinha S, Mahapatra A, Jha P, Sethi S. HLA desensitization based on results of the Luminex technique in kidney transplant - a single-center experience. Indian J Nephrol. 2021;31(5):454.
24. Toyoda M, Shin B, Ge S, Mirocha J, Thomas D, Chu M, et al. Impact of desensitization on antiviral immunity in HLA-sensitized kidney transplant recipients. J Immunol Res. 2017;2017:1-24.
25. Orandi B, Garonzik-Wang J, Massie A, Zachary A, Montgomery J, Van Arendonk K, et al. Quantifying the risk of incompatible kidney transplantation: a multicenter study. Am J Transplant. 2014;14(7):1573-80.
26. Manook M, Koeser L, Ahmed Z, Robb M, Johnson R, Shaw O, et al. Post-listing survival for highly sensitised patients on the UK kidney transplant waiting list: a matched cohort analysis. Lancet. 2017;389(10070):727-34.
27. Krishnan N, Abimbola A, Machan N, Daga S, Gopalakrishnan K, Lam F, et al. HLA antibody incompatible renal transplantation: long-term outcomes similar to deceased donor transplantation. Transplant Direct. 2021; 7(8):e732.
28. Lee J, Kim DG, Kim BS, Kim MS, Kim SI, Kim YS, et al. Early hospital readmissions after ABO- or HLA-incompatible living donor kidney transplantation. Sci Rep. 2019;9(1): 3246.
29. Kahwaji J, Sinha A, Toyoda M, Ge S, Reinsmoen N, Cao K, et al. Infectious complications in kidney-transplant recipients desensitized with rituximab and intravenous immunoglobulin. Clin J Am Soc Nephrol. 2011;6:2894-900.
30. Padmanabhan A, Ratner L, Jhang J, Duong J, Markowitz G, Vasilescu E, et al. Comparative outcome analysis of ABO-incompatible and positive crossmatch renal transplantation: a single-center experience. Transplantation. 2009; 87(12):1889-96.

CHAPTER 20

ABO-incompatible Kidney Transplantation

Pranaw K Jha, Vijay Kher

CASE VIGNETTE

Mr MP, a 50-year-old diabetic patient with hypertension and chronic kidney disease, has reached end-stage renal disease (ESRD). His blood group is O. His parents have diabetes and hence are unsuitable for donation. His wife's blood group is B and she wants to be the donor. Another prospective donor is his brother whose blood group is A. The patient's anti-B antibody titer is 256 and anti-A antibody titer is 64. During evaluation, he is also found to have donor-specific antihuman leukocyte antigen (HLA) antibody against his brother with a positive flow cytometry crossmatch while the crossmatch with his wife is negative and there are no donor-specific antibodies.

a. *What is the best treatment option for the patient? Should he remain on the waitlist or proceed with ABO-incompatible (ABOi) transplant?*
b. *Who is a better donor for him—his wife or his brother?*
c. *What are important concerns in case he opts for ABOi transplant?*
d. *Which method of extracorporeal therapy will be best in this case?*

Ans.

a. As the patient does not have any suitable donor, an ABOi transplant will be a better option than being on waitlist. The survival has been found to be better for patients undergoing an incompatible transplant rather than being on the waitlist for a compatible kidney.
b. His wife will be a better donor despite the high antiblood group titer as there are no donor-specific anti-HLA antibodies against her. The baseline antiblood group antibody titer does not have any correlation with overall graft outcome and then incidence of antibody-mediated rejections (AMRs).
c. An important concern is that if he opts for an incompatible transplant, there will be higher risk of an acute AMR leading to graft loss. A higher burden of immunosuppression and higher risk of infections are other important concerns.
d. Immunoadsorption (IA) will be the best extracorporeal method in the present case for antibody removal as it is more selective and removes only antiblood group antibodies with relatively lesser chances of bleeding-related complications (although there are no randomized trials comparing the three modalities of extracorporeal therapy). It will be more cost effective as well. The cost of IA column is more than that of the double filtration plasmapheresis (DFPP) or regular plasma exchange, but the number of sessions required will be lesser and this will also reduce the required duration of hospital stay pretransplant. The IA columns can be reused to make it more cost effective.

INTRODUCTION

Kidney transplantation is the best form of renal replacement therapy for patients with ESRD. It increases life expectancy and improves the quality of life. There is a huge demand and supply gap, and the number on transplant waitlist is ever growing. Those who are lucky enough to get a living donor often have to face the immunological barriers of blood group incompatibility and HLA incompatibility. Almost one third of the potential willing living donors get rejected due to this.[1]

HISTORY

The first successful kidney transplant was done in 1954 in Boston by Merrill et al. between identical twins.[2] The initial attempts at ABOi renal transplant were met with high failure rates and soon it was realized that blood group compatibility is an important prerequisite for a successful kidney transplant. Slapak et al. reported for the first time, use of plasmapheresis in an accidental ABOi transplant to successfully salvage the graft.[3] Alexandre et al. reported the first series of successful ABOi kidney transplants using plasmapheresis, splenectomy, and regular immunosuppression.[4] ABOi kidney transplant increased in popularity in Japan due to the absence of a deceased donor program. In the late 1990s, large series of ABOi renal transplants were reported from Japan. Soon, it gained popularity in other countries as well. At present, it constitutes almost 33% of renal transplants in Japan.[5] It has been gaining popularity in India as well over the past decade.[6-8]

CHAPTER HIGHLIGHTS

- ABO-incompatible transplant circumvents the problem of blood group incompatibility in renal transplant.
- Patient and graft outcomes are acceptable and at par with compatible transplants in long term.
- Preconditioning is needed to prevent acute AMRs.
- Unpredictable acute AMR and TMA remain an important concern.
- Efforts to minimize immunosuppression to reduce the infection and related morbidity are needed.

BLOOD GROUP COMPATIBILITIES IN TRANSPLANT—ROLE OF BLOOD GROUP ANTIGENS AND ANTIBODIES

In a conventional blood group-compatible transplant, blood group AB is a universal recipient while other blood group patients can receive kidneys from the same blood group donors or blood group O donors (universal donors). **Figure 1** shows the blood group compatibilities in a conventional transplant. Any deviation from this compatibility constitutes ABOi transplant.

Blood group antigens are present in the red blood cells (RBCs) and other tissues (kidney, pancreas, salivary gland, body fluids). There are three major blood group antigens—A, B, and H. H antigen is present in all the individuals. A- or B-allele-encoded glycosyl-transferase gene expression leads to specific carbohydrate determinant getting added to the H antigen leading to A and B blood group subtypes.[9] If a kidney is transplanted across the blood group barrier, the presence of preformed antiblood group (isoagglutinin) reacts with the blood group antigens present on the endothelium of renal vessels leading to the formation of microthrombi and subsequently hyperacute rejection.

The antiblood group antibodies are formed within the first 3–6 months of life, stabilize by 5–6 years of age, and then decline in the old age. These antibodies produced by bone

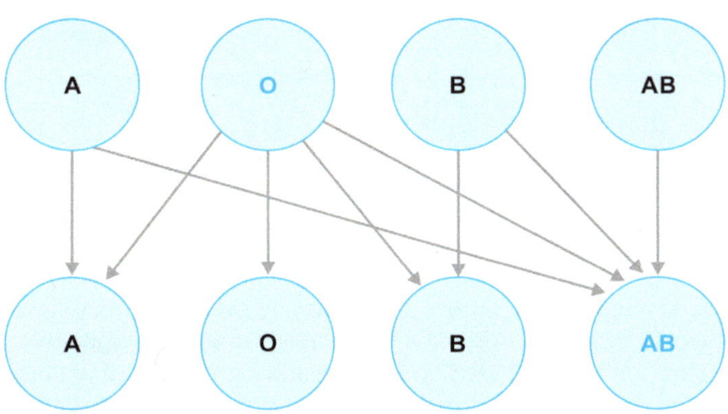

Fig. 1: Blood group compatibilities in a conventional transplant. Person with O blood group can be a universal donor, while person with AB group can be a universal recipient.

marrow and lymph gland cells are formed as cross-reactive antibodies against food and environmental antigens. Different methods of detecting these antibodies are as follows:

- *Tube method:* This method of antibody detection has been used traditionally. The RBCs and plasma were mixed with enhancement solution and allowed to incubate. This is shaken, spun, and read. A positive test is indicated by hemolysis. This test has wide variation and it is the least reproducible.
- *Column agglutination technique (the gel method):* This utilizes gel column which is impregnated with antiglobulin reagent that traps antibody-bound RBCs. The patient's serum sample with reagent RBCs is mixed with low ionic strength solution (LISS). This is placed at the top of column well and allowed to incubate. If the test is negative, the RBCs will pass to the bottom. If it is positive, it will lead to trapping of cells in the gel. A strong positive reaction manifests as large agglutinates staying at the top of the gel where the sample was originally kept. This technique has less subjective variation, and it is more reproducible than the tube technique.
- *Flow cytometry:* Here, RBCs are incubated with dithiothreitol (DTT)-treated serum. These RBCs are then stained with antihuman immunoglobulin G (IgG). Isotonic saline is added to this and the RBCs are resuspended and assessed by a flow cytometer. Flow cytometry is the most reproducible method but is more expensive and not available everywhere.
- *Solid phase assay:* Microtiter plates with wells are coated with reagent RBC stroma of known phenotype. Patient plasma and LISS are added to the well and then incubated. The plate is washed and indicator RBCs coated with anti-IgG are added. This is spun and read. A positive test is shown by a uniform layer of indicator RBCs at the bottom of the well.

Gel column agglutination test is the preferred method for antibody titer assessment due to less variability and easy availability. Tube method is an acceptable alternative.

Although almost all the preconditioning protocols include methods for antibody removal, there is a wide variation in the acceptable immediate pretransplant titer levels. The optimal pretransplant titer is still unestablished, varying from 1:4 to 1:32.[10-18] In the initial studies, Shimmura et al. showed that higher antibody titers are associated with poorer outcomes.[19] This was also observed by Gloor et al. who showed that a high preoperative titer and rapidly rising titer in the post-transplant period are associated with AMR.[20] Few studies have shown that higher titer even up to 2 weeks post-transplant can lead to AMR[21] although studies over the last decade have shown that antibody titer may not be that relevant in the modern era of immunosuppressants of tacrolimus, mycophenolate mofetil (MMF), and steroids.[22] But, overall, it is still widely believed that isoagglutinin removal is an important part of ABOi renal transplant preconditioning protocol and it should be as complete as possible.

DESENSITIZATION

In order to perform a successful ABOi transplant, desensitization (also known as preconditioning) is needed to remove the antiblood group antibodies present as well as deplete the source of antibody production. The preconditioning regime therefore consists of the following components **(Fig. 2)**:

- An extracorporeal method to remove preexisting isoagglutinin. This consists of regular plasmapheresis, DFPP, or IA. IA is the most selective method. The IA columns are coated with A or B antigen. Isoagglutinin gets adsorbed on this. Although meant for single use, these have been reused as well as higher cost is a limiting factor.[23,24] An important advantage of this method is that no substitution is required.

  In DFPP, the plasma is separated by centrifugation or membrane separation method and it is made to pass through another column which selectively removes Ig.[25] In one session of DFPP, approximately 70% and 60% of IgM and IgG, respectively, are removed.

  Regular plasmapheresis is the least selective method and consists of removal of large amount of plasma and subsequent replacement with fresh frozen plasma or albumin. Intravenous immunoglobulin (IVIg) has been regularly used post plasmapheresis and DFPP (not IA) as a part of the preconditioning regimen, although there has been concern about antibody rebound titer with the use of IVIg which can increase the number of sessions needed to achieve the desired target.[26] The number of sessions of plasmapheresis depends on the baseline titers. To reach Ab titers of <1:16, 1–2 and 2–3 sessions are required for baseline titers of <32 and 64, respectively.
- Suppression of new isoagglutinin formation by surgical splenectomy or administration of B-cell-depleting agent rituximab. As surgical splenectomy is associated with significant morbidity and mortality, it has been replaced by rituximab. Successful ABOi transplants have been reported with rituximab-free protocols as well.[16] But studies have shown better death-censored graft survival with rituximab-based regimen than without it.[27]
- Regular immunosuppression—apart from depletion therapies mentioned above, induction therapies such as interleukin 2 (IL2) receptor antagonist basiliximab or antithymocyte globulin (ATG) are used. Maintenance immunosuppression is used consisting of a calcineurin inhibitor, MMF, and steroid.

Figure 3 shows a prototype of desensitization protocol. Various desensitization protocols have been developed using combination of the above-mentioned methods **(Figs. 4A to C)**. Despite the presence of multiple protocols, superiority of one over the other has not been proven.

ACCOMMODATION

Accommodation is the process whereby despite the presence of antiblood group antibodies, the graft continues to function without any rejection. It is defined as the presence of detectable C4d deposition in the presence of normal graft function and structure as per the consensus of the American Society of Transplantation.[28]

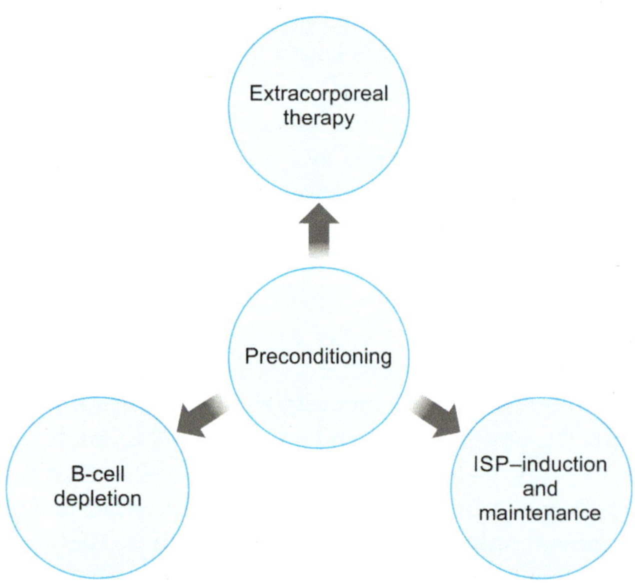

Fig. 2: Components of preconditioning (also known as desensitization) regimen in an ABO-incompatible transplant. Antiblood group antibodies are removed by extracorporeal therapy. B-cell depletion is achieved by rituximab. Regular immunosuppression (ISP) consists of calcineurin inhibitor, antiproliferative agent, and prednisolone.

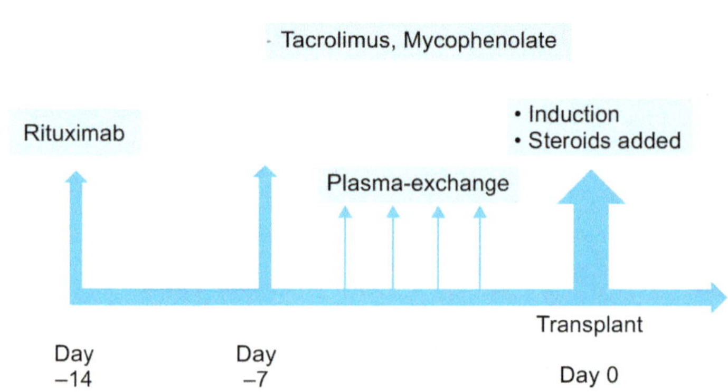

Fig. 3: A typical desensitization protocol. Rituximab is usually given 2 weeks before transplant while tacrolimus and mycophenolate mofetil are started 1 week in advance and extracorporeal antibody removal (by regular plasmapheresis/double filtration plasmapheresis/immunoadsorption) is started. Transplant is done once the target antibody titer is reached (on day 0).

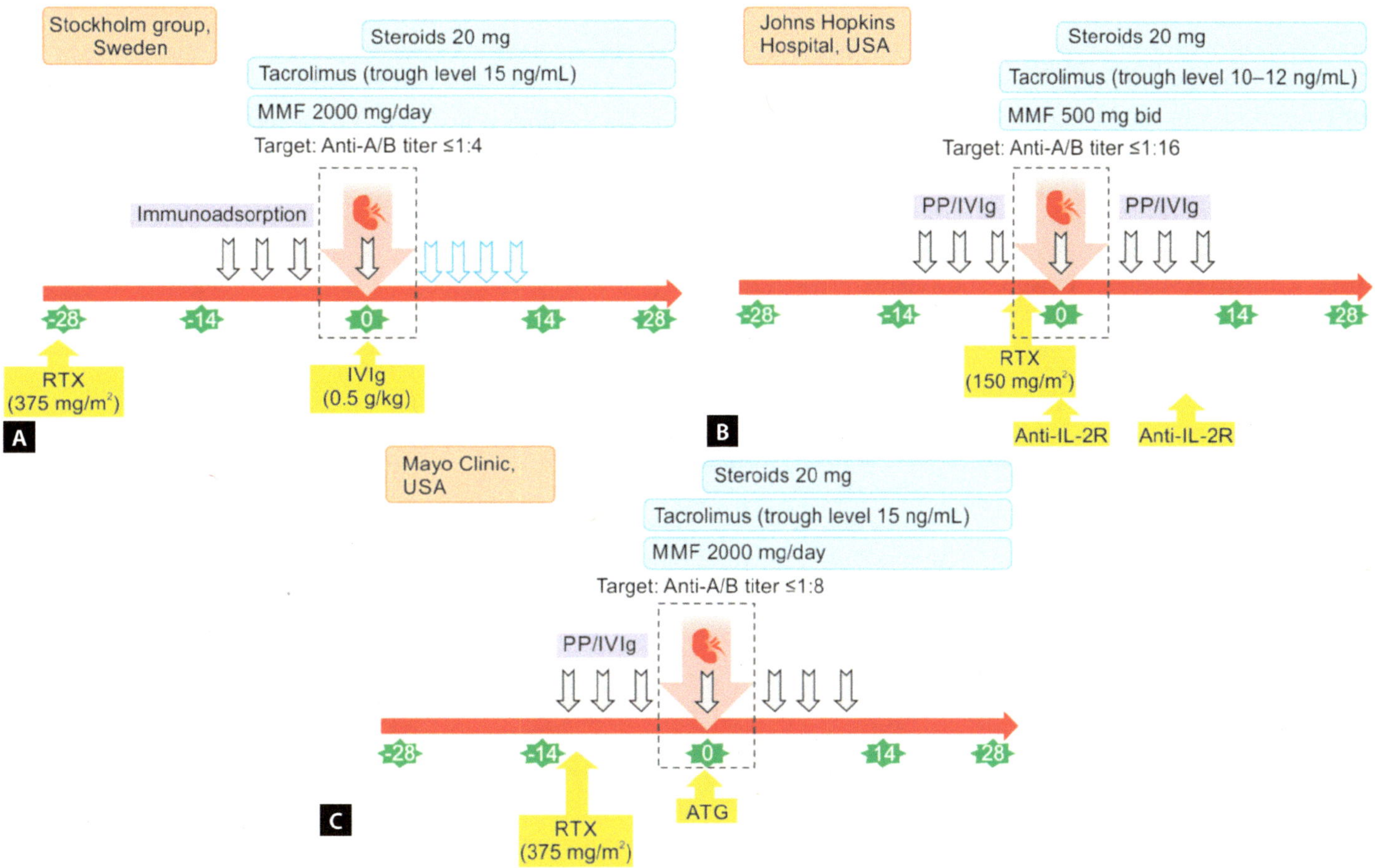

Figs. 4A to C: Various ABO-incompatible (ABOi) desensitization protocol. (ATG: antithymocyte globulin; IL-2R: interleukin-2 receptor; IVIg: Intravenous immunoglobulin; MMF: mycophenolate mofetil; PP: plasmapheresis; RTX: rituximab)
Source: Sonnenday CJ, Warren DS, Cooper M, Samaniego M, Haas M, King KE, et al. Plasmapheresis, CMV hyperimmune globulin, and anti-CD20 allow ABO-incompatible renal transplantation without splenectomy. Am J Transplant. 2004;4(8):1315-22.

The mechanism of accommodation is not clear. There are multiple hypotheses as follows **(Fig. 5)**:

- Defects in glycosyl-transferase enzyme due to ischemia reperfusion injury which lead to reduced blood group antigen expression on the donor endothelium, thereby reducing the immunogenicity.[29]
- Upregulation of complement regulatory proteins, such as CD59, which prevents the formation of final membrane attack complex of complement pathway on the graft.[30]
- A switch to IgG2 isotype of IgG. IgG2 is less effective at activating complement. It also binds and inhibits other cytotoxic isotypes.[31]
- Bcl-xl and Bcl-2 upregulation in the accommodated graft and the absence of Bax, a proapoptotic marker.[32]

The risk of acute AMR is high during the first 2 weeks of an ABOi transplant. Accommodation happens within the first 2–3 weeks, after which the graft outcomes are similar to ABO-compatible (ABOc) transplants.

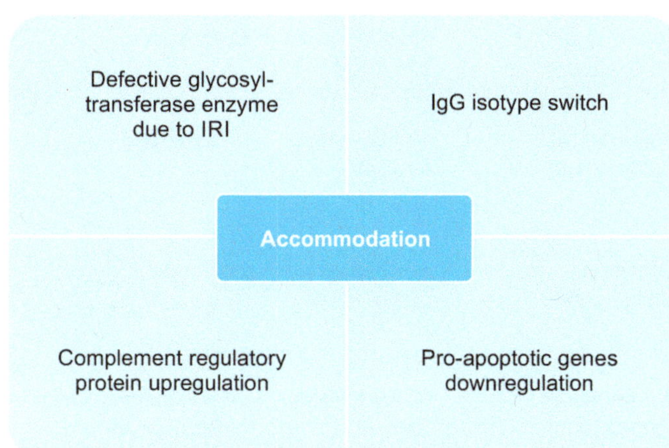

Fig. 5: Mechanism of accommodation. (IgG: immunoglobulin G; IRI: ischemia reperfusion injury)

OUTCOMES

Graft and patient outcomes of ABOi have improved over the past few decades and it is at par with ABOc transplants now barring the initial 2 weeks.[33-35] It has been shown that patients undergoing an ABOi transplant have a survival advantage when compared with those waiting to receive a potential ABOc transplant.[36] The initial drop in graft survival is due to an increased incidence of AMR in an unaccommodated graft. Once the graft is accommodated, the outcomes are comparable.

Increased incidence of infections in ABOi transplant has been a matter of concern that has been highlighted in many studies. Infection is the most important cause of patient loss in an ABOi transplant.[35,37,38] Efforts toward minimizing the immunosuppression burden and tailoring it as per the risk profile can help in reducing this. There have been studies of rituximab-free ABOi transplants with good results. Steroid-free ABOi transplants have also been tried with good success. **Table 1** shows outcomes of ABOi transplants in different settings with variable protocols.

With increasing experience and improving outcomes, more challenging ABOi transplants are being performed. Kosoku et al. reported a pilot study of ABOi transplants in 17 elderly patients (>60 years) and reported good patient and graft survival.[39] Uchida et al. reported a pilot experience of ABOi kidney transplant as a second transplant.[40]

ANTIBODY-MEDIATED REJECTIONS IN ABO-INCOMPATIBLE TRANSPLANTS

Antibody-mediated rejections in ABOi transplants are unpredictable and sudden, leading to the loss of a well-functioning graft in a matter of few hours. It has been characteristically seen in the first 2–3 weeks of the transplant

TABLE 1: Outcome of ABO-incompatible (ABOi) renal transplants.

Study/period	*No.*	*Desensitization*	*Outcomes*
Takahashi et al.[41] (1989–2001)	441 ABOi versus 1,055 ABOc	DFPP or PLEX or IA; splenectomy	• 9 years graft survival 59% in ABOi versus 57% in ABOc • Patient survival 84% in ABOi versus 88% in ABOc • Acute rejection 58% in ABOi • Infection 18.8%
Montgomery et al.[34] (1995–2010)	738 ABOi versus 77,455 ABOc	Variable	• 10 years graft survival 72.9% ABOi versus 76.1% ABOc • Patient survival 74.5% ABOi versus 75.1% ABOc • AMR 3%
Toki et al.[15] (1999–2004)	57 ABOi	DFPP/splenectomy	• 8 years graft survival 70% • Patient survival • AMR 33%
Uchida et al.[10] (1999–2010)	25 ABOi	DFPP or PLEX; splenectomy or Ritux	• Patient and graft survival 100% • AMR 8% • CMV antigenemia 48%
Genberg et al.[14] (2001–2005)	15 ABOi versus 30 ABOc	IA/Ritux/IVIg	• At 1 year graft survival 86.7% in both groups • Patient survival 100% in ABOi versus 96.7% in ABOc • AMR 0 • Infection 40%
Tyden et al.[42] (2002–2006)	60 ABOi versus 274 ABOc	IA/Ritux/IVIg	• At 61 months graft survival 97% versus 95% (ABOi vs. ABOc) • Patient survival 98% both groups • AMR 0
Wilpert et al.[12] (2004–2009)	40 ABOi versus 43 ABOc	IA/Ritux/IVIg	• Graft survival 100% in ABOi at 3.3 years versus 93% in ABOc at 1.5 years • Patient survival 98% in both groups • AMR 0 • Infection 50%
Flint et al.[16] (2005–2008)	37 ABOi versus 52 ABOc	PLEX/IVIg	• Graft survival 100% at 2.1 years • Patient survival 100% • AMR 5.4% • Infection 40.5%
Ashimine et al.[43] (2005–2009)	92 ABOi versus 228 ABOc	DFPP/splenectomy or Ritux or none	• 5 years graft survival 87% versus 97.7% (ABOi vs. ABOc)
Okumi et al.[44] (2005–2013)	144 ABOi versus 333 ABOc	DFPP/Ritux/IVIg	• Graft survival 86.9% versus 92% (ABOi vs. ABOc) • Patient survival 96.7% in ABOi versus 96.2% in ABOc • AMR 0 • Infection 29.1% in ABOi versus 19.5% in ABOc (ABOi 4 vs. 4.6 years ABOc follow-up)
Opelz et al.[27] (2005–2012)	1,420 ABOi versus 1,420 ABOc	PLEX or IA; Ritux	• 3 years graft survival 93.4% in ABOi versus 93.2% in ABOc • Patient survival 95.6% in ABOi versus 96.3% in ABOc • Acute rejection in first year 16.3% in ABOi versus 17.8% in ABOc • Infection-related hospitalization in first year 17.1% in ABOi versus 19.5% in ABOc

Contd...

Contd...

Study/period	*No.*	*Desensitization*	*Outcomes*
Speer et al.[45] (2004–2018)	48 ABOi versus 96 ABOc	IA/PLEX/Ritux/IVIg	• 8 years graft survival better in ABOi group • Patient survival similar • Death from infection higher in ABOi • AMR 2% in ABOi versus 3% in ABOc
van Agteren et al.[46] (2006–2012)	50 ABOi versus 100 ABOc	IA/Ritux/IVIg	• 5 years graft survival 90% versus 97% (ABOi vs. ABOc) • AMR 22% • Viral infection 16%
Lipshutz et al.[47] (2008–2009)	18 ABOi	PLEX/Ritux/IVIg	• Graft survival 94.4% • Patient survival 100% • AMR 0
Jha et al.[48] (2011–2020)	121 ABOi	DFPP or PLEX or IA/IVIg/Ritux	• Graft survival 94% at 2.7 years • Patient survival 93% • AMR 3% • Infection 37%
Thukral et al.[49] (2014–2015)	30 ABOi versus 30 ABOc	PLEX/IVIg/Ritux	• 1 year patient and graft survival 96.7% in both ABOi and ABOc groups • AMR 6.7% in ABOi versus 3.3% in ABOc • Infection 13.3% in ABOi versus 16.6 in ABOc group

(ABOc: ABO-compatible; AMR: antibody-mediated rejection; CMV: cytomegalovirus; DFPP: double filtration plasma exchange; IA: immunoadsorption; IVIg: intravenous immunoglobulin; PLEX: plasma exchange; Ritux: rituximab)

and does not have any correlation with the baseline antibody titer. An explosive increase in the post-transplant titer has been seen in few patients preceding the rejection, but this is not always the case. The graft biopsy shows features of AMR and thrombotic microangiopathy (TMA).[7]

Although there have been reports of successful salvage, more often than not, the graft is lost. Complements are thought to play an important role and complement inhibitor eculizumab has been used to successfully prevent and treat AMR in ABOi transplants.[50,51] However, the cost and availability of the drug are limiting factors. Other therapies that have been used to successfully treat AMR in few cases include plasmapheresis, splenectomy, IVIg, bortezomib (proteosome inhibitor), and daratumumab (anti-CD38 antibody).[16,46,47,52,53]

Dosing of Rituximab

Protocol for rituximab varies from center to center. In an analysis by Jha et al., 200 mg rituximab was given 2 weeks prior to transplant. In another study from India by Ravichandran and Kannan, rituximab was given on day 7 at a dose of 200 mg.[54]

Post-transplant Monitoring

Routine measurement of Ab titers after transplantation is not recommended as may not alter the outcomes of the transplant. Decision of post-transplant plasmapheresis should depend on presence of graft dysfunction with rising Ab titers from baseline. More data are needed to reach any consensus.[55]

Recent Literature

In a recently published systematic review and meta-analysis in Lancet on ABOi renal transplantation, higher mortality and graft loss were found in ABOi renal transplants within the first 3 years. However, long-term outcomes after 5 years showed equivalent survival rates and organ function. The results showed inferior outcomes in terms of infectious (such as polyoma nephropathy) and noninfectious complications (higher rates of bleeding events, higher surgical revisions, with more postoperative wound infections, hematomas, and lymphoceles), and graft rejection episodes.[56]

Another meta-analysis by de Weerd and Betjes showed that ABOi kidney transplantation has good outcomes but is associated with a higher risk for graft loss and lower patient survival within the first year after transplantation compared with ABOc.[35]

UNANSWERED QUESTIONS

Despite the success of ABOi transplantation over the past few decades, there are quite a few unanswered questions.

- Why only few of these transplants undergo hyperacute rejection within the initial few weeks while most of the remaining accommodate? How can one detect and prevent such rejection? Most of these rejections leading to graft loss have findings of TMA.
- What is the role of antibody titer in acute rejection? While the initial studies showed a relation between baseline antibody titer and acute rejections, the recent studies have refuted this.[19,21,22]

- What is the best cutoff of immediate pretransplant antibody titer? The acceptable titer has varied in literature.[57]
- What is an optimal preconditioning regimen which minimizes the chances of rejection and has minimum risk of infection? What is the optimum number of plasmapheresis sessions needed in pre- and post-transplant periods? The necessity of B-cell depletion therapy has been questioned and few centers have done transplants without it with good outcomes.[16,18]

A nonhuman primates model of hyperacute rejection has been developed to study mechanism of rejection, accommodation, and clinical intervention in an ABOi kidney transplant.[58]

CONCLUSION

ABO-incompatible transplantation has become an important treatment modality for patients with only blood group-incompatible donors and who do not have a suitable swap. Graft and patient outcomes have improved over the past few decades. Although unpredictable AMRs still remain the Achilles heel. More studies are needed to understand the pathophysiology of the AMR in ABOi setting so that effective therapy may be devised to prevent and treat it. Increased incidence of infection due to higher immunosuppression burden remains an important challenge.

REFERENCES

1. Segev DL, Gentry SE, Warren DS, Reeb B, Montgomery RA. Kidney paired donation and optimizing the use of live donor organs. JAMA. 2005;293(15):1883-90.
2. Merrill JP, Murray JE, Harrison JH, Guild WR. Successful homotransplantation of the human kidney between identical twins. J Am Med Assoc. 1956;160(4):277-82.
3. Slapak M, Naik RB, Lee HA. Renal transplant in a patient with major donor-recipient blood group incompatibility: reversal of acute rejection by the use of modified plasmapheresis. Transplantation. 1981;31(1):4-7.
4. Alexandre GP, Squifflet JP, De Bruyere M, Latinne D, Reding R, Gianello P, et al. Present experiences in a series of 26 ABO-incompatible living donor renal allografts. Transplant Proc. 1987;19(6):4538-42.
5. Takahashi K, Saito K. ABO-incompatible kidney transplantation. Transplant Rev (Orlando). 2013;27(1):1-8.
6. Jha PK, Bansal SB, Sethi SK, Jain M, Sharma R, Nandwani A, et al. ABO-incompatible renal transplantation in developing world—crossing the immunological (and mental) barrier. Indian J Nephrol. 2016;26(2):113-8.
7. Jha P, Nandwani A, Kher A, Bansal SB, Sethi S, Sharma R, et al. ABO-incompatible renal transplantation: the journey so far on a road less traveled. Indian J Transplant. 2018;12(3): 177-81.
8. Prabhakar A, Gang S, Hegde U, Konnur K, Patel H, Rajapurkar M. Kidney transplantation with ABO-incompatible donors: a comparison with matched ABO compatible donor transplants. Indian J Nephrol. 2021;31(4):358-64.
9. Yamamoto F, McNeill PD, Hakomori S. Genomic organization of human histo-blood group ABO genes. Glycobiology. 1995; 5(1):51-8.
10. Uchida J, Kuwabara N, Machida Y, Iwai T, Naganuma T, Kumada N, et al. Excellent outcomes of ABO-incompatible kidney transplantation: a single-center experience. Transplant Proc. 2012;44(1):204-9.
11. Tyden G, Kumlien G, Genberg H, Sandberg J, Sedigh A, Lundgren T, et al. The Stockholm experience with ABO-incompatible kidney transplantations without splenectomy. Xenotransplantation. 2006;13(2):105-7.
12. Wilpert J, Fischer KG, Pisarski P, Wiech T, Daskalakis M, Ziegler A, et al. Long-term outcome of ABO-incompatible living donor kidney transplantation based on antigen-specific desensitization. An observational comparative analysis. Nephrol Dial Transplant. 2010;25(11):3778-86.
13. Oettl T, Zuliani E, Gaspert A, Hopfer H, Dickenmann M, Fehr T. Late steroid withdrawal after ABO blood group-incompatible living donor kidney transplantation: high rate of mild cellular rejection. Transplantation. 2010;89(6):702-6.
14. Genberg H, Kumlien G, Wennberg L, Berg U, Tydén G. ABO-incompatible kidney transplantation using antigen-specific immunoadsorption and rituximab: a 3-year follow-up. Transplantation. 2008;85(12):1745-54.
15. Toki D, Ishida H, Setoguchi K, Shimizu T, Omoto K, Shirakawa H, et al. Acute antibody-mediated rejection in living ABO-incompatible kidney transplantation: long-term impact and risk factors. Am J Transplant. 2009;9(3):567-77.
16. Flint SM, Walker RG, Hogan C, Haeusler MN, Robertson A, Francis DMA, et al. Successful ABO-incompatible kidney transplantation with antibody removal and standard immunosuppression. Am J Transplant. 2011;11(5):1016-24.
17. Fuchinoue S, Ishii Y, Sawada T, Murakami T, Iwadoh K, Sannomiya A, et al. The 5-year outcome of ABO-incompatible kidney transplantation with rituximab induction. Transplantation. 2011;91(8):853-7.
18. Montgomery RA, Locke JE, King KE, Segev DL, Warren DS, Kraus ES, et al. ABO incompatible renal transplantation: a paradigm ready for broad implementation. Transplantation. 2009;87(8):1246-55.
19. Shimmura H, Tanabe K, Ishikawa N, Tokumoto T, Takahashi K, Toma H. Role of anti-A/B antibody titers in results of ABO-incompatible kidney transplantation. Transplantation. 2000;70(9):1331-5.
20. Gloor JM, Lager DJ, Moore SB, Pineda AA, Fidler ME, Larson TS, et al. ABO-incompatible kidney transplantation using both A2 and non-A2 living donors. Transplantation. 2003;75(7):971-7.
21. Tobian AA, Shirey RS, Montgomery RA, Cai W, Haas M, Ness PM, et al. ABO antibody titer and risk of antibody-mediated rejection in ABO-incompatible renal transplantation. Am J Transplant. 2010;10(5):1247-53.
22. Shimmura H, Tanabe K, Ishida H, Tokumoto T, Ishikawa N, Miyamoto N, et al. Lack of correlation between results of ABO-incompatible living kidney transplantation and anti-ABO blood type antibody titers under our current immunosuppression. Transplantation. 2005;80(7):985-8.

23. Jha PK, Tiwari AK, Sethi SK, Kher V. Reusing immunoadsorption column—making the ABO incompatible renal transplant affordable. Indian J Nephrol. 2017;27(3):241-2.
24. Tiwari V, Gupta A, Divyaveer S, Bhargava V, Malik M, Gupta A, et al. Immunoadsorption column reuse. Indian J Nephrol. 2021;31(1):33-8.
25. Jha PK, Tiwari AK, Bansal SB, Sethi SK, Ahlawat R, Kher V, et al. Cascade plasmapheresis as preconditioning regimen for ABO-incompatible renal transplantation: a single-center experience. Transfusion. 2016;56(4):956-61.
26. Kher A, Agarwal A, Jha P, Bansal D, Madken M, Narula AS, et al. Anti A/B antibody titer rebound: are we making it worse? Be aware of your intravenous immunoglobulin. Indian J Nephrol. 2018;28(5):407-9.
27. Opelz G, Morath C, Susal C, Tran TH, Zeier M, Döhler B. Three-year outcomes following 1420 ABO-incompatible living-donor kidney transplants performed after ABO antibody reduction: results from 101 centers. Transplantation. 2015;99(2):400-4.
28. Beigel JH, Tomashek KM, Dodd LE, Mehta AK, Zingman BS, Kalil AC, et al. Remdesivir for the treatment of Covid-19—final report. N Engl J Med. 2020;383(19):1813-26.
29. Takahashi K. Accommodation in ABO-incompatible kidney transplantation: why do kidney grafts survive? Transplant Proc. 2004;36(2 Suppl):193S-6S.
30. Griesemer AD, Okumi M, Shimizu A, Moran S, Ishikawa Y, Iorio J, et al. Upregulation of CD59: potential mechanism of accommodation in a large animal model. Transplantation. 2009;87(9):1308-17.
31. Kirk AD, Baldwin WM, Cascalho MI, Chong AS, Sykes M, West LJ. American society of transplantation symposium on B cells in transplantation: harnessing humoral immunity from rodent models to clinical practice. Am J Transplant. 2007;7(6):1464-70.
32. Salama AD, Delikouras A, Pusey CD, Cook HT, Bhangal G, Lechler RI, et al. Transplant accommodation in highly sensitized patients: a potential role for Bcl-xL and alloantibody. Am J Transplant. 2001;1(3):260-9.
33. Tanabe K. Japanese experience of ABO-incompatible living kidney transplantation. Transplantation. 2007;84(12 Suppl): S4-7.
34. Montgomery JR, Berger JC, Warren DS, James NT, Montgomery RA, Segev DL, et al. Outcomes of ABO-incompatible kidney transplantation in the United States. Transplantation. 2012;93(6):603-9.
35. de Weerd AE, Betjes MGH. ABO-incompatible kidney transplant outcomes: a meta-analysis. Clin J Am Soc Nephrol. 2018;13(8):1234-43.
36. Massie AB, Orandi BJ, Waldram MM, Luo X, Nguyen AQ, Montgomery RA, et al. Impact of ABO-incompatible living donor kidney transplantation on patient survival. Am J Kidney Dis. 2020;76(5):616-23.
37. Barnett AN, Manook M, Nagendran M, Kenchayikoppad S, Vaughan R, Dorling A, et al. Tailored desensitization strategies in ABO blood group antibody incompatible renal transplantation. Transplant Int. 2014;27(2):187-96.
38. Lentine KL, Axelrod D, Klein C, Simpkins C, Xiao H, Schnitzler MA, et al. Early clinical complications after ABO-incompatible live-donor kidney transplantation: a national study of Medicare-insured recipients. Transplantation. 2014;98(1):54-65.
39. Kosoku A, Uchida J, Kabei K, Nishide S, Shimada H, Iwai T, et al. Favorable outcomes of elderly ABO-incompatible kidney transplantation-pilot single center experience. Urol Int. 2018;101(4):459-66.
40. Uchida J, Kosoku A, Kabei K, Nishide S, Shimada H, Iwai T, et al. Pilot experience with ABO-incompatible kidney transplantation as a second transplant. Urol Int. 2019;102(4):441-8.
41. Takahashi K, Saito K, Takahara S, Okuyama A, Tanabe K, Toma H, et al. Excellent long-term outcome of ABO-incompatible living donor kidney transplantation in Japan. Am J Transplant. 2004;4(7):1089-96.
42. Tyden G, Donauer J, Wadstrom J, Kumlien G, Wilpert J, Nilsson T, et al. Implementation of a protocol for ABO-incompatible kidney transplantation—a three-center experience with 60 consecutive transplantations. Transplantation. 2007;83(9):1153-5.
43. Ashimine S, Watarai Y, Yamamoto T, Hiramitsu T, Tsujita M, Nanmoku K, et al. Neither pre-transplant rituximab nor splenectomy affects de novo HLA antibody production after renal transplantation. Kidney Int. 2014;85(2):425-30.
44. Okumi M, Toki D, Nozaki T, Shimizu T, Shirakawa H, Omoto K, et al. ABO-incompatible living kidney transplants: evolution of outcomes and immunosuppressive management. Am J Transplant. 2016;16(3):886-96.
45. Speer C, Kalble F, Nusshag C, da Silva LP, Schaier M, Becker LE, et al. Outcomes and complications following ABO-incompatible kidney transplantation performed after desensitization by semi-selective immunoadsorption—a retrospective study. Transpl Int. 2019;32(12):1286-96.
46. van Agteren M, Weimar W, de Weerd AE, Te Boekhorst PAW, Ijzermans JNM, van de Wetering J, et al. The first fifty ABO blood group incompatible kidney transplantations: the Rotterdam experience. J Transplant. 2014;2014:913902.
47. Lipshutz GS, McGuire S, Zhu Q, Ziman A, Davis R, Goldfinger D, et al. ABO blood type-incompatible kidney transplantation and access to organs. Arch Surg. 2011;146(4): 453-8.
48. Jha PK, Bansal SB, Rana A, Nandwani A, Kher A, Sethi S, et al. ABO-incompatible kidney transplantation in India: a single-center experience of first hundred cases. Indian J Nephrol. 2022;32(1):42-6.
49. Thukral S, Kumar D, Ray DS. Comparative analysis of ABO-incompatible kidney transplantation with ABO-compatible transplantation: a single-center experience from Eastern India. Saudi J Kidney Dis Transpl. 2019;30(1):97-107.
50. Lanfranco L, Joly M, Del Bello A, Esposito L, Cognard N, Perrin P, et al. Eculizumab for thrombotic microangiopathy associated with antibody-mediated rejection after ABO-incompatible kidney transplantation. Case Rep Transplant. 2017;2017:3197042.
51. West-Thielke P, Progar K, Campara M, Jasiak N, Gallon L, Tang I, et al. Eculizumab for prevention of antibody-mediated rejection in blood group-incompatible renal transplantation. Transplant Proc. 2018;50(1):66-9.

52. Lee JH, Lee H, Kim K, Lee SW, Song JH, Hwang SD. Acute anti-A/B antibody-mediated rejection after ABO-incompatible kidney transplantation treated with bortezomib and plasmapheresis: a case report. Transplant Proc. 2022;54(2):540-3.
53. Spica D, Junker T, Dickenmann M, Schaub S, Steiger J, Rüfli T, et al. Daratumumab for treatment of antibody-mediated rejection after ABO-incompatible kidney transplantation. Case Rep Nephrol Dial. 2019;9(3):149-57.
54. Ravichandran R, Kannan S. Long term follow-up of ABO incompatible kidney transplantation—a study from India. Open Access Lib J. 2016;3:1-5.
55. Bhalla AK, Anil Kumar BT, Chauhan M, Das P, Gandhi B, Hegde U, et al. ABO-incompatible kidney transplantation: Indian working group recommendations. Indian J Transplant 2019;13:252-8.
56. Scurt FG, Ewert L, Mertens PR, Haller H, Schmidt BMW, Chatzikyrkou C. Clinical outcomes after ABO-incompatible renal transplantation: a systematic review and meta-analysis. Lancet. 2019;393(10185):2059-72.
57. Shin M, Kim SJ. ABO incompatible kidney transplantation—current status and uncertainties. J Transplant. 2011;2011: 970421.
58. Wang J, Feng H, Zhang C, Zhong S, Wang L, Zhu L, et al. Establishment of a hyperacute rejection model of ABO-incompatible renal transplantation in nonhuman primates. Front Immunol. 2021;12:807604.

CHAPTER

21

Kidney Paired Donation in India: Status, Challenges, and Recommendations

Vivek Kute, Priti Meena, Manisha Sahay, Sanshriti Chauhan, Hari Shankar Meshram

INTRODUCTION

About one-third of the end-stage kidney disease (ESKD) patients are excluded from the live-donor kidney transplant (LDKT) program due to blood type incompatibility or positive donor-specific crossmatch, and there exists a huge disparity between transplant organs' supply and demand.[1] Thus, there is a need for other innovative approaches such as kidney paired donation (KPD), human leukocyte antigen (HLA)-incompatible kidney transplantation (KT), and ABO-incompatible KT (ABOiKT) to meet the growing demand for donor kidneys.[2-6] Rapaport first introduced the concept of KPD almost 30 years ago. South Korea, a nation with limited access to deceased donors (DD) where the majority of transplants are reliant on live-donor source, was the first country to report the establishment of a KPD program in 1991. Despite several advantages, KPD in India is associated with several challenges in implementation. In this chapter, we aim to describe the status of KPD in India, its legal aspects, challenges, and recommendations.

WHAT IS KIDNEY PAIRED DONATION?

In KPD, a living kidney donor who is otherwise incompatible with his recipient exchanges kidneys with another donor–recipient pair (DRP). This enables exchange of kidneys between ABO-incompatible and HLA-incompatible living DRPs to receive better compatible kidneys.

Several kidney exchange strategies in KPD include a conventional two-way loop exchange between two incompatible DRPs and an n-way (3,[7] 4,[8] 5,[9] 6,[10] or more pairs) loop exchange among multiple incompatible DRPs. The traditional two-way KPD match between A-to-B and B-to-A pairs is relatively easy and can be performed "manually without computer software" **(Fig. 1A)**. Furthermore, three and more pairs can also be utilized to perform multiple exchanges to benefit more patients.

Kute et al. demonstrated successful LDKT with two[11] and three-way KPD[12] **(Fig. 1B)** with desensitization in ESKD patients who were highly sensitized.

DOMINO PAIRED KIDNEY EXCHANGE

In domino KPD, a nondirected altruistic donor donates a kidney to an unintended recipient of an incompatible DRP and then the donor of that DRP (domino donor) donates kidney to another DRP or to the waiting list.[13] In LDKT, the anonymity of donors or recipients is a complex issue and is handled differently as per individual center practices. Anonymity is preserved in Europe and USA for specified indirect KPD but not in the case of countries such as Korea, Romania, and India due to practicality and to avoid mistrust.[14]

Nondirected anonymous donors (NDAD) do not mandatorily require pair matching and can initiate transplants into a KPD registry with a guarantee of at least two domino-chain transplants.[15] There are different models for multiway exchanges with NDAD, which are: (1) closed-chain donation model: a nondirected donor initiating a chain ending with donation of the final recipient's donor to a kidney transplant waiting list patient, or (2) open-chain donation model: final recipient's donor becomes a bridge donor, starting a new chain of transplants.

A fusion model proposed by Billa et al.[16] links the DD waitlist to a KPD program. This model allocates one of the DD kidneys to the first patient on DD waitlist and the other to the KPD registry, which will initiate swap transplant chain. The kidney of the last donor of this chain is donated to the second patient on DD waitlist leading to an overall three transplants from one DD instead of two transplants.

Unbalanced Kidney Paired Donation

Another strategy to increase KPD numbers is inclusion of ABO/HLA compatible pairs, who may also benefit from receiving a transplant better suited for them. This altruistically unbalanced paired donation was first proposed as a possible solution to help blood group O recipients in a KPD program. Unbalanced KPD can be attractive to otherwise compatible pairs who have a high degree of HLA mismatch

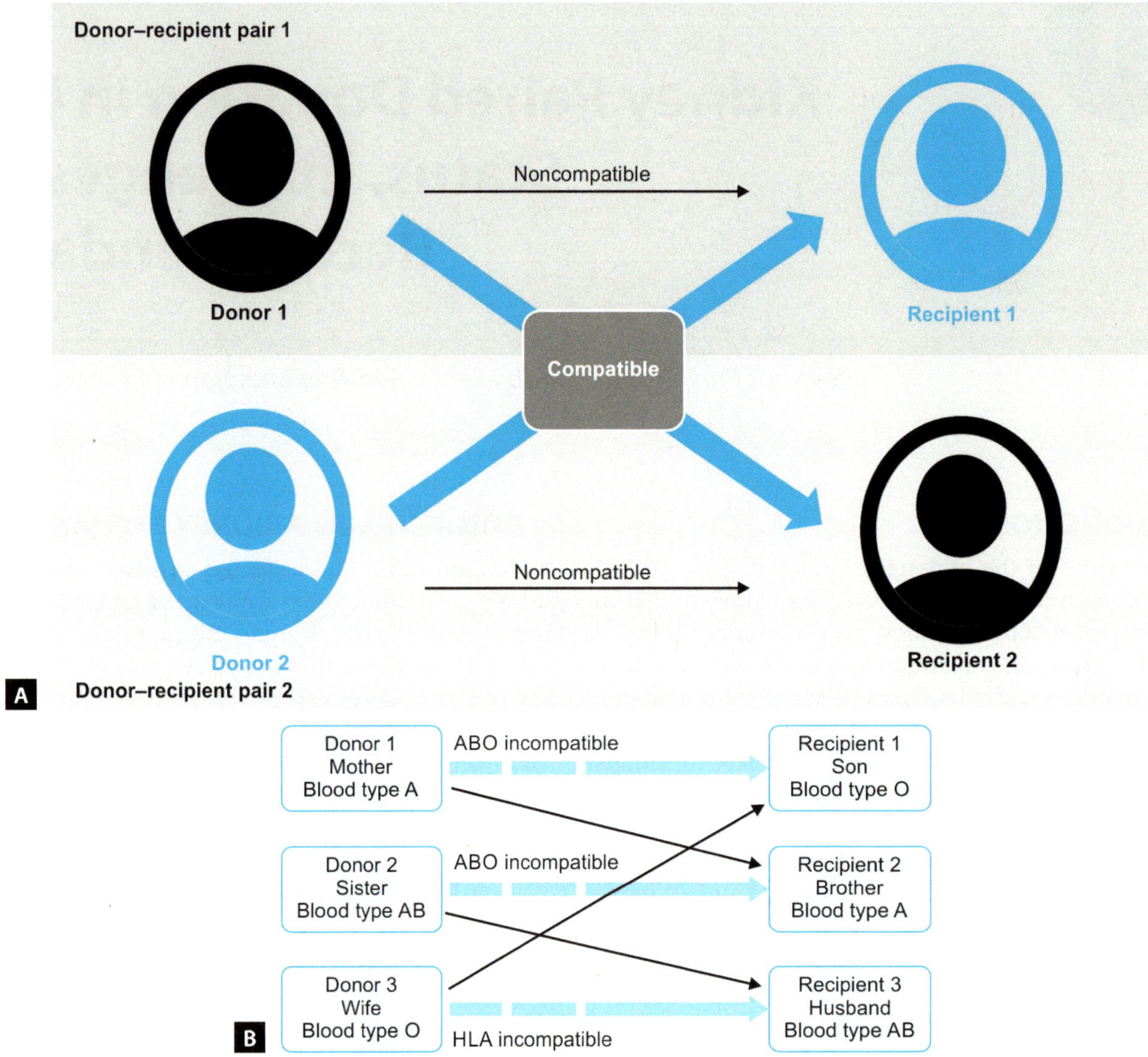

Figs. 1A and B: (A) Two-way KPD; (B) Three-way KPD. (KPD: kidney paired donation)

if the KPD allocation algorithm provides a better HLA match for the recipient in the compatible pair.

How is Matching Done?

Priority for matching depends on blood group matching, likelihood of the recipient finding donor-specific antibodies (DSA) or a cross-match negative donor in the pool. Other factors that can be used for prioritization can include the number of HLA mismatches, the donor's center to the recipient's center distance, the donor–donor or donor–recipient age difference, cytomegalovirus (CMV) and Epstein–Barr virus (EBV) mismatch status of the proposed pair, and time on dialysis. However, none of these rules out possible transplants as a timely transplant supersedes all other factors.

Advantages

Kidney paired donation is a cost-effective method that provides an opportunity to identify compatible transplants to the incompatible DRPs. Desensitization procedures used in incompatible transplants involve expensive immunological tests, plasmapheresis, immunoadsorption, use of rituximab, and excessive immunosuppressive agents, which result in increased expenses, hospitalization, higher chances of infections, and rejection and are associated with poor graft survival. KPD is cheaper than desensitization with reduced immunosuppression required; hence, it should be preferred for incompatible kidney recipients. The KPD program can potentially assist in increasing kidney donor pool in India.

INTERNATIONAL KIDNEY PAIRED DONATION PROGRAMS

Four national KPD programs of the Netherlands, UK, Canada, and Australia are managed by a country's government or national organization. In these national programs, match cycles occur every 3–4 months. In the Australian program, ABO-incompatible donor matching is now also permitted for patients with anti-A and/or anti-B titers of 1:64 or less. Computer-based ABO and virtual cross-match (negative DSA) allocation is done. Subsequently, the final decision regarding transplantation is made after the cell-dependent cytotoxicity and flow cytometry cross-matches of proposed pairs are performed. In Netherlands and Canada, donors are required to travel to the recipient center for surgery, whereas in the UK and Australia, the kidneys are transported between centers. In some other programs, the matching is done real time.

CHAPTER HIGHLIGHTS

- Adoption of new strategies in KT, such as KPD, ABOiKT, and HLA incompatible KT, is crucial to increase the kidney donor pool.
- KPD is a cost-effective method that provides an opportunity to identify compatible transplants for the incompatible donor–recipient pairs.
- KPD should be the preferred method for patients who have incompatibilities with their intended donors.
- Several factors that affect KPD outcomes remain controversial such as optimal chain length, HLA matching, use of software and registry for KPD programs, and compliance with the applicable guidelines for KPD.
- In countries such as India, the KPD program faces challenges due to issues such as legal, administrative, social, availability of deceased donors for KPD, and anonymity preservation.

CHALLENGES

There are several logistic issues in KPD. To establish KPD in India on a nationwide level, an expert and dedicated team is required. Issues such as safe and rapid transportation, an appropriate organ allocation software are needed to be resolved. There is need of government support to achieve a multicenter KPD program at state and national levels. Transplant centers should work together to reduce the waiting time for KPD. Sociocultural diversity and lack of a proper national healthcare system to support the KPD program are the other concerns. Several factors that affect KPD outcomes such as optimal chain length, HLA matching, use of software and registry for KPD programs, and compliance with the applicable guidelines for KPD still remain controversial.

In countries such as India, the KPD program faces challenges due to issues such as legal, administrative, social, availability of DDs for KPD, and anonymity preservation. There can be a risk of donor reneging too.[17] Due to certain logistic issues such as doing multiple transplants at the same time, problems such as postponement or cancelation of the transplant at the last moment can happen. These issues hinder the KPD KT and make them difficult to execute.

STATUS AND OUTCOMES IN INDIA

In India, mostly single-center KPD is practiced. The KPD program at the Institute of Kidney Diseases and Research Center, Dr. HL Trivedi Institute of Transplantation Sciences, Ahmedabad, India, has done an exemplary work by performing more than 300 KPD transplants in India.[18]

In a study by Kute et al.,[19] the impact of a single-center KPD transplant was evaluated to increase the donor pool in India. For 300 KPD transplants, two-way kidney exchange (KE) was done in 124 patients (n = 248), three-way in 14 (n = 42), four-way in 1 (n = 4), and six-way in 1 (n = 6) patients. The graft versus patient survival data at 1, 3, 5, and 10 years was 1 year: 97.6 versus 88.9%, 3-year: 94.2 versus 81.8%, 5-year: 94.2 versus 74.7%, and 10-year: 90.7 versus 68.1%.

Kute et al.[20] reported the longest kidney exchange series in India. The report included involving 10 DRPs. The results showed 100% recipient, graft, and donor survival. Donor-specific antibodies were negative in two highly sensitized recipients during the follow-up of 3 months.

A study conducted across two different centers in India showed patient survival rates at 94% and death-censored graft survival rates at 88% in patients with ABOiKT (n = 50). The rate of acute antibody-mediated rejection (AAMR) was 8%, biopsy-proven acute rejection was 22%, and infection rate was 22%.

Apex Swap Transplant Registry (ASTRA) was established in 2011 with an objective to aid patients to identify swap pairs. As on January 12, 2019, 365 registrations and 65+ transplants (two domino: five pairs and six pairs) have been performed. The process starts with identification of pairs with letters from two primary nephrologists followed by registration within ASTRA and a full evaluation for both transplant donor and recipient.[21]

In an analysis by Jha et al.,[22] 742 transplants were performed, of which 26 (3.5%) were KPD. Patients with KPD had a significantly higher number of HLA mismatches. The study showed no significant difference in patient survival and death-censored graft survival.

Pahwa et al.[23] reported results of 44 KPDs. The graft survival rate was found to be 100% at a median follow-up of 33 months.

LEGAL ISSUES IN KIDNEY PAIRED DONATION

The Transplant Human Organ and Tissue Act (THOTA) has defined the term "near relative" as daughter, son, spouse, mother, father, sister, brother, grandmother, grandfather, grandson, or granddaughter. Amendment in THOTA in 2014 permitted the authorization committee to permit KPD transplantation.[24] As of now, only first-degree near-relatives are allowed to donate kidney after due approval from the authorization committee of the hospital or district or state. The potential KPD recipient must be medically fit and eligible to receive a KT. The recipient should have a medically suitable willing living donor who is otherwise unable to donate to his intended recipient

TABLE 1: Key elements of success of kidney paired donation (KPD) program.

- KPD is a legal, cost-effective, rapidly expanding modality with good long-term outcome with a potential to increase LDKT by 25% in India[27]
- The quality and quantity of KPD matching will be superior in a national program versus single-center programs due to the availability of a large donor pool. Differences between single-center and multicenter KPD are given in **Table 2**
- Transplant surgery should be performed at the same place where evaluation and admission of the patient are done. It should be the center where the patient is willing to do follow-up after surgery. Simultaneous transplant surgery is recommended rather than sequential surgery
- Better immunological match rather than age difference between KPD donors should be the key issue in allocation
- Three-way exchange has optimum quality and quantity of matching[28]
- Computerized algorithms are encouraged over manual allocation. However, the allocation algorithm should be made simple to reduce the waiting time when the donor pool is small, e.g., in single-center programs and the absence of computer allocation system, nonanonymous manual allocation can be considered
- Standard written informed consent is must for each DRP. DRP should be informed about the expected waiting time prior to transplantation, with every attempt to reduce the waiting time, especially in cases for hard-to-match pairs
- Transplant team members, stakeholders, and policymakers should work together to expand KPD
- Potential KPD transplant centers should study the key elements of success of other successful KPD programs in India
- Formation of KPD registry is one of the principal strategies to improve the quality and quantity of KPD matching
- DRP needs to be cognizant of transcultural issues, language, and legal barrier in national program when patients and their donors may belong to different regions or states of India
- KPD rules must be framed and updated by appropriate regulatory authority
- Provision of legal clearance by a single authority is required
- All KPD activities should be directed and supervised by National Organ and Tissue Transplant Organization (NOTTO)
- NOTTO website should provide information about KPD, ABOiKT, and deceased donor kidney transplantation so that patients can make independent decisions
- All data must be entered in the National Organ and Tissue Transplant Registry as mandated under THOTA, India
- Appropriate government notification or executive orders related to KPD must be issued

(ABOiKT: ABO-incompatible kidney transplantation; DRP: donor–recipient pair; KPD: kidney paired donation; LDKT: living-donor kidney transplant; THOTA: Transplant Human Organ and Tissue Act)

because of ABO or HLA incompatibility. An informed consent is must from DRP pair and they must adhere to the regulations of the transplant program.

RECOMMENDATIONS AND SUGGESTIONS

The Indian Society of Organ Transplantation (ISOT) Clinical Practice Guideline document provides information and assists in decision-making **(Table 1)**.[25,26] The available Indian studies reported various topics such as advantages of KPD, roles and responsibilities of transplant coordinator, consent process and applicable regulatory documentation, patient evaluation in KPD, legal clearance, KPD allocation, place and timing of transplantation, and optimal number of exchanges in KPD.

Donor–recipient pairs do not choose their match. They are free to decline a match or withdraw from the KPD program at any time, for any reason.

Donor–recipient pairs are allowed to meet each other after completing all medical fitness and legal documents and before final allocation.

TABLE 2: Advantages and disadvantages of single-center versus multicenter kidney paired donation (KPD) programs.[29]

Kidney paired donation	*Single-center*	*Multicenter*
Donor pool	Less	More
Surgical team requirement	More	Less
Donor transport	Not required	Required
Shipping of kidneys	Not required	Required
Cold ischemia time	Less	More
Surgical team skills	Same	Different
Hospital atmosphere	Familiar	Unfamiliar
Follow-up	Same center	Difficult
Administrative cost	Less	More

Other steps for increasing donor pool include:

- Increased awareness of KPD[30,31]
- Multicenter, state, and national KPD programs[32-34]
- Use of compatible pairs[35-38]
- KPD with ABOiKT[39]
- Use of A2 donor to O patient
- Longer chains[40]
- KPD with HLA desensitization
- Expanding the number of acceptable mismatches
- Living and DD list exchange[41] as approved in Gujarat State Organ and Tissue Transplant Organization
- Nonsimultaneous donations in carefully selected DRP[42]
- International KPD with appropriate legal permission.[43,44]

REFERENCES

1. Kute VB, Suresh GK, Patel HV, Shah PR, Modi PR, Shah VR, et al. Expanding the donor pool for kidney transplantation in India. Indian J Transplant. 2017;3:111-6.

2. Ferrari P, Weimar W, Johnson RJ, Lim WH, Tinckam KJ. Kidney paired donation: principles, protocols and programs. Nephrol Dial Transplant. 2015;8:1276-85.
3. Kute VB, Prasad N, Shah PR, Modi PR. Kidney exchange transplantation current status, an update and future perspectives. World J Transplant. 2018;3:52-60.
4. Kute VB, Patel HV, Shah PR, Modi PR, Shah VR, Rizvi SJ, et al. Past, present and future of kidney paired donation transplantation in India. World J Transplant. 2017;7:134-43.
5. Kute VB, Vanikar AV, Shah PR, Gumber MR, Patel HV, Engineer DP, et al. Increasing access to kidney transplantation in countries with limited resources: the Indian experience with kidney paired donation. Nephrology (Carlton). 2014;19: 599-604.
6. Kher V, Jha PK. Paired kidney exchange transplantation—pushing the boundaries. Transpl Int. 2020;33(9):975-84.
7. Kute VB, Gumber MR, Shah PR, Patel HV, Vanikar AV, Modi PR, et al. Successful three-way kidney paired donation transplantation: the first Indian report. Indian J Nephrol. 2014;24:45-7.
8. Kute VB, Patel HV, Shah PR, Modi PR, Shah VR, Kasat GS, et al. Four-way kidney exchange transplant with desensitization increases access to living-donor kidney transplant: first report from India. Exp Clin Transplant. 2018;16(5):528-32.
9. Kute VB, Meshram HS, Patel HV, Engineer D, Banerjee S, Chauhan S, et al. First single-center five-way kidney exchange cycle in India. Indian J Transplant. 2021;15:338-42.
10. Kute VB, Patel HV, Varyani UT, Shah PR, Modi PR, Shah VR, et al. Six end-stage renal disease patients benefited from first non-simultaneous single center 6-way kidney exchange transplantation in India. World J Nephrol. 2016;5:531-7.
11. Kute VB, Vanikar AV, Patel HV, Shah PR, Gumber MR, Engineer DP, et al. Combining kidney paired donation with desensitization increases renal transplantation rate in highly sensitized patients. Indian J Transplant. 2013;7:109-11.
12. Kute VB, Patel HV, Shah PR, Modi PR, Shah VR, Rizvi SJ, et al. Increasing access to kidney transplantation for sensitized recipient through three-way kidney paired donation with desensitization: the first Indian report. World J Clin Cases. 2016;10:351-5.
13. Travasso C. Five patients benefit from India's first "domino" kidney swap. BMJ. 2013;347:f4260.
14. Pronk MC, Burnapp L, Reinders MEJ, Massey EK. Relinquishing anonymity in living donor kidney transplantation: lessons learned from the UK policy for anonymous donors. Transpl Int. 2022;35:10091.
15. Rees MA, Kopke JE, Pelletier RP, Segev DL, Rutter ME, Fabrega AJ, et al. A nonsimultaneous, extended, altruistic-donor chain. N Engl J Med. 2009;360(11):1096-101.
16. Billa V, Verma U, Usulumarty D, Rangaraj N, Sanap G, Kothari J, et al. A novel method to increase the kidney donor pool: a fusion model linking the deceased donor waitlist to a paired kidney exchange program. Indian J Transplant. 2018;3:187-92.
17. Cowan N, Gritsch HA, Nassiri N, Sinacore J, Veale J. Broken chains and reneging: a review of 1748 kidney paired donation transplants. Am J Transplant. 2017;17(9):2451-7.
18. Kute VB, Shah PS, Vanikar AV, Gumber MR, Patel HV, Engineer DP, et al. Increasing access to renal transplantation in India through our single-center kidney paired donation program: a model for the developing world to prevent commercial transplantation. Transpl Int. 2014;27:1015-21.
19. Kute VB, Patel HV, Shah PR, Modi PR, Shah VR, Rizvi SJ, et al. Impact of single centre kidney paired donation transplantation to increase donor pool in India: a cohort study. Transpl Int. 2017;7:679-88.
20. Kute VB, Patel HV, Modi PR, Rizvi SJ, Engineer DP, Banerjee S, et al. Paired kidney exchange in India: future potential and challenges based on the experience at a single center. Transplantation. 2021;105(5):929-32.
21. Apex Swap Transplant Registry. [online] Available from http://www.apexkidneyfoundation.org/astra/. [Last accessed May, 2022].
22. Jha PK, Sethi S, Bansal SB, Jain M, Sharma R, Phanish MK, et al. Paired kidney exchange transplantation: maximizing the donor pool. Indian J Nephrol. 2015;25:349-54.
23. Pahwa M, Saifee Y, Tyagi V, Chadha S, Jauhari H. Paired exchange kidney donation in India: a five-year single-center experience. Int Urol Nephrol. 2012;44(4):1101-5.
24. Sahay M. Transplantation of human organs and tissues act—"Simplified". Indian J Transplant. 2018;12:84-9.
25. Kute VB, Agarwal SK, Sahay M, Kumar A, Rathi M, Prasad N, et al. Kidney-paired donation to increase living donor kidney transplantation in India: guidelines of Indian Society of Organ Transplantation—2017. Indian J Nephrol. 2018; 1:1-9.
26. Kute VB, Agarwal SK, Sahay M, Kumar A, Rathi M, Prasad N, et al. Kidney-paired donation to increase living donor kidney transplantation in India: guidelines of Indian Society of Organ Transplantation—2017 (Special Article). Indian J Transplant. 2018;12:67-74.
27. Kute VB, Patel HV, Shah PR, Modi PR, Shah VR, Rizvi SJ, et al. Seventy-seven kidney paired donation transplantations at a single transplant centre in India led to an increase in living donor kidney transplantations in 2015. Clin Kidney J. 2017;10:709-14.
28. Kute VB, Patel HV, Mishra VV, Agarwal SK. Optimum chain length in kidney exchange program and the way ahead. Indian J Nephrol. 2021;31:95-6.
29. Krishnan N, Kute VB. Paired kidney exchange. In: Abraham G, Rohit A (Eds). Handbook of Renal Transplantation in Developing Countries. India: Oxford University Press; 2020.
30. Kute VB, Vanikar AV, Shah PR, Gumber MR, Patel HV, Engineer DP, et al. Ten kidney paired donation transplantation on World Kidney Day 2013: raising awareness and time to take action to increase donor pool. Ren Fail. 2013;35: 1269-72.
31. Kute VB, Gumber MR, Dhananjay KL, Vanikar AV, Yadav DK, Patel MP, et al. Living donor exchange programs in renal transplantation: a paradigm ready for broad implementation. Int Urol Nephrol. 2013;45:597-9.
32. Kute VB, Patel HV, Shah PR, Vanikar AV, Trivedi HL. National kidney paired donation program in India: challenges, solution, future direction. Nephrology (Carlton). 2015;20(6): 442.
33. Kute VB, Gumber MR, Vanikar AV, Shah PR, Patel HV, Engineer DP, et al. Comparison of kidney paired donation transplantations with living related donor kidney transplantation: implications for national kidney paired donation program. Ren Fail. 2013;35:504-8.

34. Kute VB, Vanikar AV, Shah PR, Gumber MR, Patel HV, Modi PR, et al. Facilitators to national kidney paired donation program. Transpl Int. 2013;26:e38-9.
35. Kute VB, Vanikar AV, Gumber MR, Shah PR, Patel HV, Engineer DP, et al. Successful three-way kidney paired donation with compatible pairs to increase donor pool. Ren Fail. 2014;36:447-50.
36. Varyani UT, Kute VB, Patel HV, Shah PR, Vanikar AV, Modi PR, et al. Participation of compatible donor to improve HLA matching can increase kidney transplant rate of O blood group patients. Clin Queries Nephrol. 2015;4:38.
37. Bingaman A, Kapturczak M, Murphey C, Wright F. Kidney paired donation: a single center approach to increase living donor transplantation. Clin Transpl. 2010;345-52.
38. Bingaman A, Kapturczak M, Ashlagi I, Murphey C. 400 kidney paired donor transplants at a single center; the Methodist San Antonio experience. Am J Transplant. 2017; 17(Suppl. 3).
39. Montgomery RA. Renal transplantation across HLA and ABO antibody barriers: integrating paired donation into desensitization protocols. Am J Transplant. 2010;10(3):449-57.
40. Anderson R, Ashlagi I, Gamarnik D, Roth AE. Finding long chains in kidney exchange using the traveling salesman problem. Proc Natl Acad Sci U S A. 2015;112(3):663-8.
41. Kute VB, Patel HV, Shah PR, Modi PR, Shah VR, Trivedi HL. A potential solution to make best use of living donor-deceased donor list exchange. Am J Transplant. 2016;16(12): 3580.
42. Kute VB, Patel HV, Modi PR, Rizvi SJ, Shah PR, Engineer DP, et al. Non-simultaneous kidney exchange cycles in resource-restricted countries without non-directed donation—a prospective single-center cohort study. Transpl Int. 2021; 34(4):669-80.
43. Kute VB, Patel HV, Shah PR, Modi PR, Shah VR, Rizvi SJ, et al. International kidney paired donation transplantations to increase kidney transplant of O group and highly sensitized patient: first report from India. World J Transplant. 2017;7:64-9.
44. Kute V, Jindal RM, Prasad N. Kidney paired donation program versus global kidney exchange in India. Am J Transplant. 2017;17(10):2740-1.

CHAPTER

22

Deceased Donation

22.1 Deceased Donor Care

Indira Menon, Sunil Shroff, Chacko Korula Jacob

INTRODUCTION

The year 2021 is the golden jubilee year of the first successful live donor kidney transplant in India done at Christian Medical College, Vellore, in January 1971.

Despite being high on the list of live donors, India lags far behind most countries in organ donation in brain-dead situations—a mere 0.52 per million population in comparison with Spain and Croatia at 49.61 and 34.63 per million population.[1] It is estimated that more than 0.5 million persons die in India each year of conditions where organ transplants could have helped.

The onus is on the medical community to raise awareness about organ donation and dispel myths surrounding this act of life-giving generosity. The intensive care doctors are the custodians of the organs after death, be it brain or circulatory, and have to ensure their optimal preservation for maximum benefit.

The process of care of the donor for the purpose of organ transplantation requires understanding of:

- History and evolution of organ transplantation in India
- Identification and certification of the brain-dead donor
- Counseling of family members
- Pathophysiology of brain death
- Hemodynamic and organ-specific monitoring of the donor
- Understanding the role of the transplant coordinator.

BRIEF HISTORY AND EVOLUTION OF ORGAN TRANSPLANTATION IN INDIA

The first attempts at kidney transplantation in India were from deceased donors in 1965 and 1966 by Dr PK Sen and his team at the King Edward Memorial (KEM) Hospital, Mumbai. Their team transplanted two patients with kidneys from such donors and the recipients succumbed on day 3 and 11 with a functioning graft. Later, Professor Udupa and his team at the Banaras Hindu University also attempted deceased transplantation but the recipient died within a few days.

The early challenges in deceased donation included both medical and societal issues. The team faced technical difficulties involving surgical grafting and procurement of organs from the general population. Dr Karanjavala, the urologist and surgeon-in-charge of the kidney transplant program at KEM Hospital, Mumbai, said in an article that "the toughest challenge was handling the very hostile and negative reaction that erupted from members of the medical profession and general public to the efforts at using cadaver donor organs some calling the surgery 'neo-cannibalism'." Dr Karanjavala further says this reaction led to a great setback to the cadaver program in not only Mumbai but also perhaps the rest of the country. This negativity made the deceased donation program in India a nonstarter.

It was the success of the live kidney transplantation program in India that made it a reality. The start to the program was given in 1971 by Dr Mohan Rao and Dr KV Johny from the Christian Medical College, Vellore. After this success, gradually other centers started their live kidney transplant program. The deceased donor organ transplant in India, however, became feasible only in the mid-1990s following the passage of the Transplantation of Human Organ and Tissues Act (THOTA).

First introduced in parliament in 1992, the Bill No. LIX-F 1992 underwent several modifications to finally become the Transplantation of Human Organs Bill 1994. In 2011, the government of India introduced the Transplantation of Human Organs (Amendment) Act, and its rules were passed on March 27, 2014. This in its present form is what governs organ retrieval, storage, distribution, and other aspects of organ transplantation in most states and union territories in India. The state of Tamil Nadu spearheaded both the live and the deceased donor organ transplantation program in the country. The tireless effort of nongovernment organizations and the support of the state bureaucracy helped establish procedures and protocols to implement the program and to facilitate organ sharing between hospitals.[2]

Since 2011, the number of organs available from deceased donors in India has increased and the growth of the deceased donor program in India is reflected in **Figure 1**.

The above matters are mentioned in some detail to put in perspective the topic under discussion, which is care of the deceased donor. This becomes particularly important as multiorgan donor donations and movement of organs across state borders become increasingly common and this is likely to increase even further with proactive policies, better awareness among both the public and healthcare professionals, and acceptance of the concept of brain death and organ donation.

Declaration of brain death is part of the 1994 THOTA, but it is being used only for organ donation. If the relatives refuse organ donation, there is no clarity on whether the brain-dead patient can be disconnected from life support or not. There is a need for a uniform declaration of death, and this change has to take place in the "Registration of Birth and Death Act" of 1969 by including brain death along with circulatory death.

IDENTIFYING POTENTIAL DONORS AND CERTIFYING BRAIN DEATH

All patients with severe brain injury or irreversible coma should be considered possible organ donors as early

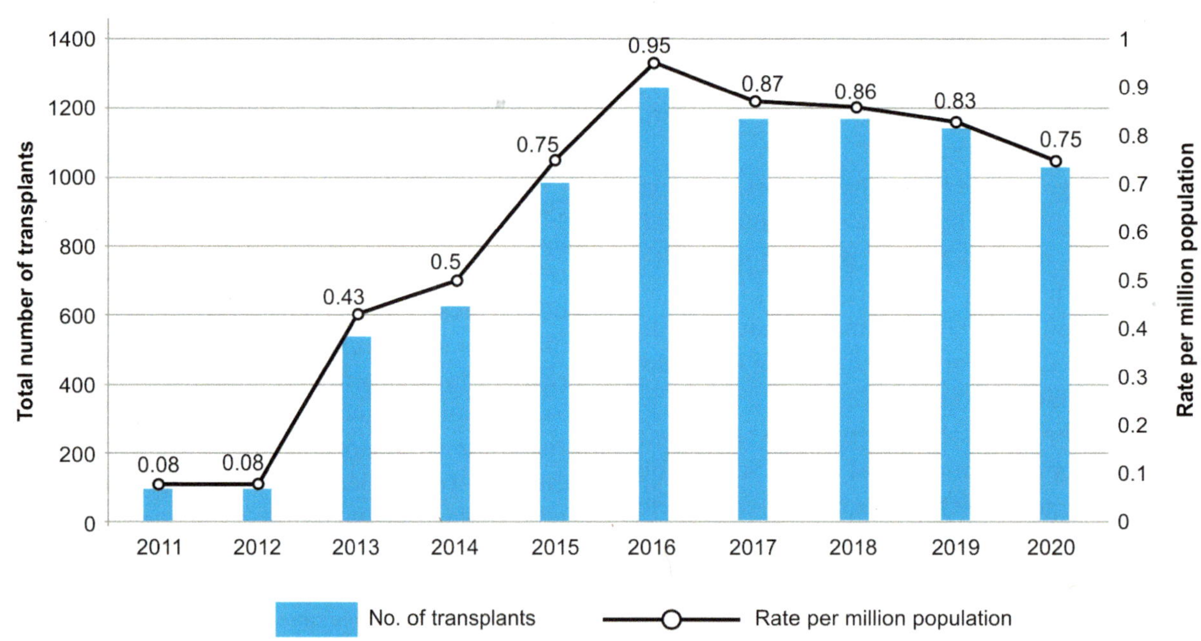

Year	Total no. of kidneys transplanted from deceased donors	Rate per million population
2011	96	0.08
2012	96	0.08
2013	542	0.43
2014	628	0.5
2015	984	0.75
2016	1,261	0.95
2017	1,169	0.87
2018	1,164	0.86
2019	1,138	0.83
2020	1,032	0.75

Fig. 1: Total kidney transplants from deceased donors (India 2011–2020).
Source: Global database on donation and transplantation (GODT) (http://www.transplant-observatory.org/)

identification of brainstem death and optimization of donor care ensure functional preservation of the retrieved organs.

Prior to testing for brainstem activity, it is mandatory that certain prerequisites are met **(Table 1)**:

- *There is a cause for the catastrophic brain injury:* Major trauma, intracranial bleed with midline shift, and subarachnoid hemorrhage or primary brain tumor.
- *The irreversibility of the condition is confirmed:*
  - Exclude medical conditions such as metabolic encephalopathy, acid–base, and electrolyte imbalances.
  - *Exclude medications causing unresponsiveness:* Sedatives, narcotics, and muscle relaxants.
    - Check drug levels or wait for the half-lives to pass.
  - *Exclude hypothermia:* The patient's body temperature should be ideally above 35°C.
- *Neuroimaging:* Computed tomography (CT)/magnetic resonance imaging (MRI)/cerebral angiography helps in diagnosis and the prognosis.

Once the above conditions have been fulfilled, clinical tests for brain death should be carried out by competent authorities.[2,3]

TABLE 1: Factors predisposing to brain death.

Prerequisite	*Details*
Proximate cause for unresponsive state that is incompatible with survival	Major trauma, intracranial bleed with midline shift, or brain tumor
Neurological imaging in order to confirm diagnosis	CT brain, MRI, and angiography
Exclusion of associated medical conditions that could account for unresponsiveness	Exclusions of severe acid–base, metabolic or electrolyte abnormalities
Exclusion of drugs causing unresponsiveness	Sedatives, narcotics, and muscle relaxants. In drug overdose, allow time for five half-lives/measure drug levels
Normal temperature	Core temperature >32°/90°

(CT: computed tomography; MRI: magnetic resonance imaging)

Testing Brainstem Activity

See **Table 2**.

Apnea Test

This definitive test is performed in the presence of *four empaneled doctors including a neurologist/neurosurgeon.*

The principle of the apnea test is to raise the partial pressure of carbon dioxide (pCO_2) levels to allow maximum stimulation of the respiratory center. To perform this test, the patient must be normothermic and hemodynamically stable [systolic blood pressure (BP) >90 mm Hg, peripheral oxygen saturation (SpO_2) >85% for >30 seconds] with or without inotropic support. Apnea testing should be aborted if these criteria are not met:

- An arterial blood gas (ABG) is taken while the patient is on mechanical ventilation with 100% O_2.
- The ventilator is then disconnected and O_2 is given at 6 L/min via a sterile tracheal catheter placed at the level of the carina.
- The authorized doctors watch for respiratory movements while the pCO_2 rises to 20 mm Hg above the initial level

TABLE 2: Assessment of brain stem death.

Brainstem reflexes	*Brainstem death testing illustrations*	*Sensory and motor cranial nerve (respectively)*	*Region tested*
Absence of pupillary response to light	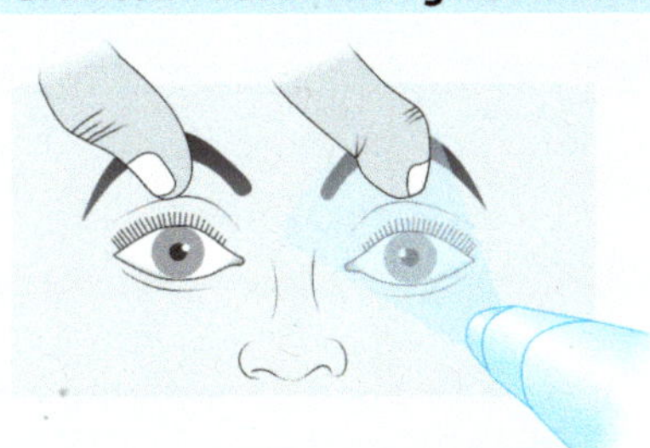	II, (III)	Upper brainstem
Absence of corneal reflexes	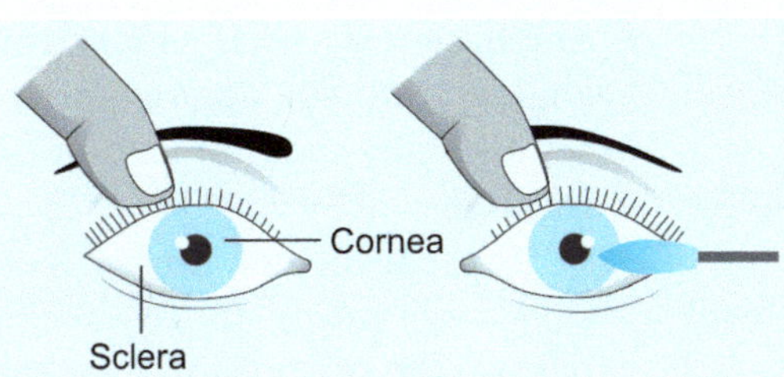	V, (VII)	Mid-upper brainstem

Contd...

Contd...

Brainstem reflexes	Brainstem death testing illustrations	Sensory and motor cranial nerve (respectively)	Region tested
Absence of cranial nerve response to pain	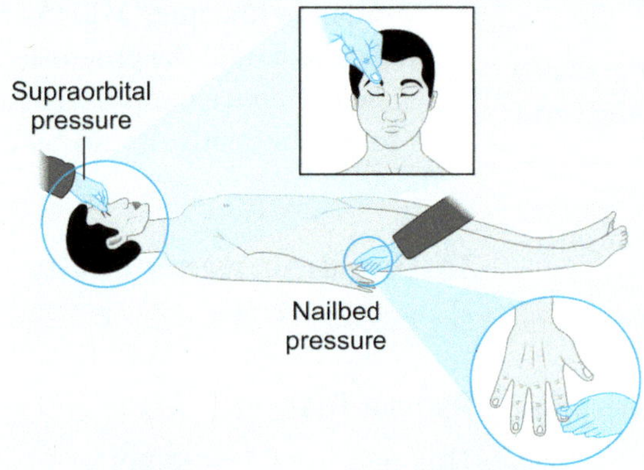	V, (VII)	Brainstem/ cerebral hemispheres (can be confused with spinal reflexes)
Absence of vestibulo-ocular reflex	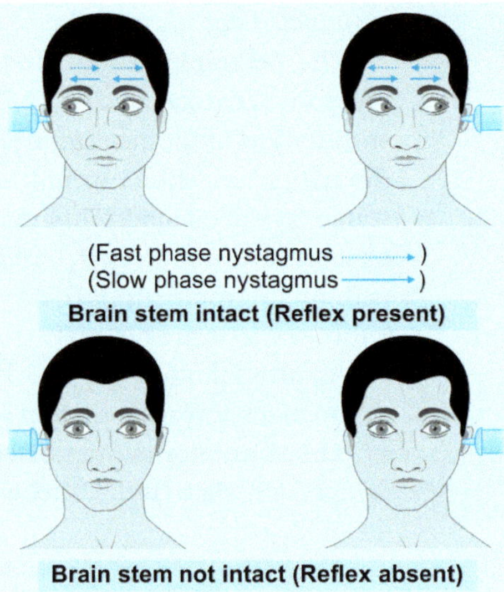	VIII, (III, VI)	Mid-brainstem
Absence of gag and cough reflexes	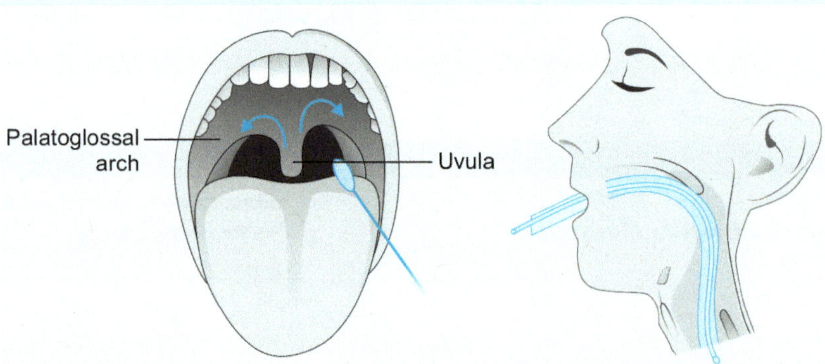	X, (IX)	Lower brainstem

Source: Brain death testing from manual for transplant coordinators—MOHAN Foundation.

or to 60 mm Hg. Partial pressure of carbon dioxide in 2 rises arterial blood ($PaCO_2$) rises by 3 mm Hg/min.[4]

- Repeating ABG after 8–10 minutes should reflect the required change.[5,6]
- Absence of respiratory effort indicates a positive apnea test and is the first certification of brain death.
- The test is repeated after 6 hours and if again positive, *the final certification of brain death is done.*

Ancillary Tests

Ancillary tests such as electroencephalography, cerebral angiography, CT angiography, transcranial Doppler, and scintigraphy can be carried out if the apnea test is not feasible.

These tests look for isoelectric electroencephalograms (EEG) recording in 18–20 channels over a 30-minute period, absence of intracerebral filling at the level of the carotid bifurcation or vertebral arteries,[6] or presence of diastolic reverberation flow with the absent forward flow. These ancillary tests cannot be used as a replacement of apnea test to confirm brain death. However, these tests do help in making the final diagnosis and sometimes can help families accept the prognosis better and hence can help with the consent process.

COUNSELING OF FAMILY MEMBERS

The most vital aspect of organ donation, counseling the family members, involves:

1. Planning
2. Explaining to the family and confirming that they have understood and accepted that their patient is dead.
3. Discussing donation.

The senior treating doctor along with the senior nurse should do the counseling. It is important to give the family adequate time to come to terms with their loss. Identify the key persons in the family and speak to them. Use positive language and explain the benefits and process of organ donation, along with a tentative timeline.[7,8]

All queries should be answered truthfully, taking the help of the regional government agencies. No financial incentives can be offered. Once the organ retrieval is completed the body should be handled with respect and dignity and the relatives informed about which organs have been harvested, without divulging information about the recipients. The pastoral care services or the transplant coordinator should provide extended support to the grieving family. While the organ transplant team may be informed about a potential donor, no member of this team should contact or interact with the donor family until consent for donation has been obtained.

PATHOPHYSIOLOGY OF BRAINSTEM DEATH

The devastating brain injury leading to brain death is accompanied by destruction of the vagal nuclei in the brainstem causing vasoplegia. This results in unchecked sympathetic stimulation (sympathetic storm) which affects various organs of the body **(Fig. 2)**.[2,9]

The cardiovascular system responds with tachycardia and rise in arterial BP. The increase in capillary bed pressure and pulmonary vasoconstriction causes endothelial damage in the lungs, with extravasation of fluid into the interstitium and release of inflammatory mediators.

Hemodynamic instability, cardiac arrhythmias, pulmonary edema, and central diabetes insipidus (CDI) could occur due to this.

Central diabetes insipidus endocrinopathy is an early sign of brain death and is associated with polyuria >3 L/day, serum sodium levels >145, and serum osmolarity > 305 mOsm.

Thyroid dysfunction manifests with increased thyroid-stimulating hormone (TSH) and low T3 but normal T4 and reverse T3 levels. It is due to peripheral inactivation of the thyroid hormone.

Hyperglycemia occurs due to relative insulin resistance and uncontrolled gluconeogenesis.

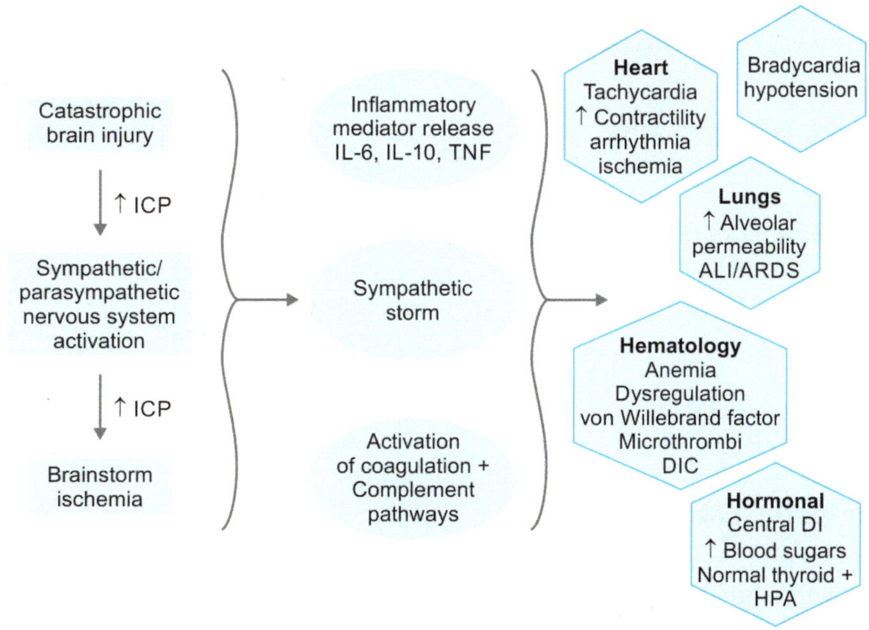

Fig. 2: Pathophysiology of brainstem death. (ALI: acute lung injury; ARDS: acute respiratory distress syndrome; DIC: disseminated intravascular coagulation; DI: diabetes insipidus; HPA: hypothalamic–pituitary–adrenal; ICP: increased intracranial pressure; IL: interleukin; TNF: tumor necrosis factor)

SPECIFIC MANAGEMENT OF THE ORGAN DONOR

It is important to stabilize the donor optimally before organ retrieval. Once the consent for organ donation is given, Kuzendorf et al.[5] noted that a longer duration of brain death (>470 minutes) improved both the kidney and the heart graft functionality and survival.[10]

Lines needed to be placed:

- Invasive arterial BP monitoring line
- Good peripheral lines/central venous catheter
- Pulmonary artery (PA) catheter is not commonly needed.

Blood samples to be sent:

- Blood grouping
- Liver function tests
- Renal function tests
- Hepatitis B/hepatitis C
- Human immunodeficiency virus (HIV)
- Cytomegalovirus (CMV) antibodies immunoglobulin G (IgG) and immunoglobulin M (IgM)
- Hepatitis B core antibody (Anti-HBc) and hepatitis B surface antibody (Anti-HBs) are extremely important.
- Complete blood count
- Serum amylase and lipase
- Store multiple vials of blood for crossmatch
- Blood for human leukocyte antigen (HLA) (some hospitals in India have started using it for organ matching).

Other tests:

- Ultrasound abdomen
    - Echocardiography—done serially to check recovery of neurologically stunned myocardium
- CT lungs (without contrast) and bronchoscopy may be needed.

Critical information the retrieval team requires:

- Past medical history—surgeries/medications/substance usage
- Blood group and body mass index (BMI)
- Virology status—HIV and hepatitis B/hepatitis C
- Hourly urine output
- BP
- Dose of inotropes
- Serum lactate and mixed venous O_2 saturation
- Any adverse hemodynamic events.

HEMODYNAMIC MANAGEMENT

Hemodynamic management is the key challenge. Profound vasodilatation and CDI lead to fluid and inotropic requirements. Euvolemia should be the goal if both kidney and lung are to be retrieved; the kidney requiring more fluid and the lung less.[4] To achieve this, various methods of hemodynamic monitoring may be considered—inferior vena cava (IVC) collapsibility, passive leg raising, and central venous pressures (still used by some centers). Insertion of PA catheters is not routinely recommended. Isotonic saline or Ringer's lactate may be given as resuscitative fluid.

Both noradrenaline and vasopressin have been associated with less graft loss and vasopressin has the dual advantage of controlling CDI if present.[5] Randomized controlled trials (RCTs) are however not available.[8] Dopamine is out of favor due to arrhythmias.

The monitoring targets are mean arterial pressure (MAP) of 65–70 mm Hg and sodium levels of 135–145 mmol/L.

Higher sodium levels are especially detrimental to liver retrieval and transplant.[5]

Severe tachycardia, which could lead to myocardial dysfunction and compromise cardiac retrieval, could be treated with esmolol infusion.[7]

Respiratory management aims to optimize gas exchange for all the organs while minimizing ventilator lung injury.[11,12] The lung protective strategy of acute respiratory distress syndrome (ARDS) management is used. Tidal volumes of 6–8 mL/kg, plateau pressures <30 mm Hg, and recruitment of atelectatic lung are to be considered. The respiratory targets are pH 7.35–7.45, minimum fraction of inspired oxygen (FiO_2) to achieve partial pressure of oxygen (PaO_2) >100, SpO_2 > 95%, and $PaCO_2$ 35–40 mm Hg. All the strategies to prevent ventilator-associated pneumonia (VAP) must be strictly adhered to.

Endocrinopathy management with universal thyroid and steroid replacement though a norm in the past is not advised as thyroid function is often normal and few RCT's have not justified their use.[13] In the case of steroids, RCTs have not replicated the results of observational studies showing better graft and recipient survival and organ procurement rates.[14] Steroids could also induce hyperglycemia, which reduces graft survival and aggravate dehydration by inducing osmotic diuresis. Blood sugars should be maintained between 140 and 180 mg/dL. In case of hemodynamic instability, one could use a lower dose of hydrocortisone infusion [50 mg intravenous (IV) bolus followed by 10 mg/hr]. Also consider thyroid hormone replacement.[15]

Central diabetes insipidus occurs in 46–86% of patients who are brain dead. It occurs early in the condition.

Evidence based drug administration is provided in **Table 3**.

DIAGNOSTIC CRITERIA FOR CENTRAL DIABETES INSIPIDUS

Central diabetes insipidus is treated with intravenous desmopressin 1–4 μg which can be repeated depending on urine volume and serum sodium levels.

TABLE 3: Evidence-based drug administration.

Hormone/drug	Dose	Remark	Evidence
Thyroid hormone Thyroxine (T4)	20 µg IV bolus 10 µg/h IV maintenance	• Precursor of T3 • Low intrinsic biological activity/slow onset Increased conversion into inactive rT3	• No RCT evidence • Observational studies—increased organ procurement
Triiodothyronine (T3)	4 µg IV bolus 3 µg/h IV maintenance	• Active hormone • Quick onset • Trigger arrhythmias	• RCTs—no benefit • Observational studies—increased organ procurement
Corticosteroid Methylprednisolone	1,000 mg IV od OR 15 mg/kg IV od OR 250 mg IV bolus 100 mg/h IV maintenance	• Monitor blood glucose levels • Take blood sample for tissue typing prior to steroid administration	• RCTs—equivocal results • Observational studies—better donor hemodynamics, increased organ procurement/better graft and recipient survival
Hydrocortisone	50 mg IV bolus 10 mg/h IV maintenance OR 300 mg/day IV	• Monitor blood glucose levels • Tissue typing sample to be taken before administration	• No RCT evidence • Observational studies—organ procurement rate same but lower vasopressor dose
Insulin	Continuous IV infusion Adjust dose to preset target blood glucose	• Frequently measure blood glucose • Avoid severe hyperglycemia and large blood glucose fluctuations	• No RCT evidence • Supported by observational studies
Desmopressin	1–4 µg IV initial	Repeat dose as per urine volume/serum Na^+	–

(IV: intravenous; RCT: randomized controlled trial; rT3: reverse T3)

TABLE 4: Diagnostic criteria for central diabetes insipidus.

Clinical feature	Diagnostic finding
Increased urine volume	Urine output >3–4 L/day or >2.5–3.0 mL/kg/h
Hypernatremia	Serum sodium concentration >145 mmol/L
Normal or increased serum osmolality	Serum osmolality >305 mmol/kg
Inappropriately dilute urine	Urine osmolality <200 mmol/kg or specific gravity <1.005

Nutritional support of the donor should continue and enteral is the preferred route.[16]

Deranged *temperature control* secondary to hypothalamic damage, vasoplegia, and drop in metabolism can lead to hypothermia causing coagulopathy and cardiac arrhythmias. Hemodynamic instability may warrant a higher body temperature but otherwise >35°C is the target. Thermal blankets, warm intravenous fluids, and heaters have been used **(Table 4)**.

Mild hypothermia has been found beneficial in renal transplants.

The spectrum of *hematological issues* in the brain-dead potential donor ranges from coagulopathy to disseminated intravascular coagulation (DIC).[17-19] About 15–25% of patients with traumatic brain injury develop DIC. RCTs have shown that restrictive transfusion is noninferior to liberal policies.

Appropriate component transfusions could be considered in donors with hemoglobin (Hb) <7 g% and in case of hemodynamic instability, tissue hypoxia, platelets <50,000, and international normalized ratio (INR) >1.5.[4,20]

Thromboprophylaxis should be continued if feasible.

Pretransplant infection screening of the donor is essential though transmission occurs in <1% of recipients.[15]

Sepsis per se is not a contraindication to organ donation provided appropriate antibiotics have been given for 48 hours at least.[5] Organs from patients with bacterial meningitis, hepatitis C, and HIV can be harvested with good results provided the recipient is treated preemptively or if based on viral load.[20-22] HIV-positive organs are given to HIV-positive recipients only.[22]

A quick reference app for organ donor optimization is available on both Google and iOS[23] and is a useful resource to remember the essential steps.

Role of the transplant coordinator: The coordinators are the unsung heroes of the whole deceased donor transplant program. Each transplant center has to have one or more trained transplant coordinators as per the 2011 amended law. Their role is vital for a viable deceased program as they interact and support the family members till the body, following organ retrieval, is transported home. They interact with the police in medicolegal cases and expedite the mandatory autopsy required. They are the glue that holds the program together.

CONCLUSION

Donor care has been standardized considerably; however, some variance in management is not unusual.[24-27] More RCTs in this field are recommended. Protection and optimal care of the donor organs are crucial to the success of transplant surgery. It is the ultimate respect to the donor and family and is the essence of critical care medicine.

REFERENCES

1. IRODaT—International Registry on Organ Donation and Transplantation. (2020). [online] Available from www.irodat.org. [Last accessed June, 2022].
2. Shroff S, Rao S, Kurian G, Suresh S. Organ donation and transplantation—the Chennai experience in India. Transplant Proc. 2007;39(3):714-8.
3. Kumar L. Brain death and care of the organ donor. J Anaesthesiol Clin Pharmacol. 2016;32(2):146-52.
4. Birtan D, Arslantas MK, Altun GT, Dincer PC, Gecegormez S, Denirel A, et al. Effect of vasoactive therapy used for brain-dead donors on graft survival after kidney transplantation. Transplant Proc. 2018;50(5):1289-91.
5. Kunzendorf U, Hohenstein B, Oberbarnscheid M, Muller E, Renders L, Schott GE, et al. Duration of donor brain death and its influence on kidney graft function. Am J Transplant. 2002;2(3):292-4.
6. Miñambres E, Ballesteros MA, Rodrigo E, García-Miguélez A, Llorca J, Ruiz JC, et al. Aggressive lung donor management increases graft procurement without increasing renal graft loss after transplantation. Clin Transplant. 2013;27(1):52-9.
7. Meyfroidt G, Gunst J, Martin-Loeches I, Smith M, Robba C, Taccone FS, et al. Management of the brain-dead donor in the ICU: general and specific therapy to improve transplantable organ quality. Intensive Care Med. 2019;45(3):343-53.
8. Consent/Authorisation Best Practice Development Group. Approaching the Families of Potential Organ Donors. NHS Blood and Transplant; 2015.
9. Zirpe K, Gurav S. Brain death and management of potential organ donor: an Indian perspective. Indian J Crit Care Med. 2019;23(Suppl. 2):S151-6.
10. Audibert G, Charpentier C, Seguin-Devaux C, Charretier PA, Grégoire H, Devaux Y, et al. Improvement of donor myocardial function after treatment of autonomic storm during brain death. Transplantation. 2006;82(8):1031-6.
11. Al-Khafaji A, Elder M, Lebovitz DJ, Murugan R, Souter M, Stuart S, et al. Protocolized fluid therapy in brain-dead donors: the multicenter randomized MOnIToR trial. Intensive Care Med. 2015;41(3):418-26.
12. Kotloff RM, Blosser S, Fulda GJ, Malinoski D, Ahya VN, Angel L, et al. Management of the potential organ donor in the ICU: Society of Critical Care Medicine/American College of Chest Physicians/Association of Organ Procurement Organizations Consensus Statement. Crit Care Med. 2015; 43(6):1291-325.
13. Beitler JR, Malhotra A, Thompson BT. Ventilator-induced lung injury. Clin Chest Med. 2016;37(4):633-46.
14. Macdonald PS, Aneman A, Jones D, Bhonagiri D. A systematic review and meta-analysis of clinical trials of thyroid hormone administration to brain dead potential organ donors. Crit Care Med. 2012;40(5):1635-44.
15. Dupuis S, Amiel JA, Desgroseilliers M, Williamson DR, Thiboutot Z, Serri K, et al. Corticosteroids in the management of brain-dead potential organ donors: a systematic review. Br J Anaesth. 2014;113(3):346-59.
16. Pinsard M, Ragot S, Mertes PM, Bleichner JP, Zitouni S, Cook F, et al. Interest of low-dose hydrocortisone therapy during brain-dead organ donor resuscitation: the CORTICOME study. Crit Care. 2014;18(4):R158.
17. Hébert PC, Carson JL. Transfusion threshold of 7 g per deciliter—the new normal. N Engl J Med. 2014;371(15): 1459-61.
18. Lisman T, Leuvenink HGD, Porte RJ, Ploeg RJ. Activation of hemostasis in brain dead organ donors: an observational study. J Thromb Haemost. 2011;9(10):1959-65.
19. Valdivia M, Chamorro C, Romera MA, Balandín B, Pérez M. Effect of posttraumatic donor's disseminated intravascular coagulation in intrathoracic organ donation and transplantation. Transplant Proc. 2007;39(7):2427-8.
20. Muller E, Barday Z, Mendelson M, Kahn D. HIV-positive to HIV-positive kidney transplantation—results at 3 to 5 years. N Engl J Med. 2015;372(7):613-20.
21. Aguilar C, Husain S, Lortholary O. Recent advances in understanding and managing infectious diseases in solid organ transplant recipients. F1000Res. 2018;7:F1000 Faculty Rev-661.
22. Fischer SA. Is this organ donor safe? Donor-derived infections in solid organ transplantation. Surg Clin North Am. 2019;9(1):117-28.
23. https://www.mohanfoundation.org/mobileapps/donoroptimisation.asp.
24. Pandit RA, Zirpe KG, Gurav SK, Kulkarni AP, Karnath S, Govil D, et al. Management of potential organ donor: Indian society of critical care medicine: position statement. Indian J Crit Care Med. 2017;21(5):303-16.
25. Joseph M. Protocol for diagnosis of brain death and maintenance for organ transplantation. [online] Available from https://www.mohanfoundation.org/organ-donation-transplant-resources/protocol-diagnosis-brain-death.asp. [Last accessed June, 2022].
26. Dictus C, Vienenkoetter B, Esmaeilzadeh M, Unterberg A, Ahmadi R. Critical care management of potential organ donors: our current standard. Clin Transplant. 2009; 23(Suppl. 21):2-9.
27. Youn TS, Greer DM. Brain death and management of a potential organ donor in the intensive care unit. Crit Care Clin. 2014;30(4):813-31.

22.2 Allocation Criteria

Jayasurya R, Sreejith Parameswaran

INTRODUCTION

The demand for kidneys far exceeds the number of available donors. It is estimated that about two lakh people develop end-stage renal disease (ESRD) in India annually.[1] Nationwide data on the number of patients waiting for kidney transplantation is unavailable in India, but data is available from some states. The state of Tamil Nadu had 6,164 patients waiting for kidney transplantation,[2] while Kerala had 1,792,[3] and Telangana had 4,954[4] patients waiting for a kidney. The global observatory data shows that India performed about 8,000 kidney transplantation operations in 2018; 85% of the kidneys were from living donors.[5] Living donor kidney transplantation usually happens between near relatives, and even when the donor is not a near relative, it is still a "directed donation." However, deceased donor organs are a scarce and precious resource. There will be multiple legitimate, deserving recipients for organs from a deceased donor, and it is essential to put in place an efficient, fair, and transparent process to procure organs from deceased donors and allocate them to deserving recipients. Therefore, countries with a deceased donor organ transplantation program need to define rules for allocating available organs.

ETHICAL PRINCIPLES RELEVANT TO ORGAN ALLOCATION

The ethical principles of "justice" and "utility" are central to the organ allocation policy. Any organ allocation system should ensure equality and fairness in the allocation of organs (justice). However, clinical and logistic issues conflict with the fair allotment of organs in many instances. Therefore, besides being "fair," the organ allocation system needs to be efficient to ensure maximum utilization of available organs (utility). Equally important are the issues of transparency and traceability. Information on all organs procured and transplanted should be made available to the general public through a government mechanism to ensure public trust and commitment to the program. It is essential to ensure traceability of the donor in the interest of the safety of the recipients in the context of potential transmission of infections through donated organs.

MODELS OF ORGAN ALLOCATION SYSTEMS

There is considerable variation in organ allocation systems used in different countries. Some countries consider deceased organs as a "national resource," whereas, in others, organ allocation is done at a regional level. The central principle of different organ allocation systems is to ensure equitable distribution of organs while ensuring the best outcomes. Most allocation systems use point-based priority systems, where points are awarded based on different factors.[6,7]

MEDICAL CRITERIA USED BY ORGAN ALLOCATION SYSTEMS

Longevity Matching

Many allocation systems use longevity-matching strategies where the life expectancy of the donor organ is matched with the recipient's life expectancy. Transplanting kidneys from young donors into older recipients may result in many such recipients dying with functioning grafts. Transplanting kidneys from donors who are old to young recipients will result in early graft failure and recipients going back to the waiting list. Longevity matching is achieved in the United Kingdom (UK) by deducting points from pairs with a significant donor–recipient age difference. In the case of older recipients, using kidneys from older donors might increase utility, but there will be additional risks for this age group with a higher risk for graft dysfunction. In the United States (US), the United Network for Organ Sharing (UNOS) introduced a significant change in 2014 for longevity matching based on two scoring systems—Kidney Donor Profile Index (KDPI) and the estimated post-transplant survival (EPTS). The scores are based on 10 donor factors and 4 recipient factors **(Table 1)**.

TABLE 1: Longevity matching in deceased donor kidney allocation in the United States.

KDPI	*EPTS*
Age	Age
Height	Dialysis time
Weight	Prior organ transplant status
Ethnicity	Diabetes status
Hypertension	
Diabetes	
Cause of death	
Serum creatinine	
Hepatitis C status	
Donation after circulatory death	

(EPTS: estimated post-transplant survival; KDPI: Kidney Donor Profile Index)

The top 20% of kidneys with the most extended predicted survival (KDPI score ≤20%) are prioritized for the top 20% of patients with the longest predicted patient survival (EPTS ≤20%). Using this system improves overall graft life (increased utility) but at the cost of prolonged waiting time for older recipients (reduced equity).

Human Leukocyte Antigen Matching

Human leukocyte antigen (HLA) matching is incorporated in allocation systems to increase utility. In UK, US, and Australia, zero mismatched kidneys are allowed for national sharing. HLA-DR matching is ranked higher than HLA-B matching in the UK, while HLA-A matching is no longer considered. In the US, other than zero mismatches, points are given only for HLA-DR matching. In Canadian provinces, HLA matching is no longer considered, whereas Eurotransplant provides points for the absence of each HLA-A, -B, and -DR mismatch. Also, Eurotransplant gives points for rare HLA.

Waiting Time

The most widely accepted factor for equity of organ allocation is waiting time. Therefore, the time since initiation of dialysis is usually considered the waiting period for organ allocation (instead of the time of registration in the waiting list).

Sensitization

Some patients have anti-HLA antibodies against many potential donors, which are expressed as calculated panel reactive antibodies (cPRA). Highly sensitized patients have limited access to transplantation. Hence, they are given priority in most organ allocation programs. Regional and national sharing of organs is allowed to increase their donor pool.

Prior Living Kidney Donors

Most allocation programs prioritize previous donors who developed ESRD after donating a kidney.

Blood Group

Kidneys are allocated to blood group identical waitlisted recipients, except for prioritization of HLA sensitization and zero mismatches. Blood group-based allocation avoids longer waiting times for O recipients. However, this results in longer waiting times for blood group B in Western countries, which is common in ethnic minorities. Blood group B (not A or AB) candidates are eligible for O donor kidneys in the UK. In the US, A2 and A2B kidneys are prioritized for preconsented B candidates, as group B recipients usually have low anti-A titers.

Medical Urgency

Most transplant programs prioritize patients who cannot receive adequate dialysis and with no further dialysis access options.

Priority for Pediatric Recipients

Most allocation programs prioritize pediatric patients because of the unique benefits of transplantation for growth and development. "Share 35" was implemented in the US in 2005 to preferentially allocate young deceased donors (<35 years old) to pediatric recipients (<18 years old). As pediatric patients usually require retransplantation, sensitization from the previous transplantation may adversely affect their prospects for second transplantation. To minimize HLA sensitization from poorly HLA-matched kidneys, different strategies are used. For example, zero mismatched and no DR mismatched kidneys are prioritized in pediatric recipients in the UK.[7]

In the following section, we briefly discuss the kidney allocation system used in the United States and the system followed in India.

UNITED STATES

Organ sharing is a nationwide system in the US by which deceased organs are allocated to potential recipients. The first US kidney allocation system was introduced in 1987. The deceased donor kidney allocation policy of the UNOS/organ procurement and transplant network (OPTN) was revised extensively in 2014.

According to the first system, the entire country was divided into 58 donor service areas (DSA) to allocate organs. Only zero mismatched kidneys were shared nationally. Since there were differences between organ supply and demand across different regions, there were significant differences in waiting times between regions. In March 2000, the health and human services department established the "final rule" for the national allocation of organ donors to reduce regional disparities. According to this, all donors were allocated based on the category of donors:

- Standard criteria donors <35 years
- Standard criteria donors >35 years
- Expanded criteria donors
- Donors after circulatory death

Within each sequence, priority was given to the groups such as zero mismatched patients, highly sensitized patients, blood group identical patients, and prior living donors. This system also had many limitations. A revised UNOS/OPTN policy was implemented in 2014 to increase the utilization of available kidneys, reduce regional variations, and improve outcomes of transplanted organs. The following parameters were considered when a donor's kidney was entered into the matching system.

- EPTS
- KDPI

- Further priority is given to the waitlisted candidates with less common blood types (blood types B and O) and high cPRA scores.
- Candidates are prioritized according to waiting list time.

For recipients >18 years of age, the calculation of waiting list time is based on the earliest of the following:

- Registration date with measured or calculated creatinine clearance <20 mL/min
- Date of starting dialysis treatment

For candidates <18 years of age, the waiting list time begins on either the date of registration or the date of initiation of dialysis, whichever is earliest.

Kidneys are allocated locally, regionally, and nationally, except for zero mismatched kidneys and highly sensitized candidates, for whom the allocation is at the national level. No points are assigned to patients based on medical urgency for the national allocation of kidneys. However, the physician can use judgment to assign medical urgency points locally.

Within a few months of implementing the revised policy, the following changes were noticed.

- There was an increase in the number of transplants for highly sensitized candidates (defined as cPRA >99%).
- There was an increase in nonlocal transplants.
- There was a decrease in the number of age mismatched kidneys (difference between donor and recipient more than 15 years).
- There was an increase in transplants for candidates aged 18–49 years and a decrease in transplants for candidates over 50 years.
- There was a decrease in pediatric transplants and decreased transplantation of zero mismatched kidneys.[7,8]

DECEASED DONOR KIDNEY ALLOCATION RULES IN INDIA

India enacted the Transplantation of Human Organs Act (THOA) in 1994, subsequently amended and updated in 2011 and 2014. The THOA legalized brain deaths in India, notified rules to regulate organ and tissue transplantation to curb commercial transplantation activities, and provided the framework for developing an organized deceased donor transplantation program. The government of India subsequently implemented the National Organ Transplant Program (NOTP) to implement the THOA, including training of the workforce and promotion of organ donation from deceased donors. Under this program, the National Organ and Tissue Transplant Organization (NOTTO) was established as a national networking organization for deceased donor organ sharing and allocation in India. Under NOTTO, there are five "Regional Organ and Tissue Transplant Organization (ROTTO)" covering the entire country under five "regions," with each ROTTO having all the states in that region under its jurisdiction. ROTTO facilitates coordination between states in sharing organs and tissues and between the states and the NOTTO. The NOTTO has framed rules for allocating deceased donor organs and tissues, which are broadly applicable to states.

An essential feature of organ allocation rules in India is categorizing transplantation centers as "government (public) sector" and "private sector." Transplantation activities, especially deceased donor organ procurement, in India predominantly happen in hospitals under the private sector, with a smaller contribution from public hospitals. Concerns about the accessibility of transplantation services at private hospitals for the underprivileged lead to "enabling" provisions in the organ allocation rules in India (justice). The provision essentially prioritizes public sector hospitals for allocating kidneys, with at least 50% of procured kidneys preferentially offered to patients waitlisted at government hospitals.[9]

The kidney allocation principles and algorithm notified by NOTTO and broadly followed by states in India are summarized in **Box 1**. The scoring system proposed (but not implemented by most Indian states) for prioritizing kidney allocation to recipients is summarized in **Table 2**.

BOX 1: Kidney allocation principles and algorithm notified by the National Organ and Tissue Transplant Organization (NOTTO).[9]

Allocation principles

1. Allocation will be done first based on the city waiting list. If no recipient is eligible in the city waiting list, then allocation will be done to the state and then to other states in the ROTTO and then to other ROTTO nationally. To minimize cold ischemia time, most donated organs should be allocated within the city or at the most state where retrieval has been done
2. Kidney from pediatric donor (<18 years) first will go to a pediatric patient. If no pediatric patient is eligible, then to an adult patient
3. Blood group O kidney will be allocated to a recipient with group O, then to next available on the waiting list of other compatible blood groups, i.e., first group A, then group B, and last group AB in that sequence
4. In the case of blood group A or B, the organ will be allocated to the same blood group failing which to blood group AB. AB will be allocated to AB only

Allocation algorithm

Once there is a call for a possible deceased donor,

Step 1: Check the blood group of the available deceased donors to follow the principle of allocation based on the blood group as above

Step 2: If there is a recipient in the "urgent list" as per accepted criteria and approved by the appropriate committee, then one of the two available kidneys will go to the urgent case. If there are two recipients in the urgent list, then allocation will be done to one patient with urgent criteria having more points in the scoring system

Contd...

Contd...

Criteria of urgent listing

In the case of a kidney transplant, an urgent list is basically for a patient on the following two principles:

1. Patient who no longer has dialysis access and thus cannot be maintained on dialysis
2. Patients with ESRD who are unlikely to get a donor with a negative crossmatch
   a. >90% panel reactive antibody

The priority/urgent list should be reviewed every 3 months by the SOTTO Kidney Transplant Advisory Committee

Step 3: Recipients requiring multi-organ transplants will get priority. If there are more than two recipients in the multi-organ recipient list, then allocation will be done to a patient having more points in the scoring system

Step 4: If there is NO urgent case and NO multi-organ recipient, then allocation will be done to a patient registered for "kidney alone" transplantation based on the status of the hospital; doing retrieval of kidneys means whether it is transplant hospital or retrieval only hospital

If transplant hospital

One kidney is used locally, and the other will be allocated. It is expected that the scoring system will also be followed by the hospital for the local allocation of the kidney

If retrieval hospital—both will be allocated

Step 5: See kidneys retrieval hospital, whether it is a government hospital or a private hospital

1. Kidney retrieved from a government hospital will be allocated as follows:
   a. First patients listed in government-ONLY hospital list, then
   b. Patients listed out of combined government and private hospital list, then
   c. Patients listed out of private-ONLY hospital list
2. Kidney retrieved from a private hospital will be allocated as follows:
   a. First patients listed in private hospitals list, then
   b. Patients listed out of combined government and private hospital list, then
   c. Patients listed out of the government hospital list

(ESRD: end-stage renal disease; ROTTO: Regional Organ and Tissue Transplant Organization; SOTTO: State Organ and Tissue Transplant Organization)

TABLE 2: Scoring system proposed for kidney allocation.[9]

Criteria for scoring	*Points allotted*
Time on dialysis	(+1) for each month on dialysis
Previous immunological graft failure within 3 months of transplantation	(+3) for each graft failure
Age of recipient	(+3) for <6 years (+2) for 6 to <12 years (+1) for 12 to <18 years
Patient on temporary vascular access	
• With failed all AV fistula sites • With failed AV graft after all failed AVF sites	(+2) (+4)
Panel reactive antibody (PRA)	(+0.5) for every 10% above 20%
Previous living donor now requiring a kidney transplant	(+5)
Near relative (as per definition of THOTA) of previous deceased donor now requiring a kidney transplant	(+5)

(AV: arteriovenous; AVF: arteriovenous fistula; THOTA: Transplantation of Human Organs and Tissues Act)

TABLE 3: The Maastricht classification of DCD.

Category	*Type*	*Circumstances*	*Typical location*
1	Uncontrolled	Dead on arrival	Emergency department
2	Uncontrolled	Unsuccessful resuscitation	Emergency department
3	Controlled	Cardiac arrest follows planned withdrawal of life sustaining treatments	ICU
4	Either	Cardiac arrest in a patient who is brain dead	ICU

(DCD: donation after circulatory death; ICU: intensive care unit)

Donation After Circulatory Death

Donation after circulatory death (DCD-earlier referred to as donation after cardiac death or donation from non-heart beating donor) refers to procurement of organs for transplantation from patients who died by circulatory criteria (Vs brain steam death). DCD may be 'controlled' or 'uncontrolled'. Procurement of organs from a patient after cardiac arrest which was unexpected and from which the patient could not be resuscitated is referred to as uncontrolled DCD. Controlled DCD refers to organ procurement after planned withdrawal of life support which has been determined to be of no benefit to a critically ill patient in the ICU **(Table 3)**.

The shortage of organ donors has prompted increasing reliance of DCD in many countries, despite it being logistically challenging and associated with more short-term complications in kidney transplantation due to higher incidence of delayed graft function. The long-term outcomes of DCD kidney transplantation are similar to donation after brain death (DBD).

In India, DCDs were performed at Ahmedabad and Chandigarh. The Institute of Kidney Diseases and Research Centre (IKDRC) at Ahmedabad performed 33 controlled DCDs between 1999 and 2012 and reported excellent outcomes with 1- and 10-year patient survival of 87.3% and

72.8%, with DGF in 31%. PGIMER, Chandigarh performed 26 kidney transplantation after DCD till December 2020. The initial experience of 9 noncontrolled DCDs were reported. Warm ischemia time was 68±15.16 minutes and cold ischemia ranged from 3.5 to 13 hours. 80% had DGF and one graft had primary nonfunction. Expansion of DCD may contribute significantly to the donor pool in India.

CONCLUSION

Different countries follow different deceased donor kidney allocation systems based on medical and logistic considerations, and such systems have evolved over the years. The primary purpose of organized organ allocation systems is to ensure equitable distribution of donor organs while ensuring the best chances of survival for transplanted recipients. India has devised its organ allocation criteria with provisions enabling better access to transplantation services for the underprivileged.

REFERENCES

1. Modi GK, Jha V. The incidence of end-stage renal disease in India: a population-based study. Kidney Int. 2006;70:2131-33.
2. TRANSTAN. Transplant Authority of Tamil Nadu. [online] Available from https://transtan.tn.gov.in/activewaitlist.php. [Last accessed February, 2022].
3. Kerala Network for Organ Sharing. [online] Available from [Last accessed February, 2022]. EGovernment of Telangana.
4. Jeevandan. [online] Available from https://jeevandan.gov.in/. [Last accessed February, 2022].
5. Global Observatory on Donation and transplantation. [online] Available from http://www.transplant-observatory.org/. [Last accessed June, 2022].
6. Wu DA, Watson CJ, Bradley JA, Johnson RJ, Forsythe JL, Oniscu GC. Global trends and challenges in deceased donor kidney allocation. Kidney Int. 2017;91(6):1287-99.
7. Lee D, Kanellis J, Mulley WR. Allocation of deceased donor kidneys: a review of international practices. Nephrology (Carlton). 2019;24(6):591-8.
8. Israni AK, Salkowski N, Gustafson S, Snyder JJ, Friedewald JJ, Formica RN, et al. New national allocation policy for deceased donor kidneys in the United States and possible effect on patient outcomes. J Am Soc Nephrol. 2014;25(8):1842-8.
9. National Organ and Tissue Transplant Organization. Allocation criteria for deceased donor kidney transplant (guidelines). [online] Available from www.notto.gov.in. [Last accessed June, 2022].

22.3 How to Set Up a Deceased Donor Program

Noble Gracious, Georgi Abraham

BACKGROUND

The burden of end-stage renal disease in India has risen dramatically in the last decade due to the increasing prevalence of risk factors such as diabetes mellitus and hypertension. The deaths attributable to chronic kidney disease (CKD) in India increased from 0.59 million in 1990 to 1.18 million in 2016.[1] The exact burden of end-stage renal disease in terms of incidence and prevalence remains elusive due to the lack of kidney failure registries at any significant administrative level. In 2015, the Million Death Study projected the annual deaths due to kidney failure to be 136,000.[2]

A systematic review estimated that in 2010, 2.6 million people received renal replacement therapy (RRT) worldwide, while the number of patients who required the RRT was estimated to be 4.9 million.[3] The treatment gap is pronounced in the low-income countries of the Asian region where a conservative estimate showed that ideally 1.9 million people should have but did not receive adequate therapy.[3] Based on the data from a survey of academic nephrology centers using the International Society of Nephrology (ISN) Global Kidney Health Atlas methodology, it was estimated that the number of patients on chronic dialysis in India was 174,478, translating into a prevalence of 129 per million population.[4]

Since RRT resources are scarce in India, the need for improvement in deceased donor (DD) transplantation is essential. **Table 1** gives the data from the International Registry in Organ Donation and Transplantation (IRODAT) registry regarding the deceased donations in India in 2020. Moreover, there are no data on the need for liver or heart transplants in the country. A well-functioning organ donation program from DD and transplantation is a felt need in the country.

TABLE 1: Deceased donation in India from the International Registry in Organ Donation and Transplantation (IRODAT) registry (2020).

Organs	No. of deceased donations	Per million population
Kidney	516	0.37
Liver	291	0.21
Pancreas	14	0.01
Heart	89	0.06
Lung	67	0.05

HISTORICAL AND LEGAL ASPECTS OF DECEASED DONATION IN INDIA

In India, the first renal transplantation was carried out at the King Edward Memorial (KEM) Hospital in Bombay in May 1965. The procedure was carried out using a cadaveric donor, and the recipient was a patient who was suffering from a hydronephroma.[5] The second kidney transplant in April 1966 was again a cadaveric donor. The transplantation surgery was carried out by the same team in a patient with chronic renal failure.[5] In the initial days of organ transplantation, the system was largely unregulated. There were many reports of organ trafficking. The law-and-order agencies uncovered large-scale organ trafficking in many parts of India.[6,7]

The current state of organ transplantation in India evolved through addressing multiple legal, moral, and ethical challenges. The first real institutionalization and standardization of the transplantation program through legalization was via the enactment of the Transplantation of Human Organs and Tissues Act (THOTA) in 1994.[8] The major objective of this legislation was to curb organ trading and promote deceased organ donation. The multiple kidney organ trading scandals across the country between 2000 and 2008 revealed some of the major loopholes in the legislation through which organized organ trade networks were getting away.[9] Multiple rounds of discussions took place, between various stakeholders, and the draft bill was submitted in 2009.

The bill was eventually passed with 43 amendments as recommended by the Parliamentary Standing Committee in 2011 with the objective of plugging the loopholes in the system, which made commercial organ trading possible.[10] The new rules were notified in 2014. The major provisions of the THOTA Act, including the amendments and the rules of 2014 declared that the deceased donation can be either after brain death (brain-stem death) or after cardiac death. Form 10 (brain death declaration form) was used for the certification of brain death. This was expected to be filled by the board of medical experts certifying brain-stem death.

According to the new legislation, the Medical Board or the Brain Death Committee was supposed to be constituted by the registered medical practitioner (RMP), which comprises a panel of four doctors: hospital administrator, resident doctor, neurologist/neurosurgeon/physician/intensivist/anesthetist, and treating doctor. An additional modification to the composition of the Medical Board was that whenever a neurologist or a neurosurgeon was unavailable, any physician, anesthetist, or intensivist nominated by the hospital administrator in charge may certify brain death.

Clinically, the complete and permanent cessation of circulation, respiration, and functions of the brain is defined as death. The cessation of vital functions (permanent stoppage of heart, respiration, and brain activity) irreversibly is the cardiopulmonary criterion for the declaration of death.[11] But in the context of organ donation, the definition of death is more nuanced. Organ donation is classified as donation after brain death (DBD) and donation after cardiac death (DCD).[12] The latter is also known as non-heart-beating donation.

One of the important factors that determine the success of a transplant is the speed and promptness with which the organ is procured after the death of the donor. Only those organs that are recently perfused can be taken up for transplantation. In the case of DBD, the donor is described as someone who has had a primary brain death, but the cardiac circulation and respiration are still intact or are maintained by medical measures, including mechanical ventilation or extracorporeal machine oxygenation (ECMO) device.[12] The donors are also known as beating-heart donors. In India, even in the initial version of the THOTA (1994), the declaration of death via brain-stem death criteria was acknowledged legally.

In the current scenario, people can opt in for the organ donation program if they want their organs to be used after death. To opt in, they need to submit a donor pledge form (self-consent form) for deceased donation (named Form 7).[8,13] In the event of brain-stem death, it is mandatory for the treating doctor to ask the primary caregiver or the individual in legal possession of the body whether the donor had made any prior authorization as specified in the self-consent form for the removal of his/her organs or tissues after death for therapeutic purposes.[8,13] If not, the primary caregiver/relative should be made aware of the option to authorize an organ donation. It should also be noted that for all practical purposes, even if the donor has authorized his organs for donation before death, the consent of a near relative or person in legal possession of the body is required.[13,14]

There are other consent forms to cover different scenarios. For example, Forms 1 and 2 deal with near-relative consent and spouse consent, respectively. In the case of consent for organ donation from a family, there is Form 8. This form is also applicable to the donation of organs involving minors. Form 9 deals with the consent for organ donation from unclaimed bodies. However, there are experts who are of the opinion that it is high time to get rid of the clause of donation from unclaimed bodies in its current form.[14] In their experience, this clause creates unnecessary fear and ambiguity, and moreover, hardly any donation has come from this category since the inception of the act.

The brain death declaration form as mentioned earlier is Form 10. Hospital registration for organ transplantation is done via Form 12, while the registration of a hospital for organ retrieval is done via Form 13. The retrieval of organs is permitted for any hospital with an intensive care unit facility (ICU) on registration with the appropriate authority, and these hospitals are categorized as nontransplant organ retrieval centers (NTORC). For registering as a retrieval center, a hospital should have an ICU facility with optimum manpower, infrastructure, and equipment to diagnose brain-stem death; maintain the brain stem, dead donor; and retrieve and transport organs and tissues (in addition to having the provision for the temporary storage of organs).[15,16] The donor family is not expected to pay any cost for the donor management, organ retrieval, organ/tissue transportation, and organ preservation. The billing is stopped once the certification is complete and the additional cost of all the steps required for optimal organ utilization is expected to be met by either the recipient, government, nongovernmental organizations (NGOs) or societies, or a combination of these institutions.[15,17]

In the case of medicolegal cases (MLC), specific protocols must be adhered to as per the THOTA. Post brain death and immediately after the consent is taken from people in legal possession of the body for organ donation, the RMP of the healthcare institution requests the Superintendent of Police (SP) or Deputy Inspector General (DIG) of the area to facilitate the timely retrieval of organs from the donor.[18] The safeguards are to ensure that the many steps involved in the transplantation process, most importantly the retrieval of organs, do not jeopardize the determination of the cause of death, and also as far as the transplant team is concerned, prevent any unnecessary delay in the retrieval of organs.[13] The retrieving doctor is expected to prepare the medical report clearly describing in detail the organs or tissues being retrieved. The postmortem notes will record these facts. This will be done by the RMP doing the postmortem.[18] Depending on state laws, it should be made clear that the designated forensic expert should make himself available at the time of organ/tissue retrieval, even if it is beyond office timings.[19]

Sometimes, if the retrieval hospital is privately owned and is not equipped to conduct postmortem, they are expected to arrange transportation of the body along with the relevant medical records and post organ/tissue retrieval to the designated postmortem center. The postmortem centers are expected to undertake the postmortem of such cases without any delay or causing any inconvenience to the donor family. The qualification required and the role of transplant coordinators in the organ donation and

Flowcharts 1A and B: (A) In the donor hospital; (B) In the recipient hospital.

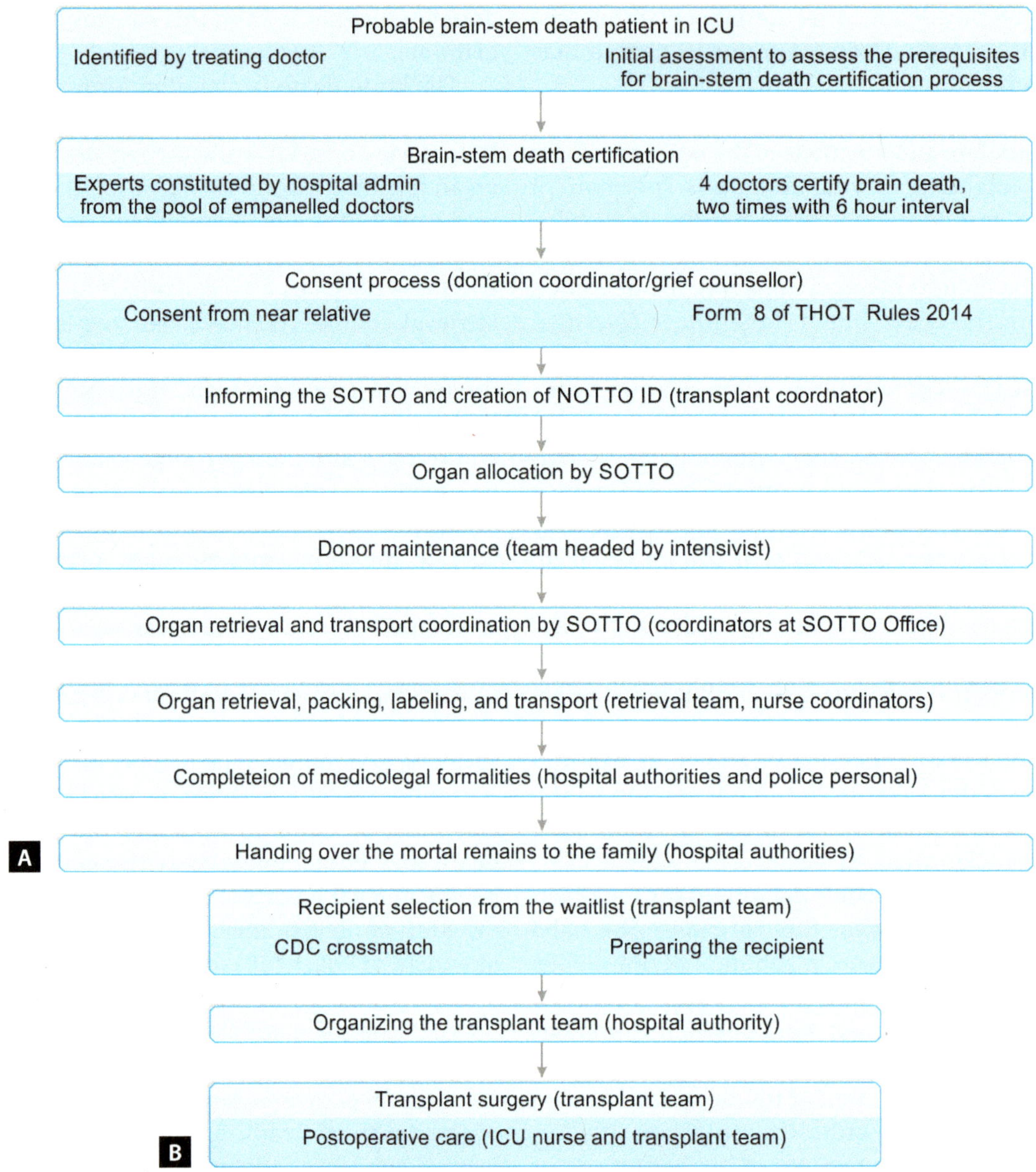

(CDC: complement-dependent cytotoxicity; ICU: intensive care unit; ID: identity document; NOTTO: National Organ and Tissue Transplant Organization; SOTTO: State Organ and Tissue Transplant Organization)

transplantation process are clearly defined in the THOTA. The transplant coordinator is a mandatory requirement for registering the hospitals as transplant centers.[13,15] The human resources required and processes involved in setting up deceased organ donation are depicted in **Flowcharts 1A and B**.

BRAIN DEATH DIAGNOSIS AND BRAIN DEATH DONATION PATHWAY

Brain-stem death is "irreversible cessation of cerebral and brain-stem function; characterized by absence of electrical activity in the brain, blood flow to the brain, and brain function as determined by clinical assessment of responses. A brain-stem dead person is dead, although his or her cardiopulmonary functioning may be artificially maintained for some time".

In the case of brain-stem death, though there is a complete and irreversible loss of all brain functions, the heart will be still beating, thus making it the right time to procure organs from the deceased's body. Therefore, today, it is an accepted notion that even if a person's heart is beating, he/she may be declared "brain-stem dead". Thus, in simple words, a person is "brain-stem dead" when all the functions of the brain cease. The brain-stem death expert committee constituted for the purpose has to satisfy themselves that the patient satisfies all the prerequisites for brain-stem death testing as listed below and proceeds to the certification process as per the protocol laid down by the state as stipulated by the law.

Prerequisites for Brain-stem Death

- Clinical or neuroimaging evidence of an acute central nervous system (CNS) catastrophe (e.g., traumatic brain injury, subarachnoid hemorrhage)
- Exclusion of complicating medical conditions that may confound clinical assessment [no severe electrolyte, acid–base, endocrine, or circulatory (i.e., shock) disturbance]
- No drug intoxication or poisoning, including any sedative drug administered in the hospital, may confound the clinical assessment
- Core temperature >36°C (97°F)
- Systolic blood pressure >100 mm Hg; vasopressors may be required.

Examination Findings

- Coma
- Absent brain-originating motor response, including response to pain stimulus above the neck or other brain-originating movements (e.g., seizures, decerebrate, or decorticate posturing)
- Absent pupillary light reflex; pupils are mid-position (3.5–4 mm)
- Absent corneal reflexes
- Absent oculocephalic (doll's eyes) and oculovestibular (caloric responses) reflexes
- Absent jaw jerk
- Absent gag reflex
- Absent cough with tracheal suctioning
- Absent sucking or rooting reflexes (in neonates)
- Apnea as demonstrated by apnea test.

Apnea Test

The apnea test is performed after all the following criteria for brain death have been met:

- Core temperature ≥36°C or 97°F
- Systolic blood pressure ≥100 mm Hg
- Eucapnia ($PaCO_2$ 35–45 mm Hg)
- Absence of hypoxia
- Euvolemic status.

The test is not valid in patients who chronically have high $PaCO_2$ values (CO_2 retainers) and in cases of neuromuscular paralysis or high cervical spinal cord lesions. In a positive apnea test, there was no respiratory response to $PaCO_2$ >60 or 20 mm Hg greater than baseline values and a final arterial pH of <7.28.

Disconnecting the ventilator is often associated with profound hypoxemia and hemodynamic instability. This can be obviated by increasing inspired oxygen before and during the test. Preoxygenation eliminates stores of respiratory nitrogen and accelerates oxygen transport through the tracheal cannula. The fraction of inspired oxygen should be 1.0 for 10 minutes, up to a maximum PaO_2 of 200 mm Hg or until the $PaCO_2$ exceeds 40 mm Hg. Ventilation frequency is reduced to eucapnia; positive end-expiratory pressure is reduced to 5 cmH_2O. Once pulse oximetry is >95%, an arterial blood gas (ABG) is obtained. The patient is then disconnected from the ventilator. Oxygen is provided by a tracheal cannula at 6 L/min; the tip should lie at the carina. Alternatives include using a T-piece system with oxygen flow at 12 L/min and using continuous positive airway pressure (CPAP) 10–20 cmH_2O, with oxygen flow at 12 L/min.

Visual observation is the standard method for detecting respiratory movement. 8–10 minutes with no observable respiratory effort is a standard observation period. $PaCO_2$ was measured just prior to reconnection to the ventilator to confirm that the target level (>60 or 20 mm Hg greater than baseline values) was achieved.

Ancillary Tests

- Four-vessel conventional cerebral angiography
- Transcranial doppler
- Magnetic resonance angiography
- Computed tomographic angiography
- Single-photon emission computed tomographic (SPECT) brain scintigraphy
- Electroencephalography
- Evoked potentials.

There are two types of donation after death resulting from two different forms of clinical determination of death **(Fig. 1)**:

1. Donation after neurological death (NDD)
2. Donation after circulatory death (DCD)

[Organ donation after medical assistance in dying (MAiD).]

Cleveland Clinic has classified deceased donors as given below:

- *Standard criteria donors (SCD):* These kidneys are from donors under the age of 50 years and do not meet any of the criteria below that are assigned to expanded criteria donors (ECD).
- *ECD:* These organs come from donors over the age of 60 or 50–59 years who also have at least two of the following criteria—history of high blood pressure, the donor passed away from a cerebrovascular accident (CVA) (stroke), or who had a creatinine higher than the normal laboratory value (1.5 mg/dL). About 15–20% of the donors in the United States meet the expanded criteria.
- *DCD:* These donors do not meet the standard criteria for brain death. Their hearts stopped before the organs were

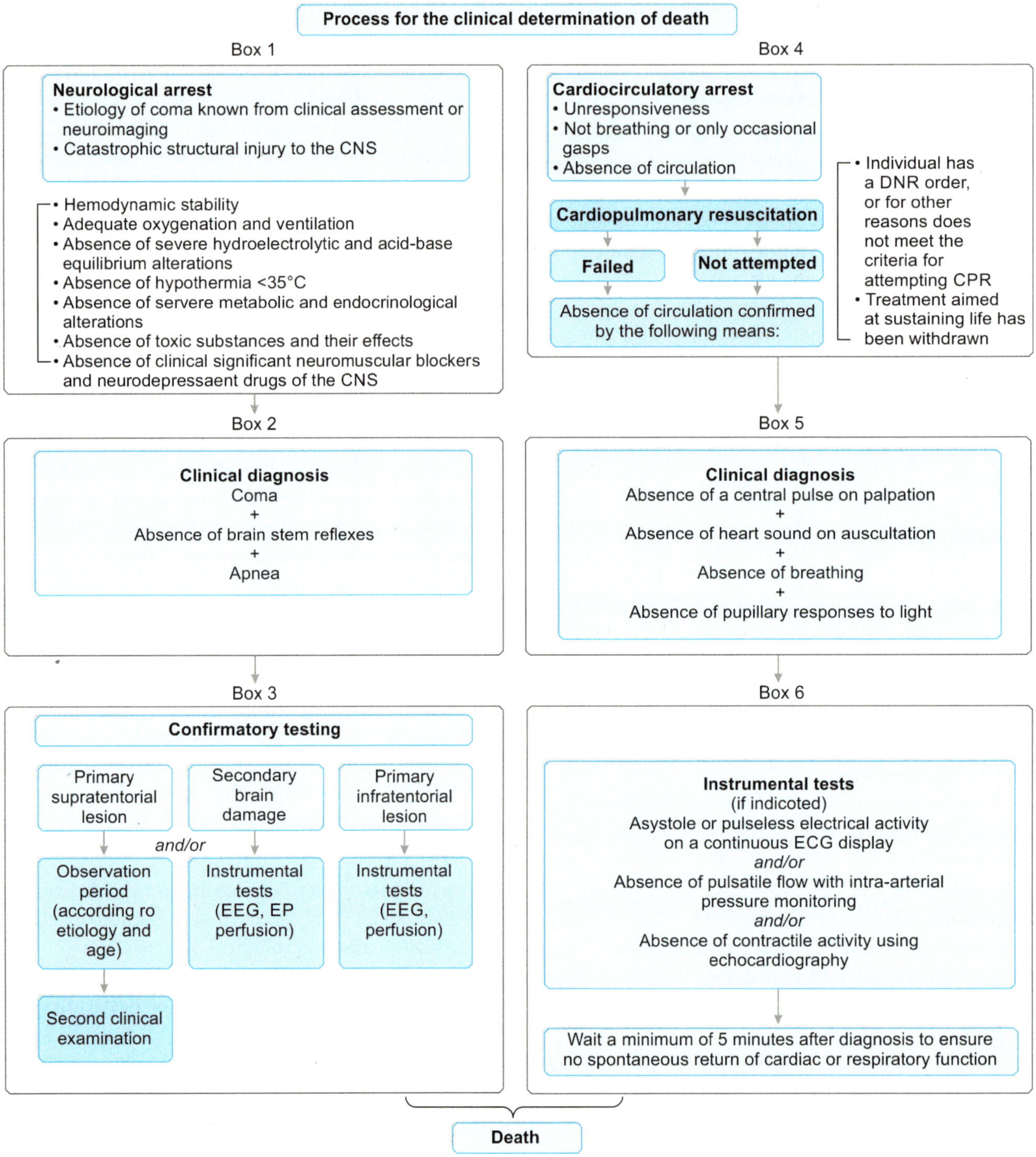

Fig. 1: Clinical determination of death: two different workflows but a common end point-death. (CNS: central nervous system; CPR: cardiopulmonary resuscitation; DNR: do not resuscitate; ECG: electrocardiogram; EEG: electroencephalogram)

removed. DCD occurs when continuing medical care is futile, and the donor patient is to be removed from all medical life-sustaining measures/supports.

- *Double-kidney transplants (duals):* During the year, we may have access to donors that are at the more extreme limit of the ECD. Research has found that using both of these kidneys in one recipient is preferable to only one.
- *Donors with high-risk social behavior:* These donors are individuals who at some point in their life practiced high-risk behavior for sexually transmitted disease, drug use, or were incarcerated. All of these donors are tested for the transmissible disease at the time of organ recovery. You will be informed of the high-risk behavior.

ORGAN DONOR MAINTENANCE

Management of the potential organ donor primarily involves the use of supportive measures to reverse or mitigate the physiological changes that occur after brain death, including potentially severe autonomic and inflammatory responses. From the author's experience, road traffic accident victims are the common source of donations in this part of the world. Other donors are partial hanging, poisoning (organophosphorus), and cobra bite envenomation victims. Donors with encephalopathy and brain death due to rabies are a contraindication for donation.

Monitoring and Electrolytes

- Monitor temperature, heart rate and rhythm, SpO_2, blood pressure, and mean arterial pressure (MAP), continuously; monitor urine output, serially.
- Insert two large-bore intravenous (IV) lines. Consider inserting a central venous catheter and/or pulmonary-artery catheter (PAC) to monitor a patient's hemodynamics (placement of PAC is particularly important in patients with an ejection fraction <45% or requiring high-dose inotropic medication). Insert an arterial line.
- Obtain echocardiogram for all potential donors. Repeat echocardiogram when the patient has stabilized if the initial echocardiogram shows significant cardiac dysfunction.
- Early flexible bronchoscopy for inspection and airway clearance
- Maintain serum Na >135 and <155 mEq/dL.
- Maintain serum K >4 and <5 mEq/dL.
- Assess serum Mg, Ca, and PO_4, and replace as needed.
- Assess serum lactate and central or mixed venous oxygen saturation.
- Correct metabolic acidosis with Na bicarbonate and mild hyperventilation. Aim for arterial pH 7.35–7.45.
- Watch for autonomic storm with hypertension.

Ventilation

- *Mode:* Typically, volume control
- *Tidal volume:* 6–8 mL/kg (use ideal predicted body weight)
- *Respiratory rate:* 8–16 breaths/min
- *Positive end-expiratory pressure (PEEP):* 5–10 cmH_2O
- *Initial FiO_2:* 100%; after stabilization, titrate down to 40%, as tolerated.

Goals of Resuscitation

- Normal core body temperature versus mild hypothermia
- MAP ≥60 mm Hg
- Central venous pressure ≤12 mm Hg
- Pulmonary artery occlusion pressure ≤12 mm Hg
- Left ventricular stroke work index >15
- Dopamine dosage <10 µg/kg/min
- Urine output ≥1 mL/kg/h
- Volume resuscitation: Replete volume with isotonic crystalloids (e.g., 0.9% saline, lactated Ringer solution, Plasma-Lyte, Normosol).

Hematological Management

- Correct abnormal international normalized ratio (INR) or partial thromboplastin time (PTT) (e.g., ≥1.5 times control) with fresh frozen plasma.
- Infuse packed red blood cells (RBC) to maintain blood hemoglobin >7 mg/dL. Higher preprocurement hemoglobin may be needed depending on the planned procedure.

Vasopressors and Inotropes

- After repletion of circulating volume, if MAP <60 mm Hg, assess whether the cause of hypotension is decreased systemic vascular resistance (SVR) or decreased cardiac output.
- Infuse arginine vasopressin as noted below for decreased SVR.
- If MAP remains <60 mm Hg and left ventricular ejection fraction (LVEF) >45%, add a vasopressor agent (e.g., norepinephrine, phenylephrine).
- If MAP remains <60 mm Hg and LVEF <45%, add an inotropic agent (e.g., dobutamine, dopamine, epinephrine).

Hormonal Resuscitation

- Consider levothyroxine (T4) for persistent hypotension after fluid repletion: a 20 µg bolus is given IV, followed by an infusion of 10 µg/h.
- Arginine vasopressin: 1 unit bolus IV, followed by continuous infusion of 0.01–0.04 units/min, adjusted to maintain MAP >60 mm Hg and urinary output 0.5–1 mL/kg/h.
- Hydrocortisone 300 mg IV, then 100 mg every 8 hours
- *Insulin:* There is no universally accepted insulin regimen. To achieve a target blood glucose range (120–180 mg/dL), avoid the use of glucose-containing IV fluids and administer insulin only when necessary.

As soon as consent is obtained for organ retrieval after brain death declaration, ensure that enough blood is retrieved from the donor for immunological testing, microbiology evaluation, and organ suitability assessment. A minimum of 20–40 mL of blood in a citrated tube, two to three small lymph nodes, and a small piece of the spleen are required for human leukocyte antigens (HLA) typing and crossmatching testing. Keep a spare blood sample in the refrigerator in case the kidney may need transportation to another hospital.

ORGAN RETRIEVAL

The coordination of retrieval surgery with different transplant hospitals is the responsibility of the State Organ and Tissue Transplant Organization (SOTTO) in consultation with the donor hospital. In our country, there are no exclusive retrieval teams, and hence, the recipient hospital has to send their transplant surgeons for organ retrieval. The multiorgan retrieval team should ensure details of the date of birth, age, gender, cause of death, blood grouping, and kidney description, including dimension, weight, any tears, and a number of blood vessels, if on a patch there should be documentation of the time of retrieval of kidney—warm ischemia time, storage, and transport. It is also the responsibility of the retrieval team to verify all the documents including the consent form and ensure that all are in order before proceeding with the organ retrieval.

ORGAN ALLOCATION

Once the brain death is certified and declared, the treating doctor in the presence of the transplant coordinator must seek the consent of a near relative of the DD. After obtaining the consent, the hospital has to inform the SOTTO about the availability of an eligible donor for the allocation purpose. The following results should be available soon after brain death has been declared, namely:

- Hepatitis B surface antigen (HbsAg)
- Anti-hepatitis C virus (HCV) antibody
- Human immunodeficiency virus (HIV) status
- Blood grouping and typing
- Kidney function
- Liver function
- Complete hemogram including coagulation profile.

A bedside ultrasound of the liver, kidney, and pancreas and two-dimensional (2D) echocardiogram and imaging of the chest must be done to assess the suitability of the organs for transplantation. These reports also have to be shared with the SOTTO for informing the transplant centers when making an organ offer. The transplant center has the prerogative to accept the organ offer on the basis of information provided through the state networking organization within the stipulated time which varies in different states.

Allocation will be done first based on the regional waiting list. If no recipient is eligible on the regional waiting list, then allocation will be done to the state and then to other states in the Regional Organ and Tissue Transplant Organization (ROTTO) and then to other ROTTO nationally through National Organ and Tissue Transplant Organization (NOTTO). In order to minimize cold ischemia time, most donated organs are allocated within the city or at the most state, where retrieval has been done. A kidney from a pediatric donor (less than 18 years) will first go to a pediatric patient. If no pediatric patient is eligible, then an adult patient will be considered. Blood group O kidney will be allocated to the recipient with group O and then to the next available on the waiting list of other compatible blood groups, i.e., first group A, then group B, and last group AB in that sequence. In the case of blood group A or B, the organ will be allocated to the same blood group failing which to blood group AB. AB will be allocated to AB only.

Liver and heart allocation is on a rotation basis to the center and the recipient hospital has to choose the appropriate recipient based on the donor characteristics and the recipient's medical status.

ACCESS TO TRANSPLANTATION

Access to transplantation involves several steps from referral to a transplant center, assessing the medical/surgical fitness to undergo a transplant and financial capability to bear the expenses of transplant surgery and postoperative care. Those who are waitlisted should also undergo periodic medical assessments to determine their readiness for transplant when the organ offer is made. This includes cardiovascular disease assessment, malignancy screening, and infectious disease screening [tuberculosis (TB), hepatitis B, hepatitis C, HIV, venereal disease research laboratory (VDRL) tests, etc.]. Complications of coronary artery disease being the predominant cause of death mandate a detailed workup and corrective measures. The recipient should be psychologically counseled regarding the need for lifestyle modification (smoking, alcohol, lack of exercise, drug addiction, alternative therapy), strict compliance with antirejection medications, need for regular transplant physician follow-up, the economics of transplant management, avoidance, and prompt treatment of infections; all ensure the success of transplantation.

PATIENT REGISTRATION AND WAITLIST MANAGEMENT

All patients who want to be on the waitlist for cadaver donors have to be registered by the concerned hospital through the online registration portal of the state organ transplant network maintained by SOTTO. A kidney advisory committee will approve registration and confirm the need for renal transplants for every newly registered patient. Once approved, the patient will be put on the active list in the system and allocation scoring for that patient will be done based on the guidelines formed, which are specific to the states. Patients should be less than or equal to 65 years of age at the time of registration. The patient should be a case of end-stage renal disease on maintenance dialysis for more than 3 months on a regular basis.

The patient should not have an absolute contraindication for renal transplant, as given under:

- Advanced untreatable cardiovascular disease
- Irreversible cerebrovascular accident
- Inoperable malignancy
- Untreatable major psychiatric illness (to be certified by a psychiatrist).

Patients should be registered ONLY in ONE hospital registered under the THOTA with the state authority. However, he/she can change the hospital at any stage, and his or her allocation scoring and seniority in the central waiting list will not change. However, his/her seniority on the waiting list of locally available kidneys with the new hospital will be applicable 1 month after the date of the change. The patient can be registered for a DD even though the patient is waiting for a living donor transplant.

IMMUNOLOGICAL SCREENING OF THE DONOR AND RECIPIENT

Screen and identify anti-HLA antibodies in a potential recipient to ensure the best graft outcome. Physical crossmatches include complement-dependent cytotoxicity (CDC) and flow cytometric crossmatches. More recently, the virtual crossmatch, using the single antigen bead (SAB) assay, has assumed much significance, particularly in the DD setting. The histocompatibility of the donor–recipient is basically decided on the CDC crossmatch in our country. HLA typing of donor and recipient is not done as a routine in DD programs in India and it does not influence the organ allocation policy at present.

PREPARING THE KIDNEY RECIPIENT ON CONTINUOUS AMBULATORY PERITONEAL DIALYSIS FOR ORGAN TRANSPLANT

Patients on continuous ambulatory peritoneal dialysis (CAPD) can be dialyzed till their entry into the operation theater, and the peritoneal cavity should be emptied by draining the effluent before transplantation. The dialysis effluent should be sent for Gram stain and culture. Every effort should be made by the recipient surgeon to prevent a peritoneal tear in case the allograft has delayed function, necessitating the continuation of peritoneal dialysis until graft recovery. If any leak of dialysis fluid is observed, peritoneal dialysis should be discontinued and the patient is switched over to hemodialysis. In the author's practice, the permanent peritoneal dialysis catheter can be removed if the allograft is functioning well soon after the transplantation. Patients with active peritonitis should not undergo DD transplantation.

GRAFT DYSFUNCTION ASSESSMENT (FIG. 2)

As with any transplantation, when tissue from a donor who is genetically different is transplanted, the recipient mounts an immune response that, if uncontrolled, results in the destruction of the graft. Immune monitoring and immunosuppression play a significant role and impact early rejection rates. Based on the timing when the rejection occurs (posttransplant), the rejection is classified as follows:

- Hyperacute (usually within 24 hours)
- Early acute (3–7 days)

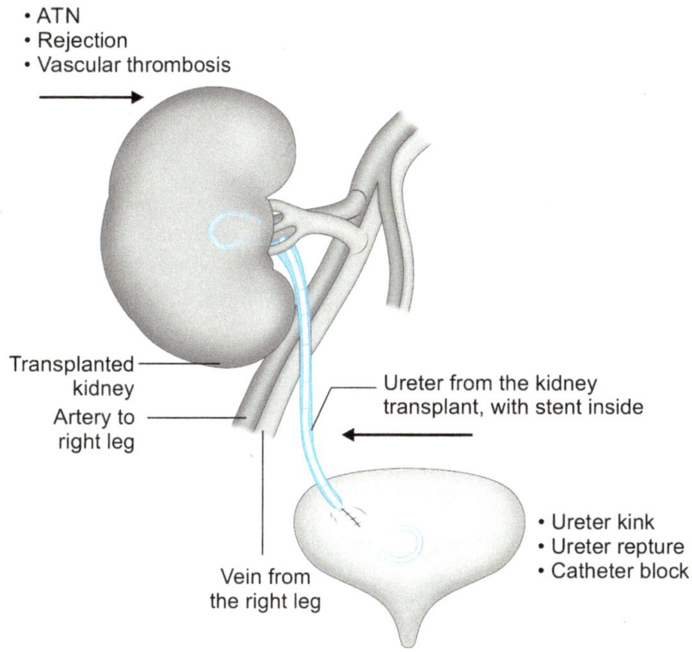

Fig. 2: Causes of allograft dysfunction in the early transplantation period. (ATN: acute tubular necrosis)

- Late acute (due to noncompliance with medications or infection)
- Chronic.

As is the practice in most centers in India, DD transplantation is performed without HLA matching and other immunological testing, optimal results, and long-term survival may be compromised. Organ retrieval and transplantation are carried out without prolonged cold ischemia time, ensuring a reduced incidence of acute tubular injury. A warm ischemia time of 30–45 minutes is optimal. The recent addition of machine perfusion, though costly, provides better graft function in the postoperative period. Strict aseptic techniques for organ retrieval and transport of the kidney are of paramount importance to prevent postoperative allograft infection. A donor with suspected sepsis should not be considered for donation. If allograft function does not recover, periodic kidney biopsies are warranted to differentiate between acute tubular injury, rejection, drug toxicity, recurrence of original disease, and graft pyelonephritis.

FROZEN SECTION OF A KIDNEY BIOPSY FROM A DECEASED DONOR

This was a donation after neurological death from a 54-year-old male patient whose serum creatinine was 1.3 mg/dL on admission, which increased to 2.5 mg/dL and decrease in urinary output. This frozen section shows no significant tubular damage due to the presence of nuclei and normal vessels and glomerulus. Hence, frozen section from the DD kidney gives valuable information regarding the viability of the organ **(Fig. 3)**.

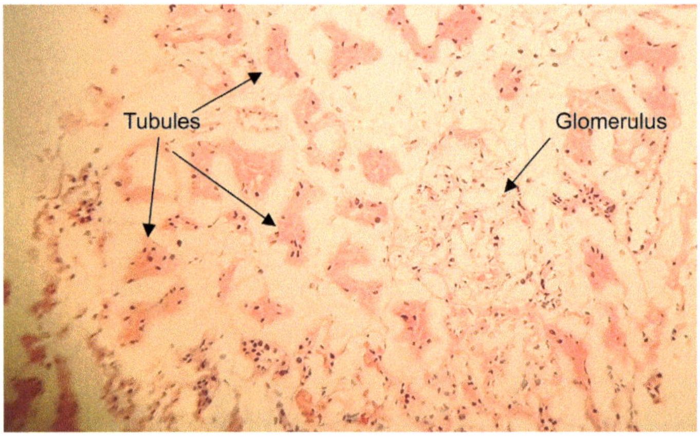

Fig. 3: Frozen section of a deceased donor (DD) kidney prior to implantation.
Courtesy: Dr Anil Tarigopula, MD.

ROLE OF STATE ORGAN AND TISSUE TRANSPLANT ORGANIZATION, REGIONAL ORGAN AND TISSUE TRANSPLANT ORGANIZATION, AND NATIONAL ORGAN AND TISSUE TRANSPLANT ORGANIZATION IN ORGAN ALLOCATION

Allocation will be done first based on the regional waiting list. If no recipient is eligible on the regional waiting list, then allocation will be done to the state and then to other states in the ROTTO and then to other ROTTO nationally through NOTTO. In order to minimize cold ischemia time, most donated organs are allocated within the city or at the most state, where retrieval has been done. All donor hospitals have to create a donor identity document (ID) in the NOTTO website, and organs will be allocated only to the patients who are already listed in the waiting list and have a valid unique NOTTO ID.

SUMMARY

Hundreds of deceased organ transplants are carried out across India every year, yet it seems that the systems in place have quite a bit of room for improvement. We have previously been unsuccessful in trying to adopt organ transplant models that have proved to be functional in developed nations. It is vital to recognize that India is vastly different from these nations in the way that we go about cultural, religious, and socioeconomic factors. Patterns of healthcare financing in the country have shown that a considerable chunk of the Indian population meets their healthcare expenditure through out-of-pocket expenses. The exhaustive steps involved in the deceased organ donation and transplant program require highly skilled personnel and reliable infrastructure at every level for smooth functioning as depicted in **Flowcharts 1A and B**. Hence, crafting a tailormade transplant program takes into consideration all the aforementioned factors, which include not only the infrastructure required for donation and transplantation but also the need for trained human resources and systems in place.

REFERENCES

1. Xie Y, Bowe B, Mokdad AH, Xian H, Yan Y, Li T, et al. Analysis of the global burden of disease study highlights the global, regional, and national trends of chronic kidney disease epidemiology from 1990 to 2016. Kidney Int. 2018;94(3):567-81.
2. Dare AJ, Fu SH, Patra J, Rodriguez PS, Thakur JS, Jha P. Renal failure deaths and their risk factors in India 2001–13: nationally representative estimates from the Million Death Study. Lancet Glob Health. 2017;5(1):e89-95.
3. Liyanage T, Ninomiya T, Jha V, Neal B, Patrice HM, Okpechi I, et al. Worldwide access to treatment for end-stage kidney disease: a systematic review. Lancet. 2015;385(9981):1975-82.
4. Jha V, Ur-Rashid H, Agarwal SK, Akhtar SF, Kafle RK, Sheriff R. The state of nephrology in South Asia. Kidney Int. 2019;95(1):31-7.
5. Acharya VN. Status of renal transplant in India—May 1994. J Postgrad Med. 1994;40(3):158.
6. Bhattacharjee Y. (2010). The downfall of India's kidney kingpin. Discover Magazine. [online] Available from https://www.discovermagazine.com/health/the-downfall-of-indias-kidney-kingpin [Last accessed July, 2022].
7. Kumar R. (2020). How maximum city Mumbai became epicentre of illegal kidney trade with 100 transplants a month. The Print. [online] Available from https://theprint.in/pageturner/excerpt/how-mumbai-became-epicentre-illegal-kidney-trade-with-100-transplants-month/351719/ [Last accessed July, 2022].
8. The Transplantation of Human Organs and Tissues Act, 1994. (1994). [online] Available from https://indiankanoon.org/doc/71680523/ [Last accessed July, 2022].
9. Delhi policeman arrested in kidney racket scandal | Reuters. Reuters. (2008). [online] Available from https://www.reuters.com/article/topNews/idINIndia-31972520080215?edition-redirect=in [Last accessed July, 2022].
10. Illegal organ transplant can attract 10-year jail. The Hindu. (2011). [online] Available from https://www.thehindu.com/news/national/illegal-organ-transplant-can-attract-10year-jail/article2351612.ece [Last accessed July 2022].
11. Sarbey B. Definitions of death: brain death and what matters in a person. J Law Biosci. 2016;3(3):743-52.
12. Rao PS, Ojo A. The alphabet soup of kidney transplantation: SCD, DCD, ECD—fundamentals for the practicing nephrologist. Clin J Am Soc Nephrol. 2009;4(11):1827-31.
13. Gracious N, Jose VR. Certification of brain stem death in India: medico-legal perspectives. Amrita J Med. 2020;16(2):71.
14. Shroff S. Twenty-five years of transplantation law in India—progress and the way forward. Indian J Transplant. 2019;13(3):151.
15. Sahay M. Transplantation of human organs and tissues Act—"Simplified." Indian J Transplant. 2018;12(2):84.
16. Pandit RA, Zirpe KG, Gurav SK, Kulkarni AP, Karnath S, Govil D, et al. Management of potential organ donor: Indian Society of Critical Care Medicine: position statement. Indian J Crit Care Med. 2017;21(5):303-16.
17. Srivastava A, Mani A. Deceased organ donation and transplantation in India: promises and challenges. Neurol India. 2018;66(2):316.
18. Navin S, Kanvinde H. Training of Trainers—Role of Police in Brain Death and Organ Donation—A Resource Manual. Mohan Foundation; 2015.
19. Mehta D, Saksena N, Mittal Y. Organ Transplant Law: Assessing Compatibility With the Right to Health [Internet]. Vidhi Center for Legal Policy; 2017. p. 65.

CHAPTER 23

Kidney Transplantation in Children

Arpana Iyengar, Arvind Bagga

CASE VIGNETTE

An 8-year-old boy was diagnosed with posterior urethral valves at 2 years of age and underwent fulguration for the same. Despite being on clean intermittent catheterization (CIC) and oxybutynin, he progressed to end-stage kidney disease (ESKD) by 7 years of age. He underwent augmentation cystoplasty and was on continuous ambulatory peritoneal dialysis for more than a year. Preparation for transplantation was initiated. The child's mother was evaluated and found to be a potential donor with no mismatches in HLA A, B or DR locus. The child underwent kidney transplantation and received induction therapy with Basiliximab followed by triple immunosuppression with tacrolimus, mycophenolate mofetil and steroids. Immediate postoperative period was uneventful and he was discharged with a stable serum creatinine of 0.5 mg/dL. He developed urinary tract infection after 2 months, despite continuing CIC and antibiotic prophylaxis. There was a rise in creatinine to a maximum of 1.8 mg/dL that reduced to 0.9 mg/L following treatment for the UTI. The boy is 10 years old now, goes to school, continuous to do CIC and maintains stable kidney function with a serum creatinine of 0.8 mg/dL.

INTRODUCTION

Kidney transplantation is the therapy of choice for children with end-stage kidney disease (ESKD) and is associated with better quality of life and lower risk of morbidity and mortality compared to other kidney replacement therapies. Patient and graft survival have significantly improved over the decades with changes in immunosuppressive protocols, operative techniques, and interventions for infection prophylaxis and monitoring. We discuss the indications, immunobiology, evaluation, monitoring, complications, management, and outcomes of transplantation in children.

CAUSES OF END-STAGE KIDNEY DISEASE AND INDICATIONS FOR TRANSPLANTATION

The chief causes of ESKD include congenital abnormalities of the kidney and urinary tract, followed by chronic glomerulonephritis and focal segmental glomerulosclerosis. Polycystic kidney diseases, nephronophthisis, Alport syndrome, congenital nephrotic syndrome, neuropathic bladder, cystinosis, and primary hyperoxaluria (PH) are also important causes.[1-3]

Indications for kidney transplantation in children include:[4]

- Symptoms of uremia not responsive to standard therapy
- Failure to thrive because of limited caloric intake
- Delayed psychomotor development and poor metabolic control, including hypervolemia, hyperkalemia, and metabolic bone disease.

Contraindications to kidney transplantation include the presence of untreated malignancy, active infections, chronic infection with human immunodeficiency virus (HIV), and progressive neurological diseases. A multidisciplinary team should carefully evaluate the option of transplantation in children with multiple congenital anomalies and severe mental retardation, with consent from ethicists and informed input from parents. Socioeconomic factors should be considered carefully before preparing infants and children for transplantation.[5] In preemptive transplantation, renal transplantation is undertaken without initiation of dialysis and is an ideal treatment option in children with good long-term outcomes. Patients who have received prolonged dialysis show a higher risk of allograft failure compared to those undergoing preemptive kidney transplantation.[6]

PRETRANSPLANT EVALUATION

The challenge of late detection of chronic kidney disease (CKD) and its comorbidities still exists as studies have observed one-third of children presenting for the first time to the nephrologist in stage III/IV, with 25% already being in stage V. This is a barrier to optimal pretransplant preparation.[3,7] Pretransplant evaluation is performed to make sure that the child can bear the surgical stress and identify any contraindications to transplantation. Evaluation includes immune evaluation with human leukocyte antigen (HLA)

CHAPTER HIGHLIGHTS

- Renal transplantation is the most effective form of renal replacement therapy in children.
- Preemptive renal transplantation in children has better graft and patient survival compared to those with a dialysis vintage of 12 to 18 months.
- Long-term challenges following transplantation are related to bacterial and viral infections, growth and medication related toxicities.
- Though the 5 years allograft survival is excellent, long-term graft survival poses challenges in low resource settings.
- Deceased organ transplantation with priority for pediatric recipients is a critical need.

and crossmatching, and optimization of anemia, cardiac function, bone disease, and nutritional status.

After clinical examination, a number of tests are performed, including blood group, HLA typing (A, B, and DR), and evaluation for preformed cytotoxic antibodies. The requirements for a transplant are a compatible blood group and a negative cytotoxic crossmatch. Serology for hepatitis (B and C) virus, HIV, cytomegalovirus (CMV), Epstein–Barr virus (EBV), varicella, and syphilis is necessary. A chest X-ray film, electrocardiogram, and echocardiogram are obtained to screen for pulmonary illnesses and structural cardiac diseases.

Urological Interventions

Evaluation of the lower urinary tract is required in patients with congenital anomalies of the kidney and urinary tract with or without obstruction. A renal ultrasound and voiding cystourethrography are mandatory to assess the lower urinary tract. When indicated, bladder evaluation might require cystoscopy and urodynamic studies. Children with small bladder capacity benefit with the use of medications (e.g., oxybutynin) that result in relaxation of the detrusor muscle. Patients with neurogenic bladder often require clean intermittent catheterization (CIC) of native bladders before and following transplantation. Bladder capacity is increased by its augmentation with segments of ileum, stomach or appendix, and creation of a permanent cutaneous conduit (Mitrofanoff) that enables the child to be continent with timely drainage through CIC.

Vesicoureteral reflux (VUR) following transplantation may result in recurrent urinary tract infections (UTIs), especially when associated with voiding dysfunction. However, in the post-transplant period, the presence of reflux per se without voiding dysfunction is not associated with subsequent graft function, hypertension, or rejection. In patients with VUR, the bladder is evaluated for obstruction, spasticity, and dysfunction. Both native dilated ureters can serve as vascularized patch grafts for augmentation cystoplasty. Transplant outcomes in patients with high-grade reflux may be disappointing due to postoperative UTI. Reimplantation prior to transplant might result in bladder wall changes that complicate transplant surgery.[8]

Nephrectomy of native kidneys is not usually necessary prior to transplantation. The indications for pretransplant nephrectomies include the need for space for the allograft (polycystic kidneys; small child receiving an adult kidney), massive proteinuria (congenital nephrotic syndrome), uncontrolled hypertension, recurrent pyelonephritis, severe polyuria (better volume control immediately post-transplant), and malignancy. Most surgeons do not prefer to do native nephrectomies during the time of transplant surgery.

Vaccination

Potential recipients should receive all age-appropriate immunizations, including hepatitis A and B, pneumococcal, and varicella vaccinations.[9,10] Live vaccines should be given at least 4 weeks prior to transplantation. Inactivated or killed vaccines can be administered 3–6 months post-transplantation.

Human Leukocyte Antigen Typing and Crossmatching

The ABO blood group and HLA are important for the survival of the allografts. ABO blood group antigens are expressed on endothelial cells. In the presence of ABO incompatibility, naturally present antibodies to these antigens may attach to antigens on the graft endothelium to cause hyperacute rejection and irreversible graft loss. HLA class I (A, B, and C) antigens are present on all nucleated cells, but not on red cells. HLA class II (DR, DQ, and DP) antigens are present on macrophages, dendritic cells, B cells, activated T lymphocytes, and tubular epithelial and endothelial cells. These antigens are expressed codominantly, with each individual inheriting one haplotype from each parent. HLA mismatches refer to a number of nonshared HLA between the donor and recipient. Children are one-haplotype matched with their parents, while siblings can be completely matched, one-haplotype matched, or completely mismatched, depending upon haplotype recombination.

Three types of crossmatch tests are important during pretransplant preparation—complement-dependent cytotoxicity (CDC), CDC-antihuman globulin HLA, and flow cytometry. The details of these investigations, including the risk of rejection, are given in **Table 1**.[11,12] The immunological risk of transplant is considered as "high risk" when the crossmatch is positive by all three methods, "intermediate risk" when flow cytometry and Luminex single antigen bead crossmatch are positive and "standard risk" when only Luminex single antigen bead assay is positive. Patients with all the above tests being negative are considered to have the least risk.

Human Leukocyte Antigen and ABO Incompatibility

HLA-DR, HLA-A, and HLA-B are important factors that influence post-transplant outcomes. Children may be sensitized (positive flow cytometry crossmatch or positive CDC crossmatch) as a consequence of repeated blood transfusions, infections, and previous events of renal transplantation. Rh matching is usually not a requirement for successful transplantation. While ABO compatibility between donor and recipient is considered a prerequisite for successful transplantation, ABO-incompatible transplants are increasingly being performed following desensitization with plasmapheresis and therapy with intravenous immunoglobulin (IVIg) and anti-CD20 monoclonal antibodies.[13,14]

TABLE 1: Types of crossmatching and immunological risk of transplant.

Parameters	*Complement-dependent cytotoxicity (CDC)*	*CDC-anti-human globulin*	*Flow cytometry*
HLA antibodies	Yes	Yes	Yes
Non-HLA antibodies	Yes	Yes	Yes
IgM antibodies	Yes	Yes	No
Antibody titer detected	Moderate to high	Moderate to low	Low
Low antibody titer detected	No	Some extent	Yes
Risk of rejection			
High	+	+	+
Intermediate	–	–	+
Standard	–	–	– (Luminex +)
Least risk	–	–	–

(HLA: human leukocyte antigen; IgM: immunoglobulin M)

PRETRANSPLANT COUNSELING

Families of recipients and donors are counseled regarding the risks of surgery and the need for lifelong follow-up. Patients are counseled regarding the risks of graft dysfunction, infections, and the importance of adherence to medications.

A number of disorders, chiefly PH1, C3 glomerulopathy (chiefly dense deposit disease), nongenetic forms of focal segmental glomerulosclerosis, and specific forms of atypical hemolytic uremic syndrome, may recur post-transplantation. Cardiac, pulmonary, dental, and psychological evaluations are required depending upon comorbidities. Growth and nutrition should be optimized as both malnutrition and obesity predispose to post-transplant complications. Clinical practice guidelines on the process of transplant evaluation are provided by Kidney Disease: Improving Global Outcomes (KDIGO).[15,16] Pediatric centers with an active transplant program are encouraged to have clearly written protocols for evaluation, monitoring, and follow-up of their patients.

INTRA- AND PERIOPERATIVE ISSUES

In infants and young children, the allograft is placed intra-abdominally. The renal artery is anastomosed to the aorta and renal vein to the inferior vena cava. In children weighing >30 kg, the graft is placed in the iliac fossa and the renal artery and vein are connected to the common or external iliac artery and vein, respectively **(Fig. 1)**. The ureter is anastomosed to the bladder using ureteroneocystostomy. Meticulous attention to aspects related to surgery is necessary to improve the short- and medium-term outcomes following transplantation.

Children need attention with regard to maintenance of hemodynamic stability during the intraoperative and perioperative periods. Intraoperative medical management includes close attention to fluid therapy, administration of immunosuppressive medication, diuretics, and antibiotics.

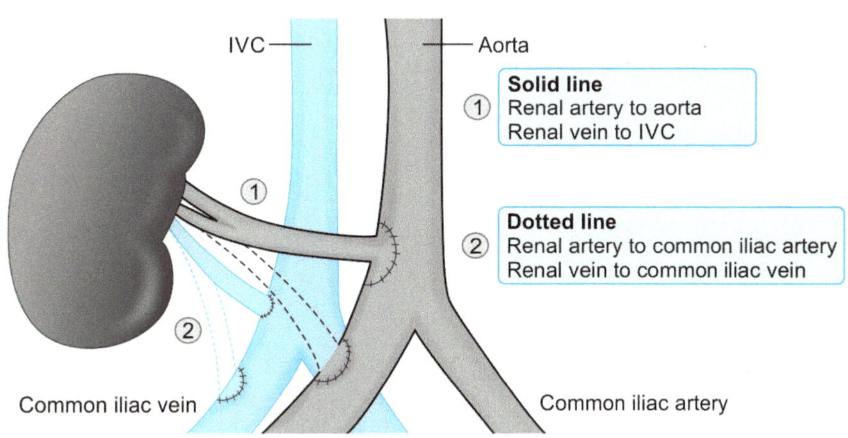

Fig. 1: Vascular anastomoses in (1) young children and (2) older children. (IVC: inferior vena cava)

Central venous pressure should be maintained at 10–15 cm of water before the aortic cross-clamps are removed to ensure good blood flow to the allograft. The adult kidney can contain up to 250 mL of blood, which may represent a large percentage of total blood volume in an infant or a small child. A low circulatory state can promote thrombosis of the allograft. Frusemide may be administered at a dose of 1–2 mg/kg to induce diuresis.

POSTOPERATIVE MANAGEMENT

Postoperative management includes close monitoring of fluid and electrolytes, immunosuppressive therapy, and anti-infective prophylaxis. In living-related transplants, the allograft kidney begins making urine almost immediately. Fluid and electrolyte management includes replacement of insensible losses and urine output with appropriate fluids, most commonly normal saline, dextrose normal saline, and occasionally N/2 saline or Ringer lactate. Close monitoring of serum electrolytes is useful for further adjustments. Common metabolic problems in the acute stage include hypokalemia, hyperglycemia, and rarely hypophosphatemia. Central venous pressure should be kept at 5–10 cm of water. A urinary catheter is left in place for 4–5 days. The duration of antibiotic administration varies in individual units.

Immunosuppression

The aim of immunosuppressive therapy in transplant recipients is to prevent or reduce sensitization to the allograft. This must be accomplished with constant attention to maintaining a balance in immunosuppression. Excess therapy results in an increased risk of infection and malignancy, while inadequate immunosuppression results in allograft rejection. Immunosuppression is initiated at the time of transplant surgery and continues through the life of the allograft. Immunosuppressive protocols, summarized in **Table 2**, are discussed below.[17]

Induction Therapy

Induction therapy is used to deplete or modulate T-cell responses at the time of antigen presentation; decrease the incidence, frequency, and severity of acute rejection; and improve survival of the allograft. The medications that are available include antithymocyte globulin (ATG), interleukin-2 receptor (IL2R) antibodies, and alemtuzumab.

Interleukin-2 receptor antagonists (basiliximab) are nonlymphocyte-depleting agents that inhibit the proliferation of activated T and B lymphocytes. Hypersensitivity reactions need to be monitored. Antithymocyte thymoglobulin (thymoglobulin, rabbit; ATGAM, horse) are polyclonal lymphocyte-depleting agents that target the HLA and other immune cell receptors resulting in cellular inactivation and depletion. Infusion-related reactions, leukopenia, and thrombocytopenia are common side effects. Alemtuzumab is a monoclonal agent targeting CD52 receptors, resulting in the depletion of T and B cells.

Infants and young children have relatively strong immune reactions, show rapid clearance of medications,

TABLE 2: Medications of the immunosuppressive protocol.

Immunosuppression	*Protocol*	*Dose*
Basiliximab	Day 0: Before transplant; 30 minutes after methylprednisolone dose Repeat dose on day 4	12 mg/m^2; IV infusion over 30 minutes <30 kg: 10 mg; >30 kg: 20 mg
Antithymocyte globulin	4–5 doses	1.5 mg/kg
Corticosteroids	Day-1: Oral prednisolone Day-0: IV methylprednisolone ~90 minutes before surgery Day-1 onward: Oral prednisolone	60 mg/m^2 10 mg/kg 60–30 mg/m^2/day till day 30 30–15 mg/m^2 till day 60 15–7.5 mg/m^2 till 6 months, taper
Cyclosporine	Day-1 onward: Oral Day-0: Evening of transplant Target 2-hour cyclosporine levels 0–3 months: 1,000–1,200 ng/mL 3–12 months: 800–1,000 ng/mL >12 months: 600–800 ng/mL	6–8 mg/kg/day in two divided doses Dose titrated to 2-hour drug levels
Tacrolimus	Day-1 onward: Oral Day-0: Evening of transplant Target trough tacrolimus levels 0–3 months: 10–12 ng/mL 3–12 months: 8–10 ng/mL >12 months: 5–8 ng/mL	0.1–0.15 mg/kg/dose twice a day Dose titrated to trough levels
Mycophenolate mofetil	Day-1 onward: Oral	600 mg/m^2/dose Reduced by 50% if receiving tacrolimus

and benefit from induction therapies. In low-risk individuals (first transplant, unsensitized recipients), most centers prefer to use either no induction or IL2R antibodies (basiliximab). Induction with basiliximab is extended in steroid avoidance protocols. Polyclonal antibody (thymoglobulin and ATG) is used in high-risk recipients, such as highly sensitized patients, retransplants, and patients with delayed graft function. These agents, including alemtuzumab, are also part of steroid withdrawal and immunosuppression minimization protocols.

Steroid Avoidance

Long-term adverse effects of steroids have resulted in steroid avoidance trials, especially in children. The KDIGO guidelines recommended that steroids can be discontinued in the first week of transplant in those with low risk and if induction therapy was administered.[18] However, there is wide variability in the use of such protocols across centers.[19] Early steroid withdrawal or avoidance is generally used following the induction therapy with mono or polyclonal antibodies, while late steroid withdrawal is undertaken when no induction therapy was used. Protocols of steroid minimization show growth-related benefits in prepubertal patients. Steroid avoidance in pediatric transplant recipients is effective in terms of graft outcomes during the first year following transplantation, and with limited adverse effects.[20]

POST-TRANSPLANT COMPLICATIONS

Delayed Graft Function

Delayed graft function is empirically defined as the need for dialysis in the first 7 days following transplantation; the condition is more common in deceased donor compared to live donor transplants. Delayed graft function has detrimental consequences on the graft, including the risk of acute rejection and lower graft survival. Intradialytic hypotension and thrombosis can potentially affect graft survival.[21] The overall incidence of delayed graft function in live-related transplantation is 1–4%, while it is 5–50% in deceased donor transplantation.[22]

The underlying pathophysiology of delayed graft function is due to ischemia (before or during organ procurement), which is aggravated by the reperfusion injury during implantation of the harvested organ in the recipient. There is tissue injury due to stimulation of various factors, e.g., inducible nitric oxide synthase and anerobic metabolism with depletion of adenosine triphosphate (ATP) that results in generation of reactive oxygen species. Inflammatory cell infiltration releases mediators, which further aggravate the injury. The consequences are detrimental and can result in acute rejection and compromised long-term graft survival.

Surgical Complications

Surgical complications include lymphocele, perirenal serous fluid collection, hematoma, urinary leaks, and ureterovesical junction obstruction. Usually, no therapy is needed. If perirenal fluid collection is massive or causes pressure on the transplanted kidney, percutaneous aspiration may be needed. Ureteral stents are used for the prevention and treatment of ureterovesical junction obstruction. Vascular complications include renal arterial and venous thrombosis, which are particularly common in infants and small children. Attention to technical details and prevention of postoperative dehydration help prevent these complications.

Acute Rejection

Acute deterioration in kidney allograft function is associated with specific pathologic changes in the graft. Acute rejection is of two types: antibody-mediated rejection (ABMR) and T cell-mediated rejection (TCMR). Hyperacute rejection could happen within minutes after the transplant due to preformed antibody or ABO incompatibility. The presence of circulating donor-specific alloantibodies, inflammation of glomeruli (glomerulitis), or peritubular capillary (peritubular capillaritis) are hallmarks of ABMR. Lymphocytic infiltration of the tubules and interstitium, and occasionally the arterial intima, is characteristic of TCMR.

Screening for rejection is done by conventional methods of measuring serum creatinine, estimated glomerular filtration rate (eGFR), and quantification of protein excretion. Periodic screening for CMV, EBV, and polyomavirus is indicated. Renal biopsy is undertaken in the event of a rise of serum creatinine. Post-transplant HLA alloantibody screening is used to characterize the type of acute rejection.

The Banff classification for rejection includes six categories of diagnosis:[23] (1) Normal biopsy or nonspecific changes, (2) antibody-mediated changes, (3) borderline acute TCMR, (4) TCMR, (5) interstitial fibrosis and tubular atrophy, and (6) other nonrejection changes.

Classification of Antibody-mediated Rejection

- *Active ABMR:* Microvascular inflammation, intimal arteritis; linear C4d staining in peritubular capillaries; donor-specific antibodies (**Figs. 2A and 2B**).
- *Chronic active ABMR:* Transplant glomerulopathy, peritubular capillary basement membrane multilayering, and intimal fibrosis; linear C4d staining in peritubular capillaries; donor-specific antibodies (**Fig. 2B**).
- *Chronic ABMR:* Transplant glomerulopathy, peritubular capillary basement membrane multilayering, and intimal fibrosis; prior diagnosis of active or chronic active ABMR; donor-specific antibodies.

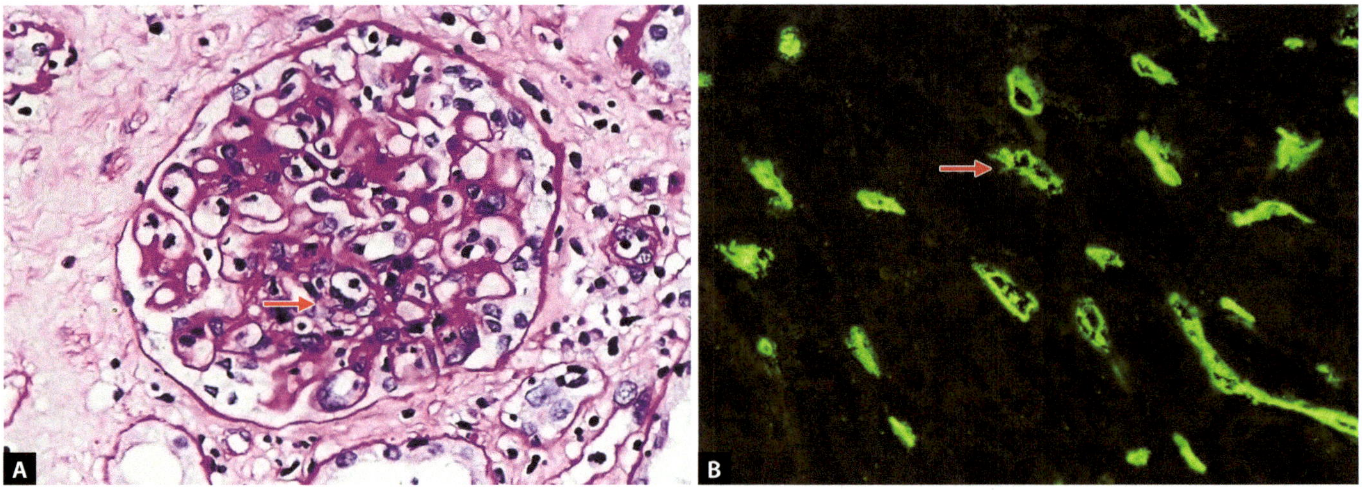

Figs. 2A and B: (A) Transplant glomerulitis in active antibody-mediated rejection: Periodic acid–Schiff (PAS) stain highlights the glomerular capillaries, which are dilated and partially obliterated by mononuclear and swollen endothelial cells (arrow); (B) C4d by immunofluorescence in a patient with acute antibody-mediated rejection. There is widespread circumferential staining of the peritubular capillaries (arrow).
Courtesy: Dr Anila Abraham, Renopath Lab, Chennai.

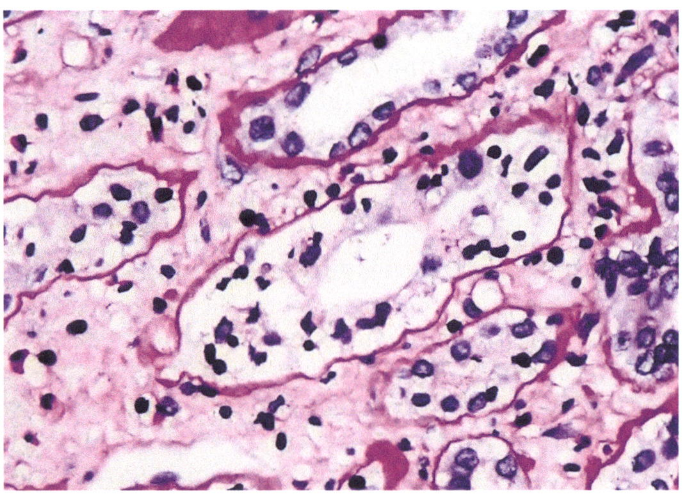

Fig. 3: Severe tubulitis in a patient with acute cell-mediated rejection. Periodic acid–Schiff (PAS) stain delineates the tubular basement membrane, allowing identification and counting of lymphocytes within the tubule.
Courtesy: Dr Anila Abraham, Renopath Lab, Chennai.

Classification of T cell-mediated Rejection

- *Active TCMR:* (1A) Moderate tubulitis with interstitial inflammation; (1B) severe tubulitis with interstitial inflammation; (2A) mild-to-moderate intimal arteritis; (2B) severe intimal arteritis; (3) transmural arteritis with/without fibrinoid necrosis **(Fig. 3)**
- *Chronic active TCMR:* (1A) Moderate tubulitis with cortical inflammation; (1B) severe tubulitis with cortical inflammation; (2) arterial intimal fibrosis with mononuclear cell inflammation **(Fig. 3)**

A summary of medications and strategies for the treatment of acute rejection are given in **Table 3**. The reader is advised to refer to recent guidelines for management.[24]

TABLE 3: Therapeutic options in the management of antibody-mediated and T cell-mediated rejection.

Antibody-mediated rejection	*T cell-mediated rejection*
• Pulse corticosteroids • Thymoglobulin • Plasma exchange • Rituximab • Bortezomib • Eculizumab	• Pulse corticosteroids; oral steroids • Thymoglobulin • Optimize immunosuppression • Alemtuzumab

Chronic Rejection

Chronic rejection is defined as impaired graft function of at least 3 months after transplant that is independent of acute rejection, drug toxicity, and recurrence of the disease. Chronic rejection results in a progressive decline in GFR in the presence of hypertension and proteinuria.[25] Histopathological features range from transplant glomerulopathy to arteriosclerosis, chronic interstitial fibrosis, and tubular atrophy. Risk factors for chronic rejection include the presence of donor-specific antibodies, recurrent acute rejection, inadequate immunosuppression, deceased donor transplantation, recurrent infections, BK virus nephropathy, and nephrotoxicity associated with calcineurin inhibitors. The management is supportive, with modification of therapy in patients with calcineurin inhibitor-associated nephrotoxicity.

Hypertension

Hypertension in the early post-transplant period is related to fluid overload and due to the use of corticosteroids and calcineurin inhibitors. Later, hypertension is seen in a majority of patients and may be related to disease of native kidneys and side effects of immunosuppressive medications. Hypertension is managed with low-sodium diet and medications, usually calcium channel or β-adrenergic blockers. Angiotensin-converting enzyme inhibitors (ACEIs) are considered useful due to their inhibitory effect on proteinuria and glomerulosclerosis, and cardioprotection. A combination of both calcium channel blockers and ACEI is satisfactory in those with severe hypertension.[26] Ambulatory blood pressure monitoring helps in the diagnosis of masked and nocturnal hypertension, both of which may contribute to cardiovascular morbidity.

Side Effects of Medications

Cosmetic side effects may be the reason for noncompliance and delayed acute rejection, particularly in adolescents. Tacrolimus is associated with nephrotoxicity, tremors, and diabetes mellitus and cyclosporine can cause nephrotoxicity, hypertension, tremors, hirsutism, and gum hyperplasia. Diarrhea, vomiting, and myelosuppression are common with MMF; patients receiving azathioprine need monitoring for myelosuppression, pancreatitis, and hepatotoxicity.

Metabolic and Hematological Complications

Metabolic complications following transplantation include hypomagnesemia, hypophosphatemia, hyperkalemia, and renal tubular acidosis. Dyslipidemia is a complication of therapy with steroids, sirolimus, and calcineurin inhibitors. Children receiving tacrolimus are at risk of hyperglycemia, with ~5% developing new-onset diabetes mellitus after transplantation (NODAT) in the long term. Other risk factors for NODAT include the use of high-dose steroids and a family history of diabetes. Strict control of diabetes is essential for long-term patient and graft survival.

Hematological complications include anemia, erythrocytosis, and thrombocytopenia. Anemia may be related to bone marrow suppression due to therapy with mycophenolate mofetil (MMF), azathioprine, or tacrolimus. Aplastic anemia can occur due to parvovirus B19 and CMV infection, and hemolytic anemia due to recurrent hemolytic-uremic syndrome. Neutropenia and thrombocytopenia might be due to underlying viral infection or secondary to immunosuppressive medication(s).

Recurrent Disease

Disease recurrence is an important complication following transplantation.[27] In children undergoing kidney transplant, 7–8% of graft loss is secondary to recurrence of which 70–80% is due to glomerulonephritis.[28] Recurrence of the primary disease may result in a high risk of graft loss (>30–50%) in focal segmental glomerulosclerosis (FSGS) (14–50%), membranoproliferative glomerulonephritis (30–100%), membranous nephropathy (50%), hemolytic-uremic syndrome (20–60%), and PH1 (80–100%). Recurrent FSGS is defined as persistent proteinuria of a urine spot protein creatinine (UPCR) ratio of ≥1 in case of a previously anuric patient or an increase of UPCR by ≥1 in patients with proteinuria at the time of transplantation. Genetic testing is important as the risk of recurrent FSGS is minimal in patients with pathogenic or likely pathogenic variants. Risk factors of recurrence include late steroid resistance (>80%), time to end-stage renal disease <48 months, and sclerosis at the time of renal biopsy. The donor should undergo genetic evaluation; heterozygous carrier of a recessive genetic disorder or those with a variant of unknown significance may be considered for transplantation, after explaining the risk of recurrence.[29]

Urological Disorders

Patients with urological problems have a higher rate of infections and urological procedures post-transplant. A study from India showed that of 44 patients with abnormal bladder who underwent renal transplantation, graft survival at 1 and 2 years was 72.7% and 59%, respectively.[8]

Infections

Infections are a major morbidity following transplantation. While bacterial infections are most commonly observed in the first month of transplantation, fungal and viral infections occur 1–6 months later. UTIs are important, especially in patients with congenital abnormalities of the urinary tract, neurogenic bladder, and bladder dysfunction.

A retrospective study in adult transplant recipients from India showed that CMV, tuberculosis, and fungal infections had a prevalence of 21.8%, 10.6%, and 23%, respectively. Pulmonary infections due *to Pneumocystis jirovecii* need early recognition and therapy. Co-trimoxazole prophylaxis, up to 6 months following transplantation, is strongly recommended. Tuberculosis can rarely develop in the first year following transplantation and that requires intensive therapy for 3 months, followed by a less intensive schedule for the next 9 months. The use of rifampicin is restricted due to its interactions with calcineurin inhibitors. Systemic mycoses due to *Aspergillus*, *Candida*, and *Cryptococcus* infections may rarely occur.

With limited access to molecular diagnostic tests, regular monitoring for CMV, EBV, and BK virus is a challenge **(Table 4)**. For details, the reader is directed to the KDIGO guidelines on hepatitis C infection in transplantation and a recent review on viral infections in pediatric transplantation.[30,31]

Growth and Nutrition

Growth failure or short stature impedes the quality of life and has an important effect on psychological development.

TABLE 4: Common viral infections following renal transplantation.

Virus	Clinical features	Diagnosis	Treatment
Cytomegalovirus	Fever, malaise invasive disease; organ dysfunction	• Pancytopenia, elevated transaminases • Blood PCR • Biopsy shows viral inclusions	Valganciclovir daily till PCR negative, followed by prophylaxis for 180 days
Epstein–Barr virus	• Infectious mononucleosis-like syndrome • Lymphoproliferative disease	• PCR for RNA load • Viral capsid or nuclear antigen • Biopsy: Nuclear inclusions	• Reduce immunosuppression • Rituximab • Chemotherapy
Hepatitis C virus	• Asymptomatic • Weight loss, jaundice • Elevated tacrolimus trough levels	• Nucleic acid testing positive • Abnormal liver function tests • Renal biopsy: Membranous or membranoproliferative glomerulonephritis	Specific antiviral therapy[30]
BK virus	• Preclinical latent phase • Clinical: Graft dysfunction sterile pyuria • Hemorrhagic cystitis • Ureteric stenosis	• Blood PCR: BK virus >4 log copies/mL • Urine PCR: >1 × 10^7 copies/mL • mRNA >6 log copies/ng total urine RNA • Urine: Decoy cells • Biopsy: Tubulointerstitial fibrosis	Reduce immunosuppression >10,000 copies/mL: CNI sparing regimen; leflunomide; intravenous immunoglobulin

(CNI: calcineurin inhibitors; mRNA: messenger ribonucleic acid; PCR: polymerase chain reaction; RNA: ribonucleic acid)

Majority of pediatric allograft recipients do not achieve normal adult height even with good graft function. Post-transplant growth is more likely to be affected in young children than in older children and adolescents. Efforts to improve nutritional intake, correct metabolic acidosis, and minimize corticosteroid therapy are necessary. Growth hormone therapy is indicated in patients with persistent short stature.[32,33]

Malignancy

The risk of malignancy is increased with the intensity and duration of immunosuppression. The chief malignancy in children is a post-transplant lymphoproliferative disorder, noted in 1–10% transplant recipients, particularly in seronegative recipients of EBV-positive donors. An increased risk of post-transplant lymphoproliferative disorder is seen in younger children and can manifest as early as the first year of transplant, or later in the second or third year. The severity ranges from infectious mononucleosis-like illness to a lymphoma-like illness. Key strategy for management includes the reduction of immunosuppression.[34]

ADULT VERSUS PEDIATRIC TRANSPLANTATION

There are many differences between adult and pediatric renal transplantation, listed in **Table 5**. The distinguishing features are the spectrum of native kidney disease, pharmacokinetics of transplant-related medications, risk of infection, issues related to growth, quality of life, and immunological basis for better graft survival. Maintaining long-term graft function is critical since the projected patient survival is several decades longer than in adults. Multidisciplinary inputs from the pediatric nephrologist, transplant surgeon, urologist, anesthetist, immunologist, dietitian, and social worker are vital in providing optimum care to children.

TRANSPLANT OUTCOMES

Data from the North American Pediatric Renal Trails Collaborative Studies (NAPRTCS) shows graft survival rates at 1, 3, and 5 as 99.5%, 97.2%, and 94.9% in living donor transplants and as 97.6%, 94.4%, and 90.1%, respectively, in deceased donor transplants.[1] Preemptive transplantation is associated with improved patient and graft survival.[1,6] Though the 1-year allograft survival rates of transplants across centers in India are quite similar to the NAPRTCS report, the outcomes at 5 years are less satisfactory.[35-41] Several factors might contribute to the disparities in transplant outcomes between the developed and the developing world.

Deceased organ transplantation programs are active only in a few states in India, and there is a need to focus on prioritized allocation criteria for children. A dedicated website (www.notto.gov.in) has been launched by the National Organ Transplant Program for providing information on organ and tissue donation, organ and tissue pledging, networking of hospitals, and establishing the national registry of organ and tissue transplantation and donation. The two important amendments made with regard to kidney transplantation under the Transplantation of Human Organs and Tissue Act (THOTA) include expansion of the definition of near relative to include grandparents and provision of swap donation.

In children, the outcomes of graft survival are comparable between deceased organs and living donor transplantation. An Indian study on 37 children, who received kidneys from adult deceased donors, showed 1-, 3-, 5-, and 10-year death-censored graft survival to be 90.4%, 86.4%, 73.3%, and 73.3%, respectively.[42]

TABLE 5: Differences between adult and pediatric renal transplantation.

Characteristics	***Adult***	***Children***
Common native kidney disease	Diabetes, hypertension	Congenital anomalies of kidneys and urinary tract, chronic glomerulonephritis
Pretransplant evaluation	Urological preparation not a common need	Need urological evaluation and preparation in selected cases
Vascular anastomoses	Mainly external iliac vessels	Involve the distal aorta and vena cava just cephalad to the bifurcation in infants; common iliac vessels in young children; external iliac vessels in adolescents
Drug pharmacokinetics	Well-established drug response and toxicity profiles	• Need higher dose immunosuppression (mg/kg) to maintain therapeutic levels • Higher drug metabolism • Varied adverse effects and toxicity profile • Need for special formulations
Physical growth	Not a relevant parameter	Important determinant of well being
Infection	Seropositive to viral infections	Seronegative to most viral infections
Graft survival	Reduces with age	• Best in children <5 years old • Adolescents are a high-risk group

CONCLUSION

Transplantation is the most effective form of kidney replacement therapy in children. With advances in immunobiology and immunosuppressants, both allograft and patient outcomes continue to improve. Main morbidities following transplantation are related to bacterial and viral infections, and growth and medication-related toxicities. Young children weighing <10 kg and those with congenital or functional disorders of the lower urinary tract pose significant medical and surgical challenges.

REFERENCES

1. Chua A, Cramer C, Moudgil A, Martz K, Smith J, Blydt-Hansen T, et al. Kidney transplant practice patterns and outcome benchmarks over 30 years: the 2018 report of the NAPRTCS. Pediatr Transplant. 2019;(8):e13597.
2. North American Pediatric Renal Trials and Collaborative Studies (2014). 2014 Annual Transplant Report. [online] Available from https://web.emmes.com/study/ped/annlrept/annualrept2014.pdf. [Last accessed June, 2022].
3. Kamath N, Iyengar AA. Chronic kidney disease (CKD): an observational study of etiology, severity and burden of comorbidities. Indian J Pediatr. 2017;84(11):822-5.
4. Davis ID, Bunchman TE, Grimm PC, Benfield MR, Briscoe DM, Harmon WE, et al. Pediatric renal transplantation: indications and special considerations. A position paper from the Pediatric Committee of the American Society of Transplant Physicians. Pediatr Transplant. 1998;2(2):117-29.
5. Iyengar A, Lewin S, Lantos JD. Considering family resources when making medical recommendations. Pediatrics. 2018;141(1):e20171198.
6. Amaral S, Sayed BA, Kutner N, Patzer RE. Preemptive kidney transplantation is associated with survival benefits among pediatric patients with end-stage renal disease. Kidney Int. 2016;90(5):1100-8.
7. Hari P, Singla IK, Mantan M, Kanitkar M, Batra B, Bagga A. Chronic renal failure in children. Indian Pediatr. 2003;40:1035-42.
8. Mishra SK, Muthu V, Rajapurkar MM, Desai MR. Kidney transplantation in abnormal bladder. Indian J Urol. 2007;23(3):299-304.
9. Kroger AT, Duchin J, Vázquez M. (2017) ACIP General Best Practice Guidelines for Immunization. Recommendations. CDC. [online] Available from https://www.cdc.gov/vaccines/hcp/acip-recs/general-recs/index.html. [Last accessed June, 2022].
10. Banerjee S, Dissanayake PV, Abeyagunawardena AS. Vaccinations in children on immunosuppressive medications for renal disease. Pediatr Nephrol. 2016;31(9):1437-48.
11. Althaf MM, Kossi ME, Jin JK, Sharma A, Halawa AM. Human leukocyte antigen typing and crossmatch: a comprehensive review. World J Transplant. 2017;7(6):339-48.
12. South AM, Grimm PC. Transplant immunodiagnostics: crossmatch and antigen detection. Pediatr Nephrol. 2016;31:897-905.
13. Jha PK, Bansal SB, Sethi SK, Jain M, Sharma R, Nandwani A, et al. ABO-incompatible renal transplantation in developing world—crossing the immunological (and mental) barrier. Indian J Nephrol. 2016;26(2):113-8.
14. Sethi SK, Bansal SB, Wadhwani N, Tiwari A, Arora D, Sharma R, et al. Pediatric ABO-incompatible kidney transplantation: evolving with the advancing apheresis technology: a single-center experience. Pediatr Transplant. 2018;22(3):e13138.
15. Lentine KL, Kasiske BL, Levey AS, Adams PL, Alberú J, Bakr MA, et al. KDIGO clinical practice guideline on the evaluation and care of living kidney donors. Transplantation. 2017;101(8S Suppl 1):S1-109.
16. Chadban SJ, Ahn C, Axelrod DA, Foster BJ, Kasiske B, Kher V, et al. KDIGO clinical practice guideline on the evaluation and management of candidates for kidney transplantation. Transplantation. 2020;104:S103.
17. Wiseman AC. Immunosuppressive medications. Clin J Am Soc Nephrol. 2016;11(2):332-43.
18. Kidney Disease: Improving Global Outcomes (KDIGO) Transplant Work Group. KDIGO clinical practice guideline for the care of kidney transplant recipients. Am J Transplant. 2009;9(Suppl 3):S1.

19. Nehus E, Liu C, Hooper DK, Macaluso M, Kim MO. Clinical practice of steroid avoidance in pediatric kidney transplantation. Am J Transplant. 2015;15(8):2203-10.
20. Puliyanda DP, Pizzo H, Rodig N, Somers MJ. Early outcomes comparing induction with antithymocyte globulin vs alemtuzumab in two steroid-avoidance protocols in pediatric renal transplantation. Pediatr Transplant. 2020;24(3):e13685.
21. Schroppel B, Legendre C. Delayed kidney graft function: from mechanism to translation. Kidney Int. 2014;86(2):251-8.
22. Grenda R. Delayed graft function and its management in children. Pediatr Nephrol. 2017;32(7):1157-67.
23. Jeong HJ. Diagnosis of renal transplant rejection: Banff classification and beyond. Kidney Res Clin Pract. 2020; 39(1):17-31.
24. Leblanc J, Subrt P, Paré M, Hartell D, Sénécal L, Blydt-Hansen T, et al. Practice patterns in the treatment and monitoring of acute T cell-mediated kidney graft rejection in Canada. Can J Kidney Health Dis. 2018;5:2054358117753616.
25. Shreshta B, Haylor J. Evolution of the concept and pathogenesis of chronic renal allograft injury: an updated review. Exp Clin Transplant. 2016;14(6):596-605.
26. Seeman T, Feber J. Should ACE inhibitors or calcium channel blockers be used for post-transplant hypertension? Pediatr Nephrol. 2020;36(3):539-49.
27. Lim WH, Shingde M, Wong G. Recurrent and de novo glomerulonephritis post renal transplantation. Front Immunol. 2019;10:1944.
28. Cosio FG, Cattran DC. Recent advances in our understanding of recurrent primary glomerulonephritis after kidney transplantation. Kidney Int. 2017;91(2):304-14.
29. Cochat P, Fargue S, Mestrallet G, Jungraithmayr T, Koch-Nogueira P, Ranchin B, et al. Disease recurrence in pediatric renal transplantation. Pediatr Nephrol. 2009;24(11):2097-108.
30. Kidney Disease: Improving Global Outcomes (KDIGO) Hepatitis C Work Group. KDIGO 2018 clinical practice guideline for the prevention, diagnosis, evaluation, and treatment of hepatitis C in chronic kidney disease. Kidney Int Suppl. 2018;8:91-165.
31. Scaggs Huang FA, Danziger-Isakov L. Infectious disease risks in pediatric renal transplantation. Pediatr Nephrol. 2019;34(7):1155-66.
32. Mehls O, Fine RN. Growth hormone treatment after renal transplantation: a promising but underused chance to improve growth. Pediatr Nephrol. 2013;28(1):1-4.
33. Ingulli EG, Mak RH. Growth in children with chronic kidney disease: role of nutrition, growth hormone, dialysis, and steroids. Curr Opin Pediatr. 2014;26(2):187-92.
34. Mynarek M, Schober T, Behrends U, Maecker-Kolhoff B. Posttransplant lymphoproliferative disease after pediatric solid organ transplantation. Clin Dev Immunol. 2013;2013: 814973.
35. Chacko B, Rajamanickam T, Neelakantan N, Tamilarasi V, John GT. Pediatric renal transplantation—a single center experience of 15 years from India. Pediatr Transplant. 2017; 11(8):844-9.
36. Vasudevan A, Iyengar A, Jose B, Phadke K. Pediatric renal transplantation: a single-center experience. Transplant Proc. 2008;40(4):1095-8.
37. Sinha A, Hari P, Guleria S, Gulati A, Dinda AK, Mehra NK, et al. Outcome of pediatric renal transplantation in north India. Pediatr Transplant. 2010;14(7):836-43.
38. Meena J, Sinha A, Hari P, Dinda AK, Khandelwal P, Goswami S, et al. Pediatric kidney transplantation: experience over two decades. Asian J Pediatr Nephrol. 2018;1(1):22-8.
39. Srivastava A, Prabhakaran S, Sureka SK, Kapoor R, Kumar A, Sharma RK, et al. The challenges and outcomes of living donor kidney transplantation in pediatric and adolescent age group in a developing country: a critical analysis from a single center of north India. Indian J Urol. 2015;31(1):33-7.
40. Phadke K, Iyengar A, Karthik S, Kumar A, Olakkengil S. Pediatric renal transplantation: the Bangalore experience. Indian Pediatr. 2006;43(1):44-8.
41. Bijalwan P, Sanjeevan KV, Mathew A, Nair TB. Outcome and complications of living donor pediatric renal transplantation: experience from a tertiary care center. Ind J Urol. 2017; 33(3):221-5.
42. Kute VB, Trivedi HL, Vanikar AV, Shah PR, Gumber MR, Patel HV, et al. Long-term outcome of deceased donor renal transplantation in pediatric recipients: a single-center experience from a developing country. Pediatr Transplant. 2012;16(6):651-7.

CHAPTER 24

Reproductive Health in Kidney Transplantation

Urmila Anandh, Swarnalatha Guditi, Divya Bajpai

INTRODUCTION

Kidney transplantation almost completely reverses the abnormal uremic physiology. Most kidney recipients hope and often succeed in becoming parents. A successful pregnancy outcome is often dependent on many clinical factors associated with the patient. Besides, advances in immunosuppressive therapy, obstetric and neonatal care has contributed significantly toward both maternity and paternity in transplant recipients.

FERTILITY IN END-STAGE KIDNEY DISEASE

End-stage kidney disease (ESKD) affects fertility in both men and women. The predominant cause of infertility in men is shown to be changes in the male sex hormone (testosterone).[1] This hormonal imbalance is the consequence of physiologic changes in the hypothalamic–pituitary–gonadal (HPG) axis.[2] Leydig cell dysfunction also contributes to profound hypogonadism in male ESKD patients.

Uremia causes direct effects on spermatogenesis and sperm function in men with advanced chronic kidney disease (CKD). Semen analysis showed decreased volume, oligoasthenozoospermia, decreased sperm viability and motility.[3] Testicular pathology showed Sertoli cell atrophy and increased fibrosis.

Infertility in young males with ESKD is often seen with congenital genitourinary developmental defects associated with congenital anomalies of kidney and urinary tract (CAKUT).[4] Ejaculatory dysfunction (ED) is also one of the important and common causes of male infertility in ESKD.[5] Uremic myopathy, nutritional deficiencies, vascular factors, and use of pharmacological agents (β-blockers, diuretics, neuromodulators) also predispose to ED in male ESKD patients.[6]

In women, the uremic pathophysiology interferes with conception in many ways. It interferes with female reproductive cycle, ovulation, and is responsible for deranged levels of reproductive hormones.[7]

Older studies have reported that women on dialysis are often amenorrheic or oligomenorrheic suggesting anovulation.[8] Recent advances in dialysis and uremia control have led to an improvement in reproductive function with 42% of women on dialysis reporting menstrual cycles.[9] Most women have low estrogen and progesterone levels leading to uterine atrophy. The normal physiology of tonic and cyclic gonadotropin secretion in dialysis women is absent. This absence of cyclicity is presumed to due a defect in the hypothalamic regulation of gonadotropin secretion.[10] Also, high follicle-stimulating hormone (FSH) levels in these patients mimic a postmenopausal state.

Another factor responsible for this deranged physiology is the increased levels of prolactin in dialysis patients. These increased levels are presumably because of increased secretion and reduced renal clearance.[11] Women on dialysis have high circulating endorphin levels because of impaired renal clearance which are implicated in anovulation.[12] The altered reproductive pathophysiology is summarized in **Figure 1**.

FERTILITY AFTER RENAL TRANSPLANTATION

The functions of the hypothalamic–pituitary–ovarian axis normalize in females after few months of kidney transplantation. Sex hormone levels tend to normalize, sexual function improves, and ovulation and menstruation return. In men, the hormonal levels are also restored. The sperm quality and spermatogenesis are also restored in the majority of patients.[13,14] In a case series from the Nizams Institute of Medical Sciences (NIMS), Hyderabad, four out of six male KTRs became fathers despite having abnormal sperm count.

However, not all men and women would experience recovery of fertility after transplantation despite the reversal of the uremic pathophysiology.[15]

EFFECT OF IMMUNOSUPPRESSION ON PREGNANCY

Paternal exposure to corticosteroids, calcineurin inhibitors (CNIs), and azathioprine (AZA) do not document an

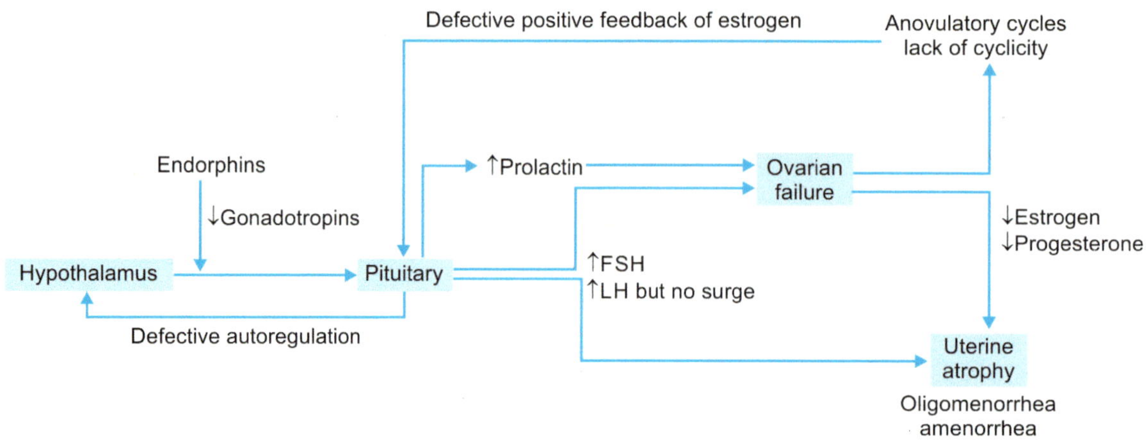

Fig. 1: Endocrine changes in women with chronic kidney disease (CKD). (FSH: follicle-stimulating hormone; LH: luteinizing hormone)

CHAPTER HIGHLIGHTS

- Reproductive function in patients with CKD is suboptimal because of altered sex hormone physiology.
- The reproductive function improves following kidney transplantation.
- With improved care, a pregnant kidney transplant recipient (KTR) hopes to undergo a successful pregnancy with minimal maternal complications.
- Fetal complications in a pregnant KTR are still common but improving continuously.
- Rigorous selection criteria and management of a pregnancy reduce the deleterious impact on allograft function.

increased risk of obstetric complications or congenital malformations.[16] The use of mammalian target of rapamycin inhibitors (m-TORi) in males has severe effects on fertility.[17] Mycophenolic acid (MPA) is teratogenic and paternal MPA exposure at the time of conception could theoretically pose a threat to the unborn child.[18]

Transplacental transfer of corticosteroids in pregnant mothers may have adverse effects on glucose metabolism and may aggravate gestational diabetes.[19] The fetus does not convert AZA to the active 6-mercaptopurine. MPA crosses the placenta and exerts adverse fetal effects causing malformations. MPA also increases the risk of miscarriage, preterm birth, and low birth weight.[18,20] Kidney Disease Improving Global Outcomes (KDIGO) and European Best Practice Guidelines advise switching from mycophenolate to AZA before pregnancy.[21] CNIs pass across the placenta, but the degree of transfer is limited. In the mother, CNIs may exacerbate hypertension.[22]

In female KTRs, an increased prevalence of hypogonadism, dysmenorrhea, ovarian cysts, and infertility has been documented with m-TORi. These drugs are teratogenic and it is advisable to discontinue when pregnancy is contemplated. However, few case reports highlight successful pregnancies with these drugs.[23]

PREGNANCY IN A KIDNEY TRANSPLANT RECIPIENT—MATERNAL AND FETAL COMPLICATIONS

CASE VIGNETTE 1

A 22-year-old KTR presented to our outpatient department (OPD) enquiring about fertility and pregnancy. She received a kidney 2 years back from her mother. Her kidney function was stable (serum creatinine –0.8 mg/dL) and she had no proteinuria. Her blood pressure was controlled with 5 mg of enalapril. She was on triple immunosuppression which included mycophenolate mofetil (MMF). After extensive counseling and discussion with the obstetric team in our hospital, she was shifted to AZA and amlodipine. Her enalapril and MMF were stopped. She was advised contraception for another 3 months at least. After a year, she became pregnant. The first two trimesters were uneventful (one episode of asymptomatic bacteriuria) and she was doing well till her 32nd week of pregnancy. A week later, she developed superimposed preeclampsia. The maternal and fetal conditions were assessed and she underwent an elective cesarean section. The baby was 1.8 kg at birth and needed neonatal intensive care for 2 days. Currently, both mother and child are doing well.

This case illustrates that more than maternal complications, fetal complications are still common in pregnant KTRs. Transplant recipients are at a higher risk of having a preterm birth.[24,25] In the UK Transplant Pregnancy Registry,[26] maternal hypertension and baseline graft dysfunction (serum creatinine of >1.7 mg/dL) were found to be risk factors for preterm birth. The incidence of low birth weight and fetal growth restriction was also higher among transplant recipients.[26,27] Published registry and in-center reports suggest a 50–64% rate of preterm delivery. Most preterm deliveries occur because of maternal and fetal compromise rather than spontaneous preterm labor.[28] The incidence of intrauterine growth retardation is as high as 30–50% in KTRs, mostly because of secondary hypertension and the propensity to develop preeclampsia as illustrated in our case.[29]

Preterm birth and low birth weight increase not only neonatal mortality but also the likelihood of long-term complications such as developmental deficits, diabetes, hypertension, and cardiovascular diseases. Live birth rate in transplant recipients is reported to be similar to nontransplant mothers.[26,27] Rates of spontaneous abortions have been found comparable to non-transplant pregnancies. The use of MPA significantly increases the risk of spontaneous abortions.[30] Rates of stillbirth are reported to be higher in transplant recipients, with maternal age being a significant predictor of the same.[31]

Data regarding maternal mortality is limited but reassuring.[32,33] However, it is important to note that there is no evidence available from the developing countries which contribute to >95% of maternal deaths worldwide. Maternal hypertension, serum creatinine (prepregnancy), and the presence of proteinuria have been consistently associated with adverse maternal outcomes.[26] Additional factors affecting outcomes are advanced maternal age, black race, and presence of diabetes.[34]

PREGNANCY AND ALLOGRAFT FUNCTION

CASE VIGNETTE 2

A 30-year-old KTR who underwent a deceased donor transplantation 6 years back followed up in the transplant OPD with a history of 3 months of amenorrhea. Her native kidney disease was lupus nephritis. Her evaluation revealed a 6-week-old conception. The mother's renal functions were stable for the last 6 years and the current creatinine was 1.0 mg/dL [estimated glomerular filtration rate (eGFR) 76 mL/min]. The serum creatinine level was unchanged from her last follow-up 6 months back. She had no proteinuria. Her hypertension was well controlled with 10 mg of amlodipine once a day. As she had expressed a desire to become pregnant, her MMF was changed to AZA 2 years back. She had an uneventful pregnancy till the 30th week when her hypertension worsened requiring three antihypertensives. She had no proteinuria and no hypoalbuminemia. At 34th week, she underwent a cesarean section because of fetal distress. There was no flare of lupus during the pregnancy. Postpartum, the antihypertensive requirement came down to baseline. At 6 weeks, her serum creatinine was 1.2 mg/dL (eGFR 61 mL/min) and her lupus was inactive. The baby was doing well.

The physiological changes in pregnancy in a KTR are often not as profound as in a normal pregnancy. The increase in GFR which is observed in nontransplant mothers is blunted in transplant recipients.[27] The rise in urine protein excretion due to hyperfiltration is greater in transplant recipients compared with nontransplant mothers.[35]

Long-term graft outcomes in mothers with a well-functioning graft preconception are reported to be comparable to nonpregnant recipients.[36,37] The presence of stable graft function with no significant proteinuria and absence of hypertension predicts better long-term graft survival postpregnancy. Also, the timing of pregnancy has an impact on graft outcomes with adverse outcomes in pregnancies during the early posttransplant period.[37]

Recent data sheds light on the changes in GFR in pregnant KTR. A study from Mayo clinic shows a decline in GFR postpregnancy compared to their prepregnancy levels. This study also looked at the histological changes in the mother. There were increased chronic vascular changes (higher cv scores) in biopsies performed postpartum. The vascular changes are thought to be worsening hypertension during pregnancy as was noted in our case. These changes in the GFR and histology, however, did not impact overall allograft survival.[38]

The rate of rejection is not increased during pregnancy. Risk factors that predict rejection are high serum creatinine at baseline, rejection episode before pregnancy, and changing levels of immunosuppressive drugs. The modification of the immunosuppressive regimen does not increase the risk of rejection.[34]

MANAGEMENT OF PREGNANCY

Preconception Counseling

Pregnancy after kidney transplantation is not without complications and hence, prepregnancy counseling for both men and women KTRs of childbearing age is recommended. This important area is often overlooked and approximately 50% of women KTRs do not receive any form of prepregnancy counseling.[39] Counseling should start at the earliest and should contain information about the timing of pregnancy, safe contraceptive methods, effect of immunosuppression and modifications required, adverse maternal and fetal outcomes, type of delivery, breastfeeding, and postpregnancy care.[40]

Timing of Conception

Though fertility returns to normal within few months of kidney transplantation, it is recommended to avoid pregnancy in the first year of transplantation. Most of the previous studies have considered it safe to conceive after the second-year posttransplantation. At this time, most women are stable at nadir doses of immunosuppression with less risk of rejection and have completed prophylactic antiviral drugs. Emerging evidence suggests that with newer immunosuppressive regimens, selected recipients can have favorable pregnancy outcomes after 1-year posttransplant.[41] Timing of pregnancy needs to be individualized in high-risk KTRs.

The American Society of Transplantation recommends avoiding pregnancy in the first year after transplantation.[25]

Besides the timing of conception, many other factors should be considered when a KTR contemplates pregnancy.

The following factors should be kept in mind by a physician when pregnancy is discussed with the transplant recipient:

- At least 6 months after transplantation
- Stable allograft function and creatinine <1.4 mg/dL
- No recent episodes of acute rejection
- Blood pressure ≤140/90 mm Hg
- No or minimal proteinuria ≤500 mg/24 hours
- Prednisone ≤15 mg/day
- AZA ≤2 mg/kg/day
- Stopping MMF and sirolimus 6 weeks prior to conception.[42]

Medical Management During Pregnancy

Mothers should be monitored both by transplant physicians and obstetricians throughout the pregnancy. The frequency of monitoring is guided by the baseline allograft function and obstetric complications, if any. Most mothers need to be seen every 2–4 weeks till near term and more frequently thereafter.[43] The visits can also be completed using telemedicine, especially in times of the pandemic.[44] Monitoring must include surveillance for hypertension, gestational diabetes, infections, and graft rejection. Unbound concentrations of tacrolimus must be monitored as they are increased during pregnancy while the whole blood concentration is reduced.[45] Maternal screening for various complications in pregnancy is described in **Table 1**.

Fetal monitoring is like that in nontransplant pregnancies. Cell-free fetal deoxyribonucleic acid (DNA) testing (to detect fetal aneuploidy) is not advised in transplant recipients because of the chimeric state due to the kidney allograft.

Vaginal delivery is the preferred mode of delivery in KTRs. Cesarean delivery should be considered only for obstetric indications. Transplant recipients have a high predisposition to cesarean delivery as compared to the general population (43–72%).[26,30] Obstetricians must be aware of the anatomy of transplanted kidney and ureter before cesarean section.

Management of Immunosuppression

As discussed earlier, immunosuppressive drugs cross the placenta to varying degrees and all carry some risks in pregnancy **(Table 2)**. A regimen combining either tacrolimus

TABLE 1: Pregnancy-related complications and their management in kidney transplant recipients.

Risks	***Management***
• *KTRs with hypertension* are at higher risk of secondary preeclampsia (PE), abortions, IUGR, low birth weight, and preterm delivery • KTRs are at an increased risk of PE[24]	• Target BP is not clearly established. BP readings <140/90 mm Hg are acceptable but overcorrection can be detrimental. Drugs are the same as in CKD • Low-dose aspirin can be used for PE prevention.[40] It is important to differentiate between PE, chronic hypertension, and rejection
• KTRs during pregnancy are at risk of *graft dysfunction* • It can be due to volume depletion, CNI toxicity, preeclampsia, rejection, or obstruction (rare)	• Detailed evaluation includes volume status assessment, urine analysis, CNI levels, and ultrasonography of graft • CNI levels are to be kept close to the prepregnancy levels • Kidney biopsy is generally safe during pregnancy
• *Graft rejection* rates are comparable to nonpregnant recipients[24,26,28] (1–2%) • Patients with hyperemesis are at risk of reduced absorption of immunosuppression	• Treatment requires augmentation of baseline immunosuppression, methylprednisolone (for cell-mediated rejection), intravenous immunoglobulin, and plasmapheresis (for antibody-mediated rejection). • There is limited data about safety of rituximab and antithymocyte globulin **(Table 2)**
• Few studies (not all) suggest higher incidence of *gestational diabetes* in recipients (up to 8%)[46] • Contributing factors include CNI use, obesity, and steroid use • Hyperglycemia during organogenesis can be associated with congenital anomalies	• Management includes optimizing steroids and CNI doses, nutrition therapy, and insulin
Infections • Pregnant recipients are prone to bacterial urinary tract infections and progression to pyelonephritis which is associated with adverse outcomes • Cytomegalovirus infection can be transmitted to fetus	• Routinely screening all pregnant transplant recipients for asymptomatic bacteriuria every 2–4 weeks is recommended. Asymptomatic bacteriuria is treated with appropriate antibiotics tailored to sensitivity results • Screening is required if clinically indicated (weak recommendation to perform surveillance testing every trimester). Diagnosed mothers to be screened for congenital CMV • There is no therapy proven safe for the treatment of CMV in pregnancy. CMV hyperimmuneglobulin can be used in selected cases

(BP: blood pressure; CKD: chronic kidney disease; CMV: cytomegalovirus; CNI: calcineurin inhibitors; IUGR: intrauterine growth retardation; KTR: kidney transplant recipient)

TABLE 2: Safety of commonly used immunosuppressive drugs in pregnancy.

Drug name	FDA category	Pregnancy considerations	Lactational considerations
Drugs which can be used			
Steroids	C	• Prednisone ≤10 mg/day is acceptable for use in pregnancy as the amount of drug reaching the fetus is ~8–10 times lower than the maternal concentration and is less than fetal endogenous production. Occasionally, association with oral clefts is reported • Increased infection risk and risk of gestational diabetes are present	Breast milk levels are 5–25% of the maternal serum levels. If higher doses are used, the infant is to be monitored for growth suppression, and hypoadrenalism
Azathioprine	D	It has shown teratogenicity in animal models but not in humans (not metabolized by fetal liver). KDIGO suggests switching from mycophenolate to azathioprine preconception. Doses >2 mg/kg/day should be avoided for the risk of congenital anomalies, hematologic toxicities, and intrauterine growth retardation	Metabolite 6-mercaptopurine (6-MP) is present in breast milk. Maintenance doses are acceptable in recipient mothers
Tacrolimus	C	It has not been associated with increased teratogenicity. However, preterm delivery, low birth weight, kidney dysfunction, transient neonatal hyperkalemia, and fetal distress are reported but causality is not established. Exacerbation of maternal hypertension and hyperglycemia can occur. KDIGO recommends use of tacrolimus in pregnant recipients with frequent monitoring of levels (see text)	It is present in breast milk, but the relative concentrations in the infant are in an acceptable range
Cyclosporine A	C	Similar to tacrolimus but more evidence is available about cyclosporine A	It is present in breast milk but the relative concentrations in the infant are in an acceptable range
Drugs to be avoided			
Mycophenolate mofetil	D	High risk of teratogenicity causing cardiovascular and cranial malformations. Recommended to discontinue at least 6 weeks prior to conception	Evidence is not available about excretion in breast milk
m-TORi	C	Very limited evidence suggests fetal harm. KDIGO guidelines suggest discontinuation in the preconception period	Evidence is not available about excretion in breast milk
Drugs with very limited evidence			
Rituximab	C, D	It crosses the placenta and can be detected in the newborn. In utero exposure to rituximab may cause fetal harm	It is present in breast milk. Data on safety is limited; however, the absorption for infant gut is considered minimal
Antithymocyte globulin (rabbit derived)	Not assigned	There is limited evidence and should be used only if benefits outweigh the risks	It is not known if antithymocyte globulin (rabbit) is excreted in breast milk
Belatacept	Not assigned	Evidence related to belatacept use in pregnancy is limited	It is not known if belatacept is present in breast milk

Note: FDA category: A, controlled human studies show no risk; B, no evidence of risk in studies; C, risk cannot be ruled out; D, positive evidence of risk; X, contraindicated in pregnancy.
(FDA: Food and Drug Administration; KDIGO: Kidney Disease Improving Global Outcomes; m-TORi: mammalian target of rapamycin inhibitors)

or cyclosporine AZA and low-dose steroids is considered safe during pregnancy. Mycophenolate and sirolimus must be stopped before conception.[46] The safety of belatacept during pregnancy is not established. Graft function must be carefully monitored for few months in all women undergoing modifications in immunosuppression. There is a concern of immunological abnormalities and neurocognitive deficits in the fetus exposed to immunosuppression in utero.[47] In NIMS, all pregnant KTRs were on triple. Immunosuppression consisting of steroids, tacrolimus, and AZA.

TABLE 3: Contraception in kidney transplant recipient (KTR).

Contraceptive method	*Issues*
Intrauterine devices (IUDs) • Nonhormonal—copper • Hormonal—levonorgestrel	• Most effective contraceptive methods. Heavy menstrual bleeding—less ideal in KTRs with anemia and coagulopathy • No ↑ risk of pelvic inflammatory disease
Combined hormonal contraception (estrogen and progestin)	• Oral contraceptive pills, dermal patches, and vaginal rings • ↑ Risk of hypertension and venous thromboembolic disease • Interaction with corticosteroids and mycophenolic acid can reduce its efficacy
Progestin-only agents	• Daily pills or depot medroxyprogesterone acetate (DMPA) as an intramuscular injection 12 weekly and subcutaneous implants which work for 3 years • Not associated with ↑ risk of thrombosis or hypertension • Decline in bone mineral density • The subcutaneous implant is not associated with bone loss, though its use has not been described in transplant patients
Barrier methods	• Prevents both pregnancy and sexually transmitted infections • Ideal for women using teratogenic immunosuppressives • Failure rates are high with barrier methods, hence should be used in conjunction with other methods

Breastfeeding in Renal Transplant Recipient

Corticosteroids, AZA, and CNIs are secreted in breast milk in minimal concentrations and do not cause any adverse effects to the baby. There are no specific trials for the safety of MMF and m-TORi and hence should be avoided during breastfeeding. The National Transplantation Pregnancy Registry has reported no specific problems related to breastfeeding in the children of recipients.[30]

CONTRACEPTION

Data suggests that most of the pregnancies in KT patients were unplanned due lack of counseling to use birth control measures to prevent high-risk pregnancies.[47,48] The maternal and fetal complications associated with unintentional pregnancies exceeds far more than with planned pregnancies with contraceptive use. Hence, it is important that all KT patients in the reproductive age group are provided with contraception counseling. There are various contraceptive methods in renal transplant recipients: Intrauterine devices (IUDs), combined hormonal contraception (CHC), and progestin-only pills. For women with uncomplicated solid organ transplants, all forms of contraceptives were classified as category 2, meaning that the advantages of using the method generally outweigh the theoretical or proven side effects.[49] The contraceptive methods and issues associated with them are discussed in **Table 3**.[50]

CONCLUSION

Many KTRs are becoming fathers and mothers. This gratifying improvement in fertility of these patients is because of advances in kidney transplantation procedures, use of appropriate immunosuppression, effective pregnancy monitoring, and advanced obstetric and neonatal care.

REFERENCES

1. Edey MM. Male sexual dysfunction and chronic kidney disease. Front Med. 2017;4:32.
2. Holley JL. The hypothalamic-pituitary axis in men and women with chronic kidney disease. Adv Chronic Kidney Dis. 2004;11:337-41.
3. Xu LG, Xu HM, Zhu XF, Jin LM, Xu B, Wu Y, et al. Examination of the semen quality of patients with uremia and renal transplant recipients in comparison with a control group. Andrologia. 2009;41:235-40.
4. Hsieh MH, Hollander A, Lamb DJ, Turek PJ. The genetic and phenotypic basis of infertility in men with pediatric urologic disorders. Urology. 2010;76:25-31.
5. Mieusset R, Fauquet I, Chauveau D, Monteil L, Chassaing N, Daudin M, et al. The spectrum of renal involvement in male patients with infertility related to excretory-system abnormalities: phenotypes, genotypes, and genetic counseling. J Nephrol. 2017;30:211-8.
6. Papadopoulou E, Varouktsi A, Lazaridis A, Boutari C, Doumas M. Erectile dysfunction in chronic kidney disease: from pathophysiology to management. World J Nephrol. 2015;4:379-87.
7. Schmidt RJ, Holley JL. Fertility and contraception in end-stage renal disease. Adv Ren Replace Ther. 1998;5:38-44.
8. Lim VS. Reproductive function in patients with renal insufficiency. Am J Kidney Dis. 1987;9:363-7.
9. Holley JL, Schmidt RJ, Bender FH, Dumler F, Schiff M. Gynecologic and reproductive issues in women on dialysis. Am J Kidney Dis. 1997;29:685-90.
10. Handelsman DQ. Hypothalamic-pituitary gonadal axis in chronic renal failure. Endocrinol Metab Clin North Am. 1993:22:145-61.
11. Sievertsen GD, Lim VS, Nakawatase E, Frohman LA. Metabolic clearance and secretion rates of human prolactin in normal subjects and in patients with chronic renal failure. J Clin Endocrinol Metab. 1980;50:846-51.
12. Ginsburg ES, Owen Jr WF. Reproductive endocrinology and pregnancy in women on hemodialysis. Semin Dial. 1993:6:105-16.

13. Holley JL, Schmidt RJ. Changes in fertility and hormone replacement therapy in kidney disease. Adv Chronic Kidney Dis. 2013;20:240-5.
14. Wang G-C, Zheng J-H, Xu L-G, Min Z-L, Zhu Y-H, Qi J, et al. Measurements of serum pituitary-gonadal hormones and investigation of sexual and reproductive functions in kidney transplant recipients. Int J Nephrol. 2010;2010:1-6.
15. Diemont WL, Vruggink PA, Meuleman EJ, Doesburg WH, Lemmens WA, Berden JH. Sexual dysfunction after renal replacement therapy. Am J Kidney Dis. 2000;35:845-51.
16. Xu L-G, Wang H-W, Peng W-L, Jin L-M, Zhu X-F, Xu H-M, et al. Marital status and fertility of 185 male renal transplant recipients in China. J Androl. 2008;29:618-21.
17. Zuber J, Anglicheau D, Elie C, Bererhi L, Timsit MO, Mamzer-Bruneel MF, et al. Sirolimus may reduce fertility in male renal transplant recipients. Am J Transplant. 2008;8:1471-79.
18. Hoeltzenbein M, Elefant E, Vial T, Finkel-Pekarsky V, Stephens S, Clementi M, et al. Teratogenicity of mycophenolate confirmed in a prospective study of the European Network of Teratology Information Services. Am J Med Genet A. 2012;158:588-96.
19. Levitz M, Jansen V, Dancis J. The transfer and metabolism of corticosteroids in the perfused human placenta. Am J Obstet Gynecol. 1978;132:363-6.
20. Constantinescu S, Coscia LA, Armenti VT. Mycophenolic acid product discontinuation prior to conception: analysis of pregnancies in kidney transplant recipients. Am J Transplant. 2016;16:228.
21. EBPG Expert Group on Renal Transplantation. European best practice guidelines for renal transplantation. Section IV: long-term management of the transplant recipient. IV.10. Pregnancy in renal transplant recipients. Nephrol Dial Transplant. 2002;17(Suppl. 4):50-5.
22. Paziana K, Del Monaco M, Cardonick E, Moritz M, Keller M, Smith B, et al. Ciclosporin use during pregnancy. Drug Saf. 2013;36:279-94.
23. Carta P, Caroti L, Zanazzi M. Pregnancy in a kidney transplant patient treated with everolimus. Am J Kidney Dis. 2012;60:329.
24. Deshpande NA, James NT, Kucirka LM, Boyarsky BJ, Garonzik-Wang JM, Montgomery RA, et al. Pregnancy outcomes in kidney transplant recipients: a systematic review and meta-analysis. Am J Transplant. 2011;11(11):2388-404.
25. McKay DB, Josephson MA, Armenti VT, August P, Coscia LA, Davis CL, et al. Reproduction and transplantation: report on the AST consensus conference on reproductive issues and transplantation. Am J Transplant. 2005;5:1592-9.
26. Sibanda N, Briggs JD, Davison JM, Johnson RJ, Rudge CJ. Pregnancy after organ transplantation: a report from the UK transplant pregnancy registry. Transplantation. 2007;83:1301-7.
27. Bramham K, Nelson-Piercy C, Gao H, Pierce M, Bush N, Spark P, et al. Pregnancy in renal transplant recipients: a UK national cohort study. Clin J Am Soc Nephrol. 2013;8(2):290-98.
28. del Mar Colon M, Hibbard JU. Obstetric considerations in the management of pregnancy in kidney transplant recipients. Adv Chronic Kidney Dis. 2007;14:168-77.
29. McKay DB, Josephson MA. Pregnancy after kidney transplantation. Clin J Am Soc Nephrol. 2008;3:S117-25.
30. Coscia LA, Constantinescu S, Moritz MJ, Frank AM, Ramirez CB, Maley WR, et al. Report from the National Transplantation Pregnancy Registry (NTPR): outcomes of pregnancy after transplantation. Clin Transpl. 2010:65-85.
31. Coscia L, Daly T, Nathan H, Armenti D, Kliniewski D, Constantinescu S, et al. Transplant pregnancy registry international. Transplantation. 2017;101:S64.
32. Levidiotis V, Chang S, McDonald S. Pregnancy and maternal outcomes among kidney transplant recipients. J Am Soc Nephrol. 2009;20(11):2433-40.
33. Rahamimov R, Ben-Haroush A, Wittenberg C, Mor E, Lustig S, Gafter U, et al. Pregnancy in renal transplant recipients: long-term effect on patient and graft survival. A single-center experience. Transplantation. 2006;81(5):660-4.
34. Stratta P, Canavese C, Giacchino F, Mesiano P, Quaglia M, Rossetti M, et al. Pregnancy in kidney transplantation: satisfactory outcomes and harsh realities. J Nephrol. 2003;16(6):792-806.
35. Davison JM. The effect of pregnancy on kidney function in renal allograft recipients. Kidney Int. 1985;27(1):74-9.
36. Sturgiss SN, Davison JM. Effect of pregnancy on the long-term function of renal allografts: an update. Am J Kidney Dis. 1995;26(1):54-6.
37. Rose C, Gill J, Zalunardo N, Johnston O, Mehrotra A, Gill JS. Timing of pregnancy after kidney transplantation and risk of allograft failure. Am J Transplant. 2016;16(8):2360-67.
38. Kattah AG, Albadri S, Alexander MP, Smith B, Parashuram S, Mai ML, et al. Impact of pregnancy on GFR decline and kidney histology in kidney transplant recipients. Kidney Int Rep. 2022;7:28-35.
39. Yildirim Y, Uslu A. Pregnancy in patients with previous successful renal transplantation. Int J Gynaecol Obstet. 2005;90:198-202.
40. Yoshikawa Y, Uchida J, Kosoku A, Akazawa C, Suganum N. Pregnancy counseling for kidney transplant recipients. Clin Mother Child Health. 2020;17:341.
41. Josephson MA, McKay DB. Women and transplantation: fertility, sexuality, pregnancy, contraception. Adv Chronic Kidney Dis. 2013;20(5):433-40.
42. Shah S, Verma P. Overview of pregnancy in renal transplant patients. Int J Nephrol. 2016;2016:4539342.
43. Cabiddu G, Spotti D, Gernone G, Santoro D, Moroni G, Gregorini G, et al. A best-practice position statement on pregnancy after kidney transplantation: focusing on the unsolved questions. The Kidney and Pregnancy Study Group of the Italian Society of Nephrology. J Nephrol. 2018;31(5):665-81.
44. Bajpai D, Shah S. COVID-19 pandemic and pregnancy in kidney disease. Adv Chronic Kidney Dis. 2020;27(5):397-403.
45. Hebert MF, Zheng S, Hays K, Shen DD, Davis CL, Umans JG, et al. Interpreting tacrolimus concentrations during pregnancy and postpartum. Transplantation. 2013;95(7):908-15.
46. Leroy C, Rigot J-M, Leroy M, Decanter C, Le Mapihan K, Parent AS, et al. Immunosuppressive drugs and fertility. Orphanet J Rare Dis. 2015;10:136.
47. Dardier V, Lacroix A, Vigneau C. Pregnancies after kidney transplant: what are the consequences for the cognitive development of children? Nephrol Ther. 2021;17(2):74-9.
48. Guazzelli CA, Torloni MR, Sanches TF, Barbieri M, Pestana JO. Contraceptive counseling and use among 197 female kidney transplant recipients. Transplantation. 2008;86:669-72.
49. Curtis KM, Tepper NK, Jatlaoui TC, Berry-Bibee E, Horton LG, Zapata LB, et al. U.S. medical eligibility criteria for contraceptive use, 2016. MMWR Recomm Rep. 2016;65:1-103.
50. Paulen ME, Folger SG, Curtis KM, Jamieson DJ. Contraceptive use among solid organ transplant patients: a systematic review. Contraception. 2010;82:102-12.

CHAPTER 25

Vaccination in Kidney Transplant Recipients

Gokulnath, Prashant C Dheerendra

CASE VIGNETTE 1

Mrs M, a 60-year-old diabetic with end stage renal disease presumed to be due to diabetic nephropathy is on waiting list for a cadaveric kidney transplantation. He is expected to receive an organ in the next few months. How will you optimize his immunity to various vaccine preventable diseases?

INTRODUCTION

The pretransplant period is an opportune time to review the vaccination of the prospective recipients and optimize their immunity to vaccine-preventable diseases, before exposure to immunosuppressive medications. Both organ failure and organ transplantation are conditions in which host immunity is depressed. Ideally, the prospective kidney transplant recipient (KTR) should receive appropriate vaccinations from an early period during chronic kidney disease (CKD). However, this is often not the case and visits to the transplant clinic must be utilized to create and execute a personalized vaccination strategy for the patients. This process must start from the first visit to the transplant clinic.

Live vaccines are contraindicated in the post-transplant period and hence it is imperative to administer them pretransplant. A minimum gap of 4 weeks is needed between live vaccine administration and kidney transplantation. For inactivated vaccines, the gap should be 2 weeks long to allow antibodies to develop.

Most inactivated vaccines are safe after kidney transplantation though data on safety and efficacy are not available for all the vaccines in this period.

Seroconversion rates following vaccination are lower in transplant recipients compared to the general population.[1] Also, antibody titers wane over time.[2] Still, vaccination has been proven to decrease the burden of infectious diseases after transplantation.

The Indian Society of Nephrology (ISN) has published guidelines for the vaccination of KTRs.[3] The society advises vaccination in KTRs to be guided by age-appropriate inactivated vaccines used for the general population of similar age. The guidelines also emphasize the vaccination of pets, household contacts, and healthcare workers to provide further protection to KTRs, by preventing transmission from them. Inactivated vaccines should be used for vaccinating contacts to prevent transmission of vaccine strains to KTRs. If only a live vaccine is available, it should be avoided and if obligatory, contact between KTRs and the vaccinated member should be avoided for 2 weeks.

HEPATITIS B

The American Society of Transplantation Infectious Diseases Community of Practice (AST IDCOP) recommends initial screening for a kidney transplant candidate with hepatitis B surface antigen (HbsAg), hepatitis B surface antibody (anti-HBs), and hepatitis B core antibody (anti-HBc).[4] All the three tests being negative identify a susceptible host with no prior infection or vaccination and indicate the need for vaccination. Anti-HBs titers >10 IU/mL denote immunity and the titers need to be repeated annually. Titers <10 IU/mL denote insufficient immunity and necessitate vaccination. In Indian recipients, consideration should be given for a booster dose when titers fall below 100 IU/mL.[3] Ideally, the vaccination has been carried out earlier in the course of CKD. Since there is a possibility that the donor might be HBsAg negative but anti-HBc positive, it is important to complete the vaccination pretransplantation.

The response to vaccination is suboptimal after transplantation and titers tend to decline with time.[2] If vaccination is needed after transplantation, it is initiated once the period of intense immunosuppression has elapsed, and the patient is on stable immunosuppression. This is generally after 3 months of transplantation. Another strategy to improve seroconversion in immunocompromised hosts is to use a double dose of the vaccine—40 μg/dose compared to 20 μg—at each inoculation.[5] The number of doses is increased to four—0, 1, 2, and a booster at 6 months—compared to three (0, 1, and 6 months) in immunocompetent adults.

CHAPTER HIGHLIGHTS

- Response to vaccination is better before transplantation, so it is important to administer the indicated vaccines in this period.
- Live vaccines should be avoided after transplantation; inactivated vaccines can be administered in this period.
- Hepatitis B, pneumococcal, influenza, varicella, and COVID-19 vaccination are obligatory for both adults and children.
- *Haemophilus influenzae* and meningococcal vaccination are important in children.
- For other diseases, general guidelines for age-matched general population should guide vaccination.
- Passive immunization using immune globulins should be administered along with vaccines when they are available and indicated.

When titers are inadequate 4 weeks after the last dose, the whole vaccination schedule can be repeated. Administering only the booster and checking titers after 4 weeks are also valid. If titers are inadequate after the booster dose, a complete revaccination series should be carried out.[6] Patients who do not mount a serological response after two full vaccination series are unlikely to seroconvert with further efforts. They must be educated about hepatitis B virus (HBV) prevention. Accelerated and granulocyte-macrophage colony-stimulating factor (GM-CSF) boosted schedules have been tried but cannot be recommended on a routine basis, especially in post-transplant patients.[7,8]

INFLUENZA

A large prospective study has shown that influenza vaccination decreases complications such as pneumonia in transplant recipients even though seroconversion rates are suboptimal.[9,10] The injectable, inactivated quadrivalent seasonal influenza vaccine is administered before the flu season begins. A live vaccine is available but should not be used. In India, late autumn (October) is the optimum time for administration. The vaccine has demonstrated efficacy even in the early post-transplant period.[11] The Kidney Disease: Improving Global Outcomes (KDIGO) recommend that the vaccine be administered at the onset of the influenza season, in all KTRs who have been transplanted at least 1 month previously.[12] A second dose after 6 months may be appropriate if influenza is still prevalent in the community.

There were concerns about the vaccine precipitating rejection, but these have not been proven.[13] In fact, registry data associate vaccination with lower rates of allograft loss and death in the first post-transplant year.[14] On the other hand, influenza itself may precipitate rejection.[15]

PNEUMOCOCCUS

All patients on dialysis and transplant recipients need to be vaccinated against *Pneumococcus*. A pneumococcal polysaccharide vaccine (PPSV) which confers immunity against 23 strains (PPSV-23) and a 13-valent pneumococcal conjugate vaccine (PCV-13) are available. Both should be used and the sequence in which they are administered as well as the duration between them is important.

Pneumococcal conjugate vaccine administration shortly after a dose of PPSV-23 might dampen the immune response.[16] PPSV administration a few months following PCV administration may lead to a higher antibody response.[17] Hence, the Advisory Committee on Immunization Practices (ACIP) recommends a gap of 1 year between PCV and PPSV in adults aged 65 years or older.[18] Preferably, the PCV vaccine is administered first in view of its probable immune-boosting effect on the PPSV. The same general guidelines apply to transplant candidates and dialysis patients except that the gap can be as less as 8 weeks.[18]

The antibody response generated by the PPSV-23 vaccine wanes over time.[19] Recommendations regarding revaccination vary, but it is a common practice to revaccinate immunocompromised patients with PPSV-23 every 5 years.

Revaccination with PCV-13 is not recommended in adult patients.

Coadministration of either vaccine with the seasonal flu vaccine is safe.[20] Pneumococcal conjugate vaccine should be separated by 4 weeks from the quadrivalent meningococcal conjugate vaccine as the latter can lead to lower pneumococcal antibody titers.[6]

VARICELLA

Primary varicella infection can cause severe disease in the transplant population. Varicella serology is checked to ascertain the immune status of the candidate. Since the varicella vaccine is a live vaccine and cannot be given after transplantation, it is important to begin the vaccination at least 2–3 months before the anticipated date of transplantation. One dose of the vaccine is administered and serology is rechecked after 4 weeks. If adequate, one can proceed with the transplantation. If inadequate, the AST IDCOP guidelines recommend a second dose and rechecking the titers 4 weeks later.[6]

Those who fail to mount an antibody response after two doses are candidates for postexposure prophylaxis (PEP) in case exposure occurs after transplantation. When urgent transplantation is needed in patients who have received varicella vaccination in the previous month, prophylaxis around the time of transplantation is warranted.

Though there are small studies suggesting that the vaccine can be safe in the post-transplant period in selected patients, use of the vaccine after transplantation should be avoided.[21] In at least one case, the vaccine strain was demonstrated to be the cause of disseminated infection.[22]

COVID-19

All KTRs and candidates should receive the COVID-19 vaccine as per local availability and guidelines. A period of 2 weeks should elapse between the last dose of vaccine and transplantation. As transplant recipients are at high risk for severe disease, those who have received two doses of the vaccine previously are candidates for a third dose.[23]

Recipients who have recovered from COVID-19 also need to get vaccinated or continue the vaccination if partially vaccinated. The ISN recommends that the vaccine dose should be delayed by 4–8 weeks after recovery from an infection.[24]

The relevance of antibody testing after vaccination is not known. Many tests are qualitative and do not quantify antibody levels. On the other hand, levels below measurable amounts can still be protective.[25] Also, there may be protective T cell-mediated immunity in the absence of an antibody response.[26]

Vaccination of the recipients is one part of action required to protect KTRs from COVID-19. Standard COVID-19 protection protocols continue to be important after vaccination. Vaccination of close contacts and healthcare providers gives another layer of protection to this susceptible population.

TETANUS, DIPHTHERIA, AND PERTUSSIS

Vaccination with the Td (tetanus and adult diphtheria) vaccine every 10 years is recommended for adults aged 18–64 years who have completed primary vaccination in their childhood. One of the doses can be of the Tdap (tetanus, diphtheria, and acellular pertussis) vaccine.[27] The same guidelines can be followed in KTRs.

One dose of Tdap vaccine during each pregnancy is recommended for female KTRs between weeks 27 and 36. If vaccination is missed during pregnancy and the KTR has not received a dose of Tdap in the past, then the dose can be given postpartum.[28]

The Tdap vaccine is contraindicated in patients who developed unexplained encephalopathy within 7 days of administration of any previous vaccine containing the pertussis component. The Td vaccine can be used instead. In adults with unstable neurological illnesses, vaccination with Tdap is deferred till the acute phase resolves.

HUMAN PAPILLOMAVIRUS

Kidney transplant recipients are at increased risk of anogenital cancers caused by the human papillomavirus (HPV).[29] Hence, vaccination is recommended for those who have not been vaccinated previously.

The 9-valent vaccine is used for vaccination of male and female KTRs who have not been vaccinated previously. Three doses are administered pretransplant at 0, 1, and 6 months. If transplantation occurs before completion of the schedule, it can be completed 3–6 months following transplantation.

Like other vaccines, seroconversion rates are lesser compared to the normal population but rates as high as 80% have been demonstrated for some HPV types.[30]

The Indian guidelines emphasize vaccination in young KTRs aged 9–13 years.[3] Catch-up vaccination can be done up to the age of 26 years.

OTHER VACCINES

Hepatitis A

Seroepidemiological studies from the All India Institute of Medical Sciences (AIIMS) have shown that almost all children above 16 years of age have protective antibodies against hepatitis A.[31] Among Indian adult patients with chronic liver disease, 97.6% have antibodies against hepatitis A virus (HAV).[31] The inactivated vaccine is advised in seronegative transplant candidates and KTRs.

Rabies

Kidney transplant recipients can receive cell culture vaccines for PEP with five doses of the vaccine—0, 3, 7, 14, and 28 days. Rabies immune globulin (RIG) should be infiltrated around the bite site in all immunosuppressed patients.[32]

Typhoid

The oral typhoid vaccine is contraindicated in KTRs. When indicated, the killed Vi polysaccharide vaccine should be used.[3]

Cholera

The oral live vaccine is contraindicated, but the killed oral vaccine can be used when indicated.[3]

Zoster

The recombinant subunit zoster vaccine can be used in KTRs and has shown significant protection from morbidity but as of now, it is unavailable in India.[6] The live attenuated vaccine is contraindicated.

Japanese Encephalitis

The inactivated Vero cell-derived vaccine can be used for vaccination in the endemic districts of India.

Yellow Fever

The live vaccine is contraindicated in KTRs. Travel to endemic areas is not advised and some countries do insist on vaccination.

CONSIDERATIONS IN PEDIATRIC PATIENTS

Children should receive all the immunizations as per the Universal Immunization Program of the Government of India in the pretransplant period. Some of the most important vaccines that children need, such as the measles, mumps, and rubella (MMR) vaccine, and the varicella vaccine are live virus vaccines. These diseases can be severe in the immunosuppressed children and hence it is important to complete them before transplantation. For example, in immunosuppressed patients, measles can have a mortality rate of 40–70%.[33] Maternal-derived antibodies provide passive immunity in the first year of life. Administering the MMR and varicella vaccines early in life elicits a weaker antibody response. In order to avoid this, the earliest age that these vaccines can be administered is 6 months.

The oral polio vaccine (OPV) administered as part of the pulse polio program is contraindicated for KTRs and their contacts and family members as it is a live vaccine.[34] The inactivated polio vaccine (IPV) can be used. The rotavirus vaccine (RVV) and Bacillus Calmette–Guérin (BCG) vaccine are both live vaccines administered early in the lives of children. Usually, vaccination has been completed by the time the child is brought for transplantation.

The PCV is a part of the Universal Immunization Program and three doses are administered at 6 weeks, 14 weeks, and 9–12 months. The PPSV vaccine is administered after 2 years of age and at least 8 weeks after the last PCV dose. Revaccination 5 years after the first dose of PPSV is recommended. The quadrivalent inactivated influenza vaccine should be administered annually as in immunocompetent children. A live influenza vaccine is available but should be avoided in KTRs.

Pediatric patients should be vaccinated with *H. influenzae* type b (Hib) conjugate vaccine as per routine schedule. Meningococcal vaccination with the quadrivalent conjugate vaccine is recommended for all adolescents aged 11–18 years. In the context of both adult and pediatric transplantation, meningococcal and Hib vaccination are important when eculizumab use is anticipated, in patients with sickle cell disease and in ABO-incompatible transplants.

PASSIVE IMMUNIZATION IN KIDNEY TRANSPLANT RECIPIENTS

Passive immunization with disease-specific immune globulins has a role in transplant candidates and recipients. A common indication is when an unvaccinated or non-immune KTR is exposed to certain pathogens. HBV, rabies, and tetanus are the common infective agents against which immune globulin is available. Varicella-zoster immune globulin is not commercially available in India. It is important to administer the immune globulins as soon as possible after exposure. Protection from infection may be incomplete, but the severity of illness is reduced. If an inactivated vaccine is available (tetanus, hepatitis B, and rabies), active and passive immunization should be administered concurrently to provide both immediate and durable protection. Of note, RIG provides the best protection when it is infiltrated around the bite site rather than at a distant locale.[32] The immune globulin and the vaccine should be administered using separate syringes at different sites. Intravenous immune globulin (IVIg) is used in case of exposure to measles since a specific immune globulin is not available.[35]

Hepatitis B immune globulin (HBIg) allowed liver transplantation to be performed in patients with HBV-related cirrhosis while preventing a recurrence in the graft.[36] Over time, nucleoside analogs have largely replaced HBIg for this indication.[37]

Table 1 summarizes the salient aspects of various vaccines relevant to KTRs.

TABLE 1: Vaccines in kidney transplant recipients.

Vaccine	*Pretransplant*	*Post-transplant*	*Comments*
Hepatitis B	Yes(I)	Yes(I)	Monitor anti-HBs; booster if <10 IU/mL
Pneumococcal	Yes(I)	Yes(I)	Both PCV and PPSV to be administered
Influenza	Yes(I)	Yes(I)	Vaccinate at the beginning of the flu season
Varicella	Yes(I)	No	To be given pretransplant; monitor serology
COVID-19*	Yes(I)	Yes(I)	Follow local guidelines
MMR	Yes(R)	No	Live vaccine
Tdap and Td	Yes(R)	Yes(R)	Administer every 10 years; important in pregnancy
Human papillomavirus	Yes(R)	Yes(R)	Important in younger patients
Haemophilus influenzae	Yes(R)	Yes(R)	Indicated in patients with sickle cell disease, eculizumab use, and ABO-incompatible transplantations
Meningococcal	Yes(R)	Yes(R)	Indicated in adolescents, ABO-incompatible transplants, eculizumab use, and sickle cell disease

Contd...

Contd...

Vaccine	Pretransplant	Post-transplant	Comments
Hepatitis A	Yes(R)	Yes(R)	
Oral polio vaccine (OPV)	Yes(R)	No	Family members should also avoid this vaccine
Injectable polio vaccine (IPV)	Yes(R)	Yes(R)	Alternative to OPV
Rotavirus	Yes(R)	No	Live vaccine
Rabies	Yes(R)	Yes(R)	Rabies immune globulin (RIG) also to be administered
Japanese encephalitis—inactivated Vero cell-derived vaccine	Yes(R)	Yes(R)	Only in endemic districts
Oral typhoid vaccine	Yes(R)	No	Live vaccine
Parenteral typhoid vaccine	Yes(R)	Yes(R)	
Oral live cholera vaccine	Yes(R)	No	
Oral killed cholera vaccine	Yes(R)	Yes(R)	
Recombinant zoster vaccine	Yes(I)	Yes(I)	Not yet available in India
Yellow fever	Yes(R)	No	Live vaccine

*COVID vaccination administered pretransplant as well as post-transplant and booster recommended. Family members and health caregivers should be vaccinated.

(I: important especially in the context of transplantation; R: routine usage as in general age-matched population; anti-HBs: hepatitis B surface antibody; MMR: measles, mumps, and rubella; PCV: pneumococcal conjugate vaccine; PPSV: pneumococcal polysaccharide vaccine; Tdap: tetanus, diphtheria, and acellular pertussis; Td: tetanus and adult diphtheria)

CONCLUSION

In conclusion, optimizing immunity of KTRs to vaccine preventable diseases is a continuous process which ideally begins in the early stages of CKD. Specific attention needs to be paid to this aspect in the immediate pretransplant period as some vaccines are contraindicated after transplantation. A well tailored plan needs to be made for each patient in order to prevent vaccine preventable disease and death.

REFERENCES

1. Krishnamurthy G, Kher V, Naik S. Immunogenicity and efficacy of hepatitis B vaccination in Indian chronic renal failure patients on hemodialysis and after renal transplantation. Nephron. 1996;74(2):424-5.
2. Moal V, Motte A, Vacher-Coponat H, Tamalet C, Berland Y, Colson P. Considerable decrease in antibodies against hepatitis B surface antigen following kidney transplantation. J Clin Virol. 2015;68:32-6.
3. Guidelines for vaccination in kidney transplant recipients. Indian J Nephrol. 2016;26(7):19.
4. Te H, Doucette K. Viral hepatitis: guidelines by the American Society of Transplantation Infectious Disease Community of Practice. Clin Transplant. 2019;33(9):e13514.
5. Stevens CE, Alter HJ, Taylor PE, Zang EA, Harley EJ, Szmuness W. Hepatitis B vaccine in patients receiving hemodialysis. Immunogenicity and efficacy. N Engl J Med. 1984;311(8):496-501.
6. Danziger-Isakov L, Kumar D, AST ID Community of Practice. Vaccination of solid organ transplant candidates and recipients: guidelines from the American Society of Transplantation Infectious Diseases Community of Practice. Clin Transplant. 2019;33(9):e13563.
7. Krishnamurthy K, John GT, Abraham P, Jacob CK. Granulocyte macrophage colony stimulating factor augmented hepatitis B vaccine protocol for rapid seroprotection in voluntary kidney donors. Indian J Med Res. 2004;119(4):162-4.
8. Engler SH, Sauer PW, Golling M, Klar EA, Benz C, Stremmel W, et al. Immunogenicity of two accelerated hepatitis B vaccination protocols in liver transplant candidates. Eur J Gastroenterol Hepatol. 2001;13(4):363-7.
9. Kumar D, Ferreira VH, Blumberg E, Silveira F, Cordero E, Perez-Romero P, et al. A 5-year prospective multicenter evaluation of influenza infection in transplant recipients. Clin Infect Dis. 2018;67(9):1322-9.
10. Blumberg EA, Albano C, Pruett T, Isaacs R, Fitzpatrick J, Bergin J, et al. The immunogenicity of influenza virus vaccine in solid organ transplant recipients. Clin Infect Dis. 1996;22(2):295-302.
11. Pérez-Romero P, Bulnes-Ramos A, Torre-Cisneros J, Gavald J, Aydillo TA, Moreno A, et al. Influenza vaccination during the first 6 months after solid organ transplantation is efficacious and safe. Clin Microbiol Infect. 2015;21(11):1040.e11-18.
12. Kidney Disease: Improving Global Outcomes (KDIGO) Transplant Work Group. KDIGO clinical practice guideline for the care of kidney transplant recipients. Am J Transplant. 2009;9(Suppl. 3):S1-155.
13. Cohet C, Haguinet F, Dos Santos G, Webb D, Logie J, Ferreira GL, et al. Effect of the adjuvanted (AS03) A/H1N1 2009 pandemic influenza vaccine on the risk of rejection in solid organ transplant recipients in England: a self-controlled case series. BMJ Open. 2016;6(1):e009264.
14. Hurst FP, Lee JJ, Jindal RM, Agodoa LY, Abbott KC. Outcomes associated with influenza vaccination in the first year after kidney transplantation. Clin J Am Soc Nephrol. 2011;6(5):1192-7.

15. Vilchez RA, McCurry K, Dauber J, Lacono A, Griffith B, Fung J, et al. Influenza virus infection in adult solid organ transplant recipients. Am J Transplant. 2002;2(3):287-91.
16. Lazarus R, Clutterbuck E, Yu LM, Bowman J, Bateman EA, Diggle L, et al. A randomized study comparing combined pneumococcal conjugate and polysaccharide vaccination schedules in adults. Clin Infect Dis. 2011;52(6):736-42.
17. Musher DM, Rueda AM, Nahm MH, Graviss EA, Rodriguez-Barradas MC. Initial and subsequent response to pneumococcal polysaccharide and protein-conjugate vaccines administered sequentially to adults who have recovered from pneumococcal pneumonia. J Infect Dis. 2008;198(7):1019-27.
18. Kobayashi M, Farrar JL, Gierke R, Britton A, Childs L, Leidner AJ, et al. Use of 15-valent pneumococcal conjugate vaccine and 20-valent pneumococcal conjugate vaccine among U.S. adults: updated recommendations of the Advisory Committee on Immunization Practices—United States, 2022. MMWR Morb Mortal Wkly Rep. 2022;71(4): 109-17.
19. Musher DM, Manof SB, Liss C, McFetridge RD, Marchese RD, Bushnell B, et al. Safety and antibody response, including antibody persistence for 5 years, after primary vaccination or revaccination with pneumococcal polysaccharide vaccine in middle-aged and older adults. J Infect Dis. 2010;201(4): 516-24.
20. Honkanen PO, Keistinen T, Kivelä SL. Reactions following administration of influenza vaccine alone or with pneumococcal vaccine to the elderly. Arch Intern Med. 1996; 156(2):205-8.
21. Weinberg A, Horslen SP, Kaufman SS, Jesser R, Devoll-Zabrocki A, Fleckten BN, et al. Safety and immunogenicity of varicella-zoster virus vaccine in pediatric liver and intestine transplant recipients. Am J Transplant. 2006;6(3):565-8.
22. Kraft JN, Shaw JC. Varicella infection caused by Oka strain vaccine in a heart transplant recipient. Arch Dermatol. 2006;142(7):943-5.
23. Werbel WA, Boyarsky BJ, Ou MT, Massie AB, Tobian AAR, Garonzik-Wang JM, et al. Safety and immunogenicity of a third dose of SARS-CoV-2 vaccine in solid organ transplant recipients: a case series. Ann Intern Med. 2021;174(9):1330-2.
24. Kute VB, Agarwal SK, Prakash J, Guleria S, Shroff S, Sharma A, et al. NOTTO COVID-19 vaccine guidelines for transplant recipients. Indian J Nephrol. 2021;31(2):89-91.
25. Tau N, Yahav D, Schneider S, Rozen-Zvi B, Sneineh MA, Rahamimov R. Severe consequences of COVID-19 infection among vaccinated kidney transplant recipients. Am J Transplant. 2021;21(8):2910-2.
26. Cucchiari D, Egri N, Bodro M, Herrera S, Risco-Zevallos JD, Casals-Urquiza J, et al. Cellular and humoral response after MRNA-1273 SARS-CoV-2 vaccine in kidney transplant recipients. Am J Transplant. 2021;21(8):2727-39.
27. Guidelines for vaccination in normal adults in India. Indian J Nephrol. 2016;26(Suppl. 1):S7-14.
28. Havers FP, Moro PL, Hunter P, Hariri S, Bernstein H. Use of tetanus toxoid, reduced diphtheria toxoid, and acellular pertussis vaccines: updated recommendations of the Advisory Committee on Immunization Practices—United States, 2019. MMWR Morb Mortal Wkly Rep. 2020;69(3):77-83.
29. Madeleine MM, Finch JL, Lynch CF, Goodman MT, Engels EA. HPV-related cancers after solid organ transplantation in the United States. Am J Transplant. 2013;13(12): 3202-9.
30. Nelson DR, Neu AM, Abraham A, Amaral S, Batisky D, Fadrowski JJ. Immunogenicity of human papillomavirus recombinant vaccine in children with CKD. Clin J Am Soc Nephrol. 2016;11(5):776-84.
31. Acharya SK, Batra Y, Bhatkal B, Ojha B, Kaur K, Hazari S, et al. Seroepidemiology of hepatitis A virus infection among school children in Delhi and North Indian patients with chronic liver disease: implications for HAV vaccination. J Gastroenterol Hepatol. 2003;18(7):822-7.
32. Rupprecht CE, Briggs D, Brown CM, Franka R, Katz SL, Kerr HD, et al. Use of a reduced (4-dose) vaccine schedule for postexposure prophylaxis to prevent human rabies: recommendations of the Advisory Committee on Immunization Practices. MMWR Recomm Rep. 2010;59(RR-2):1-9.
33. Kaplan LJ, Daum RS, Smaron M, McCarthy CA. Severe measles in immunocompromised patients. JAMA. 1992; 267(9):1237-41.
34. Nkowane BM, Wassilak SG, Orenstein WA, Bart KJ, Schonberger LB, Hinman AR, et al. Vaccine-associated paralytic poliomyelitis. United States: 1973 through 1984. JAMA. 1987;257(10):1335-40.
35. McLean HQ, Fiebelkorn AP, Temte JL, Wallace GS, Centers for Disease Control and Prevention. Prevention of measles, rubella, congenital rubella syndrome, and mumps, 2013: summary recommendations of the Advisory Committee on Immunization Practices (ACIP). MMWR Recomm Rep. 2013;62(RR-04):1-34.
36. McGory RW, Ishitani MB, Oliveira WM, Stevenson WC, McCullough CS, Dickson RC, et al. Improved outcome of orthotopic liver transplantation for chronic hepatitis B cirrhosis with aggressive passive immunization. Transplantation. 1996;61(9):1358-64.
37. Terrault NA, Lok ASF, McMahon BJ, Chang MA, Hwang JP, Jonas MM, et al. Update on prevention, diagnosis, and treatment of chronic hepatitis B: AASLD 2018 hepatitis B guidance. Hepatology. 2018;67(4):1560-99.

CHAPTER

26

Combined Liver Kidney Transplantation

Venu Madhav Thumma, Sukanya Bhrugumalla

CASE VIGNETTE

A 36-year-old male with alcohol related cirrhosis with model for end-stage liver disease (MELD) of 24 is listed for liver transplant. While on the transplant waiting list he is admitted with acute kidney injury (AKI) and hepatic encephalopathy. His serum creatinine is 5.4 mg/dL. His urine output is less than 300 mL/day and he is in metabolic acidosis with a pH of 7.23. Over the next 4 weeks, he receives regular hemodialysis, his serum creatinine decreases to 2.6 mg/dL with a urine output of about 600 mL/day. His hepatic encephalopathy has improved. The treating center has approached the regional organ allocation center for listing him for combined liver and kidney transplant. Is he a candidate for combined liver and kidney transplant?

INTRODUCTION

There is an increasing incidence of renal insufficiency in patients with chronic liver disease (CLD). Since the introduction of the Model for End-Stage Liver Disease (MELD) score, there has been an increase in the number of patients being listed for combined liver and kidney transplantation (CLKT). The criteria for listing for CLKT patients have changed over a period of time. This chapter summarizes the current concepts of CLKT.

PATHOPHYSIOLOGY

Cirrhosis causes circulatory disturbances due to splanchnic arterial vasodilatation and further causes a reduction in systemic vascular resistance. The factors involved are increased levels of nitric oxide, carbon monoxide, and endogenous cannabinoids in splanchnic circulation.[1] Initially, the cardiac output is increased to compensate the decrease in systemic vascular resistance. However, in advanced cases, there is decrease in circulatory volume as increase in cardiac output is unable to compensate. There is activation of renin–angiotensin axis and sympathetic nervous system to maintain normal arterial pressure. However, due to sodium and free water retention, ascites and eventually renal failure occur due to intrarenal vasoconstriction and hypoperfusion.[1]

ACUTE KIDNEY INJURY

Acute kidney injury (AKI) is defined by an acute increase in serum creatinine by ≥0.3 mg/dL or by ≥50% in <48 hours from a stable value in the preceding 3 months. AKI is seen in up to half of the hospitalized patients with cirrhosis.[2] AKI is often caused by an increase in existing hemodynamic disturbances and is often precipitated by a complication such as spontaneous bacterial peritonitis or variceal bleed and is reversible once the precipitating event is treated.

CHRONIC KIDNEY DISEASE

Chronic kidney disease (CKD) occurs in 3.4–13% of hospitalized patients with cirrhosis.[3] CKD can occur in CLD due to the following reasons:

- Hepatorenal syndrome (HRS)
- Hypovolemia-induced renal failure
- Parenchymal renal disease
- Drug-induced renal failure.

Traditionally, CKD was defined based on the persistent elevation of serum creatinine above 1.5 mg/dL. CKD is now defined as glomerular filtration rate (GFR) of <60 mL/min/1.73 m^2 for >3 months.[4] CKD now includes both structural kidney damage and functional kidney damage due to HRS type 2. The prevalence of CKD in cirrhosis is between 22 and 32%.[3] CKD is increasing in cirrhotic patients due to increase in the prevalence of nonalcoholic fatty liver disease (NAFLD) and better understanding of HRS type 2.

In a cohort of 78,640 cirrhotic patients on the liver transplant waiting list, the prevalence of CKD according to the new definition increased significantly from 8% in 2002 to 15% in 2017.[5] Preliver transplant AKI or CKD was associated with increased postliver transplant mortality.[5]

CHAPTER HIGHLIGHTS

- Criteria for combined liver and kidney transplantation (CLKT) in patients with both organ damage and metabolic disorders are well defined across all societies.
- Definite survival benefit is noted in patients on renal replacement therapy (RRT) at CLKT than those not on RRT.
- Better guidelines are needed for CLKT in patients with cirrhosis and acute kidney injury for optimal organ allotment.
- Early and better identification of irreversible renal dysfunction in cirrhotics is needed to prevent organ wastage and to reduce waiting time of patients listed for kidney transplant alone.

CRITERIA FOR COMBINED LIVER AND KIDNEY TRANSPLANTATION

Combined liver and kidney transplantation, as the name suggests, is the transplantation of both liver and kidney. It can be either simultaneous liver and kidney transplant (SLKT), where both liver and kidney are transplanted at the same time, or delayed, where the kidney implantation is delayed by 48–72 hours after the liver implantation. Here, the harvested kidney from the donor is kept functional using a hypothermic machine perfusion.

Another terminology that frequently crops up while discussing liver and kidney transplant is sequential liver and kidney transplantation. This is usually meant for patients where the etiology involves both organs, e.g., polycystic kidney and liver disease, but only one of the organs is transplanted as the patient does not satisfy the criteria for CLKT. Patients with borderline renal function undergoing liver transplant first become eligible for "safety cover," where they receive priority for cadaveric kidney allocation when renal function deteriorates. Another term used is kidney after liver transplant (KALT). This is typically done in patients who develop secondary renal insufficiency long after liver transplant. A patient's survival in KALT is comparable to CLKT but is inferior to renal transplant alone.

The criteria accepted for allocation of organs for CLKT are relatively uniform among patients with CKD and CLD. However, when it comes to CLD with AKI, there is inability to accurately differentiate the cause of AKI, especially HRS versus intrarenal etiology. Renal biopsy to assess structural damage to kidneys is rarely done in clinical practice due to risk of bleeding in cirrhotic patients. So, the criteria are heterogeneous among patients with cirrhosis and AKI.[6] Decrease in muscle mass in cirrhotic patients, increased volume of distribution, and increased tubular secretion can impact serum creatinine levels, thereby underestimating renal dysfunction.[6] Iothalamate clearance is a better test for the measurement of renal function;[7] however, it is not widely used. Among the various equations to find true GFR in cirrhosis patients, modified diet for renal disease-6 (MDRD-6) has been found to be the best.[8] It takes into consideration blood urea nitrogen and serum albumin, both of which are altered in liver disease. In patients with GFR < 30 mL/min/m^2, MDRD-6 is better.[8] In patients with GFR > 30 mL/min/1.73 m^2, MDRD-6 underestimates renal function.[8] Apart from this, there is difficulty in assessing reversibility of renal dysfunction. The recovery depends on the degree of renal dysfunction, need for dialysis, age, and presence of comorbidities such as diabetes and hypertension.

There is no standard allocation policy that is followed by all centers in the world. There are several criteria proposed for CLKT.[9] In a survey of 88 transplant centers, 73% used dialysis duration between 4 and 8 weeks for CLKT listing.[10]

The recent United Network for Organ Sharing (UNOS) criteria for CLKT are:[11]

- *Chronic kidney insufficiency:*
  - Patients should have GFR < 60 mL/min for the last 3 months

    and
  - Patient is on regular maintenance dialysis at the time of listing or with a GFR < 35 mL/min at the time of listing
- *Sustained AKI:*
  - 6 consecutive weeks of dialysis dependence

    or
  - Documented GFR < 25 mL/min for at least 6 weeks
- *Presence of a metabolic disease associated with development of renal failure*:
  - Hyperoxaluria
  - Atypical hemolytic uremic syndrome
  - Familial non-neuropathic systemic amyloid or methylmalonic aciduria.

They introduced the "safety net" for patients with marginal renal function who receive liver transplants alone so that they have access to early kidney transplantation should the renal function worsen after the liver transplant.[11]

BENEFITS OF COMBINED LIVER AND KIDNEY TRANSPLANTATION

- Dialysis after transplant has been shown to predict both poor survival for patients and liver grafts. Post-transplant dialysis was an independent risk factor for graft loss.[12] There is a 35% increased risk for graft loss in liver-only recipients with CKD who require dialysis after liver transplant.[12] CLKT improves the outcome of the liver graft.
- The recipient will have a single exposure to risk of anesthesia.
- There are immunological benefits for CLKT. The recipient is exposed to one set of antigens. The patients who receive liver transplant alone will have difficulty in finding suitable kidney grafts due to sensitization from previous liver transplant and blood transfusions.[13] The

liver graft among CLKT recipients confers an immunological privilege to the kidney graft, especially among recipients with preformed donor-specific anti-human leukocyte antigen (HLA) antibodies, with reduced risk of acute cellular as well as antibody-mediated rejection, and better preservation of long-term renal function compared to patients receiving kidney transplant alone.[14] The mechanism of this protection of kidney graft by the implanted liver is mediated through class I antibodies. The liver has a large surface area to absorb these antibodies. In crossmatch positive recipients of CLKT, there is decreased inflammation and endothelial cell activation.[15] There are unknown mechanisms that shift the gene expression within the kidney from proinflammatory to tissue regeneration pattern.[15]

DISADVANTAGES OF COMBINED LIVER AND KIDNEY TRANSPLANTATION

There is a proportion of patients whose native kidney recovers after CLKT. In a study by Levitsky et al.,[16] renal scans showed three functioning kidneys in a subset of patients who received CLKT. The additional benefit which can be due to kidney transplantation in CLKT recipients is unknown[17] and is difficult to assess. There are also reports of adverse outcomes after CLKT.[18] Even in patients with GFR < 45 mL/min/1.73 m^2, recovery of renal function is expected if the pretransplant dysfunction is due to HRS.

Renal allograft futility[19] is defined as "patient death or need for renal replacement therapy (RRT) at 3 months after transplantation." After CLKT, 39% experienced delayed graft function, and 20.7% had renal allograft futility.[19] Recipients with renal allograft futility had greater MELD scores, prolonged hospitalization, intraoperative base deficit, higher kidney and liver donor risk indices, prolonged kidney cold ischemia, and inferior overall survival. Multivariate predictors of renal allograft futility included pretransplant dialysis duration, kidney cold ischemia, kidney donor risk index, and recipient hyperlipidemia. The authors suggested that renal transplantation should be deferred in liver recipients at high risk of renal allograft futility.

COMBINED LIVER AND KIDNEY TRANSPLANTATION: SURGICAL OPTIONS

The liver transplant can be done by piggyback technique or standard method. After a liver transplant, the kidney can be placed in retroperitoneal or abdominal space. Intraoperative hemodialysis may be used to manage fluid shifts, continuous veno-venous hemodialysis may be used if there is hemodynamic instability. Kidney placement is often delayed in these cases or when the liver transplant takes unusually long time. Machine perfusion is used to maintain graft function in such a case.[6]

Indiana Approach[20]

Some liver transplant recipients are very sick with significant coagulopathy and may require inotropic support. The hemodynamic status may not be good for the new kidney. The raised bilirubin may crystalize in tubules of the kidneys and cause AKI.[9] In Indiana approach, liver transplantation is performed first, while the kidney graft is placed on a hypothermic pulsatile perfusion machine. Implantation of the kidney graft is delayed for 2–3 days which allows stabilization of hemodynamics and coagulopathy. Delayed kidney transplant (by >48 hours) in CLKT was associated with improved patient and graft survival.[20]

En bloc CLKT technique[21] can be used in which the liver and right kidney are procured together with the renal vein kept attached to the inferior vena cava. The splenic artery and gastroduodenal artery are recovered in a standard fashion. During backbench preparation, the donor renal artery is anastomosed to the donor splenic artery to reestablish renal circulation from the celiac axis. Arterial reconstruction is completed prior to reperfusion with anastomosis between the donor celiac axis and the recipient hepatic artery prior to reperfusion. This is done to allow the kidney to receive arterial blood at the same time as reperfusion, similar to a standard kidney transplant. The liver and kidney are reperfused simultaneously in the en bloc setting. The limitations of this technique are as follows:

- Left kidney cannot be used with this technique.
- Aberrant arteries which require reconstruction will be a challenge
- In the event of thrombosis, both grafts may be lost.

OUTCOMES OF COMBINED LIVER AND KIDNEY TRANSPLANTATION

Five-year patient survival rates among patients selected to receive CLKT range from 64 to 76%.[6]

Singal et al.[22] assessed outcomes of CLKT based on liver disease etiology. The 5-year outcomes for liver graft and kidney graft were best for primary biliary cirrhosis (82%) and least for hepatitis C virus (HCV) (66%). Follow-up renal function assessed at 1, 3, and 5 years showed poor renal function among patients receiving CLKT for HCV, nonalcoholic steatohepatitis (NASH), cryptogenic cirrhosis, and hepatitis B virus (HBV).

In a study from the United Kingdom Transplant Registry,[17] the advantage of CLKT appears to benefit only those who are on established RRT at the time of transplant. Significantly higher patient survival and liver graft survival were noted for patients on RRT at the time of transplantation undergoing CLKT in comparison to those on RRT receiving liver transplant alone. Compared to the current consensus, it seems that patients with estimated glomerular filtration rate (eGFR) <44 mL/min/1.73 m^2 do not benefit by receiving CLKT in terms of patient and liver graft survival. Only those already on RRT have a favorable survival outcome from CLKT. In this study, the data did not support CLKT approach based on eGFR alone. Patient and graft survival benefit for patients on RRT at transplantation favored CLKT as against liver transplant alone, but the renal function of the long-term survivors was not superior following CLKT. Kidney graft survival was 90.6% at 1 year, 88.7% at 3 years, and 84.0% at 5 years post-transplantation in the CLKT group.

METABOLIC INDICATIONS FOR COMBINED LIVER AND KIDNEY TRANSPLANTATION

Primary Hyperoxalurias[23]

Primary hyperoxalurias are autosomal recessive disorders that result in the overproduction of oxalate, leading to hyperoxaluria, nephrocalcinosis, and CKD. There are three types of primary hyperoxaluria:

1. *Type 1 primary hyperoxaluria:* There is deficiency of alanine-glyoxylate aminotransferase, which facilitates transamination of glyoxylate to glycine in the liver. This is the most common type of hyperoxaluria. It has a very aggressive clinical course. The median age of presentation is 5.6 years.
2. *Type 2 primary hyperoxaluria:* There is deficiency of a primarily hepatic enzyme, glyoxylate reductase-hydroxypyruvate reductase. There is accumulation of oxalate and L-glycerate. The median age of presentation is 3.2 years.
3. *Type 3 primary hyperoxaluria:* It is caused by a deficit of 4-hydroxy-2-oxoglutarate aldolase, resulting in the accumulation of oxalate. This is the mildest form.

The mean age of patients at first liver/kidney transplant is 16.5 years for type 1 and about 40 years for type 2 hyperoxaluria.

In patients with type 1 primary hyperoxaluria, doing kidney transplantation alone is associated with rapid recurrence of the disease. However, since a large amount of oxalate accumulates in the body over the years of disease, it is important to prevent rapid oxalate deposition in the renal graft. Namely, it can further lead to acute oxalate nephropathy and irreversible renal failure. In patients who undergo CLKT, there will be requirement for RRT in the perioperative period till the excess accumulated oxalate is cleared from the body. In type 1 hyperoxaluria, sequential liver and kidney transplantation can be done, where liver is transplanted first and kidney is transplanted after several months. This will decrease the oxalate production in the body prior to kidney transplantation. In approximately 30% of western primary hyperoxaluria patients, vitamin B_6 effectively lowers hepatic oxalate production. A small subset of patients shows a complete response defined as a normalization of the oxalate excretion rate. In these selected adult patients with confirmed evidence of B_6 responsiveness, isolated kidney transplant can be considered.

BIOMARKERS AND COMBINED LIVER AND KIDNEY TRANSPLANTATION

There are plasma and urine biomarkers of renal injury such as neutrophil gelatinase-associated lipocalin, kidney injury molecule-1, interleukin-18, human endothelin-1, uromodulin, epidermal growth factor, and fatty acid binding protein. These biomarkers are useful to predict recovery of renal function in patients with AKI and may be used in future allocation policies for CLKT.

CONCLUSION

The incidence of renal dysfunction in cirrhosis is progressively increasing. Literature suggests better patient and graft survival in this subgroup of patients with CLKT when compared to liver transplant alone. The indications for CLKT in metabolic diseases such as primary hyperoxaluria are well established. Consensus for CLKT in patients with CKD and cirrhosis also exists across all transplant centers. However, in the absence of a consensus for defining irreversible AKI in cirrhosis, the criteria for CLKT in this subgroup of patients vary across centers leading to wide variation in post-transplant outcomes. Though UNOS guidelines exist since 2017, this has not found wide acceptance outside the United States. Better predictors of irreversible renal dysfunction in cirrhosis are needed. In future, biomarkers and better scoring systems may be available to predict the requirement of CLKT.

REFERENCES

1. Ginès P, Schrier RW. Renal failure in cirrhosis. N Engl J Med. 2009;361(13):1279-90.
2. Wong F, O'Leary JG, Reddy KR, Garcia-Tsao G, Fallon MB, Biggins SW, et al. Acute kidney injury in cirrhosis: baseline serum creatinine predicts patient outcomes. Am J Gastroenterol. 2017;112(7):1103-10.
3. Wong F, Reddy KR, O'Leary JG, Tandon P, Biggins SW, Garcia-Tsao G, et al. Impact of chronic kidney disease on outcomes in cirrhosis. Liver Transpl. 2019;25(6):870-80.
4. Wong F, Nadim MK, Kellum JA, Salerno F, Bellomo R, Gerbes A, et al. Working Party proposal for a revised classification system of renal dysfunction in patients with cirrhosis. Gut. 2011;60(5):702-9.
5. Cullaro G, Verna EC, Lee BP, Lai JC. Chronic kidney disease in liver transplant candidates: a rising burden impacting post-liver transplant outcomes. Liver Transpl. 2020;26(4):498-506.
6. Singal AK, Ong S, Satapathy SK, Kamath PS, Wiesner RH. Simultaneous liver kidney transplantation. Transpl Int. 2019;32(4):343-52.
7. Hsu CY, Bansal N. Measured GFR as "gold standard"—all that glitters is not gold? Clin J Am Soc Nephrol. 2011;6(8):1813-4.

8. Francoz C, Nadim MK, Baron A, Prié D, Antoine C, Belghiti J, et al. Glomerular filtration rate equations for liver-kidney transplantation in patients with cirrhosis: validation of current recommendations. Hepatology. 2014;59(4):1514-21.
9. Ekser B, Contreras AG, Andraus W, Taner T. Current status of combined liver-kidney transplantation. Int J Surg. 2020; 82S:149-54.
10. Nadim MK, Davis CL, Sung R, Kellum JA, Genyk YS. Simultaneous liver-kidney transplantation: a survey of US transplant centers. Am J Transplant. 2012;12(11):3119-27.
11. Boyle G. Simultaneous liver kidney (SLK) allocation policy. [online] Available from https://optn.transplant.hrsa.gov/policies-bylaws/policies/. [Last accessed October, 2022].
12. Nagai S, Safwan M, Collins K, Schilke RE, Rizzari M, Moonka D, et al. Liver alone or simultaneous liver-kidney transplant? Pretransplant chronic kidney disease and post-transplant outcome—a retrospective study. Transpl Int. 2018; 31:1028.
13. Enestvedt CK. PRO: simultaneous liver-kidney transplantation in the current era: still the best option. Clin Liver Dis (Hoboken). 2020;16(6):266-71.
14. Taner T, Heimbach JK, Rosen CB, Nyberg SL, Park WD, Stegall MD. Decreased chronic cellular and antibody-mediated injury in the kidney following simultaneous liver-kidney transplantation. Kidney Int. 2016;89(4):909-17.
15. Taner T, Park WD, Stegall MD. Unique molecular changes in kidney allografts after simultaneous liver-kidney compared with solitary kidney transplantation. Kidney Int. 2017;91(5):1193-202.
16. Levitsky J, Baker T, Ahya SN, Levin ML, Friedewald J, Gallon L, et al. Outcomes and native renal recovery following simultaneous liver-kidney transplantation. Am J Transplant. 2012;12(11):2949-57.
17. Tinti F, Mitterhofer AP, Umbro I, Nightingale P, Inston N, Ghallab M, et al. Combined liver-kidney transplantation versus liver transplant alone based on KDIGO stratification of estimated glomerular filtration rate: data from the United Kingdom Transplant registry—a retrospective cohort study. Transpl Int. 2019;32(9):918-32.
18. Locke JE, Warren DS, Singer AL, Segev DL, Simpkins CE, Maley WR, et al. Declining outcomes in simultaneous liver-kidney transplantation in the MELD era: ineffective usage of renal allografts. Transplantation. 2008;85(7):935-42.
19. Lunsford KE, Bodzin AS, Markovic D, Zarrinpar A, Kaldas FM, Gritsch HA, et al. Avoiding futility in simultaneous liver-kidney transplantation: analysis of 331 consecutive patients listed for dual organ replacement. Ann Surg. 2017; 265(5):1016-24.
20. Ekser B, Mangus RS, Fridell W, Kubal CA, Nagai S, Kinsella SB, et al. A novel approach in combined liver and kidney transplantation with long-term outcomes. Ann Surg. 2017;265(5):1000-8.
21. Lee TC, Cortez AR, Kassam AF, Morris MC, Winer LK, Silski LS, et al. Outcomes of en bloc simultaneous liver-kidney transplantation compared to the traditional technique. Am J Transplant. 2020;20(4):1181-7.
22. Singal AK, Salameh H, Kuo YF, Wiesner RH. Evolving frequency and outcomes of simultaneous liver kidney transplants based on liver disease etiology. Transplantation. 2014;98(2):216-21.
23. Knotek M, Novak R, Jaklin-Kekez A, Mrzljak A. Combined liver-kidney transplantation for rare diseases. World J Hepatol. 2020;12(10):722-37.

CHAPTER 27

Combined Kidney Pancreas Transplantation

B Ramesh Kumar, Manisha Sahay

INTRODUCTION

Simultaneous pancreas–kidney (SPK) transplantation is an established, definitive treatment for selected diabetic patients with end-stage kidney disease (ESKD). Nearly 90% of pancreas transplants in the United States are performed as SPK transplants, with the remainder performed as sequential pancreas after kidney (PAK) transplants or pancreas transplants alone (PTA).[1,2]

EPIDEMIOLOGY

According to the International Pancreas Transplant Registry (IPTR), more than 61,000 pancreas transplants were performed worldwide between 1966 and 2020, including more than 34,000 in the United States. In the United States during 2019, 868 SPK transplants, 58 PTA, and 44 sequential PAK transplants were performed.[2-4]

While SPK transplants most often involve grafts procured from a single deceased donor following brain death, a few are simultaneous living-donor kidney and deceased-donor pancreas transplants, and some SPK transplants (3%) are performed from a deceased donor after cardiac death. Simultaneous living-donor kidney and segmental pancreas transplantation is rarely performed at present.

Pancreas after kidney typically involves transplantation of a deceased-donor pancreas graft into a recipient following either a functioning living- (most common, 80%) or deceased-donor kidney allograft. Some diabetic patients without advanced kidney disease may be candidates for PTA.

The vast majority of SPK and PAK transplants are performed in patients with type 1 diabetes, although an increasing number are performed in patients with a type 2 diabetes phenotype. According to the IPTR, approximately 21% of SPK and 14% of PAK transplants are performed in patients with a type 2 diabetes phenotype.

INDICATIONS FOR SIMULTANEOUS PANCREAS–KIDNEY OR PANCREAS AFTER KIDNEY TRANSPLANT

- Therapeutic option for patients with insulin-requiring diabetes and advanced chronic kidney disease (CKD) or ESKD. The majority of these patients receive an SPK transplant, although some will receive a sequential PAK transplant.
- Insulin-requiring diabetes with normal or near-normal kidney function may be considered for PTA if they have hypoglycemic unawareness or brittle diabetes with wild variations in blood glucose levels, and/or if their quality of life is unacceptable because of diabetes-related sequelae.
- Primarily indicated for patients with type 1 diabetes. However, SPK and PAK transplants may be performed for some patients with insulin-requiring diabetes who meet certain selection criteria and exhibit a type 2 diabetes phenotype, characterized by the presence of detectable C-peptide levels, older age of onset of diabetes (and older age at transplant), history of non-insulin-requiring diabetes preceding the need for insulin therapy, shorter duration of insulin dependence, and history of obesity.[5-7]

The above guidelines are based upon the assumption that patients with extreme insulin resistance may not be appropriate candidates for pancreas transplantation.

However, IPTR data as well as a number of single-center reports suggest that measuring C-peptide levels is largely irrelevant in terms of either patient selection or predicting outcomes.

Moreover, individual centers may have other cutoffs for SPK or PAK candidate exclusion, such as age >50 years or body mass index (BMI) >28 kg/m^2. Alternatively, other centers may transplant patients up to 65 years of age and with a BMI of 30–35 kg/m^2.

Patients qualifying for an SPK or PAK transplant are usually referred to the transplant center by a nephrologist because of stage 4/5 CKD.

Approximately 16% of SPK transplants are performed in patients prior to the initiation of dialysis therapy. Most of these patients will have advanced diabetic nephropathy, but some may have kidney disease from a condition other than diabetes.

Thus, ESKD does not have to be secondary to advanced diabetic nephropathy to qualify for either SPK or PAK transplantation if the patient has insulin-requiring diabetes. This unique situation offers the opportunity to treat both the kidney disease and the insulin-requiring diabetes successfully regardless of cause.

SELECTION OF OPTIMAL PROCEDURE

The selection of the optimal procedure for individual patients depends upon patient-specific factors and organ availability.

- For younger patients (i.e., <45 years old) with type 1 diabetes who have no other cardiac risk factors and few other comorbidities, in the absence of a living-kidney donor, *SPK transplant provides the best survival* compared with either dialysis or deceased-donor kidney transplantation alone (KTA) with advantages in:
    - Achievement of normoglycemia and insulin independence which may increase longevity and also improve the quality of life.
    - Short median waiting times of 2–3 years compared with deceased-donor KTA (4–6 years)
- However, because the 1- and 4-year mortality for waitlisted SPK transplant candidates has been reported to be 6.6 and 41.3%, respectively, performing a *living-donor KTA may be preferred if an individual is facing a long waiting time for SPK transplantation, is not doing well on dialysis, or has "stable" diabetes.* Following KTA, in the absence of sensitization, the waiting time for a PAK transplant is usually 1–2 years.
- If the candidate, on the other hand, is not yet on dialysis or has an anticipated short waiting time for SPK transplant (based upon blood type, degree of sensitization, and geographic region), then waiting for an SPK transplant is a reasonable option.

Because patients with insulin-requiring diabetes and ESKD have a high annual mortality rate on dialysis (5–10%), the shorter waiting time associated with a living-donor KTA becomes an important consideration. In addition, not all patients with insulin-requiring diabetes and ESKD qualify for SPK transplant or are even interested in receiving a pancreas transplant, particularly if they believe that their diabetes is well controlled and are not experiencing extreme glucose hypermobility, hypoglycemia unawareness, or life-threatening, sight-threatening, limb-threatening, progressive, or accelerated complications of diabetes.

OBSERVATIONS

In an analysis of the United Network for Organ Sharing (UNOS) registry from 1995 to 2010 of all adults registered for an SPK or PAK, the following observations were reported:

- 5-year patient survival was comparable between SPK and PAK (86 vs. 83%, respectively), but 10-year patient survival was higher with SPK compared with PAK (70 vs. 63%, respectively).
- 10-year kidney allograft survival rates were similar (61%) for recipients of either an SPK or a living-donor KTA. Patients who received a PAK after either living- or deceased-donor KTA had superior 10-year kidney allograft survival compared with those who did not. Kidney allograft survival rates were highest (70%) for recipients of a living-donor KTA, followed by a sequential PAK.
- 10-year pancreas allograft survival rates were 59% for SPK, 44% for PAK following living-donor KTA, and 42% for PAK following deceased-donor KTA.

These findings suggest *that both patient and kidney allograft longevity are maximized by achieving an insulin- and dialysis-free state, whether this is accomplished by either an SPK or a PAK, preferably following a living-donor KTA.*

Adding a pancreas to a kidney transplant (either simultaneously or sequentially) provides a survival advantage beyond KTA compared with all treatments available to the uremic diabetic patient.

The decision to be placed on the deceased-donor waitlist in order to receive an SPK transplant depends upon their dialysis duration and tolerability, their predicted waiting time on the list for SPK, and the severity and progression of diabetic complications. However, in general, the availability of a human leukocyte antigen (HLA)-identical (or zero HLA mismatch) living donor takes precedence over an SPK transplant because of the projected longer life span of the kidney in this setting.

Finally, when analyzing the relative value of receiving either a kidney or a pancreas transplant or both, it is apparent that a functioning kidney transplant (in the absence of a functioning pancreas transplant) is a better predictor of long-term patient survival compared with a functioning pancreas transplant (in the absence of a functioning kidney transplant). Although patients with both kidney and pancreas grafts functioning have the best longevity, a functioning living-donor KTA represents an excellent option from a life expectancy perspective.

In general, if a patient believes that diabetes is controlling their life more than they are controlling their diabetes, or if the presence of diabetes (independent of kidney failure) is self-perceived to be causing significant impairment in their overall quality of life, then either SPK or PAK transplantation should be considered as a treatment option.

For patients who have a well-functioning transplanted kidney, the decision to undergo PAK transplantation depends upon their quality of life and overall satisfaction with KTA, their willingness to undergo another surgical procedure, and/or the presence of progressive or accelerated diabetic complications.

PATIENT SELECTION

The primary determinants for recipient selection are the presence of glucose hypermobility reflecting underlying insulin deficiency, the degree of difficulty in achieving adequate glucose control, progressive diabetic complications (including CKD), degree of nephropathy (which determines the type of transplant), cardiovascular risk and iliac vascular disease, other comorbidities (e.g., substance abuse, lung or liver disease, and obesity), emotional and psychosocial stability, and overall functional and performance status. In other words, *the need for insulin therapy alone is not sufficient to qualify for any type of pancreas transplantation.*

Age

Appropriate candidates for SPK transplantation are generally younger than KTA candidates with diabetes, reflecting several factors. Patients with type 1 diabetes mellitus tend to develop ESKD at an earlier age than patients with type 2 diabetes mellitus. Additionally, long-standing diabetes contributes to a higher incidence of other complications, such as cardiovascular disease, which affects transplant candidacy. An analysis of the UNOS database, including 20,854 pancreas transplant recipients between 1996 and 2012, demonstrated that graft survival was superior in recipients 40–49 years of age, with reduced patient survival in those 50–59 years of age and poor graft and patient survival in those >60 years of age.[8] However, according to IPTR data, some patients aged 60 years and older may benefit from SPK transplantation.

We believe that highly selected patients between the ages of 50 and 65 years may benefit from SPK or PAK transplantation if they do not have significant comorbidities such as advanced cardiovascular, cerebrovascular, or peripheral vascular disease. At the other end of the recipient age spectrum, very few pancreas transplants are performed in the pediatric population (18 years or younger), particularly with advances in the early diagnosis of diabetes and kidney disease, insulin delivery systems, and glucose monitoring.

Glomerular Filtration Rate

The national pancreas allocation system requires SPK transplant candidates to meet criteria for kidney transplant listing [glomerular filtration rate (GFR) ≤ 20 mL/min *or* dialysis dependence] in order to receive credit for waiting time.

Insulin Requirement

Daily insulin requirements and serum C-peptide levels are assessed in order to determine whether the patient will likely benefit from pancreas transplantation. Since pancreas transplantation restores endogenous insulin production, patients who are insulinopenic or who have undetectable or very low C-peptide levels are most likely to benefit from the procedure.

In general, patients with insulin requirements exceeding 1 unit/kg/day may not always achieve euglycemia after pancreas transplant. In our practice, a very high daily insulin requirement suggests that the patient may have insulin resistance or anti-insulin/islet cell antibodies; such patients may be less likely to benefit from pancreas transplantation and be rendered insulin free, although no randomized studies have examined this issue. However, patients who are on peritoneal dialysis may have large insulin requirements due to the use of dextrose-containing dialysate, and their daily insulin requirements will likely decrease when peritoneal dialysis is discontinued following kidney transplantation.

Complications of insulin therapy, including the presence of hypoglycemic unawareness and frequency/severity of either hypoglycemic or hyperglycemic episodes, may increase the urgency for pancreas transplantation.

Body Mass Index

The maximum allowable BMI for SPK or PAK transplantation varies between centers but is often lower than that for KTA because pancreas transplantation requires intra-abdominal surgery, and post-transplantation wound healing and surgical complications are affected to a greater extent by an elevated BMI.[9] Most centers use a BMI threshold of 30 kg/m^2. Some centers may consider performing SPK transplants in selected patients with a BMI in the 30–35 kg/m^2 range, whereas very few pancreas transplants are ever performed in patients with a BMI > 35 kg/m^2. In some studies, increasing recipient BMI is an independent risk factor for pancreas graft loss and death in the short term, whereas obesity is a risk factor for pancreas graft loss in the long term.

At the other end of the BMI spectrum, patients with a very low BMI may have a higher mortality following SPK transplantation possibly because of associated conditions such as deconditioning, frailty, malnutrition, and sarcopenia.

Furthermore, an elevated BMI is often associated with insulin resistance and, in a single-center, retrospective series was associated with post-transplant diabetes. It is important to note, however, that in the absence of early graft loss or surgical complications, SPK transplantation in obese recipients is associated with excellent long-term outcomes.

Limited data are available with SPK transplant in patients who have previously undergone bariatric surgery. However, in those patients who remain insulin dependent following successful bariatric surgery with significant weight loss, SPK transplantation remains a viable option. In addition, many patients with obesity may benefit from structured weight loss programs and "prehab" in an attempt to improve their transplant candidacy and subsequent outcomes.

Other Criteria

In addition to age, duration of diabetes and insulin use, C-peptide levels (as a marker of endogenous insulin secretion), daily insulin requirements, and BMI, potential recipients *should be screened for tobacco and other substance use, functional capacity, presence and severity of diabetic-related complications, and additional comorbidities.*

CONTRAINDICATIONS

Although contraindications may vary by transplant center, absolute contraindications that are adopted by most centers include:

- Age >65 years
- Non-insulin-requiring diabetes
- BMI >35 kg/m^2
- Advanced cardiopulmonary disease (ejection fraction below 30%, pulmonary artery systolic pressure >50 mm Hg, or positive cardiac stress test with uncorrectable coronary artery disease)
- Heavy smoking [>1 pack/day or patients with moderate-to-severe smoking-related morbidities (coronary heart disease, symptomatic or documented cerebrovascular or peripheral vascular disease, chronic obstructive lung disease, history of noncutaneous malignancy)]
- Severe peripheral vascular (aortoiliac) disease
- Moderate-to-severe dysfunction in other (nonkidney) organ systems [lung, liver, central nervous system (CNS)] including cirrhosis, portal hypertension, advanced chronic obstructive pulmonary disease, dementia, or severe neurologic deficits
- Active malignancy with the exception of nonmelanoma skin cancer or low-grade prostate cancer
- Severe local or systemic infection
- Inadequate psychosocial support and financial resources
- Active substance addiction or abuse
- Major psychiatric illness that cannot be managed sufficiently to enable post-transplant care and safety
- Poor overall functional and performance status (severe deconditioning or malnutrition, frailty, dementia, wheelchair bound, need for chronic oxygen therapy)
- Chronic nonhealing wounds
- Projected life expectancy <5 years.

A list of commonly accepted *relative contraindications* would be:

- Age <18 or >60 years
- BMI > 30–35 kg/m^2
- Daily insulin requirement > 1 unit/kg
- Insulin requiring for <3 years
- Left ventricular ejection fraction <40%
- Recent myocardial infarction or stroke
- Pulmonary artery systolic pressure >50 mm Hg (confirmed by right heart catheterization)
- Active tobacco smoking (up to 1 pack/day or patient has mild smoking-related morbidities)
- History of major unilateral or bilateral extremity amputations
- Presence of aortoiliac or aortobifemoral bypass graft
- Symptomatic cerebrovascular or peripheral vascular disease
- Positive thrombophilia screen or history of hypercoagulability
- Peritoneal dialysis with history of multiple prior episodes of peritonitis
- History of multiple previous laparotomies
- History of previous intra-abdominal/pelvic irradiation or multiple surgical procedures
- Severe or uncontrolled orthostasis or hypotension
- Severe or uncontrolled gastroparesis
- Presence of an ostomy, feeding tube, or chronic bladder drainage catheter
- History of previous substance abuse, psychiatric illness, or noncompliance/nonadherence
- Limited psychosocial support and resources (lives alone, relies on public transportation).

PRETRANSPLANT EVALUATION

Patient selection is aided by a comprehensive medical evaluation before transplantation performed by a multidisciplinary team that confirms the diagnosis of insulin-requiring diabetes, determines the patient's ability to withstand the operative procedure and requisite chronic immunosuppression, establishes the absence of any exclusion criteria, and documents end-organ complications for future tracking following transplantation.

Potential recipients are carefully screened for coronary heart disease, congestive heart failure, peripheral vascular disease, active infections, and chronic nonhealing wounds.

All candidates for pancreas allografts should undergo an extensive pretransplant evaluation for cardiovascular disease. In general, however, the pretransplant medical evaluation for a diabetic patient is similar regardless of whether they are being considered for either SPK transplant, PAK transplant, or KTA, *with the exception that thrombophilia screening is performed prior to consideration for pancreas transplantation.*

Cardiovascular Evaluation

Probably the single most important clinical aspect of recipient selection is the overall assessment of cardiovascular risk, burden, and reserve. *Cardiovascular disease remains the most common cause of death following pancreas transplantation among diabetic patients.* Coronary heart disease, defined by prior myocardial infarction, coronary bypass, or percutaneous coronary angioplasty in the past was associated (independent of age) with a 20% 1-year mortality in SPK and PAK transplant recipients, four times greater than in diabetic recipients without a history of myocardial infarction and/or revascularization. Among such patients, traditional cardiovascular risk factors include a long duration of diabetes, hypertension, dyslipidemia, tobacco use, older age, and male gender. Nontraditional risk factors include long dialysis duration, proteinuria, and hyperparathyroidism.

The approach depends upon cardiovascular risk factors, including dialysis duration, duration of diabetes, and smoking history.

- In all candidates who are already on dialysis and who have had diabetes for more than 25 years, any smoking history, or other cardiovascular risk factors or disease (age >55 years, hypertension, history of myocardial infarction, congestive heart failure, low ejection fraction, valvular heart disease, arrhythmias, pulmonary hypertension, cerebrovascular disease, or previous major amputation), referral for formal cardiology evaluation and potential cardiac catheterization should be considered. Such patients are considered to be at especially high risk for coronary heart disease. The decision to proceed with cardiac catheterization is made in conjunction with the patient's cardiologist and nephrologist, recognizing the risk of contrast nephropathy.[10-12]
- In all candidates who are not on dialysis, have had diabetes for ≤25 years, are nonsmokers, *and* have no other cardiovascular risk factors, we perform noninvasive testing and reserve cardiac catheterization for those patients who have a positive noninvasive stress test. For patients who are able to exercise and achieve 85% maximum heart rate, we use an exercise stress test.

The requirement for catheterization in higher-risk patients is that a significant number of false-negative noninvasive stress results are observed among patients with ESKD.

Significant coronary heart disease that is not amenable to revascularization may exclude candidates from pancreas transplant consideration. It is important to note, however, that most diabetic patients with ESKD have identifiable cardiac and/or peripheral vascular disease. *It is not the presence but rather the severity of the cardiovascular disease (and if it is correctable) that determines whether the patient is an appropriate candidate for pancreas transplantation.*

In patients with smoking-related morbidities (coronary artery disease, symptomatic or documented cerebrovascular or peripheral vascular disease, chronic obstructive lung disease, history of noncutaneous malignancy), complete smoking cessation is required and should be validated by urine nicotine tests prior to transplant.

A *newer contraindication is chronic severe hypotension related to severe diabetic autonomic neuropathy or chronic dialysis, either of which may result in significant and irreversible cardiac dysfunction* because of the inability to consistently maintain a systolic pressure above 100 mm Hg, which places the transplanted pancreas at high risk for vascular thrombosis and the transplanted kidney will be at risk for ongoing ischemic damage with poor recovery of kidney function.

Evaluation of Peripheral Vascular Disease

Peripheral vascular disease is common among diabetic patients with ESKD and may prevent successful transplantation of either the kidney or the pancreas because of technical and hemodynamic considerations.

Careful examination of iliac and peripheral pulses should be done in all patients.

To identify patients with iliac calcifications, screening all diabetic patients older than 45 years of age, those with long-standing hypertension, or those with poor femoral pulses or evidence of vascular disease elsewhere (e.g., coronary heart disease or cerebrovascular disease), with a noncontrast abdominopelvic computed tomography (CT) scan should be considered.

In addition, many centers will perform carotid and iliac artery duplex ultrasonographic imaging as part of the standard evaluation for transplantation in this patient population. The diagnosis of peripheral vascular disease is difficult to establish in such patients because of the presence of medial artery calcifications that render vessels noncompressible for a standard ankle-brachial index and/or toe-brachial index.

Patients with symptoms of peripheral vascular disease (e.g., claudication), diminished pulses on exam, or abnormal imaging are referred to a vascular specialist for further assessment and testing.

Hypercoagulability Evaluation

In contrast to KTA, *the risk of pancreas thrombosis is relatively high because it is a low microcirculatory flow organ with its blood supply based on collateral circulation.* Consequently, patients with a history of thrombophilia (hypercoagulability) or those on anticoagulation represent a unique risk factor for early pancreas graft loss. In addition, diabetes may be associated with a prothrombotic state. For these reasons, thrombophilia screening on all potential pancreas transplant recipients should be done with the selective use of perioperative anticoagulation to reduce the risk of early thrombosis.[13]

Cancer Screening

Malignancy in the past 2 years, with the exception of cutaneous squamous, basal cell tumors, and early prostate cancer with low Gleason score, is another contraindication. Consultation and "clearance" may need to be obtained from an oncology specialist, but ultimately a determination will need to be made if the patient's mortality in the absence of transplantation is predicted to be higher than their risk of recurrence.

Standard cancer screening for SPK or PAK transplantation is similar to KTA and may include chest radiography, mammography, gynecologic examination, dermatology assessment (particularly with any history of skin cancer), colonoscopy, and prostate-specific antigen testing depending upon age and gender.

Infectious Disease Evaluation

Incurable or incompletely treated or unresolved active or chronic infections represent another contraindication and may include chronic active hepatitis B, hepatitis C, and uncontrolled human immunodeficiency virus (HIV).

However, in the absence of cirrhosis, adequately treated hepatitis B [hepatitis B surface antigen (HbsAg) negative] or hepatitis C virus are no longer considered contraindications to transplantation.

In the case of hepatitis C viral infection without cirrhosis, transplantation may precede treatment for hepatitis C to take advantage of organs from hepatitis C-positive donors provided that the patient has been accepted as a good candidate for anti-hepatitis C virus treatment.

In addition, HIV-infected patients with adequately controlled HIV infection, characterized by a CD4 count > 200, undetectable HIV ribonucleic acid (RNA) levels, a stable antiretroviral regimen for a minimum of 3 months, and absence of opportunistic infections in the past 12 months, may be considered acceptable for pancreas transplantation.

However, patients with chronic nonhealing wounds or osteomyelitis are not considered appropriate for transplantation.

Psychosocial Evaluation

An adequate support system with requisite resources is needed to ensure the success of transplantation. Abstinence from all illicit drugs for a minimum of 6 months and documentation of compliance are necessary. Smoking cessation is strongly encouraged and at some centers is an absolute requirement. Social alcohol and medicinal marijuana use are considered acceptable, but overuse/dependency/abuse is a contraindication. The use of narcotics for chronic pain is a risk factor that must be carefully evaluated as it has been shown to be associated with inferior outcomes. In cases of substance addiction, referral to a structured rehabilitation or cessation program may be indicated.

Functional Assessment

Severe frailty, deconditioning, malnutrition, and sarcopenia are relative contraindications to transplant; some of these patients may benefit from structured "prehab" programs.

The presence of untreatable advanced dysfunction of another major organ system or a projected life expectancy of <5 years because of other irreversible systemic illness or multiple comorbidities are additional contraindications to transplantation.

It is better to perform standard frailty or "fit" testing in all of our potential (SPK or KTA) candidates that includes grip strength, gait speed, timed repeated chair stands (get up and go test) and 6-minute walk, balance test, assessment of level of physical activity, and activities and daily level scale. This frailty instrument generates a numerical score that categorizes patients as fit, intermediately fit, or frail.[14]

In an analysis of data from the Scientific Registry of Transplant Recipients (SRTR) between 2006 and 2019, the risk of mortality progressively increased for SPK transplant recipients capable of self-care [adjusted hazard ratio (aHR) 1.18, 95% confidence interval (CI) 1.00–1.41], requiring assistance (aHR 1.31, 95% CI 1.06–1.60), and who are disabled (aHR 1.55, 95% CI 1.10–2.19), compared with that of patients with normal functioning.

CONCLUSION

- Simultaneous pancreas–kidney transplantation is an established treatment for selected diabetic patients with end-stage diabetic nephropathy. Pancreas transplants are performed as SPK transplants, sequential PAK transplants, or PTA.
- Selection of the optimal procedure for individual patients depends on patient-specific factors and organ availability:
  - For suitable candidates who are not on dialysis (or just started dialysis) and anticipate a short waiting time for SPK transplant (i.e., <2 years), we prefer an SPK rather than living-donor kidney transplant.
  - For suitable candidates who have already been on dialysis for a year or two and are anticipating a waiting time for SPK of 2 years or more, we prefer a living-donor KTA if one is available. Patients with diabetes and ESKD on dialysis have high mortality on the waiting list.
  - For patients who have a well-functioning transplanted kidney, the decision to undergo PAK transplantation depends upon the patient's quality of life and satisfaction with living-donor KTA, willingness to go through another procedure, and diabetes control and complications.
- Suitability of candidates for SPK transplantation depends upon patient-specific factors, including age, body size,

comorbidities, functional status, social support, burden of vascular disease, and cardiovascular risk profile. In order to be placed on the waiting list, potential candidates must meet certain standards based on GFR, daily insulin requirements, C-peptide levels, and BMI. Potential recipients are screened for tobacco and other substance use, functional capacity, presence and severity of diabetic-related complications, iliac and cardiac vascular disease, and additional comorbidities.

- Patient selection is aided by a comprehensive medical evaluation before transplantation performed by a multidisciplinary team that confirms the diagnosis of insulin-requiring diabetes, determines the patient's ability to withstand the operative procedure and requisite chronic immunosuppression, establishes the absence of any exclusion criteria, and documents end-organ complications for future tracking following transplantation. Potential recipients are carefully screened for coronary heart disease, congestive heart failure, peripheral vascular disease, active infections, and chronic nonhealing wounds. All candidates for pancreas allografts should undergo an extensive pretransplant evaluation for cardiovascular disease. In general, however, the pretransplant medical evaluation for a diabetic patient is similar regardless of whether they are being considered for either an SPK/PAK or a KTA.

REFERENCES

1. Redfield RR, Scalea JR, Odorico JS. Simultaneous pancreas and kidney transplantation: current trends and future directions. Curr Opin Organ Transplant. 2015;20(1):94-102.
2. Gruessner A. Updated International Pancreas Transplant Registry (IPTR) data. 2020. Personal communication.
3. Kandaswamy R, Stock PG, Gustafson SK, Skeans MA, Urban R, Fox A, et al. OPTN/SRTR 2018 Annual Data Report: pancreas. Am J Transplant. 2020;20(Suppl. s1):131-92.
4. Open Procurement & Transplantation Network. [online] Available from: https://optn.transplant.hrsa.gov/data. [Last accessed September, 2022].
5. Gruessner AC, Laftavi MR, Pankewycz O, Gruessner RWG. Simultaneous pancreas and kidney transplantation—is it a treatment option for patients with type 2 diabetes mellitus? An analysis of the International Pancreas Transplant Registry. Curr Diab Rep. 2017;17(6):44.
6. Stratta RJ, Rogers J, Farney AC, Orlando G, El-Hennawy H, Gautreaux MD, et al. Pancreas transplantation in C-peptide positive patients: does "type" of diabetes really matter? J Am Coll Surg. 2015;220(4):716-27.
7. Al-Qaoud TM, Odorico JS, Redfield 3rd RR. Pancreas transplantation in type 2 diabetes: expanding the criteria. Curr Opin Organ Transplant. 2018;23(4):454-60.
8. Siskind E, Maloney C, Akerman M, Alex A, Ashburn S, Barlow M, et al. An analysis of pancreas transplantation outcomes based on age groupings—an update of the UNOS database. Clin Transplant. 2014;28(9):990-4.
9. Neidlinger N, Singh N, Klein C, Odorico J, Munoz del Rio A, Becker Y, et al. Incidence of and risk factors for post-transplant diabetes mellitus after pancreas transplantation Am J Transplant. 2010;10(2):398-406.
10. Becker BN, Odorico JS, Becker YT, Groshek M, Werwinski C, Pirsch JD, et al. Simultaneous pancreas-kidney and pancreas transplantation. J Am Soc Nephrol. 2001;12(11):2517-27.
11. Douzdjian V, Abecassis MM, Corry RJ, Hunsicker LG. Simultaneous pancreas-kidney versus kidney-alone transplants in diabetics: increased risk of early cardiac death and acute rejection following pancreas transplants. Clin Transplant. 1994;8(3 Pt 1):246-51.
12. Manske CL, Thomas W, Wang Y, Wilson RF. Screening diabetic transplant candidates for coronary artery disease: identification of a low risk subgroup. Kidney Int. 1993;44(3): 617-21.
13. Pomero F, Di Minno MN, Fenoglio L, Gianni M, Ageno W, Dentali F. Is diabetes a hypercoagulable state? A critical appraisal. Acta Diabetol. 2015;52(6):1007-16.
14. Alhamad T, Lentine K, Anwar S, Maw T, Horwedel T, Peng J, et al. Functional capacity pre-transplantation measured by 6 minute walk test and clinical outcomes. Am J Transplant. 2016;16(Suppl. 3).

CHAPTER

28

Psychological Issues in Kidney Transplant Recipients

Surendra K Mattoo, Akhilesh Sharma, Ajaypal Singh

CASE VIGNETTE

Mr SK is a 52-year-old male working in a bank as a manager. He belongs to middle socioeconomic status, extended family, and lives in a rural area. His wife is a homemaker, elder daughter is married, and son is preparing for public services examinations after graduation. He had been very anxious and dependent on others. He smokes a few cigarettes and drinks alcohol on weekends. He has frequent arguments with wife over this. He had a family history of diabetes, hypertension, coronary artery disease, and depressive disorder. At 34 years of age, during the closing months of financial year, he would increase his alcohol intake due to increased work pressure. He had multiple episodes of depression during all these years. He had to take treatment for most of these. He was also diagnosed with hypertension at 37 years of age, but he was not adherent to lifestyle changes and medications. He started having weakness, easy fatigability, frequent nocturia, and symptoms of depression 2 years ago. He was incidentally detected to have chronic kidney disease when he decompensated after an episode of diarrhea. He was admitted to the intensive care unit (ICU) due to altered sensorium and improved after multiple dialysis. He would have episodes of panic when he would have flashbacks of ICU stay. He receives regular dialysis and has been advised for transplant. He got registered for the cadaveric transplant waitlist, but the waiting period is very long. His sister and wife got themselves checked for human leukocyte antigen (HLA) compatibility as potential live donors. Currently, he has been feeling low, hopeless, sleepless, fatigued, gets easily irritable, has stopped alcohol but is still not fully able to quit smoking. He is also on antidepressants and hypnotics. He is not able to function well and depends a lot on his subordinates. His employer bank only pays for inpatient treatment expenses, not for outpatient expenses. He avoids attending online group sessions for smoking cessation. His wife matched for a compatible donor. The transplant team started the process, and referred for psychiatric assessment.

Discussion

Donor assessment revealed that she was cognitively preserved, had no past psychiatric history, had mild anxiety, and depressive symptoms in reaction to the ongoing stressors, had good problem solving, and had social and religious coping. There was no familial pressure. She was a well-informed and unconditional donor.

The recipient had anxious-dependent personality, recurrent depressive disorder, poor coping in stress, resorted to alcohol, had poor health-related behaviors, and had poor adherence to treatment in past for diabetes, hypertension, and depression. Presently he was fully abstinent from alcohol, still using tobacco occasionally, and having depressive symptoms that could be understood in terms of physical illness and reaction to situation. He had some lack of information regarding post-transplant treatment, lifestyle changes, and expectations from transplant.

Education sessions with transplant team were carried out. Motivational enhancement for tobacco with support of nicotine replacement for 3 days worked. A plan for skill training to manage work stress in closing months and a change of seat at workplace was discussed. He opted for later and his management agreed with no financial loss. The family managed for operative and immediate postoperative expenses through employer bank. Their state government runs a plan to support post-transplant medication at a subsidized rate. The nearest center identified was Postgraduate Institute of Medical Education and Research (PGIMER) Chandigarh, with local support from the state medical college, 50 km from their residence. Transplant was successful. He had mild delirium for 3 days which was managed conservatively.

His son would accompany him initially for few months to office, and then he started managing at new post. He had cravings for cigarettes, especially in morning and evening. Follow-ups have been regular and with family support he was maintaining a healthy lifestyle. He has started spending time at local Satsang frequently. He had some symptoms of depression seasonally in March, and is being managed with light therapy and low-dose escitalopram for 1 month for the last 4 years. He has learned self-management and monitoring of insulin, blood sugar levels, and blood pressure. He had COVID-19 infection, contacted his transplant team and was admitted and managed with steroids.

INTRODUCTION

Solid organ transplantation is a well-developed field scientifically. The outcomes depend on a host of medical and psychosocial factors. A preoperative assessment of these factors for suitability of candidate as well as for optimum outcomes is practiced globally. This is necessary because the unmet need is very high, especially in developing countries such as India. Transplant is a teamwork. Pretransplant assessment of psychosocial factors, tiding over the psychosocial crisis during peritransplantation phase and for enhancing successful post-transplantation period, psychiatrists, psychologists, and medical social workers form an essential part of this team. Psychiatry in transplantation medicine is a subspecific area; it represents a psychiatric—ethical and legal judgment in different phases of the process of transplant. Transplant is a stressful journey of a patient's physical body and mind, which undergoes a lot of changes with challenges. A successful outcome of renal transplant requires resilience of not only the physical body but also the mind. In this chapter, we will discuss the psychiatric assessment with the help of a case vignette.

WHY SHOULD A PSYCHOSOCIAL ASSESSMENT BE CARRIED OUT?

Persons with chronic noncommunicable diseases have high comorbidity. Not only chronic noncommunicable diseases, such as diabetes, hypertension, and coronary artery diseases, with resultant end organ damage, such as end-stage renal disease, are highly comorbid, but they also have a higher incidence and prevalence of psychiatric disorders such as anxiety and depression than those without chronic noncommunicable diseases. Similarly, persons with mental illness have high incidence and prevalence of chronic physical illness similar to noncommunicable diseases. Persons with chronic illness and end organ damage have depression, anxiety, and hopelessness as a psychological reaction to their primary illness because of decreased functioning, disability, and poor quality of life in the pretransplant phase. This may also happen due to social role limitations and financial implications secondary to these. Psychiatric illness is common in renal transplant patients and leads to poor transplant outcome, adherence, and quality of life. It was shown that psychiatric evaluation in the pretransplantation period can predict post-transplant psychiatric adjustment.

Difficulties in getting a suitable transplant even in the developed world and much more in developing resource-limited countries such as India also contribute to it. The legal and procedural hassles, fear of rejection, and medication side effects during transplantation also contribute to it. Post-transplantation limitations, role changes, financial burdens, lifestyle changes, and medication side effects may also contribute to these. Treatment adherence, lifestyle modifications, and adaptation to new roles are the most important predictors of outcome of transplantation. Various psychosocial factors in addition to medical factors are important in treatment adherence, lifestyle modifications, and post-transplantation role adjustments, so their assessment is a must.

With due diligence, a vast majority of the clients have a successful outcome. Assessment of these factors leads to the establishment of a clear communication between client, donor, and transplant team along with family, facilitates proper informed consent, and increases therapeutic alliance. The identification of psychosocial issues leads to better preparation for the pretransplant phase and plan client-specific strategies to help optimize post-transplant adherence and outcomes **(Table 1 and Box 1)**.

For renal transplant, assessment of both recipient and donor is equally important. The donor's motivational assessment and family psychosocial assessment as well as support system assessment also predicts better selection for transplant success.

ASSESSMENT OF DONOR

It is a very big decision to donate an organ. There can be no transplant without a donor. Living donors are mostly close family members who are emotionally connected to the recipient. It is because of this connectivity that they volunteer. It is the first and foremost that psychiatric assessment of donor is carried out so that decisions can be taken in the best interest of the donor. Donors are generally of three types. The first is the "unconditional donors" who would have emotional suffering if they were not allowed to donate. They are most common and constitute the majority. The second category is the "impulsive donors, family pressured donors, and those who expect financial compensation." The third category is "altruistic donors," whose motivation is only the well-being of recipient. Here, reward for donation is personal gratification. They are not aware of the identity of recipient and vice versa. Generally, the last two groups of donors are not encouraged. They are not governed by moral commitment or feeling of loyalty toward the recipient. For this purpose, the team should initially carry out separate interviews with donor and recipient. Thereafter, joint interviews should be conducted. These interviews help the donor in becoming fully aware of their reasons for donation, at times uncovering their unconscious feeling toward recipient with the help of a psychiatrist or psychologist and lastly any unrealistic expectation of the recipient. The following crucial points should be assessed as part of donor assessment **(Box 2)**.

Finally, based upon these one needs to ascertain his capacity for informed consent.

TABLE 1: Psychiatric comorbidity in postrenal transplant patients.

Psychiatric morbidity	*Prevalence/incidence*	*Remarks*
Major depressive disorder	20–30%	• Risk higher in first year of postrenal transplant • *Risk factors:* Stress associated with physical recovery, rehabilitation, adaptation to immunosuppressive medications, and psychosocial role change
Anxiety disorder	30–40%	• PTSD symptoms result from any medical crisis during waiting period, surgery itself, and hallucinations and delusions associated with postsurgical delirium • Adjustment disorder and sleep disturbance are often reported and associated with poor quality of life
Psychotic disorder	7.5/1,000 person-years (PY) after renal transplant compared with 7.2/1,000 PY for all patients on chronic dialysis and 9.6/1,000 PY for dialysis patients aged 65 years or younger	• *Risk factors associated:* Graft loss, allograft rejection, and cadaveric donation • Psychosis associated with an increased risk of both death (AHR, 2.09; 95% CI, 1.71–2.56; $p < 0.001$) and graft loss (AHR, 1.79; 95% CI, 1.15–2.78; $p = 0.01$) • Graft loss due to noncompliance was significantly more common after psychosis (9.0 vs. 3.7% in patients not hospitalized for psychosis)
Cognitive disorder	30–50%	• Impairments in verbal memory and executive functions are most commonly reported • Often associated with mood disorders and side effects of immunosuppressive medications
Substance use disorder	17% (current substance use) 14% (current tobacco use) Current drug 0.5–3% (for cannabis abuse or dependence)	• Only 29.4% quit smoking after the transplant • Rates of SUDs are less than liver transplant patients
Delirium	0.8% in cohort studies 2–20% incidence	• Incidence increased with age and fragility (18–49 years old: 2.0%; 50–64 years old: 4.6%; 65–75 years old: 9.2%; and ≥75 years old: 13.8%) • Recipients with delirium had increased risks of ≥2-week length of stay, institutional discharge, graft loss, and mortality

(AHR: adjusted hazard ratio; CI: confidence interval; PTSD: post-traumatic stress disorder; SUD: substance use disorder)

BOX 1: Points for recipient assessment.

- High comorbidity of contributing noncommunicable diseases with psychiatric illness
- High prevalence of psychiatric illness in persons waiting for transplant
- Adherence to lifelong medications and lifestyle changes requires good psychosocial health
- Informed consent requires psychosocial competence
- Peri- and post-transplant periods may require psychosocial interventions

BOX 2: Points for donor assessment.

- Exploration of donor for his knowledge regarding impact of donation on physical, mental, social, and spiritual aspects of his health
- Exploration of donor's knowledge regarding the impact of the above said aspects on personal, familial, work related, sexual, leisure, and financial aspects of his life later
- Exploration regarding risks associated with surgical procedure
- Exploration regarding his awareness that it is possible the graft may get rejected
- Exploration regarding motivation for donation
- Exploration regarding his relationship with recipient
- Exploration regarding any coercion/pressure for donation
- Exploration regarding his current mental status and any history of mental illness
- Socioeconomic assessment
- Assessment of peer, work related, and organizational support

The donor may not understand the large amount of information and if there are gaps found, they are again educated regarding all the processes, procedures, and impact on various aspects of their life. Even after consenting, there may be residual ambivalence in some of the donors and if not resolved it may lead to adverse physical and psychosocial consequences post donation. So, motivational interviewing by a psychiatrist or psychologist can help them realize their exact reasons and then reconsider their decision. If they withdraw, then it is not told to the recipient; rather they are presented as medically unfit candidate to the recipient's family whatever may be the reason of withdrawing. Culturally validated instruments for comprehensive psychosocial assessment can aid the interviews or clinical assessments. To date, there is no universal tool available for recommendation. Socioeconomic assessment in detail is a must because donors do not get any financial assistance as per law. Preoperative recovery takes time. Long-term functioning and employment may be affected for several of them **(Box 3)**.

BOX 3: Recipient care.

Preoperative:
- Educate them properly about the process, procedures, and impact on future life
- Motivational interviewing to resolve ambivalence and to arrive at a final decision
- Use culturally valid psychometric instruments if you think they can help more
- Socioeconomic assessment and future for these in hand

Postoperative:
- Follow-up multidisciplinary planning for physical and mental wellbeing in place
- Physical rehabilitation plan
- Psychosocial interventions, such as mindfulness and cognitive behavioral therapy if required
- Peer mentoring programs, if available
- Financial supports, if they need
- Donor advocacy

BOX 4: Donor care.

Most of the donors recover well. Psychosocial assessment and interventions are to help them take informed decision without ambivalence, to tide immediate postoperative crisis, most importantly to identify those at risk for morbidity, and to help them when recipient dies/graft fails. Need for peer programs, lifelong multidisciplinary care, development of specific interventions, and advocacy is there.

Postoperative recovery is known to decrease physical as well as psychological quality of life in a minority of donors, but it improves over the next few weeks. This time, psychological support is most required as well as financial aspects need to be cared for as donor is not able to work.

Most important risk factors for this are low educational and employment status. There is evidence that during the initial few years post donation when donors face health issues, they tend to develop health-related anxiety, depressive symptoms, and future worries. This might also be true for later life. Postoperatively psychological support is required for those donors where graft rejects and/or recipient dies. Transplant teams and families of recipients generally do not take donors along in this process. They are generally not included in mourning rituals. The attitude of the recipient's family is an important determinant of the donor's psychological health after recipient's death. Currently, almost all guidelines recommend that along with physical monitoring, psychosocial well-being of the donor must be monitored post-transplant for a long duration **(Box 4)**.

ASSESSMENT OF RECIPIENT

The goal of recipient assessments is selection of candidate patients who are most likely to benefit from transplant and help them make proper informed consent. Objectives are (1) identification of risk factors, issues both social and psychological that require help before transplant and in perioperative and postoperative phases and (2) to have an individualized multidisciplinary plan in hand to manage the challenges during different phases.

BOX 5: Important points need to be assessed during the initial interview of the recipient.

- Any anger, distress, and emotional issues toward the system because of long waiting
- Knowledge, attitude, and beliefs toward transplant procedure and transplant team
- Daily activities and social support
- Expectations from transplant
- Communication and therapeutic alliance with transplant team
- Adherence and self-management of medications, appointments, lab tests, communicating warning signs, and follow-up visits
- General lifestyle and health-related behaviors
- Change in role post-transplant and caregiver burden
- Past adaptations to stressors and coping for physical, psychological, and social in nature

Evaluation of Understanding about Transplantation and Expectations

The psychiatric team carries out separate interviews with family and recipient initially followed by joint interviews. First, assess the knowledge and awareness regarding "the process, procedure, and post-transplant lifestyle changes, medication adherence and regular follow-ups, tough perioperative period, possibility of infection, graft reactions, graft rejections, chances of candidates' death, financial burden for surgery, and lifelong, caregiver burden." Second, assess what the recipient hopes to gain from surgery. Third, assess whether their expectations are realistic. Patients expect improvement in their physical health, pain, functioning, and quality of life. Transplant team expects the patient and family to understand all the above-mentioned possible surgical complications, adherence to medications, and lifestyle changes. They expect a good communication and follow-up from family and patient for reporting the danger signs, etc. If some discrepancy is found, then it can be resolved through education sessions, increasing communication between transplant team and patient party. This improved communication increases therapeutic alliance which is necessary for the post-transplant period. During the initial interview, the following points need to be assessed **(Box 5)**.

Socioeconomic Assessment

Distance from transplant care center, hospice care, socioeconomic status, caregivers support (joint vs. nuclear family and psychosocial services as tertiary level of support) all these information are useful in creating a holistic plan for a patient so that he can receive continuity of care. Provisions of various government funds regarding operative expenditure, postoperative medicinal provisions, and familial and social support post-transplantation should be explored in association with a medical/transplant social worker. All these financial, familial, and social support plans should be made in advance, especially for the post-transplant period. These have been predictors of post-transplant adherence, success, and psychiatric morbidity.

Premorbid Psychiatric State

A careful history of past psychiatric illnesses such as anxiety, mood, or psychotic disorders is very much important. Major mental disorders such as bipolar, schizophrenia, and obsessive–compulsive disorders have a spectrum of severity and significant majority have a relapsing recurring course with need for long-term or lifetime treatment and support. Such cases run a risk of relapse or recurrence in the operative period and may be nonadherent to treatment in the post-transplant phase. These disorders in the acute phase are a contraindication for transplant as the candidate may not understand the nature of process and procedures, may not give valid informed consent, and may not follow therapeutic advice. In contrast, a stable status does not constitute an absolute contraindication. This is a debatable issue in the West. However, it is seen that majority of post-transplant persons with schizophrenia achieve outcomes comparable to others. Here, the decision of the psychiatrist is very important on a case-by-case basis. It is well known that psychiatric disorders are very common in each phase of transplant, i.e., waiting patients [depression, anxiety, post-traumatic stress disorder (PTSD) following dialysis and ICU admissions], during the procedure (delirium, etc.), and post-transplantation (postoperative delirium, steroid psychosis, depression, anxiety, sleep disturbances, etc). During pretransplant assessment, it is very important to distinguish depression-like features due to medical causes and exhaustion from reactive depression as well as primary endogenous depression. So, the goal is to identify those candidates who can be managed with appropriate measures and achieve successful transplantation. Also, it is important to identify very carefully those who need to get stabilization with future plan in hand for the postoperative period. All cases need a long-term plan post-transplantation.

Assessment of Personality

The interpersonal pattern of communication, expectations, emotional expressions, and behaviors that are common in renal transplant patients who need attention are emotionally unstable—borderline and histrionic in females and obsessive–compulsive and antisocial in males. These personality factors are to be identified and a plan for long-term counseling and psychotherapy should be in place. These are predictors of poor adherence in the post-transplant period, which leads to poor quality of life. Severe personality disorders such as borderline and antisocial have been considered by some centers as absolute contraindications. A potential increased risk of nonadherence to treatment has been observed in patients with a prolonged hospitalization, psychological regression, addiction, relational difficulties, and/or diverse behavioral problems. On rare occasions following transplantation, patients are ambivalent about transplantation, which may diminish their motivation to manage the medical regimen leading to rejection and graft failure.

Assessment for Substance Misuse

A detailed history of substance use, misuse, and dependence needs to be collected. The form, content, pattern, and paraphernalia need to be assessed. These are risk factors for primary physical illness (such as diabetes, hypertension, dyslipidemia, chronic liver diseases, and viral infections) contributing to renal failure. Also, these increase chances of graft failure and post-transplant failure due to altered immune response, nonadherence to treatment, and poor lifestyle. Therefore, an appropriate motivational assessment for quitting before being considered for transplant is necessary. Harm reduction strategy and preferably long-term abstinence must be confirmed. Risk for relapse in future and a plan for continuous relapse-prevention measures and rehabilitation should be in place. Acute current dependence and harm contradict immediate candidature for transplant. Notably, the stress of the surgical procedure can lead to relapse to addictions so that the patients' ability to manage complex post-transplant medical regimens is at risk.

Body Image

There is emerging evidence that post-transplant physical recovery is influenced by recipients' perception of disease and their body. Body image improves post-transplant in comparison to those receiving hemodialysis. The transplant not only leads to anatomic and physical restoration, but psychological transplantation also takes place parallelly. After transplant, patients experience a gamut of both positive and negative emotions such as guilt, gratefulness, and fear. So, pre- and post-transplantation assessment of body image is very important along with other factors and in a minority, it may require attention and psychiatric help.

Current Mental Status

Most important before transplant is to assess the mood, feelings, thinking, hope, desire to improve and live, any morbid pattern of mood, thinking and behavior that warrants treatment and delaying procedure. Also, it is important to see whether the mood, feelings, and thinking can be understood to be normal expected reactions to the

BOX 6: Possible contraindications.

- There are both absolute and relative psychiatric contraindications for transplant
- Current active psychosis, mood episode, substance dependence, dementia, and severe and profound intellectual disability are generally regarded as absolute ones
- It is the psychiatric assessment that is required to maximize the distributive justice for those who can benefit from transplant
- For majority, depression and anxiety pre- and post-transplant can be there in mild to moderate form
- Proper assessment for their risk can help in adequate and timely management
- Personality, lifestyle including substance use, socioeconomic factors, coping, and support are most commonly encountered issues

situation. A plan in hand must be there as well for post-transplant and later period. There are situations where an urgent transplantation and urgent psychiatric assessment are required, such as where the candidate has made a suicide attempt. Here, if it is understandable as an isolated event due to circumstances, then it is generally not a contraindication. Recurrent attempts with past history and mental illness need to be treated first and require a lot of psychiatric management expertise. At times, the candidate may not be in a situation to communicate; in such cases collateral sources of information help us in assessment and making a plan.

Cognitive Functions

Chronic renal disease and its contributing noncommunicable diseases all impact higher cognitive functions. Similarly, repeated hemodialysis and medications for immunosuppression have cognitive side effects. Pretransplant assessment of cognitive functions is important to ascertain that the patient understands the process, procedure, and consequences for giving informed consent and can adhere to post-transplant lifestyle and medications. Many centers exclude persons with intellectual disability, but research has shown that persons with mild intellectual disability have comparable post-transplant quality of life. Here, dementia is an absolute contraindication but cognitive changes secondary to organ failure and resultant encephalopathy are indications for transplant **(Box 6)**.

DURING PERIOPERATIVE PERIOD

Mostly delirium occurs and occasionally a psychiatric consultation is required. Looking at the patient profile, psychiatrists can help choose safer psychotropics such as haloperidol, quetiapine, or olanzapine for severe hyperactive delirium. Looking at the complexity of the situation, it is very difficult to prevent delirium in these patients. But pretransplant assessment can guide us for some candidates who are at more than usual risk such as those with a history of delirium, old age, preexisting cognitive change, and sensory deprivations. However, there are no specific studies in post-transplant patients except one that points out that quetiapine is effective in decreasing hyperactive delirium. Delirium can start days to weeks post-transplant and can last a protracted course in some of the patients. It increases hospital stay, cost, and mortality and predicts poor quality of life in ICU patients.

POST-TRANSPLANT

In addition to some cases of protracted delirium, infections, minor graft reactions, delayed recovery and discharge cause worries, apprehensions, fear of graft rejection, sleep disturbances, and emotional reactions in patients. Generally, the in-hospital psychiatrist/psychologist takes care of them with reassurance, counseling, music, and supportive sessions. Occasionally, medications for sleep are required. Nonbenzodiazepines sedative hypnotics and melatonin can be given occasionally.

Most of the patients who are easily discharged initially have a good honeymoon period. But when they start adjusting to changed roles, limitations in lifestyle, immunosuppressants, laboratory tests and frequent precautions along with adjustment in family, work, and society, they may develop ambivalence, anxiety, depression, and sleep-related problems. Here also, the role of a psychiatrist as a part of the multidisciplinary team comes into play along with support of family, friends, work colleagues, and transplant peer groups. This is the time when our pretransplant planning comes into action. For those who resume substance and poor lifestyle with nonadherence to post-transplant advice, it becomes a challenge to manage because they deteriorate physically very rapidly. Similarly, psychological support to caregivers should be provided as and when needed.

PSYCHOLOGICAL THERAPIES FOR TRANSPLANT PATIENTS

Bibliotherapy

It involves educating the patient about his/her nature of illness, prognosis, and change of course with renal transplant, effect of transplant on patients' life at various levels. This is an ongoing process where concern and issues raised by patients are addressed simultaneously. This is the essential part of most transplant programs.

Skill Training

Most of the transplant programs include skill training to enhance coping skills of patients to overcome stress of transplantation and to improve self-management and post-transplant adherence.

Interpersonal Psychotherapy

After renal transplant, the patient may go through stages of grief due to loss of his/her previous role. By using his skills, the psychiatrist takes the patient through it and facilitates the acceptance of the new role. Individual psychotherapy has been shown to be more effective than group therapy.

Remote Intervention Therapy

When logistical challenges are present, internet-based video conferencing or mobile phone calls can be used to deliver psychotherapeutic intervention.

Others

There are no efficacy studies on the treatment for substance-use disorder specific to transplant population. Frequent follow-up with random toxicological screening, motivation enhancement therapy (MET), and relapse prevention counseling (RPC) are useful. Cognitive behavior therapy for depression and anxiety disorder is useful.

PSYCHOTROPIC USE IN RENAL TRANSPLANT PATIENTS

Stable psychiatric patients may require medications for relapse prevention, for acute exacerbations, and for occasional subsyndromal symptoms. Mostly, these are required for a short duration for patients with no past psychiatric illness who constitute majority receiving transplant. It is well planned for the first category of patients. There are some important points that need to be kept in mind for prescribing psychotropics **(Box 7)**.

BOX 7: Psychotropic prescription.

- Start when nonpharmacological measures do not work, and they are necessary after weighing risks and benefits
- Start with lower doses and go slow in accordance with creatinine clearance or estimated glomerular filtration rate
- Monotherapy should be preferred
- Drug–drug interaction to be looked for before prescribing any psychotropics
- Monitoring of plasma levels of a few drugs can be a better guide in case of renal transplant
- Adverse effects of the immunosuppressants need to be monitored regularly
- Immunosuppressants have frequent neuropsychiatric side effects
- Only few psychotropics among antidepressants, antipsychotics, and benzodiazepines are low risk for use in transplant patients.
- Drug interactions are very common between immunosuppressants and psychotropics through hepatic metabolizing enzyme cytochrome P450 3A4

SUGGESTED READING

1. Anil Kumar BN, Mattoo SK. Organ transplant and the psychiatrist: an overview. Indian J Med Res. 2015;141(4):408-16.
2. Belaiche S, Décaudin B, Dharancy S, Noel C, Odou P, Hazzan M. Factors relevant to medication non-adherence in kidney transplant: a systematic review. Int J Clin Pharm. 2017;39(3):582-93.
3. Bruns C, Giese J, Phillippi D, Moore D, Hall P. Knowledge and attitudes toward renal transplantation in individuals undergoing transplant evaluation. Prog Transplant. 2021;31(3):271-8.
4. De Pasquale C, Pistorio ML, Veroux M, Indelicato L, Biffa G, Bennardi N, et al. Psychological and psychopathological aspects of kidney transplantation: a systematic review. Front Psychiatry. 2020;11:106.
5. Goetzinger AM, Blumenthal JA, O'Hayer CV, Babyak MA, Hoffman BM, Ong L, et al. Stress and coping in caregivers of patients awaiting solid organ transplantation. Clin Transplant. 2012;26:97-104.
6. Hamedan MS, Aliha JM. Relationship between immunosuppressive medications adherence and quality of life and some patient factors in renal transplant patients in Iran. Glob J Health Sci. 2014;6(4):205-12.
7. Kofman T, Pourcine F, Canoui-Poitrine F, Kamar N, Malvezzi P, François H, et al. Safety of renal transplantation in patients with bipolar or psychotic disorders: a retrospective study. Transpl Int. 2018;31(4):377-85.
8. Kumnig M, Jowsey-Gregoire SG. Preoperative psychological evaluation of transplant patients: challenges and solutions. Transplant Res Risk Manag. 2015;7:35-43.
9. Medved V, Medved S, Skocic Hanzek M. Transplantation psychiatry: an overview. Psychiatr Danub. 2019;31(1):18-25.
10. Naqvi R. Evaluation of psychiatric issues in renal transplant setting. Indian J Nephrol. 2015;25(6):321-5.
11. Shroff S. Legal and ethical aspects of organ donation and transplantation. Indian J Urol. 2009;25(3):348-55.

ANNEXURES: PSYCHIATRIC ASSESSMENT PERFORMA FOR RENAL TRANSPLANT

Annexure 1

Name of donor: ____________________

Age/gender: ____________________

Relationship with recipient: ____________________

Education: ____________________

Employment: ____________________

Income (monthly): ____________________

Socioeconomic status: ____________________

Health insurance: ____________________

Family type: ____________________

Support systems: ____________________

Physical comorbidity: ____________________

Current medications: ____________________

Past psychiatric history and treatment: ____________________

Family history of psychiatric illness: ____________________

Personality: ____________________

Current disability and functioning: ____________________

Knowledge regarding impact of donation
(on physical, mental, social, and spiritual aspects of his health): ____________________

Knowledge regarding the impact of donation
(on personal, familial, work related, sexual, leisure, and financial aspects of his life later): ____________________

Knowledge regarding risks associated with surgical procedure: ____________________

Knowledge regarding his awareness that it is possible the graft may get rejected: ____________________

Exploration regarding motivation for donation: ____________________

Exploration regarding his relationship with recipient: ____________________

Exploration regarding any coercion/pressure for donation: ____________________

Current mental status: ____________________

Assessment of peer, work related, and organizational support: ____________________

Postoperative support (rehabilitation, treatment, advocacy, etc.): ____________________

Annexure 2

Name of donor: ______________________

Age/gender: ______________________

Relationship with recipient: ______________________

Education: ______________________

Employment: ______________________

Income (monthly): ______________________

Socioeconomic status: ______________________

Health insurance: ______________________

Family type: ______________________

Support systems: ______________________

Physical comorbidity: ______________________

Current medications: ______________________

Past psychiatric history and treatment: ______________________

Family history of psychiatric illness: ______________________

Personality: ______________________

Current disability and functioning: ______________________

Substance use: ______________________

Body image: ______________________

Cognitive functions: ______________________

Relationship with donor: ______________________

Past adaptations to stressors and coping for physical, psychological, and social in nature: ______________________

Assess any anger, distress, and emotional issues toward the system because of long waiting: ______________________

Assess knowledge, attitude, and beliefs toward transplant procedure and transplant team: ______________________

Assess daily activities and social support: ______________________

Expectations from transplant: ______________________

Communication and therapeutic alliance with transplant team: ______________________

Adherence and self-management (of medications, appointments, lab tests, communicating warning signs, and follow-up visits): ______________________

General lifestyle and health-related behaviors: ______________________

Knowledge regarding risks associated surgical procedure: ______________________

Knowledge regarding his awareness that it is possible the graft may get rejected: ______________________

Change in role post-transplant and caregiver burden: ______________________

Current mental state examination: ______________________

Knowledge of post-transplant rehabilitation plan: ______________________

Assessment of pre- and post-transplant peer, work related, and organizational support: ______________________

Assessment of post-transplant local health support and contingency plans: ______________________

CHAPTER

29

Transplantation of Human Organs and Tissues Act: Simplified

Manisha Sahay

CASE VIGNETTE

Mr X met with an accident on 1st March 2022. He was 29 years male working as a software engineer in Mumbai, India. His father Mr Y expired 3 years ago at the age of 68 years. The patient was living with his mother (54 years) and wife (27 years) and his two children. He had pledged his organs during his life and his driving license showed that he was a registered organ donor.

He was admitted to the hospital on 1st March 2022 at 6 PM with head injury and after all hospital procedures and tests he shifted to the theatre for craniotomy. His mother and wife were O+ and were ready to donate blood if required. However, his condition did not improve, and he was declared brain death on 3rd March 2022 at 9 PM.

Family members (both wife and mother) consented to organ donation. His heart, kidneys, liver and corneas were retrieved and transplanted to 6 patients as per the waiting list.

Which all forms would be relevant for this transplantation?

Form 8

For declaration cum consent

Near relative or lawful possessor of brainstem dead person (including minors)

Form 10

For certification of brainstem death

Board of medical experts certifying brainstem death

Form 7

Patient had filled form 7 during his life and his wife had a donor card

For organ or tissue pledging individual of age 18 years or above

(Hospital should have certificate of registration Form 16 and of renewal if applicable Form 17)

INTRODUCTION

Human organ and tissue transplantation was started in India in 1962. Initially, organ transplant was unregulated, and organ trafficking was rampant. The Transplantation of Human Organs Act is the primary legislation related to organ donation and transplantation in India and was passed in 1994. It was aimed at regulation of removal, storage, and transplantation of human organs for therapeutic purposes and for prevention of commercial dealings in human organs. An amendment to the act was proposed by the states of Goa, Himachal Pradesh, and West Bengal in 2009. The amendment to the act was passed by the parliament in 2011, and the rules were notified in 2014. The same was adopted by the proposing states and union territories by default and maybe adopted by other states by passing a resolution. In India, matters related to health are governed by each state. Some states are yet to adopt TA 2014 rules.

There are some differences between the act of 1995 and subsequent rules passed in 2014 **(Table 1)**.[1-4] This chapter provides a snapshot of the Transplantation of Human Organs and Tissues Act (THOTA), which is not usually a part of the nephrology textbooks. However, a good understanding is required by all involved in transplantation.

REGULATORY BODIES FOR TRANSPLANTATION

Advisory Committee

The chairperson is an administrative expert not below the rank of the Secretary to the State Government. Other members include two medical experts who have a postgraduate medical degree and at least 5 years' experience in the field of organ or tissue transplantation. The term of the members is for a period of 2 years. The advisory committee advises the appropriate authority.

Appropriate Authority

It inspects and grants registration to new hospitals for transplantation and conducts regular inspections of already registered hospitals. It can also investigate complaints regarding breaches of the act. It is conferred with the powers of a civil court and can summon any person, request documents, and issue search warrants.

TABLE 1: Key differences between transplantation of human organ act THOA 1994 and THOTA 2014.

	THOA 1994	*THOTA 2014*
Advisory committee	No	Yes
Appropriate authority	Mentioned	*Defined:* Who and what
Authorization committee	State	Included hospitals of >25 transplants/year
Video	No	Video recording
Definition of brain death	Yes	Yes
Brain death declaration team	Neurology/ neurosurgeon	Added physician, anesthetist, intensivist
Hospitals	Transplanting centers	Added nontransplant retrieval centers
Which hospital	–	Any hospital with RMP and ICU facility
Registration of hospital	Organ retrieval	Yes, for organ retrieval but not needed for tissue retrieval
Scope of donor	"Near-relative" means spouse, son, daughter, father, mother, brother, or sister	Near-relative included grandparents, grandchildren
Swap donations	No	Yes
Pledge	No	Yes Form 7
Counseling for donation	Mentioned	Mandatory
Medicolegal cases	Not defined	Simplified
Number of forms	13	21
Role of doctor	Needed for organ retrieval	Yes, for organ retrieval, not for tissue
Transplant coordinators	Mentioned	Mandatory
Organ retrieval charges	Not mentioned	Recipient/ government/NGO
Scope	Organs	Organs and tissues
Penalties	Less	More
Registries	No	Yes

(ICU: intensive care unit; NGO: nongovernment organization; RMP: registered medical practitioner; THOA: Transplantation of Human Organ Act; THOTA: Transplantation of Human Organs and Tissues Act)

Authorization Committee

All "other than near-related transplantations" (described below) or foreign transplantations are evaluated by the authorization committee. It ensures that there are no commercial dealings in transplantation.

The authorization committee maybe at the state or the hospital level. Transplantations from hospitals that do less than 25 transplants per year are referred to state committee, while hospitals that do more than 25 transplants can refer them to their own hospital authorization committee.

CHAPTER HIGHLIGHTS

- Transplantation of human organs in India is governed by rules.
- It governs both living and deceased donor transplantations.
- These were first implemented in 1994.
- The rules were last amended in 2014.
- The amended rules can help increase the donor pool.
- Grandparents as living related donors and swap transplants have been included in the amended rules.
- A basic knowledge of these rules is essential for all transplant physicians, nephrologists, urologists as well as the students.

The authorization committee consists of:

- Medical practitioner or Chief Medical Officer (CMO) or person in any other equivalent post in the major government hospital of the district who is the chairperson.
- Two senior registered medical practitioners residing in the concerned state/district and who are not part of any transplant team are members.
- Secretary of Health or Director of Health or nominee
- Two senior persons of high integrity, credibility, and social standing (if possible one female) should be members of committee. These maybe doctors, lawyers, chartered accountants, judges, police personnel, etc. The quorum of the authorization committee consists of a minimum of four members. The quorum is not complete without participation of the Chairman, the Secretary (Health) or nominee, and Director of Health Services or nominee. All "other than near-related" transplantations from hospitals that do less than 25 transplants per year are referred to this committee.

Competent Authority

Competent authority means the head of the institution or hospital carrying out transplantation or committee constituted by the head of the institution or hospital; the members of this committee should not be a part of the transplant team.

APPEAL

Any person aggrieved by the order of a regulatory body may appeal to the central government or state government as the case maybe within 30 days from receipt of the order.

FORMS

There are 21 forms described in the 2014 rules. These are given in **Table 2**. All the transplant physicians and surgeons and the hospitals performing transplants should be aware of these forms and should send the applications in a proper format to avoid delays.[5]

TABLE 2: The 21 forms in THOTA 2014.

Form	*Given by*
1. For organ or tissue donation from identified living near-related donor	Donor—him/her
2. For organ or tissue donation by living spousal donor	Spouse—him/her
3. For organ or tissue donation by other than near-relative living donor	Donor—him/her
4. For certification of medical fitness of living donor	Registered medical practitioner
5. For certification of genetic relationship of living donor with recipient	Head of Pathology Laboratory
6. For spousal living donor	Competent authority and authorization committee in case of foreigners
7. Patient had filled form 7 during his life and his wife had a donor card	For organ or tissue pledging (Individual of age 18 years or above)
8. For declaration cum consent	Near relative or lawful possessor of brainstem dead person (including minors)
9. For unclaimed body in a hospital or prison	Person in lawful possession of the unclaimed body
10. For certification of brainstem death	Board of medical experts certifying brainstem death
11. Application for approval of transplantation from living donor	Proposed recipient and the proposed living donor
12. Application for registration of hospital for organ or tissue transplant other than cornea	Head of the institution
13. Application for registration of tissue banks other than eye banks	Head of the institution
14. Application for registration of tissue banks other than eye banks	Head of the institution
15. Application for registration of eye bank, corneal transplantation center, eye retrieval center under THOTA	
16. Hospital should have certificate of registration for organ/tissue transplantation/retrieval and/or tissue banking	
17. Hospital should have certificate of registration	Appropriated authority on the letterhead
18. Certificate by the authorization committee of hospital	Issued on the letterhead
19. Certificate by competent authority for Indian near-relative, other than spouse	Issued on the letterhead
20. Verification certificate in respect of domicile status of recipient or donor	Tehsildar/authorized officer (required only for donor—other than near-relative or recipient if they do not belong to state where transplant hospital is located)
21. Certificate of relationship between donor and recipient in case of foreigners	Embassy concerned

(THOTA: Transplantation of Human Organs and Tissues Act)

TYPES OF DONORS

Living Donors

Living donors may include living-related donors, spousal donors, or other than near-related donors. For all living donations, the donor is subjected to all relevant medical tests to determine eligibility and compatibility to donate the organ. The physical and mental evaluation of the donor should be certified by the registered medical practitioner in Form 4. The permission for transplantation and the documents required vary with the type of living donor.

Near-related Donors

Near-related donors include parents, siblings, and children. In the recent 2014 rules, grandparents have also been included in the list of near-related donors. There should be documentary evidence of relationship, i.e., birth certificates, relationship certificate from Tehsildar or subdivisional magistrate or Metropolitan Magistrate or Sarpanch of the Panchayat, identity certificates such as Electors' Photo Identity Card or voters' identity card or Aadhaar card, and documentary evidence of residence of the patient and proposed donor, ration card, or passport or driving license or permanent account number card or bank account and family photograph depicting the proposed donor and the proposed recipient.

If the relationship is not established with the above documents, human leukocyte antigen matching or deoxyribonucleic (DNA) fingerprinting from a laboratory accredited with the National Accreditation Board for Testing and Calibration Laboratories should be done. The forms required to be filled in live donation include Form 1 for donor consent, Form 4 for donor fitness, Form 11 which is a joint application form, and committee permission which is given as per format given in Form 18.

Spousal Donor Transplants

Spousal donor transplants are also considered as near-related transplants where the proposed transplant is between a married couple. Documents such as marriage certificate and marriage photograph are kept for records along with the information on the number and age of children and a family photograph depicting the entire family and birth certificate of children containing the particulars of parents. For a spousal donor, the forms required thus include Form 2, Form 4 for donor fitness, and Form 11 which is a joint application form filled by the donor and recipient. The permission is granted in the format given in Form 6.

Swap Donation

In order to increase the donor pool, provision for swap donation was made in THOTA 2011. Swap donation means if in a family (family number one), donor and recipient are near related but their blood group is incompatible, i.e., donor is A+ and recipient is B+, and in another family (family number two), the donor is B+ while the recipient is A+, the donor of family number 1 can donate to recipient 2, and donor 2 can donate to recipient 1. Swap transplant should be carried out simultaneously, so there is no donor reneging. Donor reneging means that one of the donors backs out from donation. Furthermore, the donor and recipient pair in a family should be near related.

Other than Near-related Donors

This includes all donors except those under near-related donors. In these cases, the authorization committee is responsible for giving permission. Most controversies occur in this category as a rich recipient may coerce the poor donor to donate his/her organ against his will in exchange for money. There are several checks in the act to curb this organ trading. The donor–recipient interview is recorded. The joint application made by the recipient and donor is scrutinized, and a personal interview is carried out by the authorization committee. The committee has the following functions: (1) It evaluates that there is no commercial transaction between the recipient and the donor; (2) documents the reason why the donor wants to donate; (3) tries to establish the link between the donor and the recipient; (4) examines the documentary evidence of the link, for example, proof that they have lived together, etc.; examines old photographs showing the donor and the recipient together; (5) ensures that there is no middleman involved; (6) ascertains financial status of the donor and the recipient by examining appropriate evidence of their vocation and income for the previous 3 financial years and any gross disparity between the two; (7) ensures that the donor is not a drug addict; (8) ensures that the near relative or any adult person related to donor by blood or marriage is interviewed regarding awareness about his or her intention to donate an organ or tissue; (9) verifies the authenticity of the link between the donor and the recipient, and the reasons for donation, and also notes any strong views or disagreement or objection of kin. The forms required thus include Form 3 for donor consent, Form 4 for donor fitness, and Form 11 which is a joint application form and committee permission. The committee grants permission in the format given in Form 19 for other than near-related donors.

Donor or Recipient from Other States

When the living donor and/or recipient are from a state different from the state where the transplantation is to be undertaken, verification of residential status by Tehsildar or any other authorized officer of the state of domicile of donor or recipient is required as per Form 20 and a copy is marked to the appropriate authority.

Foreign Donors

All foreign transplants are dealt by the state authorization committee. In case of foreign donors donating to their relatives in India or Indian donors donating to foreigners, the transplantation is permitted only in near-related donors. In case both recipient and donor are foreigners and are coming for transplantation to India, the transplant is permitted in India with permission from a senior embassy official of the country of origin or by the government of that country who certifies the relationship between the donor and the recipient and the permission is granted in the format as outlined in Form 21.

DECEASED DONORS

Organs can be retrieved after brain death or circulatory death. Although donation after circulatory death is being practiced at Postgraduate Institute of Medical Education and Research (PGIMER), Chandigarh, it is still in infancy in India.

Brainstem death is a clinical diagnosis where the heart continues to function; however, there is cessation of functions of brain stem. The brainstem death is diagnosed by absence of brainstem reflexes and apnea test. Brainstem reflexes include pupillary reflex, corneal reflex, gag reflex, vestibulo-ocular reflex, and caloric test. The principle behind apnea test is that if the ventilator is disconnected, carbon dioxide builds to 60 mm Hg, and if the brain stem is intact, there should be stimulation of respiration. If there is no respiratory effort, the apnea test is deemed to be positive. The apnea test is repeated in a span of 6 hours. As per the law, the brain death certification is done by a panel of four doctors: (1) hospital administrator; (2) registered medical practitioner appointed by Superintendent; (3) neurologist/neurosurgeon/physician, intensivist, critical care specialists, or anesthetist; and (4) treating doctor. Brain death certification is mandated by law even if there is no organ donation so that the public gets used to the idea of brainstem death. Brain death certification should be uncoupled from organ donation.

Some people may wish to donate their organs after death, and they can pledge their organs for therapeutic purpose during their lifetime by filling in the pledge form, which is mentioned in Form 7 of the THOTA 2014 rules in the presence of two or more witnesses (at least one of whom is a near relative of such person). Some people may not be aware of the option of organ donation and may not have pledged their organs when alive. Hence, it is mandatory for the medical practitioner to ask the near relative or person in lawful possession of the body of a person admitted to the intensive care unit (ICU) that whether the donor had signed the pledge form. If not, the relative should be made aware of the option of organ donation. Even if the donor has pledged his organs before death, the consent of near relative or person in lawful possession of the body is also required.

If the relative consents to organ donation, then the brain death certificate should be signed and appropriate forms should be filled. The forms required for donation from a brain-dead donor include Forms 8 and 9.

The committee grants permission in the format given in Form 10. The cost for maintenance of the cadaver (brainstem-dead-declared person) and retrieval of organs or tissues is not borne by the donor family but is borne by the recipient or institution or government or nongovernment organization or society as decided by the respective state government.

PROCEDURE FOR DONATION OF ORGAN OR TISSUE IN MEDICOLEGAL CASES

In medicolegal cases (MLCs), after the brainstem death declaration and consent, the registered medical practitioner of the hospital requests the Superintendent of Police or Deputy Inspector General of the area either directly or through the police post located in the hospital to facilitate timely retrieval of organs from the donor, and a copy of such a request is sent to the designated postmortem doctor of area. The medical report is prepared at the time of retrieval by the retrieving doctor and is taken on record in postmortem notes by the registered medical practitioner doing postmortem so that determination of the cause of death is not jeopardized. The registered medical practitioner should be present at the time of organ or tissue retrieval, even after office hours. In case the retrieval hospital is not conducting the postmortem, they arrange transportation of the body along with medical records, after organ retrieval, to the designated postmortem center, and the postmortem center undertakes the postmortem of such cases on priority, even beyond office timing, so that the body is handed over to the relatives with least inconvenience.

QUALIFICATIONS

Qualifications of transplant surgeons and cornea and tissue retrieval technicians have been defined in the act and rules.

REGISTRATION OF HOSPITALS

Registration of hospitals and tissue banks workforce, facilities required for the registration of a hospital as a transplant center, and infrastructure, equipment requirements and guidelines, and standard operating procedures for tissue banks have been outlined in the act.

For registering a new hospital for transplantation, an application for registration should be filled as specified in Form 12, Form 13, Form 14, or Form 15, depending on organ, tissue, or eye bank. The application along with the specified fee should be submitted to the appropriate authority. The form includes details of the geographic location of the hospital, connectivity, staff, equipment, laboratories, blood bank details, and biomedical waste management. After inspection, the permission is given in the format of Form 17. The permission is valid for 5 years.

Some hospitals may wish to contribute to organ donation but do not have facilities for organ transplantation. Such hospitals are known as nontransplantation organ retrieval centers. Any hospital having ICU facilities along with workforce, infrastructure, and equipment as required to diagnose and maintain the brainstem-dead person and to retrieve and transport organs and tissues, including the facility for their temporary storage, can register as a retrieval center.

Registration is also mandatory for nongovernmental organizations, registered societies, and trusts working in the field of organ or tissue removal, storage, or transplantation.

TRANSPLANT COORDINATORS

As per the THOTA 2014 rules, all organ retrieval and transplanting centers should have a transplant coordinator. The prerequisites to become a transplant coordinator are specified in the act. Some organizations, e.g., MOHAN foundation, provide training to the coordinators. In Telangana, Osmania General Hospital in collaboration with Jeevandan Program has been given the task of providing certificate courses for the transplant coordinators **(Fig. 1)**. In a deceased donor program, the transplant coordinators are involved at each step of the process and coordinate brain death declaration, organ retrieval, packaging of organs, help in form filling, and even help with the last rites of the donor. The organ transplant program requires coordination between multiple doctors, laboratory personnel and police personnel, and more than one hospital. Hence, the role of a transplant coordinator is very important. They provide help even in living donor programs.

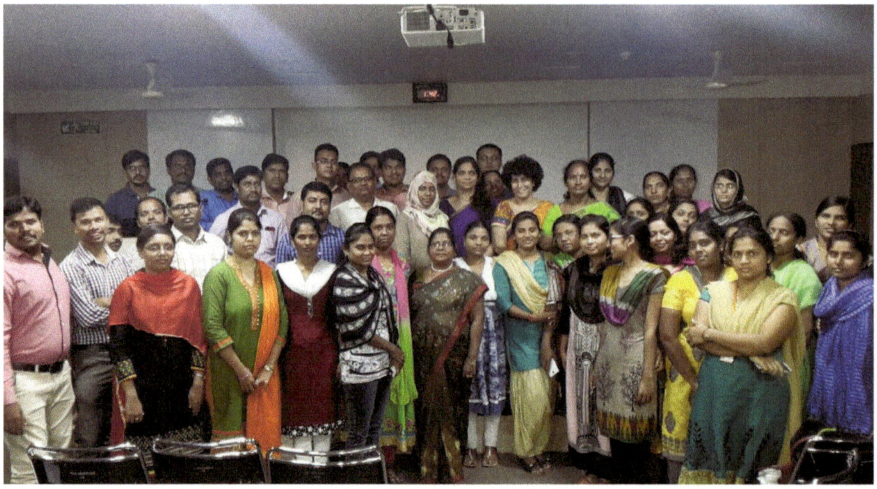

Fig. 1: Transplant coordinators in Osmania General Hospital, Telangana, in collaboration with Jeevandan Program.

PENALTIES

In order to curb illegal, unethical, and commercial organ trading, the act has defined penalties for the removal of organ without authority. These include financial penalties, imprisonment, or suspension of license.

NATIONAL, REGIONAL, AND STATE REGISTRIES AND NETWORKING

The act provides for the establishment and maintenance of registries. These are being done at national and regional levels. The transplantation and tissue organizations work at a three-tier level.

- *National Organ and Tissue Transplant Organization (NOTTO):* It is currently located at Safdarjung Hospital in New Delhi. NOTTO is a national-level organization set up under the Directorate General of Health Services, Ministry of Health and Family Welfare, Government of India. The national network division of NOTTO functions as an apex center for coordinating all activities and networking for procurement and distribution of organs and tissues and maintaining registry of organs and tissues donation and transplantation in the country. The website for NOTTO is www.notto.nic.in.
- *Regional Organ and Tissue Transplant Organization (ROTTO):* It is at the regional level and coordinates transplantation-related activities in the region.
- *State Organ and Tissue Transplant Organization (SOTTO):* It is at the state level and coordinates activities. Some state-level organizations include Jeevandan in Telangana, TRANSTAN in Tamil Nadu, Kerala Network for Organ Sharing (KNOS) in Kerala, Jeevasarthakathe in Karnataka, Zonal Transplant Coordination Center (ZTCC) in Maharashtra, and Rajasthan Network for Organ Sharing (RNOS) in Rajasthan. These have their own websites and maintain data about the transplants and donations done in their respective states and are important sources of transplant and organ donation data. State units should be linked to hospitals, organ- or tissue-matching laboratories, and tissue banks within their area and also to regional and national networking organizations.

The act lays emphasis on the development of national and regional networking. Presently, some states have their own data entry platforms, and data integration between these platforms is a challenge. Going forward, all state, regional, and national registries should be on a common platform. This will provide an excellent repository of patients waiting for transplant, patients transplanted, and transplant outcomes. Also donor details (live or deceased), including all demographic, clinical, laboratory, and follow-up data would be captured. Analysis of this data would help to identify the factors associated with poor outcomes. In addition, it would help in matching of organ donors and recipients and provide the option of a best possible match using big data analysis. As each region may have its own unique needs, the local centers should also be given some autonomy to fine-tune the policies according to the local needs.

ORGAN ALLOCATION

As organ supply from deceased donors is limited and demand is huge, there is a policy for organ allocation to the most suitable candidate. Organs are allocated in the following order:

1. Those who do not have any suitable living donor among near relatives
2. Those who have a suitable living donor available among near relatives, but the donor has refused in writing to donate
3. Those who have a suitable living donor available and who have also not refused to donate in writing

The sequence of allocation of organs shall be in the following order: (1) State list, (2) regional list, (3) national list, (4) person of Indian origin, and (5) foreigner.

CONCLUSION

The transplantation act has evolved over the last few decades to its present form. The latest rules are available on the website of Indian Society of Organ Transplantation as well. As transplant physicians and surgeons, we should make ourselves aware of the existent rules. Even the students in the transplant program should be made aware of these guidelines. This will go a long way in avoiding legal hassles in day-to-day transplant practice.

REFERENCES

1. Government of India. (1994). Transplantation of Human Organs Act, 1994. Central Act 42. [online] Available from https://legislative.gov.in › sites › files › A1994-42 [Last accessed 21 March, 2022].
2. Gazette—Transplantation of Human Organs Rules. (GSR NO. 51(E), dr 4-2-1995) [As amended vide GSR 571(E), dt31-7-2008]. (1995). [online] Available from https://main.mohfw.gov.in/sites/default/files/Amendment%202008.pdf [last accessed 21 March, 2022].
3. Transplantation of Human Organs (Amendment) Act, 2011. [online] Available from https://www.india.gov.in/transplantation-human-organs-amendment-act-2011. [Last accessed May, 2018].
4. The Gazette of India. Extraordinary Transplantation of Human Organs and Tissues Rules (THOT) Ministry of Health and Family Welfare Notification. Part 2. Sec 3. New Delhi: The Gazette of India; 2014.
5. Sahay M. Transplantation of human organs and tissues act—"Simplified". Indian J Transplant. 2018;12:84-9.

Index

Page numbers followed by *b* refer to box, *f* refer to figure, *fc* refer to flowchart, and *t* refer to table

D

H

M

N

O

P

Q

R